HANDBOOK OF
NEURODEVELOPMENTAL AND GENETIC DISORDERS
IN CHILDREN

Handbook of Neurodevelopmental and Genetic Disorders in Children

SECOND EDITION

EDITED BY

Sam Goldstein
Cecil R. Reynolds

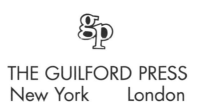

THE GUILFORD PRESS
New York   London

© 2011 The Guilford Press
A Division of Guilford Publications, Inc.
72 Spring Street, New York, NY 10012
www.guilford.com

Printed in the United States of America

This book is printed on acid-free paper.

Last digit is print number: 9 8 7 6 5 4 3 2 1

The authors have checked with sources believed to be reliable in their efforts to
provide information that is complete and generally in accord with the standards
of practice that are accepted at the time of publication. However, in view of the
possibility of human error or changes in behavioral, mental health, or medical
sciences, neither the authors, nor the editor and publisher, nor any other party who
has been involved in the preparation or publication of this work warrants that the
information contained herein is in every respect accurate or complete, and they are
not responsible for any errors or omissions or the results obtained from the use of such
information. Readers are encouraged to confirm the information contained in this
book with other sources.

Library of Congress Cataloging-in-Publication Data

Handbook of neurodevelopmental and genetic disorders in children / edited by Sam
Goldstein, Cecil R. Reynolds.–2nd ed.
      p. ; cm.
   Includes bibliographical references and index.
   ISBN 978-1-60623-990-2 (hardcover : alk. paper)
   1. Developmental disabilities—Genetic aspects—Handbooks, manuals,
etc.   2. Developmental neurobiology—Handbooks, manuals, etc.   3. Genetic
disorders in children—Handbooks, manuals, etc.   4. Pediatric neuropsychology—
Handbooks, manuals, etc.   I. Goldstein, Sam.   II. Reynolds, Cecil R.
   [DNLM: 1. Mental Retardation.   2. Child Development Disorders,
Pervasive.   3. Child.   4. Congenital Abnormalities.   5. Genetic Diseases,
Inborn.   6. Mental Disorders.   WS 107 H2365 2011]
   RJ506.D47H36 2011
   618.92′8588042—dc22

                                                        2010024244

For Allyson and Ryan,
and for the thousands of children and families
with whom I have had the privilege to work
—S. G.

To Julia, always
—C. R. R.

About the Editors

Sam Goldstein, PhD, is Assistant Clinical Instructor in the Department of Psychiatry at the University of Utah School of Medicine and Affiliate Research Professor of Psychology at George Mason University. As a neuropsychologist, he specializes in child development, school psychology, and traumatic brain injuries. Dr. Goldstein is also Clinical Director of the Neurology, Learning, and Behavior Center in Salt Lake City, where he provides assessment, case management, and treatment for individuals experiencing diverse neuropsychological impairments throughout the lifespan. He holds Fellow and Diplomate status in organizations spanning many disciplines. Dr. Goldstein is Editor-in-Chief of the *Journal of Attention Disorders* and serves on the editorial boards of six journals. He is the author or editor of over 30 books and more than 100 scholarly publications.

Cecil R. Reynolds, PhD, is Emeritus Professor of Educational Psychology, Professor of Neuroscience, and Distinguished Research Scholar at Texas A&M University. He maintained a clinical practice treating trauma victims and individuals with traumatic brain injury for 25 years before retiring from clinical work. Dr. Reynolds is past president of the National Academy of Neuropsychology (NAN) and of the American Psychological Association (APA) Divisions of Evaluation, Measurement, and Statistics; Clinical Neuropsychology; and School Psychology. He has been an editor or associate editor of several journals, is currently editor-in-chief of *Psychological Assessment*, and serves on the editorial boards of 11 journals. He is the author or editor of over 50 books and more than 300 scholarly publications; is a creator of numerous widely used psychological tests of behavior, cognition, and personality; and has received many awards from NAN, APA, and other organizations.

Contributors

Angela Giacoletti Argento, PhD, Department of Physical Medicine and Rehabilitation, University of Michigan, Ann Arbor, Michigan

David A. Baker, PsyD, Department of Pediatric Behavioral Health, Primary Children's Medical Center, Salt Lake City, Utah

Barbara C. Banz, MS, Department of Psychology, Colorado State University, Fort Collins, Colorado

Bonnie J. Baty, MS, Department of Pediatrics, Division of Medical Genetics, University of Utah, Salt Lake City, Utah

Thomas L. Bennett, PhD, Center for Neurorehabilitation Services, and Department of Psychology, Colorado State University, Fort Collins, Colorado

Brandi Berry, MA, Department of Educational Psychology, University of Nebraska–Lincoln, Lincoln, Nebraska

Erin D. Bigler, PhD, Departments of Psychology and Neuroscience, Brigham Young University, Provo, Utah

Michael B. Brown, PhD, Department of Psychology, East Carolina University, Greenville, North Carolina

Robert T. Brown, PhD, Department of Psychology, University of North Carolina at Wilmington, Wilmington, North Carolina

Ronald T. Brown, PhD, Departments of Public Health, Psychology, and Pediatrics, Temple University, Philadelphia, Pennsylvania

Jennifer L. Bruno, PhD, Department of Psychiatry and Behavioral Sciences, Stanford University School of Medicine, Stanford, California

John C. Carey, MD, Department of Pediatrics, Division of Medical Genetics, University of Utah, Salt Lake City, Utah

Suzanne B. Cassidy, MD, Genetic Medicine Central California, Fresno, California

Gina B. Christopher, PhD, Department of Educational Psychology, University of Texas at Austin, Austin, Texas

Blythe Corbett, PhD, Vanderbilt Kennedy Center, Department of Psychiatry, Vanderbilt University, Nashville, Tennessee

Sean Cunningham, MS, Neurology, Learning, and Behavior Center, Salt Lake City, Utah

Brian P. Daly, PhD, Department of Public Health, Temple University, Philadelphia, Pennsylvania

Deana B. Davalos, PhD, Department of Psychology, Colorado State University, Fort Collins, Colorado

Mario Gaspar De Alba, MD, Center for Development and Learning, University of North Carolina at Chapel Hill, Chapel Hill, North Carolina

Melissa L. DeVries, PhD, Neurology, Learning, and Behavior Center, Salt Lake City, Utah

Elisabeth M. Dykens, PhD, Vanderbilt Kennedy Center and Department of Psychology and Human Development, Vanderbilt University, Nashville, Tennessee

Phyllis Anne Teeter Ellison, EdD, Department of Educational Psychology, University of Wisconsin–Milwaukee, Milwaukee, Wisconsin

Jami Givens, MA, Department of Educational Psychology, University of Nebraska–Lincoln, Lincoln, Nebraska

Sam Goldstein, PhD, Neurology, Learning, and Behavior Center, Salt Lake City, Utah

Joan Gunther, PsyD, MIND Institute, Department of Psychiatry and Behavioral Sciences, University of California at Davis, Sacramento, California

Randi J. Hagerman, MD, MIND Institute, Department of Pediatrics, University of California at Davis, Sacramento, California

Julie Hammer, PhD, Center for Development and Learning, University of North Carolina at Chapel Hill, Chapel Hill, North Carolina

Heather Cody Hazlett, PhD, Department of Psychiatry, University of North Carolina at Chapel Hill, Chapel Hill, North Carolina

Stephen R. Hooper, PhD, Center for Development and Learning, University of North Carolina at Chapel Hill, Chapel Hill, North Carolina

Maile Ho-Turner, PhD, Honolulu, Hawaii

Joseph E. Hornyak, MD, PhD, Department of Physical Medicine and Rehabilitation, University of Michigan, Ann Arbor, Michigan

Alicia Hughes, PhD, Department of Psychology, Temple University, Philadelphia, Pennsylvania

Randy W. Kamphaus, PhD, College of Education, Georgia State University, Atlanta, Georgia

Valerie Van Horn Kerne, MA, Department of Educational Psychology, University of Texas at Austin, Austin, Texas

Shelli R. Kesler, PhD, Department of Psychiatry and Behavioral Sciences, Stanford University School of Medicine, Stanford, California

Lori A. Long, MA, Division of Advanced Studies in Learning, Technology, and Psychology in Education, Mary Lou Fulton Institute and Graduate School of Education, Arizona State University, Tempe, Arizona

Melissa J. Mathews, MA, Department of Clinical Psychology, University of Massachusetts, Amherst, Amherst, Massachusetts

Joan W. Mayfield, PhD, Our Children's House at Baylor, Dallas, Texas

William M. McMahon, MD, Department of Psychiatry, University of Utah School of Medicine, Salt Lake City, Utah

Kathleen K. McMillan, MEd (retired), Jacksonville Schools, Jacksonville, North Carolina

Kathryn N. North, MD, Department of Pediatrics, University of Sydney, Sydney, Australia, and Children's Hospital at Westmead, Westmead, New South Wales, Australia

Nancy L. Nussbaum, PhD, Department of Educational Psychology, College of Education, University of Texas at Austin, Austin, Texas

Jonathan M. Payne, PsyD, Institute for Neuroscience and Muscle Research, Children's Hospital at Westmead, Westmead, New South Wales, Australia

Steven R. Pliszka, MD, Division of Child and Adolescent Psychiatry, University of Texas at San Antonio, San Antonio, Texas

M. Paige Powell, PhD, Psychology Service, Department of Pediatrics, Baylor College of Medicine, Texas Children's Hospital, Houston, Texas

Dawn Reinemann, PhD, Holy Family Memorial, Manitowoc, Wisconsin

Cecil R. Reynolds, PhD, private practice, Bastrop, Texas

Russell P. Saneto, DO, PhD, Division of Pediatric Neurology, Departments of Neurology and Pediatrics, Seattle Children's Hospital, University of Washington, Seattle, Washington

Timothy Schulte, PsyD, Department of Graduate Psychology, James Madison University, Harrisonburg, Virginia

Adam Schwebach, PhD, Neurology, Learning, and Behavior Center, Salt Lake City, Utah

Laura Shank, PsyD, Department of Physical Medicine and Rehabilitation, University of Michigan, Ann Arbor, Michigan

Julien T. Smith, PhD, Children's Neurodevelopmental Services, Inc., Salt Lake City, Utah

Susan M. Swearer, PhD, Department of Educational Psychology, University of Nebraska–Lincoln, Lincoln, Nebraska

Anthony Swentosky, MS, Department of Psychology, University of Rhode Island, Kingston, Rhode Island

Genevieve Verdi, MEd, Department of Psychology, University of Rhode Island, Kingston, Rhode Island

Susan E. Waisbren, PhD, Department of Psychiatry, Children's Hospital, Harvard Medical School, Boston, Massachusetts

Cixin Wang, PhD, Department of Educational Psychology, University of Nebraska–Lincoln, Lincoln, Nebraska

Seth A. Warschausky, PhD, Department of Physical Medicine and Rehabilitation, University of Michigan, Ann Arbor, Michigan

Lisa L. Weyandt, PhD, Department of Psychology, University of Rhode Island, Kingston, Rhode Island

Timothy B. Whelan, PhD, Neuropsychology Service, Baystate Medical Center, Springfield, Massachusetts

Elizabeth Wilde, PhD, Cognitive Neuroscience Laboratory, Baylor College of Medicine, Houston, Texas

David L. Wodrich, PhD, ABPP, Division of Advanced Studies in Learning, Technology, and Psychology in Education, Mary Lou Fulton Institute and Graduate School of Education, Arizona State University, Tempe, Arizona

Preface

Thirteen years ago, we entertained the idea of creating a handbook as a desk reference for practicing neuropsychologists and members of related professions, to cover the broad spectrum of neurodevelopmental and genetic disorders in children. At the time, no such volume existed. In 1999, with the assistance and support of our esteemed colleagues, we were able to publish the first edition of this volume. We are pleased that this volume has been so well received and is in the small company of volumes for which second editions are completed.

This text grew out of our mutual interest in educating our students and fellow clinicians about the powerful role played by genetics in shaping the development and lives of many children. It was our intent that the text would serve as a ready and comprehensive reference, assisting clinicians to understand, evaluate, and ultimately help children with neurodevelopmental and genetic disorders.

In our daily work as scientist-practitioners, we actively blend research, training, and clinical practice. As we participate in, read, and review current research, our clinical practice—what we do and how we do it—changes. As we train our students, our self-perceptions, our ideas, and our clinical practice are sharpened. The pace at which these processes take place has continued to increase since the first edition of this volume was published. Society has increasingly acknowledged the powerful biological bases for many childhood problems. Since the publication of the first edition of this volume, the lay and professional communities have slowly worked toward balancing the contributions of biology and experience in their understandings of children's development and outcome. As the eminent neuropsychologist John Weery noted years ago, biology is not destiny. The longitudinal work of Emmy Werner and others has demonstrated that even problems with significant biological bases can be and are affected greatly in their outcome by environmental consequences. We recognize as clinicians that biology very powerfully influences the neurodevelopment and behavior of many children with such problems as attention-deficit/hyperactivity disorder, learning disabilities, and anxiety disorders. However, we continue to believe strongly that the daily lives of all children are equally powerful in shaping the consequences of those conditions. The individual child's day-to-day life within the family, in the school, and on the playground—not whether he or she demonstrates certain symptoms or diagnoses—is what determines his or her ultimate life course.

The dramatic and rapid growth in medicine, psychology, and education is greatly improving our ability to prepare all children, even those with significant differences, for their adult lives. Clinicians in the next 50 years will increasingly be expected to possess expertise not just in diagnosis and intervention, but in the medical and biological phenomena that have an impact on children's growth and development. We are very pleased with the breadth and scope of this second edition. We have added several new chapters, and many of our contributors have graciously updated and rewritten the chapters they contributed to the first edition.

ACKNOWLEDGMENTS

We wish to thank our colleagues for their scholarly and thoughtful contributions to this second edition. We also wish to thank Kathleen Gardner for her editorial organization, management, and secretarial skills, and Rochelle Serwator, Senior Editor at The Guilford Press, for her guidance, support, and friendship.

SAM GOLDSTEIN, PhD
CECIL R. REYNOLDS, PhD

Contents

PART III. DISORDERS WITH BROADER-SPECTRUM EFFECTS

Contents xvii

As human beings, our greatness lies not so much in being able to remake the world—that is the myth of the atomic age—as in being able to remake ourselves.

—MOHANDAS GANDHI

Most intellectuals today have a phobia of any explanation of the mind that invokes genetics.

—STEPHEN PINKER

I think I have discovered the secret of life—you just hang around until you get used to it.

—CHARLES M. SCHULZ

PART I
Background

CHAPTER 1

Introduction

SAM GOLDSTEIN
CECIL R. REYNOLDS

Neuropsychology is the study of brain–behavior relationships, and a clinical neuropsychologist is a clinician who applies the results of knowledge in this area to diagnosis and treatment of neurodevelopmental disorders, among other central nervous system (CNS) disturbances (e.g., CNS diseases, traumatic brain injury, cerebrovascular accidents, etc.). Clinical neuropsychology as practiced today traces its roots principally to the 1940s, although the influence of earlier practitioners such as A. R. Luria is clearly evident. As a clinical discipline, therefore, it is relatively young, but it is a burgeoning specialty within the broader discipline of psychology.

As part of our preparation for the first edition of this text, we completed a MEDLINE search over a 4-year period from January 1993 through July 1997, which yielded over 6,000 peer-reviewed research studies concerning chromosomal and genetic disorders in children. Over 4,000 studies published during the very same period of time were identified as specifically dealing with the neuropsychological evaluation and treatment of children. Yet only 42 studies dealing with both issues were found in this database. Even given the relative youth of the field, this seemed too few papers. However, the nature of the studies and their appearance in mainstream medical and psychological journals indicated the need for even broader perspectives and interdisciplinary approaches to the diagnosis and treatment of children's neurodevelopmental disorders (ironically, at a time when the politics and costs of health care were giving rise to the managed care model, which promotes singularity of treatment!).

A review of these 42 studies, which may not necessarily have represented all published studies dealing with these two issues, revealed the increasing importance of a simultaneous view and understanding of these two issues for neuropsychologists, physicians, and other medical and mental health professionals. For example, Mazzocco and Holden (1996) provided a neuropsychological profile of females with the fragile X permutation. Devenny and colleagues (1996) provided a longitudinal study of individuals with Down syndrome, and in doing so, defined the neurocognitive changes in this population over four decades. Lanoo, De-Paepe, Leroy, and Thiery (1996) provided data reflecting a profile characterized by difficulty with sustained visual attention and problems with visual construction, over and above the visual acuity problems and other phenomena associated with Marfan syndrome. Davalos and colleagues (1996) offered a neuropsychological profile reflecting a pattern of mild mental retardation, constructional apraxia, and expressive language impairment in a group of children presenting with proportionate short stature, delayed bone age, and peculiar faces. These children were subsequently identified as experiencing Floating–Harbor syndrome. And Ross, Stefanatos, Roeltgen, Kushner, and Cutler (1995) offered a longitudinal study providing a profile of neurocognitive changes in females with Turner syndrome.

As part of our work for this second edition, we completed a number of new searches from January 2004 to January 2009. We began with a Google search using the keyword "genetic disorders," which identified over 17 million citations. We then searched Google Scholar with the keyword "chromosome disorders," which produced over 5 million citations. Searching MEDLINE with the "chromosome disorders" keyword resulted in approximately 37,000 references. Finally, we identified 201 new studies dealing with neuropsychological evaluation during this time period, but fewer than two dozen new studies, dealing with both genetic disorders and neuropsychological evaluation. These studies are very similar in breadth and scope to studies published earlier. For example, a number of researchers have examined the neuropsychological characteristics of specific genetic disorders (Adams et al., 2007; Azzam et al., 2005). Other researchers have examined risk factors (Gothelf et al., 2007), as well as familial characteristics (Gambardella et al., 2008; Veltman et al., 2005).

When the contributions of genetics to more common and diverse childhood problems, such as learning disabilities and attention-deficit/hyperactivity disorder (ADHD), are examined along with the genetic role in many lower-incidence problems, the importance of understanding and beginning to develop a cohesive genetic–environmental model becomes clear immediately. As Rutter (1997) has noted,

> Quantitative genetic research has been most informative in showing the importance of genetic influences on virtually all forms of human behavior. Behavior has to have a biological basis and it is necessary that we understand how the biology functions. Equally the same research has been crucial in its demonstration that environmental influences are also ubiquitous. (p 396)

NATURE AND NURTURE

There are few topics as inflammatory, polemic, or controversial in psychology and related sciences as the so-called "nature–nurture controversy." Briefly stated, this controversy revolves around whether human development and human behavior (both overt and covert) are determined by human beings' genetic constitution (nature) or by the environment (nurture) in which people grow and develop. Few, if indeed any, contemporary scientists approach this question in such simplistic terms. The arguments now tend to center around the relative contributions of nature and nurture to human development and behavior, and the mechanisms of interaction and plausibility of transaction between them. It is also acknowledged that for specific human attributes, the answers will vary.

A *genotype* may be considered the raw material and blueprints (genes and chromosomes) provided through the melding of the parental genotypes. Except in the case of monozygotic twins and cloning, no two human genotypes are alike. The human organism then grows and develops in a unique environment to produce the visible, assessable, acting *phenotype*—the expression of the genotype in the unique environment. Attributes known to be "genetically determined" can often be altered in the course of development or even later in life. Height, known to have strong heritability in the human population, can be altered dramatically in an individual by manipulation of diet. As subsequent chapters of this volume indicate, many outcomes for some genetic disorders are entirely dependent on, or at least strongly determined by, changes in environment. Phenylketonuria (PKU) is a classic example. When phenylalanines are eliminated from the diet of youngsters with PKU, the outcomes for intellect, school adjustment, and other behavioral variables are all much improved. Even behaviors as complex as adult sexual behaviors and preference, which are strongly genetically influenced, can be altered by significant changes in maternal stress levels at particular times during pregnancy (for a review, see Houshyar & Kaufman, 2005). There are certain critical periods during gestation when hormonal releases affect cell migration and organ development in a preprogrammed fashion. Mothers under very high levels of stress may alter those hormonal release patterns in ways that affect adult sexual behavior in their offspring. It seems that few components of human behavior are too simple to be influenced by environment, or too complex to be related to the genotype. The complexity of the interaction and potential transaction is virtually incomprehensible when we recall that no two combinations of genotype and environment have been or ever will be identical.

To many scientists, ourselves included, it does appear that as our skills, insights, and techniques of investigation continue to grow in number and in sophistication, we learn that our biology has a more pronounced impact on our behavior than we would prefer to believe. Even at the extremes of the hereditary influences argued by some scientists, there is much room for change, intervention, and environmental influence.

Take the controversial case of the heritability of human intelligence. The debate about this begins with differences of opinion about the very nature of the phenomenon (for a review, see Naglieri & Goldstein, 2009). Moreover, the extremes of the various scientific arguments place the nature–nurture contributions to intelligence at 80% and 20% and at 20% and 80%, respectively (e.g., see Herrnstein & Murray, 1994; Jensen, 1980; Reynolds & Brown, 1984). One may argue urgently for relative contribution and interaction within these two extremes, but even in the most extreme genetic view (i.e., the view that 80% of the variance in human intelligence is genotype variation), two propositions remain inescapable:

1. Heritability statistics only apply to groups, and the genetic influence on intelligence for an individual may be more or less than the group heritability.
2. Even if 80% of an individual's intellectual level is genetically determined, changes in intellectual level as a function of environmental influences and transaction may be enormous.

The latter proposition requires some elaboration. Psychological variables such as intelligence and personality are measured in interval scales of measurement, which have no true zero point denoting the absence of the trait, such as zero reflects on a ratio scale of measurement. With a true zero point, the actual amount of a characteristic (e.g., height) can be determined, and such statements as "A height of 6 feet is twice a height of 3 feet" are accurate. However, interval scales, having no true zero point, begin measurement at the midpoint of a characteristic's distribution—the only point we can locate definitively. We then measure outward toward the two ends of a distribution, each of which is asymptotic to its axis. That is, we do not know where intelligence begins or ends, and an IQ of 100 does not reflect twice the intelligence of an IQ of 50. Herein lies the clinician's opportunity to intervene and potentially create meaningful results, even under the adversity of strong genetic determination. To increase an individual's intellectual level by a full 20% may mean an increase of 10, 20, 30, 40, or even more points on a psychometric scale. The same may hold true for other human characteristics that present as complex behavioral phenomena.

As subsequent chapters of this book describe, many genetic disorders have high degrees of variable expressivity, often (but not always) for unknown reasons. We believe many of these reasons to be treatment-related, or at least associated with biological and environmental interplay. Early involvement of clinicians who understand brain–behavior relationships is necessary if children with neurodevelopmental disorders are to have the maximum developmental opportunities. All of this may be taken to mean that although genetics or biology may be destiny, it need not be.

The human brain represents the product of a construction project that has been going on for 6 billion years. In its physical form and function, the brain represents millions upon millions of trial-and-error adaptive adjustments. Consisting of an estimated 100 billion neurons and many more glial cells organized into thousands of regions, the human brain governs body function and movement in a seamlessly integrated manner; even more importantly, it regulates cognition. Not surprisingly, although the brains of different species may not look exactly alike, they all work according to the same principles and mechanisms. These neurons and glial cells communicate via a nearly infinite number of synaptic connections, yet the entire organ in a human being weighs only about 3 pounds. Gram for gram, the human brain delivers an array of motoric, behavioral, cognitive, and emotional capacities that is nearly impossible to fathom in light of its size. Because the brain is the center of our consciousness and being, it is fitting that an increasing scientific literature is being devoted to understanding and facilitating its development and operation—in particular, to appreciating the developmental disorders and conditions that adversely affect children's transition into adulthood.

Cortical development is genetically preprogrammed in many ways. Not all genetic disorders have a full phenotypic impact at the same time. Environments may also alter the timing of development and change as well. As Bigler and Clement (1997) note so well, the process of maturation greatly complicates the evaluation of neurodevelopmental disorders in children and adolescents. The effects of the interaction between age and genetic expressivity of a disorder with CNS implications adds to the complexity of all tasks with such children. A common change in CNS development may have radically different implications and outcomes, even in adulthood, if the age of occurrence is varied.

OBJECTIVES OF THIS VOLUME

Clinicians of the 21st century will need to possess a working knowledge of genetics as well as neuropsychology. Yet, even as we publish the second edition of this volume, the science of what we choose to term *behavioral genetics* remains in its infancy, as our literature review reflects. The 21st century clinician will exemplify the biopsychosocial model of the future. Clinicians will continue to be called upon to assess the relationship between brain function and behavior. They will be asked to assess function by skills (e.g., the skills necessary to read efficiently). They will be asked to plan treatment, to monitor that treatment, and to assess progress. As increasing information is gathered

concerning the influence of human genetics upon behavior, clinicians will be increasingly called upon to guide mental health, medical, and educational professionals in blazing new trails to improve the quality of life for children and adults with genetic disorders affecting their behavior and development. Clinicians who work with children must be knowledgeable about developmental psychology as well.

The primary objective of this expanded second edition, as of the first edition, is to provide readers with a stand-alone compendium concerning the impact of genetics on neurodevelopment in children. In planning this second edition, we have continued to recognize that this primary mission entails creating a text similar in breadth and scope to those handbooks of neuropsychology that are familiar to each of us. The goal of those texts, as of this one, is to provide a comprehensive set of resource materials that will be available to readers as needed, organized in a framework that is understandable and immediately useful in clinical practice. Clinical child neuropsychologists and related professionals today and in the future must be scientist-practitioners; to do so effectively requires a special type of literature.

We have divided the text into three sections. Part I, "Background," offers our view of the role of neuropsychology in the assessment, treatment, and management of children with neurobehavioral and genetic disorders. In Chapter 2, the role of neuropsychology in the assessment of these populations is discussed. Chapter 3 is an overview providing readers with a basic model for understanding genetics, as well as up-to-date information concerning current trends and research in the field of human genetics. Chapter 4 then examines current research concerning the use of neuroimaging to determine structural and biochemical differences in children with genetic disorders. Finally, psychosocial issues related to emotional, educational, familial, and behavioral problems are reviewed and discussed in Chapter 5. This information lays a firm foundation for the following discussions of specific genetic disorders in children. A working understanding of this information is essential for all practicing clinicians.

Part II of the volume two contains chapters dealing with seven disorders or groups of disorders that have accepted, though as yet not completely identified, genetic etiologies. These disorders have a common theme, in that they primarily affect learning and behavior; thus topics that often do not find their way into genetics and neurobehavioral texts are included. The disorders covered here are learning disabilities; ADHD; oppositional, conduct, and aggressive disorders; Tourette syndrome; anxiety disorders; mood disorders; and autism spectrum disorders. These chapters, as well as those in Part III, provide readers with an overview of current genetic, behavioral, and developmental issues; guides to assessment; and discussions of treatment, care, and management.

Part III is by far the lengthiest section: It contains 17 chapters offering overviews of lower-incidence disorders in the general population. In this second edition, we have expanded this section by adding several new chapters. Clinicians can expect to see increasing numbers of children with these problems, especially within medical settings. Furthermore, the increasing recognition of the impact such impairments have upon children's functioning at school has now paved the way for many of these children to receive specialized services within school settings. Thus these problems are also likely to be faced more and more often by school psychologists, school nurses, and other educational staff members. The approach to educating children with such disorders can and usually does have a major impact on the quality of their lives. As an example, consider children with Down syndrome. In the not very distant past, children with Down syndrome children were rarely seen in public, and most were treated through residential placements in state facilities designed for children with severe developmental disorders. However, not all children with Down syndrome also have mental retardation, and most of those who do have intellectual impairment in the mild to moderate range. Decades of research have shown that children with Down syndrome are best educated in a public school setting with maximum exposure to the normal school environment. Social and behavioral outcomes in particular are superior for these children when they are educated in public schools, according to a least-restrictive-environment model, as opposed to the isolation and restricted nature of an institutional setting. Increasingly, knowledge about the neuropsychological functioning of children with neurodevelopmental disorders and about ways to facilitate their development is intertwined with the public school systems of our nation—and for good reason, for this is increasingly where the children are educated.

CONCLUSION

The path to success in life is neither simple nor easy for the majority of youth in the new millennium. Given the medical community's increasing ability to address the health needs of children with complex genetic and neurodevelopmental disorders, their subsequent increased survival rates, the increased public recognition of these disorders, and the greater availability of organized support for children whose genetic disorders primarily affect learning and development, the path to success for these children has perhaps become somewhat less convoluted and rocky. Ye the increasing educational, social, and family pressures placed upon children constitute an entirely new set of burdens for all youth. Neuropsychologists and related medical, mental health, and educational professionals will play an increasing role in shaping the life path for children with genetic and neurodevelopmental disorders.

Although the liabilities of these children are of most interest to many professionals, their assets and tenacity in some cases must also be well defined and understood. Several longitudinal studies over the past few decades have set out to develop an understanding of these assets and their related processes. In particular, the complex interaction of protective and risk factors with is being examined, the goal of developing a model to apply this knowledge in clinical practice (Rutter & Quinton, 1984; Werner & Smith, 2001). These studies and others have made major contributions in two ways. First, they have identified resources across children's lives that predict successful adjustment for those exposed to adversity; second, they have begun the process of clarifying ways in which these protective factors promote adaptation (Wyman, Sandler, Wolchik, & Nelson, 2000). Some of these processes can serve to protect against the negative effects of neurodevelopmental and genetic disorders, while others simply act to enhance development, regardless of the presence of disability.

Knowledgeable professionals offer their patients, clients, and students a powerful sense of hope by providing accurate information, understanding, and support. It is true that much remains to be uncovered and understood concerning the impact of genetics and the interaction of genetics with the environment in shaping the lives of children. However, identification through careful assessment, intervention and accommodation through implementation of thoughtful treatment, and the provision of support will make a significant positive difference for children with genetic and neurodevelopmental disorders.

REFERENCES

Adams, H. R., Kwon, J., Marshall, F. J., De Blieck, E. A., Pearce, D. A., & Link, J. W. (2007). Neuropsychological symptoms of juvenile onset Batten disease: Experiences from two studies. *Journal of Child Neurology, 22,* 621–627.

Azzam, A., Lerner, D. M., Peters, K. F., Wiggs, E., Rosenstein, D. L., & Biesecker, L. G. (2005). Psychiatric and neuropsychological characterization of Palaster–Hall syndrome. *Clinical Genetics, 67,* 87–92.

Bigler, E. B., & Clement, P. F. (1997). *Diagnostic clinical neuropsychology.* Austin: University of Texas Press.

Davalos, I. P., Figuera, L. E., Bobadilla, L., Martinez-Martinez, R., Matute, E., Partida, M. D., et al. (1996). Floating–Harbor syndrome: A neuropsychological approach. *Genetic Counseling, 7,* 283–288.

Devenny, D. A., Silverman, W. P., Hill, A. L., Jenkins, E., Sersen, E. A., & Wisniewski, K. E. (1996). Normal aging in adults with Down's syndrome: A longitudinal study. *Journal of Intellectual Disability Research, 40,* 208–221.

Gambardella, S. P., Coppola, A., DiBonaventura, C., Bovo, G., Boaretto, F., Ciampa, E. G., et al. (2008). Familial mesial temporal lobe epilepsy: A clinical and genetic study of 15 Italian families. *Journal of Neurology, 255,* 16–23.

Gothelf, D., Feinstein, C., Thompson, T., Gu, E., Penniman, L., Van Stone, E., et al. (2007). Risk factors for emergence of psychotic disorders in adolescents with 22q11. 2 deletion syndrome. *American Journal of Psychiatry, 164,* 663–669.

Herrnstein, R., & Murray, H. (1994). *The bell curve.* New York: Free Press.

Houshyar, S., & Kaufman, J. (2005). Resiliency in maltreated children. In S. Goldstein & R. B. Brooks (Eds.), *Handbook of resilience in children* (pp. 181–202). New York: Kluwer Academic/Plenum Press.

Jensen, A. R. (1980). *Perspectives on bias in mental testing.* New York: Plenum Press.

Lanoo, E., DePaepe, A., Leroy, B., & Thiery, E. (1996). Neuropsychological aspects of Marfan syndrome. *Clinical Genetics, 49,* 65–69.

Mazzocco, M. M., & Holden, J. J. (1996). Neuropsychological profiles of three sisters homozygous for the fragile X permutation. *American Journal of Medical Genetics, 64*(2), 323–328.

Naglieri, J., & Goldstein, S. (2009). Understanding the strengths and weaknesses of intelligence and achievement. In J. Naglieri & S. Goldstein (Eds.), *Practitioner's guide to assessing intelligence and achievement* (pp. 2–10). Hoboken, NJ: Wiley.

Reynolds, C. R., & Brown, R. T. (1984). Bias in mental testing: An introduction to the issues. In R. T. Brown & C. R. Reynolds (Eds.), *Perspectives on bias in mental testing* (pp. 1–26). New York: Plenum Press.

Ross, J. L., Stefanatos, G., Roeltgen, D., Kushner, H., & Cutler, G. B. (1995). Ulrich–Turner syndrome: Neurodevelopmental changes from childhood through adolescence. *American Journal of Medical Genetics, 58,* 74–82.

Rutter, M. L. (1997). Nature–nurture integration: The example of anti-social behavior. *American Psychologist, 52,* 390–398.

Rutter, M. L., & Quinton, D. (1984). Long-term follow-up of women institutionalized in childhood: Factors promoting good functioning in adult life. *British Journal of Developmental Psychology, 18,* 225–234.

Veltman, M. W., Thompson, R. J., Craig, E. E., Dennis, N. R., Roberts, S. C., Moore, V., et al. (2005). A paternally inherited duplication in the Prader–Willi/Angelman syndrome critical region: A case and family study. *Journal of Autism and Developmental Disorders, 35,* 117–127.

Werner, E. E., & Smith, R. S. (2001). *Journeys from childhood to midlife: Risk, resilience, and recovery.* Ithaca, NY: Cornell University Press.

Wyman, P. A., Sandler, I., Wolchik, S., & Nelson, K. (2000). Resilience as cumulative competence promotion and stress protection: Theory and intervention. In D. Cicchetti, J. Rappaport, I. Sandler, & R. Weissberg (Eds.), *The promotion of wellness in children and adolescents* (pp. 148–167). Washington, DC: Child Welfare League of America.

CHAPTER 2

Neuropsychological Assessment in Genetically Linked Neurodevelopmental Disorders

CECIL R. REYNOLDS
JOAN W. MAYFIELD

Children in general have always posed special problems in clinical assessment and evaluation, and even more so from a psychometric standpoint. Infancy and childhood are the times of the greatest (and most rapid) breadth and depth of change in the human lifetime. This alone presents a significant challenge to those who would assess a child's status in order to make predictions about a child's future and about interventions that may be required to facilitate growth and development. Children who are developing normally or with only mild levels of disability can be difficult to assess accurately, for reasons related to the maturity of their language development, motor development, social skills, and attention, concentration, and memory skills. As the extent of disability increases, accurate assessment becomes ever more challenging.

Moreover, certain developmental periods pose special problems. During infancy in particular, a child's very limited language and motor skills prevent a thorough assessment of cognitive functions and higher cortical development. A pediatric neurologist can get a reasonable estimate, but only at a gross level, of neurodevelopmental status from a neurological examination that focuses on reflexes, muscle tone, and a review of cranial nerve functions. The neuropsychologist can add some additional details about higher cortical functions (i.e., thinking, reasoning, intellectual development, and language development), but our measures, even the most sophisticated (e.g., Bayley, 2005), remain crude. Except for very low levels of performance, scores on such instruments are relatively poor predictors of adult status. Little in the way of localization of function can be accomplished, and higher cortical systems of brain function are rarely assessed well. In these early years, we clinicians are often left with an unsatisfactory feeling about what we have accomplished with such assessments. However, an assessment at even these early stages by a neuropsychologist makes significant contributions to diagnosis and treatment.

With infants changing so rapidly, it is imperative to have carefully constructed standards of normality if developmental problems are to be detected accurately. Minor variants of normal development need not be diagnosed as disorders, nor should significant problems be overlooked. It is in this context that psychometric testing has the most to offer. Psychologists are accustomed to using norm-referenced tests, such as the Bayley Scales of Infant and Toddler Development, Third Edition (Bayley, 2005). Such tests have carefully constructed normative reference tables that define normal variations in development, typically considered as within two standard deviations of the mean of a normally functioning reference group. Tests constructed specifically for use with infants, despite involving such observation (as opposed to demand performances, as with older children and adults), compare relevant functions of infants to the distribution of the same functions for infants developing normally. Such quantitative approaches are a necessity for accurate diagnosis during times of rapid change. Informal or subjective observations and ratings place far too many cognitive demands on the clinician to produce consistent, reliable results.

Neuropsychological testing is thus important to establish the presence of a cognitive disorder. Since neuropsychological testing is norm-referenced by chronological age, progress can be monitored via repeated or serial testing, and changing patterns of symptomatology can be detected. The effectiveness (or lack thereof) of interventions can be documented as well, and changes can be made as indicated.

These same quantitative procedures are useful throughout childhood and adolescence, when cognitive development continues to be rapid and is often uneven. Quantitative tracking of change, and the detection of change through psychometric methods providing age-corrected deviation scaled scores, are necessities.

MONITORING AND MANAGING SYMPTOM EXPRESSION

All of the various disorders addressed in this volume are believed to have some degree of genetic linkage, and some of these linkages are stronger and more obvious than others. However, they all show what is termed *variable expressivity* (i.e., the number and/or the severity of the symptoms defining the disorder vary across individuals). The variability of symptom expression must be monitored and will have clear treatment implications.

The interaction between the genetic basis of a disorder on the one hand, and the individual's environmental circumstances and other biological predispositions (which may or may not be affected by the genetics of the primary disorder) on the other, will also alter the severity of symptoms. Phenylketonuria (PKU), for example, is an entirely genetic disorder. Yet the treatment compliance of both the family and the individual, along with the child's temperament, predisposition for intellectual development, and numerous other factors, will act to determine the cognitive symptoms displayed. This will have implications for whether special education programming for mental retardation, specific learning disabilities, or even serious emotional disturbance is required. Although dietary treatment is always indicated for PKU, one cannot assume what other treatments will be necessary. Rather, periodic formal neuropsychological testing should be conducted to detect cognitive changes that may require additional forms of intervention, and that may even provide some suggestive data about a patient's dietary compliance. Assessment of behavior and affect through norm-referenced, age-corrected methods (e.g., Reynolds & Kamphaus, 2004) are also necessary, as individuals with genetic disorders are commonly at increased risk of developing emotional and behavioral problems (see also Warzak, Mayfield, & McAllister, 1996).

There is no cure or elimination of all symptoms for the disorders treated in this volume. Rather, most viable treatments center on symptom management. Neuropsychological and psychological assessment has two primary roles to play beyond assisting in diagnosis. The first, as noted above, is the evaluation of the severity of symptom expression; the second is the assessment of treatment effects through careful psychometric monitoring of changes in symptom expression.

Historically, neuropsychological evaluations were conducted with adults with known brain damage or injury, to determine lateralization or localization of lesion or injury. As Lezak (1995) points out, "[the] rapid evolution [of such evaluations] in recent years reflects a growing sensitivity among clinicians to the practical problems of identification, assessment, care, and treatment of brain damaged patients" (p. 7)—a comment that pertains as well to any patient with a compromised central nervous system (CNS), especially if higher cortical functions are involved. Neuropsychologists are often asked to provide information concerning prognosis for recovery, functional ability, and course of treatment. However, the practice of neuropsychology has broadened to include the need to clarify conditions where brain damage or CNS compromise has not been identified; in these cases, evaluations provide additional information for differential diagnoses, which result in more effective treatment planning.

As neuropsychologists gained more knowledge about brain–behavior relationships, they applied their knowledge to adults without known brain damage. After this, they turned their attention to problems of earlier development, which ultimately provided an understanding of brain–behavior functioning in children (Reitan & Wolfson, 1974). We agree that "child clinical neuropsychology has emerged as an important theoretical, empirical, and methodological perspective for understanding and treating developmental, psychiatric, psychosocial, and learning disabilities in children and adolescents" (Teeter & Semrud-Clikeman, 1997, p. 1). In more recent years, school psychologists have become more versed in neuropsychology and its application to children with neurodevelopmental and genetic disorders as well (e.g., D'Amato, Fletcher-Janzen, & Reynolds, 2005; Miller, 2010).

The remaining purposes of this chapter are to give a functional definition of neuropsychology, to provide information concerning the necessary components of a neuropsychological evaluation, and to discuss their relationship to treatment. An overview of neuropsychological assessment processes is then presented, both historically and in the context of current practices that incorporates the basic components of evaluation and encourages integrative, comprehensive assessment of CNS compromise. Furthermore, the chapter provides information concerning why children and adolescents are referred for neuropsychological evaluations, and how the results of such evaluations are relevant to their educational needs (in terms of effective remediation techniques, educational placement, and parental expectations).

WHAT IS NEUROPSYCHOLOGY?

Neuropsychology is the study of brain–behavior relationships. It requires acceptance of the idea that the brain, working as an interdependent, systemic network, controls and is all-inclusively responsible for behavior. Although this premise seems simple enough now, radical behavioral psychology in the 1960s and early 1970s ignored the brain, leading some to espouse the view that the brain was irrelevant to learning and behavior.

Neuropsychological assessment examines the relationship between brain functioning and behavior through tests that tap specific domains of functioning—typically much more specific domains than those that are represented on general tests of intelligence, such as attention, memory, forgetting, sensory functions, constructional praxis, and motor skills (Farmer & Peterson, 1995; Hynd & Reynolds, 2005; Reitan & Wolfson, 1985). Neuropsychologists examine the functioning of the brain based on behavioral expression, and are able to determine whether a brain dysfunction exists or whether atypical patterns of neocortical development are present.

A neurologist looks at the anatomical construction of the brain. Working in conjunction with neurologists, neuropsychologists are able to determine the functional sequelae of CNS dysfunction. Neurologists use advanced neuroimaging techniques, including various forms of magnetic resonance imaging (MRI), positron emission tomography (PET), and single-photon emission computed tomography (SPECT) of brain regions. Working in conjunction with neurologists, neuropsychologists focus on behavior and cognition in order to offer educational help and remediation strategies to teachers, counselors, and parents. Clinical neuropsychologists deal with a variety of issues as caregivers seek to understand the educational and psychological needs of children and youth who are coping with neurological deficits. Parents frequently want to know what they can do to provide the optimal learning environment to help their children reach their full potential. They seek to understand the specific deficits experienced by the children. On the basis of a child's medical, family, and developmental history, as well as the specific behavioral and educational concerns, a neuropsychological assessment is designed and conducted.

Although this chapter discusses specific neuropsychological tests and batteries of tests, neuropsychology is not a set of techniques. Rather, it is a way of thinking about behavior, often expressed as test scores; in essence, it is a paradigm for understanding behavior.

COMPONENTS OF A NEUROPSYCHOLOGICAL EVALUATION

A neuropsychological evaluation of a child will differ in design from that of an adult. Of necessity, it will include educational and behavioral measures that may not be necessary with adults. The most common neuropsychological batteries and approaches will thus need to be supplemented in specific ways, depending on the referral questions posed. The following nine general guidelines should nevertheless prove useful and are derived from a variety of sources, including our own practices, the general teachings of Lawrence C. Hartlage, and other specific sources—in particular, Rourke, Bakker, Fisk, and Strang (1983), which we find to be remarkably current.

1. *All (or at least a significant majority) of a child's educationally relevant cognitive skills or higher-order information-processing skills should be assessed.* This will often involve an assessment of general intellectual level *(g)* via a comprehensive IQ test, such as a Wechsler scale, the Kaufman Assessment Battery for Children, Second Edition (KABC-II; Kaufman & Kaufman, 2004), or the Reynolds Intellectual Assessment Scales (RIAS; Reynolds & Kamphaus, 2003). Efficiency of mental processing as assessed by strong measures of *g* is essential to provide a baseline for interpreting all other aspects of the assessment process. Assessment of basic academic skills (including reading, writing, spelling, and math) will be necessary, along with tests such as the Test of Memory and Learning—Second Edition (TOMAL-2; Reynolds & Voress, 2007), which also have the advantage of including performance-based measures of attention

and concentration. Problems with memory, attention, concentration, and new learning are the most common of all complaints following CNS compromise and are frequently associated with more chronic neurodevelopmental disorders (e.g., learning disabilities, attention-deficit/hyperactivity disorder [ADHD]).

2. *Testing should sample the relative efficiency of the right and left hemispheres of the brain.* Asymmetries of performance are of interest on their own, but different brain systems are involved in each hemisphere, and these have differing implications for treatment. Even in a diffuse injury such as anoxia, it is possible to find greater impairment in one portion of an individual's brain than in another. Specific neuropsychological tests like those of Halstead and Reitan or the Luria–Nebraska Neuropsychological Battery—Children's Revision (LNNB-CR; Golden, 1986) are useful here, along with measures of verbal and nonverbal memory processes. In neurodevelopmental disorders, uneven development often occurs.

3. *Testing should sample both anterior and posterior regions of cortical function.* The anterior portion of the brain is generative and regulatory, whereas the posterior region is principally receptive. Deficits and their nature in these systems will have a great impact on treatment choices. Many common tests, such as tests of receptive (posterior) and expressive (anterior) vocabulary, may be applied here, along with a systematic and thorough sensory perceptual examination and certain specific tests of motor function. In conjunction with point 2 above, this allows for evaluation of the integrity of the four major quadrants of the neocortex: right anterior, right posterior, left anterior, and left posterior.

4. *Testing should determine the presence of specific deficits.* Any specific functional problems a child is experiencing must be determined and assessed. In addition to such problems being of importance in the assessment of children with neurodevelopmental disorders, traumatic brain injury (TBI), stroke, and even some toxins can produce very specific changes in neocortical function that are addressed best by the neuropsychological assessment. Similarly, research with children with leukemia suggests the presence

of subtle neuropsychological deficits following chemotherapy—deficits that may not be detected by more traditional psychological measures. Certain transplant patients will display specific patterns of deficits as well. Neuropsychological tests tend to be less g-loaded as a group and to have greater specificity of measurement than many common psychological tests. Noting areas of specific deficits is important in both diagnosis and treatment planning.

5. *Testing should determine the acuteness versus the chronicity of any problems or weaknesses found.* The "age" of a problem is important to diagnosis and to treatment planning. When a thorough history is combined with the pattern of test results obtained, it is possible, with reasonable accuracy, to distinguish chronic neurodevelopmental disorders such as dyslexia or ADHD from new, acute problems resulting from trauma, stroke, or disease. Particular care must be taken in developing a thorough, documented history when such a determination is made. Rehabilitation and habilitation approaches take differing routes in the design of intervention and treatment strategies, depending on the age of the child involved and the acuteness or chronicity of the problems evidenced. As children with neurodevelopmental disorders age, symptoms will wax and wane as well, and distinguishing new from old symptoms is important when treatment recommendations are being made.

6. *Testing should locate intact complex functional systems.* The brain functions as a series of interdependent, systemic networks often referred to as *complex functional systems.* Multiple systems are affected by CNS problems, but some systems are almost always spared except in the most extreme cases. It is imperative in the assessment process to locate strengths and intact systems that can be used to overcome the problems the child is experiencing. Treatment following CNS compromise involves habilitation and rehabilitation, with the understanding that some organic deficits will represent permanently impaired systems. As the brain consists of complex, interdependent networks of systems that produce behavior, the ability to ascertain intact systems is crucial to enhancing the probability of designing successful treatment. Identification of in-

tact systems also suggests the potential for a positive outcome to parents and teachers, as opposed to fostering low expectations and fatalistic tendencies on identification of brain damage or dysfunction.

7. *Testing should assess affect, personality, and behavior.* Neuropsychologists sometimes ignore their roots in psychology and focus on assessing the neural substrates of a problem. However, CNS compromise will results in changes in affect, personality, and behavior. Some of these changes will be transient, some will be permanent, and (because children are growing and developing beings) some will be dynamic. Some of these changes will be direct (i.e., the results of CNS compromise at the cellular and systemic levels), and others will be indirect (i.e., reactions to loss or changes in function, or to how others respond to and interact with the individual). A thorough history, including times of onset of problem behaviors, can assist in determination of direct versus indirect effects. As mentioned earlier, comprehensive approaches such as the Behavior Assessment System for Children, Second Edition (BASC-2; Reynolds & Kamphaus, 2004), which contain behavior rating scales, omnibus personality inventories, and direct observation scales, seem particularly useful. Notably, the BASC-2 has added scales to assess executive functions more thoroughly, as a reflection of the increasing knowledge base regarding the importance of brain–behavior relationships in general and executive functions in particular. Such behavioral changes will also require intervention, and intervention will be not necessarily be the same if the changes noted are direct versus indirect or if premorbid behavior problems were evident.

8. *Test results should be presented in ways that are useful in school settings, not just to acute care or intensive rehabilitation facilities, or to physicians.* Schools are a major context in which children with chronic neurodevelopmental disorders must function, and, as noted above, school psychologists are increasingly recognizing the role of neuropsychology in school-based interventions for children with neurodevelopmental and genetic disorders. Children who have sustained insult to the CNS (e.g., TBI, stroke) will eventually return to a school or similar

educational setting. This will be where the greatest long-term impact on a child's outcome after CNS compromise will be seen and felt. Results should speak to academic and behavioral concerns, reflecting what a child needs to be taught next in school, how to teach to the child's strengths through the engagement of intact complex functional systems, how to motivate the child, and how to manage positive behavioral outcomes. For a child with TBI, additional information regarding the potential for recovery and the tenuousness of evaluation results immediately postinjury need to be communicated, as does the need for reassessment of both the child and the intervention program at regular intervals. The changing nature of symptoms in a neurodevelopmental disorder must be followed and explained to those who believe that symptom expressivity is within an affected individual's control; such beliefs are all-too-common problems, especially in cases of ADHD, Tourette syndrome, XXY syndrome, and temporal lobe seizure disorder, and even in more common psychopathological disorders (e.g., depression).

9. *If consulting directly with a school system, an evaluator must be certain that the testing and examination procedures are efficient.* School systems, which are where one finds children, do not often have the resources for funding the types of diagnostic workups neuropsychologists prefer. Therefore, when one is consulting with a school system, it is necessary to be succinct and efficient in planning a neuropsychological evaluation. If the school can provide the results of a very recent intellectual and academic assessment, as well as of a behavioral assessment, this can be then integrated into the neuropsychological assessment. If a recent intellectual and academic assessment has not been completed, it may be cost-efficient for qualified school district personnel to complete this portion of the assessment for later integration with other data obtained and interpreted by the neuropsychologist. For children in intensive rehabilitation facilities or medical settings, it may be appropriate for school personnel to participate in the evaluation prior to discharge. This collaborative involvement can facilitate program planning with the receiving school district and is preferable to eliminating needed components of the neuropsychological evaluation.

ASSESSMENT APPROACHES AND INSTRUMENTS

There are two major conceptual approaches to neuropsychological assessment. In the first approach, a standard battery of tasks designed to identify brain impairment is used. The Halstead–Reitan Neuropsychological Test Battery for Older Children (for ages 9–14) and the Reitan–Indiana Neuropsychological Test Battery for Children (for ages 5–8) are the most commonly used batteries. "The second approach to neuropsychological assessment of children favors the use of a flexible combination of traditional psychological and educational tests. The composition of this battery varies depending on a number of child variables, including the age, history, functioning level, and presenting problem of the particular child" (Telzrow, 1989, p. 227). The major theoretical premise of both the Halstead–Reitan and the Reitan–Indiana batteries is the proposition that behavior has an organic basis (i.e., the brain controls behavior), and thus that performance on behavioral measures can be used to assess brain functioning (Bigler, 1996; Dean, 1985; Grant & Adams, 1986). In order to infer brain functioning based on behavioral measures, it was necessary to validate these measures on children with known brain damage (Nussbaum & Bigler, 1989).

The Halstead–Reitan Neuropsychological Test Battery for Older Children (for ages 9–14; see Table 2.1) was adapted from the original Halstead–Reitan Neuropsychological Test Battery, which was designed for adults. The two batteries share much of the same equipment and many of the same tests; however, there are some changes in the children's battery. The Tactual Performance Test uses a 6-hole board instead of the 10-hole board. On the Speech Sounds Perception Test, the child underlines the *correct* sound from three alternatives instead of four. The Category Test has been reduced from 208 slides to 168 slides. Likewise, Parts A and B of the Trail Making Test (Trails A and B) have been reduced in length.

The Trail Making Test is one of the most sensitive of all these tasks to the presence of CNS dysfunction, but did not localize dysfunction as well as was previously believed. Subsequently, Reynolds (2002) devel-

TABLE 2.1. Halstead–Reitan Neuropsychological Test Battery for Older Children (Ages 9–14)

Test administered	Function or skills assessed	Hypothesized localization
Lateral Dominance Aphasia Screening Test	Language	Language items relate to left hemisphere; constructional items relate to right hemisphere
Finger Tapping Test	Motor	Frontal lobe
Grip Strength	Motor	Frontal lobe
Sensory-Perceptual Examination	Sensory-perceptual	
Tactile Perception Test		Contralateral parietal lobe
Auditory Perception Test		Temporal lobe
Visual Perception Test		Visual pathway; visual fields
Tactile Form Recognition		Parietal lobe
Fingertip Writing Perception Test		Peripheral nervous system; parietal lobe
Finger Localization Test		Unilateral errors implicate contralateral parietal lobe—can also occur with bilateral errors
Rhythm Test	Alertness and concentration	Global
Speech Sounds Perception Test	Alertness and concentration	Global; anterior left hemisphere
Trail Making Test		
Part A	Visual–spatial	Global
Part B	Reasoning	Global
Tactual Performance Test		
Total Time	Motor	Frontal lobe
Memory	Immediate memory	Global
Localization	Immediate memory	Global
Category Test	Reasoning	Global; sensitive to right frontal lobe dysfunction in older children

Note. Data from Reitan and Wolfson (1985).

oped the Comprehensive Trail-Making Test (CTMT), which contains five trails. The CTMT has enhanced features to make the tasks even more sensitive to frontal and executive deficits in particular, and is normed for ages 8 years, 0 months to 74 years, 11 months. Trail 1 of the CTMT is similar to that of Trails A of the original Trail Making Test, as the examinee must connect numbers circles in numerical order. This task assesses sustained attention, as well as basic sequencing and visual–spatial scanning skills. Trails 2 requires the examinee to connect numbers in ascending order while ignoring simple distractors (empty circles). Trails 3 builds on Trails 2 by including simple distractors (empty circles), as well as complex distractors (circles with line drawings inside). Trails 4 and 5 require cognitive flexibility. On Trails 4, the examinee is required to connect numbers and number words. Trails 5 requires the examinee to connect numbers

and letters in an alternating sequence (similar to Trails B of the TMT), while also being presented with empty distractor circles. The CTMT meets rigorous standards in the areas of reliability and validity. All internal-consistency values of the five CTMT trails meet or exceed a value of .70, and the reliability value of the Composite Index score is .92 (Reynolds, 2002). A recent study by Armstrong, Allen, Donohue, and Mayfield (2008) provided support for the CTMT's utility in assessment of TBI.

Further modifications have been made with the Reitan–Indiana Neuropsychological Test Battery (for ages 5–8; see Table 2.2). Trails A and B, Speech Sounds Perception Test, and Rhythms have been omitted. Numerous tests have been added: Matching Pictures, Matching V's and Figures, Star Drawing, Concentric Square, Target Test, Marching Test, Color Form Test, and Progressive Figures. On the Category Test, the

TABLE 2.2. Reitan–Indiana Neuropsychological Test Battery for Children (Ages 5–8)

Test administered	Function or skill assessed	Hypothesized localization
Lateral Dominance Aphasia Screening Test	Language	Language items relate to left hemisphere; constructional items relate to right hemisphere
Finger Tapping Test	Motor	Frontal lobe
Grip Strength	Motor	Frontal lobe
Matching Pictures	Visual–spatial	Global right hemisphere
Matching V's and Figures	Visual–spatial	Association areas
Concentric Square and Star Drawing	Visual–spatial	Global right hemisphere
Target Test	Visual–spatial	Association areas
Marching Test	Motor	Global
Color Form Test		
Reasoning	Global	Global
Progressive Figures	Alertness and concentration	Global
Sensory-Perceptual Examination	Sensory-perceptual	
Tactile Perception Test		Contralateral parietal lobe
Auditory Perception Test		Temporal lobe
Visual Perception Test		Visual pathway; visual fields
Tactile Form Recognition		Parietal lobe
Fingertip Writing Perception Test		Peripheral nervous system; parietal lobe
Finger Localization Test		Unilateral error implicate contralateral parietal lobe—can also occur with bilateral errors
Tactual Performance Test		
Total Time	Motor	Frontal lobe
Memory	Immediate memory	Global
Localization	Immediate memory	Global
Category Test	Reasoning	Global; sensitive to right frontal lobe dysfunction in older children

Note. Data from Reitan and Wolfson (1985).

number of items has been further reduced to 80, and the number caps have been replaced with color caps. The same 6-hole board is used for the Tactual Performance Test as that used for the Halstead–Reitan version; however, the board is placed horizontally rather than vertically. The Aphasia Screening Test uses the same booklet, but some of the items have been omitted and replaced with more age-appropriate items. Because young children have difficulty manipulating the manual finger tapper, an electric tapper was developed for the Finger Tapping Test.

Right–left differences, dysphasia and related deficits, and cutoff scores that differentiate nondisabled children from children with brain damage for each battery are used to determine the score on the Neuropsychological Deficit Scale, which is the child's level of performance. Based on normative comparisons, raw scores are weighted as "perfectly normal" (score = 0), "normal" (score = 1), "mildly impaired" (score = 2), or "significantly impaired" (score = 3). Separate tables are available for the test results of older children and younger children.

In contrast to the use of standard batteries, the process approach uses a flexible battery of developmental and psychological tests, which permits the clinician to select tasks appropriate to the specific referral question, functioning levels, and response limitations of the child. Client variables such as "age, gender, handedness, familial handedness, educational and occupational background, premorbid talents, patient's and family's medical, neurological, and psychiatric history, drug or alcohol abuse, use of medications (past and present), etiology of the central nervous system (CNS) dysfunction, and laterality and focus of the lesion" (Kaplan, 1990, p. 72) all provide valuable information in developing the assessment. Furthermore, this process provides an analysis of the child's neuropsychological assets, rather than focusing on a diagnosis or a specific localization of brain impairment, for which the standardized batteries have been noted. The flexible-battery approach purportedly translates more directly into educational and vocational interventions, and a major goal of conducting a neuropsychological assessment is to aid in the planning of such interventions. Finally, since this method uses more traditional educational and psychological tests that are more familiar to school personnel, this assessment is more directly applicable to school settings. Schools provide the most affordable and available habilitation and rehabilitation opportunities for children with neuropsychological impairment; therefore, it is imperative that the assessment data be transferred into these settings (Telzrow, 1989). A major concern about the process approach is the difficulty in establishing validity for the innumerable versions of batteries used, as interpretations may not be uniform or reliable. This issue has been addressed inadequately thus far.

REASON FOR REFERRAL

Children are initially referred to neuropsychologists for a variety of reasons. If a child has a congenital brain defect, the child is frequently brought to a neuropsychologist early in his or her development, particularly if developmental delays, language deficits, or behavioral problems are observed. Depending on the results of the neuropsychological evaluation, the child may qualify for early intervention programs or other special programs through the public school system.

In other cases, as a child grows, parents may seek a diagnosis of ADHD as they cope with the child's problems at home and at school because of "hyperness" or "inability to sit still." At this time the neuropsy-

chologist seeks to discover the cause of the inattentiveness—whether it is truly ADHD or a learning disability, developmental delay, or psychiatric problem that is causing the behavior problems exhibited by the child.

A child who has experienced a TBI is frequently referred for a neuropsychological evaluation to determine the extent of the brain injury in terms of the child's cognitive strengths, weaknesses, and reentry into the school environment. On the basis of this evaluation, the neuropsychologist makes appropriate recommendations to the parents and school.

Even when the parents are unable to define specific referral questions, the driving forces behind the majority of neuropsychological referrals are problems in the educational setting. Teachers are often unprepared to address these difficulties and do not understand the specific learning problems of children with brain dysfunction. No two brain dysfunctions or injuries are the same. Two children can experience the same type of injury and still require different modifications in the classroom. Parents as well as teachers are looking for answers—ways to teach their children and to provide appropriate educational opportunities. A neuropsychological evaluation helps to furnish that information; it provides data for answering the question "So what do we do now?" after a diagnosis has been made. The information gained from a neuropsychological evaluation enables the neuropsychologist to make recommendations concerning attention, learning and memory, intellectual functioning, cognitive strengths and weaknesses, problem-solving abilities, and so forth to the parents and the educators.

TEACHING TO THE CHILD'S STRENGTHS

One of the primary reasons for conducting a neuropsychological evaluation is not to determine "what has been impaired," but rather to determine "what has been spared." Educators and parents supply numerous examples of what a child is unable to do: "He cannot follow instructions," "She can't remember anything," "He cannot read." Very seldom does a referral source approach an evaluation with a list of the activities or skills that the child is able to accomplish with ease and proficiency. But whether or not the source realizes it at the time of the referral, such a list contains the very information that is urgently needed for the child to move forward in the educational process. It is essential that we teach to the child's strengths instead of his or her weaknesses. As pointed out by Reynolds (1981b), teaching to a child's weaknesses focuses on brain areas that are damaged or dysfunctional. When teaching methods focus on cortical areas that are not intact, the child's potential for failure is increased, and this is harmful to the child. Reynolds has also pointed out that research on these remedial practices (referred to as *deficit-centered models* of remediation) has found them to be ineffective.

In contrast, teaching to a child's strengths has a number of advantages. This method may be especially helpful for children who are resistant to focused remediation of weaknesses (Rourke et al., 1983). When self-confidence is low or when a failure syndrome emerges as a result of frustration, a strength-centered approach should be adopted. Second, teaching to the child's strengths may reduce the possibility of the child's falling farther and farther below peers in academic areas. Finally, Luria (1966) suggested that recovery of function following cortical damage can be achieved "by the replacement of the lost cerebral link by another which is still intact" (p. 55). "For example, a child with an impaired auditory system could be taught to differentiate simple sounds using visual or nonverbal images" (Teeter & Semrud-Clikeman, 1997, p. 364). More details on strength-centered models of remediation may be found in Reynolds and Hickman (1987).

OTHER INFORMATION NEEDED FOR ASSESSMENT

When a child is initially referred to a neuropsychologist, the child's history is the first critical piece of information. This history should include prenatal, perinatal, developmental, and medical history. It is also important to include familial information about educational or learning problems, discipline, and family structure. If the child has had a TBI or illness, age of onset, duration of illness of injury, and time since illness or trauma all provide important information.

A child's school history provides invaluable information as well. The child's grades and other school records allow the neuropsychologist to look at trends in the student's educational process, and they provide a means of comparing the student's abilities with those of peers. School transcripts may also be helpful in evaluating individual motivational factors, study habits, and daily classroom performance. IQ tests or other standardized academic tests (e.g., the most recent editions of the Woodcock–Johnson battery, the Wide Range Achievement Test, and the Wechsler Individualized Achievement Test) provide standardized scores, which give further information about a child's cognitive and academic strengths and weaknesses. If a student has been receiving special services, one cannot assume that the existing services will meet the child's present needs; these services may need to be expanded or modified to meet the actual needs of the child.

On the basis of the historical information obtained, the trained neuropsychologist conducts a structured interview, which culminates in a list of referral questions and specific concerns about the child.

HABILITATION AND REHABILITATION CONSIDERATIONS

When one is making recommendations for rehabilitation of the child with a focal injury or TBI, several additional considerations are evident. It is important to determine what type of functional system is impaired. Impaired systems may, for example, be modality-specific or process-specific. The nature or characteristics of the impairments must be elucidated before an intelligent remedial plan can be devised.

The number of systems impaired should be determined. In addition, because children may not be able to work on everything at once, a system of priorities should be devised so that the impairments with the most important impact on overall recovery are the first and most intensely addressed. The degree of impairment, a normative question, will be important to consider in this regard as well. At times this will require the neuropsychologist to reflect on the indirect effects of a child's disorder or injury, as an impaired or dysfunctional system may adversely affect other systems that are without true direct organic compromise.

As noted earlier, the quality of the neuropsychological strengths that exist will also be important; this tends to be more of an ipsative than a normative determination. Certain strengths are more useful than others as well. Preserved language and speech are of great importance, for example, whereas an intact sense of smell (an ability often impaired in TBI) is of less importance in designing treatment plans and outcome research. Even more important to long-term recovery are intact planning and concept formation skills. The executive functioning skills of the frontal lobes take on greater and greater importance with age, and strengths in these areas are crucial to long-term planning (as are weaknesses). These will change with age, however, as the frontal lobes become increasingly prominent in behavioral control after age 9 years, again through puberty, and continuing into the 20s.

BASES FOR EDUCATIONAL MODIFICATIONS

After the neuropsychologist makes his or her assessment and recommendations, the school personnel and the parents hold a multidisciplinary team meeting. The purposes of this meeting are to make appropriate modifications in the classroom that will enable the child to reach his or her academic potential, and to develop an individualized education program (IEP) for the child. In many cases, educational modifications that teachers are currently using in their regular classrooms (e.g., small groups, modified assignments, individualized instruction) are the only modifications needed. Cohen (1991) suggests developing active learning situations, slowing down, assuring that lesson tasks address the appropriate deficits, teaching the process of the activity, teaching students to become more independent, and developing strategies that can be used in various situations. In other cases, the needed modifications include scheduling or placement issues that involve much more than the regular classroom setting. Placement options include the regular classroom, with no provision or support in the classroom; modified regular education, which could in-

clude a lighter course load or special tutorial sessions; a collapsed or half-day schedule; or special education services ranging from part-time to full-time. Class size may also be a consideration. Homebound or residential education programming may be yet another option. Fatigue is common during recovery from a head injury or stroke, and a schedule that allows for a structured rest time may also be a needed option (Cohen, 1991).

Educational support materials, such as computers, calculators, audio recorders, writing aids, positioning equipment, or augmentative communication devices, may be essential equipment in providing an appropriate educational environment. The use of such classroom aids should be implemented in consultation with the occupational therapist, physical therapist, and neuropsychologist, and should be included on the IEP.

Throughout this process, school personnel must collaborate with the child's parents. Open communication and cooperation between the parents and the school will assure the parents that their requests, apprehensions, and concerns will be addressed, and that their child will be provided with the most appropriate education. The neuropsychologist and school personnel can also make appropriate recommendations for the parents. With this information, the parents are able to formulate appropriate guidelines for behaviors and expectations for their child's educational potential.

MEMORY AND LEARNING

In cases of TBI, including closed head injury, problems with memory and attention are the most common, frequent complaints at all age levels. However, memory and learning problems seem to characterize nearly any CNS disorders in which higher cortical systems are involved (e.g., see Gillberg, 1995; Knight, 1992; Reynolds & Bigler, 1997). Table 2.3 provides a listing of the primary neurodevelopmental disorders in which the clinician can anticipate memory and learning deficits. The approach to assessment proffered herein would seem to require an assessment of children's memory and immediate learning skills. The neuropsychological batteries primarily in use with children, even when accompanied by a thorough as-

TABLE 2.3. Primary Neurodevelopmental Disorders in Which Memory and Learning Are Likely to Be Compromised

Attention-deficit/hyperactivity disorder (ADHD)	*In utero* toxic exposure (e.g., neonatal cocaine addiction, fetal alcohol syndrome)	Neurofibromatosis
Autism		Prader–Willi syndrome
Cerebral palsy	Juvenile Huntington disease	Rett syndrome
Down syndrome	Juvenile parkinsonism	Schizophrenia
Endocrine disorders	Learning disability	Seizure disorders
Extremely low birthweight	Lesch–Nyhan syndrome	Tourette syndrome
Fragile X syndrome	Mental retardation	Turner syndrome
Hydrocephalus	Myotonic dystrophy	Williams syndrome
Hypoxic–ischemic injury	Neurodevelopmental abnormalities affecting brain development (e.g., anencephaly, microcephaly, callosal dysgenesis)	XXY syndrome
Inborn errors of metabolism (e.g., phenylketonuria [PKU], galactosemia)		XYY syndrome

Note. Based on Reynolds and Bigler (1997).

sessment of intellect (as they should be), provide only a brief screening of memory and learning skills. Comprehensive assessment of children's memory and learning skills is a relatively recent phenomenon: The first comprehensive batteries for evaluating memory in children were not published until the 1990s (Reynolds & Bigler, 1994; Sheslow & Adams, 1990). By contrast, adult batteries, notably the Wechsler Memory Scale, have been available since the 1930s. Nevertheless, memory assessment in children was seen as important in evaluating children's skills at least as early as the work of Binet in the 1890s, and at least one measure of short-term memory appears in every Wechsler scale and most other major intelligence tests (e.g., the various Kaufman batteries, the McCarthy scales, and the various versions of the Detroit Tests of Learning Aptitude). A brief review of the neurobiology of memory shows why it is so crucial to assess memory when organic deficiencies are suspected.

Basic Neurobiology of Memory

Attention leaves tracks or traces within the brain that become memory. *Memory*, as commonly conceived of, is the ability to recall some event or information of various types and forms. Biologically, memory functions at two broad levels: the level of the individual cell and a systemic level. With the creation of memories, changes occur in individual cells (e.g., see Cohen, 1993; Diamond, 1990; Scheibel, 1990), including alterations in cell membranes and synaptic physiology.

At the systemic level, there exists a division of sorts in the formation of memory and memory storage. There is considerable evidence for distributed storage of associative memory throughout the cortex, which may even occur as a statistical function (Cohen, 1993). At the same time, evidence indicates more localized storage of certain memories and localized centers for memory formation and for classical and operant conditioning.

The medial aspect of the temporal lobe—particularly the hippocampus and its connecting fibers within the other limbic and paralimbic structures—is particularly important in the development of associative memory. The limbic system (with emphasis on the posterior hippocampal regions) also mediates the development of conditioned responses, and some patients with posterior hippocampal lesions may not respond to operant paradigms in the absence of one-to-one reinforcement schedules. Damage to or anomalous development of either the medial temporal lobe and its connecting fibers, or the midline structures of the diencephalon, typically results in the difficulties in formation of new memories (anterograde amnesia); however, it may also disrupt recently formed memories preceding the time of injury (retrograde amnesia). Various regions within the limbic and paralimbic structures have stronger roles in formation of certain types of memory, and simple conditioned memories may occur at a subcortical level. Through all the interactions of these systems, related mechanisms of attention, particularly in the brainstem and the frontal lobes, are brought to bear and will influence memory formation directly and indirectly. Memory is a complex function of the interaction of brain systems (with unequal contributions), and damage to one or more of many structures may impair the ability to form new memories.

In right-handed individuals, there is a tendency for damage to, or abnormal developmental patterns within, the left temporal lobe and adjacent structures to affect verbal and sequential memory more strongly. Damage to the cognate areas of the right hemisphere affects visual and spatial memory more adversely.

Through distributive storage of memory, the entire brain participates in memory functioning. The recall of well-established memories tends to be one of the most robust of neural functions, whereas the formation of new memories, sustained attention, and concentration tend to be the most fragile of neural functions. Neurological dysfunction of most types is associated with a nonspecific lessening of memory performance, along with disruptions of attention and concentration; this is of greater consequence when temporolimbic, brainstem, or frontal lobe involvement occurs. However, a variety of psychiatric disturbances, especially depression, may also suppress fragile anterograde memory systems. A careful analysis of memory, forgetting, affective states, history, and comprehensive neuropsychological test results may be necessary before one can conclude that memory disturbances are organic in origin, especially in the complex case of neurodevelopmental disorders.

Assessing Memory

The two most widely regarded and recommended memory batteries for children are the Wide Range Assessment of Memory and Learning (WRAML2; Sheslow & Adams, 2003) and the Test of Memory and Learning (TOMAL-2; Reynolds & Voress, 2007). The WRAML2 consists of nine subtests divided equally into three scales, Verbal Memory, Visual Memory, and Learning, followed by brief delayed-recall tasks to assess rapidity of the decay of memory. The original WRAML represented a substantial improvement over existing measures of memory in children when it appeared in

1990, but it still provided a somewhat limited scope of assessment. To increase the breadth and depth of assessment of memory and learning functions in children with a coordinated battery of diverse tasks, Reynolds and Bigler (1994) developed the original TOMAL. The TOMAL-2 continues to provide professionals with a standardized measure of different memory functions of children and adolescents from the age of 5. The many well-normed, reliable subtests of the TOMAL-2 provide examiners with the maximum flexibility in evaluating various referral questions and the choice of the most comprehensive assessments available. The individual subtests also have good reliability and specificity of measurement.

Test of Memory and Learning—Second Edition

The TOMAL-2 is a comprehensive battery of memory and learning tasks normed for used with children, adolescents, and adults from the age of 5 years, 0 months through 59 years. The TOMAL-2 has the broadest range of memory tasks available in a standardized memory battery (Hartman, 2007). The core battery consists of eight subtests (four verbal and four nonverbal), whose scores contribute to the Verbal Memory Index and Nonverbal Memory Index, which can be combined to derive a Composite Memory Index. A Delayed Verbal Recall Index is also available; this requires a repeat recall from two subtests of the core battery administered 30 minutes after the first administration. Six supplementary subtests (four verbal, two nonverbal) can be used to provide a broader, even more comprehensive assessment of memory. A supplementary subtest may be substituted for a core subtest when a core subtest cannot be given, is spoiled, or is inappropriate for a particular examinee.

As noted above, memory may behave in unusual ways in an impaired brain, and traditional content approaches to memory may not be useful. The TOMAL-2 thus provides alternative groupings of the subtests into five supplementary indexes: Attention/Concentration, Sequential Recall, Free Recall, Associative Recall, and Learning (Reynolds & Voress, 2007).

Table 2.4 gives the names of the subtests and summary scores, along with their met-

TABLE 2.4. Core and Supplementary Subtests and Indexes Available for the Test of Memory and Learning—Second Edition (TOMAL-2)

Index	Subtests	M	SD
Core composite indexes[a]			
Verbal Memory		100	15
	Memory for Stories	10	3
	Word Selective Reminding	10	3
	Object Recall	10	3
	Paired Recall	10	3
Nonverbal Memory		100	15
	Facial Memory	10	3
	Abstract Visual Memory	10	3
	Visual Sequential Memory	10	3
	Memory for Locations	10	3
Supplementary composite indexes			
Verbal Delayed Recall		100	15
	Memory for Stories Delayed	10	3
	Word Selective Reminding Delayed 10	3	
Attention/Concentration[b]		100	15
	Digits Forward	10	3
	Letters Forward	10	3
	Manual Imitation	10	3
	Digits Backward	10	3
	Letters Backward	10	3
Sequential Recall[b]		100	15
	Visual Sequential Memory	10	3
	Digits Forward	10	3
	Letters Forward	10	3
	Manual Imitation	10	3
Free Recall[c]		100	15
	Facial Memory	10	3
	Abstract Visual Memory	10	3
	Memory for Location 10	3	
Associative Recall[c]		100	15
	Memory for Stories	10	3
	Paired Recall	10	3
Learning[b]		100	15
	Word Selective Reminding	10	3
	Object Recall	10	3
	Paired Recall	10	3
	Visual Selective Reminding	10	3

[a]The eight Verbal Memory and Nonverbal Memory subtests make up the Composite Memory Index.
[b]Requires at least one supplementary subtest.
[c]Is derived entirely from core subtests.

rics. The TOMAL-2 subtests are scaled to the familiar metric of a mean of 10 and a standard deviation of 3 (range = 1–20). Composite or summary scores are scaled to a mean of 100 and a standard deviation of 15. All scaling was done using the method of continuous norming and is described in detail in Reynolds and Voress (2007).

A skilled examiner can administer the core TOMAL-2 battery in less than 30 minutes. However, the learning curve is quite steep, and it is not unusual for an examiner to require 60 minutes to complete the entire assessment during the first two to three administrations. After that, most examiners can complete the core battery in 30–35 minutes. Another 25–35 minutes are required to administer all of the supplementary subtests once the examiner has mastered administering the tasks. The subtests are briefly described in Table 2.5.

The TOMAL-2 subtests systematically vary the format of both presentation and response, so as to sample verbal, visual, and motoric modalities and combinations of these. Multiple trials to a criterion are provided on several subtests, including the Selective Reminding subtests, so that learning or acquisition curves may be derived. Multiple trials (at least five are necessary, according to Kaplan [1996], and the TOMAL-2 provides up to eight) are provided on the Selec-

TABLE 2.5. Description of TOMAL-2 Subtests

Core

- *Memory for Stories.* A verbal subtest requiring recall of a short story read to the examinee. Provides a measure of meaningful and semantic recall, and is also related to sequential recall in some instances.

- *Facial Memory.* A nonverbal subtest requiring recognition and identification from a set of distractors: black-and-white photos of various ages, both genders, and various ethnic backgrounds. Assesses nonverbal meaningful memory in a practical fashion and has been extensively researched. Sequencing of responses is unimportant.

- *Word Selective Reminding.* A verbal free-recall task in which the examinee learns a word list and repeats it; the examinee is only reminded of words left out in each trial. Tests learning and immediate recall functions in verbal memory. Trials continue until mastery is achieved or until six trials have been attempted. Sequence of recall is unimportant.

- *Abstract Visual Memory.* A nonverbal task assessing immediate recall for meaningless figures where order is unimportant. The examinee is presented with a standard stimulus and is required to recognize the standard from any of six distractors.

- *Object Recall.* The examiner presents a series of pictures, names them, has the examinee recall them, and repeats this process until mastery is achieved or until five trials have been attempted. Verbal and nonverbal stimuli are thus paired, and recall is entirely verbal, creating a situation found to interfere with recall for many individuals with learning disabilities but to be neutral or facilitative for individuals without disabilities

- *Visual Sequential Memory.* A nonverbal task requiring recall of the sequence of a series of meaningless geometric designs. The ordered designs are shown, followed by a presentation of a standard order of the stimuli, and the examinee indicates the order in which they originally appeared.

- *Paired Recall.* A verbal paired-associates task on which the examinee is required to recall a list of word pairs when the first word of each pair is provided by the examiner. Both easy and hard pairs are used.

- *Memory for Location.* A nonverbal task that assesses spatial memory. The examinee is presented with a set of large dots distributed on a page and is asked to recall the locations of the dots in any order.

Supplementary

- *Digits Forward.* A standard verbal number recall task. Measures low-level rote recall of a sequence of numbers.

- *Visual Selective Reminding.* A nonverbal analogue to Word Selective Reminding, where examinees point to specified dots on a card, following a demonstration by the examiner, and are reminded only of dots recalled incorrectly. Trials continue until mastery is achieved or until five trials have been attempted.

- *Letters Forward.* A language-related analogue to common digit span tasks, using letters as the stimuli in place of numbers.

- *Manual Imitation.* A psychomotor, visually based assessment of sequential memory. The examinee is required to reproduce a set of ordered hand movements in the same sequence as presented by the examiner.

- *Digits Backward.* This is the same basic task as Digits Forward, except that the examinee recalls the numbers in reverse order.

- *Letters Backward.* A language-related analogue to the Digits Backward task, using letters as the stimuli instead of numbers.

tive Reminding subtests to allow an analysis of the depth of processing. In the Selective Reminding format (wherein examinees are reminded only of stimuli "forgotten" or unrecalled), when items once recalled are unrecalled by an examinee on later trials, problems are revealed in the transference of stimuli from working memory and immediate memory to more long-term storage. Cueing is also provided at the end of certain subtests, to add to the examiner's ability to probe depth of processing.

Subtests are included that sample sequential recall (which tends strongly to be mediated by the left hemisphere, especially temporal regions; e.g., see Lezak, 1995) and free recall in both verbal and visual formats to allow localization. To assess more purely right-hemisphere functions, tests of pure spatial memory are included; these are very difficult to confound via verbal mediation.

Well-established memory tasks (e.g., recalling stories) that correlate well with school learning are also included, along with tasks more common to experimental neuropsychology that have high (e.g., Facial Memory) and low (e.g., Visual Selective Reminding) ecological salience. Some subtests employ highly meaningful material (e.g., Memory for Stories), whereas others use highly abstract stimuli (e.g., Abstract Visual Memory).

Aside from allowing a comprehensive review of memory function, the purpose of such a factorial array of tasks across multiple dimensions is to allow a thorough, detailed analysis of memory function and of the sources of any memory deficits that may be discovered. The task of the neuropsychologist demands subtests that have great specificity and variability of presentation and response, and that sample all relevant brain functions, in order to solve the complex puzzle of dysfunctional brain–behavior relationships. Kaufman (1979) first presented a detailed model for analyzing test data in a comprehensive format (later elaborated; Kaufman, 1994), which likens the task of the clinician to that of a detective. The thoroughness, breadth, and variability of the TOMAL-2 subtests, coupled with their excellent psychometric properties, make the TOMAL-2 ideal for use in a model of "intelligent testing" and particularly in the analysis of brain–behavior relationships associated with memory function.

ASSESSMENT OF BRAIN–BEHAVIOR RELATIONSHIPS THROUGH LURIAN PROCESSING MODELS

The previously reviewed approaches to assessing brain–behavior relationships focus on specificity of aptitudes or mental skills (i.e., their relative distinctiveness from one another) as a model for their assessment. Processing models of brain function focus more heavily on the manipulative demands of a mental task than on the content demands. Cognitive tasks can thus be grouped according to these processing demands for more reliable and detailed assessment, leading to conclusions about brain function with direct implications for intervention (e.g., see Hartlage & Reynolds, 1981; Kamphaus & Reynolds, 1987; Reynolds, 1981a, 1981b).

Lurian Theories

From a clinical perspective, the neuropsychological models of information processing espoused by Luria are of the greatest utility. "Alexander R. Luria's theory of higher cortical function has received international acclaim. His conceptual schemes of the functional organization of the brain are probably the most comprehensive currently available" (Adams, 1985, p. 878). Much of Luria's work elaborated and extended the earlier work of Sechenov (1863/1965) and Vygotsky (1978).

Luria defined mental processes in terms of two sharply delineated groups, *simultaneous* and *successive*, following Sechenov's suggestions. The first process involves the integration of elements into simultaneous groups. Luria further qualified Sechenov's original meaning, indicating that simultaneous processing means the synthesis of successive elements (arriving one after the other) into simultaneous spatial schemes, whereas successive processing means the synthesis of separate elements into successive series.

Luria (1966) divided the brain into three blocks. Block One consists of the brainstem and reticular system and is responsible principally for regulating level of consciousness, arousal, and the overall tone of the cortex. Block Two consists of the parietal, occipital, and temporal lobes of the brain (the lobes posterior to the central sulcus) and is responsible for receiving and encoding sensory input. Block Three consists of those regions of the brain anterior to the central sulcus (the frontal lobes and the prefrontal regions) and is responsible for the self-regulation of behavior, including such variables as attention, planning and execution of behavior, and other tasks generally referred to as *executive functions*. In Luria's model, various zones and regions of the brain interact in a transactional manner to produce complex behavior; thus the functional localization of complex mental tasks is seen as dynamic, defying efforts at highly specific anatomical localization. Luria's approach lends itself to strength-centered intervention models, wherein the clinician actively seeks intact complex functional systems within the brain that can be used to habilitate and facilitate learning, rather than to models focusing on remediating dysfunctional or damaged brain systems (e.g., see Reynolds, 1981b, 1997; Riccio & Reynolds, 1998).

Two neuropsychological batteries for children are based primarily on Luria's theory of brain function. The first to be published was the Kaufman Assessment Battery for Children (K-ABC; Kaufman & Kaufman, 1983), followed soon thereafter by the Luria–Nebraska Neuropsychological Battery—Children's Revision (LNNB-CR; Golden, 1986). A second edition of the K-ABC is now available (the KABC-II; Kaufman & Kaufman, 2004). Each of these batteries has a stronger focus on process than the typical neuropsychological test per se, with the possible exception of the TOMAL-2, but the TOMAL-2 focuses on memory processes more specifically.

Kaufman Assessment Battery for Children, Second Edition

The original K-ABC was designed and standardized for use with children ages 2½ years through 12½ years and was divided into three scales, closely following a Lurian model: the Sequential Processing Scale, the Simultaneous Processing Scale (these two were summed to provide a global score, the Mental Processing Composite), and the Achievement Scale (a measure of previously acquired information). The K-ABC was a useful scale for applications in the neuropsychological evaluation of children. Detailed discussions of its use in neuropsychology are provided in Kamphaus and Reynolds

(1987), Reynolds and Kamphaus (1997), and Reynolds, Kamphaus, Rosenthal, and Hiemenz (1997). The KABC-II (Kaufman & Kaufman, 2004), normed for ages 3 years through 18 years, maintains this utility and expands its assessment as a function of the Luria model, with the addition of a Planning Ability Scale.

In both the K-ABC and the KABC-II, the Kaufmans define mental processes in a manner similar to Luria's and provide a standardized assessment of these functions. *Simultaneous processing* here refers to the mental ability to integrate input simultaneously in order to solve a problem correctly. Simultaneous processing frequently involves spatial, analogical, or organizational abilities (Kaufman & Kaufman, 1983, 2004), as well as problems solved through the application of visual imagery. The Gestalt Closure and the Triangles (an analogue of Wechsler's Block Design task) subtests of the KABC-II are prototypical measures of simultaneous processing. To solve these items correctly, one must mentally integrate the components of the design to "see" the whole. Such a task seems to match up nicely with Luria's qualifying statement about the synthesis of separate elements into spatial schemes (e.g., in Triangles, the larger pattern of triangles, which may form squares, rectangles, or larger triangles). Whether the tasks are spatial or analogical in nature, the unifying characteristic of simultaneous processing is the mental synthesis of the stimuli to solve the problem, independent of the sensory modality of the input or the output.

Sequential processing, on the other hand, emphasizes the arrangement of stimuli in sequential or serial order for successful problem solving. In every instance, each stimulus is linearly or temporally related to the previous one (Kaufman & Kaufman, 1983, 2004), creating a form of serial interdependence within the stimulus. The KABC-II includes subtests that tap various modalities of sequential processing. Hand Movements involves visual input and a motor response; Number Recall involves auditory input with a response involving the auditory output channel only; and Word Order involves the visual channel for input and an auditory response. Therefore, the mode of presentation or mode of response is not what determines the scale placement of a task; rather, the mental processing demands of the task are important (Kaufman & Kaufman, 1983, 2004). By providing systematic variation of modality of input and modality of response, the KABC-II provides a clinical vehicle for locating intact complex functional systems, as well as for specifying where any potential breakdown may have occurred in a faulty functional system. Qualitative evaluation of a child's performance on the KABC-II can be most useful in such instances and can lead to more effective rehabilitation plans.

New to the KABC-II is the Planning Ability Scale. This scale consists of two subtests, Pattern Reasoning and Story Completion, wherein the examinee has to use inductive reasoning to determine the plan of a series of either abstract/geometric shapes or meaningless pictures (Pattern Reasoning) or to determine the missing elements in a set of pictures that tell a story (Story Completion). The plan must be deduced, and the examinee then completes the premeditated sequence. Although these subtests are strong measures of overall cognitive function, it is not yet clear from data in the KABC-II manual that they differentiate Planning Ability as a separate construct. However, the Sequential and the Simultaneous Processing Scales are very useful from a Lurian perspective.

No one with an intact brain uses only a single type of information processing to solve problems. These two methods of information processing are constantly interacting (even in the so-called "split brain" following commissurotomy), although one approach will often take a lead role in processing. Which method of processing takes the lead role can change according to the demands of the problem or (as is the case with some individuals) can persist across problem type, forming habitual modes of processing. In fact, any problem can be solved through either method of processing, but in most cases one method is clearly superior to another. What makes the KABC-II a valuable tool is that the two mental processing scales are primarily, not exclusively, measures of sequential or simultaneous processing. "Pure" scales (i.e., scales measuring only one process) do not exist. Careful observation of a child's performance, which should be the order of the day during any evaluation, will be particularly important to any neuropsychological assessment or neuropsychological

interpretation of KABC-II test results; observation in many cases will be a primary source of information regarding which mental processes a child has invoked on any given task, regardless of its scale.

An equally important component of the KABC-II is the Knowledge Scale (formerly the Achievement Scale, with a few changes). This scale measures abilities that serve to complement the mental processing scales. Performance on the KABC-II Knowledge Scale, like that on the K-ABC Achievement Scale, is viewed as an estimate of children's success in the application of their mental processing skills to the acquisition of knowledge from the environment (Kaufman, Kamphaus, & Kaufman, 1985). This scale contains measures of what have been identified traditionally as verbal intelligence, general information, and acquired school skills. Keeping in mind that it is not possible to separate entirely what individuals know (achievement) from how well they think (intelligence), the Kaufmans have attempted to differentiate the two variables more clearly than traditional measures of intelligence generally do. From a clinical-neuropsychological standpoint, the KABC-II allows one to assess information-processing skills without as much contamination from prior learning. Measurement of children's academic skills, however, is a traditional component of the comprehensive neuropsychological assessment. The inclusion of the Knowledge Scale in the KABC-II affords the opportunity to observe the application of processing skills to complex learning tasks, to assess functional academic levels, and to estimate long-term memory ability.

Majovski (1984) noted the high degree of fit between Luria's theory and the original K-ABC, and recommended that the test be used as an integral part of a neuropsychological battery for children (see also Spreen & Strauss, 1991). It is a good complement to nearly any choice of neuropsychological instruments. Majovski found the K-ABC particularly useful in contrasting problem-solving skills with acquisition of facts and in evaluating how a child solves a particular problem.

When young children (below age 6) are being assessed, the KABC-II should be the neuropsychologist's test of choice for measuring intellectual skill. The KABC-II mental processing subtests are child-oriented and much briefer than (but with comparable reliability to) those of its major competitor, the Wechsler Preschool and Primary Scale of Intelligence—Third Edition (Wechsler, 2002). For assessing mental processes, the KABC-II model seems far superior to other measures of intelligence, since it is far less dependent on prior learning and exposure to the mainstream Anglo culture (e.g., see Kamphaus & Reynolds, 1987). When one is assessing the intellectual processes of non-native English speakers, the independence of the KABC-II mental processing scales is particularly important, so as not to confound cultural experiences and cultural dependence of test items with neuropsychological processing (e.g., see Ardila, Roselli, & Puente, 1994). A growing body of literature shows the appropriateness of the KABC-II across a broad range of U.S. ethnic minorities.

Support for use of the KABC-II model in the context of neuropsychological assessment also comes from a variety of sources in cerebral specialization research. In a comprehensive review of research concerning the lateralization of human brain functions, Dean (1984) concluded that the original K-ABC is well suited to clinical use and in research with children.

It has been proposed that sequential processing and simultaneous processing are lateralized to the left and right hemispheres, respectively (e.g., Reynolds, 1981b). Many other dichotomies have been suggested. Some find the research on cerebral specialization difficult to coalesce. Indeed, the many seeming contradictions in the results of cerebral specialization studies have prompted at least one pair of leading researchers to remark some decades ago: "[To] say that the field of hemispheric specialization is in a state of disarray and that the results are difficult to interpret is an understatement. The field can best be characterized as chaotic" (Tomlinson-Keasey & Clarkson-Smith, 1980, p. 1). On the other hand, reviews by Dean (1984) and Reynolds (1981a) noted some consistencies, especially when one focuses on process specificity and not the content of the task stimulus, consistencies upheld by research of subsequent decades.

For the vast majority of individuals, the left cerebral hemisphere appears to be specialized for linguistic, propositional, serial, and analytic tasks, and the right hemisphere for more nonverbal, oppositional, synthetic, and holistic tasks. The literature includes a large number of studies of hemispheric specialization that have attempted to provide anatomical localization of performance on specific, yet higher-order, complex tasks. Much of the confusion in the literature stems from the apparently conflicting data in many of these studies. However, Luria's principle of dynamic functional localization, and the knowledge that any specific task can potentially be performed through any of the brain's processing modes, should give some insight into the conflicting results that appear in the literature. In this regard, it is most important to remember that cerebral hemispheric asymmetries of function are process-specific and not stimulus-specific. Shure and Halstead (1959) noted early in this line of research that manipulation of stimuli is at the root of hemispheric differences—a notion that is well supported by subsequent empirical research (e.g., Ornstein, Johnstone, Herron, & Swencionis, 1980) and thought (e.g., Reynolds, 1981a, 1981b). The confusion of the content and sensory modality through which stimuli are presented with the process by which they are manipulated, particularly in the secondary and tertiary regions of each lobe of the neocortex, seems to be at the root of the chaos. How information is manipulated while in the brain is not dependent on its modality of presentation and not necessarily dependent on its content, though the latter may certainly be influential. The variations in content and in method of presentation of the tasks that make up the scales of the KABC-II allow one to tease out any modality or content effects that may nevertheless occur for a specific child, though clearly the emphasis of the KABC-II is on process, not content.

We think that a process-oriented explanation provides a better organizing principle than does a focus on content. The "content-driven" attempts at explaining hemispheric differences fail to recognize the possibilities for processing any given set of stimuli or particular content in a variety of processing modes. Bever (1975) emphasized this point and elaborated on two modes of information processing that are of interest here because of their similarity to simultaneous and sequential cognitive processes.

The KABC-II also taps most of the functions identified by Dean (1984) in his review of the literature on cerebral specialization, with the exceptions of depth, haptic, and melodic perceptions. These skills are assessed by other traditional neuropsychological batteries, although such tasks are virtually nonexistent for the very young child. Careful observation may still provide insight into neuropsychological processing deficits, especially if one pays particular attention to the manner in which errors are made. Qualitative and quantitative data are complementary, not interchangeable; Kaufman's (1994) philosophy of "intelligent testing" is just as crucial to neuropsychological assessment as to any other area of clinical evaluation.

Finally, the KABC-II offers, with a variety of supplementary subtests, assessment according to the Cattell–Horn–Carroll model of intelligence. This will be of less interest to the neuropsychologist, but it broadens the appeal of the KABC-II in a variety of circumstances.

Luria–Nebraska Neuropsychological Battery—Children's Revision

The LNNB-CR (Golden, 1986) is a downward extension of the Luria–Nebraska Neuropsychological Battery for adults. Originally, in its research form, it was administered down to age 5, but reliable performance could only be obtained beginning at age 8 (Golden, 1997). After age 12, the adult battery is used.

There are 11 scales on the LNNB-CR, and each is listed and described in Table 2.6. As Golden (1997) describes, the LNNB-CR lends itself to three levels of interpretation: scale, item, and qualitative. Each of the 11 scales yields a T-score, and the resulting profile has been the subject of significant empirical work. However, the items within these scales vary in modality and other demand characteristics, and an analysis of item scores is also used. Finally, Luria was a renowned clinician and approached patients individually; Golden (1986) thus designed the LNNB-CR to allow qualitative analysis as a supplement to the typical Western psychological approach of quantitative analysis of performance on the various scales. As Table 2.6 indicates, the LNNB-CR has some scales and items where process is the dominant feature, but others where content and learned behavior predominate. Careful review of LNNB-CR performance at all three levels (scale, item, and qualitative) is not just possible but necessary. In a qualita-

TABLE 2.6. Scales of Luria–Nebraska Neuropsychological Battery—Children's Revision (Ages 8–12)

Scales	Description of abilities assessed
Motor Skills	Motor speed, complex coordination, imitation of motor movements, constructural praxis
Rhythm	Attention, perceiving and repeating rhythmic patterns, analyzing groups of tones
Tactile	Finger localization, arm localization, two-point discrimination, movement discrimination, shape discrimination, stereognosis, verbal–tactile integration
Visual	Visual recognition, visual discrimination, spatial perception
Receptive Speech	Following simple commands, comprehending verbal directions, decoding phonemes, naming
Expressive Language	Reading and repeating words and simple sentences, naming object from description, using automated speech, discerning missing words
Writing	Analyzing letter sequences, spelling, writing from dictation, copying
Reading	Letter and word calling, sentence and paragraph reading, nonsense syllable reading
Arithmetic	Simple calculation, number writing, number recognition (Arabic and Roman)
Memory	Verbal and visual memory, some interference tasks
Intelligence	Vocabulary, verbal reasoning, picture interpretation, social reasoning, deduction, scanning

tive analysis, an examiner is more concerned with wrong answers than with correct ones and analyzes the nature of the errors committed by the examinee. For example, was the inability to write to dictation caused by a visual–motor problem; a visual-perceptive deficit; a failure of comprehension; or a planning, attention, or execution problem? Only through careful observation and a review of successful tasks can these questions be answered. Examiners must have extensive experience with normal individuals, however, to avoid overinterpretation. This process of interpretation at multiple levels continues to be consistent with Kaufman's (1979, 1994) philosophy of "intelligent testing" and is advisable for use with all assessment devices discussed herein. However, the LNNB-CR was devised with these approaches in mind, making it more amenable to multilevel analysis. A revision of the LNNB-CR is underway that is intended to expand the scale from its currently very limited age range, extending it downward to age 5 years. This will certainly make the battery more useful for children with various neurodevelopmental disorders.

Boston Process Approach

Another, newer effort at evaluating process in neuropsychological assessment is known as the Boston Process Approach (BPA) and is described in detail in Kaplan (1988, 1990). This model also tries to integrate quantitative and qualitative approaches to interpretation and analysis of performance on various cognitive tasks. The BPA alters the format of items on traditional tests such as the various Wechsler scales, and BPA versions of the Wechsler Intelligence Scale for Children—Third Edition and the Wechsler Adult Intelligence Scale—Third Edition are available. Additional, supplementary tests have been devised specifically for the BPA over many years, including the Boston Naming Test, the Boston Diagnostic Aphasia Examination, and the California Verbal Learning Test, along with others. As with other methods of assessment, examiners are advised to use BPA assessments in conjunction with history and interview data and observations of the patient.

The strength of the BPA lies in its flexibility, which enables a neuropsychologist to tailor the assessment to the referred problem. There is quite a bit of research on individual aspects of the BPA (e.g., see White & Rose, 1997), but research on the BPA as a whole is lacking. The modifications made to well-designed, carefully standardized tests such as the Wechsler scales also have unpredictable and at times counterintuitive outcomes in patient examination (e.g., Slick et al., 1996). Slick and colleagues (1996) found that changes made to the BPA version of the Wechsler Adult Intelligence Scale—Revised caused a substantial number of individuals to earn lower scores on the modified items than on the corresponding standardized versions of the items, even though the intent of the modification was in part to make the items easier. This could easily draw a clinician into overinterpretation and overdiagnosis of pathology. Slick and colleagues correctly conclude that whenever changes are made to standardized instruments, comprehensive norms are required under the new testing conditions. They also conclude that clinical interpretation of such modified procedures prior to the development and purveyance of the norms is questionable from an ethical standpoint.

The lack of good normative or reference data has been a long-term problem for neuropsychological assessment (e.g., see Reynolds, 1997). This causes a variety of problems related to test interpretation, not the least of which involve understanding the relationship of status variables such as gender, ethnicity, and socioeconomic status to test performance. The BPA, because of its principal strengths, also makes inordinate cognitive demands on the examiner. Until the BPA's normative and data integration problems are solved, it is recommended here primarily only as a research approach (albeit a most promising one). It may be useful now, but only to a small group of clinicians with extensive, supervised training in its use from one of its progenitors.

CONCLUDING REMARKS

There are many methods and models of neuropsychological assessment. The field of pediatric neuropsychology is young as clinical disciplines go. Controversies continue over the training and credentialing of neuropsychologists as well. However, the field has proven itself to be of value in contributing to patient care, and thereby it will continue to grow and even thrive. Clinicians must recognize that patient care is the ultimate goal and must provide carefully integrated, treatment-relevant data. A clinician writing a report on a child's neuropsychological examination should pay particular attention to the following suggestions:

1. *Write reports that go beyond a simple descriptive presentation of test data and findings.* A clinician should integrate data across the history and across data sources. Data should be interpreted for the reader.

2. *Write professionally.* A clinician should use proper grammar and formal language structures in presenting reports.

3. *Use language that is easily understood.* Reports on children will be used in many arenas, and writing a child's neuropsychological report in such a way as to be interpretable only by a physician or another neuropsychologist does not facilitate treatment. The report of the neuropsychologist is of no value if it cannot be understood. Reports should be cognitively accessible to school personnel (including teachers, counselors, and school psychologists), rehabilitation staff (e.g., occupational therapists, speech therapists, physical therapists), and parents, in addition to referring physicians.

4. *Write reports about children, not about tests.* Too often the neuropsychological evaluation of a child reads like a test recital (i.e., test after test is presented, and the child's performance is noted). No data integration is attempted, and it is common to find contradictory statements in such rote reports. Parents often interpret such impersonal reports as lacking in concern or interest for their child.

5. *Draw diagnostic conclusions.* Whenever possible, the examining clinician should proffer a diagnostic summary for consideration of other sources. Diagnosis is treatment-relevant and should be noted.

6. *Describe treatment implications of neuropsychological findings.* Although no one clinician can reasonably be expected to know all treatment implications of a set of findings, clinicians should note, to the extent of their knowledge, treatment implications of the findings of their own examinations. Neuropsychological results may indicate a need for specific interventions (e.g., neurocognitive therapy, speech therapy) or for specific methods of intervention within a known class (e.g., reading instruction via phonics vs. whole language; inefficacy of certain behavior therapies in the face of particular neuropsychological findings).

Neuropsychologists have much of value to offer in the care of children with neurodevelopmental disorders. Data and recommendations related to symptom expressivity, new problems, effectiveness of treatment, and possible behavioral interventions are some of their most valuable offerings. In this age of cost containment, it is crucial to provide useful, scientifically supported conclusions that contribute to treatment and other facets of patient care, and to maximize the benefit of the neuropsychological examination for the child.

REFERENCES

Adams, K. (1985). Review of the Luria–Nebraska Neuropsychological Battery. In J. V. Mitchell (Ed.), *Ninth mental measurements yearbook*. Lincoln, NE: Buros Institute of Mental Measurement.

Ardila, A., Roselli, M., & Puente, A. (1994). *Neuropsychological evaluation of the Spanish-speaker.* New York: Plenum Press.

Armstrong, C. M., Allen, D, N., Donohud, B., & Mayfield, J. (2008). Sensitivity of the Comprehensive Trail Making Test to traumatic brain injury in adolescents *Archives of Clinical Neuropsychology, 23,* 351–358.

Bayley, N. (2005). *Bayley Scales of Infant and Toddler Development—Third Edition.* San Antonio, TX: Harcourt Assessment.

Bever, T. G. (1975). Cerebral asymmetries in humans are due to the differentiation of two incompatible processes: Holistic and analytic. In D. Aronson & R. Reiber (Eds.), *Developmental psycholinguistics and communication disorders.* New York: New York Academy of Sciences.

Bigler, E. D. (1996). Bridging the gap between psychology and neurology: Future trends in pediatric neuropsychology. In E. S. Batchelor, Jr., & R. S. Dean (Eds.), *Pediatric neuropsychology* (pp. 27–54). Needham Heights, MA: Allyn & Bacon.

Cohen, R. A. (1993). *The neuropsychology of attention.* New York: Plenum Press.

Cohen, S. B. (1991). Adapting educational programs for students with head injuries. *Journal of Head Trauma Rehabilitation, 6*(1), 47–55.

D'Amato, R. C., Fletcher-Janzen, E., & Reynolds, C. R. (Eds.). (2005). *Handbook of school neuropsychology*. Hoboken, NJ: Wiley.

Das, J. P., Kirby, J. R., & Jarman, R. F. (1979). *Simultaneous and successive cognitive processes*. New York: Academic Press.

Dean, R. S. (1984). Functional lateralization of the brain. *Journal of Special Education, 8*, 239–256.

Dean, R. S. (1985). Foundation and rationale for neuropsychological bases of individual differences. In L. Hartlage & K. Telzrow (Eds.), *Neuropsychology of individual differences* (pp. 7–39). New York: Plenum Press.

Diamond, M. C. (1990). Morphological cortical changes as a consequence of learning and experience. In A. B. Scheibel & A. F. Wechsler (Eds.), *Neurobiology of higher cognitive function* (pp. 1–12). New York: Guilford Press.

Farmer, J. E., & Peterson, L. (1995). Pediatric traumatic brain injury: Promoting successful school reentry. *School Psychology Review, 24*(2), 230–243.

Gillberg, C. (1995). *Clinical child neuropsychiatry*. Cambridge, UK: Cambridge University Press.

Golden, C. J. (1986). *Manual for the Luria–Nebraska Neuropsychological Battery—Children's Revision*. Los Angeles: Western Psychological Services.

Golden, C. J. (1997). The Nebraska-Neuropsychological Children's Battery. In C. R. Reynolds & E. Fletcher-Janzen (Eds.), *Handbook of clinical child neuropsychology* (2nd ed., pp. 237–251). New York: Plenum Press.

Grant, I., & Adams, K. M. (Eds.). (1986). *Neuropsychological assessment of neuropsychiatric disorder* (2nd ed.). New York: Oxford University Press.

Hartlage, L. C., & Reynolds, C. R. (1981). Neuropsychological assessment and the individualization of instruction. In G. W. Hynd & J. E. Obrzut (Eds.), *Neuropsychological assessment of the school-aged child* (pp. 355–378). New York: Grune & Stratton.

Hartman, D. E. (2007). Test review: Wide Range Assessment of Memory and Learning–2 (WRAML-2). Wredesigned and weally improved. *Applied Neuropsychology, 14*(20), 138–140.

Hynd, G. W., & Reynolds, C. R. (2005). School neuropsychology: The evolution of a specialty in school psychology. In R. C. D'Amato, E. Fletcher-Janzen, & C. R. Reynolds (Eds.), *Handbook of school neuropsychology* (pp. 3–14). New York: Wiley.

Kamphaus, R. W., & Reynolds, C. R. (1987). *Clinical and research applications of the K-ABC*. Circle Pines, MN: American Guidance Service.

Kaplan, E. (1988). A process approach to neuropsychological assessment. In T. Boll & B. K. Bryant (Eds.), *Clinical neuropsychology and brain function: Research, measurement, and practice*. Washington, DC: American Psychological Association.

Kaplan, E. (1990). The process approach to neuropsychological assessment of psychiatric patients. *Journal of Neuropsychiatry, 2*(1), 72–87.

Kaplan, E. (1996). *Discussant*. Symposium on assessment of children's memory at the annual meeting of the National Association of School Psychologists, Atlanta, GA.

Kaufman, A. S. (1979). *Intelligent testing with the WISC-R*. New York: Wiley-Interscience.

Kaufman, A. S. (1994). *Intelligent testing with the WISC-III*. New York: Wiley-Interscience.

Kaufman, A. S., Kamphaus, R. W., & Kaufman, N. L. (1985). The Kaufman Assessment Battery for Children: K-ABC. In C. S. Newark (Ed.), *Major psychological assessment instruments*. Boston: Allyn & Bacon.

Kaufman, A. S., & Kaufman, N. L. (1983). *K-ABC interpretation manual*. Circle Pines, MN: American Guidance Service.

Kaufman, A. S., & Kaufman, N. L. (2004). *Kaufman Assessment Battery for Children, Second Edition*. Bloomington, MN: Pearson Assessments.

Knight, R. G. (1992). *The neuropsychology of degenerative brain diseases*. Hillsdale, NJ: Erlbaum.

Lezak, M. D. (1995). *Neuropsychological assessment* (3rd ed.). New York: Oxford University Press.

Luria, A. R. (1966). *Human brain and psychological processes*. New York: Harper & Row.

Majovski, L. (1984). The K-ABC: Theory and applications for child neuropsychological assessment and research. *Journal of Special Education, 18*, 266–268.

Miller, D. C. (Ed.). (2010). *Best practices in school neuropsychology*. New York: Wiley.

Nussbaum, N. L., & Bigler, E. D. (1989). Halstead–Reitan Neuropsychological Test Batteries for Children. In C. R. Reynolds & E. Fletcher-Janzen (Eds.), *Handbook of clinical child neuropsychology* (pp. 181–192). New York: Plenum Press.

Ornstein, R., Johnstone, J., Herron, J., & Swiencionis, C. (1980). Differential right hemisphere engagement in visuospatial tasks. *Neuropsychologia, 18*, 49–64.

Reitan, R. M., & Wolfson, D. (1974). *Clinical neuropsychology: Current status and applications*. Washington, DC: Winston.

Reitan, R. M., & Wolfson, D. (1985). *The Halstead–Reitan Neuropsychological Battery: Theory and clinical interpretation*. Tucson, AZ: Neuropsychological Press.

Reynolds, C. R. (1981a). Neuropsychological assessment and the habilitation of learning: Considerations in the search for the aptitude x treatment interaction. *School Psychology Review, 10*, 343–349.

Reynolds, C. R. (1981b). The neuropsychological basis of intelligence. In G. W. Hynd & J. E. Obrzut (Eds.), *Neuropsychological assessment of the school-aged child* (pp. 87–124). New York: Grune & Stratton.

Reynolds, C. R. (1997). Measurement and statistical problems in neuropsychological assessment of children. In C. R. Reynolds & E. Fletcher-Janzen (Eds.), *Handbook of clinical child neuropsychology* (2nd ed., pp. 180–203). New York: Plenum Press.

Reynolds, C. R. (2002). *Comprehensive Trail-Making Test*. Austin, TX: PRO-ED.

Reynolds, C. R., & Bigler, E. D. (1994). *Manual for the Test of Memory and Learning*. Austin, TX: PRO-ED.

Reynolds, C. R., & Bigler, E. D. (1997). Clinical neuropsychological assessment of child and adolescent memory with the Test of Memory and Learning. In C. R. Reynolds & E. Fletcher-Janzen (Eds.), *Handbook of clinical child neuropsychology* (2nd ed., pp. 296–319). New York: Plenum Press.

Reynolds, C. R., & Hickman, J. A. (1987). Remediation, deficit-centered models of. In C. R. Reynolds & L. Mann (Eds.), *Encyclopedia of special education* (pp. 1339–1342). New York: Wiley-Interscience.

Reynolds, C. R.., & Kamphaus, R. W. (1997). The Kaufman Assessment Battery for Children: Development, structure, and applications in neuropsychology. In A. Horton, D. Wedding, & J. Webster (Eds.), *The neuropsychology handbook* (2nd ed., Vol. 1, pp. 291–330). New York: Springer.

Reynolds, C. R., & Kamphaus, R. W. (2003). *Reynolds Intellectual Assessment Scales*. Lutz, FL: Psychological Assessment Resources.

Reynolds, C. R., & Kamphaus, R. W. (2004). *Behavior Assessment System for Children, Second Edition*. Bloomington, MN: Pearson Assessments.

Reynolds, C. R., Kamphaus, R. W., Rosenthal, B., & Hiemenz, J. (1997). Applications of the Kaufman Assessment Battery for Children (K-ABC) in neuropsychological assessment. In C. R. Reynolds & E. Fletcher-Janzen (Eds.), *Handbook of clinical child neuropsychology* (2nd ed., pp. 252–269). New York: Plenum Press.

Reynolds, C. R., & Voress, J. K. (2007). *Test of Memory and Learning—Second Edition*. Austin, TX: PRO-ED.

Riccio, C. A., & Reynolds, C. R. (1998). Neuropsychological assessment of children. In M. Hersen & A. Bellack (Series Eds.) & C. R. Reynolds (Vol. Ed.), *Comprehensive clinical psychology: Vol. 4. Assessment* (pp. 267–302). New York: Elsevier Science.

Rourke, B. P., Bakker, D. J., Fisk, J. L., & Strang, J.

D. (1983). *Child neuropsychology*. New York: Guilford Press.

Scheibel, A. B. (1990). Dendritic correlates of higher cortical function. In A. Scheibel & A. Wechsler (Eds.), *Neurobiology of higher cognitive function* (pp. 239–270). New York: Guilford Press.

Sechenov, I. (1965). *Reflexes of the brain*. Cambridge, MA: MIT Press. (Original work published 1863)

Sheslow, D., & Adams, W. (1990). *Wide Range Assessment of Memory and Learning*. Wilmington, DE: Jastak Associates.

Sheslow, D., & Adams, W. (2003). *Wide Range Assessment of Memory and Learning, Second Edition*. Lutz, FL: Psychological Assessment Resources.

Shure, G. H., & Halstead, W. (1959). Cerebral lateralization of individual processes. *Psychological Monographs: General and Applied, 72*(12).

Slick, D., Hopp, G., Strauss, E., Fox, D., Pinch, D., & Stickgold, K. (1996). Effects of prior testing with the WAIS-R NI on subsequent retest with the WAIS-R. *Archives of Clinical Neuropsychology, 11*(2), 123–130.

Spreen, O., & Strauss, E. (1991). *A compendium of neuropsychological tests*. London: Oxford University Press.

Teeter, P. A., & Semrud-Clikeman, M. (1997). *Child neuropsychology: Assessment and intervention for neurodevelopmental disorders*. Needham Heights, MA: Allyn & Bacon.

Telzrow, C. F. (1989). Neuropsychological applications of common educational and psychological tests. In C. R. Reynolds & E. Fletcher-Janzen (Eds.), *Handbook of clinical child neuropsychology* (pp. 227–246). New York: Plenum Press.

Tomlinson-Keasey, C., & Clarkson-Smith, L. (1980). *What develops in hemispheric specialization?* Paper presented at the annual meeting of the International Neuropsychological Society, San Francisco.

Vygotsky, L. S. (1978). *Mind in society*. Cambridge, MA: Harvard University Press.

Warzak, W. J., Mayfield, J. W., & McAllister, C. (1996, November). *Integrating neuropsychological and behavioral data to develop comprehensive assessment strategies in brain injured individuals*. Paper presented at the 30th Annual Convention of the Association for Advancement of Behavior Therapy, New York.

Wechsler, D. (2002). *Wechsler Preschool and Primary Scale of Intelligence—Third Edition*. San Antonio, TX: Psychological Corporation.

White, R. F., & Rose, F. E. (1997). The Boston Process Approach: A brief history and current practice. In G. Goldstein & T. Incagnoli (Eds.), *Contemporary approaches to neuropsychological assessment* (pp. 171–212). New York: Plenum Press.

CHAPTER 3

Neurodevelopmental Disorders and Medical Genetics

An Overview

BONNIE J. BATY
JOHN C. CAREY
WILLIAM M. McMAHON

The entrance of the discipline of medical genetics into the care of persons with neurodevelopmental disorders is a relatively recent but highly significant event. The application of the principles of genetics to medicine is crucial because of the important role of genes in the causation of human developmental disorders. In addition, a precise diagnosis of a genetic condition or syndrome is important to the person diagnosed, his or her family, and the practitioner caring for the individual. Moreover, parents of individuals with disabilities and differences frequently ask questions about the chance of a disorder's occurring in future pregnancies.

Medical genetics has only recently emerged as a bona fide specialty in organized medicine. In the 1960s, the fields of biochemical genetics, clinical cytogenetics, and dysmorphology developed and paved the way for the delineation of this discipline. Now, with the recently publicized advances in the mapping and cloning of human disease genes, interest in genetics and its roles in human disorders is commonplace; indeed, these have become topics of everyday conversations. The purpose of this chapter is to summarize the body of knowledge and principles of medical genetics needed for the discussion of the neurodevelopmental disorders presented in this book. The first section of the chapter provides an overview of basic concepts in human genetics. The second section comprises a primer on the principles of medical genetics. The chapter closes with a brief discussion of the concept of behavioral phenotypes in dysmorphic syndromes and genetic conditions.

BASIC CONCEPTS IN MEDICAL GENETICS

Genomic Structure

The influence of genetics as we currently know it is primarily the result of research accomplished during the last 50 years of the 20th century. The basic foundation of the field of genetics is the understanding of genomic structure. The *genome* is the term applied to the total complement of deoxyribonucleic acid (DNA). DNA molecules are organized into approximately 30,000 units (*genes*). Alterations in these genes, either alone or in combination with alterations in other genes, can produce the diseases that we call *genetic disorders*. Genes are strips of DNA that are the functional and physical units of heredity, passed from parent to offspring. Most genes contain the information for making a specific protein product. They are organized in a microscopically visible set of structures called *chromosomes*. The basic biology of DNA and chromosomes was established in the 1950s and 1960s; thus most of our knowledge of the molecular, chromosomal, and even biochemical bases of human diseases has been acquired in just the past 50–60 years.

Each human cell—with the exception of a few cell types, notably the *gametes* (i.e., sperm or egg cells)—contains 23 pairs of different chromosomes for a total of 46 chromosomes. One member of each pair is derived from an individual's father, while the other is derived from the mother. One pair of chromosomes is designated as sex chromosomes, consisting of XX in a female and XY in a male. XX indicates that females have two sex chromosomes with the same sequence of genes, while XY indicates that males have two sex chromosomes with a different sequence of genes, forming the basis for the unique features of X-linked inheritance. The remaining 22 pairs of chromosomes are called *autosomes* and are numbered from 1 to 22. A gamete or germ cell is different from a somatic cell, in that it contains only one chromosome from each pair. The reader is referred to basic texts of biology and genetics that discuss cell division and meiosis in more detail (e.g., Jorde, Carey, & Bamshad, 2010).

Types of Genetic Disorders

Genetic disorders in humans are classified into four major groups:

1. *Chromosome disorders*. In these conditions, the entire chromosome or segments of a chromosome are missing or duplicated. They are divided into conditions of abnormal number (*aneuploidy*) and conditions of abnormal structure. Human chromosome disorders are diagnosed by performing a *karyotype* (chromosome study) of a body tissue—usually blood, but almost any tissue in which cells can grow can be utilized. The resulting chart of the chromosomes is called a *karyogram*. A number of disorders, such as the Down, Klinefelter, and 22q11 deletion syndromes, have missing or extra chromosomal material as their biological basis. Some of the important concepts that relate to chromosome syndromes are discussed below.

2. *Monogenic (Mendelian) conditions*. These are disorders in which a single gene or pair of genes contains a *mutation* (alteration of DNA structure) that is the primary cause of the disease. They are divided into *autosomal dominant, autosomal recessive*, and *X-linked* conditions. The term *Mendelian* derives from Gregor Mendel, the 19th-century scientist who established the basic laws of heredity in his studies of plants.

3. *Multifactorial or polygenic disorders*. These are conditions caused by a combination of multiple effects, either multiple genes (hence the term *polygenic*) or gene–environment interactions. Epidemiological and family studies indicate that there is a genetic basis for these conditions, but the conditions do not follow the simple, regular rules of inheritance established for single-gene disorders (Mendel's laws). Many human diseases fall into this less well-defined category. These include neurodevelopmental disorders such as attention-deficit/hyperactivity disorder (ADHD) (Acosta, Arcos-Burgos, & Muenke, 2004; Faraone, 2004) and learning disabilities (Chapman, Raskind, Thomson, Berninger, & Wijsman, 2003; Francks, MacPhie, & Monaco, 2002; Plomin & Walker, 2003), as well as psychiatric disorders such as autism spectrum disorders and bipolar disorders (Fisch, 2008; Sherman et al., 1997; Smalley, 1997).

4. *Mitochondrial disorders*. This group of disorders includes a relatively small number of diseases caused by alterations of the small cytoplasmic mitochondrial chromosome.

The chromosome, monogenic, and multifactorial disorders, as well as their principles, are reviewed in some detail in this chapter. Although a discussion of mitochondrial disorders is important in any review of genetic diseases, these conditions are not covered in detail here. The reader is referred to recent texts on medical genetics for more detail on mitochondrial disorders (Gelehrter, Collins, & Ginsberg, 1998; Jorde et al., 2010; Nussbaum, McInnes, & Willard, 2007).

Table 3.1 summarizes the various types of human genetic disorders defined above, with examples in each category. This table also lists three other features of inheritance—*mosaicism, genomic imprinting*, and *anticipation*, which are defined and discussed later in this chapter. All of the concepts in

TABLE 3.1. Types of Human Genetic Disorders

Inheritance	Exemplary disorders
Traditional	
Chromosome	Down syndrome, Klinefelter syndrome
Monogenic/Mendelian	Neurofibromatosis type 1, fragile X syndrome
Multifactorial/polygenic	Learning disabilities, autism spectrum disorders, schizophrenia
Nontraditional	
Mitochondrial	Kearns–Sayre syndrome, MELAS[a]
Mosaicism	Turner syndrome, fragile X syndrome
Genomic imprinting	Prader–Willi and Angelman syndromes
Anticipation	Fragile X syndrome, Huntington disease

Note. [a]MELAS, mitochondrial encephalopathy and stroke-like episodes.

the table are also discussed in the chapters on individual conditions.

Population Prevalence of Human Genetic Disorders

Although genetic disorders are often thought of as rare and exotic, these conditions constitute an important cause of human mortality and morbidity. The most common causes of infant mortality as of the mid-1980s were congenital malformations, most of which have some genetic basis. About one-third of children with developmental disabilities have a congenital malformation or other genetic condition as the primary etiology of the problem. By the 1970s, 50% of all deaths in childhood were found to be attributable to genetic causes (Jorde et al., 2010). At least 50% of sensory disabilities are caused by genetic mechanisms (Morton & Nance, 2006). Twelve percent of adult hospital admissions are for genetic causes (Rimoin, Connor, Pyeritz, & Korf, 2007) and 10% of the chronic diseases (heart problems, diabetes, arthritis) that occur in adult populations have a significant genetic component (Weatherall, 1985).

The calculation of incidence and prevalence figures for genetic disorders is very complex. Difficulties in establishing disease registries and standardization in diagnosis and recording practices make estimates challenging. Various investigations that have attempted to estimate the frequency of monogenic disorders, chromosome disorders, and congenital malformations derive figures of about 3–7% for the likelihood that an individual will develop one of these well-established genetic disorders during his or her lifetime. These figures, however, do not include cases of common adult diseases such as schizophrenia, diabetes mellitus, and cancer, all of which have some genetic basis (Jorde et al., 2010). Moreover, most epidemiologists would not classify human disease as purely environmental/acquired or purely genetic. Rather, causation of human disease represents a continuum. At one end of the spectrum are those disorders that are strongly determined by genes, especially monogenic and chromosome disorders; at the other end are those that are strongly determined by environment. However, there is now increasing evidence that many infectious diseases or even types of resistance to infectious diseases (e.g., resistance to HIV) have a genetic basis (Cheung, Wynhoven, & Harrigan, 2004; Quirk, McLeod, & Powderly, 2004), and thus most diseases are multifactorial in the strict sense of the word.

Types of Genetic Services

With the development of medical genetics as a specialty in mainstream medicine, clinical genetic services have become an integral part of the health care delivery system in North America and Europe, where most university medical centers have a program or clinic in genetics. In addition, medical genetics services are becoming more common in other countries. The percentage of clinical genetics posters presented at the American Society of Human Genetics meetings from countries outside North America and Europe has increased remarkably from the 1990s to the present. The major objective of clinical genetic programs is to provide genetic diagnosis and counseling services for the referred patient population.

The cornerstone of medical genetics is the art and science of genetic counseling. Although the term *counseling* implies that this service is in the domain of mental health or psychotherapy, genetic counseling in fact is a marriage of human genetics and behavioral science. In 1975, the American Society of Human Genetics adopted a definition that was proposed by an assigned working group:

> Genetic counseling is a communication process which deals with the human problems associated with the occurrence, or the risk of occurrence, of a genetic disorder in a family. This process involves an attempt by one or more appropriately trained persons to help the individual or family to: (1) comprehend the medical facts including the diagnosis, probable cause of the disorder, and available management; (2) appreciate the way heredity contributes to the disorder and the risk of occurrence in specified relatives; (3) understand alternatives for dealing with the risk of reoccurrence; (4) choose a course of action which seems to them appropriate in the view of their risk, their family goals, and their ethical and religious standards and act in accordance with that decision, and (5) to make the best possible adjustment to the disorder in the affected family member and/ or to the risk of recurrence of that disorder. (Ad Hoc Committee on Genetic Counseling, 1975, p. 241)

This definition illustrates the complex tasks presented to the practitioner of medical genetics. The first task involves establishing the diagnosis and discussing the natural history and management of the disorder in question. The second task requires an understanding of the basic tenets of medical genetics. The third and fourth objectives of the genetic counseling process underlie the primary differentiation between the genetic model suggested here and the traditional biomedical approach. Here the tasks involve a discussion of reproductive options and a facilitation of decision making, respectively. Implicit in the definition is the notion of respect for the family members' autonomy and for their perception of the risk. The final task of the genetic counseling process involves helping the family cope with the condition, its impact, and its potential heritability. All of the tasks require strong communication skills to enable the family to understand and process complicated medical and personal information and to utilize the information in a way that enhances their health and quality of life.

The 1975 definition was drafted during an early period in the establishment of medical genetics as a service. Because of this, the National Society of Genetic Counselors (NSGC Definition Task Force, 2006) has published a more contemporary definition of genetic counseling, which simplifies and broadens the definition and addresses current practice:

> Genetic counseling is the process of helping people understand and adapt to the medical, psychological and familial implications of genetic contributions to disease. This process integrates the following:
>
> - Interpretation of family and medical histories to assess the chance of disease occurrence or recurrence.
> - Education about inheritance, testing, management, prevention, resources and research.
> - Counseling to promote informed choices and adaptation to the risk or condition. (p. 79)

The practice of clinical genetics involves a diverse array of services. A genetics program or clinic provides diagnosis, management, genetic counseling, and consultation. These occur in a variety of settings, including university outpatient clinics, community clinics, hospital wards, and specialty clinics, often with a multidisciplinary team approach. For example, medical geneticists are often involved in organizing or coordinating team clinics for such disorders as Turner syndrome, neurofibromatosis type 1 (NF1), and sickle cell disease. Multidisciplinary clinics have improved medical care for individuals with genetic disorders and birth defects by providing better access to services, greater likelihood of multidisciplinary consensus in medical decision making, concentrated expertise among a group of practitioners, less redundancy of services, and the ability to offer unusual services (e.g., direct access to research protocols, support groups and emergency coverage). Genetic services also include prenatal screening, which is presently done in conjunction with obstetricians and perinatologists. Moreover, genetic practitioners are closely involved with the development, orchestration, and delivery of genetic screening programs, which serve prenatal, neonatal, and general populations. Genetic practitioners also provide presymptomatic or predictive genetic testing, which enables family members at risk for specific gene mutations in their family to learn whether or not they have a gene mutation that will predict or predispose them to genetic disease. From this development, the specialty of cancer genetics emerged within the field in the last decade. Traditionally, genetic conditions have few treatment options available. However, this is gradually changing with the advent of therapies involving enzyme replacement (e.g., for mucopolysaccharidoses) and gene therapy (e.g., for severe combined immunodeficiency deficiency), in addition to more traditional therapies such as pharmacological treatment (e.g., growth hormone for Turner syndrome) and nutritional management (e.g., a special diet for Prader–Willi syndrome). Genetic services are beginning to include treatment centers. The various types of clinical genetic services are discussed in detail elsewhere (Donnai, 2002; Read & Donnai, 2007; Rimoin et al., 2007).

An essential aspect of evaluation in a clinical genetic setting is the documentation of family history. It is now considered standard for practitioners evaluating a person with a potential genetic disorder to construct an accurate family history (*pedigree*) and place it in the patient's chart. The NSGC has developed recommended standards for symbols to be used in the construction of a pedigree to document this important data set (Bennett, 1999; Bennett et al., 1995; see *www. nsgc.org/client_files/consumer/family_history_logos.pdf for family-friendly instructions*).

PRINCIPLES OF MEDICAL GENETICS: A PRIMER

In this section, the basic principles of medical genetics required to understand the biological basis of the syndromes described in this book are summarized. Our goal here is not to provide a comprehensive summary of the science, but rather to highlight the important points. The key terms important in

clinical discussion of these genetic disorders are emphasized throughout the discussion (see also Jorde et al., 2010; Rimoin et al., 2007).

Chromosome Disorders

Figure 3.1 is a standard *karyogram*, showing the chromosome arrangement of a normal male. Note that the chromosomes are paired and numbered from 1 to 22. There are dark and light areas (*bands*) on each chromosome. Each chromosome is lined up in a standard way, with the *centromere* (central constriction) representing a landmark. The shorter of the two longitudinal chromosome segments is called the *p arm*, and the longer one is called the *q arm*. The chromosomes are grouped according to the size and location of the centromere. Chromosomes 1 through 3 have a centrally placed centromere (*metacentric*), while chromosomes 4 and 5 have a *submetacentric* construction. Details of the standard banding/numbering system are available in many genetic texts. Figure 3.2 shows two chromosome diagrams (*idiograms*) and their designated bands.

Most chromosome studies done in a clinical setting utilize a *Giemsa-banding* (*G-banding*) technique, which averages about 550 bands on all 23 pairs of chromosomes. A more recently developed technique called *high-resolution banding* (HRB) stops the cell in an early part of the cell cycle and allows for more extended chromosomes, and thus for more bands (average about 650). HRB techniques allow for the recognition of more subtle chromosome disorders. For example, research using HRB in the early 1980s demonstrated that some patients with Prader–Willi syndrome had a subtle but definite missing piece (deletion) of the uppermost band on the long arm of chromosome 15. However, HRB was not sensitive enough to pick up the deletion seen in individuals with Williams syndrome. In this situation, the diagnosis of the characteristic deletion of Williams syndrome requires a newer technique combining DNA fluorescent probes with HRB of chromosomes. This technique, called *fluorescent in situ hybridization* (FISH), is of significance because it is now the technique of choice for detecting the subtle deletions of Prader–Willi, Angelman, Williams, and 22q11.2 deletion syndromes. Also, it is sometimes utilized to

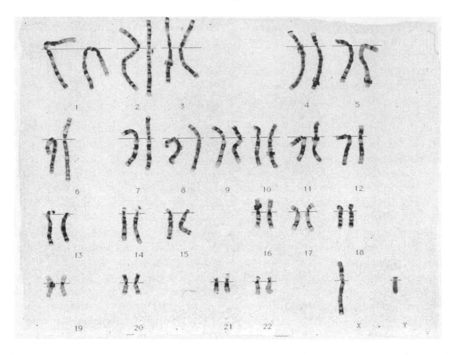

FIGURE 3.1. G-banded karyogram from a normal male. Note that there are 23 pairs of chromosomes arranged in a specific, orderly array. The autosomes are numbered from 1 through 22, and the sex chromosomes are conventionally placed at the bottom right-hand portion of the karyotype. The individual pattern of G-bands determines the chromosome. (Courtesy of Dr. Art Brothman, University of Utah Health Sciences Center)

pick up more subtle submicroscopic deletions in relatively well-known deletion syndromes, such as 5p or 4p deletion syndrome. Figure 3.3 is a black-and-white photograph of FISH in a patient with the 22q11.2 deletion syndrome. This important condition is the most common autosomal deletion syndrome in humans.

A special application of the FISH technique is called *subtelomeric FISH analysis*. The tips of chromosomes are called *telomeres*. It has been shown (de Vries, Winter, Schinzel, & van Ravenswaaij-Arts, 2003; Flint & Knight, 2003) that about 5–10% of undiagnosed individuals with mental retardation and other signs of multisystem involvement have a deletion close to the tip of a chromosome (the subtelomeric region). Some of these deletions coincide with known deletion syndromes (e.g., 4p deletion syndrome), and others are in regions without previously described syndrome associations. An even newer technique, called *comparative genomic hybridization* (CGH) *microarray analysis*, detects small deletions and dupli-

cations (but not rearrangements) throughout the genome. The technique uses an array of small, regular-spaced, cloned segments of DNA from all the chromosomes. CGH has become the principal approach in screening an individual with a neurodevelopmental condition and no medical diagnosis for a subtle chromosome abnormality (such as small deletions or duplications) (Edelman & Hirschhorn, 2009). Figure 3.4 is a black-and-white photograph of a microarray analysis. Laboratory tests have become clinically available that combine a microarray assay with a conventional karyotype, followed by confirmation of abnormal results using FISH probes. Because the deletions and duplications detected with these powerful new tools are usually smaller than previously described imbalances, genotype–phenotype data are needed to provide clinical prediction. These techniques have enabled practitioners to diagnose a higher percentage of individuals with clinical symptoms suggesting a chromosomal condition, including many individuals whose tests were negative when previous techniques were used (Edelman & Hirschhorn, 2009).

As mentioned above, chromosome disorders can be divided into disorders of chromosome number and structure. Disorders of chromosome number are those conditions in which there is either an entire extra chromosome or a missing chromosome. Down syndrome (trisomy 21) involves the presence of an extra chromosome 21 (usually the entire chromosome) and represents the prototypical chromosome condition of abnormal number (see Hazlett, Hammer, Hooper, & Kamphaus, Chapter 19, this volume). Turner syndrome (monosomy X) and Klinefelter syndrome (47,XXY) represent other disorders of abnormal chromosomal number (see Powell & Schulte, Chapter 13, and Hazlett, De Alba, & Hooper, Chapter 20, this volume).

Disorders of abnormal structure involve conditions where a segment of a chromosome is either missing (*deletion*) or extra (*duplication*). The terms *partial monosomy* and *partial trisomy*, respectively, are also utilized. The most common deletion syndromes include 5p deletion (also known as *cri du chat* syndrome), 4p deletion (Wolf–Hirschhorn syndrome), and 18q deletion. Although the letter p or q refers to the particular chromosomal arm, that designation does not tell one where the actual deletion is; the banding number is also needed. A more comprehensive discussion of chromosome biology is available in most textbooks of human and medical genetics.

In the 1980s, as noted above, a number of chromosome deletion syndromes involving very subtle deletions were described. These have come to be known as the *microdeletion syndromes*. Prader–Willi, Angelman, and Williams syndromes all fall into this category. Because the deletions are subtle and are thought to affect a potentially definable cluster of neighboring genes, the microdeletion syndromes are sometimes referred to as *contiguous-gene syndromes*. Prader–Willi and Angelman syndromes are prototypical

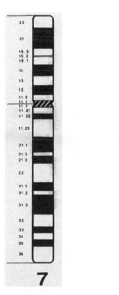
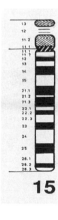

FIGURE 3.2. Idiograms at the 550-band resolution for chromosomes 7 and 15, two important chromosomes for neurobehavioral disorders. Chromosome 7 is a typical *submetacentric* chromosome (i.e., the centromere is off center). The part of the chromosome on the shorter side is called the *short arm* or *p arm*; the part on the longer side is called the *long arm* or *q arm*. Chromosome 15 is called an *acrocentric* chromosome; the centromere is near one end, and the short arm contains the *satellite material*. Note that the band numbers move consecutively away from the centromere, and the chromosome arms are divided broadly into segments and then into individual bands. Chromosomes are numbered by segment and then by band. The region that is deleted in the Prader–Willi syndrome is the 15q11–13 region. The region that is deleted in Williams syndrome is the 7q11.2 region. (Courtesy of Dr. Art Brothman, University of Utah Health Sciences Center)

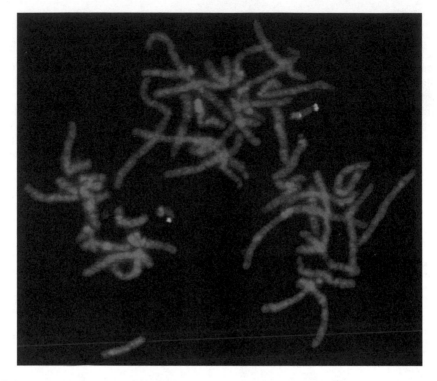

FIGURE 3.3. An abnormal FISH study of an individual with a 22q11.2 deletion. The normal chromosome 22 shows two signals, while the other chromosome 22 (lower left) is missing a signal. Thus there is a missing piece of DNA in the critical region consistent with this syndrome. (Courtesy of Dr. Art Brothman, University of Utah Health Sciences Center)

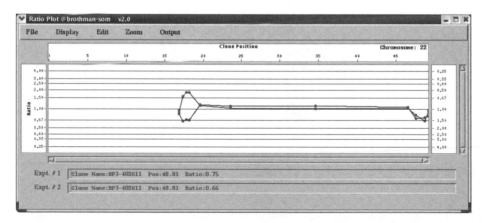

FIGURE 3.4. Ratio plot of chromosome 22, showing deletion at the DiGeorge locus (22q11.2) on the left of the plot where the two lines separate. Each clone is shown by a dot along the line and signifies that the clone is deleted. (Courtesy of Dr. Art Brothman, University of Utah Health Sciences Center)

for the group and are discussed further in the section below on nontraditional inheritance.

From a clinical point of view, chromosome disorders are associated with characteristic syndromes. In each of these conditions there is a recognizable and relatively reproducible pattern of physical manifestations, minor anomalies, and sometimes major congenital malformations, often consistent enough to be recognized by the experienced clinician. The syndrome thus represents the manifestations that we actually observe physically or clinically (*phenotype*). The concept of phenotype is contrasted with the term *genotype*, which refers to the individual's genetic constitution. For example, the phenotype in Down syndrome is the constellation of physical findings first described by Dr. J. Langdon Down; the genotype is the chromosomal constitution of 47,XY +21. (About 90–95% of persons with Down syndrome have the chromosomal finding of trisomy 21, while the remaining 5–10% have other structural changes; see Hazlett et al., Chapter 19, this volume.)

One of the clinical decisions that often confronts the practitioner is when to order a chromosome analysis. The most common reason for such a study is to confirm the presence of a well-established chromosome disorder, such as Down or Turner syndrome. Since autosomal chromosome disorders produce syndromic patterns of multiple anomalies, usually with intellectual disability, a karyotype is indicated in a person who has this type of clinical picture. Thus, in the evaluation of an individual with developmental delay or a neurodevelopmental disorder, a chromosome study is obviously indicated when a person has multiple major and minor anomalies or features different from those of his or her family background. The question of doing a karyotype in a person who has an intellectual disability or developmental delay without dysmorphic signs or minor anomalies is somewhat more controversial. However, since the dysmorphic features can often be quite subtle even in established syndromes (e.g., 5p deletion/*cri du chat* syndrome and 17p deletion/Smith–Magenis syndrome), most geneticists seriously consider doing a karyotype for any individual with developmental delay or intellectual disability (Curry et al., 1997). Since microarray analysis is capable of detecting very small

imbalances, with correspondingly subtle physical features, most clinicians currently order microarray analysis for individuals with these "nondistinctive" findings. Many clinicians have also considered doing a karyotype for any individual with autism who has no associated medical diagnosis. This is because of the recognition of the inverted duplication 15 syndrome, where the clinical signs are quite subtle (Battaglia et al., 1997). The yield of chromosome studies looking for this finding or for other chromosome disorders in large populations of individuals with autism but with no medical diagnosis is currently under investigation in the United States and Europe (Edelman & Hirschhorn, 2009), and this testing can be pursued on a case-by-case basis. It is important to order both a high-resolution karyotype and FISH when one is considering one of the specific microdeletion syndromes (i.e., Prader–Willi, Angelman, Williams, or 22q11 deletion syndrome).

Another reason for a chromosome study is to study a parent when a child has a disorder of chromosome structure. Here one is looking for a chromosome rearrangement (e.g., translocation, inversion). There are a number of other indications for performing chromosome studies that are not as relevant to the neurodevelopmental arena and are not discussed in detail here; these include recurrent miscarriages, an undiagnosed stillborn infant, concern about one of the chromosomal instability syndromes, and diagnosis of certain malignancies. Comprehensive discussions of these indications are available in the texts cited earlier in the chapter.

Monogenic Disorders

Monogenic disorders are those conditions resulting from a *mutation* (change in a gene), either in a single allele or both alleles of a gene. Prior to the 1980s, the notion of a monogenic disorder was one that involved an assumption. Now that the genes for over 2,000 human disorders have been mapped to a chromosomal location, or in many cases identified (cloned) (see the Online Mendelian Inheritance in Man [OMIM] website, discussed below), the notion of the gene is no longer a theoretical construct.

Monogenic disorders, also known as Mendelian conditions, can be divided into autosomal dominant, autosomal recessive, and X-linked conditions. The determination of the inheritance pattern was known long before the new DNA technology became available; it was based on interpretation of pedigree structure. Thus, when a condition was recognized to occur through generations in a vertical fashion, the assumption was usually made that the condition was an autosomal dominant disorder. This was the logic that permitted the recognition of NF1 as an autosomal dominant condition long before the gene was identified in 1990. (NF1 is utilized in this section to illustrate principles.)

The concept of an *autosomal dominant* gene means that one allele in each gene pair possesses a mutation, while the other is a normal *(wild-type) allele*. In recent years many of these mutations have been determined at the molecular level for many conditions. When a person has an autosomal dominant mutation, the chance of transmitting the mutation to offspring is one in two (or 50%) with each pregnancy. The pedigree structure will often be multigenerational because inheriting the trait from one parent is sufficient to cause the condition. Figure 3.5 shows a typical autosomal dominant pedigree in a family with NF1. Note that there is transmission in this particular family history from a father to a son (i.e., male-to-male transmission), confirming that this is an autosomal trait and not an X-linked trait. (In an X-linked trait, a male cannot transmit the trait to a male offspring because the

father transmits his Y to a son and his X to a daughter.) In many autosomal dominant traits, a condition starts off with a person called the *progenitor*. In that situation it is assumed that there is a *de novo* (new) mutation in the gene. Thus, in many autosomal dominant conditions there will be no family history because the particular person in question is the progenitor for the disorder. This is often the case in NF1, where in the clinical setting about 50% of all patients who present to a medical genetics clinic have their disorder because of a de novo mutation. (The other 50% inherit the gene from one of their parents.) This illustrates the point that the absence of any family history of a condition by no means excludes genetic causation. In fact, in X-linked and autosomal recessive conditions (where there is often no family history) as well, the belief that the lack of family history mitigates against a genetic disorder is inaccurate.

An *autosomal recessive* disorder is one in which both alleles in a gene pair have a mutation. In an autosomal recessive pedigree, each parent is assumed to carry a mutant copy of the gene, and thus the parents are called *carriers* or *heterozygotes*. The term *homozygote* is used when a person has two mutant alleles or two normal alleles. Because of the *segregation pattern* (the genotypes inherited by the offspring) that occurs in recessive situations, the chance that a family in which both parents are carriers will have a child with the recessive condition is one in

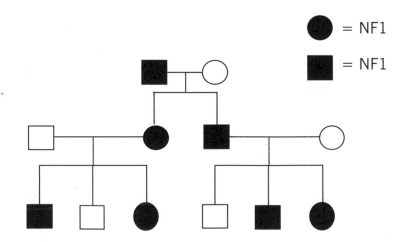

FIGURE 3.5. This family pedigree illustrates the typical inheritance pattern of an autosomal dominant trait, NF1. Note the transmissions from a father to a son.

four (25%) with each pregnancy. Most inborn errors of metabolism, such as most of the mucopolysaccharidoses (see M. Brown, Chapter 15, this volume), are inherited in an autosomal recessive fashion. These biochemical conditions represent disorders of intermediary metabolism, and a homozygous deficiency of an enzyme accounts for each such disorder. Moreover, the hemoglobinopathies, including sickle cell anemia (see Smith & Baker, Chapter 18, this volume), are also inherited in an autosomal recessive fashion. A comprehensive discussion of the principles of population genetics that are important in any discussion of autosomal recessive diseases can be found in the textbooks cited earlier.

The third type of disorder transmitted in a Mendelian fashion is an *X-linked* disorder. The X-linked disorders are conditions that from pedigree structures (and now DNA technology) are known to be mutations on the X chromosome. In this situation, a female (who typically has two X chromosomes) will "carry" the gene for the condition and may or may not express it, while the male (who only has a single X) will almost invariably express the condition. Again, just as in autosomal dominant disorders, some individuals who have an X-linked disorder may have it because of a new mutation of the gene on the X chromosome. Figure 3.6 shows a typical X-linked pedigree of a family with fragile X syndrome seen in a clinical setting (see Hagerman, Chapter 14, this volume). Other conditions of significance in the neurodevelopmental arena with X-linked inheritance include Hunter syndrome (see M. Brown, Chapter 15, this volume), Lesch–Nyhan syndrome (see Wodrich & Long, Chapter 23, this volume), and X-linked aqueductal stenosis/hydrocephalus. In addition to fragile X syndrome, several other X-linked conditions can cause intellectual disability and neurodevelopmental disorders (Stevenson, Schwartz, & Schroer, 1999).

Decisions about patterns of inheritance are complex and often controversial in the field of medical genetics. Knowledge of the genetic basis for many conditions is now being acquired through recent developments in DNA technology. In some cases, this has led us to recognize that a single clinical condition can be caused by multiple mutations (some genes have several hundred different mutations), and in some cases can have multiple modes of inheritance. For example, retinitis pigmentosa mutations are associated with both dominant and recessive modes of inheritance in different families. Detailed discussions of the evidence for inheritance patterns of human diseases and phenotypes are available in the classic multivolume text *Mendelian Inheritance in Man*. V. A. McKusick, the author, is regarded as the father of medical genetics, and has produced 12 editions of this seminal work. One is now able to look up conditions or phenotypes and discover key and recent citations on clinical and genetic aspects as well as molecular biology (McKusick, 1998). Moreover, this work is currently available online through the World Wide Web (*www.ncbi.nlm.nih.gov/omim*) at no cost. This is an incomparable and invaluable resource for current knowledge about the genetic and molecular basis of almost any condition. The 12th print edition (McKusick, 1998) included 8,587 entries; as of May 2009, the online version (OMIM) listed 12,777 loci. Another online resource that is especially useful for clinical information—including differential diagnosis, diagnostic tests, detailed genetic information, management, and family support groups—is GeneTests (*www.ncbi.nlm.nih.gov/sites/GeneTests/?db=GeneTests*).

Genotype–Phenotype Relationships: Basic Tenets

Although the discussion thus far seems to be relatively straightforward, the actual evaluation of a patient with a potential genetic condition is not so clear-cut. As mentioned above, an abnormality of chromosome structure or a gene mutation produces a phenotype that is recognizable and often discrete. However, the relationship between the gene alteration and the disease state is complex, as there is marked variability in the clinical picture, regardless of the genotype. Various conditions seem to have their own intrinsic degree of variability. For these reasons, geneticists over the past century have developed concepts that explain the often fuzzy relationship between genotype and phenotype. These concepts are discussed in the following paragraphs.

Expressivity is a term utilized in genetics to refer to the variability in clinical severity

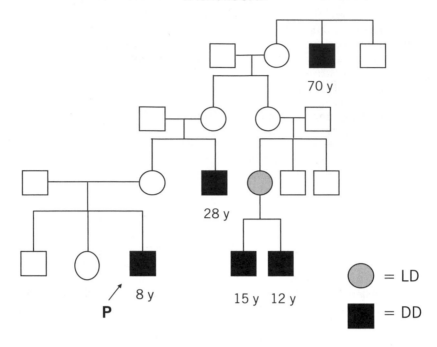

FIGURE 3.6. A typical family pedigree of an X-linked condition, fragile X syndrome. Note that one female is mildly affected, and there is no male-to-male transmission. LD, learning disabilities; DD, developmental delay.

seen in a given condition. Various members of the same family with a certain genetic trait have exactly the same mutation, yet the degree of involvement can range from minimal to severe. The study of the clinical aspects of NF1 illustrates this point (see Payne & North, Chapter 17, this volume). About 50–70% of patients with NF1 only have *café au lait* spots or dermal neurofibromas, and their disorder is of mild significance. Approximately 30–50% of patients have one of the many listed serious manifestations of NF1, including optic pathway tumors, neurofibrosarcomas, or scoliosis. Even within the same multigenerational kindred, there will be marked variability. This discussion also applies to Noonan syndrome (see Teeter Ellison, Chapter 16, this volume). Again, even within the same pedigree, there will be marked variability in the clinical signs (short stature, pulmonic stenosis, etc.), even though all patients will have at least the facial features.

Penetrance is the frequency of expression of a genotype. Some individuals who carry a gene mutation in a Mendelian disorder will have no observed clinical signs of the condi-

tion, while others with the same mutation will have clinical signs. Penetrance is usually expressed as the ratio of individuals with the mutation and symptoms to all individuals with the mutation. The absence of any signs of such a disorder will give the impression that the gene in question has skipped a generation. The concept of incomplete penetrance or lack of penetrance is an attempt to explain the clinical picture where the genotype and phenotype do not match, as one would expect. All of the monogenic conditions described in this book essentially have 100% penetrance. For example, in NF1, individuals who have the trait have some cutaneous or eye signs of NF1—usually by the age of 5, but certainly by the age of 20 years. Sometimes it may be difficult to exclude the presence of the gene in a young child, but usually by adulthood, the *café au lait* spots, dermal neurofibromas, and Lisch nodules of the iris have made their appearance. In examination of NF1 pedigrees, one does not see examples of three-generation pedigrees where the gene mutation has skipped. On the other hand, in tuberous sclerosis, there have been cases reported in which there are two affected offspring of normal, unaffected parents. This particular pedigree structure could be described as incomplete penetrance; however, one does not see three generations of people with tuberous sclerosis where the person in the middle generation lacks any signs. Most geneticists currently think that families with siblings affected with tuberous sclerosis and unaffected parents represent *germ-line mosaicism* (i.e., mutation occurring in multiple gametes and not in somatic cells, putting the parents at increased risk for recurrence). Mosaicism is now thought to occur more often than previously recognized. In Table 3.1 it is listed as one of the nontraditional modes of inheritance, and it is discussed further below.

The concepts of expressivity and penetrance are critical in the evaluation of family histories of complex diseases such as depressive disorders and learning disabilities. In such kindreds, it is typical to have multiple affected family members with intervening relatives who do not express the condition (nonpenetrance) or express it partially (variable expressivity). In these cases, we are not only dealing with variable expression of a single gene, but often multiple genes and/ or environmental factors. We often think of these genes as conferring a susceptibility to the condition.

Age is an important factor in the concepts of both expressivity and penetrance. For many conditions, symptoms are age-specific. This means that the phenotype changes with age and may be harder to recognize at some ages than others. Examples are coarsening of facial features in mucopolysaccharidoses as storage material accumulates in the body, the development of adrenal tumors in multiple endocrine neoplasia, and dilation of the aortic root in Marfan syndrome. Thus symptoms vary not only between family members, but in individuals throughout the life cycle. It also means that penetrance is sometimes calculated as an age-specific curve.

The concept of *heterogeneity* presently has a number of usages in medical genetics. The traditional concept is *genetic heterogeneity*, in which a certain phenotype (e.g., retinitis pigmentosa or cataracts) is known to be caused by different genetic alterations (i.e., autosomal dominant, autosomal recessive, or X-linked). With the recent advances in DNA technology, the existence of genetic

heterogeneity has been proven. For example, in tuberous sclerosis, some families with this autosomal dominant gene map to chromosome 16 and have a mutation of a certain tumor suppressor gene, whereas other families map to chromosome 9 and have the disorder because of mutations of a different gene. This can be referred to as either *locus heterogeneity* or genetic heterogeneity. The term is also used to refer to a mixture of phenotypes as well. For example, when it was recognized in the 1980s that bilateral acoustic neuromas were not seen in classical NF, the notion of phenotypic heterogeneity of the NFs was proposed. Even before the two separate genes were mapped and cloned, clinicians and scientists were referring to multiple forms of NF. Now the terms NF1 and NF2 are used for the classic condition (NF1) and for bilateral acoustic neuromas (NF2).

The concept of *pleiotropy* refers to the idea that diverse manifestations in different organs and systems can have a single-gene cause. Again, NF1 illustrates this concept nicely. In this syndrome one sees manifestations that at first glance do not seem to be tied together pathogenically (i.e., *café au lait* spots, neurofibromas, optic pathway tumors, learning disabilities, skeletal findings, etc.). The notion here is that a single gene has multiple roles in development and cell biology, and thus that a mutation in this gene has multiple effects. In the case of NF1, the common denominator is presumably in the control of cells derived from the developing neural crest of the embryo. To give another example, the pleiotropic manifestations of Noonan syndrome include the characteristic face, short stature, pectus excavatum, and pulmonic stenosis. Again, this diverse array of effects appears to be due to the single mutation. The concept of pleiotropy is important in understanding how a gene produces the phenotype (i.e., its pathogenesis) and the idea of a syndrome.

As mentioned in various places in the chapter, *mutation* refers to the specific alteration of the DNA molecule in a particular condition. In recent years, with the advances in DNA technology, the specific mutations that cause many disorders have been detected. For example, after the gene for NF1 was identified in 1990, about 10% of individuals with NF1 had a detectable mutation. In the other 90%, scientists were not technically able to find the gene alteration, presumably because of the size of the NF1 gene. Since 1990, because of new techniques, laboratory scientists have been able to detect the disease-causing mutations in 95% of NF1 patients (Messiaen et al., 2000). Of note is the fact that about 80% of the mutations are ones in which the gene is basically inactivated (i.e. there is simply one operating gene, while the other is not operating). In some cases the entire gene is deleted, while in others a small deletion of only a few nucleotides is present. Most cases are caused by a single nucleotide change that either results in a shortened protein or affects function of the protein. In other conditions, the specific type and location of gene mutations affect the phenotype. For example, Apert syndrome is due to relatively specific mutations of a gene that encodes a protein called fibroblast growth factor receptor 2 (Webster & Donoghue, 1997). This is a cell receptor protein that sits on the outside of a cell and, when signaled by a growth factor, sends a message to the nucleus of the cell. It is now known that Apert syndrome is due to mutations of the gene that alter the extracellular portion of this growth factor receptor. Mutations of other parts of this same gene produce different phenotypes and cause recognized syndromes that have manifestations overlapping with those of Apert syndrome, but are considered different and distinct clinical syndromes (Reardon et al., 1994; Wilkie et al., 1995). These other syndromes, which include Crouzon and Pfeiffer syndromes, are not discussed here in detail.

In summary, the area of genotype–phenotype correlation is a timely topic. Ideally, better understanding of how mutations in specific genes produce specific phenotypes will clarify the pathogenesis of human diseases of this nature.

Recently Delineated Concepts: Nontraditional Inheritance

As mentioned above, the concepts of variability, pleiotropy, and heterogeneity were created to explain observed relationships between genotypes and phenotypes. In the 1980s and 1990s, a number of newer, nontraditional categories of inheritance were recognized. One of these, *mosaicism*, has been mentioned above. In mosaicism, there are two cell lines—either one that is normal and one that contains a gene or chromosome mutation, or two that are abnormal. More rarely, mosaic individuals have more than two cell lines. In many cases, a normal cell line makes the phenotype milder. Other concepts proposed in the 1990s include *genomic imprinting* and *anticipation*. These concepts have altered thinking about the clinical and genetic aspects of several important conditions. These concepts are discussed below, as they relate to two of the conditions described in this text (i.e., Prader–Willi and fragile X syndromes), as well as to Angelman syndrome.

The principle of *genomic imprinting* challenged the central dogma of genetics that arose from Mendel's experiments with peas. Originally it was thought that a trait was inherited from a mother or a father, and that the parent of origin made no difference. However, it has become increasingly apparent that in some genes the parent of origin does make a difference and has an effect on phenotype and disease manifestation. In imprinting, the expression of a gene is influenced by the parental origin of the gene, and the activity level depends on this origin. The concept of genomic imprinting in humans is best illustrated by Prader–Willi and Angelman syndromes. As mentioned earlier, it has been known since the early 1980s that a microdeletion on chromosome 15 in the upper portion of the long arm could produce Prader–Willi syndrome (see Dykens, Cassidy, & DeVries, Chapter 25, this volume). A similar deletion was recognized in some patients with Angelman syndrome. (Angelman syndrome is a condition of profound developmental disability, seizure disorder, muscle tone abnormalities, small head size, and a characteristic face.) If a deletion arises on the paternal chromosome 15, the offspring will develop Prader–Willi syndrome; if the deletion arises on the maternal chromosome 15, the offspring will develop Angelman syndrome. Thus there is a definite parent-of-origin effect. It is now clear that a gene (or genes) within the crucial segment of chromosome 15 is normally only active on the paternal chromosome and not the maternal one (the maternal copy is said to be *imprinted*). In a case when the critical gene (or genes) is deleted on the paternal chromosome and thus inactivated, this deletion results in Prader–Willi syndrome. Conversely, the gene for Angelman syndrome has also been identified, and the logic is the reverse. Although most cases of Prader–Willi syndrome and Angelman syndrome are *sporadic* (i.e., without a family history), this parent-of-origin effect results in some unusual pedigrees that would not at first glance fit any of the simple rules of single-gene disorders discussed above (see Jorde et al., 2010).

Another concept that is classified as nontraditional is *anticipation*. Since the early part of the 20th century, it has been observed that some genetic diseases display an earlier age of onset and have more severe expression in later generations of the family tree. Such disorders are said to exhibit anticipation. Until recently, most investigators felt that this was probably a bias of ascertainment and not a real biological phenomenon. In the early 1990s, the genes for a number of conditions were identified through the positional cloning approach. These included fragile X syndrome (see Hagerman, Chapter 14, this volume), myotonic dystrophy, and Huntington disease. These conditions share a unique mutation mechanism, that of the expanded DNA repeat; they have thus been labeled the *trinucleotide repeat-expansion disorders*. There are repeat sequences of DNA nucleotides that are normally present in all individuals; persons with repeat-expansion disorders have an increased number of these nucleotide repeat sequences. Such an expansion affects the way the DNA works, or the amount or function of the protein, and therefore it produces the disease. There is also a correlation with repeat size and phenotype: Larger repeat sizes are associated with more severe symptoms and/or earlier onset. Repeats in the expanded range are unstable and tend to get larger in offspring. For example, in fragile X syndrome, expanded cytosine–guanine–guanine repeats are associated with methylation of a cytosine–guanine dinucleotide) island, which appears to "turn off" the gene. Thus for these conditions triplet repeat expansions explain the phenomenon of anticipation and give it a biological basis. Like genomic imprinting, this phenomenon provides the biological and molecular basis for observations in family histories that were discrepant with the known rules of Mendelian inheritance.

DNA Technology and Linkage

The tools and strategies to localize a particular gene for a Mendelian disorder to its particular chromosome (or chromosomes) arose in the late 1970s and early 1980s. The combination of the development of DNA probes, complicated computer programs, and restriction endonucleases laid the groundwork for the application of this technology. Before this, the biological bases for the overwhelming majority of genetic disorders (except the biochemical disorders) were almost entirely unknown. One could speculate that a condition like NF1 was due to some disorder of neural crest biology, or that Apert syndrome was due to a developmental disorder of the skeleton, but the real basis of the pleiotropy in each case was unclear. For this reason, the concept that one can map a gene by utilizing the incredible and well-known variation in DNA structure arose. The concept of linkage analysis is based on the idea that an individual's normal DNA variations cosegregate with the disease genes in question. By using complicated computer programs and previously linked DNA probes, one can map a gene. Once a disease gene is mapped, the first step toward being able to isolate the causative gene is accomplished. The isolation of the gene for a condition is referred to as *gene identification* or *cloning*. If the basic structure of the DNA is known, one can then derive the amino acid sequence and the peptide structure. The strategy, once called *reverse genetics* and now referred to as *positional cloning*, has been highly successful since the 1980s in identifying important disease genes. The first gene mapped by this approach was the gene for Huntington disease. In the late 1980s, the genes for cystic fibrosis, Duchenne muscular dystrophy, and NF1 were mapped and then cloned. Another important refinement of linkage analysis introduced in the 1990s is the use of *single-nucleotide polymorphisms*. This type of DNA variation is ubiquitous in the genome and enabled mapping at much smaller intervals of DNA, thus enabling more rapid localization of genes. The process of identifying human genes has been aided by the Human Genome Project, a massive, government-funded biological project that succeeded in mapping the entire human genome between 1990 and 2003 (see the National Human

Genome Research Institute website, *www. nhgri.nih.gov*). Correlation of the detected mutations with specific phenotypes is now ongoing for all conditions in which there has been gene identification.

Figure 3.7 illustrates this paradigm. First, families with a particular dominant or recessive condition are collected. If, by chance, some patients have an associated chromosomal rearrangement that suggests a gene location, the success rate in mapping the gene is improved. Once a gene is mapped, linkage testing in the clinical arena is available. For example, in familial cases of NF1, the families that are interested in prenatal diagnosis or early-infancy diagnosis (often before any *café au lait* spots have developed) now have this option. Once a gene has been mapped or localized, perusal of the existing gene map may show *candidate genes* in the same region that may be the basis for the disorder in question. This approach was used to clone the gene responsible for Apert syndrome. Once the gene for a related but different condition called Crouzon syndrome (referred to above) was mapped to chromosome 10, and a candidate gene on chromosome 10 was discovered that encodes fibroblast growth factor

receptor 2, mutations were detected in patients with Crouzon syndrome. The logical hypothesis was that perhaps different mutations of the same gene cause related disorders, including Apert syndrome. This turned out to be the case, and it is now known that the gene for fibroblast growth factor receptor 2 is the causative gene in Apert syndrome (Webster & Donoghue, 1997). As mentioned above, this paradigm was also successful in mapping and cloning the important gene in fragile X syndrome. At present, if a person is recognized to have fragile X syndrome and this is confirmed on a molecular basis, DNA testing can be offered to other members of the family who are at risk. Direct mutation testing for the expanded repeat of fragile X syndrome is currently available in most clinical molecular laboratories in North America (see Hagerman, Chapter 14, this volume). With the increased use of faster technology that shortens the time between mapping and cloning a gene, direct mutation testing has become the norm for clinical testing. Interestingly, although new techniques have revolutionized the availability of clinical tests once biological samples are available, the process is still just as dependent on astute

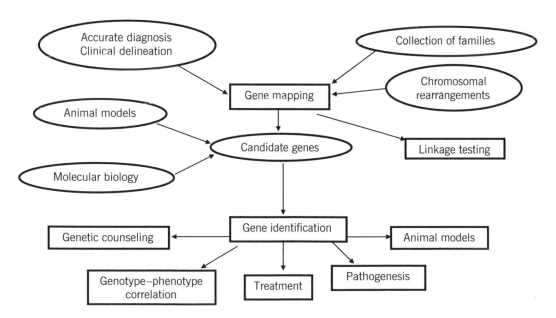

FIGURE 3.7. The gene-cloning paradigm: The chronology of the mapping and identifying of a disease gene, with its resulting consequences. Note that mapping a gene results in the possibility that linkage testing can be used in the clinical arena. Cloning a gene creates the potential for understanding pathogenesis and perhaps orchestrating strategies for treatment and prevention.

clinicians' reporting and collecting blood samples from families affected with genetic disorders.

The ultimate aim of this strategy is to understand the molecular pathogenesis of these single-gene conditions. If the protein is detected and its role in cell biology is sorted out, then investigators can begin to propose treatments that can alter or modify the sequence of events in the cell pathway in question. For example, the gene for NF1 is a tumor suppressor gene that is involved in signal transduction within the cell. The encoded protein, neurofibromin, is known to slow down growth within the cell. Thus, if a mutation occurs, the expected brakes on cell growth will not be present and will predispose a person to develop benign or malignant tumors. If one could figure out how to alter some of the elements of the pathway, then perhaps one could prevent the occurrence of benign or malignant tumors in NF1.

Multifactorial Inheritance

Multifactorial inheritance refers to the important group of disorders that have an inherited component involving more than one gene and/or gene–environment interactions. These include such important neurodevelopmental disorders as learning disabilities, Tourette syndrome, mood disorders, and autism spectrum disorders (see the appropriate chapters of this volume). It has been challenging to delineate the genetic components of these conditions because of the difficulty in describing discrete phenotypes, unraveling the effects of multiple genes and environmental factors, and determining genetic heterogeneity. Genes influencing these conditions may operate by any of the mechanisms described for Mendelian (single-gene) conditions, and a given condition may involve genes with different modes of inheritance. Because of the complexity of these conditions, geneticists have developed mathematical models to study genetic effects in these disorders. Some of the important concepts related to multifactorial inheritance are discussed in the following paragraphs.

Multifactorial conditions are often thought of in the context of a normal curve of *susceptibility*, with both genes and the environment capable of contributing susceptibility. There may be a *threshold* above

which symptoms are expressed (*penetrance* of the condition is the percentage above the threshold). This threshold may be different for males and females. Figure 3.8 shows a liability distribution for a multifactorial disease in a population. These conditions are usually common, and often are mixtures of multiple conditions with similar or identical phenotypes (*genetic heterogeneity*). In many cases, Mendelian conditions have been identified and "pulled out" of the more general category (e.g., fragile X and Rett syndromes are subsets of autism; fragile X, Turner, Noonan, and Williams syndromes, as well as NF1 and sickle cell anemia, are subsets of ADHD).

The analytical tools that have been most useful in the analysis of multifactorial conditions are *twin concordance studies* (measuring the frequency of the condition in identical and fraternal twins); large-scale family studies with *linkage analysis* (matching disease status to known DNA markers) and *segregation analysis* (observation of proportion of affected offspring); and the use of computer models to compute *heritability* (estimate of the proportion of cases attributed to genetic factors) and the likelihood of major-gene and other models. For most multifactorial conditions, we have not delineated models that provide risk figures for families; therefore, recurrence risks are generally derived from empirical data from family studies, taking into account gender of the proband and degree of relationship. Since most of these conditions also have environmental triggers, it will be important to study these factors as well.

Diagnostic Principles

For many of the genetic disorders described in this chapter and in this text, clinicians and investigators have set forth criteria that allow a practitioner to arrive at a secure diagnosis. The idea of developing these criteria arose in the 1980s as gene linkage studies progressed. It became clear to both clinicians and scientists that in order for anyone to attempt to map a gene, there had to be a consensus on who was affected and who was not. The diagnostic criteria for NF1 illustrate this principle. In 1987, at a National Institutes of Health (NIH) conference on NF1 and NF2, criteria were proposed

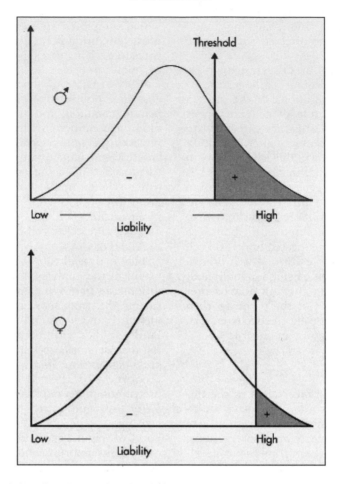

FIGURE 3.8. A liability distribution for a multifactorial disease in a population. To be affected with the disease, an individual must exceed the threshold on the liability distribution. This figure shows two thresholds, a lower one for males and a higher one for females. From Jorde, Carey, Bamshad, and White (2003). Copyright 2003 by C.V. Mosby, Inc. Reprinted by permission.

for making the diagnosis of this condition. Table 3.2 presents these criteria. The basic premise is that if a patient's manifestations fulfill the required items, a clinician can settle upon a highly secure diagnosis of the condition (NIH Consensus Development Conference, 1988). Diagnostic criteria are not widely available or established for many other genetic conditions. However, in certain circumstances (e.g., Apert syndrome) diagnostic criteria are not really necessary, since the distinctiveness of the pattern is clear-cut. For conditions in which the diagnosis can be made on a molecular basis (e.g., Prader–Willi syndrome), diagnostic checklists or criteria are not needed as much for diagnosis, but are still useful to help a clinician decide who

needs to be evaluated. The concept of diagnostic criteria is emphasized here simply to underscore the subjective nature and occasional difficulty of arriving at the diagnosis of a genetic disorder or syndrome. This concept is further discussed below in regard to syndromes (and, later, to behavioral phenotypes). Diagnosis is often considerably more difficult for multifactorial conditions (e.g., see discussion in Goldstein, Schwebach, & Cunningham, Chapter 6, this volume).

Syndrome Diagnosis

The term *syndrome* is utilized in a specific way in the field of medical genetics. It refers to a recognizable and consistent pat-

TABLE 3.2. NIH Consensus Statement: Diagnostic Criteria for NF1

The diagnostic criteria for NF1 are met in an individual if two or more of the following are found:

- Six or more *café au lait* macules of over 5 mm in greatest diameter in prepubertal individuals and over 15 mm in greatest diameter in postpubertal individuals.
- Two or more neurofibromas of any type or one plexiform neurofibroma.
- Freckling in the axillary or inguinal regions.
- Optic glioma.
- Two or more Lisch nodules (iris hamartomas).
- A distinctive osseous lesion such as sphenoid dysplasia or thinning of the long bone cortex with or without pseudoarthrosis.
- A first-degree relative (parent, sibling or offspring) with NF1 by the above criteria.

Note. From NIH Consensus Development Conference (1988).

tern of multiple manifestations known to have a specific etiology. The cause is usually a mutation of a single gene, a chromosome alteration, or an environmental agent. In other words, a syndrome is a specific complex phenotype that has a single cause. The notion of syndrome is related closely to the concept of pleiotropy, described earlier. The diagnosis of malformation or developmental syndromes in general is a challenge, as over 1,000 syndromes involving multiple congenital anomalies are listed in catalogs and diagnostic computer programs (see Jones, 2006; Hennekam, Allanson, & Krantz, 2009).

In addition to knowledge of the more common disorders, the clinician who approaches the area of syndromology needs knowledge and skill in the recognition of minor anomalies of structure, which often provide phenotypic clues for a diagnosis. Thus, for example, diagnosing Williams syndrome can be difficult in early childhood or infancy unless one is familiar with the physical characteristics of the face in the context of the developmental condition. Even such signs as curly hair and characteristic voice are part of the component manifestations that are helpful in diagnosis. Since no individual feature or manifestation is obligatory in almost any syndrome, one has to be familiar with the clinical variability in order to secure the diagnosis. The diagnosis of a chromosome syndrome can often be straightforward if

the clinician has the appropriate index of suspicion; ordering the chromosome study confirms the diagnosis. As mentioned earlier, if one is considering a microdeletion syndrome, the appropriate chromosome study (including FISH) needs to be performed. By contrast, if the condition in question possesses relatively consistent features (e.g., as the multiple *café au lait* spots of NF1), and diagnostic criteria are available to establish the diagnosis, the diagnostic reasoning process can be fairly straightforward. Conditions familiar in childhood may be harder to recognize in adulthood, as the typical features may change with age; thus it is important to obtain information about how phenotype changes with age.

One of the important points in this discussion is that the concept of a syndrome encompasses a multiplicity of manifestations, most of which are variable within the constellation. In chromosome syndromes in general, and in the syndromes discussed in this book in particular, some disorder of development is likely to be present. In that sense, intellectual disability (mental retardation) is accepted widely as a component manifestation of many of these syndromes. In the same sense, alterations in cognition, personality, and behavior can be variable manifestations in many of these syndromes, just like the more clearly defined manifestation of intellectual disability. This point is the essence of the concept of *behavioral phenotype*, which is discussed below.

Environmental Syndromes

In addition to syndromes of single-gene or chromosome etiology, there exist several syndromes caused by teratogenic agents. A *teratogen* is an agent external to the fetus that induces structural malformations, growth deficiency, or functional alterations during prenatal development. Although teratogens cause only a small percentage of developmental disabilities and birth defects, they are an important group because of the potential for prevention. In the neurobehavioral arena, the most important and common condition is fetal alcohol syndrome (FAS). This condition has a recognizable pattern of malformation consisting of prenatal growth deficiency (low birthweight and birth length), postnatal growth deficiency (short stature, failure to thrive), microcephaly, and a characteristic pattern of minor facial anomalies (Streissguth, Clarren, & Jones, 1985; Thackray & Tifft, 2001). Although at first glance the facial anomalies may seem nonspecific, taken together they are diagnostic of FAS. These facial alterations include short palpebral fissures (small eyelids on horizontal measurement), short upturned nose, long philtrum (distance from nasal septum to upper lip), and relatively thin upper lip. The facial gestalt of older children with FAS is quite characteristic, and a clinician who has experience with the disorder can make a secure clinical diagnosis in the context of maternal alcohol abuse. The full syndrome occurs in 10–40% (depending on the study) of infants whose mothers drink excessively and abuse alcohol (Stratton, Howe, & Battaglia, 1996). While the issue of whether moderate or less frequently used amounts of alcohol cause adverse effects is controversial and not clear-cut, there is no question that maternal alcoholism is a significant risk factor for this recognizable syndrome.

One of the component manifestations of FAS is neurodevelopmental difficulty. A majority of children with FAS have learning disabilities, but some have enough developmental delay to be diagnosed as having intellectual disability/mental retardation. In addition to this, a behavioral phenotype has been proposed in the literature (Mattson & Riley, 1998; Stratton et al., 1996). This particular behavioral profile includes attention deficits, hyperactivity, an unusual degree of memory loss, and conduct problems (a deficiency in a person's awareness of the consequences of his or her actions). Although none of these components of the behavioral profile are specific, when taken together in the context of full FAS they appear to represent a consistent manifestation of the overall pattern.

Some of the other teratogenic syndromes are known to involve developmental difficulties, but all require additional investigation before any firm conclusions can be drawn. For instance, some children with the fetal valproate syndrome have been said to have autism (Christianson, Chesler, & Kromberg, 1994), but this requires further investigation. Children with fetal hydantoin and isotretinoin syndromes have also been recognized to have developmental disabilities, but further

study on the learning profile is also needed. Little is known about the adult phenotypes in the teratogenic syndromes.

Benefits of Diagnosis

Often the diagnosis of a neurodevelopmental disorder or dysmorphic syndrome is relegated to the area of the exotic. However, as has been emphasized throughout this chapter, diagnosis is important for the individual, the family, and their medical practitioners. Table 3.3 summarizes the benefits of making the diagnosis of a genetic condition or syndrome. These can be illustrated in the diagnosis of Williams syndrome. Once a diagnosis has been established, and the deletion of the elastin gene has been confirmed with FISH, recurrence risk counseling can occur; if a parent does not have Williams syndrome (which is usually the case), the deletion is certainly de novo, and the recurrence risk approaches that of the background risk. Prenatal diagnosis with the FISH technique is possible in future pregnancies but is prob-

---

TABLE 3.3. Benefits of Diagnosis in a Genetic Condition or Syndrome

- *Recurrence chance in genetic counseling.* The recognition of an established disorder of known etiology provides information on cause and genetic aspects of the condition, including chance of recurrence, reproductive options, and identification of at-risk relatives.

- *Prediction of prognosis.* Each disorder has its own particular natural history and outcome. Knowledge of the degree of disability that occurs on average is often helpful to families.

- *Appropriate laboratory testing and screening.* Precise diagnosis can eliminate the need for many tests frequently considered in the evaluation of an individual with a developmental disorder. Appropriate screening can be planned according to natural history.

- *Guidelines for management.* Knowledge of the natural history of a syndrome allows for the establishment of guidelines for routine care, including suggestions for educational and vocational interventions.

- *Family support.* In some families, the knowledge of a condition helps in dealing with the uncertainty of the situation. A diagnosis provides a biological basis for a condition, as well as an entrée to support groups, specialty clinics, and other services.

ably not necessary, given the low recurrence risk in sporadic cases. An individual with Williams syndrome has a 50% risk of having a child with Williams syndrome with each pregnancy and can consider a range of reproductive options, including prenatal diagnosis. Depending on the individual's developmental status, parenting skills must also be considered. When other relatives are at increased risk for the condition, it is also important to recommend genetic counseling for other at-risk family members to preserve their reproductive choices.

In addition, the diagnosis helps the clinician in stating some predictions about prognosis—especially the neurodevelopmental outcome, but also the natural history of the condition. Individuals with Williams syndrome need a cardiac evaluation, due to a 60% occurrence of heart defects (especially supravalvular aortic stenosis). In addition, a higher index of suspicion for hearing loss, visual difficulties, urinary tract infections, and hypertension should occur, and this should further modify the primary care practitioner's health supervision plan. Clinicians have developed management guidelines, also referred to as *anticipatory guidance*, for common genetic conditions (e.g., Cassidy & Allanson, 2010). These guidelines are usually organized by the age of the individual. A diagnosis makes it possible to avoid unnecessary laboratory testing. A person with Williams syndrome who has developmental delay should not require any metabolic testing or neuroimaging—tests that are frequently done in the diagnostic evaluation of a individual with this presentation. Moreover, knowledge of the natural history of the developmental profile in Williams syndrome at least allows for some initial steps in planning educational and vocational interventions. Although it is certainly true that a "cookbook"-type plan cannot be laid out, there is a profile of strengths and weaknesses in individuals with Williams syndrome that can help the educator or therapist. Finally, making a diagnosis of a specific condition often helps a family with the experience of uncertainty, as often a general diagnosis of a developmental disability conveys a sense of meaninglessness and confusion. A diagnosis of a particular syndrome, even an uncommon one, gives a biological basis for (and often credibility to) the individual's diffi-

culties. For many families, the diagnosis is the entrée to a support group and specialty clinics with concentrated expertise (e.g., for Williams syndrome, a support group's website is *www.williams-syndrome.org*). When families participate in support groups and specialty clinics, this provides pools of patients who often volunteer for studies of genotype–phenotype correlations, which in turn improves patient care. Also, although it seems self-evident that individuals with special needs should be able to obtain services based on those needs, in practice a diagnosis often entitles these persons and their caregivers to services previously denied without a diagnosis.

One important new area of diagnosis is predictive or presymptomatic diagnosis. *Presymptomatic diagnosis* is a diagnosis based on DNA testing before symptoms are present. An example of presymptomatic diagnosis is testing for Huntington disease (HD). The genetic test is fairly straightforward, using a polymerase chain reaction assay to determine the number of cytosine–adenine–guanine repeats in the *HTT* gene. Individuals with 40 or more CAG repeats develop the symptoms of HD. The disease typically manifests itself in a person's 30s or 40s, and includes progressive chorea and dementia, with death typically occurring 10–15 years after diagnosis. It is an autosomal dominant condition, so children of a gene mutation carrier have a 50% risk of developing the condition, with age-specific penetrance that reaches 100% by late adulthood. Testing is generally only done in centers that offer a protocol including genetic counseling, neurological examination, and psychiatric evaluation and support. There are complex psychosocial and ethical issues involved in presymptomatic testing for HD. Psychosocial issues include the availability of life-altering testing when no effective treatments are currently available; complex family issues, including survivor guilt; and the risk of adverse psychological reactions in both counselees who test positive and those who test negative. Ethical issues include the nonavailability of testing without counseling, the possibility of insurance discrimination, testing in minors, and testing in situations where one family member's results reveal those of another family member. Testing in childhood is not recommended unless the child has definite neurological symptoms such as chorea or rigidity.

Predictive diagnosis is similar to presymptomatic diagnosis, but in this case the test predicts a susceptibility rather than certainty of symptoms. An example of predictive diagnosis is testing for multiple endocrine neoplasia, type 2. This condition poses a risk in childhood for adrenal malignancies, and screening and treatment are available. Thus childhood testing is recommended.

BEHAVIORAL PHENOTYPES IN MEDICAL GENETICS

The term *behavioral phenotype* has been used for the last 20 years in the fields of child psychiatry and medical genetics to refer to the neurobehavioral aspects of a condition. There is no consensus on its definition, and it is used by different people to mean different things. Turk and Hill (1995) provide an excellent summary of the issues in their review. These authors assert that "a number of conditions, recognizable by a common physical phenotype, single gene defect or chromosomal abnormality, seem also to have a constellation of behaviors or cognitive anomalies which are characteristic" (p. 105). Flint and Yule (1994) take a stricter view of this concept and require that before the term is used, there must be a distinctive behavior that occurs in almost every case and rarely in other conditions. However, we agree with Turk and Hill that this more restrictive view is not applicable to the inclusion of nonbehavioral manifestations in the definition of syndromes. For example, the atrioventricular canal defect seen in 20–30% of individuals with Down syndrome is relatively characteristic, as almost two-thirds of individuals with this defect have Down syndrome. However, there are clearly other causes of this defect other than trisomy 21, and not all patients with Down syndrome have it. Similarly, only about 20% of individuals with Turner syndrome have a left-sided obstructive lesion of the heart, and the overwhelming majority of cases who have this heart lesion do not have Turner syndrome. Thus, as illustrated here, most clinicians would not require the physical defects of the heart to occur completely consistently and specifically before including them as part of the syndrome. The same

concept then, we propose, should hold true for behavioral components.

In the literature, the term *behavioral phenotype* is used without necessarily clarifying whether it refers to a psychological/cognitive profile, a behavioral disorder, or a personality trait (Turk & Hill, 1995). In this context, we propose a modification of the definition of the term suggested by Turk and Hill. We posit that *a behavioral phenotype is a profile of behavior, cognition, or personality that represents a component of the overall pattern seen in many or most individuals with a particular condition or syndrome.* Although the profile may not be specific, it is consistent in the syndromic pattern. The challenge for the next decades (as stated in many of the chapters in this book) is continued documentation of these parameters with state-of-the-art tools. The diagnosis of a dysmorphic syndrome needs to be rigorous and clear-cut, and the documentation of the neurodevelopmental and neuropsychological profile demands the same current strategies. At present, a glance through review papers, like those of Turk and Hill (1995) and Flint and Yule (1994), gives one the impression that there is not much specificity to the behavioral patterns described in the literature reviewed. However, this perusal is not very different from one's first glance through a catalog of listed facial features and minor anomalies in chromosome syndromes. Yet the consistency in the facial features of individuals of the same age with chromosome disorders illustrates the reproducibility of these syndromes. Recognition of facial features and documentation of their pattern are often difficult without tools for quantification. These same kinds of issues apply to documentation in the neurobehavioral realm, especially in the profiles of behavioral disorders and personality traits. The principles are the same; just as the facial features differ from those of the family background in such conditions as Williams syndrome and Down syndrome, there is an alteration of the biological basis of behavior and personality beyond the family background in these conditions. Shalev and Hall (2004) have recently proposed a behavioral pattern profile. This tool consists of 12 categories of behavioral features and is intended to facilitate a standardized collection of behavioral data in a clinical setting.

Table 3.4 lists dysmorphic syndromes that have been found to have a relatively specific or characteristic behavioral profile. The chromosomal location or identified gene is listed as well. The reader is referred to the above-cited review papers. Moreover, the chapters in this text summarize the behavioral profiles of several of these syndromes.

A behavioral phenotype is generally defined by beginning with a sample of subjects with a specific dysmorphic syndrome and then studying specific cognitive, affective, or behavioral characteristics, as compared to those of a relevant control group. Some syndromes, such as Williams and Prader–Willi syndromes, have been associated with chromosomal regions as well as with behavioral patterns. A complementary approach has made use of several large affected families, extensive cognitive testing, and DNA markers to find linkages for components of a complex cognitive phenotype—developmental dyslexia. In six large families containing 94 adults affected with reading disability (documented in childhood), defective phonological awareness was linked to markers on chromosome 6, and defective single-word reading was linked to chromosome 15 (Grigorenko et al., 1997). Success in using genet-

ics to dissect this complex phenotype first required careful study of the reading disability phenotype through state-of-the-art cognitive science (Pennington, 1997). Future progress in understanding genotype–phenotype relationships in neurobehavioral disorders such as autism (Fisch, 2008) or Tourette syndrome is likely to rely on an interplay of approaches from psychology, genetics, neuroimaging, and other disciplines.

CONCLUSION

The field of medical and molecular genetics has blossomed in the last two decades, with a concomitant interest in genetics among primary care practitioners and specialists in other fields. The basic paradigm provides the potential for a newer understanding of human disease pathogenesis, similar to the advances made in infectious diseases and immunology in the early 20th century. The principles necessary to apply this approach in the clinical setting can be mastered with some effort and are valuable in the care of patients with neurodevelopmental disorders. The diagnosis of genetic disorders and syndromes is of vital importance to

TABLE 3.4. Dysmorphic Syndromes Thought to Have a Characteristic Behavioral Phenotype

Syndrome	Cause
Chromosome	
Williams syndrome	7q1 microdeletion
Velocardiofacial/DiGeorge syndrome	22q11 deletion
Prader–Willi syndrome	15q11–13 microdeletion[a]
Angelman syndrome	15q11–13 microdeletion[a]
Smith–Magenis syndrome	17p11 microdeletion
Down syndrome	Trisomy 21
Klinefelter syndrome	47,XXY
Monogenic	
Neurofibromatosis type 1 (NF1)	Mutation in *NF1* gene at 17q11.2
Noonan syndrome	Mutation in *PTPN11* gene at 12q24.1 (plus at least four other genes—genetically heterogeneous)
Fragile X syndrome	Mutation in *FMR1* gene at Xq27.3
Rett syndrome	Mutation in MECP2 gene on Xq28
de Lange syndrome	Mutation in *NIPBL* gene on 5p13.1
Environmental	
Fetal alcohol syndrome (FAS)	Maternal alcohol abuse
Fetal valproate syndrome	Maternal use of valproate

[a]Imprintable genes (see text). See also Dykens, Cassidy, and DeVries (Chapter 25, this volume).

patients, their families, and care providers. The relatively recently proposed concept of behavioral phenotype fits quite well into the paradigm of medical genetics. Ongoing work utilizing current techniques in phenotype analysis, medical genetics, and neuropsychology will be necessary to delineate the behavioral profiles, specific or nonspecific, of various syndromes. An understanding of the biological basis of the neurodevelopmental aspects in these genetic conditions can provide fresh insight into well-known and common symptomatic disorders, such as learning disabilities and autism.

REFERENCES

Acosta, M. T., Arcos-Burgos, M., & Muenke, M. (2004). Attention deficit/hyperactivity disorder (ADHD): Complex phenotype, simple genotype? *Genetics in Medicine, 6*(1), 1–15.

Ad Hoc Committee on Genetic Counseling. (1975). Report to the American Society of Human Genetics. *American Journal of Human Genetics, 27,* 240–242.

Battaglia, A., Gurrieri, F., Bertini, E., Bellacosa, A., Pomponi, M. G., Paravatou-Petsotas, M., et al. (1997). The inv dup(15) syndrome: A clinically recognizable syndrome with altered behavior, mental retardation, and epilepsy. *Neurology, 48,* 1081–1086.

Bennett, R. L. (1999). *The practical guide to the genetic family history.* New York: Wiley-Liss.

Bennett, R. L., Steinhaus, K. A., Uhrich, S. B., O'Sullivan, C. K., Resta, R. G., Lochner-Doyle, D,, et al. (1995). Recommendations for standardized human pedigree nomenclature. *American Journal of Human Genetics, 56,* 745–752.

Cassidy, S., & Allanson, J. (2010). *Management of genetic syndromes* (3rd ed.). Hoboken, NJ: Wiley-Blackwell.

Chapman, N. H., Raskind, W. H., Thomson, J. B., Berninger, V. W., & Wijsman, E. M. (2003). Segregation analysis of phenotypic components of learning disabilities: II. Phonological decoding. *American Journal of Medical Genetics, Part B (Neuropsychiatric Genetics), 121B,* 60–70.

Cheung, P. K., Wynhoven, B., & Harrigan, P. R. (2004). 2004: Which HIV-1 drug resistance mutations are common in clinical practice? *AIDS Review, 6*(2), 107–116.

Christianson, A. L., Chesler, N., & Kromberg, J. G. R. (1994). Fetal valproate syndrome: Clinical and neuro-developmental features in two sibling pairs. *Developmental Medicine and Child Neurology, 36,* 361–369.

Curry, C. J., Stevenson, R. E., Cunniff, C., Augh-

ton, D., Byrne, J., Carey, J. C., et al. (1997). Evaluation of mental retardation: Recommendations of a consensus conference. *American Journal of Human Genetics, 72,* 468–477.

de Vries, B. B. A., Winter, R., Schinzel, A., & van Ravenswaaij-Arts, C. (2003). Telomeres: A diagnosis at the end of the chromosomes. *Journal of Medical Genetics, 40,* 385–398.

Donnai, D. (2002). Genetic services. *Clinical Genetics, 61*(1), 1–6.

Edelman, L., & Hirschhorn, K. (2009). Clinical utility of array CGH for detection of chromosome imbalances associated with mental retardation and multiple congenital anomalies. *Annals of the New York Academy of Sciences, 1151,* 157–166.

Faraone, S. V. (2004). Genetics of adult attention-deficit/hyperactivity disorder. *Psychiatric Clinics of North America, 27*(2), 303–321.

Fisch, G. S. (2008). Syndromes and epistemology: Is autism a polygenic disorder? *American Journal of Medical Genetics, Part A, 146A*(17), 2203–2212.

Flint, J., & Knight, S. (2003). The use of telomere probes to investigate submicroscopic rearrangements associated with mental retardation. *Current Opinion in Genetics and Development, 13,* 310–316.

Flint, J., & Yule, W. (1994). Behavioural phenotypes. In M. Rutter, E. Taylor, & L. A. Hersov (Eds.), *Child and adolescent psychiatry: Modern approaches.* Oxford, UK: Blackwell Scientific.

Francks, C., MacPhie, I. L., & Monaco, A. P. (2002). The genetic basis of dyslexia. *Lancet Neurology, 1*(8), 483–490.

Gelehrter, T. D., Collins, F. S., & Ginsberg D. (1998). *Principles of medical genetics* (2nd ed.). Baltimore: Williams & Wilkins.

Grigorenko, E. L., Wood, F. B., Meyer, M. S., Hart, L. A., Speed, W. C., Shuster A., et al. (1997). Susceptibility loci for distinct components of developmental dyslexia on chromosomes 6 and 15. *American Journal of Human Genetics, 60,* 27–39.

Hennekam, R. C. M., Allanson, J., & Krantz, I. (2009). *Gorlin's syndromes of the head and neck* (5th ed.). New York: Oxford University Press.

Jones, K. L. (2006). *Smith's recognizable patterns of human malformation* (6th ed.). Philadelphia: Elsevier Saunders.

Jorde, L. B., Carey, J. C., & Bamshad, M. (2010). *Medical genetics* (4th ed.). Philadelphis: Mosby/Elsevier.

Jorde, L. B., Carey, J. C., Bamshad, M., & White, R. L. (2003). *Medical genetics* (3rd ed.). St. Louis, MO: Mosby.

Mattson, S. N., & Riley, E. P. (1998). A review of the neurobehavioral deficits in children with fetal alcohol syndrome or prenatal exposure to alcohol. *Alcoholism: Clinical and Experimental Research, 22*(2), 279–294.

McKusick, V. A. (1998). *Mendelian inheritance in man* (12th ed.). Baltimore: Johns Hopkins University Press.

Messiaen, L., Callens, T., Mortier, G., Beysen, D., Vandenbroucke, I., Van Roy, N., et al. (2000). Exhaustive mutation analysis of the *NF1* gene allows identification of 95% of mutations and reveals a high frequency of unusual splicing defects. *Human Mutation, 15,* 541–555.

Morton, C. C., & Nance, W. E. (2006). Newborn hearing screening—a silent revolution. *New England Journal of Medicine, 354*(20), 2151–2164.

National Institutes of Health (NIH) Consensus Development Conference. (1988). Neurofibromatosis. *Archives of Neurology, 45,* 575–578.

The National Society of Genetic Counselors' [NSGC] Definition Task Force: Resta, R., Biesecker, B. B., Bennett, R. L., Blum, S., Hahn, S. E., Strecker, M. N., et al. (2006) A new definition of genetic counseling: National Society of Genetic Counselors' Task Force report. *Journal of Genetic Counseling, 15*(2), 77–83.

Nussbaum, R. L., McInnes, R. R., & Willard, H. F. (2007). *Thompson and Thompson's genetics in medicine* (7th ed.). Philadelphia: Saunders/Elsevier.

Pennington, B. F. (1997). Using genetics to dissect cognition. *American Journal of Human Genetics, 60,* 13–16.

Plomin, R., & Walker, S. O. (2003). Genetics and educational psychology. *British Journal of Educational Psychology, 73*(Pt. 1), 3–14.

Quirk, E., McLeod, H., & Powderly, W. (2004). The pharmacogenetics of antiretroviral therapy: A review of studies to date. *Clinical Infectious Diseases, 39*(1), 98–106.

Read, A., & Donnai, D. (2007). *The new clinical genetics.* Bloxham, UK: Scion.

Reardon, W., Winter, R. M., Rutland, P., Pulleyn, L. J., Jones, B. M., & Malcolm, S. (1994). Mutations in the fibroblast growth factor receptor 2 gene cause Crouzon syndrome. *Nature Genetics, 8*(1), 98–103.

Rimoin, D. L., Connor, J. M., Pyeritz, R. E., &

Korf, B. R. (Eds.). (2007). *Emery and Rimoin's principles and practice of medical genetics* (5th ed.). Philadelphia: Churchill Livingstone.

Shalev, S. A., & Hall, J. G. (2004). Behavioral pattern profile: A tool for the description of behavior to be used in the genetics clinic. *American Journal of Medical Genetics, 128A,* 389–395.

Sherman, S. L., DeFries, J. C., Gottesman, I. I., Loehlin, J. C., Meyer, J. M., Pelias, M. Z., et al. (1997). Behavioral genetics '97: ASHG statement recent developments in human behavioral genetics: Past accomplishments and future directions. *American Journal of Human Genetics, 60,* 1265–1275.

Smalley, S. L. (1997). Behavioral genetics '97: Genetic influences in childhood-onset psychiatric disorders: Autism and attention-deficit/hyperactivity disorder. *American Journal of Human Genetics, 60,* 1276–1282.

Stevenson, R. E., Schwartz, C. C., & Schroer, R. J. (1999). *X-linked mental retardation.* Oxford, UK: Oxford University Press.

Stratton, K., Howe, C., & Battaglia, F. (1996). *Fetal alcohol syndrome: Diagnosis, epidemiology and treatment.* Washington, DC: National Academy Press.

Streissguth, A. P., Clarren, S. K., & Jones, K. L. (1985). Natural history of the fetal alcohol syndrome: A 10-year follow-up of eleven patients. *Lancet, ii,* 85–91.

Thackray, H. M., & Tifft, C. (2001). Fetal alcohol syndrome. *Pediatrics in Review, 22,* 47–55.

Turk, J., & Hill, P. (1995). Behavioural phenotypes in dysmorphic syndromes. *Clinical Dysmorphology, 4,* 105–115.

Webster, M., & Donoghue, D. J. (1997). FGFR activation in skeletal disorders: Too much of a good thing. *Trends in Genetics, 13,* 178–182.

Weatherall, D. J. (1985). *The new genetics and clinical practice* (2nd ed.). Oxford, UK: Oxford University Press.

Wilkie, W. O., Slaney, S. F., Oldridge, M., Poole, M. D., Ashworth, G. J., Hockley, A. D., et al. (1995). Apert syndrome results from localized mutations of FGFR2 and is allelic with Crouzon syndrome. *Nature Genetics, 9,* 165–172.

CHAPTER 4

Neuroimaging and Genetic Disorders

SHELLI R. KESLER
ELIZABETH WILDE
JENNIFER L. BRUNO
ERIN D. BIGLER

Neuroimaging methods allow safe and effective measurement of *in vivo* neurobiological status and are widely used to study brain–behavior relationships in children, as well as adults. Neuroimaging studies can provide insight regarding the specific neural systems that subserve the cognitive deficits associated with various syndromes and pathologies, including genetic disorders. Since the first edition of this volume was published, there have been significant advances in neuroimaging technology, stimulating a substantial increase in gene–brain–behavior research. Whereas previously we were only able to include neuroanatomical or brain morphological information associated with various childhood genetic syndromes, there have since been multiple studies involving measurements of functional brain activation, white matter pathway coherence, and neurometabolites.

Structural or volumetric magnetic resonance imaging (MRI) can provide three-dimensional, high-resolution images for qualitatively identifying gross pathology, as well as quantitative, tissue-specific (white matter, gray matter, and cerebrospinal fluid [CSF]) brain volume measurements (Kennedy, Haselgrove, & McInerney, 2003). Functional MRI (fMRI) allows *in vivo* assess-ment of brain function by detecting blood flow differences (Logothetis, 2008), but it can be challenging in children with genetic disorders that are associated with significant intellectual disability, due to the increased cognitive-behavioral demands of fMRI acquisition. White matter pathway coherence and fiber tracking are made possible by diffusion tensor imaging (DTI), which relies on water diffusion near myelinated axons (Hua et al., 2009) and provides measures of microstructural integrity (e.g., fractional anisotropy [FA]). MR susceptibility-weighted imaging (SWI) uses both phase and magnitude images to provide increased visualization of brain tumors, microbleeds, and other vascular abnormalities, as well as diffuse axonal injury associated with trauma and neurodegenerative pathologies (Sehgal et al., 2006; Thomas et al., 2008). MR spectroscopy (MRS) can detect neurometabolite levels, which putatively provide metrics of neuronal and axonal integrity, membrane turnover, and neurotransmitter function (Gujar, Maheshwari, Bjorkman-Burtscher, & Sundgren, 2005). It is now even possible to use functional neuroimaging techniques, including fMRI, to measure brain activation in real time (deCharms, 2008). All of these MR methods significantly improve the sensitivity and specificity with which researchers can identify neurodevelopmental mechanisms and trajectories associated with the cognitive-behavioral phenotypes of various genetic disorders. These data are vital for guiding, developing, and even implementing syndrome-specific treatments and interventions.

The above-mentioned neuroimaging methods all rely on MR physics and principles. They are implemented by using powerful magnetic fields and radiofrequency pulses to manipulate the nuclear magnetic resonances of hydrogen atoms, which are abundant in human tissue. MR techniques are noninvasive, though some involve the injection of contrast agents to enhance certain image targets. Unlike computed tomography (CT), MRI does not use radiation and is therefore a very low-risk procedure. However, patients with ferrous metal implants or biomedical devices cannot undergo MR techniques. Several sources are available that describe the details of MR neuroimaging techniques such as fMRI, DTI, and MRS, including works by Huettel, Song, and McCarthy (2008), Filippi (2009), Jezzard, Matthews, and Smith (2003), Mori (2007), and Gujar and colleagues (2005). Other neuroimaging techniques, including single-photon emission computed tomography, positron emission tomography (PET), and near-infrared spectroscopy, have also been utilized to provide valuable information regarding neurobiological status in various populations. These are described in Huettel and colleagues (2008) and Jezzard and colleagues (2003). Although these other imaging methods are sometimes used to assess children with genetic disorders, the primary imaging tool for this purpose is MR, and thus MR-based techniques are the focus of this chapter. Only the most recent neuroimaging findings from studies of childhood genetic disorders that involve pediatric human participants are discussed.

Genetic technologies have also advanced significantly in the past 10-plus years, allowing identification of new syndromes and further specification of gene products and their functions in the brain and other organs. Comprehensive information regarding human genes and their phenotypes is available on the World Wide Web via the Online Mendelian Inheritance in Man (OMIM) database, developed by scientists at Johns Hopkins University School of Medicine. Despite the growing number of genetic syndromes that are being identified, this chapter focuses on the most common genetic disorders affecting children. The chapter also briefly discusses neuroimaging findings from certain multifactorial syndromes that may have genetic underpinnings resulting in inherited vulnerability for the syndrome. These syndromes include attention-deficit/hyperactivity disorder (ADHD) and pervasive developmental disorders (PDDs), such as autism. OMIM numbers for individual syndromes are included when applicable.

CRANIOFACIAL SYNDROMES

Apert Syndrome (OMIM #101200)

Apert syndrome is characterized by craniosynostosis, which causes facial abnormalities and can affect the development of the brain, leading to cognitive impairments. Imaging studies of children with Apert syndrome suggest an increased incidence of ventriculomegaly, hypoplasia of the corpus callosum, cavum vergae, hypoplasia of the septum pellucidum, arachnoid cysts, and hydrocephalus (Collmann, Sorensen, & Krauss, 2005; Quintero-Rivera et al., 2006; Yacubian-Fernandes et al., 2004, 2005) (Figure 4.1).

Down Syndrome (OMIM #190685)

Resulting from trisomy of chromosome 21, Down syndrome is the most common cause of intellectual impairment. Children with Down syndrome are at increased risk for reduced total brain volumes (Pinter, Eliez, Schmitt, Capone, & Reiss, 2001b) and for smaller regional volumes, including those of the hippocampus and cerebellum (Pinter, Brown, et al., 2001; Pinter, Eliez, et al., 2001). Subcortical gray matter volumes may be enlarged (Pinter, Eliez, et al., 2001). Atrophy of the corpus callosum has also been noted (Kieslich, Fuchs, Vlaho, Maisch, & Boehles, 2002; Murphy, Brenner, & Ann Lynch, 2006) (Figure 4.2). An MRS study of children with Down syndrome demonstrated decreased levels of N-acetylaspartate (NAA) and glutamine/glutamate in the frontal lobes (Smigielska-Kuzia & Sobaniec, 2007).

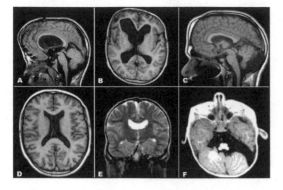

FIGURE 4.1. Apert syndrome: Ventriculomegaly and corpus callosum hypoplasia—MRI sagittal plane and T1 acquisition (A), and axial plane and T1–inversion recovery (IR) acquisition (B). Cavum vergae and arachnoid cyst in the posterior fossa—MRI in sagittal plane and T1 acquisition (C), and axial plane and T1-IR acquisition (D). Septum pellucidum hypoplasia—MRI in coronal plane and T2 acquisition (E). Arachnoid cyst in posterior fossa—MRI in axial plane and T1-IR acquisition (F). From Yacubian-Fernandes et al. (2005). Copyright 2005 by Arquivos de Neuro-Psiquiatria. Reprinted by permission.

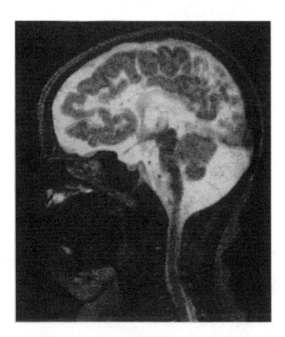

FIGURE 4.2. Down syndrome: General brain atrophy, callosal dysplasia, cerebellar hypoplasia (sagittal T2-weighted MRI). From Kieslich, Fuchs, Vlaho, Maisch, and Boehles (2002). Copyright 2002 by Sage Publications. Reprinted by permission.

Velocardiofacial Syndrome (OMIM #192430)

Velocardiofacial syndrome (VCFS) is a relatively common congenital disorder associated with cardiac and facial abnormalities, as well as learning disabilities and significant risk for serious neuropsychiatric disorders, including schizophrenia (Gothelf, 2007). Neuroimaging studies have demonstrated reduced total brain volumes (Bird & Scambler, 2000; Eliez, Antonarakis, Morris, Dahoun, & Reiss, 2001; Eliez, Schmitt, White, & Reiss, 2000) and reduced regional brain volumes, including those of the thalamus (Bish, Nguyen, Ding, Ferrante, & Simon, 2004), hippocampus (Debbane, Schaer, Farhoumand, Glaser, & Eliez, 2006; Deboer, Wu, Lee, & Simon, 2007; Kates et al., 2006), cerebellum (Bish et al., 2006; Eliez, Schmitt, White, Wellis, & Reiss, 2001), superior temporal gyrus (Eliez, Blasey, Schmitt, et al., 2001), parieto-occipital region (Campbell et al., 2006), corpus callosum (Machado et al., 2007; Shashi et al., 2004), and posterior fusiform gyrus (Glaser et al., 2007). Caudate asymmetry and enlargement have been repeatedly observed in children with VCFS (Campbell et al., 2006; Eliez, Barnea-Goraly, Schmitt, Liu, & Reiss, 2002; Kates et al., 2004; Sugama et al., 2000). Kates and colleages (2006) also demonstrated amygdalar enlargement. Simon and colleagues (2005) found a profile of reduced and enlarged regional gray matter, CSF, and white matter volumes, as well as increased and decreased white matter FA, using voxel-based morphometry and DTI. Kates and colleagues also demonstrated reduced white matter volumes in parietal and temporal regions associated with VCFS (Kates et al., 2001), as well as in frontal regions (Kates et al., 2004). Cortical thickness and shape abnormalities have been consistently noted in children with VCFS (Bearden et al., 2007; Gothelf, Schaer, & Eliez, 2008). fMRI studies suggest an altered pattern of frontal and parieto-occipital activation during working memory (Kates et al., 2007) (Plate 4.1), as well as altered activation of the left parietal regions during arithmetic (Eliez, Blasey, Menon, et al., 2001) and response inhibition tasks (Gothelf et al., 2007).

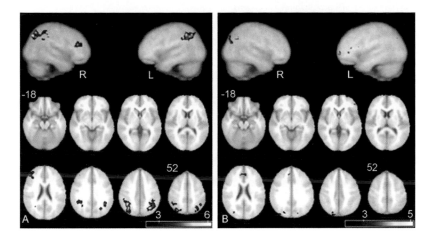

PLATE 4.1. (A) During a nonspatial working memory fMRI task, controls displayed significantly greater activation in the right middle and inferior frontal gyri (Brodmann areas [BA] 45, 46, and 48), the left and right inferior and superior parietal lobules (BA 7, 39, and 40), and the left and right occipital lobes (BA 19) than children with VCFS did. (B) Participants with VCFS displayed significantly greater activation in the left orbitofrontal cortex (BA 11), the right cingulate (BA 32), and the right cuneus and occipital cortex (BA 19) than controls did. Superior–inferior distance from the anterior commisure–posterior commisure line is indicated in both panels. The bar is a visual representation of the range of z values present in this activation map. From Kates et al. (2007). Copyright 2007 by Elsevier. Reprinted by permission.

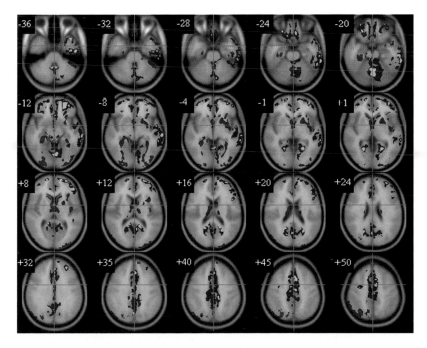

PLATE 4.2. Relative reductions (blue/pink) and increases (red/yellow) in gray matter volume in children with WS versus controls (cluster threshold = .05, p = .003, confidence interval = ± 2.1) corrected for gender and total gray volume). The maps are oriented so that the right side of the brain is shown on the left side of each panel. The z coordinate for each row of axial slices in the standard space of Talairach and Tournoux is given in millimeters. From Campbell et al. (2009). Copyright 2009 by Elsevier. Reprinted by permission.

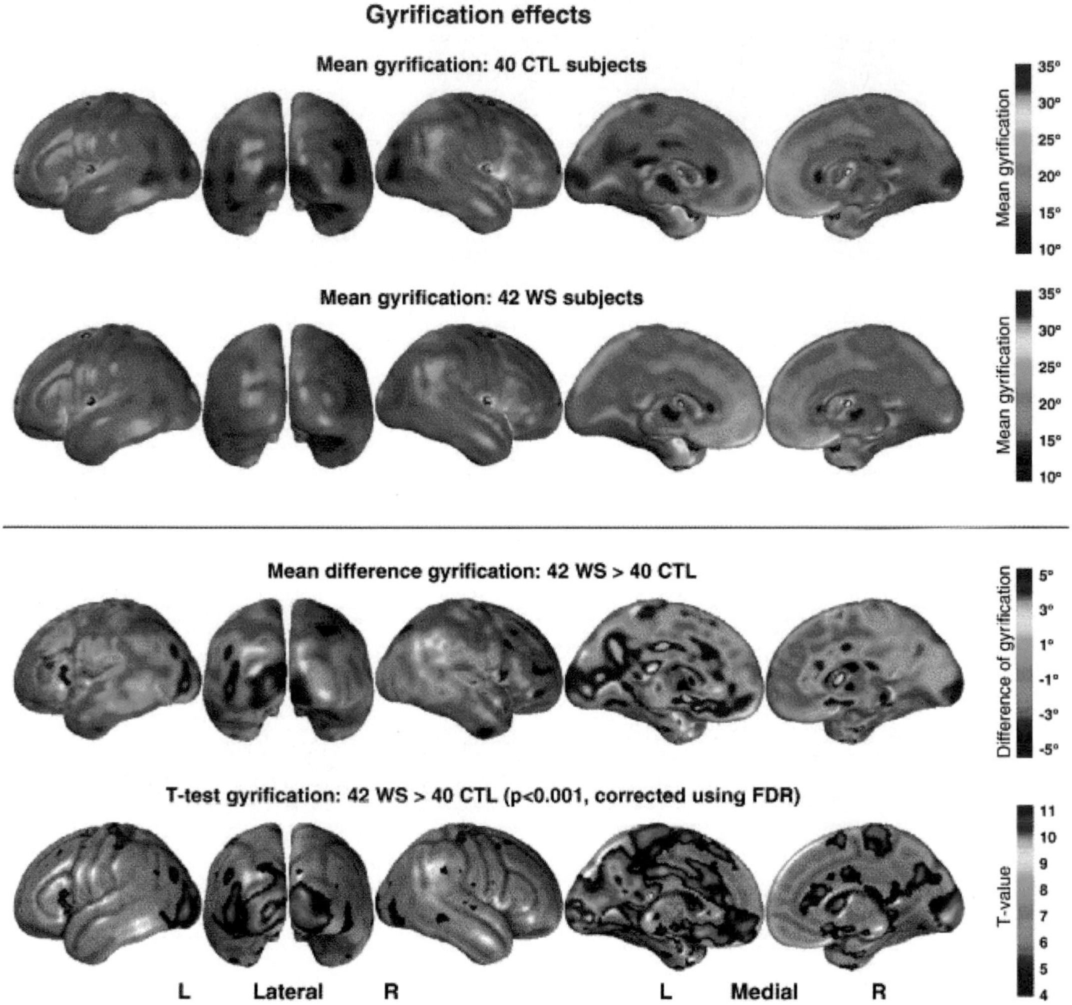

Gyrification effects

Mean gyrification: 40 CTL subjects

Mean gyrification: 42 WS subjects

Mean difference gyrification: 42 WS > 40 CTL

T-test gyrification: 42 WS > 40 CTL (p<0.001, corrected using FDR)

L   Lateral   R   L   Medial   R

PLATE 4.3. Gyrification effects in children and adults with WS. The two upper rows reveal the average distribution of local gyrification in healthy controls (CTL) and individuals with WS. Curvature values are expressed in degrees, with blue and purple colors indicating regions of lower gyrification, while yellow and red indicate areas of higher gyrification. The third row demonstrates the mean differences between participants with WS and healthy controls. Areas with higher gyrification in persons with WS appear in yellow and red, whereas blue and purple indicate higher gyrification in control subjects. The last row illustrates regions of significantly increased gyrification in persons with WS compared to normal controls (threshold $p < 0.001$; corrected for multiple comparisons using false discovery rate). From Gaser et al. (2006). Copyright 2006 by Elsevier. Reprinted by permission.

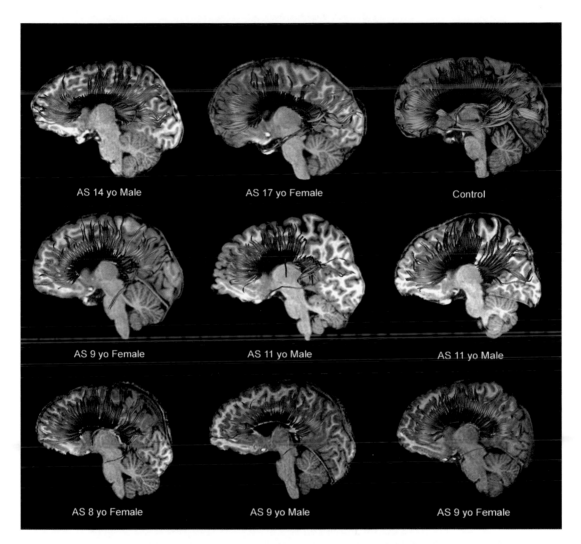

AS 14 yo Male   AS 17 yo Female   Control

AS 9 yo Female   AS 11 yo Male   AS 11 yo Male

AS 8 yo Female   AS 9 yo Male   AS 9 yo Female

PLATE 4.4. DTI tractography of the corpus callosum overlaid on T1-weighted MRI scans. The expected pattern of corpus callosum tractography is demonstrated in the typically developing control individual in the top right corner. Eight individuals with AS demonstrate abnormalities in pattern or paucity of "streamlines" generated by tractography. Green color indicates fibers coursing in an anterior-to-posterior direction; red color indicates fibers coursing in a right-to-left direction; and blue color represents fibers coursing in a superior-to-inferior direction.

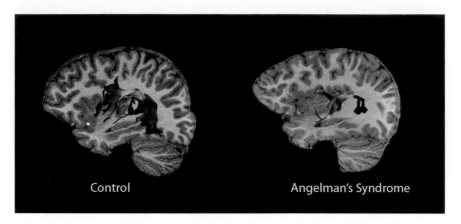

PLATE 4.5. DTI tractography of the left arcuate fasciculus in an age- and gender-matched control child versus a child with AS, demonstrating marked reduction in the fiber pattern detected via tractography.

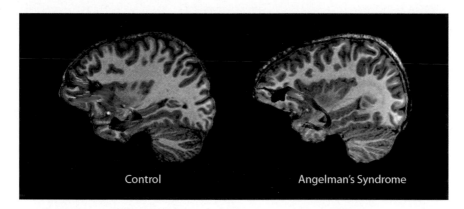

PLATE 4.6. DTI tractography of the left uncinate fasciculus in an age- and gender-matched control child versus a child with AS, demonstrating marked reduction in the fiber pattern detected via tractography.

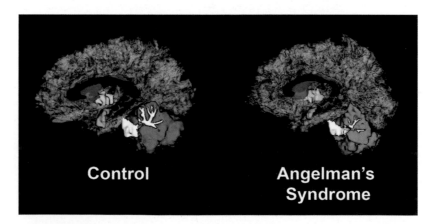

PLATE 4.7. Three-dimensional rendering of the relative volumes of structures found to differ in a cohort of children with AS versus age- and gender-comparable control children. Structures such as the cerebellum, amygdala, corpus callosum, and basal ganglia are highlighted.

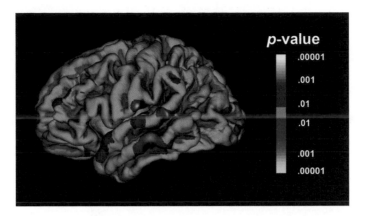

PLATE 4.8. Blue areas represent regions of significant cortical thinning in a cohort of children with AS versus age- and gender-comparable control children, located primarily in the temporal lobes. Red areas represent areas of increased cortical thickness in the children with AS, and are located in the frontal lobes.

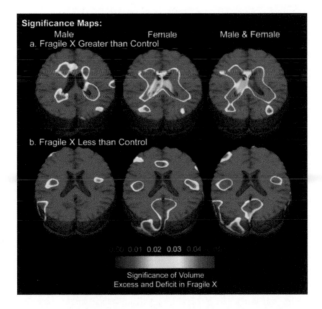

PLATE 4.9. Significance maps for group differences in local brain volume between individuals with FXS and controls. Significant volume differences between persons with FXS and healthy controls are shown for males (left panels in a and b), for females (middle panels in a and b), and for all subjects (right panels in a and b). In all maps, the persons with FXS have significant excess volumes in the ventricle and caudate regions (blue colors in panel a). Panel b shows that subjects with FXS have significant volume deficits in medial occipital regions and some temporal lobe regions. From A. D. Lee et al. (2007). Copyright 2007 by Elsevier. Reprinted by permission.

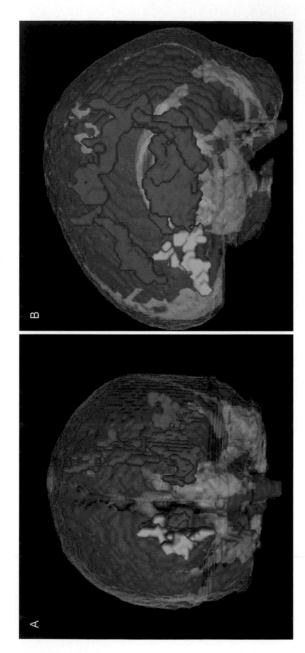

PLATE 4.10. A three-dimensional representation of aberrant white matter tracts in TS (left frontoparietal cluster is shown in blue; right prefrontal cluster is shown in green; bilateral internal capsule cluster is shown in red), as derived from FA maps positioned within a transparent, volumetrically rendered average image of all participants with TS. A, anterior view; B, sagittal view. From Holzapfel, Barnea-Goraly, Eckert, Kiesler, and Reiss (2006). Copyright 2006 by the Society for Neuroscience. Reprinted by permission.

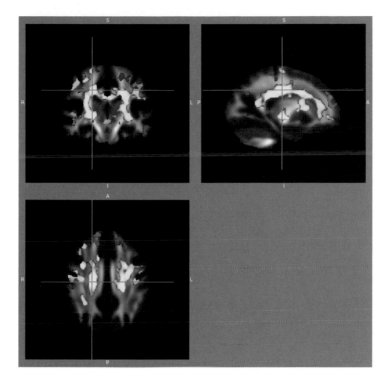

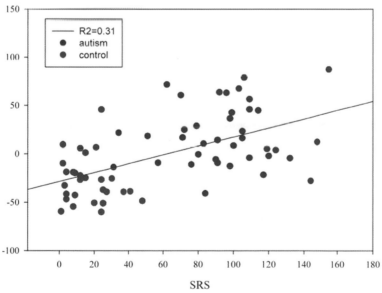

PLATE 4.11. (Top) Voxel-based DTI findings related to differences in social responsiveness based on SRS scores, as shown in the regression plot comparing DTI findings and SRS ratings (bottom). As expected, SRS scores clearly differentiate most subjects with autism from typically developing controls; in terms of DTI findings, these are expressed in white matter regions of the CC, STG, and temporal stem, to highlight some of the major differences. From Petrella, Mattay, and Doraiswamy (2008). Copyright 2008 by the Radiological Society of North America. Reprinted by permission.

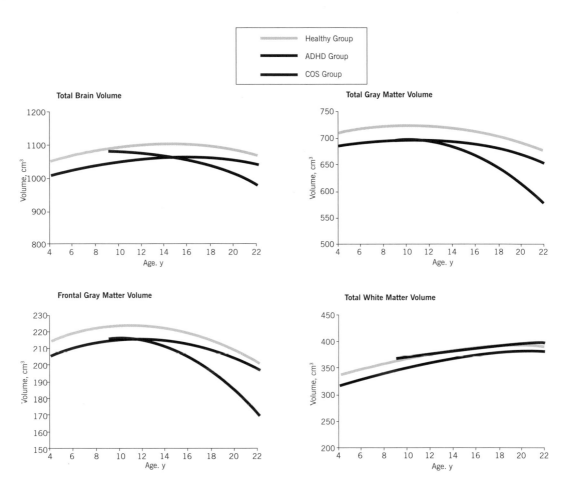

PLATE 4.12. Different brain development trajectories in typically developing children, those with ADHD, and those with childhood-onset schizophrenia (COS). From Gogtay, Giedd, and Rapoport (2002). Copyright 2002 by the American Medical Association. Reprinted by permission.

Williams Syndrome (OMIM #194050)

Williams syndrome (WS) is a neurogenetic disorder characterized by facial, cardiac, and other physical abnormalities as well as neurocognitive impairments, particularly in visual–spatial skills (Reiss et al., 2004). WS has been associated with a reduction in brain volume (Faravelli et al., 2003; Reiss et al., 2004) and with regional abnormalities in the parietal lobe volumes (Boddaert et al., 2006; Campbell et al., 2009) (see Paterson & Schultz, 2007, for a review). In addition to parieto-occipital volume reductions, Campbell and colleagues (2009) demonstrated decreased basal ganglia, left putamen/globus pallidus, thalamus, and right posterior cingulate gyrus volumes. They also noted significantly increased gray matter in the frontal lobes, anterior cingulate gyrus, left temporal lobe, and bilateral anterior cingulate white matter (Plate 4.2). Reiss and colleagues (2004) also demonstrated enlarged volumes in amygdala, superior temporal gyrus, orbital prefrontal cortex, and dorsal anterior cingulate. Cerebellar enlargement may be present very early in children with WS (Jones et al., 2002). WS may be associated with reductions in corpus callosum thickness (Luders et al., 2007) and volume (Tomaiuolo et al., 2002) as well as abnormalities in gyrification and sulcal morphometry (Faravelli et al., 2003; Gaser et al., 2006; Van Essen et al., 2006) (Plate 4.3). fMRI studies of children with WS indicate reduced prefrontal–striatal activation during response inhibition (Mobbs, Eckert, Mills, et al., 2007), reduced temporal lobe and increased right amygdala activation during auditory processing of music and noise (Levitin et al., 2003), and significantly reduced visual and parietal cortex activation during global visual processing (Mobbs, Eckert, Menon, et al., 2007).

IMPRINTING DISORDERS

Angelman Syndrome (OMIM #105830)

Symptoms associated with Angelman syndrome (AS) include functionally severe developmental delay; movement or balance disorder (usually ataxia of gait and/or tremulous movement of limbs); and behavioral uniqueness, including any combination of frequent laughter/smiling, apparent happy demeanor, and easily excitable personality. In addition, there is often delayed, disproportionate growth in head circumference, usually resulting in microcephaly (≤ 2 standard deviations of normal fronto-occipital circumference by age 2 years), which is more pronounced in individuals with 15q11.2–13 deletions. Seizures, usually with an onset before 3 years of age, are common. Characteristic abnormal electroencephalographic patterns are also often evident in the first 2 years of life.

Individuals with AS are generally thought to have normal brain imaging studies, although occasional abnormalities have been reported. The most common conventional MRI or CT change, when any is detected, is mild cortical atrophy and/or mildly delayed myelination of cerebral white matter (Harting et al., 2009; Leonard et al., 1993). Several studies using more advanced imaging applications such as PET have reported developmental dysregulation of gamma-aminobutyric acid type A (GABA(A)) in the cerebellar cortex and cerebellum of patients with various genotypic expressions of AS, but these studies are limited by small sample sizes, given the uncommon nature of the disorder (Asahina et al., 2008; Holopainen et al., 2001).

Recent studies using additional advanced neuroimaging techniques, including DTI, quantitative MRI, and magnetization transfer imaging, have revealed abnormalities in deletion-positive individuals with AS (Peters et al., 2008). Despite apparently normal imaging on conventional sequences, DTI revealed reduced FA and increased apparent diffusion coefficient (ADC) in white matter pathways involving the frontal, temporal, parietal, and limbic areas in patients with AS relative to control children (Peters et al., 2008). Plate 4.4 illustrates DTI tractography of the corpus callosum in a group of children and adolescents with AS in contrast to a typically developing adolescent, highlighting aberrant fiber patterns or paucity of fibers in the individuals with AS. The arucate and uncinate fasciculi reveal additional notable differences (Plate 4.5 and 4.6) that may relate to deficits in language, cognition, and behavior. Quantitative MRI has also highlighted reduced volumes in several regions, including the cerebellum, cerebrum, basal ganglia, and corpus callosum, in individuals with AS in comparison to age- and gender-comparable typically developing children (Plate 4.7), as well as subtle cortical thinning in temporal, frontal, and occipital regions, primarily in the left hemisphere (Plate 4.8) (Peters et al., 2009). It has not yet been determined whether these abnormalities are present in other molecular subtypes of AS.

Prader–Willi Syndome (OMIM #176270)

Patients with Prader–Willi syndrome (PWS) have a deletion in an imprinted region on paternal chromosome 15 (15q11–13), a maternal disomy for this segment, or (rarely) a chromosomal imprinting center deletion that gives rise to suppression of the equivalent paternal genes. It is characterized by a complex clinical picture that involves cognitive impairment; behavioral abnormalities such as hyperphagia, seeking and hoarding food, and eating of nonfood substances; poor impulse control; impaired responses to somatic pain; and physical manifestations including short stature, obesity, and hypogonadism. Studies of patients with PWS have highlighted pituitary abnormalities, including a reduction in pituitary height or a complete absence of the posterior pituitary bright spot in some patients, implicating central hypothalamic–pituitary dysfunction that may be related to the clinical phenotype (Iughetti et al., 2008; Miller et al., 2008). In addition, conventional MRI studies have revealed intracranial abnormalities in individuals with PWS, including ventriculomegaly, decreased volume of brain tissue in the parieto-occipital lobe, Sylvian fissure polymicrogyria, incomplete insular closure (Miller et al., 2007), and white matter lesions (Miller et al., 2006). Quantitative MRI studies have additionally demonstrated smaller cerebellar volumes in patients with PWS than in sibling controls (Miller et al., 2009).

Advanced imaging studies utilizing DTI in small samples of patients with PWS have demonstrated higher diffusivity in the left frontal white matter and the left dorsomedial thalamus, whereas reduced FA was demonstrated in the posterior limb of the internal capsule bilaterally, the right frontal white matter, and the splenium of the corpus callosum (Yamada, Matsuzawa, Uchiyama, Kwee, & Nakada, 2006).

PET studies have revealed altered GABA(A) receptor number or composition, predominantly in the cingulate, frontal, and temporal neocortices and insula, in a small sample of patients with PWS as compared to a control sample (Lucignani et al., 2004). PET studies using [18F]fluorodeoxyglucose in children with PWS have revealed decreased glucose metabolism in the right superior temporal gyrus and left cerebellar vermis—regions that are associated with taste perception/food reward and cognitive and emotional function, respectively. Increased metabolism was observed in the right orbitofrontal, bilateral middle frontal, right inferior frontal, left superior frontal, and bilateral anterior cingulate gyri, right temporal pole, and left uncus—regions that are involved in cognitive functions related to eating or obsessive–compulsive behavior (Kim et al., 2006). Finally, fMRI studies have demonstrated increased activation in the hypothalamus and orbitofrontal cortex—components of neural circuits known to be involved in hunger and motivation—in response to high- versus low-calorie foods and in comparison to controls (Dimitropoulos & Schultz, 2008). In another study, individuals with PWS had an increased blood-oxygen-level-dependent response in the ventromedial prefrontal cortex compared with normal-weight controls when viewing pictures of food; this finding supports the possibility that an increased reward value for food may underlie the excessive hunger in PWS, and also supports the significance of the frontal cortex in modulating the response to food (Miller et al., 2007).

INHERITED METABOLIC DISORDERS

Phenylketonuria (OMIM #261600)

Phenylketonuria (PKU) is an autosomal recessive disorder caused by a multiplicity of mutations mapped to chromosome 12q22–24.1. Most cases of PKU are caused by a deficiency of phenylalanine hydroxylase (classic type), but a deficiency of dihydropteridine reductase may also be implicated more rarely (malignant type). These deficiencies result in the production of compounds that are toxic to the developing brain. PKU may present in the first year of life with insufficient growth, retarded development, irritability, vomiting, eczema, musty urine, and body odor.

Upon conventional imaging, diffuse signal irregularites including white matter abnormalities (particularly on T2-weighted and fluid-attenuated inversion recovery [FLAIR] imaging) suggestive of delayed or defective myelination are often reported in patients with PKU, particularly in the parietal periatrial or periventricular white matter (Leuzzi et al., 2007), though lesions extending to frontal or subcortical white matter may be apparent in more severely affected patients. Subcortical cyst-like lesions may also be apparent. Calcification in the basal ganglia, including the globi pallidi, and frontal subcortical regions may appear on CT or T1-weighted MRI. Adherence to a strict diet may lead to resolution of these abnormalities to varying degrees in some patients after a few months on MRI (Cleary et al., 1995).

MRS findings may hold particular clinical value in the diagnosis and therapeutic monitoring of PKU, as MRS is able to detect elevated brain concentrations of phenylalanine in the affected white matter (Leuzzi et al., 2000). Given the involvement of myelin, diffusion-weighted imaging and DTI may contribute additional information to assessing and monitoring the white matter changes in patients with PKU (Ding et al., 2008; Kono et al., 2005; Peng, Tseng, Chien, Hwu, & Liu, 2004; Vermathen et al., 2007), particularly in patients whose white matter appears normal on conventional imaging or whose abnormalities are not as obvious.

Adrenoleukodystrophy (OMIM #300100)

Adrenoleukodystrophy (ALD) is a disorder characterized by adrenal insufficiency and rapid demyelination of cerebral white matter and is caused by mutation in the ALD gene on chromosome Xq28. Parieto-occipital white matter is the most commonly affected area of brain tissue, but damage may be present or progress into other white matter regions as well (Figure 4.3).

Because the course of this disease is particularly aggressive (death may ensue in 3–5

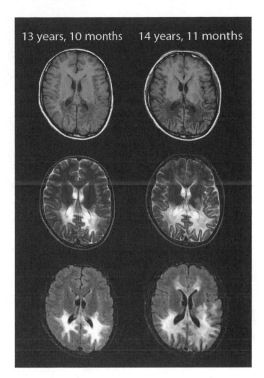

FIGURE 4.3. Conventional imaging (top, T1-weighted; middle, T2-weighted; bottom, FLAIR) demonstrating the classic pattern of parieto-occipital abnormalities in an adolescent with ALD. The progression of the disease is evident within a 1-year span of time, such that the T2-weighted and FLAIR images demonstrate involvement of the frontal lobes, in addition to more extensive involvement in the parieto-occipital areas by the second time point.

years after onset of symptoms), and because treatments such as hematopoietic stem cell transplantation (HSCT) may lead to stabilization or reversal of clinical and MRI abnormalities (see Figure 4.4) if performed at an early stage of the disease (Aubourg et al., 1990; Baumann et al., 2003; Shapiro et al., 2000), advanced imaging modalities such as MRS and DTI have recently been investigated to provide information for decision making with respect to HSCT and other potential treatments. For example, MRS has been shown to be more sensitive than MRI in detecting metabolic abnormalities, axonal damage or loss, and incipient demyelination, even in normal-appearing white matter (Kruse et al., 1994; Pouwels et al., 1998; Salvan et al., 1999), and has been used to predict lesion progression (Eichler et al.,

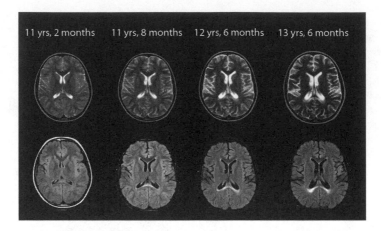

FIGURE 4.4. Conventional serial imaging (top, T2-weighted; bottom, FLAIR) from a child with ALD who is a sibling of the adolescent represented in Figure 4.3. This child was diagnosed much earlier in the course of his disease than his sibling and received HSCT just after the initial imaging. Although subtle progression of the disease is evident over time in both the T2-weighted and FLAIR images in the splenium of the corpus callosum, the relative lack of progression of the disease is evident in this child, as compared to the more typical course represented in Figure 4.3.

2002). In addition, DTI may assist in defining the extent of white matter involvement, predicting disease activity and progression, and characterizing affected white matter areas. Initial observations suggest that reduced ADC values at the leading edge of a white matter lesion may predict rapid progression of the disease (Melham & Golay, 2005).

Neuronal Ceroid Lipofuscinosis (OMIM #256730 and Others)

Neuronal ceroid lipofuscinosis (NCL) is inherited as an autosomal recessive trait, and is a progressive and fatal lysosomal storage disease characterized by the accumulation of ceroid lipofuscin in neuronal and extraneuronal cells. Clinical features include mental and motor deterioration, loss of vision, seizures, ataxia, and myoclonus. There are several variants, but the infantile type (NCL1) may be particularly aggressive in the early years.

Conventional MRI in several variants of NCL commonly demonstrates diffuse cerebral and cerebellar atrophy, T2-hyperintensity of the lobar white matter, and thinning of the cerebral cortex (Autti, Raininko, Vanhanen, & Santavuori, 1996; D'Incerti, 2000; Sayit et al., 2002; Seitz et al., 1998) (Figure 4.5). Hypointensity in the thalamus has also

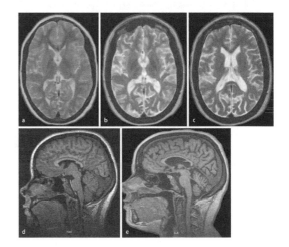

FIGURE 4.5. MR images of a patient with juvenile NCL (NCL3) show visually detectable progressive cerebral and cerebellar atrophy. T2-weighted axial image (a) and T1-weighted sagittal image (d) at the age of 12 years show normal CSF spaces. T2-weighted axial images (b, c) and T1-weighted sagittal image (e) at the age of 17 years demonstrate enlarged lateral and third ventricles as well as enlarged cerebral sulci (b, c). Note that the corpus callosum is very thin and the vermis is reduced (e). Note also that the signal intensity of the thalamus is inhomogeneous (b). From Autti, Hämäläinen, Mannerkoski, Van Leemput, and Aberg (2008). Copyright 2008 by Springer. Reprinted by permission.

been reported (Autti et al., 1996, 1997; Seitz et al., 1998; Vanhanen, Raininko, Autti, & Santavuori, 1995), though not consistently (Petersen, Handwerker, & Huppertz, 1996).

Advanced imaging in combination with conventional MR may again play a role in monitoring and therapeutic intervention, as MRS has detected abnormal findings before clinical manifestations of the disease and also has shown progressive deterioration of neurometabolism after onset (Vanhanen et al., 2004). In addition, it may help to differentiate NCL from other neurometabolic disorders (Seitz et al., 1998).

Sickle Cell Disease (OMIM #603903)

Sickle cell disease (SCD) is a recessive genetic disorder, which is caused by a point mutation resulting in the substitution of valine for glutamic acid at the sixth position in the beta chain of hemoglobin. Cerebral ischemic injury is perhaps the most devastating cerebral complication of SCD, though significant complications can occur in many organs. Neuroimaging abnormalities in SCD are related to the greater likelihood of vascular lesions and strokes in these patients, most prominently involving the periventricular regions of the brain (see Figure 4.6). The majority of children with SCD who develop stroke have arteriopathy affecting the terminal internal carotid artery or proximal middle cerebral artery. The mechanism of stenosis is purportedly as follows. The anemia resulting from the disease produces increased vascular flow on the luminal wall; this may in turn create a hyperplasia due to noninflammatory response. This thickening produces a stenosis, which increases the velocity of flow through the stenosis until thrombosis or embolus leads to occlusion. These infarctions are classically located deep within the white matter of the centrum ovale and are seen as a series of bright areas on T2-weighted and FLAIR imaging (Zimmerman, 2005). Other factors contributing to the pathogenesis of SCD-related imaging abnormalities include severe anemia, hypoxia, and acute medical events (Debaun, Derdeyn, & McKinstry, 2006). Medium- or small-vessel disease may result from these mechanisms, and the resulting vascular lesions may be clinically significant or "silent." When severe occlusive disease occurs, collateral blood vessels may arise from the posterior circulation's posterior cerebral artery branches, creating a moyamoya-like condition on arteriography.

In addition to MRI, diffusion-weighted imaging has become widely used clinically, due to its sensitivity in demonstrating acute infarction (Zimmerman, 2005). Transcranial Doppler has also been used to examine changes in blood flow, which has therefore rendered this technique an important initial step in screening patients at risk for SCD-related cerebrovascular disease (Abboud et al., 2004; Kwiatkowski et al., 2009). MR angiography has also been employed routinely at some institutions in the evaluation of cerebral vessel stensosis in patients with SCD (Kwiatkowski et al., 2009; Silva et al.,

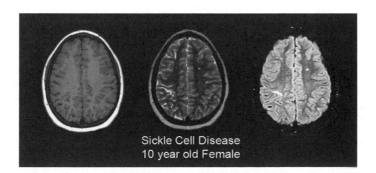

Sickle Cell Disease
10 year old Female

FIGURE 4.6. Conventional imaging (T1-weighted, T2-weighted, FLAIR) representing two classic patterns of cerebrovascular disease in a 10-year-old child with SCD. A medium-vessel infarct is evident in the right parietal area, resulting in atrophy and increased CSF. Classic small-vessel disease is also evident in the right and left frontal areas.

2009; Zimmerman, 2005). Additional advanced imaging techniques such as arterial spin labeling have been used with varying levels of success in monitoring cerebrovascular disease and evaluating novel treatment strategies in SCD (Helton et al., 2009).

Tay–Sachs Disease (OMIM #272800)

Tay–Sachs disease is a variant of juvenile GM2 gangliosidosis, a group of autosomal recessive inherited neurodegenerative diseases caused by deficiency of lysosomal beta-hexosaminidase, resulting in GM2 ganglioside accumulation in the brain. Tay–Sachs classically presents with progressive neurological deterioration that initially affects motor and spinocerebellar functioning; it commonly includes gait disturbance, speech problems, and incoordination, and may also include muscle wasting, weakness, seizures, behavioral and psychiatric disturbances, and dysphagia (Maegawa et al., 2006).

The most consistent imaging finding for individuals with Tay–Sachs disease on conventional imaging is moderate to severe cerebellar atrophy (Maegawa et al., 2006; Neudorfer et al., 2005). Mild generalized atrophy and subcortical white matter changes have also been reported, which may precede cerebellar atrophy (Maegawa et al., 2006; Neudorfer et al., 2005). Though MRS studies have only been performed in small samples of individuals with Tay–Sachs disease, there are reports that changes in metabolites on MRS were closely linked to clinical features and may prove useful for the evaluation of neuronal changes in children with this disease (Aydin, Bakir, Tatli, Terzibasioglu, & Ozmen, 2005; Imamura, Miyajima, Ito, & Orii, 2008; Maegawa et al., 2006).

X-Linked Syndromes

Fragile X Syndrome (OMIM #300624)

Fragile X syndrome (FXS) is caused by an expansion of repeated trinucleotides within the FMR1 gene on the X chromosome, resulting in disrupted production of the fragile X mental retardation protein (FMRP). The syndrome is associated with cognitive, emotional, social, and behavioral dysfunction and affects both sexes, though males have significantly worse outcome (Reiss & Dant, 2003). Neuroimaging findings have demonstrated reduced volumes in the prefrontal, anterior cingulate, superior temporal, insular, posterior cerebellum, amygdala, and hippocampal regions, as well as increased volumes in caudate, hypothalamic, and fusiform areas, when compared with findings for controls (Gothelf, Furfaro, 2008; Hoeft et al., 2008; A. D. Lee et al., 2007) (Plate 4.9). A DTI study in females with FXS reported lower FA values in frontostriatal and parietal sensory–motor white matter pathways (Barnea-Goraly et al., 2003). Haas and colleagues (2009) demonstrated similar white matter anomalies in males with FXS by showing greater relative white matter fiber density in the left ventral frontostriatal pathway than that of controls. In addition, lower dorsolateral prefrontal cortex choline/creatine levels have been demonstrated in males with FXS than in controls (Kesler, Lightbody, & Reiss, 2009). fMRI studies highlight aberrant neurofunction in left orbitofrontal cortex (Tamm, Menon, Johnston, Hessl, & Reiss, 2002), ventrolateral prefrontal cortex (Hoeft, Hernandez, et al., 2007), cingulate, basal ganglia, and hippocampus (Menon, Leroux, White, & Reiss, 2004) during various response inhibition tasks; in right middle frontal gyrus and left cerebellum during a math task (Rivera, Menon, White, Glaser, & Reiss, 2002); in hippocampus and basal forebrain during a memory task (Greicius, Boyett-Anderson, Menon, & Reiss, 2004); in fusiform gyrus and left superior temporal gyrus during a face and gaze discrimination task (Garrett, Menon, MacKenzie, & Reiss, 2004); in the anterior cingulate cortex and caudate nucleus during an emotion recognition task (Hagan, Hoeft, Mackey, Mobbs, & Reiss, 2008); and in the left insula, left amygdala, and bilateral prefrontal cortices during an eye gaze discrimination task (Watson, Hoeft, Garrett, Hall, & Reiss, 2008).

Klinefelter Syndrome

Klinefelter syndrome (KS) is a disorder characterized by sex chromosome aneuploidy (47,XXY) that affects males. It is associated with language-based learning disorders and with executive, social, and motor planning difficulties, but spatial abilities are preserved (Giedd et al., 2007). Individuals with KS were found to have smaller total cerebral volumes than those of age-matched male controls, as well as smaller lobar volumes in all lobes except parietal white matter. In contrast, the lateral ventricles in individuals with KS were shown to be significantly larger than those of age-matched male controls (Giedd et al., 2007). More localized gray matter volume reductions have been observed in the insula, amygdala, hippocampus, cingulate, temporal, and occipital gyri in KS (Giedd et al., 2006; Rose et al., 2004; Shen et al., 2004). KS is associated with thinner cortex in the left inferior frontal, left motor, left inferior parietal, and bilateral temporal regions (Giedd et al., 2007). MR case reports of individuals with a more severe variant of the syndrome (49,XXXXY) demonstrate some of the findings listed above, in addition to the presence of white matter disease (Hoffman, Vossough, Ficicioglu, & Visootsak, 2008).

Rett Syndrome (OMIM 312750)

Children with Rett syndrome typically demonstrate normal early development, followed by severe neurodevelopmental decline, apraxia, and autistic-like behaviors (Chahrour & Zoghbi, 2007). Rett syndrome primarily occurs in females, although certain mutations of the associated X-linked MECP2 gene are believed to cause syndromic features in boys (Kankirawatana et al., 2006; Leonard et al., 2001). The first morphometric MR studies showed significantly reduced cerebral volumes with a greater decrease of gray matter in comparison to white matter, particularly in the frontal regions, and disproportionally reduced caudate and midbrain volumes (Chang, Huang, & Huang, 1998; Reiss et al., 1993; Subramaniam, Naidu, & Reiss, 1997). Dunn and colleagues (2002) also demonstrated reduced basal ganglia volumes including caudate and thalamus. A more recent study utilizing multimodal volumetric MR techniques showed reduced total brain volumes affecting both gray and white matter, as well as decreased gray matter volumes in the bilateral parietal lobe, right cingulate, right middle occipital, left middle frontal, and bilateral pre- and postcentral gyri (Cart-

er et al., 2008). Many of the recent neuroimaging studies have focused on neurochemical changes using MRS and have consistently demonstrated decreased NAA and increased choline on average throughout the brain (Gokcay, Kitis, Ekmekci, Karasoy, & Sener, 2002; Horska et al., 2000, 2009; Naidu et al., 2001). Others have noted specific regional vulnerabilities, including decreased NAA in the frontal lobe (Horska et al., 2000; Khong, Lam, Ooi, Ko, & Wong, 2002; Naidu et al., 2001); decreased NAA in the insula, hippocampus (Horska et al., 2000; Naidu et al., 2001), and cingulate gyrus white matter (Pan, Lane, Hetherington, & Percy, 1999); and increased glutamate in cingulate gray matter (Pan et al., 1999) and left frontal white matter (Horska et al., 2009).

Turner Syndrome

Turner syndrome (TS) results from complete or partial X monosomy in females and is associated with short stature, gonadal dysgenesis, and other physical features, as well as executive and visual–spatial function deficits (Kesler, 2007). Volumetric MR studies have consistently indicated parietal lobe abnormalities in children and adolescents with TS (Brown et al., 2002, 2004). In addition, TS has been associated with abnormalities of occipital lobe and cerebellar morphology (Brown et al., 2002; Fryer, Kwon, Eliez, & Reiss, 2003). Amygdala, superior temporal gyrus, and orbitofrontal volumes may be enlarged compared to those of controls (Good et al., 2003; Kesler et al., 2003; Kesler, Garrett, et al., 2004; Rae et al., 2004), while hippocampal and corpus callosum volumes are reduced (Fryer et al., 2003; Kesler, Garrett, et al., 2004). Several fMRI studies have demonstrated frontoparietal deficits associated with spatial orientation (Kesler et al., 2004b), working memory (Haberecht et al., 2001; Hart, Davenport, Hooper, & Belger, 2006), arithmetic (Kesler, Menon, & Reiss, 2006), and response inhibition (Tamm, Menon, & Reiss, 2003). A recent DTI study illustrated significantly reduced structural connectivity (e.g., FA) among frontal, striatal, and parietal regions, whereas parietotemporal connectivity was enhanced (Holzapfel, Barnea-Goraly, Eckert, Kesler, & Reiss, 2006) (Plate 4.10).

INHERITED ATAXIAS

Friedreich Ataxia (OMIM #229300)

Friedreich ataxia is the most common of the inherited ataxias and the most consistently diagnosed during childhood. Symptoms include gait ataxia and speech impairments. Studies utilizing qualitative MRI methods have indicated atrophy of the cerebellum (Mantovan et al., 2006; Mateo et al., 2004), subcortical regions, and frontal lobe (Mantovan et al., 2006). A quantitative regional MRI study demonstrated reduced volume, altered shape, and iron accumulation in the dentate nuclei of the cerebellum (Boddaert et al., 2007). An fMRI study indicated an abnormal pattern of cortical activation associated with finger movements (Mantovan et al., 2006).

NEUROCUTANEOUS SYNDROMES

Sturge–Weber Syndrome (OMIM #185300)

Sturge–Weber syndrome, also referred to as encephalotrigeminal angiomatosis, is characterized by skin abnormalities (e.g., port wine marks), meningeal angiomas, seizures, developmental delays, and calcification of cerebral tissue (Pascual-Castroviejo, Pascual-Pascual, Velazquez-Fragua, & Viano, 2008). Diffuse cerebral atrophy is a common MRI finding (Adams, Aylett, Squier, & Chong,

2009; Ergun, Okten, Gezercan, & Gezici, 2007; Hu et al., 2008). Gray and white matter volumes may be reduced in the brain regions surrounding angiomas, with frontal and temporal white matter volumes being particularly vulnerable (Pfund et al., 2003). MRS studies suggest abnormal NAA and choline levels in frontal tissue, despite normal DTI and qualitative MRI findings (Batista et al., 2008; Sijens et al., 2006). A study including DTI revealed abnormal FA in left parietal white matter (Juhasz et al., 2007), and MR SWI studies have demonstrated abnormalities in gyrification patterns and gray–white matter junction (Hu et al., 2008; Juhasz et al., 2007).

Tuberous Sclerosis Complex (OMIM #191100)

Tuberous sclerosis complex (TSC) is a multisystem genetic disorder characterized by skin abnormalities (e.g., hypomelanotic macules), seizures, and intellectual disability. MRI findings frequently include cortical tubers, transmantle dysplasia, subependymal nodules, giant cell astrocytomas, white matter anomalies, hemimegalencephaly, cortical dysplasia, and schizencephaly (Arca, Pacheco, Alfonso, Duchowny, & Melnick, 2006; Christophe et al., 2000; O'Callaghan et al., 2008) (Figure 4.7). Eluvathingal and colleagues (2006) also noted a high incidence of cerebellar lesions in children with TSC.

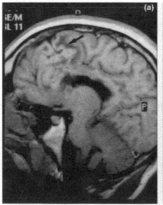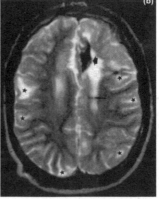

FIGURE 4.7. MRI scans of a 17-year-old male with TSC, showing numerous cortical tubers (stars), infolded cortical dysplasia (as deep distortion of the normal cortical architecture) (thin arrows), and dystrophic calcification as signal void in b (thick arrow). From Christophe et al. (2000). Copyright 2000 by Elsevier. Reprinted by permission.

Neurofibromatosis (OMIM #162200, Type 1; OMIM #101000, Type 2)

Neurofibromatosis (NF) is an autosomal dominant disorder in which tumors grow in nerve tissues of the brain as well as cells under the skin. MRI studies reveal multiple hyperintensities, or unidentified bright objects (UBOs), corresponding to lesions in the basal ganglia, thalamus, brainstem, hippocampus, cerebellum (Lopes Ferraz Filho, et al., 2008), and corpus callosum (Mimouni-Bloch, Kornreich, Kaadan, Steinberg, & Shuper, 2008), as well as optic gliomas (Hsieh, Wu, Wang, Chin, & Chen, 2007). Using DTI, Alkan and colleagues (2005) demonstrated significantly increased ADC values within UBOs in the frontal lobe, parieto-occipital region, cerebellar white matter, globus pallidus, hippocampus, thalamus, and midbrain in children with NF1; ADC values were also significantly increased even in normal-appearing hippocampal and thalamic tissues. ADC is another index of microstructural integrity in brain tissues. fMRI studies of children with NF1 have indicated significantly altered patterns of prefrontal, temporal, parietal, and occipital activation associated with phonological and visual–spatial processing (Billingsley et al., 2003, 2004). An MRS study demonstrated significantly increased choline and myo-inositol levels in normal-appearing frontal and parietal white matter, as well as significantly decreased NAA in normal-appearing frontal white matter (Alkan et al., 2003).

MULTIFACTORIAL SYNDROMES

In the nosology of childhood neuropsychiatric disorders, problems of diagnostic classification and specificity exist for complex disorders with potential multiple etiologies and overlap in symptoms and behaviors, especially in terms of their genetics and the role that neuroimaging may play in defining each disorder. In contrast to disorders discussed elsewhere in this chapter (e.g., X-linked syndromes, where distinct genetic bases for the behavioral and neuropsychological phenotype of each disorder are well known), complex neuropsychiatric disorders are much more ambiguous with respect to

genetics and etiology; hence we use the term *multifactorial syndromes* in this section. For example, the *Diagnostic and Statistical Manual of Mental Disorders*, fourth edition (DSM-IV; American Psychiatric Association, 1994) lists pervasive developmental disorders (PDDs) as a general category encompassing a broad spectrum of disorders first diagnosed in infancy, childhood, or adolescence, including autistic disorder, Rett's disorder (although more is known about the genetics of this disorder than when DSM-IV came out in 1994; see Matijevic, Knezevic, Slavica, & Pavelic, 2009), childhood disintegrative disorder, Asperger's disorder, and the catch-all diagnosis of PDD not otherwise specified (PDD-NOS). For each of these disorders, although the phenotypic behaviors may be specific enough to identify and label with behavioral characteristics (as has been done in the DSM-IV classifications), specific etiologies are not well understood and are assumed to be multiple.

Pervasive Developmental Disorders

The multifactorial nature of the PDDs is exemplified by autism and can be readily appreciated by viewing Figure 4.8, taken from Geschwind and Levitt (2007). There is no single path that consistently leads to autism, and without a specified etiology, understanding this disorder (or any PDD) from a neurobiological perspective is challenging. However, recent genetic studies are beginning to demonstrate genes that may be participating in this complex disorder (see Bayou, M'Rad, Ahlem, Bechir Helayem, & Chaabouni, 2008; Bishop, 2009; Levitt & Campbell, 2009). Because nearly two-thirds of the genes in the human genome are related to brain function in some fashion (Petrella, Mattay, & Doraiswamy, 2008), it becomes obvious why the neurodevelopmental processes that lead to any of the multifactorial disorders are exceedingly complex; nonetheless, the search for candidate genes for autism has revealed some most interesting findings. For example, Glessner and colleagues (2009) recently observed that genes that potentially regulate synaptic function and neuronal connectivity among diverse brain regions may play a role in autism. This observation has direct implications for how

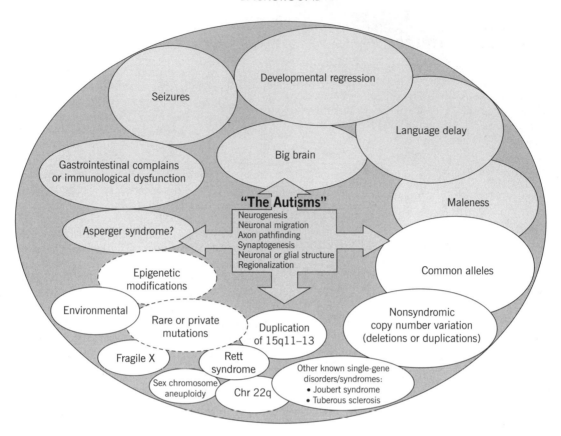

FIGURE 4.8. This diagram shows the multifactorial nature of what may be the basis for the autism spectrum disorders. Such complexity makes it impossible to focus on a single factor in the study of autism, and underscores the need to consider such complexities in neuroimaging and neuropsychological outcome studies of this disorder. From Geschwind and Levitt (2007). Copyright 2007 by Elsevier. Adapted by permission.

neuroimaging should be used to examine potential anomalies in attempting to improve our understanding of autism.

Indeed, from a neuroimaging standpoint, the role that connectivity plays appears to be critical in understanding all of the multifactorial syndromes, not just autism. However, there are two core features of autism—impairment in communication and social behavior—that can be the target of neuroimaging investigations of connectivity. Figure 4.9 shows three coronal views of the brain, all at approximately the same level, in three different subjects, all males and about 14 years of age: one with autism, one with traumatic brain injury (TBI), and one age-matched, healthy, typically developing control. The reader is asked to view these brains and decide which one is the brain of the child with autism. It is relatively easy to pick

out the scan image in the middle as that of the child who suffered a severe TBI because there are clearly noticeable differences: The ventricles are dilated, prominent cortical sulci are visible, and the hippocampi are withered. However, which of the other two scan images is that of the child with autism? It is impossible to tell simply by viewing the images. The typical image of the brain of the child with autism appears normal (Bigler et al., 2003). So if gross appearance reveals no universally distinguishing feature that identifies a child with autism, the abnormalities of autism must be found within the neural organization of the brain—its microanatomy and neural integrity.

Currently the best method to noninvasively assess the microanatomy of the living brain is DTI (Lainhart, Lazar, Bigler, & Alexander, 2006), which has been used in

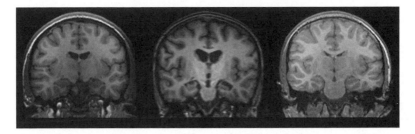

FIGURE 4.9. Three coronal MRI sections are depicted, all from males approximately 14 years of age. The middle one is obviously abnormal, with dilated ventricles and with cortical and hippocampal atrophy. The one on the viewer's right is from a child with autism, and the control child is on the viewer's left. These comparisons are shown merely to demonstrate that the typical MRI findings in children with autism reflect no gross abnormality and cannot be distinguished from those of typically developing controls simply through visual inspection. This indicates that more refined neuroimaging analyses, such as DTI, are necessary to uncover the complex neural aberrations that may underlie autism.

several investigations of autism (see reviews by Muller, 2007; White, Nelson, & Lim, 2008). This research has focused on connectivity within the brains of individuals with autism versus typically developing controls. Among many candidate areas to investigate, there are two logical places to begin examining brain connectivity in individuals with autism—the corpus callosum (CC) and the superior temporal gyrus (STG). The CC is used since it is the largest brain commissure and houses the major white matter pathways that integrate the two cerebral hemispheres (Sullivan & Pfefferbaum, 2006); the STG is used because it not only is involved in communication (i.e., auditory processing and receptive language), but participates in social cognition and human behavioral interaction (Paul et al., 2007; Pelphrey & Carter, 2008). Several studies that have used DTI to examine these brain regions have found significant differences in these regions between subjects with autism and typically developing controls. Firsts, these studies have suggested a significant difference in the organization of white matter within the STG (Bigler et al., 2007; J. E. Lee et al., 2007). This has implications for disorganization of language function: The normal language circuitry is not properly in place in individuals with autism, and this also likely disrupts the normal integration of information necessary for social-emotional processing. Furthermore, DTI studies specific to the CC show that it may be slightly smaller in autism, with potentially disorganized white matter connectivity (Alexander et al., 2007; Lee et al.,

2009). This probably disrupts the integration between the two hemispheres, which is also necessary for normal social-emotional functioning and the integration of verbal and nonverbal information.

Using DTI, an example of these abnormal areas of white matter development in autism is given in Plate 4.11 (Petrella et al., 2008), which shows the relationship of scores on the Social Responsiveness Scale (SRS; Constantino, 2005)—an index of social interactive behavior, reciprocity, and reactivity—to differences in the CC and white matter of the temporal lobe, including the STG and temporal stem. Notice in this illustration that SRS scores differentiate individuals with autism from typically developing individuals, and that increased problems with social responsiveness relate to DTI-detected white matter differences. Also note in this illustration how widespread the white matter differences are.

Interestingly, disorders in the PDD category are associated with another multifactorial set of disorders classified by DSM-IV as attention-deficit and disruptive behavior disorders. ADHD is the most common of these and is often a component of PDDs (Sinzig, Walter, & Doepfner, 2009) and many other neuropsychiatric disorders (Galanter & Leibenluft, 2008; Nijmeijer et al., 2008). Gogtay, Giedd, and Rapaport (2002) have shown a number of neuroanatomical differences in brain size and structure in children with ADHD, particularly in frontal lobe development (see also Castellanos et al., 2002; Kelly, Margulies, & Castellanos, 2007). A summary of these findings is provided in

Plate 4.12, which shows different developmental trajectories among typically developing children, children with ADHD, and children with childhood-onset schizophrenia. These and similar studies suggest that there are likely to be critical stages in these disorders where brain development, connectivity, and/or cellular pruning are disrupted, and that these disruptions probably relate to the behavioral phenotypic expression of the disorders.

Tourette Syndrome

Another multifactorial disorder is Tourette syndrome, characterized by the occurrence of irresistible, stereotyped, unwanted, and unplanned movements and/or vocalizations (tics). Symptoms frequently begin as early as 6–7 years of age, often peaking in intensity in adolescence (Swain, Scahill, Lombroso, King, & Leckman, 2007). From a neuropsychiatric perspective, obsessive–compulsive disorder (OCD) and ADHD have a very high comorbidity with Tourette syndrome (Plessen, Royal, & Peterson, 2007; Singer, 2005) and probably share aberrant neural sytems associated with impulse control, motor control, and executive functioning. Because the presence of tics is central to Tourette syndrome, but it also shares features with ADHD and OCD, various theories about dysfunctional frontostriatal pathways have been proposed; contemporary neuroimaging studies support such dysfunction for all of these disorders (MacMaster, O'Neill, & Rosenberg, 2008). For example, Church and colleagues (2009) have shown by using fMRI methods that regulatory or control networks are different in persons with Tourette syndrome compared to typically developing controls. Neuroimaging has also shown the expected involvement of dopaminergic nuclei (including the substantia nigra and ventral tegmental areas) in Tourette syndrome, in association with the abnormal tic behavior (Gilbert et al., 2006; Wong et al., 2008).

It has long been assumed that inherited vulnerabilities predispose individuals to develop neuropsychiatric disorders, and that when such inherited vulnerabilities interact with particular adverse environmental circumstances or stressors, the neuropsychiatric disorders emerge (State, Lombroso, Pauls, & Leckman, 2000). Likewise, it has long been assumed that environmental stressors during childhood adversely affect brain development and predispose individuals to develop neuropsychiatric disorders (van Winkel, Stefanis, & Myin-Germeys, 2008). A host of unknown genetic and environmental factors are probably involved in all disorders that can be categorized as multifactorial syndromes. One of the early models for gene–environment interaction dealt with alcoholism and other substance abuse (see Alterman & Tarter, 1983). This type of outcome was relatively easy to understand within these rather blatant models of developmental psychopathology because children being raised by parents with addiction problems experience multiple sets of adverse circumstances: heritability of the disorder, potential gestational effects of substance abuse during conception and pregnancy, and the adverse effects on parenting resulting directly or indirectly from the parents' alcoholism/drug addiction. However, neuroimaging has opened entirely new avenues of investigation that are becoming incredibly informative about how dynamic the relationship among heritability, brain development, and parental psychopathology may be, and how this extends beyond the older models of substance-abusing parents and dysfunctional environment. For example, a recent study by Choi, Jeong, Rohan, Polcari, and Teicher (2009) used DTI to examine white matter integrity in young adults exposed to parental verbal abuse. In the group exposed to such abuse, there were changes in white matter connectivity in several limbic regions of the brain, compared to matched typically developed young adults. Such findings suggest that adverse environmental effects may disrupt normal neural development in brain areas associated with emotional health and well-being. It is likely that such disruption of normal brain development in childhood results in greater susceptibility to the development of later psychiatric disorder, particularly if there is already increased genetic susceptibility.

Personality Disorders

Another multifactorial disorder with complex genetic and environmental influences occurs within the spectrum of difficulties defined in DSM-IV as personality disorders (Goodman, New, & Siever, 2004; Mc-Closkey et al., 2009). These disorders were originally assumed to be the quintessential, prototypical disorders illustrating psychodynamic influences in the emergence of psychopathology (Goldstein, 1989). However, neuroimaging has clearly demonstrated that borderline personality disorder (BPD) can also be characterized by underlying neuroanatomical differences (see White et al., 2008) and complex gene–environment interactions (Kendler et al., 2008). Several investigations have now shown disrupted brain connectivity (particularly between frontal and limbic areas) in BPD, using a variety of neuroimaging techniques (Grant et al., 2007; Koenigsberg et al., 2009; Rusch et al., 2007; Volpe et al., 2008). Needless to say, there appear to be structural and functional abnormalities in the brain in individuals with all forms of DSM-IV-identified personality disorders (Harenski, Kim, & Hamann, 2009).

It is likely that the combination of neuroimaging studies, genetic research, and a better understanding of how environmental influences alter brain development will become most informative about particular vulnerabilities, as well as what brings about wellness in developing children. Such improvements will undoubtedly improve our understanding of all the multifactorial syndromes.

THE CENTRAL THEME: GENE–BRAIN–BEHAVIOR RELATIONSHIPS

The central theme of the discussion above is that genetic aberrations are often associated with altered neurodevelopment, affecting brain structure, function, and/or biochemistry. Furthermore, brain abnormalities tend to result in cognitive-behavioral deficits, as many of the studies cited above have demonstrated. For example, decreased left frontal white matter NAA was higher in children with Rett syndrome who had seizures than in those without, as well as in patients with higher clinical severity scores (Carter et al., 2008). Lower inferior parietal lobe FA may correspond to impaired arithmetic ability in VCFS (Barnea-Goraly, Eliez, Menon, Bammer, & Reiss, 2005). Increased cortical atrophy was associated with increased clinical severity ratings in children with Sturge–Weber syndrome (Kelley, Hatfield, Lin, & Comi,

2005). These are just a few examples. The use of such neuroimaging predictors in multivariate models can significantly improve the accuracy of prognosis. Studies attempting to predict outcomes in various populations show that neuroimaging measures are able to explain 30–82% of the variance, which in some cases exceeds the percentages explained by currently available alternative methods (Hoeft, Veno, et al., 2007; Richardson et al., 2004).

Gene–brain–behavior relationships can also guide the development of treatments for cognitive-behavioral symptoms in genetic disorders. For example, researchers noted abnormalities in the basal ganglia and hippocampi of individuals with FXS (Greicius et al., 2004; Reiss & Dant, 2003). These regions contain cholinergic pathways that are associated with executive function and memory—areas of significant dysfunction in FXS (Reiss & Dant, 2003; Sarter, Bruno, & Givens, 2003; Sarter & Parikh, 2005). In addition, choline appears to be significantly reduced in the executive prefrontal cortex of individuals with FXS (Kesler et al., 2009). Based on the combination of neuroimaging data and research regarding the influence of the FMR1 gene on cholinergic neurons, clinical investigators initiated a drug trial of donepezil to augment acetylcholine function in individuals with FXS. The results of this trial included significantly improved executive function and decreased problem behaviors (Kesler et al., 2009). Though this study involved a very small sample and an open-label design, it illustrates the potential of neuroimaging research for contributing to syndrome-specific interventions.

CONCLUSIONS

Many genetic disorders are associated with abnormal neurodevelopment. These alterations in neurobiological status are often related to cognitive-behavioral deficits. Advancing neuroimaging technologies allow for increasing specificity and sensitivity in the identification of neural systems subserving the cognitive deficits associated with these genetic syndromes. Such data significantly improve clinical outcome prognosis accuracy and can provide biological targets for syndrome-specific treatment development.

References

Abboud, M. R., Cure, J., Granger, S., Gallagher, D., Hsu, L., Wang, W., et al. (2004). Magnetic resonance angiography in children with sickle cell disease and abnormal transcranial Doppler ultrasonography findings enrolled in the STOP study. *Blood, 103*(7), 2822–2826.

Adams, M. E., Aylett, S. E., Squier, W., & Chong, W. (2009). A spectrum of unusual neuroimaging findings in patients with suspected Sturge–Weber syndrome. *American Journal of Neuroradiology, 30*(2), 276–281.

Alexander, A. L., Lee, J. E., Lazar, M., Boudos, R., DuBray, M. B., Oakes, T. R., et al. (2007). Diffusion tensor imaging of the corpus callosum in autism. *NeuroImage, 34*(1), 61–73.

Alkan, A., Sarac, K., Kutlu, R., Yakinci, C., Sigirci, A., Aslan, M., et al. (2003). Proton MR spectroscopy features of normal appearing white matter in neurofibromatosis type 1. *Magnetic Resonance Imaging, 21*(9), 1049–1053.

Alkan, A., Sigirci, A., Kutlu, R., Ozcan, H., Erdem, G., Aslan, M., et al. (2005). Neurofibromatosis type 1: Diffusion weighted imaging findings of brain. *European Journal of Radiology, 56*(2), 229–234.

Alterman, A. I., & Tarter, R. E. (1983). The transmission of psychological vulnerability: Implications for alcoholism etiology. *Journal of Nervous and Mental Disease, 171*(3), 147–154.

American Psychiatric Association. (1994). *Diagnostic and statistical manual of mental disorders* (4th ed.). Washington, DC: Author.

Arca, G., Pacheco, E., Alfonso, I., Duchowny, M. S., & Melnick, S. J. (2006). Characteristic brain magnetic resonance imaging (MRI) findings in neonates with tuberous sclerosis complex. *Journal of Child Neurology, 21*(4), 280–285.

Asahina, N., Shiga, T., Egawa, K., Shiraishi, H., Kohsaka, S., & Saitoh, S. (2008). [(11)C]flumazenil positron emission tomography analyses of brain gamma-aminobutyric acid type A receptors in Angelman syndrome. *Journal of Pediatrics, 152*(4), 546–549.

Aubourg, P., Blanche, S., Jambaque, I., Rocchiccioli, F., Kalifa, G., Naud-Saudreau, C., et al. (1990). Reversal of early neurologic and neuroradiologic manifestations of X-linked adrenoleukodystrophy by bone marrow transplantation. *New England Journal of Medicine, 322*(26), 1860–1866.

Autti, T. H., Hämäläinen, J., Mannerkoski, M., Van Leemput, K. V., & Aberg, L. E. (2008). JNCL patients show marked brain volume alterations on longitudinal MRI in adolescence. *Journal of Neurology, 255*, 1226–1230.

Autti, T., Raininko, R., Santavuori, P., Vanhanen, S. L., Poutanen, V. P., & Haltia, M. (1997). MRI of neuronal ceroid lipofuscinosis: II. Postmortem MRI and histopathological study of the brain in 16 cases of neuronal ceroid lipofuscinosis of juvenile or late infantile type. *Neuroradiology, 39*(5), 371–377.

Autti, T., Raininko, R., Vanhanen, S. L., & Santavuori, P. (1996). MRI of neuronal ceroid lipofuscinosis: I. Cranial MRI of 30 patients with juvenile neuronal ceroid lipofuscinosis. *Neuroradiology, 38*(5), 476–482.

Aydin, K., Bakir, B., Tatli, B., Terzibasioglu, E., & Ozmen, M. (2005). Proton MR spectroscopy in three children with Tay–Sachs disease. *Pediatric Radiology, 35*(11), 1081–1085.

Barnea-Goraly, N., Eliez, S., Hedeus, M., Menon, V., White, C. D., Moseley, M., et al. (2003). White matter tract alterations in fragile X syndrome: Preliminary evidence from diffusion tensor imaging. *American Journal of Medical Genetics, Part B, Neuropsychiatric Genetics, 118B*(1), 81–88.

Barnea-Goraly, N., Eliez, S., Menon, V., Bammer, R., & Reiss, A. L. (2005). Arithmetic ability and parietal alterations: a diffusion tensor imaging study in velocardiofacial syndrome. *Brain Research: Cognitive Brain Research, 25*(3), 735–740.

Batista, C. E., Chugani, H. T., Hu, J., Haacke, E. M., Behen, M. E., Helder, E. J., et al. (2008). Magnetic resonance spectroscopic imaging detects abnormalities in normal-appearing frontal lobe of patients with Sturge–Weber syndrome. *Journal of Neuroimaging, 18*(3), 306–313.

Baumann, M., Korenke, G. C., Weddige-Diedrichs, A., Wilichowski, E., Hunneman, D. H., Wilken, B., et al. (2003). Haematopoietic stem cell transplantation in 12 patients with cerebral X-linked adrenoleukodystrophy. *European Journal of Pediatrics, 162*(1), 6–14.

Bayou, N., M'Rad, R., Ahlem, B., Bechir Helayem, M., & Chaabouni, H. (2008). Autism: An overview of genetic aetiology. *Tunisie Medicale, 86*(6), 573–578.

Bearden, C. E., van Erp, T. G., Dutton, R. A., Tran, H., Zimmermann, L., Sun, D., et al. (2007). Mapping cortical thickness in children with 22q11.2 deletions. *Cerebral Cortex, 17*(8), 1889–1898.

Bigler, E. D., Mortensen, S., Neeley, E. S., Ozonoff, S., Krasny, L., Johnson, M., et al. (2007). Superior temporal gyrus, language function, and autism. *Developmental Neuropsychology, 31*(2), 217–238.

Bigler, E. D., Tate, D. F., Neeley, E. S., Wolfson, L. J., Miller, M. J., Rice, S. A., et al. (2003). Temporal lobe, autism, and macrocephaly. *American Journal of Neuroradiology, 24*(10), 2066–2076.

Billingsley, R. L., Jackson, E. F., Slopis, J. M., Swank, P. R., Mahankali, S., & Moore, B. D. (2003). Functional magnetic resonance imaging of phonologic processing in neurofibromatosis 1. *Journal of Child Neurology, 18*(11), 731–740.

Billingsley, R. L., Jackson, E. F., Slopis, J. M., Swank, P. R., Mahankali, S., & Moore, B. D.

(2004). Functional MRI of visual–spatial processing in neurofibromatosis, type I. *Neuropsychologia, 42*(3), 395–404.

Bird, L. M., & Scambler, P. (2000). Cortical dysgenesis in 2 patients with chromosome 22q11 deletion. *Clinical Genetics, 58*(1), 64–68.

Bish, J. P., Nguyen, V., Ding, L., Ferrante, S., & Simon, T. J. (2004). Thalamic reductions in children with chromosome 22q11.2 deletion syndrome. *NeuroReport, 15*(9), 1413–1415.

Bish, J. P., Pendyal, A., Ding, L., Ferrante, H., Nguyen, V., McDonald-McGinn, D., et al. (2006). Specific cerebellar reductions in children with chromosome 22q11.2 deletion syndrome. *Neuroscience Letters, 399*(3), 245–248.

Bishop, D. V. (2009). Genes, cognition, and communication: insights from neurodevelopmental disorders. *Annals of the New York Academy of Sciences, 1156*, 1–18.

Boddaert, N., Le Quan Sang, K. H., Rotig, A., Leroy-Willig, A., Gallet, S., Brunelle, F., et al. (2007). Selective iron chelation in Friedreich ataxia: Biologic and clinical implications. *Blood, 110*(1), 401–408.

Boddaert, N., Mochel, F., Meresse, I., Seidenwurm, D., Cachia, A., Brunelle, F., et al. (2006). Parieto-occipital grey matter abnormalities in children with Williams syndrome. *NeuroImage, 30*(3), 721–725.

Brown, W. E., Kesler, S. R., Eliez, S., Warsofsky, I. S., Haberecht, M., Patwardhan, A., et al. (2002). Brain development in Turner syndrome: A magnetic resonance imaging study. *Psychiatry Research, 116*(3), 187–196.

Brown, W. E., Kesler, S. R., Eliez, S., Warsofsky, I. S., Haberecht, M., & Reiss, A. L. (2004). A volumetric study of parietal lobe subregions in Turner syndrome. *Developmental Medicine and Child Neurology, 46*(9), 607–609.

Campbell, L. E., Daly, E., Toal, F., Stevens, A., Azuma, R., Catani, M., et al. (2006). Brain and behaviour in children with 22q11.2 deletion syndrome: A volumetric and voxel-based morphometry MRI study. *Brain, 129*(Pt. 5), 1218–1228.

Campbell, L. E., Daly, E., Toal, F., Stevens, A., Azuma, R., Karmiloff-Smith, A., et al. (2009). Brain structural differences associated with the behavioural phenotype in children with Williams syndrome. *Brain Research, 1258*, 96–107.

Carter, J. C., Lanham, D. C., Pham, D., Bibat, G., Naidu, S., & Kaufmann, W. E. (2008). Selective cerebral volume reduction in Rett syndrome: A multiple-approach MR imaging study. *American Journal of Neuroradiology, 29*(3), 436–441.

Castellanos, F. X., Lee, P. P., Sharp, W., Jeffries, N. O., Greenstein, D. K., Clasen, L. S., et al. (2002). Developmental trajectories of brain volume abnormalities in children and adolescents with attention-deficit/hyperactivity disorder. *Journal*

of the American Medical Association, 288(14), 1740–1748.

Chahrour, M., & Zoghbi, H. Y. (2007). The story of Rett syndrome: From clinic to neurobiology. *Neuron, 56*(3), 422–437.

Chang, Y. C., Huang, C. C., & Huang, S. C. (1998). Volumetric neuroimaging in children with neurodevelopmental disorders—mapping the brain and behavior. *Zhonghua Minguo Xiaoerke Yixue Zazhi, 39*(5), 285–292.

Choi, J., Jeong, B., Rohan, M. L., Polcari, A. M., & Teicher, M. H. (2009). Preliminary evidence for white matter tract abnormalities in young adults exposed to parental verbal abuse. *Biological Psychiatry, 65*(3), 227-234.

Christophe, C., Sekhara, T., Rypens, F., Ziereisen, F., Christiaens, F., & Dan, B. (2000). MRI spectrum of cortical malformations in tuberous sclerosis complex. *Brain and Development, 22*(8), 487–493.

Church, J. A., Fair, D. A., Dosenbach, N. U., Cohen, A. L., Miezin, F. M., Petersen, S. E., et al. (2009). Control networks in paediatric Tourette syndrome show immature and anomalous patterns of functional connectivity. *Brain, 132*(Pt. 1), 225–238.

Cleary, M. A., Walter, J. H., Wraith, J. E., White, F., Tyler, K., & Jenkins, J. P. (1995). Magnetic resonance imaging in phenylketonuria: Reversal of cerebral white matter change. *Journal of Pediatrics 127*(2), 251–255.

Collmann, H., Sorensen, N., & Krauss, J. (2005). Hydrocephalus in craniosynostosis: A review. *Child's Nervous System, 21*(10), 902–912.

Constantino, J. N. (2005). *Social Responsiveness Scale.* Los Angeles: Western Psychological Services.

Debaun, M. R., Derdeyn, C. P., & McKinstry, R. C., III. (2006). Etiology of strokes in children with sickle cell anemia. *Mental Retardation and Developmental Disabilities Research Reviews, 12*(3), 192–199.

Debbane, M., Schaer, M., Farhoumand, R., Glaser, B., & Eliez, S. (2006). Hippocampal volume reduction in 22q11.2 deletion syndrome. *Neuropsychologia, 44*(12), 2360–2365.

Deboer, T., Wu, Z., Lee, A., & Simon, T. J. (2007). Hippocampal volume reduction in children with chromosome 22q11.2 deletion syndrome is associated with cognitive impairment. *Behavioral Brain Functions, 3*, 54.

deCharms, R. C. (2008). Applications of real-time fMRI. *Nature Reviews Neuroscience, 9*(9), 720–729.

Dimitropoulos, A., & Schultz, R. T. (2008). Food-related neural circuitry in Prader–Willi syndrome: Response to high- versus low-calorie foods. *Journal of Autism and Developmental Disorders, 38*(9), 1642–1653.

D'Incerti, L. (2000). MRI in neuronal ceroid lipofuscinosis. *Neurological Sciences, 21*(3, Suppl.), S71–S73.

Ding, X. Q., Fiehler, J., Kohlschutter, B., Wittkugel, O., Grzyska, U., Zeumer, H., et al. (2008). MRI abnormalities in normal-appearing brain tissue of treated adult PKU patients. *Journal of Magnetic Resonance Imaging, 27*(5), 998–1004.

Dunn, H. G., Stoessl, A. J., Ho, H. H., MacLeod, P. M., Poskitt, K. J., Doudet, D. J., et al. (2002). Rett syndrome: Investigation of nine patients, including PET scan. *Canadian Journal of Neurological Sciences, 29*(4), 345–357.

Eichler, F. S., Barker, P. B., Cox, C., Edwin, D., Ulug, A. M., Moser, H. W., et al. (2002). Proton MR spectroscopic imaging predicts lesion progression on MRI in X-linked adrenoleukodystrophy. *Neurology, 58*(6), 901–907.

Eliez, S., Antonarakis, S. E., Morris, M. A., Dahoun, S. P., & Reiss, A. L. (2001). Parental origin of the deletion 22q11.2 and brain development in velocardiofacial syndrome: A preliminary study. *Archives of General Psychiatry, 58*(1), 64–68.

Eliez, S., Barnea-Goraly, N., Schmitt, J. E., Liu, Y., & Reiss, A. L. (2002). Increased basal ganglia volumes in velo-cardio-facial syndrome (deletion 22q11.2). *Biological Psychiatry, 52*(1), 68–70.

Eliez, S., Blasey, C. M., Menon, V., White, C. D., Schmitt, J. E., & Reiss, A. L. (2001). Functional brain imaging study of mathematical reasoning abilities in velocardiofacial syndrome (del22q11.2). *Genetics in Medicine, 3*(1), 49–55.

Eliez, S., Blasey, C. M., Schmitt, E. J., White, C. D., Hu, D., & Reiss, A. L. (2001). Velocardiofacial syndrome: Are structural changes in the temporal and mesial temporal regions related to schizophrenia? *American Journal of Psychiatry, 158*(3), 447–453.

Eliez, S., Schmitt, J. E., White, C. D., & Reiss, A. L. (2000). Children and adolescents with velocardiofacial syndrome: A volumetric MRI study. *American Journal of Psychiatry, 157*(3), 409–415.

Eliez, S., Schmitt, J. E., White, C. D., Wellis, V. G., & Reiss, A. L. (2001). A quantitative MRI study of posterior fossa development in velocardiofacial syndrome. *Biological Psychiatry, 49*(6), 540–546.

Eluvathingal, T. J., Behen, M. E., Chugani, H. T., Janisse, J., Bernardi, B., Chakraborty, P., et al. (2006). Cerebellar lesions in tuberous sclerosis complex: Neurobehavioral and neuroimaging correlates. *Journal of Child Neurology, 21*(10), 846–851.

Ergun, R., Okten, A. I., Gezercan, Y., & Gezici, A. R. (2007). Sturge–Weber syndrome accompanied with multiple congenital intracranial lesions. *Acta Neurochirurgica (Wien), 149*(8), 829–830 (discussion, 830).

Faravelli, F., D'Arrigo, S., Bagnasco, I., Selicorni, A., D'Incerti, L., Riva, D., et al. (2003). Oligoyric microcephaly in a child with Williams syndrome.

American Journal of Medical Genetics, Part A, 117A(2), 169–171.

Filippi, M. (2009). *fMRI techniques and protocols.* New York: Springer.

Fryer, S. L., Kwon, H., Eliez, S., & Reiss, A. L. (2003). Corpus callosum and posterior fossa development in monozygotic females: A morphometric MRI study of Turner syndrome. *Developmental Medicine and Child Neurology, 45*(5), 320–324.

Galanter, C. A., & Leibenluft, E. (2008). Frontiers between attention deficit hyperactivity disorder and bipolar disorder. *Child and Adolescent Psychiatric Clinics of North America, 17*(2), 325–346.

Garrett, A. S., Menon, V., MacKenzie, K., & Reiss, A. L. (2004). Here's looking at you, kid: Neural systems underlying face and gaze processing in fragile X syndrome. *Archives of General Psychiatry, 61*(3), 281–288.

Gaser, C., Luders, E., Thompson, P. M., Lee, A. D., Dutton, R. A., Geaga, J. A., et al. (2006). Increased local gyrification mapped in Williams syndrome. *NeuroImage, 33*(1), 46–54.

Geschwind, D. H., & Levitt, P. (2007). Autism spectrum disorders: Developmental disconnection syndromes. *Current Opinion in Neurobiology, 17*(1), 103–111.

Giedd, J. N., Clasen, L. S., Lenroot, R., Greenstein, D., Wallace, G. L., Ordaz, S., et al. (2006). Puberty-related influences on brain development. *Molecular Cellular Endocrinology, 254–255*, 154–162.

Giedd, J. N., Clasen, L. S., Wallace, G. L., Lenroot, R. K., Lerch, J. P., Wells, E. M., et al. (2007). XXY (Klinefelter syndrome): A pediatric quantitative brain magnetic resonance imaging case–control study. *Pediatrics, 119*(1), e232–e240.

Gilbert, D. L., Christian, B. T., Gelfand, M. J., Shi, B., Mantil, J., & Sallee, F. R. (2006). Altered mesolimbocortical and thalamic dopamine in Tourette syndrome. *Neurology, 67*(9), 1695–1697.

Glaser, B., Schaer, M., Berney, S., Debbane, M., Vuilleumier, P., & Eliez, S. (2007). Structural changes to the fusiform gyrus: A cerebral marker for social impairments in 22q11.2 deletion syndrome? *Schizophrenia Research, 96*(1–3), 82–86.

Glessner, J. T., Wang, K., Cai, G., Korvatska, O., Kim, C. E., Wood, S., et al. (2009). Autism genome-wide copy number variation reveals ubiquitin and neuronal genes. *Nature, 459*, 569–573.

Gogtay, N., Giedd, J., & Rapoport, J. L. (2002). Brain development in healthy, hyperactive, and psychotic children. *Archives of Neurology, 59*(8), 1244–1248.

Gokcay, A., Kitis, O., Ekmekci, O., Karasoy, H., & Sener, R. N. (2002). Proton MR spectroscopy in Rett syndrome. *Computerized Medical Imaging and Graphics, 26*(4), 271–275.

Goldstein, W. N. (1989). Update on psychodynamic thinking regarding the diagnosis of the borderline patient. *American Journal of Psychotherapy, 43*(3), 321–342.

Good, C. D., Lawrence, K., Thomas, N. S., Price, C. J., Ashburner, J., Friston, K. J., et al. (2003). Dosage-sensitive X-linked locus influences the development of amygdala and orbitofrontal cortex, and fear recognition in humans. *Brain, 126*(Pt. 11), 2431–2446.

Goodman, M., New, A., & Siever, L. (2004). Trauma, genes, and the neurobiology of personality disorders. *Annals of the New York Academy of Sciences, 1032,* 104–116.

Gothelf, D. (2007). Velocardiofacial syndrome. *Child and Adolescent Psychiatric Clinics of North America, 16*(3), 677–693.

Gothelf, D., Furfaro, J. A., Hoeft, F., Eckert, M. A., Hall, S. S., O'Hara, R., et al. (2008). Neuroanatomy of fragile X syndrome is associated with aberrant behavior and the fragile X mental retardation protein (FMRP). *Annals of Neurology, 63*(1), 40–51.

Gothelf, D., Hoeft, F., Hinard, C., Hallmayer, J. F., Stoecker, J. V., Antonarakis, S. E., et al. (2007). Abnormal cortical activation during response inhibition in 22q11.2 deletion syndrome. *Human Brain Mapping, 28*(6), 533–542.

Gothelf, D., Schaer, M., & Eliez, S. (2008). Genes, brain development and psychiatric phenotypes in velo-cardio-facial syndrome. *Developmental Disabilities Research Reviews, 14*(1), 59–68.

Grant, J. E., Correia, S., Brennan-Krohn, T., Malloy, P. F., Laidlaw, D. H., & Schulz, S. C. (2007). Frontal white matter integrity in borderline personality disorder with self-injurious behavior. *Journal of Neuropsychiatry and Clinical Neuroscience, 19*(4), 383–390.

Greicius, M. D., Boyett-Anderson, J. M., Menon, V, & Reiss, A. L. (2004). Reduced basal forebrain and hippocampal activation during memory encoding in girls with fragile X syndrome. *NeuroReport, 15*(10), 1579–1583.

Gujar, S. K., Maheshwari, S., Bjorkman-Burtscher, I., & Sundgren, P. C. (2005). Magnetic resonance spectroscopy. *Journal of Neuro-Ophthalmology, 25*(3), 217–226.

Haas, B. W., Barnea-Goraly, N., Lightbody, A. A., Patnaik, S. S., Hoeft, F., Hazlett, H., et al. (2009). Early white-matter abnormalities of the ventral frontostriatal pathway in fragile X syndrome. *Developmental Medicine and Child Neurology, 51*(8), 593–599.

Haberecht, M. F., Menon, V., Warsofsky, I. S., White, C. D., Dyer-Friedman, J., Glover, G. H., et al. (2001). Functional neuroanatomy of visuospatial working memory in Turner syndrome. *Human Brain Mapping, 14*(2), 96–107.

Hagan, C. C., Hoeft, F., Mackey, A., Mobbs, D., & Reiss, A. L. (2008). Aberrant neural function during emotion attribution in female subjects with fragile X syndrome. *Journal of the American Academy of Child and Adolescent Psychiatry, 47*(12), 1443–1454.

Harenski, C. L., Kim, S. H., & Hamann, S. (2009). Neuroticism and psychopathy predict brain activation during moral and nonmoral emotion regulation. *Cognitive, Affective, and Behavioral Neuroscience, 9*(1), 1–15.

Hart, S. J., Davenport, M. L., Hooper, S. R., & Belger, A. (2006). Visuospatial executive function in Turner syndrome: functional MRI and neurocognitive findings. *Brain, 129*(Pt. 5), 1125–1136.

Harting, I., Seitz, A., Rating, D., Sartor, K., Zschocke, J., Janssen, B., et al. (2009). Abnormal myelination in Angelman syndrome. *European Journal of Paediatric Neurology, 13*(3), 271–276.

Helton, K. J., Paydar, A., Glass, J., Weirich, E. M., Hankins, J., Li, C. S., et al. (2009). Arterial spin-labeled perfusion combined with segmentation techniques to evaluate cerebral blood flow in white and gray matter of children with sickle cell anemia. *Pediatric Blood Cancer, 52*(1), 85–91.

Hoeft, F., Hernandez, A., Parthasarathy, S., Watson, C. L., Hall, S. S., & Reiss, A. L. (2007). Fronto-striatal dysfunction and potential compensatory mechanisms in male adolescents with fragile X syndrome. *Human Brain Mapping, 28*(6), 543–554.

Hoeft, F., Lightbody, A. A., Hazlett, H. C., Patnaik, S., Piven, J., & Reiss, A. L. (2008). Morphometric spatial patterns differentiating boys with fragile X syndrome, typically developing boys, and developmentally delayed boys aged 1 to 3 years. *Archives of General Psychiatry, 65*(9), 1087–1097.

Hoeft, F., Ueno, T., Reiss, A. L., Meyler, A., Whitfield-Gabrieli, S., Glover, G. H., et al. (2007). Prediction of children's reading skills using behavioral, functional, and structural neuroimaging measures. *Behavioral Neuroscience, 121*(3), 602–613.

Hoffman, T. L., Vossough, A., Ficicioglu, C., & Visootsak, J. (2008). Brain magnetic resonance imaging findings in 49,XXXXY syndrome. *Pediatric Neurology, 38*(6), 450–453.

Holopainen, I. E., Metsahonkala, E. L., Kokkonen, H., Parkkola, R. K., Manner, T. E., Nagren, K., et al. (2001). Decreased binding of [11C]flumazenil in Angelman syndrome patients with GABA(A) receptor beta3 subunit deletions. *Annals of Neurology, 49*(1), 110–113.

Holzapfel, M., Barnea-Goraly, N., Eckert, M. A., Kesler, S. R., & Reiss, A. L. (2006). Selective alterations of white matter associated with visuospatial and sensorimotor dysfunction in Turner syndrome. *Journal of Neuroscience, 26*(26), 7007–7013.

Horska, A., Farage, L., Bibat, G., Nagae, L. M.,

Kaufmann, W. E., Barker, P. B., et al. (2009). Brain metabolism in Rett syndrome: Age, clinical, and genotype correlations. *Annals of Neurology, 65*(1), 90–97.

Horska, A., Naidu, S., Herskovits, E. H., Wang, P. Y., Kaufmann, W. E., & Barker, P. B. (2000). Quantitative 1H MR spectroscopic imaging in early Rett syndrome. *Neurology, 54*(3), 715–722.

Hsieh, H. Y., Wu, T., Wang, C. J., Chin, S. C., & Chen, Y. R. (2007). Neurological complications involving the central nervous system in neurofibromatosis type 1. *Acta Neurologica Taiwan, 16*(2), 68–73.

Hu, J., Yu, Y., Juhasz, C., Kou, Z., Xuan, Y., Latif, Z., et al. (2008). MR susceptibility weighted imaging (SWI) complements conventional contrast enhanced T1 weighted MRI in characterizing brain abnormalities of Sturge–Weber syndrome. *Journal of Magnetic Resonance Imaging, 28*(2), 300–307.

Hua, K., Oishi, K., Zhang, J., Wakana, S., Yoshioka, T., Zhang, W., et al. (2008). Mapping of functional areas in the human cortex based on connectivity through association fibers. *Cerebral Cortex, 19*(8), 1889–1895.

Huettel, S. A., Song, A. W., & McCarthy, G. (2008). *Functional magnetic resonance imaging* (2nd ed.). Sunderland: Sinauer Associates.

Imamura, A., Miyajima, H., Ito, R., & Orii, K. O. (2008). Serial MR imaging and 1H-MR spectroscopy in monozygotic twins with Tay–Sachs disease. *Neuropediatrics, 39*(5), 259–263.

Iughetti, L., Bosio, L., Corrias, A., Gargantini, L., Ragusa, L., Livieri, C., et al. (2008). Pituitary height and neuroradiological alterations in patients with Prader–Labhart–Willi syndrome. *European Journal of Pediatrics, 167*(6), 701–702.

Jezzard, P., Matthews, P. M., & Smith, S. M. (2003). *Functional MRI: An introduction to methods.* Oxford, UK: Oxford University Press.

Jones, W., Hesselink, J., Courchesne, E., Duncan, T., Matsuda, K., & Bellugi, U. (2002). Cerebellar abnormalities in infants and toddlers with Williams syndrome. *Developmental Medicine and Child Neurology, 44*(10), 688–694.

Juhasz, C., Haacke, E. M., Hu, J., Xuan, Y., Makki, M., Behen, M. E., et al. (2007). Multimodality imaging of cortical and white matter abnormalities in Sturge-Weber syndrome. *American Journal of Neuroradiology, 28*(5), 900–906.

Kankirawatana, P., Leonard, H., Ellaway, C., Scurlock, J., Mansour, A., Makris, C. M., et al. (2006). Early progressive encephalopathy in boys and MECP2 mutations. *Neurology, 67*(1), 164–166.

Kates, W. R., Burnette, C. P., Bessette, B. A., Foley, B. S., Strunge, L., Jabs, E. W., et al. (2004). Frontal and caudate alterations in velocardiofacial syndrome (deletion at chromosome 22q11.2). *Journal of Child Neurology, 19*(5), 337–342.

Kates, W. R., Burnette, C. P., Jabs, E. W., Rutberg, J., Murphy, A. M., Grados, M., et al. (2001). Regional cortical white matter reductions in velocardiofacial syndrome: A volumetric MRI analysis. *Biological Psychiatry, 49*(8), 677–684.

Kates, W. R., Krauss, B. R., Abdulsabur, N., Colgan, D., Antshel, K. M., Higgins, A. M., et al. (2007). The neural correlates of non-spatial working memory in velocardiofacial syndrome (22q11.2 deletion syndrome). *Neuropsychologia, 45*(12), 2863–2873.

Kates, W. R., Miller, A. M., Abdulsabur, N., Antshel, K. M., Conchelos, J., Fremont, W., et al. (2006). Temporal lobe anatomy and psychiatric symptoms in velocardiofacial syndrome (22q11.2 deletion syndrome). *Journal of the American Academy of Child and Adolescent Psychiatry, 45*(5), 587–595.

Kelley, T. M., Hatfield, L. A., Lin, D. D., & Comi, A. M. (2005). Quantitative analysis of cerebral cortical atrophy and correlation with clinical severity in unilateral Sturge–Weber syndrome. *Journal of Child Neurology, 20*(11), 867–870.

Kelly, A. M., Margulies, D. S., & Castellanos, F. X. (2007). Recent advances in structural and functional brain imaging studies of attention-deficit/hyperactivity disorder. *Current Psychiatry Reports, 9*(5), 401–407.

Kendler, K. S., Aggen, S. H., Czajkowski, N., Roysamb, E., Tambs, K., Torgersen, S., et al. (2008). The structure of genetic and environmental risk factors for DSM-IV personality disorders: A multivariate twin study. *Archives of General Psychiatry, 65*(12), 1438–1446.

Kennedy, D. N., Haselgrove, C., & McInerney, S. (2003). MRI-based morphometric analysis of typical and atypical brain development. *Mental Retardation and Developmental Disabilities Research Reviews, 9*(3), 155–160.

Kesler, S. R. (2007). Turner syndrome. *Child Adolescent Psychiatric Clinics of North America, 16*(3), 709–722.

Kesler, S. R., Blasey, C. M., Brown, W. E., Yankowitz, J., Zeng, S. M., Bender, B. G., et al. (2003). Effects of X-monosomy and X-linked imprinting on superior temporal gyrus morphology in Turner syndrome. *Biological Psychiatry, 54*(6), 636–646.

Kesler, S. R., Garrett, A., Bender, B. G., Yankowitz, J., Zeng, S. M., & Reiss, A. L. (2004). Amygdala and hippocampal volumes in Turner syndrome: A high-resolution MRI study of X-monosomy. *Neuropsychologia, 42*, 1971–1978.

Kesler, S. R., Haberecht, M. F., Menon, V., Warsofsky, I. S., Dyer-Friedman, J., Neely, E. K., et al. (2004). Functional neuroanatomy of spatial orientation processing in Turner syndrome. *Cerebral Cortex, 14*(2), 174–180.

Kesler, S. R., Lightbody, A. A., & Reiss, A. L. (2009). Cholinergic dysfunction in fragile X syndrome and potential intervention: A preliminary 1H MRS study. *American Journal of Medical Genetics, Part A, 149A*(3), 403–407.

Kesler, S. R., Menon, V., & Reiss, A. L. (2006). Neuro-functional differences associated with arithmetic processing in Turner syndrome. *Cerebral Cortex, 16*(6), 849–856.

Khong, P. L., Lam, C. W., Ooi, C. G., Ko, C. H., & Wong, V. C. (2002). Magnetic resonance spectroscopy and analysis of MECP2 in Rett syndrome. *Pediatric Neurology, 26*(3), 205–209.

Kieslich, M., Fuchs, S., Vlaho, S., Maisch, U., & Boehles, H. (2002). Midline developmental anomalies in Down syndrome. *Journal of Child Neurology, 17*(6), 460–462.

Kim, S. E., Jin, D. K., Cho, S. S., Kim, J. H., Hong, S. D., Paik, K. H., et al. (2006). Regional cerebral glucose metabolic abnormality in Prader–Willi syndrome: A 18F-FDG PET study under sedation. *Journal of Nuclear Medicine, 47*(7), 1088–1092.

Koenigsberg, H. W., Siever, L. J., Lee, H., Pizzarello, S., New, A. S., Goodman, M., et al. (2009). Neural correlates of emotion processing in borderline personality disorder. *Psychiatry Research, 172*(3), 192–199.

Kono, K., Okano, Y., Nakayama, K., Hase, Y., Minamikawa, S., Ozawa, N., et al. (2005). Diffusion-weighted MR imaging in patients with phenylketonuria: Relationship between serum phenylalanine levels and ADC values in cerebral white matter. *Radiology, 236*(2), 630–636.

Kruse, B., Barker, P. B., van Zijl, P. C., Duyn, J. H., Moonen, C. T., & Moser, H. W. (1994). Multislice proton magnetic resonance spectroscopic imaging in X-linked adrenoleukodystrophy. *Annals of Neurology, 36*(4), 595–608.

Kwiatkowski, J. L., Zimmerman, R. A., Pollock, A. N., Seto, W., Smith-Whitley, K., Shults, J., et al. (2009). Silent infarcts in young children with sickle cell disease. *British Journal of Haematology, 146*(3), 300–305.

Lainhart, J. E., Lazar, M., Bigler, E. D. & Alexander, A. (2006). *The brain during life in autism: Advances in neuroimaging research*. New York: Nova Science.

Lee, A. D., Leow, A. D., Lu, A., Reiss, A. L., Hall, S., Chiang, M. C., et al. (2007). 3D pattern of brain abnormalities in fragile X syndrome visualized using tensor-based morphometry. *NeuroImage, 34*(3), 924–938.

Lee, J. E., Bigler, E. D., Alexander, A. L., Lazar, M., DuBray, M. B., Chung, M. K., et al. (2007). Diffusion tensor imaging of white matter in the superior temporal gyrus and temporal stem in autism. *Neuroscience Letters, 424*(2), 127–132.

Lee, J. E., Chung, M. K., Lazar, M., DuBray, M. B., Kim, J., Bigler, E. D., et al. (2009). A study of diffusion tensor imaging by tissue-specific, smoothing-compensated voxel-based analysis. *NeuroImage, 44*(3), 870–883.

Leonard, C. M., Williams, C. A., Nicholls, R. D., Agee, O. F., Voeller, K. K., Honeyman, J. C., et al. (1993). Angelman and Prader–Willi syndrome: A magnetic resonance imaging study of differences in cerebral structure. *American Journal of Medical Genetics, 46*(1), 26–33.

Leonard, H., Silberstein, J., Falk, R., Houwink-Manville, I., Ellaway, C., Raffaele, L. S., et al. (2001). Occurrence of Rett syndrome in boys. *Journal of Child Neurology, 16*(5), 333–338.

Leuzzi, V., Bianchi, M. C., Tosetti, M., Carducci, C. L., Carducci, C. A., & Antonozzi, I. (2000). Clinical significance of brain phenylalanine concentration assessed by in vivo proton magnetic resonance spectroscopy in phenylketonuria. *Journal of Inherited Metabaolic Disease, 23*(6), 563–570.

Leuzzi, V., Tosetti, M., Montanaro, D., Carducci, C., Artiola, C., Carducci, C., et al. (2007). The pathogenesis of the white matter abnormalities in phenylketonuria: A multimodal 3.0 tesla MRI and magnetic resonance spectroscopy (1H MRS) study. *Journal of Inherited Metabolic Disease, 30*(2), 209–216.

Levitin, D. J., Menon, V., Schmitt, J. E., Eliez, S., White, C. D., Glover, G. H., et al. (2003). Neural correlates of auditory perception in Williams syndrome: An fMRI study. *NeuroImage, 18*(1), 74–82.

Levitt, P., & Campbell, D. B. (2009). The genetic and neurobiologic compass points toward common signaling dysfunctions in autism spectrum disorders. *Journal of Clinical Investigation, 119*(4), 747–754.

Logothetis, N. K. (2008). What we can do and what we cannot do with fMRI. *Nature, 453*, 869–878.

Lopes Ferraz Filho, J. R., Munis, M. P., Soares Souza, A., Sanches, R. A., Goloni-Bertollo, E. M., & Pavarino-Bertelli, E. C. (2008). Unidentified bright objects on brain MRI in children as a diagnostic criterion for neurofibromatosis type 1. *Pediatric Radiology, 38*(3), 305–310.

Lucignani, G., Panzacchi, A., Bosio, L., Moresco, R. M., Ravasi, L., Coppa, I., et al. (2004). GABA A receptor abnormalities in Prader–Willi syndrome assessed with positron emission tomography and [11C]flumazenil. *NeuroImage, 22*(1), 22–28.

Luders, E., Di Paola, M., Tomaiuolo, F., Thompson, P. M., Toga, A. W., Vicari, S., et al. (2007). Callosal morphology in Williams syndrome: A new evaluation of shape and thickness. *NeuroReport, 18*(3), 203–207.

Machado, A. M., Simon, T. J., Nguyen, V., McDonald-McGinn, D. M., Zackai, E. H., & Gee, J. C. (2007). Corpus callosum morphology and ventricular size in chromosome 22q11.2 deletion syndrome. *Brain Research, 1131*(1), 197–210.

MacMaster, F. P., O'Neill, J., & Rosenberg, D. R. (2008). Brain imaging in pediatric obsessive-compulsive disorder. *Journal of the American Academy of Child and Adolescent Psychiatry, 47*(11), 1262–1272.

Maegawa, G. H., Stockley, T., Tropak, M., Banwell, B., Blaser, S., Kok, F., et al. (2006). The natural history of juvenile or subacute GM2 gangliosidosis: 21 new cases and literature review of 134 previously reported. *Pediatrics, 118*(5), e-550–e1562.

Mantovan, M. C., Martinuzzi, A., Squarzanti, F., Bolla, A., Silvestri, I., Liessi, G., et al. (2006). Exploring mental status in Friedreich's ataxia: A combined neuropsychological, behavioral and neuroimaging study. *European Journal of Neurology, 13*(8), 827–835.

Mateo, I., Llorca, J., Volpini, V., Corral, J., Berciano, J., & Combarros, O. (2004). Expanded GAA repeats and clinical variation in Friedreich's ataxia. *Acta Neurologica Scandinavica, 109*(1), 75–78.

Matijevic, T., Knezevic, J., Slavica, M., & Pavelic, J. (2009). Rett syndrome: From the gene to the disease. *European Neurology, 61*(1), 3–10.

McCloskey, M. S., New, A. S., Siever, L. J., Goodman, M., Koenigsberg, H. W., Flory, J. D., et al. (2009). Evaluation of behavioral impulsivity and aggression tasks as endophenotypes for borderline personality disorder. *Journal of Psychiatric Research, 43*, 915–925.

Melham, E. R., & Golay, X. (2005). Physiological MR of the pediatric brain: Overview. In J. H. Gillard, A. D. Waldman, & P. B. Barker (Eds.), *Clinical MR neuroimaging: Diffusion, perfusion and spectroscopy* (pp. 647–673). New York: Cabridge University Press.

Menon, V., Leroux, J., White, C. D., & Reiss, A. L. (2004). Frontostriatal deficits in fragile X syndrome: Relation to FMR1 gene expression. *Proceedings of the National Academy of Sciences USA, 101*(10), 3615–3620.

Miller, J. L., Couch, J. A., Schmalfuss, I., He, G., Liu, Y., & Driscoll, D. J. (2007). Intracranial abnormalities detected by three-dimensional magnetic resonance imaging in Prader–Willi syndrome. *American Journal of Medical Genetics, Part A, 143*(5), 476–483.

Miller, J. L., Couch, J., Schwenk, K., Long, M., Towler, S., Theriaque, D. W., et al. (2009). Early childhood obesity is associated with compromised cerebellar development. *Developmental Neuropsychology, 34*(3), 272–283.

Miller, J. L., Goldstone, A. P., Couch, J. A., Shuster, J., He, G., Driscoll, D. J., et al. (2008). Pituitary abnormalities in Prader–Willi syndrome and early onset morbid obesity. *American Journal of Medical Genetics, Part A, 146A*(5), 570–577.

Miller, L., Kranzler, J., Liu, Y., Schmalfuss, I., Theriaque, D. W., Shuster, J. J., et al. (2006). Neurocognitive findings in Prader–Willi syndrome and early-onset morbid obesity. *Journal of Pediatrics, 149*(2), 192–198.

Mimouni-Bloch, A., Kornreich, L., Kaadan, W., Steinberg, T., & Shuper, A. (2008). Lesions of the Corpus callosum in children with neurofibromatosis 1. *Pediatric Neurology, 38*(6), 406–410.

Mobbs, D., Eckert, M. A., Menon, V., Mills, D., Korenberg, J., Galaburda, A. M., et al. (2007). Reduced parietal and visual cortical activation during global processing in Williams syndrome. *Developmental Medicine and Child Neurology, 49*(6), 433–438.

Mobbs, D., Eckert, M. A., Mills, D., Korenberg, J., Bellugi, U., Galaburda, A. M., et al. (2007). Frontostriatal dysfunction during response inhibition in Williams syndrome. *Biological Psychiatry, 62*(3), 256–261.

Mori, S. (2007). *Introduction to diffusion tensor imaging.* Oxford, UK: Elsevier.

Muller, R. A. (2007). The study of autism as a distributed disorder. *Mental Retardation and Developmental Disabilities Research Reviews, 13*(1), 85–95.

Murphy, A. M., Brenner, C., & Ann Lynch, S. (2006). Agenesis of the corpus callosum with interhemispheric cyst, hepatic haemangioma and trisomy 21. *Clinical Dysmorphology, 15*(3), 149–151.

Naidu, S., Kaufmann, W. E., Abrams, M. T., Pearlson, G. D., Lanham, D. C., Fredericksen, K. A., et al. (2001). Neuroimaging studies in Rett syndrome. *Brain and Development, 23*(Suppl. 1), S62–S71.

Neudorfer, O., Pastores, G. M., Zeng, B. J., Gianutsos, J., Zaroff, C. M., & Kolodny, E. H. (2005). Late-onset Tay–Sachs disease: Phenotypic characterization and genotypic correlations in 21 affected patients. *Genetics in Medicine, 7*(2), 119–123.

Nijmeijer, J. S., Minderaa, R. B., Buitelaar, J. K., Mulligan, A., Hartman, C. A., & Hoekstra, P. J. (2008). Attention-deficit/hyperactivity disorder and social dysfunctioning. *Clinical Psychology Review, 28*(4), 692–708.

O'Callaghan, F. J., Martyn, C. N., Renowden, S., Noakes, M., Presdee, D, & Osborne, J. P. (2008). Subependymal nodules, giant cell astrocytomas and the tuberous sclerosis complex: A population-based study. *Archives of Disease in Childhood, 93*(9), 751–754.

Pan, J. W., Lane, J. B., Hetherington, H., & Percy, A. K. (1999). Rett syndrome: 1H spectroscopic imaging at 4.1 tesla. *Journal of Child Neurology, 14*(8), 524–528.

Pascual-Castroviejo, I., Pascual-Pascual, S. I., Velazquez-Fragua, R., & Viano, J. (2008). Sturge–Weber syndrome: Study of 55 patients. *Canadian Journal of Neurological Sciences, 35*(3), 301–307.

Paterson, S. J., & Schultz, R. T. (2007). Neurodevelopmental and behavioral issues in Williams syndrome. *Current Psychiatry Reports, 9*(2), 165–171.

Paul, L. K., Brown, W. S., Adolphs, R., Tyszka, J. M., Richards, L. J., Mukherjee, P., et al. (2007). Agenesis of the corpus callosum: Genetic, developmental and functional aspects of connectivity. *National Reviews Neuroscience, 8*(4), 287–299.

Pelphrey, K. A., & Carter, E. J. (2008). Charting the typical and atypical development of the social brain. *Development and Psychopathology, 20*(4), 1081–1102.

Peng, S. S., Tseng, W. Y., Chien, Y. H., Hwu, W. L., & Liu, H. M. (2004). Diffusion tensor images in children with early-treated, chronic, malignant phenylketonuria: Correlation with intelligence assessment. *American Journal of Neuroradiology, 25*(9), 1569–1574.

Peters, S. U., Bacino, C. A., Chu, Z., Merkley, T., Traipe, E., Adapa, A., et al. (2009). *Phenotypic characterization in Angelman syndrome using advanced neuroimaging techniques.* Paper presented at the meeting of the American College of Medical Genetics, Tampa, FL.

Peters, S. U., Bacino, C. A., Chu, Z., Yallampalli, R., Hunter, J. V., & Wilde, E. A. (2008). *Neuroanatomical abnormalities and white matter alterations predict the overall phenotype in Angelman syndrome.* Paper presented at the Angelman's Syndrome Foundation Scientific Symposium, Boston.

Petersen, B., Handwerker, M., & Huppertz, H. I. (1996). Neuroradiological findings in classical late infantile neuronal ceroid-lipofuscinosis. *Pediatric Neurology, 15*(4), 344–347.

Petrella, J. R., Mattay, V. S., & Doraiswamy, P. M. (2008). Imaging genetics of brain longevity and mental wellness: The next frontier? *Radiology, 246*(1), 20–32.

Pfund, Z., Kagawa, K., Juhasz, C., Shen, C., Lee, J. S., Chugani, D. C., et al. (2003). Quantitative analysis of gray- and white-matter volumes and glucose metabolism in Sturge–Weber syndrome. *Journal of Child Neurology, 18*(2), 119–126.

Pinter, J. D., Brown, W. E., Eliez, S, Schmitt, J. E., Capone, G. T., & Reiss, A. L. (2001). Amygdala and hippocampal volumes in children with Down syndrome: A high-resolution MRI study. *Neurology, 56*(7), 972–974.

Pinter, J. D., Eliez, S., Schmitt, J. E., Capone, G. T., & Reiss, A. L. (2001). Neuroanatomy of Down's syndrome: A high-resolution MRI study. *American Journal of Psychiatry, 158*(10), 1659–1665.

Plessen, K. J., Royal, J. M., & Peterson, B. S. (2007). Neuroimaging of tic disorders with co-existing attention-deficit/hyperactivity disorder. *European Child and Adolescent Psychiatry, 16*(Suppl. 1), 60–70.

Pouwels, P. J., Kruse, B., Korenke, G. C., Mao, X., Hanefeld, F. A., & Frahm, J. (1998). Quantitative proton magnetic resonance spectroscopy of childhood adrenoleukodystrophy. *Neuropediatrics, 29*(5), 254–264.

Quintero-Rivera, F., Robson, C. D., Reiss, R. E., Levine, D., Benson, C. B., Mulliken, J. B., et al. (2006). Intracranial anomalies detected by imaging studies in 30 patients with Apert syndrome. *American Journal of Medical Genetics, Part A, 140A*(12), 1337–1338.

Rae, C., Joy, P., Harasty, J., Kemp, A., Kuan, S., Christodoulou, J., et al. (2004). Enlarged temporal lobes in Turner syndrome: An X-chromosome effect? *Cerebral Cortex, 14*(2), 156–164.

Reiss, A. L., & Dant, C. C. (2003). The behavioral neurogenetics of fragile X syndrome: Analyzing gene–brain–behavior relationships in child developmental psychopathologies. *Development and Psychopathology, 15*(4), 927–968.

Reiss, A. L., Eckert, M. A., Rose, F. E., Karchemskiy, A., Kesler, S., Chang, M., et al. (2004). An experiment of nature: Brain anatomy parallels cognition and behavior in Williams syndrome. *Journal of Neuroscience, 24*(21), 5009–5015.

Reiss, A. L., Faruque, F., Naidu, S., Abrams, M., Beaty, T., Bryan, R. N., et al. (1993). Neuroanatomy of Rett syndrome: A volumetric imaging study. *Annals of Neurology, 34*(2), 227–234.

Richardson, M. P., Strange, B. A., Thompson, P. J., Baxendale, S. A., Duncan, J. S., & Dolan, R. J. (2004). Pre-operative verbal memory fMRI predicts post-operative memory decline after left temporal lobe resection. *Brain, 127*(Pt. 11), 2419–2426.

Rivera, S. M., Menon, V., White, C. D., Glaser, B., & Reiss, A. L. (2002). Functional brain activation during arithmetic processing in females with fragile X syndrome is related to FMR1 protein expression. *Human Brain Mapping, 16*(4), 206–218.

Rose, A. B., Merke, D. P., Clasen, L. S., Rosenthal, M. A., Wallace, G. L., Vaituzis, A. C., et al. (2004). Effects of hormones and sex chromosomes on stress-influenced regions of the developing pediatric brain. *Annals of the New York Academy of Sciences, 1032*, 231–233.

Rusch, N., Weber, M., Il'yasov, K. A., Lieb, K., Ebert, D., Hennig, J., et al. (2007). Inferior frontal white matter microstructure and patterns of psychopathology in women with borderline personality disorder and comorbid attention-deficit hyperactivity disorder. *NeuroImage, 35*(2), 738–747.

Salvan, A. M., Chabrol, B., Lamoureux, S., Confort-Gouny, S., Cozzone, P. J., & Vion-Dury, J. (1999). In vivo brain proton MR spectroscopy in a case of molybdenum cofactor deficiency. *Pediatric Radiology, 29*(11), 846–848.

Sarter, M., Bruno, J. P., & Givens, B. (2003). Attentional functions of cortical cholinergic inputs: what does it mean for learning and memory? *Neurobiology of Learning and Memory, 80*(3), 245–256.

Sarter, M., & Parikh, V. (2005). Choline transporters, cholinergic transmission and cognition. *Nature Reviews Neuroscience, 6*(1), 48–56.

Sayit, E., Yorulmaz, I., Bekis, R., Kaya, G., Gumuser, F. G., Dirik, E., et al. (2002). Comparison of brain perfusion SPECT and MRI findings in children with neuronal ceroid-lipofuscinosis and in their families. *Annals of Nuclear Medicine, 16*(3), 201–206.

Sehgal, V., Delproposto, Z., Haddar, D., Haacke, E. M., Sloan, A. E., Zamorano, L. J., et al. (2006). Susceptibility-weighted imaging to visualize blood products and improve tumor contrast in the study of brain masses. *Journal of Magnetic Resonance Imaging, 24*(1), 41–51.

Seitz, D., Grodd, W., Schwab, A., Seeger, U., Klose, U., & Nagele, T. (1998). MR imaging and localized proton MR spectroscopy in late infantile neuronal ceroid lipofuscinosis. *American Journal of Neuroradiology, 19*(7), 1373–1377.

Shapiro, E., Krivit, W., Lockman, L., Jambaque, I., Peters, C., Cowan, M., et al. (2000). Long-term effect of bone-marrow transplantation for childhood-onset cerebral X-linked adrenoleukodystrophy. *Lancet, 356*, 713–718.

Shashi, V., Muddasani, S., Santos, C. C., Berry, M. N., Kwapil, T. R., Lewandowski, E., et al. (2004). Abnormalities of the corpus callosum in nonpsychotic children with chromosome 22q11 deletion syndrome. *NeuroImage, 21*(4), 1399–1406.

Shen, D., Liu, D., Liu, H., Clasen, L., Giedd, J., & Davatzikos, C. (2004). Automated morphometric study of brain variation in XXY males. *NeuroImage, 23*(2), 648–653.

Sijens, P. E., Gieteling, E. W., Meiners, L. C., Sival, D. A., Potze, J. H., Irwan, R., et al. (2006). Diffusion tensor imaging and magnetic resonance spectroscopy of the brain in a patient with Sturge–Weber syndrome. *Acta Radiologica, 47*(9), 972–976.

Silva, G. S., Vicari, P., Figueiredo, M. S., Carrete, H., Jr., Idagawa, M. H., & Massaro, A. R. (2009). Brain magnetic resonance imaging abnormalities in adult patients with sickle cell disease: Correlation with transcranial Doppler findings. *Stroke, 40*(7), 2408–2412.

Simon, T. J., Ding, L., Bish, J. P., McDonald-McGinn, D. M., Zackai, E. H., & Gee, J. (2005). Volumetric, connective, and morphologic changes in the brains of children with chromosome 22q11.2 deletion syndrome: An integrative study. *NeuroImage, 25*(1), 169–180.

Singer, H. S. (2005). Tourette's syndrome: From behaviour to biology. *Lancet Neurology, 4*(3), 149–159.

Sinzig, J., Walter, D., & Doepfner, M. (2009). Attention deficit/hyperactivity disorder in children and adolescents with autism spectrum disorder: Symptom or syndrome? *Journal of Attention Disorders, 13*, 117–126.

Smigielska-Kuzia, J., & Sobaniec, W. (2007). Brain metabolic profile obtained by proton magnetic resonance spectroscopy HMRS in children with Down syndrome. *Advances in Medical Science, 52*(Suppl. 1), 183–187.

State, M. W., Lombroso, P. J., Pauls, D. L., & Leckman, J. F. (2000). The genetics of childhood psychiatric disorders: A decade of progress. *Journal of the American Academy of Child and Adolescent Psychiatry, 39*(8), 946–962.

Subramaniam, B., Naidu, S., & Reiss, A. L. (1997). Neuroanatomy in Rett syndrome: Cerebral cortex and posterior fossa. *Neurology, 48*(2), 399–407.

Sugama, S., Bingham, P. M., Wang, P. P., Moss, E. M., Kobayashi, H., & Eto, Y. (2000). Morphometry of the head of the caudate nucleus in patients with velocardiofacial syndrome (del 22q11.2). *Acta Paediatrica, 89*(5), 546–549.

Sullivan, E. V., & Pfefferbaum, A. (2006). Diffusion tensor imaging and aging. *Neuroscience and Biobehavioral Reviews, 30*(6), 749–761.

Swain, J. E., Scahill, L., Lombroso, P. J., King, R. A., & Leckman, J. F. (2007). Tourette syndrome and tic disorders: A decade of progress. *Journal of American Academy of Child and Adolescent Psychiatry, 46*(8), 947–968.

Tamm, L., Menon, V., Johnston, C. K., Hessl, D. R., & Reiss, A. L. (2002). fMRI study of cognitive interference processing in females with fragile X syndrome. *Journal of Cognitive Neuroscience, 14*(2), 160–171.

Tamm, L., Menon, V., & Reiss, A. L. (2003). Abnormal prefrontal cortex function during response inhibition in Turner syndrome: Functional magnetic resonance imaging evidence. *Biological Psychiatry, 53*(2), 107–111.

Thomas, B., Somasundaram, S., Thamburaj, K., Kesavadas, C., Gupta, A. K., Bodhey, N. K., et al. (2008). Clinical applications of susceptibility weighted MR imaging of the brain—a pictorial review. *Neuroradiology, 50*(2), 105–116.

Tomaiuolo, F., Di Paola, M., Caravale, B., Vicari, S., Petrides, M., & Caltagirone, C. (2002). Morphology and morphometry of the corpus callosum in Williams syndrome: A T1-weighted MRI study. *NeuroReport, 13*(17), 2281–2284.

Van Essen, D. C., Dierker, D., Snyder, A. Z., Raichle, M. E., Reiss, A. L., & Korenberg, J. (2006). Symmetry of cortical folding abnormalities in Williams syndrome revealed by surface-based analyses. *Journal of Neuroscience, 26*(20), 5470–5483.

van Winkel, R., Stefanis, N. C., & Myin-Germeys,

I. (2008). Psychosocial stress and psychosis: A review of the neurobiological mechanisms and the evidence for gene–stress interaction. *Schizophrenia Bulletin, 34*(6), 1095–1105.

Vanhanen, S. L., Puranen, J., Autti, T., Raininko, R., Liewendahl, K., Nikkinen, P., et al. (2004). Neuroradiological findings (MRS, MRI, SPECT) in infantile neuronal ceroid-lipofuscinosis (infantile CLN1) at different stages of the disease. *Neuropediatrics, 35*(1), 27–35.

Vanhanen, S. L., Raininko, R., Autti, T., & Santavuori, P. (1995). MRI evaluation of the brain in infantile neuronal ceroid-lipofuscinosis. Part 2: MRI findings in 21 patients. *Journal of Child Neurology, 10*(6), 444–450.

Vermathen, P., Robert-Tissot, L., Pietz, J., Lutz, T., Boesch, C., & Kreis, R. (2007). Characterization of white matter alterations in phenylketonuria by magnetic resonance relaxometry and diffusion tensor imaging. *Magnetic Resonance Medicine, 58*(6), 1145–1156.

Volpe, U., Federspiel, A., Mucci, A., Dierks, T., Frank, A., Wahlund, L. O., et al. (2008). Cerebral connectivity and psychotic personality traits: A diffusion tensor imaging study. *European Archives of Psychiatry and Clinical Neuroscience, 258*(5), 292–299.

Watson, C., Hoeft, F., Garrett, A. S., Hall, S. S., & Reiss, A. L. (2008). Aberrant brain activation during gaze processing in boys with fragile X syndrome. *Archives of General Psychiatry, 65*(11), 1315–1323.

White, T., Nelson, M., & Lim, K. O. (2008). Diffusion tensor imaging in psychiatric disorders. *Topics in Magnetic Resonance Imaging, 19*(2), 97–109.

Wong, D. F., Brasic, J. R., Singer, H. S., Schretlen, D. J., Kuwabara, H., Zhou, Y., et al. (2008). Mechanisms of dopaminergic and serotonergic neurotransmission in Tourette syndrome: Clues from an in vivo neurochemistry study with PET. *Neuropsychopharmacology, 33*(6), 1239–1251.

Yacubian-Fernandes, A., Palhares, A., Giglio, A., Gabarra, R. C., Zanini, S., Portela, L., et al. (2004). Apert syndrome: analysis of associated brain malformations and conformational changes determined by surgical treatment. *Journal of Neuroradiology, 31*(2), 116–122.

Yacubian-Fernandes, A., Palhares, A., Giglio, A., Gabarra, R. C., Zanini, S., Portela, L., et al. (2005). Apert syndrome: Factors involved in the cognitive development. *Arquivos de Neuro-Psiquiatrica, 63*(4), 963–968.

Yamada, K., Matsuzawa, H., Uchiyama, M., Kwee, I. L., & Nakada, T. (2006). Brain developmental abnormalities in Prader–Willi syndrome detected by diffusion tensor imaging. *Pediatrics, 118*(2), e442–e448.

Zimmerman, R. A. (2005). MRI/MRA evaluation of sickle cell disease of the brain. *Pediatric Radiology, 35*(3), 249–257.

CHAPTER 5

Integrative Developmental Neuropsychology

A General Systems and Social-Ecological Approach to the Neuropsychology of Children with Neurogenetic Disorders

TIMOTHY B. WHELAN
MELISSA J. MATHEWS

The development of children with neurodevelopmental and genetic disorders occurs, as it does for all children, in a dynamic web of exchange. As neuropsychologists, our focus has traditionally been on the pathophysiology of the nervous system and its consequences expressed cognitively, academically, motorically, affectively, and so forth. Our expertise is thus unique in attempting to grasp the meaning of relationships between the brain and behavior, and yet we are at risk of painting clinical portraits of children that are too narrow or monochromatic unless we constantly consider influences at other levels of functioning. In this chapter, selected aspects of the literature on children, illness, and psychosocial functioning are discussed and illustrated with case material.

To set the stage, it is important to emphasize that the prevalence of adjustment difficulties among children with disabling medical conditions is high. It was known as early as the 1980s that these children are at 1½ to 3 times greater risk for behavioral, social, and psychological maladjustment than their healthy peers (Perrin, 1986; Pless, 1984). Results of epidemiological and other studies indicate that children with chronic illness experience lower academic achievement, greater absenteeism, and increased behavioral difficulties such as nervousness and aggression (Butler & Haser, 2006; Hinton, De Vivo, Fee, Goldstein, & Stern, 2004; Howe, Feinstein, Reiss, Molock, & Berger, 1993; Moleski, 2000; Palmer, Reddick, & Gajjar, 2007; Pless & Roghmann, 1971; Rutter, Tizard, & Whitmore, 1970).

Furthermore, when the affected organ—the brain—is itself the organ most intimately related to the capacity to adjust, the prognosis for successful coping drops still further. Rutter, Graham, and Yule (1970) reported from the classic Isle of Wight study that the occurrence of psychiatric disorders among children with non-neurological chronic disease was 11.6%; among those with epilepsy and no other pathology, it was 37.5%; and among children and adolescents with epilepsy associated with organic brain disease, it was 58.3%. Breslau (1985) also noted a higher prevalence of psychological adjustment difficulties among children with brain-based disease than among either healthy children or those with other systemic diseases. More specifically, it has been shown that children with brain-related disorders exhibit higher rates of internalizing disorders than do their nondisabled peers, accompanied by increasing anxiety and social avoidance as they age into adolescence (Estes, Dawson, Sterling, & Munson, 2007; Kuusikko et al., 2008). Children with brain-based developmental disorders and comorbid intellectual disorders may also be at increased risk for externalizing behavior problems, including aggression, hyperactivity, irritability, and self-injurious behaviors (Estes et al., 2007; McClintock, Hall, & Oliver, 2003; Summers, Houlding, & Reitzel, 2004).

A word of caution is nevertheless in order, however: Some seemingly pathological behaviors may actually be adaptive in those with chronic illness (Drotar & Bush, 1985; Van Dongen-Melman & Sanders-Woudstra, 1986). Moreover, not all children are negatively affected, and resiliency may be equally impressive (Stabler, 1988).

OVERARCHING CONCEPTS

It is not unusual in the fields of psychology and medicine to organize a conceptual framework for understanding disease and health within general systems theory—a general science of *wholeness*, examining sets of elements standing in interrelationship (Bertalanffy, 1968). Within this theory, the human organism exists as a hierarchy of systems ranging from the molecular level of the biological realm, to larger organ systems, to cognitive and intrapsychic levels, and on to family and social spheres. It is assumed that these systems are interrelated, that events at one level of the hierarchy have effects up and down the system, and that the system maintains a state of homeostasis during periods of stress or stability. Therefore, because changes at one level have ramifications at many other levels, one may elect to treat the experience of dysphoria by selectively inhibiting serotonin reuptake, or to utilize behavioral techniques with patients who have painful spinal degeneration.

This conceptualization was the basis for seminal writings by George Engel (1977, 1980), which led health care practitioners to the reconceptualization of disease as a biopsychosocial phenomenon, and one can see this influence in the earlier literature on families with illness (Gochman, 1985; Kerns & Curley, 1985; Kerns & Turk, 1985; Leventhal, Leventhal, & Van Nguyen, 1985) and clinical health psychology (Millon, Green, & Meagher, 1982).

In addition to consideration of a general systems organization of the individual, it is important to link our understanding to the developmental psychology of families and children. Bronfenbrenner (1979) has written about *social ecology*, defined as "the study of the relation between the developing human being and the settings and contexts in which that person is actually involved" (Kazak, 1989, p. 26). According to Kazak, who has applied these theories in families of chronically ill children—including children with physical disabilities (Kazak, 1986), phenylketonuria (Kazak, Reber, & Smitzer, 1988), and AIDS (Kazak, 1989)—the presumption in social ecology is that the child is at the center of concentric spheres of influence, with nearby rings representing family, school, and neighborhood, and with more distant impact coming from social values and culture. Again, the impact of events is bidirectional: The child is influenced by the family, for instance, and the family is influenced by the child. Thus, if the father of an adolescent boy with Duchenne muscular dystrophy whose muscles have wasted to the point of personal immobility throws himself into his office work, this may immediately affect the son and his mother, who become occupied with more intimate personal care.

MODELS

As the literature focusing on particular influences such as those described above expanded, some researchers began to assemble models incorporating these various specific of thought. The disability–stress–coping model (Wallander & Varni, 1992; Wallander, Varni, Babani, Banis, & Wilcox, 1989) identifies both risk and resistance factors. Among the former are qualities specific to the disease, such as diagnosis, visibility, and brain involvement. Resistance factors are both within the individual (e.g., competence and effectance motivation) and within the social ecology (e.g., family environment, social support).

In addition to perspectives from social learning and attribution theories, concepts of intrinsic motivation are important. It is generally assumed that humans naturally strive for effective interaction with their environment, and that successful mastery produces feelings of efficacy and competence. These feelings in turn lead to further efforts to master additional tasks (Stipek & Weisz, 1981). However, the situation may not always be so straightforward. In an examination of perceptions of competence among children with genetically based neuromuscular disease, perceptions of physical competence were more closely related to general self-worth than to actual neuropsychological measures of motor output, suggesting that children may make distorted appraisals of components of their functioning in the service of maintaining positive global self-perceptions (Whelan, 1986). In addition, a child's overall perception of psychosocial competence may be largely motivated by striving to maintain global positive self-perceptions. In a study of pediatric patients with cancer in Taiwan (Chao, Chen, Wang, Wu, & Yeh, 2003), parents' views of the children differed from the children's views of themselves. The children perceived no change in terms of academics, friends, temper, and mood; however, parents perceived their children as having a decrease in positive mood and number of friends. The implication is that children with specific neurodevelopmental disorders and chronic illnesses may not follow patterns of intrinsic motivation established in groups of healthy children.

Perhaps the most encompassing of the efforts to organize specific functional components of study is the transactional stress and coping model of adjustment to childhood illness developed by Thompson, Gil, Burbach, Keith, and Kinney (1993a, 1993b), Thompson, Gustafson, Hamlett, and Spock (1992a, 1992b), and Thompson and Gustafson (1996), which is derived from Bronfenbrenner's (1977) ecological–systems theory. As shown in Figure 5.1 and as explained in detail by Thompson, Gustafson, George, and Spock (1994), typical demographic variables are noted, as are unique disease factors. Cognitive processes and coping methods are emphasized, as is family functioning.

Any model of child clinical neuropsychology requires additional complexity because processes of development must be taken into account (Whelan & Walker, 1997). The child is conceptualized on multiple levels standing

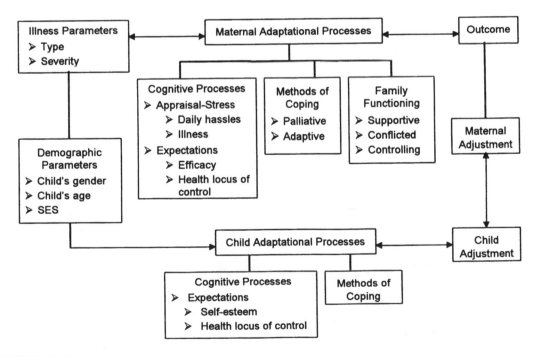

FIGURE 5.1. Transactional stress and coping model of adjustment to chronic illness. From Thompson, Gustafson, George, and Spock (1994). Copyright 1994 by Plenum Publishing Corporation. Reprinted by permission.

in interrelationship, with the hierarchy of systems set in temporal motion. Bernstein and Waber (1990) have also written in this vein on their goal in developmental neuropsychological assessment "not to diagnose deficits in a child, but rather to construct a *Child–World System* that characterizes the reciprocal relationship of the developing children and the world in which that child functions" (p. 312). Their approach was derived from the systemic traditions of Luria and Vygotsky, as well as the Wernerian approach most thoroughly elaborated in neuropsychology by Edith Kaplan. Bernstein and Waber's model considers manifestations of neurological and cognitive structures; neurological and psychological timetables of development; alternative mechanisms (pathways and strategies); and context (including the role of experience and environmental interactions). Any attributions of difficulty are thus shifted from the child to the system, and temporal/developmental processes are considered central.

This shift in thinking—from an individual child with a neurological or genetic disorder to the dysfunction of systems within and surrounding the child—is difficult to maintain. After all, professional training and individual academic interests tend to draw us as clinicians toward specific domains of expertise in our practices. Moreover, there are powerful societal influences on professional thinking and on the thinking of others in the child's social ecology. As described by Resnick (1984a) decades ago, to understand the sociological destiny of those with disability, it is necessary to understand the genesis of attitudes and expectations surrounding them. Resnick reviewed an extensive literature indicating a number of significant, though unfortunate, trends with implications for psychological health, school success, and vocational life. First, children in general may prefer interactions with able-bodied peers rather than with disabled children, and this bias may increase as they get older (Ryan, 1981; Voeltz, 1980; Weinberg, 1976; Weinberg & Santana, 1978). Second, teachers may hold negative attitudes toward disabled students (Good & Brophy, 1978; Martinek & Karper, 1981). Third, there are persistent biases against employment of persons with disabilities (Bender, 1981; Conley, 1973). Such findings

contribute to the concept of *handicapism*, a social experience involving prejudice, stereotype, and discrimination. In essence, says Resnick, there is a social construction of the reality of the disabled individual, in which people and events are "instantaneously assessed in their compatibility or discordance with the mainstream values" (1984a, p. 33). Moreover, parents and professionals may inadvertently occupy an important place in this social construction, as well-intentioned professional assistance sometimes places an identified patient in a position of continual dependence and gratitude within a larger culture that values self-reliance and independence (Sanders, 2006; Smith, English, & Vasek, 2002).

Furthermore, a dilemma exists in regard to the societal doctrine of normality, where certain behaviors and physical characteristics are acceptable and where occurrences outside these bounds are regarded as deviant (Whelan & Walker, 1997). This point of view may not be necessary or helpful for children who are born with genetic or neurodevelopmental disorders, since such children may have always viewed their so-called "deficits" as part of their identity. "Handicap" is thus defined from an "outsider's perspective" (Shontz, 1982), and "insiders" may not perceive that there is anything about their condition to overcome (Massie, 1985). The critical question within such an individual's system shifts to this: How does the individual achieve a complete sense of fulfillment, given his or her uniqueness? The following section considers a child's development, adjustment, and coping in the context of the previously mentioned biopsychosocial models.

CRITICAL VARIABLES

Throughout the 1970s and 1980s, researchers were accumulating data indicating that a conceptual grasp of the nature of coping and adjustment of children with chronic illness encompasses a broad array of factors (see Thompson & Gustafson, 1996, for a detailed review of this research). In the mid-1970s, Monat and Lazarus (1977, p. 3) developed the notion that *stress* is a situation "in which environmental demands, internal demands, or both tax or exceed the adaptive resources of an individual, social system, or tissue system." Researchers began to consider the ways in which children may adjust to these stresses when they involve illness. For example, Pless and Pinkerton (1975) described the concepts of *coping style* and *self-concept* as central to psychological adjustment to illness. They placed these concepts against a backdrop including family characteristics, the social environment, the type of illness, and so forth. Thus not only were they considering biological factors in illness; they were implying that other sections of the child's hierarchy of systems and the social environment in which they exist are important in adaptation. These domains in turn are available as potential targets of intervention.

Adjustment to stress also came under scrutiny, and what clinical psychologists had typically considered defense mechanisms began to be seen in a different, more positive light. Even earlier (Kroeber, 1964), parallels were drawn between more pathological *ego defense mechanisms* (isolation, projection, repression) and *coping mechanisms* (objectivity, empathy, suppression), the latter implying more active and effective attempts to deal with conflict. Lazarus (1983) struggled especially with the conditions under which people may deceive themselves; he tried to distinguish *classical denial* (the negation of impulse, feeling, thought, or external reality) from *partial denial* (a temporary suspension of belief during periods of health crisis). Moreover, he considered it possible that denial may reduce distress when there is no direct action one can take to improve the situation at one point in a disease process, whereas at another point it may be critical to perceive dysfunction accurately in order to take available steps to remedy or rehabilitate the situation.

Apart from traditional models of psychological adjustment, cognitive and developmental psychologists were contributing to the field. For instance, as ideas of self-worth and self-concept were explored, some studies reported that children with chronic illness were negatively affected (e.g., Lineberger, Hernandez, & Brantley, 1984). In contrast, others (e.g., Kellerman, Zeltzer, Ellenberg, Dash, & Rigler, 1980; Simmons et al., 1985) reported no significant group differences between ill and healthy children. In general, though, ill children with neurological involvement seemed at risk for poorer self-concept and lower self-esteem (Lindemann & Stranger, 1981). Below, we discuss those critical variables in the child's biopsychosocial environment—coping, self-concept, school, friends, and family.

Self-Concept, Adjustment, and Coping in the Disabled Child

Not all research suggests that children with chronic illness are at risk for poor self-concept and lowered self-esteem. In a sample of disabled adults, adolescents, and children in India, Ittyerah and Kumar (2007) found that children's self-concept was more positive than that of adolescents and adults. In addition, the correlation between participant ratings of real self and ideal self was high for all age groups. Interestingly, positive self-concepts were related more to internal factors (e.g., healthy coping mechanisms, ways of thinking about their disease), whereas negative self-concepts were related to uncontrollable external factors (e.g., poverty, negative treatment by others).

Furthermore, risk for poor self-concept and self-esteem may depend on a variety of factors particular to the individual, such as gender (Shields, Murdoch, Loy, Dodd, & Taylor, 2006) and level of pain experienced as a result of the disease process (Russo, Miller, Haan, Cameron, & Crotty, 2008). In a meta-analysis regarding the self-concept of children with cerebral palsy (Shields et al., 2006), female children appeared to be at somewhat greater risk than their male counterparts. Poor self-perceptions may spill over into many areas of life, including physical appearance, social acceptance, and athletic and academic competence. Therefore, it may be especially important to be vigilant for these symptoms in young girls with developmental disorders such as cerebral palsy. Furthermore, the experience of pain contributes to lower feelings of academic and behavioral competence than in those children who do not suffer from pain (Russo et al., 2008).

It is difficult to understand those coping and adjustment factors that may be particular to a child without considering them in terms of their environmental contexts. In subsequent sections, we attempt to outline those factors important to a child's development and coping. Individual characteristics and family variables working together may be predictive of outcomes (Majnemer & Mazer, 2004; Schuengel et al., 2006), influencing coping and adjustment beyond the medical facets of the disability.

Venning, Eliot, Wilson, and Kettler (2008) examined qualitative data regarding children's subjective experience of their chronic illness, and outlined some basic principles related to well-being and coping for chronically ill children. First, they found that the experience of a chronic illness contributed to children's sense of both personal and social discomfort, including feeling different from those around them, feeling misunderstood, and wanting to avoid others. Second, these children reported feeling unable to live normally, due to feelings of uncertainty about life and difficulty participating in activities. However, some positive aspects were found, in that the children reported feeling that they had grown personally from the experience (e.g., greater understanding and concern for others), and that in some cases there were rewards such as strengthening the family unit and learning to manage the disease. Regarding facilitation of the children's coping ability, Venning and colleagues found that children might want help adjusting to the diagnosis. Specifically, these children reported needing information about their condition and needing support from others. Cultivating effective coping strategies, accepting, normalizing, and finding meaning in their experience may therefore be helpful in promoting children's adjustment to a chronic disease process.

Social Adjustment and Peer Relationships

Peer support is important because it promotes psychological health and adjustment (Varni, Katz, Colegrove, & Dolgin, 1994; Varni, Rubenfeld, Talbot, & Setoguchi, 1989). In their extensive review of the literature, Thompson and Gustafson (1996, p. 130) concluded that "children with chronic physical illness are at risk for difficulties in social adjustment and peer relationships as well as school adjustment and performance. These difficulties may vary as a function of illness type, with children with illnesses that affect the CNS being at particular risk." Furthermore, children with neurodevelopmental disorders are more likely to exhibit poor social competence that persists over time (Cunningham, Thomas, & Warschausky, 2007; Guralnick, Hammond, Connor, & Neville, 2006). This results in loneliness, being selected for fewer peer interactions, having fewer friends, and feeling less validated and cared for in the friendships they do have (Bauminger, Shulman, & Agam, 2004; Cunningham et al., 2007; Hall & MacGregor, 2000).

With increasing cognitive impairment and comorbid medical issues, social interaction and communication difficulties may increase (Voorman et al., 2006) because the ability to interpret social situations and solve problems may be disrupted (Warschausky, Argento, Berg, & Hurvitz, 2003). Thus comorbid cognitive and medical issues may constitute a predictor of peer relationships in children with neurodevelopmental conditions, whereas this may not be so for children without disabilities (Thomas, Warschausky, Golin, & Meiners, 2008). Higher levels of functioning may provide some protective benefit in social relationships. High-functioning children with autism often report feeling as close to their friends as typically developing children, and report levels of self-concept similar to those of normally developing children in many areas of their lives (e.g., academic ability, appearance, conduct, general self-worth; Bauminger & Kasari, 2000; Bauminger et al., 2004). Greater feelings of self-worth and decreased feelings of loneliness were reported if children also reported higher perceptions of companionship, intimacy, and closeness. Given that children with disabilities often experience loneliness, developing friendships could be key to self-esteem development and maintenance (Bauminger & Kasari, 2000; Bauminger et al., 2004).

When a disease is visibly disfiguring, the consequences may become more dire, with these children being at greater risk of being treated poorly by their peers (Hearst, 2007; Hunt, Burden, Hepper, Stevenson, & Johnston, 2006; Shaw, 1981). The dynamic interplay between the child and the environment is evident in a series of case studies by Hearst (2007). In early childhood, the formation of reciprocal peer relationships is a critical task of development; however, this may be quite difficult for children with a visible disability. The challenge of forming relationships continues into middle childhood with the development of increased cognitive capabilities and awareness. At this stage, children become much more evaluative and self-critical. Bidirectionally, children with a visible disfigurement may become much more critical of themselves at the same time that teasing and bullying begin to increase in frequency.

Targets for Intervention

Children's own attitudes, as well as the attitudes of parents, teachers, and principals, were predictive of whether typically developing fourth- and fifth-grade children would include children with physical disabilities in interactions (Roberts & Lindsell, 1997). These findings not only reflect the bidirectional nature of the biopsychosocial environment, but suggest a potential avenue for intervention. When paraprofessionals are trained to facilitate social interaction between students with severe disabilities and their nondisabled peers, immediate increases in interactions between students occur (Causton-Theoharis & Malmgren, 2005). Encouraging social interaction may have positive benefits for both disabled children and those who are developing normally, which may result in improved social behaviors (Roeyers, 1996). Furthermore, training peers to recognize when a classmate is attempting to communicate with them, teaching them strategies to facilitate the communication and interaction, and instructing them to distribute those efforts over the day resulted in greater positive social interaction for children with moderate developmental disabilities (Goldstein, English, Shafer, & Kaczmarek, 1997). Typically developing children who had more frequent interactions with disabled children displayed higher acceptance and understanding of the children with disabilities (Diamond, 2001). Given that children with developmental disorders are at risk for poor social interactions, it may be useful to focus recommendations on those factors that help increase the probability of success in their environment. Early intervention may be critical, given that a child's interactional patterns tend to remain stable; if they are positive from the beginning, they are likely to remain so over time (Guralnick et al., 2006).

Coping within the Family Unit

Coping within families involves multifaceted, multidirectional interactions among all family members, each influencing the others. Parents of disabled children often report more distress than parents without disabled children do (Yau & Li-Tsang, 1999); however, many families are resilient and report adaptive, pleasant family functioning (Li-Tsang, Yau, & Yuen, 2001; Wilgosh, Scorgie, & Fleming, 2000). In a study utilizing the biopsychosocial approach, parents of children with cystinosis (Spilkin & Ballantyne, 2007) reported both positive and negative aspects in family life. For example, they found that parents saw their children as having an active role in the family, and that the average family unit as a whole was relatively happy. However, many stresses were also reported, such as worry, feeling too much responsibility, and feeling that family life was dictated by the demands of the children with cystinosis.

The picture with regard to sibling relationships and sibling adjustment suggests that family factors are also important. Overarching parent and family factors (e.g., stress, communication, and family cohesiveness) may be predictive of sibling relationships and sibling adjustment (Giallo & Gavidia-Payne, 2006), over and above peer influences (Bellin & Rice, 2007). Furthermore, the degree of conflict experienced within a sibling relationship may influence psychological state (e.g., depression, anxiety), potentially placing the healthy sibling at risk for adverse psychological outcomes (Stocker, Burwell, & Briggs, 2002; Verte, Hebbrecht, & Royers, 2006). However, siblings who characterized their relationship as warm and caring typically experienced more positive outcomes (Kim, McHale, Crouter, & Osgood, 2007; Seltzer, Greenberg, Krauss, Gordon, & Judge, 1997).

The interface between child and maternal adjustment may be especially significant in determining the outcome of the entire family system. Mothers of children with chronic illness may experience higher levels of negative affect, maladjustment, and depression than mothers of healthy children do (Berge, Patterson, & Rueter, 2006; Cadman, Rosenbaum, Boyle, & Offord, 1991; Wallander,

1993). Spilkin and Ballantyne (2007) found that mothers were more likely to endorse the feeling that the children's illness was negatively affecting their families. Mothers were also more likely than fathers to report feelings of worry and the view that the disease was having specific negative consequences for family time and finances. Furthermore, mothers and fathers may have difficulty with different aspects of the illness, which may contribute to reductions in marital satisfaction. Fathers reported more stress regarding father–child interactions, maladaptive behavior, and perceived lack of support, whereas mothers reported feeling more stress about specific aspects of the children's disease (Macias, Saylor, Haire, & Bell, 2007). However, the picture regarding marital satisfaction is mixed, with some studies finding greater marital satisfaction (Kazak, 1987; Taanila, Kokkonen, & Jaervelin, 1996) and some studies finding no differences (Seltzer & Greenberg, 2001). In a meta-analysis, Risdal and Singer (2004) found a small but significant effect for the impact of having a child with a disability on marital adjustment and satisfaction, as it placed slightly more strain on the marital relationship.

In other words, these findings suggest that a child's adjustment is affected by the experiences of maternal stress, relationships with other family members, and the family's environmental support system—a notion directly derived from social-ecological theory. Thompson and colleagues have utilized this model to understand the functioning of children with cystic fibrosis, sickle cell disease, and spina bifida. In the end, after considering the host of models that have now been proposed, Thompson and Gustafson (1996, p. 156) suggested that "stress processes, social support, and parenting are currently the most prominent intervention targets."

Elements of Adaptive and Maladaptive Coping in the Family

In 1977, Moos and Tsu developed a *life crisis* model of adjustment to childhood illness, in which the outcome of crisis precipitated by illness involves cognitive appraisals of the meaning of the illness; adaptive tasks (i.e., dealing with symptoms of the illness and its treatments, maintaining emotional balance and interpersonal relationships); and various aspects of coping skills involving defenses and problem solving. They considered all levels of a systems hierarchy, including physical and illness-related factors, personal background, and social and environmental factors. These elements contribute to a set of adaptive tasks, such as dealing with stress associated with the condition itself and its treatment, maintaining relationships with caregivers, managing distressing emotions, preserving family and social relationships, and anticipating the future.

Moos and Tsu (1977) described coping skills as involving multiple factors, including minimizing the seriousness of the situation, seeking information and support, emphasizing problem-solving skills, and finding meaning in the illness. More recent research discusses these concepts in terms of family coherence, which may also have consequences for a child's health outcomes. Optimal family functioning depends on comprehending the dynamic, shifting responsibilities that will be a part of managing chronic illness in the family. In addition to understanding the difficulties inherent in this position, family members must be able to shift and adapt their own coping strategies to meet these changing dynamics (Spilkin & Ballantyne, 2007). Families high in coherence have the ability to reframe life situations in positive terms (Kelso, French, & Fernandez, 2005; Lee, Lee, Park, Song, & Park, 2004; Walsh, 2003) and believe that they can anticipate and adapt to life events. Of course, this may be commensurate with the severity of a child's disease process and the resources truly available to a family.

With regard to coherence, some patterns were evident in those families ranked as high, medium, and low in coherence (Retzlaff, 2007). All families described an initial crisis phase and feelings that were commensurate with crisis. However, those low in coherence experienced the crisis longer and showed no definitive shift into more adaptive ways of functioning. Families high in coherence eventually began to rely on themselves to manage their situation; however, self-reliance was facilitated by positive social experiences and strong family relationships, allowing them to shift their worldviews and focus on more positive aspects of their lives.

Those lower in coherence tended to focus mostly on the negative stressors.

Similar to a life crisis approach is one that sets a family systems model within a post-traumatic stress framework (Gudmundsdottir, Gudmundsdottir, & Elklit, 2006), given that chronic illnesses may threaten the life and physical ability of the child with the disability. Specifically, Gudmundsdottir and colleagues (2006) looked at those risk (e.g., illness characteristics, dependence for self-care, and psychosocial factors) and resistance (e.g., individual characteristics, social environment, and coping abilities) factors proposed in Wallander and Varni's (1998) disability–stress–coping model of adaptation to chronic illness. The experience of memories as traumatic strongly predicted overall psychological distress and was the only predictor of a measure of overall impact on the family. However, coping ability (i.e., how the process was evaluated and managed) influenced which memories were experienced as traumatic.

In light of the relationship among coping, trauma, distress, and family impact, it is important to consider those factors that contribute to successful coping within families. Retzlaff (2007) studied those factors facilitating adaptive coping and adjustment in families of children with Rett syndrome. He found that many elements described by these families belonged to one of two categories—stressors and resources. Stressors were frequently of the following types: emotional, disease-related, uncertainty, social rejection, lack of access to experts, and social comparison with families of healthy children. Resources facilitating adjustment included material resources, access to information about the disease, and support in the couple, family, social, and professional environments. In addition, changes in families' worldviews were seen as beneficial, and similar results have been found in several other studies (Kelso et al., 2005; King et al., 2005; Poehlman, Clements, Abbeduto, & Farsad, 2005). The take-home message appears to be that successful coping is facilitated by support within the immediate family, the extended family, society, and the medical community. Increased ability to change one's world view and reframe the situation may be aided by these psychosocial factors.

DIAGNOSIS IN SYSTEMS AND SEQUENCES

Adam, the only child of an intact marriage, was born following a full-term pregnancy complicated by maternal dehydration in the first 4 months, which required several hospitalizations. There was no maternal medication or substance abuse. He was delivered following a 37-hour labor, and although there was some meconium staining, there was no need for intensive care. However, at 1 week of age he developed a fever of 105°F with gastrointestinal distress, and the distress persisted. At age 6 months, he was diagnosed with transient hypogammaglobulinemia and *Clostridium difficile*, but treatment did not relieve his chronic diarrhea, pain, and sleep disturbance. He was fed by nasogastric tube and was intermittently hospitalized for 4 years. Additional problems developed, including apnea, very occasional partial and generalized seizures, stroke-like episodes, irregular heart rate, stomach and leg pain, labile emotions, and unpredictable and sometimes markedly dysregulated behaviors. Apart from primary nighttime enuresis, developmental motor and language milestones were met in a timely way. Adam was diagnosed at an early age with an intestinal pseudo-obstruction, and he had a bowel resection. Only shortly before neuropsychological assessment at age 13, muscle biopsies were found to be consistent with mitochondrial myopathy in both mother and child. A gastrostomy tube had recently been placed, and a psychotherapist was consulted in regard to Adam's behavior problems and in order to assist him with relaxation in the face of pain.

It might seem that a child with such a lengthy history of intense medical difficulties, even though an encompassing diagnosis was exceptionally elusive, would receive supportive services without debate or hesitation; however, this was not initially the case. Prior to the diagnosis of mitochondrial myopathy, the combination of vague somatic complaints such as belly or diffuse limb pain, disruptive behavior, and efforts to retreat from the demands of the classroom because of fatigue were suspected to represent a psychiatric condition. More malignant was the suggestion by some health care professionals that this was a case of Munchausen syndrome by proxy. That accusation polarized the situation dramatically: The school system became suspicious and withholding, and the parents became horrified that they were accused of causing their son's symptoms. Suits and charges were considered; the family system reached a point at which instructional efforts (many of which were entirely appropriate) were rejected as unhelpful; and Adam was increasingly drawn away from school.

With the formal diagnosis of mitochondrial myopathy in both Adam and his mother, the parents were no longer accused. They embraced the disorder publicly, with Adam becoming a regional poster child, and with his mother becoming the subject of local newspaper articles on the disorder. The mother continued to believe that her own life was precarious, though this was medically unlikely. Neuropsychological evaluation was able to define the direction of academic modifications acceptable to both the school system and the family, and Adam's functioning in school improved. Interestingly, the family soon withdrew from psychotherapy, which could have helped them negotiate ongoing threats to the adjustment of each individual.

In this case, when all the many influences on Adam within family and social systems recognized his illness, he got better. The improvements did not result from more closely targeted medical treatments at a biological level; rather, the framework of expectations changed, promoting alterations in system relationships and a shift in affect. In a curious way, impotence, guilt, and rage were diminished when the etiology of Adam's compromises changed from a psychological to a genetic realm, and the psychological health of the family system improved when the family members organized around this rare illness. In the sense of social ecology, the family had reached a new state of homeostasis—one seeming more functional to the outsider, though still constrained within what Resnick (1984a, p. 41) has described as the "public relations representative" role, in which the individual or family members have placed upon them(selves) a constant burden of explaining and interpreting.

It should be pointed out that diagnosis is not a one-time event. Kupst and colleagues (1984) have studied different temporal reactions to the diagnosis of a child with cancer, as initial anxiety over the meaning of the diagnosis evolves during the course of actual treatment. Also, familiarity with a diagnosis may result in a more advanced conceptual understanding; for example, a preschooler may apply more sophisticated causal reasoning to a cold than to a newly diagnosed neurological disorder (Siegel, 1988). Similarly, there are developmental considerations in children's understanding of the nature of a genetic or neurodevelopmental disorder, and an extensive literature within pediatric psychology advises health care professionals to take the nature of cognitive functioning in a Piagetian sense into account when they are conveying medical diagnostic and treatment information to children of different ages (Brodie, 1974; Campbell, 1975; Mechanic, 1964; Neuhauser, Amsterdam, Hines, & Steward, 1978; Palmer & Lewis, 1976).

Specific information concerning stages of child cognitive functioning in a pediatric context may be found in Perrin and Gerrity (1981), Whitt, Dykstra, and Taylor (1979), and Bibace and Walsh (1979). In some ways, one can trace children's movement toward more systemic thinking when it comes to their own health. Thus a child functioning at a preoperational level (between ages 2 and 7) may consider illness prevention and recovery to be associated with a rigid set of rules surrounding immediate and concrete perceptions of experience—avoiding the touch of friends, for instance, or staying in bed. Later, with the emergence of formal operations, illness may be conceptualized not only in terms of internal organs whose malfunctions are manifested in external symptoms, but also in terms of psychological events as disease symptoms and causes of internal dysfunction; the etiology of headache, for example, may include too much worry. The concepts of neurodevelopmental and genetic disorders may be especially difficult to communicate when they affect academic adjustment, and many parents and professionals have found the books by Mel Levine (1990, 1993) especially helpful.

PATTERNS OF FAMILY INTERACTION

Susan was a 10-year-old girl with a rare variant of a rare disorder, leukodystrophy, which had resulted in a broad set of impairments.

She became progressively ataxic, often using a wheelchair, but still able to walk slowly and to participate in swimming. Purposeful movements could precipitate striking titubation. There were concerns about early optic atrophy and the development of horizontal nystagmus. Her seizures were under control, but she was struggling to manage abrupt moments of bowel urgency, especially given her motoric difficulties with self-toileting. Her cognitive functioning dropped to the range of mild intellectual disability, and she was placed in a substantially separate special educational setting. The prognosis for this leukodystrophy was grave—gradually progressive and devastating neurological compromises, and a greatly restricted lifespan.

Such disturbances in the growth and development of a child are terrible in and of themselves, as the expressions of a still-forming nervous system in increasing disarray because of progressive white matter disease. At issue in the context of this chapter are the various other influences in the ecology of Susan's life. Susan developed symptoms of anxiety and marked dependence on her mother, and she made increasing demands on her. The mother was the only one she permitted to assist her in toileting, and if she was unavailable (at school, for instance), Susan would not eat beforehand. Separation became difficult. Indeed, she was demanding ever more complex nighttime rituals: She wouldn't go to sleep unless certain lights were on; her mother not only had to be holding Susan's hand, but also had to be facing her daughter with her eyes open until Susan fell asleep; and she was expected to be in the same position when Susan woke. The mother and father had discontinued attending a support group for parents of children with academic special needs because their situation was so profoundly different from that of the other parents.

In considering this system from a traditional neuropsychological point of view, one might focus on Susan herself and on the nature of her cognitive and motor impairments. And, in fact, she did participate with motoric benefit in experimental drug trials coordinated at a national level for the treatment of leukodystrophy. At another level in the system hierarchy, however, she had developed symptoms of an anxiety disorder with an obsessive–compulsive quality,

as well as a measure of almost omnipotent control over parental behaviors. There were minimal efforts to target these symptoms with psychotropic medication because of the potential for negative side effects in a child with great medical complexity. Efforts thus became psychotherapeutic, assisting Susan in decreasing her fears and apprehensions— some of which were primitive, vague, and nameless, but probably connected with fears of death. For the mother, there were efforts to reframe "caring" as taking on the frightening task of letting her daughter "suffer" limit setting, in the service of ultimately acquiring greater autonomy in some things as she became more dependent in others. Nevertheless, it was not the parents' goal to establish a typical set of boundaries and roles in parent–child or marital relationships, simply because they felt they had precious little remaining time with Susan and did not wish to spend it in active conflict. Thus in many ways the family had reached a point of homeostasis. As Kazak (1989, p. 26) points out, the construct of *homeostasis* may be used to appraise patterns of family interaction that serve to maintain a sense of stability. In other words, "reactions that tend to be viewed as maladaptive (i.e., overprotectiveness, enmeshed family relationships, denial) may actually function to maintain a protective homeostasis for the family."

On the other hand, as Kazak (1989) adds, a family system may become too harmful to its members; abuse must be dealt with as an indicator of a family system gone astray, rather than simply as a homeostatic variant. Interventions leading to a new steady state must be implemented, as in the following case.

Gail was a child adopted in infancy by enormously caring parents with gentle temperaments; the adoptive father was a minister and academic at an exclusive liberal arts college. It wasn't long, however, before it was clear that the child's tempo and style of interpersonal interaction were markedly different from the parents.' Gail ultimately developed severe attention-deficit/hyperactivity disorder with highly impulsive features, as well as comorbid symptoms of oppositional defiant disorder. The contrast between parents and child was sharp, and before these diagnoses were made and interventions were implemented, the situation had deteriorated into regular and routine outbursts of harsh, abusive physical punishment of Gail by the father. His image of himself as a progressive-minded humanitarian was shattered as he was pressed beyond the heretofore unsuspected limits of his capacity to manage the situation. The presumption was that this child with a genetically based disorder was being raised by parents who did not share her biology and whose style was so different as to be nearly irreconcilable. Even though a combination of medications, behavioral and psychotherapeutic interventions, and respite greatly diminished the misfit between parents and child, the father still needed to take daily refuge in books and music within his library, which was specially constructed for soundproofing and inaccessibility. In this way, a new homeostasis was created.

Every disease has a natural history, and the capacity of a child's family system to adjust may be a function of the interplay between normal developmental challenges and the nature of the disease's impact. One of the most poignant accounts of this interaction may be found in Resnick (1984b, p. 302):

> While his age cohorts were arguing with parents over the length of their hair, he needed help washing his; while they were resisting doing assigned chores, he was unable to perform any; while they were battling curfews, he needed not only permission, but physical assistance in order to be out. Instead of sharing his peers' increased independence from parents and others, symbolized by mild acting out behaviors, this patient could merely fantasize his acting out, with his illness providing a constant reminder of his chronic dependent status.

As stated earlier, some research has proposed stages of parental adjustment, which at some points and in some families may include the experiences of fear, shock, numbness or detachment, relief, helplessness, denial, sadness or depression, anxiety, and guilt (Drotar, Baskiewicz, Irvin, Kennell, & Klaus, 1975; Hobbs, Perrin, & Ireys, 1985; McCollum, 1981). Readers are referred to Whelan and Walker (1997) for further discussion of these issues within families.

Whereas the field of clinical psychology has often focused on such painful human conditions, it is also possible to consider alternatives, and hope is one. This is a construct with a complex religious and philosophical history: Hope was among the evils in Pandora's box in Greek tradition, and it is a virtue and central theme of the Judeo-Christian message (Menninger, 1963). In more contemporary times, researchers have attempted to operationalize the meaning of hope (Petiet, 1983). It can be classified as a coping mechanism incorporating a realistic appraisal of current circumstances, a future orientation, expectant cognition, optimistic affect, and resultant motivation. As such, hope is seen as a desirable state during medical procedures and rehabilitation (Brackney & Westman, 1992; Brody, 1981; Lillis & Prophit, 1991; Rabkin, Williams, Neugebauer, Reimien, & Goetz, 1990; Ruvelson, 1990).

SOCIAL CULTURE

Information concerning contemporary cultural issues influencing the functioning of children with neurodevelopmental or genetic disorders is available elsewhere; a focus on specific cultures is too broad for the scope of this chapter. We briefly consider cultural factors here in terms of broad-system issues, with the understanding that conceptualizing a child in terms of his or her culture necessarily requires understanding each individual child and family in their own context within their culture. For example, genetic disorders may express themselves according to the culture in which they arise. As a particular instance, in many U.S. cities, a family with Duchenne muscular dystrophy—a relentlessly progressive and ultimately fatal neuromuscular disorder that has an X-linked pattern of inheritance—may be looked upon as pathologically irresponsible if the mother continues to have children, despite genetic counseling concerning the probability of having another affected son. Most families with this disorder in mainstream U.S. culture are therefore relatively small, with few affected individuals. By contrast, in San Antonio, Texas, which has a high density of families with ties to the traditions of the Catholic Church and of Mexico, large families with many affected individuals across the generations may be more common and more likely to be viewed with a charitable eye.

One of the best examples of writing concerning cultural/sociological issues and their political/economic correlates in the care of children with chronic illness is the edited volume by Hobbs and Perrin (1985). In it they organize representative chapters on specific conditions, including some with clear neurodevelopmental consequences (e.g., neuromuscular disease, sickle cell disease, and spina bifida). The direction of that text, as well as of another by Hobbs and colleagues (1985) and of work by Nelson (1984), Resnick (1984a), Silber (1984), and Strax and Wolfson (1984), extends to public policy. These writings probe such topics as health care expenditure, integrating federal programs at the state level, defining parental opportunity costs and other economic costs of disabling conditions, the role of ethics and values in shaping public policy, and preparing professionals for new roles.

The last issue—preparing professionals for new roles—deserves a personal comment. Decades ago, one of us (Whelan) began to lament to colleagues who were supervising doctoral psychology trainees in the same teaching hospital that there was a creeping trend away from a "pure" opportunity for teaching neuropsychological theory and clinical technique, and toward inclusion of more emphasis on the politics of health care delivery. As we in the community of health care providers continue to find our way in the shifting culture of professional politics and managed care, our relationships to our field and to our patients fluctuate, and we remain challenged in our practice and teaching to advocate for excellent patient care within redefined roles and product lines. At this level, we ourselves are in our patients' hierarchy of systems, and they are in ours.

Summary

In this chapter, the professional literature has been reviewed in a highly selective fashion, with the intent of providing the reader with some of the "industry standard" reference points for understanding psychosocial contributions to the development of emotional, educational, and behavioral problems in children with neurodevelopmental and genetic disorders. As well, some specific topics and clinical examples have been included that represent unique personal interests. The field appears robust, not only given its state at the moment, but also in historical context; clearly, the empirical research being derived from existing descriptive models of the ways in which children adjust to illness is much more integrated and detailed than it was when the first edition of this book appeared. Clinically, too, there has been a movement toward improved integration of information from traditional clinical psychology and neuropsychology with practices derived from developmental pediatric psychology and (because of the typical ecology of children) from school psychology. This type of cross-fertilization suggests a productive future and holds promise for continued efforts at excellence in professional practice.

Acknowledgment

We wish to acknowledge the creative and intellectually challenging input of Muireann McNulty in the development of this chapter.

References

Bauminger, N., & Kasari, C. (2000). Loneliness and friendship in high-functioning children with autism. *Child Development, 71,* 447–456.

Bauminger, N., Shulman, C., & Agam, G. (2004). The link between perceptions of self and of social relationships in high-functioning children with autism. *Journal of Developmental and Physical Disabilities, 16,* 193–214.

Bellin, M. H., & Rice, K. M. (2009). Individual, family, and peer factors associated with the quality of sibling relationships in families of youths with spina bifida. *Journal of Family Psychology, 23,* 39–47.

Bender, L. F. (1981). 1980 presidential address to the American Academy for Cerebral Palsy and Developmental Medicine. *Developmental Medicine and Child Neurology, 23,* 103–108.

Berge, J. M., Patterson, J. M., & Rueter, M. (2006). Marital satisfaction and mental health of couples with children with chronic health conditions. *Families, Systems, and Health, 24,* 267–285.

Bernstein, J. H., & Waber, D. P. (1990). Developmental neuropsychological assessment. In A. A. Boulton, G. B. Baker, & M. Hiscock (Eds.), *Neuropsychology: Vol. 17. Neuromethods* (pp. 311–371). Clifton, NJ: Humana Press.

Bertalanffy, L. von. (1968). *General systems theory.* New York: Braziller.

Bibace, R., & Walsh, M. E. (1979). Developmental stages in children's conceptions of illness. In G.

C. Stone, F. Cohen, & N. E. Adler (Eds.), *Health psychology* (pp. 285–301). San Francisco: Jossey-Bass.

Brackney, B. E., & Westman, A. S. (1992). Relationships among hope, psychosocial development, and locus of control. *Psychological Reports, 70*, 864–867.

Breslau, N. (1985). Psychiatric disorder in children with physical disabilities. *Journal of the American Academy of Child Psychiatry, 24*, 87–94.

Brodie, B. (1974). View of healthy children toward illness. *American Journal of Public Health, 64*, 1156–1159.

Brody, H. (1981). Hope. *Journal of the American Medical Association, 246*, 1411–1412.

Bronfenbrenner, U. (1977). Toward an experimental ecology of human development. *American Psychologist, 32*, 513–531.

Bronfenbrenner, U. (1979). *The ecology of human development*. Cambridge, MA: Harvard University Press.

Butler, R. W., & Haser, J. K. (2006). Neurocognitive effects of treatment for childhood cancer. *Mental Retardation and Developmental Disabilities, 12*, 184–191.

Cadman, D., Rosenbaum, P., Boyle, M., & Offord, D. R. (1991). Children with chronic illness: Family and parent demographic characteristics and psychosocial adjustment. *Pediatrics, 87*, 884–889.

Campbell, J. D. (1975). Illness is a point of view: The development of children's concepts of illness. *Child Development, 46*, 92–100.

Causton-Theoharis, J., & Malmgren, K. (2005). Increasing peer interactions for students with severe disabilities via paraprofessional training. *Exceptional Children, 71*(4), 431–444.

Chao, C., Chen, S., Wang, C., Wu, Y., & Yeh, C. (2003). Psychosocial adjustment among pediatric cancer patients and their parents. *Psychiatry and Clinical Neurosciences, 57*, 75–81.

Conley, R. W. (1973). *The economics of mental retardation*. Baltimore: Johns Hopkins University Press.

Cunningham, S. D., Thomas, P. D., & Warschausky, S. (2007). Gender differences in peer relations of children with neurodevelopmental conditions. *Rehabilitation Psychology, 52*, 331–337.

Diamond, K. (2001). Relationships among young children's ideas, emotional understanding, and social contact with classmates with disabilities. *Topics in Early Childhood Special Education, 21*(2), 104–113.

Drotar, D., Baskiewicz, A., Irvin, N., Kennell, J., & Klaus, M. (1975). The adaptation of parents to the birth of an infant with a congenital malformation: A hypothetical model. *Pediatrics, 56*, 710–717.

Drotar, D., & Bush, M. (1985). Mental health issues and services. In N. Hobbs & J. M. Perrin (Eds.), *Issues in the care of children with chronic illness* (pp. 514–550). San Francisco: Jossey-Bass.

Engel, G. (1977). The clinical application of the biopsychosocial model. *American Journal of Psychiatry, 137*, 535–544.

Engel, G. (1980). The need for a new medical model: The challenge for biomedicine. *Science, 196*, 129–136.

Estes, A. M., Dawson, G., Sterling, L., & Munson, J. (2007). Level of intellectual functioning predicts patterns of associated symptoms in school-age children with autism spectrum disorder. *American Journal on Mental Retardation, 112*, 439–449.

Giallo, R., & Gavidia-Payne, S. (2006). Child, parent and family factors as predictors of adjustment for siblings of children with a disability. *Journal of Intellectual Disability Research, 50*, 937–948.

Gochman, D. S. (1985). Family determinants of children's concepts of health and illness. In D. Turk & R. Kerns (Eds.), *Health, illness, and families* (pp. 23–50). New York: Wiley.

Goldstein,, H., English, K. Shafer, K., & Kaczmarek, L. (1997). Interaction among preschoolers with and without disabilities: Effects of across-the-day peer intervention. *Journal of Speech, Language, and Hearing Research, 40*, 33–48.

Good, T., & Brophy, J. (1978). *Looking in classrooms*. New York: Holt, Rinehart & Winston.

Gudmundsdottir, H. S., Gudmundsdottir, D. B., & Elklit, A. (2006). Risk and resistance factors for psychological distress in Icelandic parents of chronically ill children: An application of Wallander and Varni's disability–stress–coping model. *Journal of Clinical Psychology in Medical Settings, 13*, 299–306.

Guralnick, M., Hammond, M., Connor, R., & Neville, B. (2006). Stability, change, and correlates of the peer relationships of young children with mild developmental delays. *Child Development, 77*(2), 312–324.

Hall, L., & McGregor, J. (2000). A follow-up study of the peer relationships of children with disabilities in an inclusive school. *Journal of Special Education, 34*(3), 114–126.

Hearst, D. (2007). Can't they like me as I am?: Psychological interventions for children and young people with congenital visible disfigurement. *Developmental Neurorehabilitation, 10*, 105–112.

Hinton, V. J., De Vivo, D. C., Fee, R., Goldstein, E., & Stern, Y. (2004). Investigation of poor academic achievement in children with Duchenne muscular dystrophy. *Learning Disabilities Research and Practice, 19*, 146–154.

Hobbs, N., & Perrin, J. M. (Eds.). (1985). *Issues in the care of children with chronic illness*. San Francisco: Jossey-Bass.

Hobbs, N., Perrin, J. M., & Ireys, H. T. (1985).

Chronically ill children and their families. San Francisco: Jossey-Bass.

Howe, G. W., Feinstein, C., Reiss, D., Molock, S., & Berger, K. (1993). Adolescent adjustment to chronic physical disorders: I. Comparing neurological and non-neurological conditions. *Journal of Child Psychology and Psychiatry, 14,* 1153–1171.

Hunt, O., Burden, D., Hepper, P., Stevenson, M., & Johnston, C. (2006). Self-reports of psychosocial functioning among children and young adults with cleft lip and palate. *Cleft Palate-Craniofacial Journal, 43,* 598–605.

Ittyerah, M., & Kumar, N. (2007). The actual and ideal concept in disabled children, adolescents, and adults. *Psychology and Developing Societies, 19,* 81–112.

Kazak, A. E. (1986). Families with physically handicapped children: Social ecology and family systems. *Family Process, 25,* 265–281.

Kazak, A. E. (1987). Families with disabled children: Stress and social networks in three samples. *Journal of Abnormal Child Psychology, 15,* 137–146.

Kazak, A. E. (1989). Families of chronically ill children: A systems and social-ecological model of adaptation and challenge. *Journal of Consulting and Clinical Psychology, 57,* 25–30.

Kazak, A. E., Reber, M., & Snitzer, A. (1988). Childhood chronic disease and family functioning: A study of phenylketonuria. *Pediatrics, 81,* 224–230.

Kellerman, J., Zeltzer, L., Ellenberg, L., Dash, J., & Rigler, D. (1980). Psychological effects of illness in adolescence. *Journal of Pediatrics, 97,* 126–131.

Kelso, T., French, D., & Fernandez, M. (2005). Stress and coping in primary caregivers of children with a disability: A qualitative study using the Lazarus and Folkman process model of coping. *Journal of Research in Special Education Needs, 5,* 3–10.

Kerns, R., & Curley, A. (1985). A biopsychosocial approach to illness and the family: Neurological diseases across the life span. In D. Turk & R. Kerns (Eds.), *Health, illness, and families* (pp. 146–182). New York: Wiley.

Kerns, R., & Turk, D. (1985). Behavioral medicine and the family: Historical perspectives and future directions. In D. Turk & R. Kerns (Eds.), *Health, illness, and families* (pp. 338–353). New York: Wiley.

Kim, J.-Y., McHale, S. M., Crouter, A. C., & Osgood, D. W. (2007). Longitudinal linkages between sibling relationships and adjustment from middle childhood through adolescence. *Developmental Psychology, 43,* 960–973.

King, G. A., Zwaigenbaum, L., King, S., Baxter, D., Rosenbaum, P., & Bates, A. (2005). A qualitative investigation of changes in the belief systems of families of children with autism or Down syndrome. *Child: Care, Health, and Development, 32,* 353–369.

Kroeber, T. C. (1964). The coping functions of ego mechanisms. In R. W. White (Ed.), *The study of lives* (pp. 178–198). New York: Atherton.

Kupst, M. J., Schulman, J. L., Maurer, H., Honig, G., Morgan, E., & Fochman, D. (1984). Coping with pediatric leukemia: A two-year follow-up. *Journal of Pediatric Psychology, 9,* 149–163.

Kuusikko, S., Pollock-Wurman, R., Jussila, K., Carter, A. S., Mattila, M. L., Ebeling, H., et al. (2008). Social anxiety in high-functioning children and adolescents with autism and Asperger syndrome. *Journal of Autism and Developmental Disorders, 38,* 1697–1709.

Lazarus, R. S. (1983). The costs and benefits of denial. In S. Breznetz (Ed.), *Denial of stress.* New York: International Universities Press.

Lee, I., Lee, E.-O., Park, Y. S., Song, M., & Park, Y. H. (2004). Concept development of family resilience: A study of Korean families with a chronically ill child. *Journal of Clinical Nursing, 13,* 636–645.

Leventhal, H., Leventhal, E., & Van Nguyen, T. (1985). Reactions of families to illness: Therapeutic models and perspectives. In D. Turk & R. Kerns (Eds.), *Health, illness, and families* (pp. 108–145). New York: Wiley.

Levine, M. (1990). *Keeping a head in school.* Cambridge, MA: Educators.

Levine, M. (1993). *All kinds of minds.* Cambridge, MA: Educators.

Lillis, P. P., & Prophit, P. (1991). Keeping hope alive. *Nursing, 21,* 65–67.

Lindemann, J. E., & Stranger, M. E. (1981). Progressive muscle disorders. In J. E. Lindemann (Ed.), *Psychological and behavioral aspects of physical disability* (pp. 273–300). New York: Plenum Press.

Lineberger, H. P., Hernandez, J. T., & Brantley, H. T. (1984). Self-concept and locus of control in hemophiliacs. *International Journal of Psychiatry in Medicine, 14,* 243–251.

Li-Tsang, C. W. P., Yau, M.K.-S., & Yuen, H. K. (2001). Success in parenting children with developmental disabilities: Some characteristics, attitudes, and adaptive coping skills. *British Journal of Developmental Disabilities, 47,* 61–71.

Macias, M. M., Saylor, C. F., Haire, K. B., & Bell, N. L. (2007). Predictors of paternal versus maternal stress in families of children with neural tube defects. *Children's Health Care, 36,* 99–115.

Majnemer, A., & Mazer, B. (2004). New directions in the outcome evaluation of children with cerebral palsy. *Seminars in Pediatric Neurology, 11,* 11–17.

Martinek, T. J., & Karper, W. B. (1981). Teachers' expectations for handicapped and non-handicapped children in mainstreamed physical education classes. *Perceptual and Motor Skills, S3*, 327–330.

Massie, R. K. (1985). The constant shadow: Reflections on the life of a chronically ill child. In N. Hobbs & J. Perrin (Eds.), *Issues in the care of children with chronic illness*. San Francisco: Jossey-Bass.

McClintock, K., Hall, S., & Oliver, C. (2003). Risk markers associated with challenging behaviours in people with intellectual disabilities: A meta-analytic study. *Journal of Intellectual Disability Research, 47*, 405–416.

McCollum, A. T. (1981). *The chronically ill child: A guide for parents and professionals*. New Haven, CT: Yale University Press.

Mechanic, D. (1964). The influence of mothers on their children's health attitudes and behaviors. *Pediatrics, 33*, 444–453.

Menninger, K. (1963). *The vital balance*. New York: Viking Press.

Millon, T., Green, C., & Meagher, R. (Eds.). (1982). *Handbook of clinical health psychology*. New York: Plenum Press.

Moleski, M. (2000). Neuropsychological, neuroanatomical, and neurophysiological consequences of CNS chemotherapy for acute lymphoblastic leukemia. *Archives of Clinical Neuropsychology, 15*, 603–630.

Monat, A., & Lazarus, R. S. (Eds.). (1977). *Stress and coping: An anthology*. New York: Columbia University Press.

Moos, R. H., & Tsu, U. D. (1977). The crisis of physical illness: An overview. In R. H. Moos (Ed.), *Coping with physical illness* (pp. 3–21). New York: Plenum Press.

Nelson, R. P. (1984). Political and financial issues that affect.the chronically ill adolescent. In R. W. Blum (Ed.), *Chronic illness and disabilities in childhood and adolescence* (pp. 1–15). Orlando, FL: Grune & Stratton.

Neuhauser, C., Amsterdam, B., Hines, P., & Steward, M. (1978). Children's concepts of healing: Cognitive development and locus of control factors. *American Journal of Orthopsychiatry, 48*, 335–341.

Palmer, S. L., Reddick, W. E., & Gajjar, A. (2007). Understanding the cognitive impact on children who are treated for medulloblastoma. *Journal of Pediatric Psychology, 32*, 1040–1049.

Palmer, B., & Lewis, C. (1976). Development of health attitudes and behaviors. *Journal of School Health, 46*, 401–402.

Perrin, J. M. (1986). Chronically ill children: An overview. *Topics in Early Childhood Education, 5*, 1–11.

Perrin, J. M., & Gerrity, P. S. (1981). There's a demon in your belly: Children's understanding of illness. *Pediatrics, 67*, 841–849.

Petiet, C. A. (1983). *Hope: The major predictor of positive resolution after marital loss*. Paper presented at the 91st Annual Conference of the American Psychological Association, Anaheim, CA.

Pless, I. B. (1984). Clinical assessment: Physical and psychological functioning. *Pediatric Clinics of North America, 31*, 33–45.

Pless, I. B., & Pinkerton, P. (1975). *Chronic childhood disorders: Promoting patterns of adjustment*. Chicago: Year Book Medical.

Pless, I. B., & Roghmann, K. J. (1971). Chronic illness and its consequences: Observations based on three epidemiologic surveys. *Journal of Pediatrics, 79*, 351–359.

Poehlmann, J., Clements, M., Abbeduto, L., & Farsad, V. (2005). Family experiences associated with a child's diagnosis of fragile X or Down syndrome: Evidence for disruption and resilience. *Mental Retardation, 43*, 255–267.

Rabkin, J. G., Williams, J. B. W., Neugebauer, R., Remien, R. H., & Goetz, R. (1990). Maintenance of hope in HIV-spectrum homosexual men. *American Journal of Psychiatry, 147*, 1322–1327.

Resnick, M. (1984a). The social construction of disability and handicap in America. In R. W. Blum (Ed.), *Chronic illness and disabilities in childhood and adolescence* (pp. 29–46). Orlando, FL: Grune & Stratton.

Resnick, M. (1984b). The teenager with cerebral palsy. In R. W. Blum (Ed.), *Chronic illness and disabilities in childhood and adolescence* (pp. 299–326). Orlando, FL: Grune & Stratton.

Retzlaff, R. (2007). Families of children with Rett syndrome: Stories of coherence and resilience. *Families, Systems, and Health, 25*, 246–262.

Risdal, D., & Singer, G. H. S. (2004). Marital adjustment in parents of children with disabilities: A historical review and meta-analysis. *Research and Practice for Persons with Severe Disabilities, 29*, 95–103.

Roberts, C. M., & Lindsell, J. S. (1997). Children's attitudes and behavioural intentions towards peers with disabilities. *International Journal of Disability, Development, and Education, 44*, 133–145.

Roeyers, H. (1996). The influence of nonhandicapped peers on the social interactions of children with a pervasive developmental disorder. *Journal of Autism and Developmental Disorders, 23*, 303–320.

Russo, R. N., Miller, M. D., Haan, E., Cameron, I. D., & Crotty, M. (2008). Pain characteristics and their association with quality of life and self concept in children with hemiplegic cerebral palsy identified from a population register. *Clinical Journal of Pain, 24*, 335–342.

Rutter, M., Graham, P., & Yule, W. (1970). *A neuropsychiatry study in childhood* (Clinics in Developmental Medicine Nos. 35 and 36). London: Spastics International/Heinemann Medical.

Rutter, M., Tizard, J., & Whitmore, K. (1970).

Education, health, and behavior: Psychological and medical study of childhood development. London: Longman.

Ruvelson, L. (1990). The tense tightrope: How patients and their therapists balance hope and hopelessness. *Clinical Social Work Journal, 18,* 145–155.

Ryan, K. M. (1981). Developmental differences in reactions to the physically disabled. *Human Development, 24,* 240–256.

Sanders, K. Y. (2006). Overprotection and lowered expectations of persons with disabilities: The unforeseen consequences. *Work, 27,* 181–188.

Schuengel, C., Voorman, J., Stolk, J., Dallmeiher, A., Vermeer, A., & Becher, J. (2006). Self-worth, perceived competence, and behavior problems in children with cerebral palsy. *Disability and Rehabilitation, 28,* 1251–1258.

Seltzer, M. M., & Greenberg, J. S. (2001). Life course impacts of parenting a child with a disability. *American Journal of Mental Retardation, 106,* 265–286.

Seltzer, M. M., Greenberg, J. S., Krauss, M. W., Gordon, R. M., & Judge, K. (1997). Siblings of adults with mental retardation or mental illness: Effects on lifestyle and psychological well-being. *Family Relations, 46,* 395–405.

Shaw, W. C. (1981). The influence of children's dentofacial appearance on their social attractiveness as judged by peers and lay adults. *American Journal of Orthodontics, 79,* 399–415.

Shields, N., Murdoch, A., Loy, Y., Dodd, K. J., & Taylor, N. F. (2006). A systematic review of the self-concept of children with cerebral palsy compared with children without disability. *Developmental Medicine and Child Neurology, 48,* 151–157.

Shontz, F. C. (1982). Adaptation to chronic illness. In T. Millon, C. Green, & R. Meagher (Eds.), *Handbook of clinical health psychology* (pp. 153–172). New York: Plenum Press.

Siegel, M. (1988). Children's knowledge of contagion and contamination as causes of illness. *Child Development, 59,* 1353–1359.

Silber, T. (1984). Ethical considerations in the care of the chronically ill adolescent. In R. W. Blum (Ed.), *Chronic illness and disabilities in childhood and adolescence* (pp. 17–27). Orlando, FL: Grune & Stratton.

Smith, S. G., English, R., & Vasek, D. (2002). Student and parent involvement in the transition process for college freshmen with learning disabilities. *College Student Journal, 36,* 491–504.

Spilkin, A., & Ballantyne, A. (2007). Behavior in children with a chronic illness: A descriptive study of child characteristics, family adjustment, and school issues in children with cystinosis. *Families, Systems, and Health, 25,* 68–84.

Stabler, B. (1988). Perspectives on chronic childhood illness. In B. H. Melamed, K. A. Matthews, D. K. Rauth, B. Stabler, & N. Schneiderman (Eds.), *Child health psychology.* Hillsdale, NJ: Erlbaum.

Stipek, D., & Weisz, J. R. (1981). Perceived personal control and academic achievement. *Review of Educational Research, 51,* 101–137.

Stocker, C.M., Burwell, R. A., & Briggs, M. L. (2002). Sibling conflict in middle childhood predicts children's adjustment in early adolescence. *Journal of Family Psychology, 16,* 50–57.

Strax, T., & Wolfson, S. (1984). Life-cycle crisis of the disabled adolescent and young adult: Implications for public policy. In R. W. Blum (Ed.), *Chronic illness and disabilities in childhood and adolescence* (pp. 47–57). Orlando, FL: Grune & Stratton.

Summers, J. A., Houlding, C. M., & Reitzel, J. M. (2004). Behavior management services for children with autism/PDD: Program description and patterns of referral. *Focus on Autism and Other Developmental Disabilities, 19,* 95–101.

Taanila, A., Kokkonen, J., & Jaervelin, M.-R. (1996). The long-term effects of children's early-onset disability on marital relationships. *Developmental Medicine and Child Neurology, 38,* 567–577.

Thomas, P. D., Warschausky, S., Golin, R., & Meiners, K. (2008). Direct parenting methods to facilitate the social functioning of children with cerebral palsy. *Journal of Developmental and Physical Disabilities, 20,* 167–174.

Thompson, R. J., Gil, K. M., Burbach, D. J., Keith, B. R., & Kinney, T. R. (1993a). Psychological adjustment of mothers of children and adolescents with sickle cell disease: The role of stress, coping methods, and family functioning. *Journal of Pediatric Psychology, 18,* 549–559.

Thompson, R. J., Gil, K. M., Burbach, D. J., Keith, B. R., & Kinney, T. R. (1993b). Role of child and maternal processes in the psychological adjustment of children with sickle cell disease. *Journal of Consulting and Clinical Psychology, 61,* 468–474.

Thompson, R. J., & Gustafson, K. E. (1996). *Adaptation to chronic childhood illness.* Washington, DC: American Psychological Association.

Thompson, R. J., Gustafson, K. E., George, L. K., & Spock, A. (1994). Change over a 12–month period in the psychological adjustment of children and adolescents with cystic fibrosis. *Journal of Pediatric Psychology, 19,* 189–203.

Thompson, R. J., Gustafson, K. E., Hamlett, K. W., & Spock, A. (1992a). Psychological adjustment of children with cystic fibrosis: The role of child cognitive processes and maternal adjustment. *Journal of Pediatric Psychology, 17,* 741–755.

Thompson, R. J., Gustafson, K. E., Hamlett, K. W., & Spock, A. (1992b). Stress, coping, and family functioning in the psychological adjustment of mothers of children with cystic fibrosis. *Journal of Pediatric Psychology, 17*, 573–585.

Van Dongen-Melman, J. E., & Sanders-Woudstra, J. A. (1986). Psychological aspects of childhood cancer: A review of the literature. *Journal of Child Psychology and Psychiatry, 27*, 145–180.

Varni, J. W., Katz, E. R., Colegrove, R., & Dolgin, M. (1994). Percieved social support and adjustment of children with newly diagnosed cancer. *Journal of Developmental and Behavioral Pediatrics, 15*, 20–26.

Varni, J. W., Rubenfeld, L.A., Talbot, D., & Setoguchi, Y. (1989). Determination of self-esteem in children with congenital/acquired limb deficiencies, *Journal of Developmental and Behavioral Pediatrics, 10*, 13–16.

Venning, A., Eliot, J., Wilson, A., & Kettler, L. (2008). Understanding young people's experience of chronic illness: A systematic review. *International Journal of Evidence-Based Healthcare, 6*, 321–336.

Verte, S., Hebbrecht, L., & Royers, H. (2006). Psychological adjustment of siblings of children who are deaf or hard of hearing. *Volta Review, 106*, 89–110.

Voeltz, L. M. (1980). Children's attitudes toward handicapped peers. *American Journal of Mental Deficiency, 84*, 455–464.

Voorman, J. M., Dallmeijer, A. J., Schuengel, C., Knol, D. L., Lankhorst, G. J., & Becher, J. G. (2006). Activities and participation of 9- to 13-year-old children with cerebral palsy. *Clinical Rehabilitation, 20*, 937–948.

Wallander, J. L. (1993). Special section editorial: Current research on pediatric chronic illness. *Journal of Pediatric Psychology, 18*, 7–10.

Wallander, J. L., & Varni, J. W. (1992). Adjustment in children with chronic physical disorders: Programmatic research on a disability–stress–coping model. In A. M. La Greca, L. Siegel, J. L. Wallander, & C. E. Walker (Eds.), *Stress and coping in child health* (pp. 279–298). New York: Guilford Press.

Wallander, J. L., & Varni, J. W. (1998). Effects of pediatric chronic physical disorders on child and family adjustment. *Journal of Child Psychology and Psychiatry, 39*, 29–46.

Wallander, J. L., Varni, J. W., Babani, L., Banis, H. T., & Wilcox, K. T. (1989). Family resources as resistance factors for psychological maladjustment in chronically ill and handicapped children. *Journal of Pediatric Psychology, 14*, 157–173.

Walsh, F. (2003). Family resilience: A framework for clinical practice. *Family Process, 42*, 1–18.

Warschausky, S., Argento, A., Berg, M. L., & Hurvitz, E. (2003). Neuropsychological status and social problems solving in children with congenital and acquired brain dysfunction. *Rehabilitation Psychology, 48*, 250–254.

Weinberg, N. (1976). Social stereotyping of the physically handicapped. *Rehabilitation Psychology, 23*, 115–124.

Weinberg, N., & Santana, R. (1978). Comic books: Champions of the disabled stereotype. *Rehabilitation Literature, 15*, 25–33.

Whitt, J. K., Dykstra, W., & Taylor, C. (1979). Children's conceptions of illness and cognitive development. *Clinical Pediatrics, 18*, 327–339.

Whelan, T. (1986). *Neuropsychological performance, reading achievement, and perceptions of competence in boys with Duchenne muscular dystrophy.* Paper presented at the 14th Annual Meeting of the International Neuropsychological Society, Denver, CO.

Whelan, T., & Walker, M. (1997). Coping and adjustment of children with neurological disorder. In C. Reynolds & E. Fletcher-Janzen (Eds.), *Handbook of clinical child neuropsychology* (2nd ed., pp. 688–711). New York: Plenum Press.

Wilgosh, L., Scorgie, K., & Fleming, D. (2000). Effective life management in parents of children with disabilities: A survey replication and extension. *Developmental Disabilities Bulletin, 28*, 1–14.

Yau, K. M., & Li-Tsang, C. W. P. (1999). Adjustment and adaptation in parents of children with developmental disability in two-parent families: A review of the characteristics and attributes. *British Journal of Developmental Disabilities, 45*, 38–51.

PART II

Disorders Primarily Affecting Learning and Behavior

CHAPTER 6

Learning Disabilities

SAM GOLDSTEIN
ADAM SCHWEBACH
SEAN CUNNINGHAM

Learning disabilities (LD), including reading disabilities, are the most prevalent group of neurobehavioral disorders served in the public schools (U.S. Department of Education, 1994). Researchers find that it is difficult to estimate the prevalence of LD in adults, however (Corley & Taymans, 2002). A genetic component to these disabilities has been found (Astrom, Wadsworth, & De Fries, 2007; Kovas, Haworth, Dale, & Plomin, 2007; Kovas, Haworth, Petrill, & Plomin, 2007; Kovas & Plomin, 2007); therefore, a chapter addressing the neurobehavioral and genetic aspects of LD is an appropriate topic for inclusion in this text. Unlike most other genetic disorders, LD do not constitute a single, relatively well-defined entity or syndrome. Rather, they encompass an extremely heterogeneous group of problems with diverse characteristics that can result from a variety of biological influences, including genetic factors, environmental insults to the brain, and possibly (as recent research on brain development suggests) extreme lack of early environmental stimulation. As a result, the multifaceted field of LD is complex and often contentious, with many competing theories, definitions, diagnostic procedures, and suggested avenues of intervention.

Within the framework of this chapter, it is not possible to describe adequately or attempt to integrate the many competing viewpoints and claims surrounding the construct of LD. This task has admirably been undertaken by other writers in the field, who have approached LD from a broad historical perspective as well as from the viewpoint of best current practices (Lerner, 1993; Mercer, 1991; Swanson, Harris, & Graham, 2003; Torgesen, 1991). This chapter approaches LD from biomedical, neuropsychological, and information-processing perspectives.

THE CONCEPT

LD as a category of human exceptionality evolved from observations of physicians and educators as they studied and attempted to assist children with brain injuries. Alfred Strauss and Laura Lehtinen published their classic work *Psychopathology and Education of the Brain-Injured Child* in 1947. In 1966, Clements, as head of a task force sponsored by the U.S. Department of Health, Education and Welfare, strongly supported use of the term *minimal brain dysfunction*, which became popularized as MBD (Mercer, 1991).

The terms *minimal brain injury* or MBD were used to describe children of normal intelligence who appeared similar to some individuals with known brain injury, in that they exhibited a combination of hard or soft signs of neurological deficiency concomitantly with educational and sometimes behavioral disorders. MBD was believed to be responsible for observed deficits in processes such as auditory and visual perception, symbol learning, short- and long-term memory, concept formation and reasoning, fine and gross motor functions, and integrative functions—deficits resulting in disorders of receptive and expressive language, reading, writing, mathematics, physical skill development, and interpersonal adjustment. In addition, behavioral traits such as distractibility, impulsivity, perseveration, and disinhibition were often found in children with MBD (Cruickshank, Bentzen, Ratzeburg, & Tannhauser, 1961; Fletcher, Shaywitz, & Shaywitz, 1999; Gardner, 1973; Johnson & Myklebust, 1967). Thus, from the first, the field of LD centered around a medical model, with the term MBD being applied to an extremely heterogeneous group of individuals.

Johnson and Myklebust (1967) discussed the limitations of extant terminologies. They suggested that *minimal* was inappropriate to describe individuals whose resulting disabilities had a much greater than minimal impact on their learning functions, and that the words *brain injury* or *brain dysfunction* were viewed as too stigmatizing by many affected individuals and their parents.

In 1963, at a national organizing conference of concerned parents and professionals held in Chicago, Samuel Kirk proposed use of the term *learning disabilities* (LD) (Lerner, 1993). This term was quickly accepted by parents and continued to gain ascendance when federal and state governments adopted it at the time special education services were expanded to include students of average or better intelligence with otherwise unexplained academic learning problems (Mercer, 1991; U.S. Office of Education, 1977). Kirk viewed LD from a psycholinguistic perspective: He proposed that underlying specific deficiencies in central nervous system (CNS) functioning result in deficits in psychoneurological learning processes, which in turn explain observed LD. Drawing on the psycholinguistic-process model of Charles Osgood, Kirk described LD according to learning channels (auditory–verbal or visual–motor), learning levels (rote or conceptual), and specific processes (perception, reception, memory, integration, expression, etc.) (Kirk & Kirk, 1971). More recently, Naglieri and Das (2002), drawing on Luria's model of intellectual processes, have described four critical processes essential for effective learning. Luria's PASS model involves planning, attention, simultaneous processing, and successive processing. Weaknesses in various combinations of these processes have been associated with specific LD (Naglieri & Das, 2002).

Although the view of LD as neurologically based process deficits remained widespread, during the 1970s a behavioral approach to the topic was promulgated. Process deficits were roundly criticized as hypothetical constructs that could not validly or reliably be diagnosed and that had little or no demonstrable relationship to effective interventions (Hammill & Larsen, 1974, 1996; Larsen, Parker, & Hammill, 1982). Proponents of this view advocated criterion-referenced or curriculum-based assessment of a multitude of specific skills, and interventions based on a detailed analysis of the component parts of each skill to be taught/learned, along with ecological analysis and modification of the learning environment. Well-designed and group-validated approaches to curriculum instruction were held to be appropriate and effective for all students, including slow learners, without reference to supposed internal processing deficits or disabilities. This approach, now referred to as *response to intervention*, has become increasingly popular and frequently advocated within special education programs in public schools.

While debate raged, a third approach to understanding and assisting those with LD added a new dimension. Based on research centered at the University of Virginia (Hallahan, 1980) and the University of Kansas (Schumaker, Deshler, Alley, & Warner, 1983), cognitive learning models were applied to the understanding and treatment of LD. Within a cognitive framework, learners are viewed as directing their own learning by focusing on topics and skills that are personally meaningful and by developing active strategies for information acquisition. One outgrowth of cognitive theory has been the holistic or constructivist approach to teaching and learning, including whole-language methods of reading instruction. Although the tenets of cognitive theory have been applied to the population with LD in a number of ways, a major emphasis has been on helping students to develop more reflective, accurate, and efficient approaches to learning tasks (i.e., learning how to learn). Students are taught to consciously employ self-monitoring strategies and effective learning/study strategies. This model, which emphasizes a focus on *how* students learn versus *what* students learn, may have influenced the scientific discipline away from more deficit-based conceptualizations of LD (Wong, 1987).

PREVALENCE

Determining prevalence rates, or the frequency of occurrence, of LD in the population might at first glance appear to be a relatively straightforward process. However, since prevalence rates for any disease or disability are dependent on having a clear-cut definition of the disorder under consideration, and since there is no consensually accepted or experimentally validated definition of LD, the process of determining the prevalence of LD is a quagmire. At the present time, prevalence figures for this nondefinitive disorder or group of disorders cannot be determined precisely and are essentially broad estimates. However, "the DSM-IV-Text Revision does acknowledge that the prevalence of different LD types is difficult to establish because many studies focus on the prevalence of Learning Disorders in general without careful separation into specific Disorders of Reading, Mathematics, or Written Expression" (Corley & Taymans, 2002, p. 55; see American Psychological Association, 2000).

Important considerations regarding the determination of LD prevalence were presented by MacMillan (1993) and Lyon (1996). In a discussion of operationalizing disability definitions MacMillan described *prevalence rate* as referring to the total percentage of the population that is affected by a disorder, while *detection rate* refers to the number of known or identified cases. For LD, prevalence and detection rates may, and indeed probably do, differ. Depending on the stringency of identification criteria, prevalence estimates for LD have varied from as low as 1% to as high as 30% of the school-age population (Lerner, 1993). Mercer (1991) suggested that approximately 1.5% of students might have severe specific LD, while the inclusion of students with mild LD could raise that figure to about 4% or 5%. Other studies focusing on a specific classification of LD have identified 5–8% of school-age children as exhibiting arithmetic disabilities (Geary, 2003) and 5–17.5% as having dyslexia (Shaywitz, 1998). The number of children thought to have some type of LD extends to 4.6 million, only half of whom are receiving special education services (Pastor & Reuben, 2008). The most recent national estimates indicate that 6–9.7% of children suffer from LD (Pastor & Reuben, 2008).

Many factors are associated with what some view as the burgeoning or even epidemic identification rate for LD. These factors can be divided into four groups: those related to definition/classification, available diagnostic instrumentation, systems operation, and sociopolitical realities. The four factors are discussed in detail here because they are central to some of the most important and persistently ineluctable issues in the field of LD.

As mentioned above, the primary factors underlying the widely varying prevalence estimates for LD are lack of a clear-cut definition and lack of classification procedures derived from coherent theory. Lyon (1996) stated: "Valid prevalence estimates depend on a set of criteria for identification that are clear, observable, measurable, and agreed upon" (p. 58). Although research-based theory building in terms of definition and classification is proceeding apace in the areas of phonologically based reading disorders and nonverbal learning disabilities (NLD) (Torgesen, 1993), for the broad field of LD this remains a distant goal. As noted earlier, the concept of LD is multifaceted. Diverse views are engendered by a wide array of associated medical and pedagogical disciplines, including neurology, psychology, neuropsychology, speech and language pathology, optometry, occupational and physical therapy, and education, as manifested through university research, regular education, special education, and private clinical assessment/tutoring. Each profession has its own set of theoretical considerations, methodologies, and predilections. In addition, there is much variability within professional orientations. For example, among public school special education programs, the criteria for designating students as having LD vary widely. Mercer, Forgnone, and Wolking (1976) and Mercer, King-Sears, and Mercer (1990) documented the range of definitions of LD and the lack of agreement in the diagnostic criteria adopted by state boards of education across the United States. The concept of IQ–achievement discrepancy, which is presently the central feature of LD diagnosis in public schools, is operationalized differently by different states, with arbitrary cutoff points for both intellectual level and achievement level. One result of this highly flexible decision making is that the percentage of children designated as having LD differs from state to state, varying from 2.85% to 9.43%—a threefold difference (Reschly & John, 2004).

Another factor affecting the detection rate for LD is the availability of an appropriate range of reliable and valid assessment measures. Although there is much criticism of IQ–achievement discrepancy as the basis for determining presence or absence of LD (Lyon, 1996; MacMillan, 1993; Mather & Roberts, 1994; Stanovich, 1993; Toth & Siegel, 1994; Zigmond, 1993), intelligence and achievement will probably always be essential constructs for understanding individuals with LD, and therefore must be measured as accurately as possible. In addition, to the extent that types of LD are viewed as reflecting specific process deficits or information-processing deficiencies, there must be a variety of well-standardized instruments for quantifying processing strengths and weaknesses. For a given individual, it may be important to assess any of the following: phonemic awareness, phonological segmentation, grammatical and semantic comprehension, rapid automatic naming (quick label retrieval), digit/sentence repetition, oral expression, tactile perception, directional perception, spatial organization, social perception, verbal and nonverbal concept formation, concrete and abstract problem solving, processing speed, and motor coordination in its many forms. Although

there are measures available to assess these constructs, their specificity, adequacy, quality of standardization, and breadth of dissemination are highly variable. The development of psychometrically sound diagnostic instruments remains a primary goal; it will reduce misidentification and eventually have a positive impact on our understanding of the prevalence of LD, as well as specific subtypes of LD.

A third important (though somewhat overlooked) factor affecting LD prevalence rates consists of what MacMillan (1993) has termed *system identification variables*. This factor overlaps to some degree with the fourth factor, the effects of sociopolitical realities. Broadly, system identification encompasses the ecological processes within families, schools, and clinics that increase or decrease the likelihood of a given individual's being referred for evaluation and classified as having LD. Family system variables affecting whether parents seek LD assessment for a child, or whether an individual seeks assessment for him- or herself, may include socioeconomic status (SES), family values regarding educational attainment for males versus females, the presence or absence of comorbid conditions that create additional functional difficulties, the presence or absence of medical insurance coverage, and so forth. Variables within educational systems that influence the prevalence of LD include the educational philosophy of the school system, financial incentives for identification, the nature and quality of basic education provided for all students, class size, training of regular class teachers to accept and deal with diversity, availability of other types of supportive services for students and teachers, training/competence of special education diagnosticians, and the like. LD prevalence rates are also affected by sociopolitical factors, such as increased attention to learning disabilities as a result of public awareness and political advocacy; ambiguity in the definitions and overlap of disability categories; and the social desirability of an LD classification rather than a classification of intellectual disability or mental retardation (Keogh, 1993; MacMillan, 1993). In addition, MacMillan (1993, citing Zigler & Hodapp, 1986) has suggested that for LD "the ratio of detected to undetected cases may (and probably does) vary by age, IQ level, racial group, gender, and socioeconomic status" (p. 143).

Within school populations, data have been gathered on the prevalence of LD by age, race, and gender. A report from the U.S. Department of Education (2007) presented data showing that 1.22% of the students in kindergarten were receiving special education services for LD, whereas 6.49% of fifth graders were receiving such services. Lerner (1993, citing U.S. Department of Education, 1991) reported that the number of children with LD served in special education at each age level increases rapidly from 6 years to 9 years, peaks and levels off for children ages 10–12, and then gradually declines to age 18. Thus it appears that the majority of children with LD are first identified during their primary and intermediate years of elementary school, and that far fewer students are first identified during secondary school. Lerner (1993) has also suggested that the decrease in the number of students with LD served during their teen years may partially be accounted for by the number of teenagers with LD who drop out of school.

The U.S. Office of Civil Rights has been concerned about the number of students from racial and ethnic minority groups who are identified as having disabilities and enrolled in special education. A 1994 survey by that office (cited by Reschly, 1996) reported that a total of 8% of African American students, 6.5% of European American students, and 5.6% of Hispanic students were enrolled in special education under the categories of mild mental retardation, severe emotional disability, and LD. Although African American students may be overrepresented and Hispanic students underrepresented overall, according to this survey the percentage of students from each group categorized as having LD was relatively constant at 5.0% of African Americans, 5.0% of European Americans, and 4.7% of Hispanics.

The prevalence of LD by gender has long been a topic of discussion and concern. Lerner (1993, citing U.S. General Accounting Office, 1981) reported that of the special education students classified as having LD at that time, approximately 72% were boys and 28% were girls. Research studies of individuals with reading disability have typically estimated that the gender ratio of males to females ranges from 2:1 to 5:1

(Huston, 1992). Various explanations have been suggested to account for the preponderance of males with reading disability—for example, genetic factors, factors associated with differences in prenatal brain development, sex-linked differences in hemispheric specialization, postnatal maturational differences, and system identification variables (Kelley, 1993; Pennington, 2009; Thomson, 1990). Research on genetic factors as explanations for these sex differences has been equivocal, with some studies finding no differential genetic etiology between males and females in the development of reading difficulties (Hawke, Wadsworth, & De Fries, 2006). Although some of the variation in male–female prevalence or severity of reading disability can probably be attributed to biological differences, findings from three of the universities in the LD Research Network indicate that nearly equal numbers of males and females manifest dyslexia (Lyon, 1996; Kolata, 1990; Shaywitz, Shaywitz, Fletcher, & Escobar, 1990). Moreover, recent studies have found that there are confounds in the research examining sex differences in the prevalence of dyslexia, making it appear as if more males suffer from the disorder (Berninger, Nielsen, Abbott, Wijsman, & Raskind, 2008).

When prevalence estimates are determined through research-based epidemiological studies in which every child in a given cohort of children is assessed for reading disability, the ratio of males to females is close to 1:1; when estimates are determined through prevalence figures for school-identified or clinic-identified populations based on teacher or parent referral, the ratio of males to females is much higher. System identification variables resulting in gender-based ascertainment bias appear to account for the majority of this difference. As is true for boys in general, boys with reading difficulty display more behavioral problems, including regulation of activity level, than do girls. Since their functional difficulties are more readily perceived as problematic, more boys than girls are referred for assessment, and consequently more are classified to receive special education services (Shaywitz et al., 1990).

Studies of adopted children have shown that diagnoses of LD are four to five times more frequent in this group than in an equivalent group of nonadoptees (Kenny, Baldwin, & Mackie, 1967; Silver, 1970, 1989). Because information about the biological parents of adoptees is often limited or confidential, it is difficult to determine the reasons for the high rate of LD among adopted children.

ETIOLOGY

Background: Neurobiological Findings

From the time of the earliest medical reports describing cases of dyslexia, researchers have viewed LD as stemming from CNS dysfunction, more precisely, from dysfunction of specific portions of the cerebral cortex (Doris, 1986; Huston, 1992). This longstanding presumption is being reinforced and validated by modern cognitive neuroscience. Language-specific processing in areas of the brain surrounded by the sylvian fissure has been associated with a variety of language functions. The temporoparietal cortex receives projections containing but not limited to visual and auditory information. The posterior superior temporal gyrus or Wernicke's area is associated with a variety of language functions, particularly involving comprehension. However, it is probably oversimplistic to describe temporoparietal areas as those responsible for the reception of language and frontal regions as those responsible for expressive language. It is more likely that a distributed network is responsible for full coherence of the language system (Joseph, Nobel, & Eden, 2001).

Positron emission tomography (PET) and functional magnetic resonance imaging (fMRI) have been used extensively to extend our understanding of how specific components of learning map onto the brain (Ghilardi et al., 2000; Grahn, Parkinson, & Owen, 2009; Hubert at al., 2007; Rumsey et al., 1997; Thiel, 2003). As these techniques have become more refined and technologically advanced, our understanding of structural differences implicated in LD has progressed. Despite their limitations, these techniques have revealed much about structures of the brain associated with visual word form (Fritch, Friston, Liddle, & Frackowiak, 1991), orthography (Flowers, Wood, & Nailer, 1991), phonology (Rumsey et al.,

1997), and semantics (Pugh et al., 1996). However, a great deal of variability has been found within and between studies, such that multiple sites within similar regions of the brain have been implicated in these processes (Poeppel, 1996). Moreover, very few functional neuroimaging studies have been conducted specifically with children, in part due to the fact that PET requires the application of radioactive material. At least one study using fMRI has mapped language dominance in children with partial epilepsy, finding results similar to those observed in adults (Hertz-Pannier et al., 1997). Readers interested in an extended discussion of learning and brain imaging are referred to Berninger (2004).

Environmental Factors

The various types of LD have traditionally been viewed as neurological deficits intrinsic to genetic and other biological factors within individuals, and not as problems of environmental origin. However, research has documented the intimate connection between environment and neuroanatomical development (Dawson & Fischer, 1994; Hutenlocher, 1991). The pervasive effects of early environmental programming on the formation and pruning of neural networks, and the theoretical relationship of this process to the occurrence of neurologically based specific LD, are areas that are only beginning to be considered.

The prenatal, perinatal, and postnatal environmental factors associated with brain development and brain injury are best viewed at present as potential causes of LD, due to uncertainties and inconsistences in the relationships among age at onset, the severity of the circumstance or condition, the degree of transient or permanent brain dysfunction, and the broad range of possible effects on learning. For example, clinical studies have documented cases in which major structural deficits (even loss of an entire brain hemisphere) result in few observable signs of LD, whereas many individuals with severe LD have no obvious structural deficits (Bigler, 1992; Satz, 1990). In addition, confounding variables such as SES, parenting style, and early interventions mediate the degree to which a neurological abnormality will result in impaired learning. In many cases of LD, environmental etiology is presumably not a factor. However, in some cases an environmental cause is directly known or fairly certain; in other cases the environmental contribution to etiology is cloudy, involving a subtle interplay of potential factors that may be undocumented or unknown.

Genetic Factors

In the last 40 years, experimental research has provided strong support for genetic factors in some forms of LD. The familial occurrence of reading, spelling, and writing disabilities has been investigated with a variety of methodologies, such as study of family history and pedigree analysis, determination of concordance rates among identical and fraternal twins, comparison of linear regression in reading scores between identical and fraternal twins, and chromosomal analysis of family members.

The earliest widely cited family pedigree study of reading disorder, conducted by Hallgren in 1950 (cited in Pennington, 2009), consisted of a statistical analysis of dyslexia in 112 families. Among first-degree relatives (parents and siblings of an identified child), the risk for co-occurrence of this disorder was 41%, which is much higher than the usual prevalence estimates for the general population of 5–10%. Huston (1992), reporting on Hallgren's study, indicated that of the 112 families, in 90 families one parent had dyslexia; in 3 families both parents had dyslexia; and in 19 families neither parent had dyslexia. Although Hallgren's study has been criticized for methodological flaws, later studies carried out with greater technical precision, such as that of Finucci, Guthrie, Childs, Abbey, and Childs (1976), have found similar familial rates in the range of 35–45%. Finucci (1978) also published a critical review of the early investigations of dyslexia and genetics. More recent studies continue to provide considerable evidence that dyslexia and even dysgraphia have a developmental, genetic influence (Raskind, 2001).

The Colorado Family Reading Study, begun in 1973, compared the reading abilities of 125 children with reading disability (probands) and their family members to 125 matched control children without reading disability and their family members. The total number of subjects in this study was 1,044, making it an extensive family study. The results clearly demonstrated that reading disorders are familial in nature. Scores for siblings of proband subjects were significantly lower than scores for siblings of control subjects on measures of both reading and symbol-processing speed. A similar pattern of significant results was observed for the parents of probands and controls. An interesting finding was that, on average, brothers of probands exhibited significantly more reading impairment than sisters of probands did. Similarly, fathers of probands were, on average, less skilled readers than mothers of probands; however, the score difference between fathers and mothers was less than the score difference between male and female siblings (De Fries, 1991). Although reading disabilities have now conclusively been shown to be familial in nature, familial occurrence suggests but does not demonstrate genetic heritability. Empirical investigations to ascertain the genetic inheritance of LD, specifically reading disability, have included concordance studies of twins, multiple-regression studies of twins, segregation analysis studies, and chromosomal linkage studies.

Comparisons of pairs of identical and fraternal twins have been used to investigate the genetic component of reading disability in the same way that other twin studies have researched the heritability of intelligence and a variety of other personal characteristics. Many twin studies have employed a comparison of concordance rates to test for genetic etiology. A pair of twins is *concordant* for reading disability if both twins have the disability; if just one twin has a reading disability, the pair is *discordant*. Identical twins have an identical genetic makeup, while fraternal twins share about 50% of heritable variation (LaBuda & De Fries, 1990). To the extent that reading disability is genetically determined, the concordance rate for pairs of identical twins should be considerably higher than for pairs of fraternal twins when at least one member of each identical and fraternal pair has been identified as having a reading disability.

Two of the earlier reports of concordance rates for reading disability in twins were those of Hermann (1959) and Zerbin-Rudin (1967). Both of these researchers pooled the findings of smaller previous studies, possibly with some overlap in their reporting of cases. The concordance rates reported by both authors were nearly identical. Their combined data, as reported by Huston (1992), showed an average of 100% concordance for 29 identical twin pairs and about 34% concordance for 67 fraternal twin pairs.

Due to technical differences in the method for determining concordance rates, different authors sometimes report different concordance figures for the same study; that is, some authors report *pairwise* concordance rates, and others report *probandwise* concordance rates. The first method counts each concordant twin pair one time. The latter method considers each member of a concordant pair as a separate research subject, and therefore counts each concordant pair twice. Using probandwise concordance increases the percentage of concordance for both identical and fraternal twin pairs (LaBuda & De Fries, 1990). For example, in the Zerbin-Rudin (1967) study, a pairwise concordance rate for fraternal twin pairs was 34% (12 of 34 cases) as reported by Huston (1992); however, the probandwise concordance rate for those same twin pairs was 52% (24 [12 + 12] of 46 [34 + 12]) cases, as reported by De Fries (1991).

Bakwin (1973) studied 31 pairs of identical and 31 pairs of fraternal twins, finding 84% pairwise concordance for identical twin males and 83% for identical twin females. Interestingly, the pairwise concordance rate for male fraternal twins was 42%, while the rate for female fraternal twins was just 8%. Bakwin also investigated the environmental factors of birthweight and birth order as predictors of reading disability, but found no significant differences between twins with typical reading ability and twins with reading disability on these variables.

Stevenson, Graham, Fredman, and McLoughlin (1987) conducted a large-scale study of the reading and spelling abilities of 285 pairs of 13-year-old twins, who were divided into several subgroups according to type and severity of skill deficiencies. In contrast to other concordance studies of twins, these authors reported relatively similar pairwise concordance rates for identical and fraternal twin pairs (32% and 21%, respectively). Their findings suggest a fairly low level of heritability for reading disorder.

However, with IQ controlled for, Stevenson and colleagues found a strong genetic influence on spelling ability.

The most technologically sound large-scale twin study, the Colorado Twin Study, was begun in 1982 as part of the Colorado Reading Project. With IQ controlled for (Verbal or Performance IQ = 90 or above) and other types of selection criteria in place, the Colorado Study examined reading disability in 101 pairs of identical twins and 114 pairs of fraternal twins. The pairwise concordance rate of 52% for identical twins was lower than for most earlier studies, while the rate for fraternal twins was fairly typical at 33% (LaBuda & De Fries, 1990). Although there is some variation in the concordance figures generated by different studies, on the whole they do provide strong evidence for a genetic factor in the etiology of reading disability.

In the search for the genetic mechanisms underlying reading disability, two primary strategies have been employed: chromosomal linkage studies and segregation analysis. Working from phenotype (clinical manifestation of disability) to genotype (underlying genetic substrate of disability), segregation analysis involves testing all members of affected families for the presence of a reading disorder and then fitting the data to potential models of genetic transmission (e.g., autosomal dominant, autosomal recessive, codominant, or polygenetic models). Pennington and colleagues (1991) after performing segregation analysis on four subject samples, found support for a major-gene model, in which dyslexia in some families is transmitted by one or more dominant or partially dominant genes. They also found support for genetic heterogeneity (i.e., multiple genetic mechanisms in the transmission of dyslexia). Further research with more sophisticated segregation analysis has also pointed toward a major-dominant-gene effect, which occurs frequently (57% of the population) and which, when present, increases an individual's liability for reading problems (Gilger, Vorecki, De Fries, & Pennington, 1994). However, this putative gene is of low penetrance, such that only 3% of individuals having one or two copies of the defective allele demonstrated reading deficits greater than 1.96 standard deviations below the population mean. Nonaffected individuals (43% of the population) with two normal alleles and no copies of the defective allele had an extremely low probability ($p =$ .0027) of being classified as having a reading disability. Genetic links to reading disabilities have been complicated by studies finding that although alleles in specific genes have been linked to reading disabilities, the genes themselves do not contribute (Smith et al., 2001).

Working from genotype to phenotype, linkage studies have been conducted to identify the specific chromosomes and the genetic loci on those chromosomes that are associated with dyslexia. Through cytogenic studies of families in which several persons are identified as having dyslexia, the search for a gene or genes that may cause dyslexia can be narrowed. Smith, Pennington, Kimberling, and Ing (1990) and De Fries and Gillis (1993) have summarized the complex principles of linkage analysis, which involve investigating both the link between marker genes and the disability gene on a chromosome, and the link between that chromosome and the phenotypic occurrence of reading disability.

The pioneering linkage study of Smith, Kimberling, Pennington, and Lubs (1983) found evidence in some families for a link between reading disability and a marker on chromosome 15p. A later study with a larger number of subjects provided additional support for this finding (Smith et al., 1990) and further suggested that the apparent linkage was present in approximately 15–20% of families with multiple cases of reading disability.

A second possible genetic locus for reading disability in families not linked to chromosome 15 was suggested by the observation of the co-occurrence of dyslexia and disorders of the immune system that are coded to the human leukocyte antigen (HLA) region of chromosome 6 (Geschwind & Behan, 1982; Pennington, Smith, Kimberling, Greene, & Haith, 1987; Smith, Kimberling, & Pennington, 1991). Subsequent research to test this hypothesis (Cardon et al., 1994) studied linkage in two independent samples, 126 sibling pairs and 50 fraternal twin pairs, in which at least one member of each pair had a reading disability. Analyses of the reading performance of pairs genotyped for DNA markers localized the reading disability trait to a small region within chromosome 6, between markers D6S109 and D6S1260 (Turic et al., 2003). Other evidence points to the KIAA0319 gene on chromosome 6 as influencing reading ability and susceptibility to dyslexia (Paracchini et al., 2008). In addition, chromosome 15 and the region including D15S146 and D15S994 on chromosome 15 have been linked to reading disabilities (Morris et al., 2000; Schumacher et al., 2008).

A high prevalence of reading disability is found in individuals with abnormalities in sex chromosome karyotypes—the most common of which is the 47,XXY karyotype in males (Klinefelter syndrome), occurring in approximately 1 of 700 to 1 of 1,000 births (Berkow & Fletcher, 1992; Pennington, Bender, Puck, Salbenblatt, & Robinson, 1982). Although such abnormalities are not frequent occurrences in the population with LD, the strong association between some sex chromosome anomalies and reading disorders provides additional evidence for the genetic heterogeneity of reading disability.

There is evidence that reading disability per se is not inherited, but that genetic variations influence specific subskills connected to the reading process. Olson, Wise, Conners, Rack, and Fulker (1989) found significant heritability for a phonological coding task, but not for an orthographic coding task. Pauls (1996) reported genetic linkage studies of individuals with dyslexia and their family members, in which the individuals were assigned to one of four research groups according to the primary deficient process evident in their reading difficulty: phonological segmentation, nonword reading, rapid naming, and single-word identification. Similar to previous findings, phonological segmentation showed linkage to the HLA region of chromosome 6. There was no evidence for a connection between word identification and chromosome 6; however, there was some evidence that the word identification phenotype was tied to a variation in the same portion of chromosome 15 that was first implicated by Smith and colleagues (1983).

In summary, family studies, concordance studies of twins, and multiple-regression studies of twins have shown that reading disabilities run in families, that they are heritable, and that the heritable component is approximately 50%. Presently, segregation analyses point to genetic transmission via the effect of a partially dominant or dominant major gene. Genetic linkage studies have provided strong evidence that in some families and participant populations studied, reading disability is linked to chromosome 6p or chromosome 15p. Both segregation analyses and linkage analyses have led to the conclusion that phenotypic reading disability is genotypically heterogeneous; that is, increased susceptibility to reading disability can be produced by multiple genetic profiles. Furthermore, preliminary evidence suggests that within a single individual, the component processes of reading may be influenced by separate genes at different loci.

SUBTYPING

Although public agencies have primarily chosen to define LD in terms of a discrepancy between achievement and IQ-based estimates of potential achievement, this statistical definition does little to facilitate an understanding of the underlying processes that contribute to successful—and, in this case, unsuccessful—achievement. Although it has been suggested that LD is a broad, nonspecific symptom for which cause must be identified, it has yet to be demonstrated that different causes lead to different types of LD or, for that matter, require different treatments.

The work of Boder (1973) and Bakker (1979), though over 30 years old, exemplifies efforts to classify and identify LD on the basis of educational criteria. Boder described three subtypes of children with reading disabilities: (1) a *dysphonetic* group, lacking word analysis skills and having difficulty with phonetics; (2) a *dyseidetic* group, experiencing impairment in visual memory and discrimination; and (3) a mixed *dysphonetic–dyseidetic* group. The dysphonetic group included two-thirds of those identified as having reading disabilities, with the dyseidetic group constituting approximately 10%. Bakker described *L-type* and *P-type* dyslexias. Children with L-type dyslexia read quickly but made errors of omission, additions, and word mutilation. Those with P-type dyslexia tended to work slowly and to make time-consuming errors involving fragmentations and repetitions.

Among the interesting and promising attempts to define LD are studies involving multivariate analysis. These studies have found that differences between good and poor readers may reflect impairment in minor skills such as oral word rhyming, vocabulary, discrimination of reversed figures, speed of perception for visual forms, and sequential processing (Doehring, 1968). In 1979, Petrauskas and Rourke utilized a factor-analytic method to describe the difficulties of a group of children with deficient reading. They found that these readers' problems fell statistically into four subtypes: (1) primarily verbal problems, (2) primarily visual problems, (3) difficulty with conceptual flexibility and linguistic skills, and (4) no identified specific weakness. The first two groups correspond with the dysphonetic and dyseidetic groups in Boder's analysis. The third may reflect weaker intellectual skills, while the fourth may in fact reflect the long-standing clinical perception that certain children experience achievement problems that may be secondary to non-neurological factors (e.g., emotional disorder).

Mattis, French, and Rapin (1975) identified three distinct subgroups of children with LD, based on a factor analysis. These included (1) children struggling to read as the result of language problems; (2) children with articulation and graphomotor problems affecting academic achievement; and (3) children with visual–spatial or perceptual disorder. The third group displayed better verbal than nonverbal intellectual abilities. Almost 80% of the impaired children fell in the first two groups. Denckla (1972, 1977) reported similar statistics, noting that approximately 16% of children with LD experienced some type of visual–spatial or perceptual–motor problem.

Thus there is a strong tendency among factor-analytic studies to find a large group of children with problems related to verbal weaknesses and a smaller but significant group related to perceptual weaknesses. Joschko and Rourke (1985), based on an analysis of the Wechsler Intelligence Scale for Children, found a clear distinction between children with learning problems stemming from verbal weaknesses and those whose problems stemmed from nonverbal weaknesses.

Satz and Morris (1981) found five distinct groups of children with reading disabilities, again falling along this verbal–nonverbal continuum. These included (1) children with language impairment; (2) those with specific language problems related to naming; (3) those with mixed global language and perceptual problems; (4) those with perceptual–motor impairment only; and (5) an expected group similar to that reported by Petrauskas and Rourke (1979), in which no significant impairments were identified. Some researchers have hypothesized that this last group of children simply has not experienced adequate education to develop essential achievement skills, while others, as noted earlier, suggest an emotional basis for this group of children's problems. Using cluster analysis of a neuropsychological battery, Phillips (1983) identified a fairly similar profile of five subtypes of children with LD, including individuals with normal test scores, auditory processing problems, difficulty with receptive and expressive language, spatial weaknesses, and a global pattern of low test scores.

Rourke (1989) concluded that cluster-analytic studies have identified some association between learning delay and a wide variety of perceptual, linguistic, sequential, and cognitive skills. This finding has been reinforced by the work of others over a 50 year period (see Benton, 1975). According to Swartz (1974), a pattern consisting of depressed scores on four Wechsler subtests, the so-called "ACID" pattern (an acronym for Arithmetic, Coding, Information, and Digit Span subtest), characterizes the weaknesses of most children with LD. Although this view is held by many others (see, e.g., Kaufman, 1997), not all children with LD display this pattern. Children who do, however, are thought to have a particularly poor prognosis for academic performance in reading, spelling, and arithmetic (Ackerman, Dykman, & Peters, 1977). Some researchers have suggested that in a population of children with LD demonstrating this pattern, one subgroup experiences particularly poor auditory–verbal memory and sequencing, while a second group experiences poor visual–spatial abilities. This distinction is similar to that described by Joschko and Rourke (1985). However, Joschko and Rourke reported a further distinction in the ACID pattern by

age between a younger group (5–8 years old) and an older group (9–15 years old). On the basis of an extensive neuropsychological battery, these authors found a distinct pattern of differences resulting in four subtypes. Joschko and Rourke noted that "although the ACID subtypes generated in this research do not differ significantly in terms of level of academic performance, the plots of the factor score profiles for each of the reliable subtests indicate that they have qualitatively different ability profiles which may have practical applications" (p. 77). However, even these authors noted that effective remediation has not been clearly tied to this manner of ability profiling.

The inclusion of LD among the disorders evaluated and diagnosed by the medical and mental health community has been considered an adjunct to formal psychiatric, psychological, or neuropsychological evaluation. However, as it has been recognized that children with LD appear more likely than others to develop psychiatric problems, efforts have been made to refine the clinical diagnosis of learning impairments. The *Diagnostic and Statistical Manual of Mental Disorders*, fourth edition, text revision (DSM-IV-TR) lists four academic skill disorders (American Psychiatric Association, 2000): reading disorder, mathematics disorder, disorder of written expression, and learning disorder not otherwise specified. All four diagnoses require the collection of standardized test data indicating performance substantially below what would be expected from the individual's age, intelligence, and educational experience. According to these loosely definitive criteria, the problem must also interfere with the child's academic performance or activities of daily living. The "not otherwise specified" category reflects LD as an isolated weakness—for example, difficulty with spelling independent of other written language problems. DSM-IV-TR also contains a diagnosis of developmental coordination disorder, reflecting weak gross or fine motor skills that may interfere with academic achievement or daily living but are not due to a specific medical condition. Readers interested in an extensive discussion of subtypes of LD in childhood are referred to Silver and Hagin (1990) or Swanson and colleagues (2003).

A Neuropsychological Model for Assessment

The consensus in current factor-analytic research is that there are two broad groups of skills necessary for efficient learning:

1. *Auditory–verbal processes.* Weaknesses in these areas result in reading disorders and other language-based learning problems.
2. *Visual–motor and perceptual processes.* Weaknesses in these areas may result in reading problems but more likely affect handwriting, mathematics, and certain social skills.

Tables 6.1 and 6.2 present models for conceptualizing these skills and examples of these skills, respectively, in 2 × 2 grids. The model conceptualizes learning skills on rote/automatic and conceptual levels, linguistically and visually.

As it has also been demonstrated that there is a significant but small group of children experiencing achievement problems in the absence of weaknesses in either of these skill sets, professionals are also urged to consider the impact of other factors related to achievement: an environment conducive to learning; problems with attention and impulse control; self-concept as a learner; and other emotional (e.g., depression/anxiety) and behavioral (oppositional defiant disorder, conduct disorder) problems (Goldstein & Mather, 1998).

As Tables 6.1 and 6.2 suggest, language-based types of LD are directly related to impaired language skills, especially those related to phonological processes (Bishop & Adams, 1990; Pennington, 2009; Scarborough, 1990, 1998). A solid body of emerging research suggests that impairments in the capacity to process information sequentially may form the basis of impairments in phonological processing (Naglieri & Das, 2002). Furthermore, for many children, poor comprehension results from poor rote language skills such as inability to distinguish similar sounds, which then leads to poor auditory discrimination and weak phonetics. Problems with verbal short-term memory are also common among individuals with reading impairments. Memory requires phonological skill. Poor readers may experience problems recalling letters, digits, words, or phrases in exact sequence. The majority of children with language-based LD struggle to master basic foundational academic skills; others are capable of learning to read, but when the curriculum begins to accelerate in third or fourth grade and they must read to learn, they struggle as the result of weak conceptual linguistic skills. It is also not surprising that related language-based skills such as spelling and writing are impaired in children with reading disabilities. For many, spelling is even more impaired than reading (Snowling & Hulme, 1991).

Weaknesses in visual–motor skills tend to cause problems with arithmetic and handwriting, often independent of associated reading disability. Included in problems for this group of children are difficulties involving social awareness and judgment. These problems do not appear to be primarily language-based and have been referred to col-

TABLE 6.1. A Model for Conceptualizing Categories of Academic Skills

Auditory–verbal	Visual–motor
Conceptual	
Verbal conceptual skills	Visual, nonverbal conceptual skills
Rote/automatic	
Auditory motor skills	Letter perception
Auditory perception	Spatial organization and nonverbal integration
Rote auditory sequential memory	Rote visual sequential memory and retrieval
Rote and association memory and retrieval	Motor sequencing and fine motor control

Note. Adapted from table prepared by Sally Ingalls. Copyright 1991 by the Neurology, Learning, and Behavior Center, Salt Lake City, Utah. Adapted by permission.

TABLE 6.2. A Model of Conceptualizing Specific Academic and Daily Living Skills

Auditory–verbal	Visual–motor

Conceptual

Auditory–verbal	Visual–motor
• Language semantics: Word meanings, definitions, vocabulary • Listening comprehension: Understanding and memory of overall ideas • Specificity and variety of verbal concepts for oral or written expression • Verbal reasoning and logic	• Social insight and reasoning: Understanding strategies of games, jokes, motives of others, social conventions, tact • Mathematical concepts: Use of 0 in +, –, ×; place value; money equivalencies; missing elements; etc. • Inferential reading comprehension: Getting the main idea, drawing conclusions • Understanding relationship of historical events across time; understanding scientific concepts • Structuring ideas hierarchically; outlining skills • Generalization abilities • Integrating material into a well-organized report

Rote/automatic

Auditory–verbal	Visual–motor
• Early speech; naming objects • Auditory processing; clear enunciation of speech; pronouncing sounds or syllables in correct order • Naming colors • Recalling birthdate, phone number, address, etc. • Saying alphabet and other lists (days, months) in order • Easily selecting and sequencing words with proper grammatical structure for oral or written expression • Discriminating sounds, especially vowels, auditorily; blending sounds to form words; distinguishing words that sound alike (e.g., mine/mind) • Labeling and retrieval of letters, sounds, common syllables, sight words (b/d, her/here) • Phonic spelling • Listening and reading comprehension involving short-term memory, especially for rote facts • Mathematical labeling and retrieval: Counting sequentially; labeling numbers (e.g., 16/60); memory for facts about numbers and sequences of steps for computation (e.g., long division) • Recalling names, dates, and historical facts • Learning and retaining new scientific terminology	• Assembling puzzles and building with construction toys • Social perception and awareness of environment • Time sense: Doesn't ask, "Is this the last recess?" • Remembering and executing correct sequence for tying shoes • Easily negotiating stairs; climbing on play equipment; learning athletic skills; riding bike • Executing daily living skills such as pouring without spilling, spreading a sandwich, dressing self correctly • Using the correct sequence of strokes to form manuscript or cursive letters • Eye–hand coordination for drawing, assembling art projects, and handwriting • Directional stability for top–bottom and left–right tracking • Copying from board accurately • Viewing visual symbols accurately, visual discrimination, directionality, recognizing shapes or forms of words • Spelling: Visual memory for the nonphonetic elements of words

Note. Adapted from table prepared by Sally Ingalls. Copyright 1991 by the Neurology, Learning, and Behavior Center, Salt Lake City, Utah. Adapted by permission.

lectively in the neuropsychology literature as *nonverbal learning disabilities* (NLD) (Pennington, 2009; Rourke, 1989). Children with this pattern have been reported to experience problems with spatial organization, attention to visual detail, procedural skills, and mathematics; problems in shifting psychological set from one operation to another; graphomotor weaknesses; poor factual memory; and poor judgment and reasoning (Rourke, 1985). Neuropsychologists can re-liably conclude that children with NLD experience greatest deficits in visual-perceptual and organizational skills, psychomotor coordination, and complex-tactile perceptual abilities (Harnadek & Rourke, 1994). Finally, it is also suspected that individuals with NLD experience greater internalizing problems related to depression and anxiety than those with language-based LD do. It is unclear whether this pattern contributes to or is a consequence of NLD.

In their PASS model, Naglieri and Das (2002) note characteristic weaknesses in planning and attention processes for youth diagnosed with attention-deficit/hyperactivity disorder (ADHD) receiving diagnoses of ADHD, isolated weaknesses in planning for youth with mathematics LD, and isolated weaknesses in successive processes for youth with phonics-based reading disability. Readers interested in the PASS model are referred to Naglieri (1999).

EVALUATING LD IN THE CONTEXT OF A COMPREHENSIVE NEUROPSYCHOLOGICAL EVALUATION

A number of volumes provide thorough, in-depth models for assessment of LD with myriad tests and batteries. Interested readers are referred to Reynolds and Fletcher-Janzen (2008), Goldstein (1997), and Mather and Goldstein (2008). Because of space limitations, we only briefly review assessment measures in this section. The basic task facing the professional is to answer questions concerning underlying neuropsychological skills essential to learning; both assets and liabilities must be identified. Screening of basic academic skills must also be completed. In many situations, the neuropsychologist can rely upon data collected at school to provide these basic achievement measures. The most widely used battery of such measures, the Woodcock–Johnson III Tests of Achievement (Woodcock, McGrew, & Mather, 2001), is the most comprehensive. It offers by far the most thorough, well-developed assessment of academic skills, and its factor-analytic model fits well with this chapter's discussion of the underlying neuropsychological deficits contributing to LD. Subtest analysis often reveals patterns consistent with verbal, visual, rote, or conceptual weaknesses. Although achievement–intelligence discrepancies are most widely used to identify LD, the issue of high-IQ individuals with average achievement identified as having LD continues to be controversial. An age–achievement discrepancy nonetheless is a good target for the neuropsychologist; a standard deviation and a half below the age mean can be used as a cutoff.

In the absence of a comprehensive battery such as the Woodcock–Johnson III, it is recommended that neuropsychologists address collection of basic achievement data as follows:

1. *Reading.* A measure should be used to obtain single-word reading, reflecting phonetic skills and sight word achievement. An estimate of the ability to read within context and comprehend what is read should also be obtained. Instruments such as the Woodcock–Johnson III Tests of Achievement (Woodcock et al., 2001), the Gilmore (Gilmore & Gilmore, 1968), the Gray Oral Reading Test—Fourth Edition (Wiederholt & Bryant, 2001) or the Test of Reading Comprehension—Fourth Edition (Brown, Wiederholt, & Hammill, 2008) can provide clinicians with these data.

2. *Spelling.* Estimates of sight word memory for spelling and phonetic ability can be analyzed qualitatively with the Wide Range Achievement Test–4 (Wilkinson & Robertson, 2006).

3. *Mathematics.* The Wide Range Achievement Test–4 (Wilkinson & Robertson, 2006) or the Key Math–3 Diagnostic Assessment (Connolly, 2007) can be utilized to generate observations of conceptual versus rote sequential mathematics skills.

4. *Written language.* Written language skills of thematic maturity, vocabulary, capacity to organize ideas, grammar, punctuation, and general execution can be assessed with the Story Composition subtest from the Test of Written Language—Third Edition (Hammill & Larsen, 2009).

COMORBID DISORDERS

Caron and Rutter (1991) have reviewed the concept of psychiatric comorbidity and summarized different scenarios for the existence of either true or artificial comorbidity. As discussed by Lyytinen (1995), the term *comorbidity*, broadly applied, may refer to (1) the co-occurrence of two or more presumably separate neurocognitive disorders; (2) the co-occurrence of two or more independent conditions that are mediated by a common genetic or environmental etiology; (3) conditions, possibly related, that share the same or overlapping risk factors; (4) conditions that co-occur because of the secondary effects of one disorder on the other; (5) comorbid characteristics that combine to define a meaningful syndrome; and (6) conditions that result from interactive combinations of the other five states. The frequently observed comorbid conditions associated with LD illustrate all six types of comorbidity, although in a given instance the specific forms of comorbidity may be questionable or undetermined because of present empirical limitations. In addition, an apparent comorbidity may be a function of the current definitions of LD and the other disorder(s) under consideration or of the diagnostic procedures used for classification, rather than representing a true comorbidity. In addition, it may be unclear whether a given characteristic (e.g., psychosocial deficit) is an integral part of an LD pattern or whether that characteristic constitutes an associated comorbid condition (Lyytinen, 1995).

ADHD is probably the DSM-IV-TR diagnostic category that has the highest rate of comorbidity with LD. Among children diagnosed as having LD, the reported rate of ADHD has generally ranged from 15% (Shaywitz, Fletcher, & Shaywitz, 1992, cited in Lyon, 1996) to as high as 85% (Safer & Allen, 1976); most studies, such as that of Shaywitz and Shaywitz (1987), report a comorbidity figure between 30% and 40%. There have been conflicting views about whether LD and ADHD are independent disorders or whether they are manifestations of the same underlying brain dysfunction. James and Selz (1997) have suggested that due to methodological flaws in accumulated research, this question has not been fully resolved; however, many experts have concluded that although they frequently co-occur, there is strong evidence for the separateness of LD and ADHD (Barkley, 2006; Goldstein, 1997; Pennington, Grossier, & Welsh, 1993; Shaywitz, Fletcher, & Shaywitz, 1995; Silver, 1990). After reviewing several possible mechanisms for the comorbidity of ADHD with dyslexia, Pennington (2009) has suggested that in most cases dyslexia leads to ADHD as a secondary symptom, but that in a small percentage of cases there may be genetic correlation between the two disorders. In examining LD–ADHD comorbidity in twin data, Light, Pennington, Gilger, and De Fries (cited in Lyytinen, 1995) concluded that shared genetic influences account for a substantial portion of the covariance between dyslexia and ADHD.

It is widely believed that both LD and ADHD are comorbid to a greater than average degree with other categories of psychiatric disorders, such as conduct disorder, anxiety disorders, and depression. To date, few methodologically sound studies of populations with well-defined LD have evaluated this premise. Porter and Rourke (1985), using the parent interview Personality Inventory for Children (Wirt, Lachar, Klinedinst, & Seat, 1977) identified four distinct personality patterns or subtypes as characterizing the majority of the children with LD in their study. Of those classified, 44% displayed balanced, well-adjusted social-emotional functioning; 26% exhibited marked internalizing psychological disturbances (depression, anxiety, low social skills); 13% displayed roughly normal personality functioning, but with a high degree of somatic concerns; and 17% exhibited behavioral disturbance reflected in hyperkinetic, aggressive, and antisocial behaviors. Three studies that used the Minnesota Multiphasic Personality Inventory to assess emotional functioning in adults with LD (Balow & Blomquist, 1965; Gregg, Hoy, King, Moreland, & Jagota, 1992; Spreen, 1998, cited by Hooper & Olley, 1996) were consistent in reporting more maladjustment and serious psychopathology (depression, anxiety, social withdrawal, phobias, acting-out tendencies, disorganized thoughts, etc.) in the adults with LD than in their normal counterparts. In contrast, Lamm and Epstein (1992) found few differences in degree of psychopathology between individuals with LD and control subjects who were assessed via a structured rating scale. As reviewed by James and Selz (1997), the emotional consequences of LD may vary by subtype, but conflicting results have been reported. The most widely referenced psychopathology by subtype is the association of significant internalizing problems (including social isolation, anxiety, depression, and suicide) with NLD, or, as it is often termed, right-hemisphere-based LD (Bigler, 1989; Hooper & Olley, 1996; James & Selz, 1997; Rourke, 1989; Voeller, 1986).

"Psychosocial adjustment difficulties frequently are assumed to be the major social-emotional manifestation of learning disabilities" (Hooper & Olley, 1996, p. 170). Two of the earlier and persistent voices underscoring the need for a sociological perspective on LD were those of Kronick (1974, 1976) and Bryan (1974, 1978, 1991). Kronick explored ways in which difficulties with attention, concentration, perception, inference, labeling of emotions, and communication of feelings interfer with identity formation, disrupt family relationships, and produce interactional dysfunction. Bryan (1991) provided a comprehensive review of research on the attitudes of children and adolescents with LD toward themselves, their social competence, their communicative competence, and teachers' judgments of their school behavior. In all areas, with the exception of knowledge of social norms, the students with LD were found to be less socially competent than their normally achieving classmates. Voeller (1986) described children with NLD who often failed to perceive social cues and thus had difficulty correctly interpreting their social environment. These children tended to push and crowd their peers, get into arguments or fights with peers, and have difficulty maintaining friendships. They were frequently considered "strange" or "weird" by their classmates.

Adolsecents with LD are statistically at increased risk for juvenile delinquency and substance abuse, but no causal link has been established between LD and either of these conditions (Morrison & Cosden, 1997). The reported prevalence of LD among juvenile offenders generally ranges from 35% to 65%, but these figures cannot be accepted at face value, due to the methodological limitations of the research. No specific prevalence figures for substance abuse among adolescents with LD were located. The risk for both juvenile delinquency and substance abuse is increased when LD is accompanied by hyperactivity and/or conduct disorder (Morrison & Cosden, 1997).

A number of hypotheses have been proposed to account for the link between LD and juvenile delinquency or substance abuse. The most frequently offered explanations suggest the following: Low self-esteem and stresses associated with school failure lead to delinquency or substance abuse; youth with LD are more susceptible to delinquent acts as a result of impulsivity, limited understanding of cause and effect, or poor social judgment; and young offenders with LD lack the strategic planning skills to avoid being caught or to conceal their behavior when being questioned by legal authorities. A study by Waldie and Spreen (1993) provided some support for the susceptibility hypothesis that for those with LD, comorbid juvenile delinquency is linked to impulsivity and poor judgment. For reviews of the literature on LD, juvenile delinquency, and substance abuse, see Chitsabesan and Bailey (2006), Grigorenko (2006), and Katsiyannis, Ryan, Zhang, and Spann (2008).

After reviewing relevant literature, Polloway, Smith, and Patton (1984) concluded that the social skill deficits observed in children with LD persists into adulthood. In a group of 93 adults diagnosed with LD at the Learning Disabilities Clinic at Northwestern University, 25% expressed concerns about social difficulties (Blalock & Johnson, 1987). Their social problems included difficulties in making and keeping friends, as well as problems related to their specific disabilities (e.g., following and participating in conversational exchanges, locating addresses, dancing, playing cards or word games, writing personal notes and letters, etc.). In general, the adults with NLD experienced the greatest social problems and social isolation, but they were not always aware of their social handicaps.

The frequently cited comorbidity of psychopathology and psychosocial difficulties with LD may result from several different direct or indirect mechanisms or from a dynamic combination of mechanisms. As described by Hooper and Olley (1996), these mechanisms may include the following:

(1) Behavioral disruption that arises directly from abnormal brain activity; (2) heightened exposure to failure, frustration, and social stigma due associated disablties; (3) the possible effects of brain damage or anomalous neurodevelopment on subsequent temperament and personality development; (4) adverse family reactions ranging from overprotection to scapegoating; (5) the individual's own reaction to being handicapped and its effect on his or her actual capacity to cope and compete; and (6) possible adverse effects from treatments themselves (e.g., lack of or poor treatment for specific learning problems) that may restrict normal activities and socialization. (p. 164)

Although individuals with LD are increased risk for psychopathology and psychosocial deficits, there is wide variation in their patterns of social-emotional adjustment, and group findings do not dictate individual outcomes. The majority of children and adults with LD do not exhibit significant emotional disorders and function well in society. Morrison and Cosden (1997) view LD as a risk factor that in and of itself does not predict positive or negative outcomes. They propose that other internal and environmental risk–protective factors interact with the presence of LD to mediate nonacademic outcomes such as emotional adjustment, adolescent problems (e.g., dropping out of school, juvenile delinquency, substance abuse), and adult adaptation. Although the present discussion of social-emotional development and adjustment in persons with LD has been limited in scope, Mercer (1991) and Bender (1994) provide more extensive reviews of these issues.

Two additional types of comorbidity with LD are mentioned here. First, one diagnostic category or subtype of LD may be viewed as comorbid with another. Since reading is an essential educational tool, and since 80% of children identified as having LD have difficulty acquiring reading skills (Lerner, 1993), reading disability or dyslexia is often considered a child's primary deficit, with co-occurring deficits in other skill areas (e.g., mathematics or graphomotor production) considered secondary or comorbid deficits. It is possible for two distinct patterns or subtypes of LD to co-occur; for example, deficits in phonemic awareness and processing can co-occur with deficits in visual–spatial perception and spatial organization, affecting one or more academic skill areas. However, two co-occurring academic deficits (e.g., reading disability and math disability) may actually be manifestations of a single pattern of neurocognitive deficit with a shared information-processing bottleneck that impedes acquisition of skills in both academic areas (Lyytinen, 1995). Lyytinen cites two companion articles (Ackerman & Dykman, 1995; Räsänen & Ahonen, 1995) that examine the co-occurrence of reading and mathematics disorders. Light and De Fries (1995) assessed the genetic and environmental etiologies of comorbid reading and math deficits in identical and fraternal twin pairs. Their data indicated that approximately 26% of observed reading deficit was due to genetic factors that also influenced math performance.

A final category of comorbidity involves LD patterns that are observed in association with specific disorders or genetic syndromes (e.g., Klinefelter syndrome, Turner syndrome, fragile X syndrome, Tourette syndrome, neurofibromatosis, etc.). LD is a frequent concomitant of syndromes associated with sex chromosome aberrations. In Klinefelter syndrome (47,XXY in males), affected individuals are of normal intelligence but frequently demonstrate specific deficits in Verbal IQ, auditory processing, efficient use of language, and reading (Berkow & Fletcher, 1992). Turner syndrome (complete or partial absence of one X chromosome, usually observed in females) affects cognitive and learning processes to a variable degree. A typical phenotypic presentation involves characteristics associated with NLD, such as visual–spatial deficits, weakness in numerical and mathematical understanding, and social learning deficits (Mazzacco, 1996). Additional information about the patterns of learning abilities and LD that accompany specific genetic disorders is presented in other chapters of this text.

Comorbidity in neurocognitive disorders and LD is a complex topic that has received considerable emphasis in the research literature (e.g., Lyytinen, 1995). Future investigations of comorbidity will assist practitioners to view individuals with LD from a more holistic perspective. This should result in greater intervention efforts aimed at modifying the nonacademic risk factors that impede successful long-term outcomes, and at enhancing the protective factors that enhance such outcomes. Furthermore, explorations of comorbidity among LD categories or subtypes will contribute to the all-important process of defining more distinct and empirically defensible LD subtypes. Subtypes of LD comorbid with other conditions have been identified in the contemporary empirical literature (Hendriksen et al., 2007). For instance, recent studies have examined comorbidity of LD with ADHD and autism (Barnard, Muldoon, Hasan, O'Brien, & Stewart, 2008; Karande et al., 2007).

INTERVENTIONS

Since views differ regarding the nature and etiology of LD, views also differ about what constitutes appropriate and effective interventions for individuals with LD. Lyon and Moats (1988) have discussed critical issues in the instruction of students with LD. Numerous authors, representing different theoretical orientations and instructional paradigms, have presented intervention methodologies developed or adapted for pupils with LD. These include the psycholinguistic-process or specific-abilities approach (Johnson & Myklebust, 1967; Kirk & Kirk, 1971); behavioral approaches, including direct instruction and data-based instruction (Lindsley, 1971; Lovitt, 1984; Marston & Tindal, 1995; Wendling & Mather, 2008; White, 1986); cognitive approaches, including constructivism and instruction in learning strategies (Deshler & Lenz, 1989; Mercer, Jordan, & Miller, 1994; Swanson, 1993; Wong et al., 1991; Wong, Graham, Hoskyn, & Berman, 2008); and neuropsychological approaches (D'Amato, Fletcher-Janzen, & Reynolds, 2005; Hooper, Willis, & Stone, 1996; Rourke, Fisk, & Strang, 1986). Mercer (1991) and Lerner (1993) have provided lucid discussions of these instructional approaches and their application to individuals with LD. Mercer and Mercer (1993), Mather (1991), Mather and Jaffe (2002), Lerner (1993), and Mather and Goldstein (2008) outline a broad array of specific teaching strategies and techniques that have been utilized successfully with atypical learners, including those with LD.

Research has led to better development of causal theories of LD and to promising avenues of intervention for the LD subtypes or specific information-processing weaknesses explicated by those theories. According to Torgesen (1993), "The two most completely developed current causal theories of learning disabilities are the nonverbal learning disabilities syndrome ... and the theory of reading disabilities involving limitations in phonological processing" (p. 158).

A great deal of attention and research has been directed toward understanding phonological processing skills and their relation to the development of reading skills (Lyon, 1996; Pennington, 1991; Shaywitz, 1996; Stanovich, 1993; Stanovich & Siegel, 1994; Torgesen, Wagner, & Rashotte, 1994; Wagner & Torgesen, 1987). A number of well-designed longitudinal studies have documented the efficacy of instruction in phonological awareness and/or phonemic analysis and synthesis for the initial development of reading skills and for improving reading in children with reading disabilities (Ball & Blachman, 1988; Blachman, Ball, Black, & Tangel, 1994; Hatcher, Hulme, & Ellis, 1994; Lundberg, Frost, & Petersen, 1988; Storch & Whitehurst, 2002).

At the conclusion of their research report, Hatcher and colleagues (1994) suggest that children differ in their ability to acquire phonological competence, and pose the question of how best to facilitate acquisition of underlying phonological skills. In this critical area of instruction, research-based practices have emerged. Torgesen, Wagner, and Rashotte (1997) have discussed approaches to the prevention and remediation of phonologically-based reading disabilities. Hatcher, Hulme, and Snowling (2004) compared three theoretically based approaches to reading instruction and found that for children at risk of reading failure, direct instruction in phonemic awareness and phoneme–grapheme correspondence had a beneficial effect on the development of reading skills, whereas typically developing children did not require the same explicit instruction to make gains in reading. Research with the Auditory Discrimination in Depth program (Lindemood & Lindemood, 1969) showed that intensive instruction led to significant gains in reading and spelling skills for 281 subjects ages 5–55 years (Truch, 1994). Employing a different approach, Merzenich and colleagues (1996) acoustically modified speech to train sound discrimination abilities in children with language-based learning impairments. Subjects engaged in highly motivating discrimination tasks with speech stimuli altered by a computer algorithm, which stretched the duration or increased the volume of sound elements critical to the discrimination process. After a few weeks' instruction, children in the study markedly improved their ability to discriminate phonemes and recognize both brief and fast sequences of speech stimuli. They also showed significant improvement in language comprehension abilities. Although acoustically modified speech is a logically conceived and an exciting intervention concept, experts in the field of dyslexia and LD, as reported by Travis (1996), have suggested caution in regard to its potential benefits. More recent research has raised further doubts about the efficacy of this intervention (Watson et al., 2003).

Just as well-designed research can validate intervention practices and techniques for LD, it can also identify methods that are contraindicated for many students with LD. In education as a whole and in special education, there continues a great debate about the relative merits of code-oriented versus whole-language approaches to reading instruction (Foorman, 1995). From the available research, most professionals in the field of LD have concluded that when used as the primary mode of instruction, the whole-language method is less effective than structured, explicit instruction in phonics for children with reading disabilities (Iverson & Tunmer, 1993; Learning Disabilities Association, 1995; Liberman & Liberman, 1992; Pressley, 2006; Pressley & Rankin, 1994; Shapiro, 1992; Stanovich, 1994; Torgesen et al., 1994).

SUMMARY

A neuropsychological perspective on LD provides an understanding of the underlying forces that affect rate and level of achievement across academic domains. An increasing body of research is demonstrating not only that brain structures and function influence learning, but that, in a bidirectional manner, achievement over time changes the brain. Neuropsychological assessment has increasingly been utilized in academic settings. A neuropsychological perspective provides an understanding of the reasons why some children struggle academically; pediatric professionals must be well versed in these issues, as well as in general academic assessment and school issues. This chapter has provided an overview of the literature concerning the history, etiology, definition, and evaluation of LD, and of efforts to accelerate achievement for youth with LD.

REFERENCES

Ackerman, P. T., Dykman, R. A., & Peters, J. E. (1977). Teenage status of hyperactive and non-hyperactive learning disabled boys. *American Journal of Orthopsychiatry, 47,* 577–596.

American Psychiatric Association. (2000). *Diagnostic and statistical manual of mental disorders* (4th ed., text rev.). Washington, DC: Author.

Astrom, R. L., Wadsworth, S. J., & De Fries, J. C. (2007). Etiology of the stability of reading difficulties: The longitudinal twin study of reading disabilities. *Twin Research and Human Genetics, 10,* 434–439.

Bakker, D. J. (1979). Hemisphere differences and reading strategies: Two dyslexias? *Bulletin of the Orton Society, 29,* 84–100.

Bakwin, H. (1973). Reading disability in twins. *Developmental Medicine and Child Neurology, 15,* 184–187.

Ball, E. W., & Blachman, B. A. (1988). Phoneme segmentation training: Effect on reading readiness. *Annals of Dyslexia, 38,* 208–225.

Balow, B., & Blomquist, M. (1965). Young adults ten to fifteen years after severe reading disability. *Elementary School Journal, 66,* 44–48.

Barkley, R. A. (2006). *Attention-deficit hyperactivity disorder: A handbook for diagnosis and treatment.* New York: Guilford Press.

Barnard, L., Muldoon, K., Hasan, R., O'Brien, G., & Stewart, M. (2008). Profiling executive dysfunction in adults with autism and comorbid learning disability. *Autism, 12,* 125–141.

Beers, M. H., Porter, R. S., & Jones, T. V. (Eds.). (2006). *The Merck manual of diagnosis and therapy* (18th ed.). Hoboken, NJ: Wiley.

Bender, W. N. (Ed.). (1994). Social-emotional development: The task and the challenge [Special issue]. *Learning Disability Quarterly, 17*(4).

Benton, A. L. (1975). Developmental dyslexia: neurological aspects. In W. J. Friedlander (Ed.), *Advances in neurology* (Vol. 17, pp. 1–47). New York: Raven Press.

Berninger, V. W. (2004). The reading brain in children and youth: A systems approach. In B. Y. L. Wong (Ed.), *Learning about learning disabilities* (pp. 197–248). San Diego, CA: Elsevier Academic Press.

Berninger, V. W., Nielsen, K. H., Abbott, R. D., Wijsman, E., & Raskind, W. (2008). Gender differences in severity of writing and reading disabilities. *Journal of School Psychology, 46,* 151–172.

Bigler, E. D. (1989). On the neuropsychology of suicide. *Journal of Learning Disabilities, 22,* 180–185.

Bigler, E. D. (1992). The neurobiology and neuropsychology of adult learning disorders. *Journal of Learning Disabilities, 25,* 488–506.

Bishop, D. V., & Adams, C. (1990). A prospective

study of the relationship between specific language impairment, phonological disorders and reading disabilities. *Journal of Child Psychology and Psychiatry, 31*(7), 1027–1050.

Blachman, B. A., Ball, E., Black, R., & Tangel, D. (1994). Kindergarten teachers develop phoneme awareness in low-income inner-city classrooms: Does it make a difference? *Reading and Writing: An Interdisciplinary Journal, 6*, 1–17.

Blalock, J. W., & Johnson, D. J. (1987). Primary concerns and group characteristics. In D. J. Johnson & J. W. Blalock (Eds.), *Adults with learning disabilities: Clinical studies* (pp. 31–45). New York: Grune & Stratton.

Boder, E. (1973). Developmental dyslexia: A diagnostic approach based on three atypical reading patterns. *Developmental Medicine and Child Neurology, 15*, 663–687.

Brown, V. L., Wiederholt, J. L., & Hammill, D. D. (2008). *Test of Reading Comprehension—Fourth Edition* (TORC-4). San Antonio, TX: Pearson.

Bryan, T. H. (1974). Peer popularity of learning disabled children. *Journal of Learning Disabilities, 7*, 261–268.

Bryan, T. H. (1978). Social relationships and verbal interaction of learning disabled children. *Journal of Learning Disabilities, 11*, 107–115.

Bryan, T. H. (1991). Social problems and learning disabilities. In B. Y. L. Wong (Ed.), *Learning about learning disabilities* (pp. 195–229). San Diego, CA: Academic Press.

Cardon, L. R., Smith, S. D., Fulker, D. W., Kimberling, W. J., Pennington, B. F., & De Fries, J. C. (1994). Quantitative trait locus for reading disability in chromosome 6. *Science, 266*, 276–279.

Caron, C., & Rutter, M. (1991). Comorbidity in childhood psychopathology: Concepts, issues, and research strategies. *Journal of Child Psychology and Psychiatry, 32*, 1063–1080.

Chitsabesan, P., & Bailey, S. (2006). Mental health, educational, and social needs of young offenders in custody and in the community. *Current Opinion in Psychiatry, 19*, 355–360.

Connolly, A. J. (2007). *Key Math–3 Diagnostic Assessment*. San Antonio, TX: Pearson.

Corley, M., & Taymans, J. (2002). Adults with learning disabilities: A review of the literature. In J. Comings & B. Garner (Eds.), *Annual review of adult learning and literacy: A project of the National Center for the Study of Adult Learning and Literacy* (Vol. 3, pp. 44–83). San Francisco: Jossey-Bass.

Cruickshank, W. M., Bentzen, F. A., Ratzeburg, R. H., & Tannhauser, M. T. (1961). *A teaching method for brain-injured and hyperactive children*. Syracuse, NY: Syracuse University Press.

D'Amato, R. C., Fletcher-Janzen, E., & Reynolds, C. R. (Eds.). (2005). *Handbook of school neuropsychology*. New York: Wiley.

Dawson, G., & Fischer, K. W. (Eds.). (1994).

Human behavior and the developing brain. New York: Guilford Press.

De Fries, J. C. (1991). Genetics and dyslexia: An overview. In M. Snowling & M. Thomson (Eds.), *Dyslexia: Integrating theory and practice* (pp. 3–20). London: Whurr.

De Fries, J. C., & Gillis, J. J. (1993). Genetics of reading disability. In R. Plomin & G. E. McClearn (Eds.), *Nature, nurture, and psychology* (pp. 163–194). Washington, DC: American Psychological Association.

Denckla, M. B. (1972). Clinical syndromes in learning disabilities: The case for splitting versus lumping. *Journal of Learning Disabilities, 5*, 401–406.

Denckla, M. B. (1977). The neurological basis of reading disability. In F. G. Roswell & G. Natchez (Eds.), *Reading disability: A human approach to learning*. New York: Basic Books.

Deshler, D. D., & Lenz, B. K. (1989). The strategies instructional approach. *International Journal of Disability, Development and Education, 36*, 203–224.

Doehring, D. G. (1968). *Patterns of impairment in specific reading disability*. Bloomington: Indiana University Press.

Doris, J. (1986). Learning disabilities. In S. J. Ceci (Ed.), *Handbook of cognitive, social, and neuropsychological aspects of learning disabilities* (Vol. 1, pp. 3–53). Hillsdale, NJ: Erlbaum.

Finucci, J. M. (1978). Genetic considerations in dyslexia. In H. R. Myklebust (Ed.), *Progress in learning disabilities* (Vol. 4, pp. 41–63). New York: Grune & Stratton.

Finucci, J. M., Guthrie, J. T., Childs, A. L., Abbey, H., & Childs, B. (1976). The genetics of specific reading disability. *Annals of Human Genetics 40*, 1–23.

Fletcher, J. M., Lyon, G. R., Fuchs, L. S., & Barnes, M. A. (2006). *Learning disabilities: From identification to intervention*. New York: Guilford Press.

Fletcher, M., Shaywitz, S. E., & Shaywitz, B. A. (1999). Comorbidity of learning and attention disorders: Separate but equal. *Pediatric Clinics of North America, 46*, 885–897.

Flowers, D. L., Wood, F. B., & Nailer, C. E. (1991). Regional cerebral blood flow correlates of language processes in reading disability. *Archives of Neurology, 48*, 637–643.

Foorman, B. R. (1995). Research on the great debate: Code-oriented versus whole-language approaches to reading instruction. *School Psychology Review, 24*, 376–392.

Fritch, D., Friston, K. J., Liddle, P. F., & Frackowiak, R. S. J. (1991). A PET study of word finding. *Neuropsychologia, 29*, 1137–1148.

Gardner, R. A. (1973). *MBD: The family book about minimal brain dysfunction*. New York: Aronson.

Geary, D. C. (2003). Learning disabilities in arithmetic: Problem-solving differences and cognitive deficits. In H. L. Swanson, K. R. Harris, & S. Graham (Eds.), *Handbook of learning disabilities* (pp. 199–212). New York: Guilford Press.

Geschwind, N., & Behan, P. (1982). Left handedness: Association with immune disease migraine and developmental learning disorder. *Proceedings of the National Academy of Sciences USA, 79,* 5097–5100.

Ghilardi, M., Ghez, C., Dhawan, V., Moeller, J., Mentis, M., Nakamura, T., et al. (2000). Patterns of regional brain activation associated with different forms of motor learning. *Brain Research, 871,* 127–145.

Gilger, J. W., Vorecki, I. B., De Fries, J. C., & Pennington, B. F. (1994). Commingling and segregation analysis of reading performance in families of normal reading problems. *Behavior Genetics, 24,* 345–355.

Gilmore, J. V., & Gilmore, E. C. (1968). *Gilmore Oral Reading Test.* New York: Harcourt, Brace.

Goldstein, S. (1997). *Managing attention and learning disorders in late adolescence and adulthood.* New York: Wiley.

Goldstein, S., & Mather, N. (1998). *Overcoming underachieving: An action guide to helping your child succeed in school.* New York: Wiley.

Grahn, J. A., Parkinson, J. A., & Owen, A. M. (2009). The role of the basal ganglia in learning and memory: Neuropsychological studies. *Behavioural Brain Research, 199,* 53–60.

Gregg, N., Hoy, C., King, M., Moreland, C., & Jagota, M. (1992). The MMPI-2 profile of adults with learning disabilities in university and rehabilitation settings. *Journal of Learning Disabilities, 25,* 386–395.

Grigorenko, E. L. (2006). Learning disabilities in juvenile offenders. *Child and Adolescent Psychiatric Clinics of North America, 15,* 353–371.

Hallahan, D. P. (Ed.). (1980). Teaching exceptional children to use cognitive strategies. *Exceptional Education Quarterly, 1,* 1–102.

Hammill, D. D., & Larsen, S. C. (1974). The effectiveness of psychologistic training. *Exceptional Children, 41,* 5–14.

Hammill, D. D., & Larsen, S. C. (2009). *Test of Written Language—Fourth Edition (TOWL-4).* Austin, TX: PRO-ED.

Harnadek, M. C. S., & Rourke, B. P. (1994). Principal identifying features of the syndrome of nonverbal learning disabilities in children. *Journal of Learning Disabilities, 27,* 144–154.

Hatcher, P. J., Helme, C., & Snowling, M. J. (2004). Explicit phoneme training combined with phonic reading instruction helps young children at risk of reading failure. *Journal of Child Psychology and Psychiatry, 45,* 338–358.

Hatcher, P. J., Hulme, C., & Ellis, A. W. (1994). Ameliorating early reading failure by integrating the teaching of reading and phonological skills: The phonological linkage hypothesis. *Child Development, 65,* 41–57.

Hawke, J. L., Wadsworth, S. J., & De Fries, J. C. (2006). Genetic influences on reading difficulties in boys and girls: The Colorado twin study. *Dyslexia: An International Journal of Research and Practice, 12,* 21–29.

Hendriksen, J. G. M., Keulers, E. H., Feron, F. J., Wassenberg, R., Jolles, J., & Vles, J. S. H. (2007). Subtypes of learning disabilities: Neuropsychological and behavioural functioning of 495 children referred for multidisciplinary assessment. *European Child and Adolescent Psychiatry, 16,* 517–524.

Hermann, K. (1959). *Reading disability: A medical study of word-blindness and related handicaps.* Springfield, IL: Thomas.

Hertz-Pannier, L., Gaillard, W. D., Mott, S. H., Cuenod, C. A., Bookheimer, S. Y., Weinstein, S., et al. (1997). Non-invasive assessment of language dominance in children and adolescents with functional MRI: A preliminary study. *Neurology, 48,* 1003–1012.

Hooper, S. R., & Olley, J. G. (1996). Psychological comorbidity in adults with learning disabilities. In N. Gregg, C. Hoy, & A. F. Gay (Eds.), *Adults with learning disabilities: Theoretical and practical perspectives* (pp. 162–183). New York: Guilford Press.

Hooper, S. R., Willis, W. G., & Stone, B. H. (1996). Issues and approaches in the neuropsychological treatment of children with learning disabilities. In E. S. Batchelor & R. S. Dean (Eds.), *Pediatric neuropsychology: Interfacing assessment and treatment for rehabilitation* (pp. 211–247). Boston: Allyn & Bacon.

Hubert, V., Beaunieux, H., Chételat, G., Platel, H., Landeau, B., Danion, J., et al. (2007). The dynamic network subserving the three phases of cognitive procedural learning. *Human Brain Mapping, 28,* 1415–1429.

Huston, A. M. (1992). *Understanding dyslexia: A practical approach for parents and teachers.* Lanham, MD: Madison Books.

Hutenlocher, P. (1991, September 26). *Neural plasticity.* Paper presented at the Brain Research Foundation Women's Council, University of Chicago.

Iverson, S., & Tunmer, W. E. (1993). Phonological processing skills and the Reading Recovery program. *Journal of Educational Psychology, 85,* 112–126.

James, E. M., & Selz, M. (1997). Neuropsychological bases of common learning and behavior problems. In C. R. Reynolds & E. Fletcher-Janzen (Eds.), *Handbook of clinical child neuropsychology* (2nd ed., pp. 157–179). New York: Plenum Press.

Johnson, D., & Myklebust, H. (1967). *Learning*

disabilities: Educational principles and practices. New York: Grune & Stratton.

Joschko, M., & Rourke, B. P. (1985). Neuropsychological subtypes of learning-disabled children who exhibit the ACID pattern on the WISC. In B. P. Rourke (Ed.), *Neuropsychology of learning disabilities: Essentials of subtype analysis* (pp. 65–88). New York: Guilford Press.

Joseph, J., Noble, K., & Eden, G. (2001). The neurobiological basis of reading. *Journal of Learning Disabilities, 34,* 566–579.

Karande, S., Satam, N., Kulkarni, M., Sholapurwala, R., Chitre, A., & Shah, N. (2007). Clinical and psychoeducational profile of children with specific learning disability and co-occurring attention-deficit hyperactivity disorder. *Indian Journal of Medical Sciences, 61,* 639–647.

Kasiyannis, A., Ryah, J. B., Zhang, D., & Spann, A. (2008). Juvenile delinquency and recidivism: The impact of academic achievement. *Reading and Writing Quarterly: Overcoming Learning Difficulties, 24,* 177–196.

Kaufman, A. S. (1997). *Intelligent testing with the WISC-III* (4th ed.). New York: Wiley.

Kavale, K. A., & Forness, S. R. (2003). Learning disability as a discipline. In H. L. Swanson, K. R. Harris, & S. Graham (Eds.), *Handbook of learning disabilities* (pp. 76–93). New York: Guilford Press.

Kelley, D. B. (1993). Androgens and brain development: Possible contributions to developmental dyslexia. In A. M. Galaburda (Ed.), *Dyslexia and development: Neurobiological aspects of extraordinary brains* (pp. 21–41). Cambridge, MA: Harvard University Press.

Kenny, T., Baldwin, R., & Mackie, J. B. (1967). Incidence of minimal brain injury in adopted children. *Child Welfare, 46,* 24–29.

Keogh, B. K. (1993). Linking purpose and practice: Social-political and developmental perspectives on classification. In G. R. Lyon, D. B. Gray, J. F. Kavanaugh, & N. A. Krasnegor (Eds.), *Better understanding learning disabilities: New views from research and their implications for education and public policies* (pp. 311–323). Baltimore: Brookes.

Kirk, S. A., & Kirk, W. D. (1971). *Psycholinguistic learning disabilities: Diagnosis and remediation.* Urbana: University of Illinois Press.

Kolata, G. (1990, August 22). Studies dispute view of dyslexia, finding girls as afflicted as boys. *New York Times,* pp. Al, B9.

Kovas, Y., Haworth, C. M. A., Dale, P., & Plomin, R. (2007). The genetic and environmental origins of learning abilities and disabilities in the early school years. *Monographs of the Society for Research in Child Development, 72*(3), 1–160.

Kovas, Y., Haworth, C. M. A., Petrill, S., A., & Plomin, R. (2007). Mathematical ability of 10–year-old boys and girls: Genetic and environmental

etiology of typical and low performance. *Journal of Learning Disabilities, 40,* 554–567.

Kovas, Y., & Plomin, R. (2007). Learning abilities and disabilities: Generalist genes, specialist environments. *Current Directions in Psychological Science, 16,* 284–288.

Kronick, D. (1974). Some thoughts on group identification and social needs. *Journal of Learning Disabilities, 7,* 144–147.

Kronick, D. (1976). The importance of a sociological perspective toward learning disabilities. *Journal of Learning Disabilities, 9,* 115–119.

LaBuda, M. C., & De Fries, J. C. (1990). Genetic etiology of reading disability: Evidence from a twin study. In G. T. Pavlidis (Ed.), *Perspectives on dyslexia: Vol. 1. Neurology, neuropsychology, and genetics* (pp. 47–76). New York: Wiley.

Lamm, O., & Epstein, R. (1992). Specific reading impairments: Are they to be associated with emotional difficulties? *Journal of Learning Disabilities, 25,* 605–615.

Larsen, S. C., Parker, R. M., & Hammill, D. D. (1982). Effectiveness of psycholinguistic training: A response to Kavale. *Exceptional Children, 49,* 60–66.

Learning Disabilities Association. (1995, July–August). Thyroid function and learning disabilities: Is there a connection? *Learning Disabilities Association Newsbriefs, 30*(4), 17.

Lerner, J. W. (1993). *Learning disabilities: Theories, diagnosis, and teaching strategies* (6th ed.). Boston: Houghton Mifflin.

Liberman, I. Y., & Liberman, A. M. (1992). Whole language versus code emphasis: Underlying assumptions and their implications for reading instruction. In P. B. Gough, L. C. Ehri, & R. Treiman (Eds.), *Reading acquisition* (pp. 343–365). Hillsdale, NJ: Erlbaum.

Light, J. G., & De Fries, J. C. (1995). Comorbidity of reading and mathematics disabilities: Genetic and environmental etiologies. *Journal of Learning Disabilities, 28,* 96–106.

Lindemood, C., & Lindemood, P. (1969). *Auditory discrimination in depth.* Boston: Teaching Resources.

Lindsley, O. R. (1971). Precision teaching in perspective: An interview. *Teaching Exceptional Children, 3,* 114–119.

Lovitt, T. C. (1984). *Tactics for teaching.* Columbus, OH: Merrill.

Lundberg, I., Frost, J., & Petersen, O. (1988). Effects of an extensive program for stimulating phonological awareness in preschool children. *Reading Research Quarterly, 23*(3), 263–283.

Lyon, G. R. (1996). Learning disabilities. *The Future of Children, 6*(1), 54–76.

Lyon, G. R., & Moats, L. (1988). Critical issues in the instruction of the learning disabled. *Journal of Consulting and Clinical Psychology, 56,* 830–835.

Lyytinen, H. (1995). Comorbidity and developmental neurocognitive disorders. *Developmental Neuropsychology, 11*(3), 269–273.

MacMillan, D. L. (1993). Development of operational definitions in mental retardation: Similarities and differences with the field of learning disabilities. In G. R. Lyon, D. B. Gray, J. F. Kavanaugh, & N. A. Krasnegor (Eds.), *Better understanding learning disabilities: New views from research and their implications for education and public policies* (pp. 117–152). Baltimore: Brookes.

Marston, D., & Tindal, R. (1995). Performance monitoring. In A. Thomas & J. Grimes (Eds.), *Best practices in school psychology—III* (pp. 597–608). Washington, DC: National Association of School Psychologists.

Mather, N. (1991). *An instructional guide to the Woodcock–Johnson Psycho-Educational Battery—Revised.* Brandon, VT: Clinical Psychology.

Mather, N., & Goldstein, S. (2008). *Learning disabilities and challenging behaviors* (2nd ed.). Baltimore: Brookes.

Mather, N., & Jaffee, L. E. (2002). *Woodcock–Johnson III: Reports, recommendations, and strategies.* New York: Wiley.

Mather, N., & Roberts, R. (1994). Learning disabilities: A field in danger of extinction? *Learning Disabilities Research and Practice, 9*(1), 49–58.

Mattis, S., French, J., & Rapin, I. (1975). Dyslexia in children and young adults: Three independent neuropsychological syndromes. *Developmental Medicine and Child Neurology, 17,* 150–163.

Mazzacco, M. (1996). Social and academic learning disabilities in children with identified genetic syndromes. In G. R. Lyon (Chair), *Critical discoveries in learning disabilities: A summary of findings by NIH research programs in learning disabilities.* Workshop conducted at the International Conference of the Learning Disability Association, Dallas, TX.

Mercer, C. D. (1991). *Students with learning disabilities* (4th ed.). New York: Macmillan.

Mercer, C. D., Forgnone, C, & Wolking, W. D. (1976). Definitions of learning disabilities used in the United States. *Journal of Learning Disabilities, 9,* 376–386.

Mercer, C. D., Jordan, K. & Miller, S. P. (1994). Implications of constructivism, for teaching math to students with moderate to mild disabilities. *Journal of Special Education, 28,* 290–306.

Mercer, C. D., King-Sears, P., & Mercer, A. R. (1990). Learning disabilities definitions and criteria used by state education departments. *Learning Disabilities Quarterly, 13,* 141–152.

Mercer, C. D., & Mercer, A. R. (1993). *Teaching students with learning problems* (4th ed.). New York: Maxwell Macmillan.

Merzenich, M. M., Jenkins, W. M., Johnston, P., Schreiner, C., Miller, S. L., & Tellal, P. (1996). Temporal processing deficits of language learning-impaired children ameliorated by training. *Science, 271,* 77–81.

Morris, D. W., Robinson, L., Turic, D., Duke, M., Webb, V., Milham, C., et al. (2000). Family-based association mapping provides evidence for a gene for reading disability on chromosome 15q. *Human Molecular Genetics, 9,* 843–848.

Naglieri, J. A. (1999). *Essentials of CAS assessment.* New York: Wiley.

Naglieri, J. A., & Das, J. P. (2002). Practical implications of general intelligence and PASS cognitive processes. In R. J. Sternberg & E. L. Grigorenko (Eds.), *The general factor of intelligence: How general is it?* (pp. 855–884). Mahwah, NJ: Erlbaum.

Olson, R. K., Wise, B., Conners, F., Rack, J., & Fulker, D. (1989). Specific deficits in component reading and language skills: Genetic and environmental influences. *Journal of Learning Disabilities, 22,* 339–348.

Paracchini, S., Steer, C. D., Buckingham, L. L., Morris, A. P., Ring, S., Scerri, T., et al. (2008). Association of the KIAA0319 dyslexia susceptibility gene with reading skills in the general population. *American Journal of Psychiatry, 165,* 1576–1584.

Pastor, P. N., & Reuben, C. A. (2008). Diagnosed attention deficit hyperactivity disorder and learning disability: United States, 2004–2006. *Vital and Health Statistics, 10*(237).

Pauls, D. L. (1996, March). Genetic linkage studies. In G. R. Lyon (Chair), *Critical discoveries in learning disabilities: A summary of findings by NIH research programs in learning disabilities.* Workshop conducted at the Learning Disability Association International Conference, Dallas, TX.

Pennington, B. F. (2009). *Diagnosing learning disorders: A neuropsychological framework* (2nd ed.). New York: Guilford Press.

Pennington, B. F., Bender, B., Puck, M., Salbenblatt, J., & Robinson, A. (1982). Learning disabilities in children with sex chromosome anomalies. *Child Development, 53,* 1182–1192.

Pennington, B. F., Gilger, J. W., Pauls, D., Smith, S. A., Smith, S., & De Fries, J. C. (1991). Evidence for major gene transmission of developmental dyslexia. *Journal of the American Medical Association, 266,* 1527–1534.

Pennington, B. F., Grossier, D., & Welsh, M. C. (1993). Contrasting cognitive deficits in attention deficit hyperactivity disorder versus reading disability. *Developmental Psychology, 29,* 511–523.

Pennington, B. F., Smith, S. D., Kimberling, W. J., Greene, P. A., & Haith, M. M. (1987). Left handedness and immune disorders in familial dyslexics. *Archives of Neurology, 44,* 634–639.

Petrauskas, R., & Rourke, B. P. (1979). Identification of subgroups of retarded readers: A neuropsychological multivariate approach. *Journal of Clinical Neuropsychology, 1*, 17–37.

Phillips, G. W. (1983). Learning the conversation concept: A meta-analysis (Doctoral dissertation, University of Kentucky). *Dissertation Abstracts International, 44*, 1990B.

Poeppel, D. (1996). A critical review of PET studies of phonological processing. *Brain and Language, 55*, 317–351.

Polloway, E. A., Smith, J. D., & Patton, J. R. (1984). Learning disabilities: An adult development perspective. *Learning Disability Quarterly, 7*, 179–186.

Porter, J. E., & Rourke, B. P. (1985). Socioemotional functioning of learning-disabled children: A subtypal analysis of personality patterns. In B. P. Rourke (Ed.), *Neuropsychology of learning disabilities: Essentials of subtype analysis* (pp. 237–251). New York: Guilford Press.

Pressley, M. (2006). *Reading instruction that works: The case for balanced teaching.* New York: Guilford Press.

Pressley, M., & Rankin, J. (1994). More about whole language methods of reading instruction for students at risk for early reading failure. *Learning Disabilities Research and Practice, 9*(3), 157–168.

Pugh, K. R., Shaywitz, B. A., Shaywitz, S. E., Constable, R. T., Skudlarski, P., Fulbright, R. K., et al. (1996). Cerebral organization of component processes in reading. *Brain: A Journal of Neurology, 119*, 1221–1238.

Raskind, W. H. (2001). Current understanding of the genetic basis of reading and spelling disability. *Learning Disability Quarterly, 24*, 141–157.

Reschly, D. J. (1996). Identification of students with disabilities. *The Future of Children, 6*(1), 40–53.

Reschly, D. J., & John, L. (2004). State SLD identification policies and practices. *Learning Disability Quarterly, 27*, 197–213.

Reynolds, C., & Fletcher-Janzen, E. (Eds.). (2008). *Handbook of clinical child neuropsychology* (3rd ed.). New York: Springer.

Rourke, B. P. (Ed.). (1985). *Neuropsychology of learning disabilities: Essentials of subtype analysis.* New York: Guilford Press.

Rourke, B. P. (1989). *Nonverbal learning disabilities: The syndrome and the model.* New York: Guilford Press.

Rourke, B. P., Fisk, T. L., & Strang, J. D. (1986). *Neuropsychological assessment of children: A treatment-oriented approach.* New York: Guilford Press.

Rumsey, J. M., Horowitz, B., Donahue, B. C., Nace, K., Maisog, J. M., & Andreason, P. (1997). Phonologic and orthographic components of word recognition: A PET-rCBF study. *Brain, 120*, 739–759.

Satz, P. (1990). Developmental dyslexia: An etiological reformulation. In G. T. Pavlidis (Ed.), *Perspectives on dyslexia: Vol. 1. Neurology, neuropsychiatry, and genetics* (pp. 3–26). New York: Wiley.

Satz, P., & Morris, R. (1981). Learning disability subtypes: A review. In F. J. Priozzolo & M. C. Wittrock (Eds.). *Neuropsychological and cognitive processing in reading.* New York: Academic Press.

Scarborough, H. S. (1990). Very early language deficits in dyslexic children. *Child Development, 61*, 1728–1743.

Scarborough, H. S. (1998). Early identification of children at risk for reading disabilities. In B. K. Shapiro, P. J. Accardo, & A. J. Capute (Eds.), *Specific reading disability: A view of the spectrum* (pp. 75–119). Timonium, MD: York Press.

Schumaker, J. B., Deshler, D. D., Alley, G. R., & Warner, M. M. (1983). Toward the development of an intervention model for learning disabled adolescents: The University of Kansas Institute. *Exceptional Child Quarterly, 4*, 45–74.

Schumacher, J., König, I. R., Schröder, T., Duell, M., Plume, E., Propping, P., et al. (2008). Further evidence for a susceptibility locus contributing to reading disability on chromosome 15q15–q21. *Psychiatric Genetics, 18*, 137–142.

Shapiro, H. R. (1992). Debatable issues underlying whole language philosophy: A speech pathologist's perspective. *Language, Speech, and Hearing Services in Schools, 23*, 308–311.

Shaywitz, B. A., Fletcher, J. M., & Shaywitz, S. E. (1995). Defining and classifying learning disabilities and attention deficit/hyperactive disorder. *Journal of Child Neurology, 10*(Suppl. 1), S50–S57.

Shaywitz, S. E. (1996). Dyslexia. *Scientific American, 275*(5), 98–104.

Shaywitz, S. E. (1998). Current concepts: Dyslexia. *New England Journal of Medicine, 338*(5), 307–312.

Shaywitz, S. E., & Shaywitz, B. A, (1987). Attention deficit disorder: Current perspectives. *Pediatric Neurology, 3*, 129–135.

Shaywitz, S. E., Shaywitz, B. A., Fletcher, J. M., & Escobar, M. D. (1990). Prevalence of reading disability in boys and girls: Results of the Connecticut Longitudinal Study. *Journal of the American Medical Association, 264*, 998–1002.

Silver, A. A., & Hagin, R. A. (1990). *Disorders of learning in childhood.* New York: Wiley.

Silver, L. B. (1970). Frequency of adoption in children with neurological learning disability syndrome. *Journal of Learning Disability, 3*, 306–310.

Silver, L. B. (1989). Frequency of adoption of children and adolescents with learning disabilities. *Journal of Learning Disabilities, 22*, 325–327.

Silver, L. B. (1990). Attention deficit-hyperactivity disorder: Is it a learning disability or a related disorder? *Journal of Learning Disabilities, 23*, 394–397.

Smith, S. D., Kelley, P. M., Askew, J. W., Hoover, D.

M., Deffenbacher, K. E., Gayan, J., et al. (2001). Reading disability and chromosome 6p21. 3: Evaluation of MOG as a candidate gene. *Journal of Learning Disabilities, 34,* 512–519.

Smith, S. D., Kimberling, W. J., & Pennington, B. F (1991). Screening for multiple genes: Influencing dyslexia. *Reading and Writing, 3,* 285–298.

Smith, S. D., Kimberling, W. J., Pennington, B. F., & Lubs, H. A. (1983). Specific reading disability: Identification of an inherited form through linkage analysis. *Science, 219,* 1345–1347.

Smith, S. D., Pennington, B. F., Kimberling, W. J., & Ing, P. S. (1990). Genetic linkage analysis with specific dyslexia: Use of multiple markers to include and exclude possible loci. In G. T. Pavlidis (Ed.), *Perspectives on dyslexia: Vol. 1. Neurology, neuropsychology, and genetics* (pp. 77–89). New York: Wiley.

Snowling, M., & Hulme, C. (1991). Speech processing and learning to spell. In W. Ellis (Ed.), *All language and the creation of literacy.* Baltimore: Orton Dyslexia Society.

Stanovich, K. E. (1993). The construct validity of discrepancy definitions of reading disability. In G. R. Lyson, D. B. Gray, J. F. Kavanaugh, & N. A. Krasnegor (Eds.), *Better understanding learning disabilities: New views from research and their implications for education and public policies* (pp. 273–307). Baltimore: Brookes.

Stanovich, K. E. (1994). Constructivism in reading education. *Journal of Special Education, 28,* 259–274.

Stanovich, K. E., & Siegel, L. S. (1994). Phenotypic performance profile of children with reading disabilities: A regression-based test of the phonological–core variable–difference model. *Journal of Educational Psychology, 86,* 24–53.

Stevenson, J., Graham, P., Fredman, G., & McLoughlin, V. (1987). A twin study of genetic influence on reading and spelling ability and disability. *Journal of Child Psychology and Psychiatry, 28,* 229–247.

Storch, S. A., & Whitehurst, G. J. (2002). Oral language and code-related precursors to reading: Evidence from a longitudinal structural model. *Developmental Psychology, 38,* 934–947.

Strauss, A., & Lehtinen, L. (1947). *Psychopathology and education of the brain-injured child.* New York: Grune & Stratton.

Swanson, H. L., Harris, K. R., & Graham, S. (Eds.). (2003). *Handbook of learning disabilities.* New York: Guilford Press.

Swartz, G. A. (1974). *The language-learning system.* New York: Simon & Schuster.

Thiel, C. (2003). Cholinergic modulation of learning and memory in the human brain as detected with functional neuroimaging. *Neurobiology of Learning and Memory, 80,* 234–244.

Thomson, M. (1990). *Developmental dyslexia* (3rd ed.). London: Whurr.

Torgesen, J. K. (1991). Learning disabilities: Historical and conceptual issues. In B. Y. L. Wong (Ed.), *Learning about learning disabilities* (pp. 3–37). San Diego, CA: Academic Press.

Torgesen, J. K. (1993). Variations on theory in learning disabilities. In G. R. Lyon, D. B. Gray, J. F. Kavanaugh, & N. A. Krasnegor (Eds.), *Better understanding learning disabilities: New views from research and their implications for education and public policies* (pp. 153–170). Baltimore: Brookes.

Torgesen, J. K., Wagner, R. K., & Rashotte, C. A. (1994). Longitudinal studies of phonological processing and reading. *Journal of Learning Disabilities, 27,* 276–286.

Torgesen, J. K., Wagner, R. K., & Rashotte, C. A. (1997). Approaches to prevention nad remediation of phonologically based reading disabilities. In B. A. Blachman (Ed.), *Foundations of reading acquisition and dyslexia: Implications for early intervention* (pp. 287–304). Mahwah, NJ: Erlbaum.

Toth, G., & Siegel, L. S. (1994). A critical evaluation of the I.Q.-achievement discrepancy-based definitions of dyslexia. In K. P. vanden Bos, L. S. Siegel, D. J. Bakker, & D. L. Share (Eds.), *Current directions in dyslexia research* (pp. 45–70). Lisse, The Netherlands: Swets & Zeitlinger.

Travis, J. (1996). Let the games begin. *Science News, 149,* 104–106.

Truch, S. (1994). Stimulating basic reading processes using Auditory Discrimination in Depth. *Annals of Dyslexia, 44,* 60–80.

Turic, D., Robinson, L., Duke, M., Morris, D. W., Webb, V., Hamshere, M., et al. (2003). Linkage disequilibrium mapping provides further evidence of a gene for reading disability on chromosome 6p21. 3–22. *Molecular Psychiatry, 8,* 176–185.

U.S. Department of Education. (1994). *Sixteenth annual report to Congress.* Washington, DC: Author.

U.S. Department of Education. (2007). *Demographic and school characteristics of students receiving special education in the elementary grades.* Washington, DC: Author.

U.S. Office of Education. (1977). Assistance to states for education of handicapped children. Procedures for evaluating specific learning disabilities. *Federal Register, 42,* G1082–G1085.

Voeller, K. K. S. (1986). Right-hemisphere deficit syndrome in children. *American Journal of Psychiatry, 143,* 1004–1009.

Wagner, R. K., & Torgeson, J. K. (1987). The nature of phonological processing and its causal role in the acquisition of reading skills. *Psychological Bulletin, 101*(2), 192–212.

Waldie, K., & Spreen, O. (1993). The relationship between learning disabilities and persisting delinquency. *Journal of Learning Disabilities, 26,* 417–423.

Watson, C. S., Kidd, G. R., Horner, D. G., Connell, P. E. J., Lowther, A., Eddins, D. A., et al. (2003). Sensory, cognitive and linguistic factors in the early academic performance of elementary school children: The Benton–I.U. project. *Journal of Learning Disabilities, 36*(2), 165–197.

Wendling, B. J., & Mather, N. (2008). *Essentials of evidence-based academic interventions.* New York: Wiley.

White, O. R. (1986). Precision teaching—precision learning. *Exceptional Children, 52,* 522–534.

Wilkinson, G. S., & Robertson, G. J. (2006). *Wide Range Achievement Test (4th ed.) (WRAT-4).* Lutz, FL: Psychological Assessment Resources.

Wirt, R. D., Lachar, D., Klinedinst, J. E., & Seat, P. D. (1977). *Multidimensional assessment of child personality: A Manual for the Personality Inventory for Children.* Los Angeles: Western Psychological Services.

Wong, B. Y., Graham, L., Hoskyn, M., & Berman, J. (2008). *The ABCs of learning disabilities* (2nd ed.). Burlington, MA: Elsevier.

Wong, B. Y., Wong, R., Darlington, D., Jones, W., et al. (1991). Interactive teaching: An effective way to teach revision skills to adolescents with learning disabilities. *Learning Disabilities Research and Practice, 6,* 117–127.

Wong, B. Y. L. (1987). How did the results of medicognitive research impact on the learning disabled individual? *Learning Disability Quarterly, 10,* 189–195.

Woodcock, R., McGrew, K. S., & Mather, N. (2001). *Woodcock–Johnson III Tests of Achievement.* Itasca, IL: Riverside.

Zerbin-Rudin, E. (1967). Congenital word-blindness. *Bulletin of the Orton Society, 17,* 47–55.

Zigmond, N. (1993). Learning disabilities from an educational perspective. In G. R. Lyon, D. B. Gray, J. F. Kavanaugh, & N. A. Krasnegor (Eds.), *Better understanding learning disabilities: New views from research and their implications for education and public policies* (pp. 251–272). Baltimore: Brookes.

CHAPTER 7

Attention-Deficit/Hyperactivity Disorder

SAM GOLDSTEIN

The childhood cognitive and behavioral problems categorized as disorders of attention, impulsivity, and hyperactivity have presented a clinical challenge for neuropsychologists over the past 60 years. The symptom constellation referred to as attention deficit disorder (ADD) or attention-deficit/hyperactivity disorder (ADHD) (American Psychiatric Association [APA], 2000) has become one of the most widely researched areas in childhood and adolescence, with an increasing emphasis on research throughout the adult lifespan. Problems arising from this constellation of symptoms have constituted the most chronic childhood behavior disorder over nearly 40 years (Wender, 1975) and the largest single source of referrals to mental health centers (Barkley, 2006; Castle, Aubert, Verbrugge, Khalid, & Epstein, 2007; Gadow, Sprafkin, & Nolan, 2001).

ADHD is among the most common disorders of childhood. It is estimated that it affects between 5% and 8% of the population throughout life. Estimates vary, with the APA (2000) suggesting a prevalence of 3–7%. Statistics vary depending on populations studied, thresholds, and definitional criteria (Sherman, Iacono, & McGue, 1997). In clinic-referred settings, males outnumber females 6:1. In epidemiological studies of community-based settings, the ratio is 3:1 (for a review, see Barkley, 2006). The incidence of diagnosis continues to increase, with a 70% increase in the diagnosis of children and nearly a 100% increase in the diagnosis of adults between 2000 and 2003 (Centers for Disease Control and Prevention [CDC], 2005)—a pattern that has continued (Castle et al., 2007). It is now estimated that between 4% and 8% of the population has received a diagnosis of ADHD (CDC, 2005; Cuffe, Moore, & McKeown, 2005). Female adults are the fastest-growing group (Medco Health Solutions, 2005). Studies using broad-based definitions of ADHD find a prevalence of nearly 16% in adults, whereas studies using narrower definitions report a rate of 3–4% (Faraone & Biederman, 2005). Prevalence has also been reported to be higher in populations of individuals with other impairments (Altfas, 2002).

Even as professionals utilize the current diagnostic criteria involving symptoms of inattention, hyperactivity, and impulsivity, research data increasingly suggest that for the majority of affected children, impulsivity and impaired executive functions represent core deficits (for reviews, see Barkley, 2006; Goldstein & Naglieri, 2006; Goldstein & Schwebach, 2005). Children with ADHD typically experience difficulty in all aspects and situations of their lives. Their behavior is often uneven, unpredictable, and inconsistent. Professionals evaluating ADHD today must be concerned not only with the core symptoms of this disorder and their direct, immediate impact on children, but with the significant secondary impact these problems have upon children's current and future lives, as well as the lives of their family members. In particular, an increasing body of research is demonstrating the increased vulnerability of adults with ADHD to psychiatric, emotional, cognitive, academic, vocational, substance, and antisocial problems (Barkley, Fischer, Smallish, & Fletcher, 2004; Barkley & Gordon, 2002; Cuffe et al., 2009; Murphy, Barkley, & Bush, 2002; Rabiner, Anastophoulos, Costello, Hoyle, & Swartzwelder, 2008; Robin, Tzelepis, & Bedway, 2008; Sprafkin, Gadow, Weiss, Schneider, & Nolan, 2007).

The controversy and at times confusion concerning various aspects of ADHD may in part result from the tradition of viewing this disorder as a unitary phenomenon with a single cause. Voeller (1991) suggests that rather than viewing ADHD as a single behavioral abnormality with associated comorbidities, it may be better to conceptualize ADHD as a "cluster of different behavioral deficits, each with a specific neuro-substrate of varying severity occurring in variable constellations and sharing a common response to psychostimulants" (p. S4). There is no doubt, however, that the cluster of symptomatic problems constituting the diagnosis of ADHD represents a distinct disorder from others of childhood and adulthood (Accardo, Blondis, & Whitman, 1990; Biederman et al., 1996; Mrug et al., 2009). A significant percentage of affected youth continue to demonstrate the condition into adulthood, often underreporting their symptoms and impairment relative to observers' reports (Barkley et al., 2004). The consensus among researchers and clinicians is that the core symptoms of ADHD affect a significant minority of our population. For affected individuals, however, ADHD represents a poor fit between societal expectations and these individuals' abilities to meet those expectations. This phenomenon is distinct from other disorders of childhood and adulthood, and can be reliably evaluated and effectively treated.

TOWARD A WORKING DEFINITION OF ADHD

From a neuropsychological perspective, the concept of attention as an executive function has gained increasing popularity. Sustained mental effort, self-regulation, planning, execution, and maintenance are considered measures of executive functioning (Daigneault, Braun, & Whitaker, 1992). These executive functions are impaired in individuals with ADHD (Biederman et al., 2008). Nearly 20 years ago, Mirskey, Anthony, Duncan, Ahearn, and Kellam (1991) developed a neuropsychological model of attention involving four basic concepts: the ability to focus, execute, sustain or code, and shift. Eight traditional assessment measures of attention were used in a factor-analytic study to arrive at this model.

Increasingly, there is a consensus that ADHD represents a problem of faulty performance rather than faulty input. It is not so much that this population of individuals does not know what to do, but that they do not do what they know consistently. It is a problem of inconsistency rather than inability (Goldstein & Goldstein, 1998). Even in their adaptive skills, this pattern of difference between possessing a skill and using it efficiently has been well defined for individuals with ADHD (Stein, 1997).

It is quite likely that attention as a theoretical or laboratory-measured concept is quite different from the symptom of inattention as it is defined for ADHD. Nonetheless, prior to a review of the currently accepted ADHD diagnostic criteria and related issues, a brief discussion of attention as a theoretical construct is valuable.

Attention is considered a generic term used to designate a group of hypothetical mechanisms that collectively serve a function for the organism (Mesulam, 1985). In 1798, Alexander Crighton provided the earliest known reference to attention. In his two-volume work summarizing the available knowledge from throughout the world on the human mind and mental illness, the chapter titled "On Attention and Its Diseases" was apparently the first formal effort in the scientific literature to define attention, and in particular to describe the adverse processes that occur when human beings struggle with attention. Crighton defined attention as a process by which "an object of external sense or of thought occupies the mind in such a degree that a person does not receive a clear perception from any other one" (p. 254). This theme was also reflected but not cited in George Still's three published lectures before the Royal Society of Medicine in the journal *Lancet* in 1902. Still based his comments on observations of more than 26 patients who were studied relatively intensely.

Beginning with James (1890), researchers have identified attentional processes as essential prerequisites for higher cognitive functions. Hypothetical models of the development of attention have included a stagewise model (Blondis, Snow, Stein, & Roizen, 1991), as well as a model of a maturational process similar to the maturation of other executive or intellectual skills (Hagen & Hale, 1973). Although Posner and Snyder (1975) described attention as a complex field of study, others have suggested that attentional skills can be operationally and statistically defined with some confidence (Gordon & McClure, 1983). Skinner (1953) defined attention as a functional relationship between stimuli and response. His belief was that attention is not a thing, entity, or mental function, but is a description of a set of relations between stimuli or events and responses to them. Gibson and Radner (1979) defined attention as the ability to perceive the environment in relation to a specific goal. Posner (1987) suggested that attention may consist of automatic versus conscious aspects. Fuster (1989) provided a concept of inhibition interference in his neuropsychological model of executive function related to attention. All of these theories, including Titchener's (1924) description of attention as a pattern of consciousness, appear to be an extension of James's (1890) characterization of attention as bimodal. James hypothesized that attention is either passive, reflective, nonvoluntary, and effortless, or active and voluntary. James defined *sustained attention* as the active and voluntary type, which is dependent on repeated redirection of focus toward the object of attention and on resistance to attractions that coexist in the process.

Finally, Picano, Klusman, Hornbestel, and Moulton (1992) conducted a factor analysis that suggested three factors for attention. The first factor accounted for 35% of the variance and involved skills related to visual–motor scanning and shifting abilities. The capacity to divide attention appeared to be key to this task. The second factor accounted for 16% of the variance and reflected immediate attention and conceptual tracking consistent with the ability to repeat digits both forward and backward. The third factor accounted for 13.5% of the variance, reflecting sustained, effortful processing consistent with distractibility tasks. This breakdown is consistent with factor analyses by other investigators (Shum, MacFarland, & Bain, 1990).

As the fifth edition of the *Diagnostic and Statistical Manual of Mental Disorders* (DSM-5) is not expected to be published until 2013, it is important for professionals to possess a working understanding of ADHD based on current knowledge. In other words, it is important to possess a working understanding of the DSM-IV-TR diagnostic criteria for ADHD, a practical understanding of the symptoms' impact upon an individual's functioning, and a diagnostic strategy. The traditional disease model is not relevant to the definition of ADHD (Ellis, 1985). ADHD is more like obesity or intelligence: Individuals differ not in having or not having the traits, but in the degree of manifestation. ADHD symptoms are multidimensional rather than unitary (Guevremont, DuPaul, & Barkley, 1993). However, there continues to be discussion as to which dimensions represent the most clearly distinguishing deficits of the disorder. The frequency and severity of symptoms fluctuate across settings, activities, and caregivers (Tarver-Behring, Barkley, & Karlsson, 1985; Zentall, 1984). Neuropsychological profiles have also been demonstrated to differ between subtypes (Chabildas, Pennington, & Willcutt, 2001). However, these differences have not lent themselves to a differential diagnosis. There is a general consensus, however, that symptoms of ADHD fall into two broad factors: symptoms related to the behavioral manifestation of faulty attention, and those related to hyperactivity and impulsivity (Crystal, Ostrander, Chen, & August, 2001; Faraone, Biederman, & Friedman, 2000). Symptoms of hyperactivity and impulsivity appear to co-occur at such a high frequency that it is difficult to separate them on a factor-analytic basis. However, research has demonstrated subtype differences in neuropsychological profiles and patterns of comborbidity (Eiraldi, Power, & Nezu, 1997). It is also important for neuropsychologists to recognize that at times the lines blur between the symptoms and consequences or impairments of ADHD. Thus a diagnostic strategy for ADHD should include identifying not only the symptoms, but thr skills and life areas hypothesized to be directly impaired by the symptoms (Gordon et al., 2006). Having the symptoms without negative consequences would in fact preclude the diagnosis of ADHD according to DSM-IV-TR criteria.

The DSM-IV diagnostic criteria published (APA, 1994) represented an effort to move forward and correct the mistaken notion that ADHD represents a unipolar disorder. The field studies for the ADHD diagnosis were more comprehensive and better structured than previous efforts. The DSM-IV-TR (APA, 2000) criteria are identical to the DSM-IV criteria; readers are referred to DSM-IV-TR for the complete list. Since DSM-III, each succeeding diagnostic protocol has focused increasingly on the issue of impairment. Impairment has been and will continue to be a critical linchpin in making the diagnosis of ADHD, but is not well explained by symptom severity (Gordon et al., 2006). The measurement of neuropsychological processes may also be considered as part of the DSM-5 criteria for ADHD (Naglieri & Das, 2006).

Of the 276 children diagnosed with ADHD in the DSM-IV field studies, 55% had the combined type, 27% the inattentive type, and 18% the hyperactive–impulsive type (Lahey et al., 1994). Fewer than half (44%) of those with the hyperactive–impulsive type of ADHD received a DSM-III diagnosis of ADD with hyperactivity; these two diagnoses, therefore, only partially overlapped. The hyperactive–impulsive group had fewer symptoms of inattention than the children with the combined type did. They also had fewer symptoms of hyperactive–impulsive problems, suggesting that the hyperactive–impulsive type represents a less severe variant of the disorder. The hyperactive–impulsive group contained 20% females, the combined group 12%, and the inattentive group 27%. This latter number corresponds with neuropsychologists' perceptions that

females more often demonstrate the inattentive type of ADHD (Biederman et al., 2002). This overrepresentation has not been well explained by any theoretical model (Silverthorn, Frick, Kuper, & Ott, 1996), nor is it understood why preliminary research suggests that females with ADHD may be less likely than males to demonstrate executive function deficits (Seidman et al., 1997). The hyperactive–impulsive population was also younger than the other two groups in the field studies. Moreover, they had fewer disruptive symptoms of oppositional defiant disorder or conduct disorder than those with the combined type of ADHD.

A number of researchers have demonstrated the validity of the DSM-IV/DSM-IV-TR diagnostic conceptualization for ADHD, utilizing a variety of clinical and laboratory measures. Such research has included a full battery of neuropsychological tests (Brand, Das-Smaal, & De Jonge, 1996; Halperin et al.,1993; Harrier & DeOrnellas, 2005), reversal and memory tasks (O'Neill & Douglas, 1996), executive function tasks (Clark, Prior, & Kinsella, 2000; Geurts, Verte, Oosterlaan, Royers, & Sergeant, 2005; Hart & Harter, 2001), and neurological evaluation (Luk, Leung, & Yuen, 1991). The general consistency of symptoms, comorbidity, and related findings among large, well-controlled clinic and epidemiological studies suggest that the conceptualization of ADHD in DSM-IV and DSM-IV-TR has been fairly well refined. Nonetheless, these criteria continue to focus excessively on inattention as the primary problem for the disorder, limiting the focus on the impact of impulsivity as the core deficit. This perpetuates a number of major misconceptions, including the notion that the inattentive type of ADHD represents a subtype of the combined disorder (Anastopoulos, Barkley, & Shelton, 1994). Increasing research suggests that it does not. It is more likely that the inattentive type represents a distinct disorder, primarily reflecting difficulty in attending to repetitive, effortful tasks and problems with organization. Carlson and Mann (2002) described children with the inattentive type of ADHD (as distinct from the combined type) as possessing hypoactivity, lethargy, and a lack of ability to stay focused. The problems this group experiences may very well be the result of faulty skills as opposed to inconsistent or inadequate use of skills. Emerging data are also raising questions about the lack of stability of DSM-IV-TR ADHD subtypes over time as children mature (Lahey, Pelham, Loney, Lee, & Wilcutt, 2005).

A PRACTICAL DEFINITION OF ADHD

In clinical settings, it is suggested that neuropsychologists apply a practical definition of ADHD as a means of translating history and test data into functional behavior. Such a process may also assist parents and educators in understanding the children they live with and educate; it provides a logical framework within which to evaluate and understand the seemingly illogical pattern of behavior this group of children exhibits. The practical definition contains five components, with the first, impulsivity, considered to be the major contributing force in shaping the other four components. These components are briefly presented below. The interested reader is referred to Goldstein and Goldstein (1998) for an extended review.

1. *Impulsivity.* Children with ADHD have difficulty thinking before they act. They do not efficiently weigh consequences before acting and do not reasonably consider the consequences of their past behavior. They struggle to follow rule-governed behavior (Barkley, 2006), due to their problems with separating experience from response, thought from emotion, and action from reaction. In the heat of the moment, their limited capacity for self-control is quickly overwhelmed by their immediate need to act.

2. *Inattention.* Children with ADHD have difficulty remaining on task and focusing their attention, in comparison to children without ADHD of similar chronological age. A more precise review of the available literature, however, suggests that their problems do no occur during highly motivating or interesting tasks, but rather when tasks are repetitive, effortful, uninteresting, and not of the children's choosing. In these circumstances the children's inability to inhibit their desire to move off this task is limited, and thus they find themselves doing anything else that appears to be more interesting or less effortful. Although this pattern is true to some extent for everyone on a di-

mensional basis, these children represent the extreme of what is observed.

3. *Overarousal.* Due to their lack of inhibition, children with ADHD tend to be excessively restless, overactive, and easily aroused emotionally. The speed and intensity with which they move to the extreme of their emotions are much greater than those of their same-age peers.

4. *Difficulty with gratification.* Children with ADHD, due to their lack of inhibition, require immediate, frequent, predictable, and meaningful rewards. They experience difficulty in working toward a long-term goal, and thus often require brief, repeated payoffs rather than a single long-term reward. They also do not appear to respond to rewards in the same manner as other children do (Haenlein & Caul, 1987); that is, rewards do not appear to be effective in changing their behavior on a long-term basis. Moreover, they appear to require more trials to consistently demonstrate mastery over behaviors that are within their repertoires. This may be the result of a faulty ability to develop a self-cueing process necessary to know what to do and when to do it. Because of their impulsivity, their behavior may remain consequentially bound.

It also appears that these children, because of their behavior, frequently receive more negative reinforcement than others. Thus they are victims both of their temperaments, which make it difficult for them to persist, and of their reinforcement histories, which reinforce them for starting but often not for finishing tasks. It is important to keep in mind that these children like rewards and do not like punishments; in this respect, they are similar to everyone else. Nonetheless, over time they learn to respond to demands placed upon them by the environment when an aversive stimulus is removed contingent upon performance, rather than when they are promised a future reward.

5. *Emotions and locus of control.* Due to their impulsivity, children with ADHD often appear to be on a roller-coaster ride of emotions throughout their childhood. When they are happy, they are so happy people tell them to calm down. When they are unhappy, they are so unhappy people tell them to calm down. They may learn that their emotions are not valued and often lead them into trouble. They may also be more prone to de-

velop an external locus of control, to project blame onto others, and to be unwilling to recognize and accept the role they play in their own behavior. They appear more vulnerable to certain personality problems, especially those related to antisocial difficulty, in part because of these qualities combined with their life experiences. They may be more prone to depression as well, in part due to the lack of balance between successful and unsuccessful experiences on a day-in-and-day-out basis.

Increasingly, these core problems have been considered under the umbrella of concepts such as self-regulation (Goldstein & Brooks, 2007), executive functioning (Barkley, 2008), or planning (Goldstein & Naglieri, 2006). Regardless of the overall concept or term used to describe these processes, it would appear that ADHD represents a constellation of symptoms and consequent impairments resulting from inefficiency in goal-directed behavior. Children with ADHD struggle to formulate goals and plans efficiently, to sequence them temporally, and to execute them, as well as to evaluate and reevaluate outcomes in light of the intended objectives.

GENETICS AND OTHER ETIOLOGICAL CONSIDERATIONS

The genetic contribution to ADHD has been postulated by a number of authors since the early 1990s (Hechtman, 1993; Rutter et al., 1990; Stevenson, 1992; Swanson et al., 2000). There is no single gene that causes ADHD, but several genes are likely to enhance susceptibility (Faraone & Khan, 2006). The underlying genetic mechanism has been suggested to be associated with a single dopamine transporter gene (Cook et al., 1995); with variations in the DRD4 (La-Hoste et al., 1996) and DRD5 (Lowe et al., 2004) receptor genes; and with a variation in the DAT1 transporter gene (Winsberg & Comings, 1999). There is also evidence that the gene synaptosomal protein of 25 kilodaltons (SNAP-25), a gene that controls synaptic vesicle transmission, may also in contribute in part to ADHD (Faraone & Kahn, 2006). Furthermore, it has been suggested that the trait locus for reading disability on

chromosome 6 identified by Cardon and colleagues (1994) may be a locus for ADHD as well (Warren et al., 1995). Faraone and colleagues (2005), following an analysis of 20 twin studies, computed a heritability of 76% for ADHD. Moreover, it would appear that some of these genes interact with the environment in such a way that the remaining 24% contributed by the environment is still quite genetically significant.

A recent report of a genome-wide association scan of ADHD notes that earlier studies have converged in agreement that genes contribute substantially to the development of ADHD. However, despite numerous linkage and candidate gene studies, a strongly consistent and replicable association has not been identified (Neale et al., 2008). To search for ADHD susceptibility genes, Neale and colleagues (2008) genotyped approximately 600,000 gene segments in 958 ADHD-affected family trios. This led them to analyze nearly half a million gene splices in nearly 3,000 individuals constituting over 900 complete trios, using the ADHD diagnosis as phenotype. None of the association tests achieved genome-wide significance, suggesting that larger samples may be required to identify the true risk loci for ADHD.

Eaves, Silberg, and Hewitt (1993) note two complementary approaches to the genetic analysis of ADHD. The first, a dimensional approach, involves the study of a normal trait or range of activity; it assumes that ADHD is at one end of the continuum or trait. The second, a categorical approach, is based on studying children of families who meet diagnostic criteria; it assumes that ADHD is a discrete disorder (Faraone, Biederman, Chen, & Krifcher, 1992). It is important for neuropsychologists to recognize that dimensional approaches have been found to predict life outcome better than categorical approaches (Fergusson & Horwood, 1992).

Among investigators taking the dimensional approach, Willerman (1973) found the heritability of scores on an activity questionnaire to be 0.77 for a sample of 54 monozygotic and 39 dizygotic twin pairs. However, Goodman and Stevenson (1989) reported a heritability estimate of greater than 1.00 in a sample of 285 twin pairs. This finding appeared to be due to an extremely low dizygotic correlation. Corresponding dizygotic correlations for father and teacher reports were much higher, resulting in heritability estimates from 0.48 to 0.68. A subsequent twin study by Thapar, Hervas, and McGuffin (1995), using the same three activity items used by Goodman and Stevenson, confirmed the low dizygotic correlation in maternal ratings; Thapar and colleagues suggested that the role of reciprocal sibling interactions may be different in dizygotic versus monozygotic twins, or that mothers may exaggerate differences between their dizygotic twins. The low dizygotic correlation may, however, be unique to these specific questions about activity level. Edelbrock, Rende, Plomin, and Thompson (1995) reported correlations (predominantly from mothers' ratings) of .86 for monozygotic twins and .29 for dizygotic twins, giving a heritability estimate of 0.66. Zahn-Waxler, Schmitz, Fulker, Robinson, and Emde (1996) obtained a very similar estimate (0.72). However, somewhat lower heritability values were obtained from fathers' and teachers' ratings, and the correlations between raters was low.

Employing the categorical or diagnostic approach, Goodman and Stevenson (1989) demonstrated a probandwise concordance rate of 51% in 39 monozygotic twin pairs and 30% in 54 dizygotic twin pairs, yielding a heritability estimate of 0.64. De Fries and Fulker (1985, 1988), utilizing a statistical method developed by Gillis, Gilger, Pennington, and De Fries (1992), estimated the heritability of ADHD as 0.91 ± 0.36 for twins participating in a research project.

The issue of phenotypic definition, as indicated by the variation in estimates of siblings' risk (53%, 25%, or 17%, depending on whether the behavior is defined as hyperactivity, ADD, or ADHD), speaks to the complexity of relating phenotype to genotype (Biederman, Faraone, Keenan, Knee, & Tsuang, 1990; Biederman et al., 1992; Safer, 1973; Faraone et al., 1992). Levy, Hay, McStephen, Wood, and Waldman (1997), studying a cohort of 1,938 families with twins and siblings ages 4–12 years recruited from the Australian National Health and Medical Research Council Twin Registry, reported that ADHD is best viewed as the extreme of behavior that varies genetically throughout the entire population, rather than as a disorder with discrete determinants. In this study, as in others, heritability estimates for

monozygotic twins were significantly higher than for dizygotic twins. As Levy and colleagues note, ADHD has an exceptionally high heritability compared with other behavioral disorders. These authors reported that 82% of monozygotic twins and 38% of dizygotic twins met an eight-symptom ADHD cutoff for proband concordances.

Studies linking polymorphisms in the dopaminergic system to ADHD (Comings, Wu, & Chiu, 1996) and the DRD4 receptor polymorphisms to dimensional aspects of impulsivity (Benjamin et al., 1996; Ebstein et al., 1996) suggest that the polymorphisms identified to date do not account for all of the relevant heritable variation. The findings of Sherman and colleagues (1997) suggest that future molecular genetic studies of ADHD may yield more information defining ADHD as a disorder composed of two quantitatively, continuously distributed dimensions—inattention and hyperactivity–impulsivity—rather than a homogeneous categorical disorder.

Recently Faraone and colleagues (2008) genotyped nearly 6,000 single-nucleotide polymorphisms across a genome of over 1,000 individuals from families with children diagnosed with ADHD. They then performed two nonparametric linkage analyses on these families: (1) an affected-sibling-pair linkage analysis on 217 families with 601 siblings diagnosed with ADHD; and (2) a variance-components linkage analysis, using the number of ADHD symptoms as the phenotype, on 260 families with 1,100 phenotypic siblings. From these analyses, the authors concluded that their findings of an absence of regions of significant or suggestive linkage indicate that there are probably no genes of large effect contributing to the ADHD phenotype. It has further been demonstrated that the gender differences found in ADHD could be sexually dimorphic. Biederman, Kim, and colleagues (2008) found some evidence suggesting this to be the case. Genetic associations for ADHD appeared stronger when stratified by gender and in the same direction as indicated by previous neurobiological studies. Associations were stronger in males for two candidate genes (COMT and SLC6A4), and stronger in females for two others (SLC6A2 and MAOA). Furthermore, these authors reported a statistically significant gender effect for COMT.

The etiology of ADHD must also be considered in relation to other genetic disorders and to teratogens. Fragile X syndrome, Turner syndrome, Tourette syndrome, neurofibromatosis, sickle cell anemia, phenylketonuria, Noonan syndrome, and Williams syndrome are all chromosomal and genetic abnormalities in which attentional problems and ADHD have been reported (Hagerman, 1991; Mautner, Kluwe, Thakker, & Laerk, 2002). Bastain and colleagues (2002) suggest that expensive laboratory tests for genetic disorders are not indicated unless a genetic disorder is suspected because of family history, clinical signs, or low IQ. Exposure to various toxins (e.g., alcohol and cocaine exposure *in utero*, lead and vapor abuse), perinatal complications, medical problems (e.g., hypothyroidism, encephalitis), and even radiation therapy secondary to leukemia have all been reported as responsible for creation of inattention and impulsivity problems (for reviews, see Barkley, 2006; Goldstein & Goldstein, 1998). ADHD and depressive symptoms are commonly identified after pediatric traumatic brain injury, but may predate the trauma (Bloom et al., 2001).

The neurobiology of ADHD implicates impairment in brain structure—particularly differences in size of certain structures, interacting with metabolic differences (Zametkin & Rapoport, 1987). In efficient brain metabolism in prefrontal and cingulate regions, as well as in the right thalamus caudate, hippocampus, and cerebellum, has been reported in adults with ADHD (Zametkin, Nordahl, & Gross, 1990). Regional abnormalities of glucose metabolism demonstrated by positron emission tomography studies generally demonstrate a fundamental biological difference between individuals with and without ADHD. Castellanos and colleagues (1996) suggest that connections among the right prefrontal cortex, caudate, and cerebellum reflect the brain's so-called "braking system"—a system that operates inefficiently in individuals with ADHD. Semrud-Clikeman and colleagues (2000) found reversed caudate asymmetry on magnetic resonance imaging scans of 10 males diagnosed with ADHD. They noted that findings in the right prefrontal cortex, cerebellum, and basal ganglia appeared to be associated with behavioral measures of inattention and inhibition. Children with

ADHD were found in another study to be unable to active the caudate nucleus, suggesting core abnormality in this function for ADHD (Vaiyda et al., 2005). These authors concluded that children with ADHD experience reduced engagement of a frontostriatal–temporoparietal network when engaging in inhibitory tasks.

DEVELOPMENTAL COURSE AND COMORBIDITY

Although the core problems children with ADHD experience reflect similar difficulty with impulsivity, inattention, and hyperactivity, each child's presentation is unique in terms of the manifestation of these problems and associated comorbid factors (Goldstein & Goldstein, 1998). As an increasing body of scientific data is generated concerning the developmental course and adult outcome of children with ADHD, it appears that the comorbid problems they develop predict their life outcomes better than the diagnosis of ADHD itself does. ADHD in isolation appears to best predict school struggles, difficulty meeting expectations without the home setting, and possible mild substance abuse as an adult. However, it does not predict the significant negative emotional, behavioral, and personality outcomes that have been reported.

Infants who have been noted to demonstrate difficult temperament do not handle changes in routines well. They exhibit a low frustration threshold and a high intensity of response (Carey, 1970; Chess & Thomas, 1986; Thomas & Chess, 1977). In follow-up studies of such infants, as many as 70% develop school problems (Terestman, 1980). These infants appear at greater risk than others of receiving a diagnosis of ADHD. It is also important to note that these difficult infants exert a significant negative impact on their developing relationships with caregivers—relationships that are critical in predicting children's life outcomes (Houshyar & Kaufman, 2005; Katz, 1997).

Although early symptoms of ADHD may be viewed as transient problems of young children, research data suggest that ignoring these signs results in the loss of valuable treatment time. At least 60–70% of children later diagnosed with ADHD could have been identified by their symptoms during the preschool years (Cohen, Sullivan, Minde, Novack, & Helwig, 1981). Young children manifesting symptoms of ADHD are more likely to present with speech and language problems (Baker & Cantwell, 1987), and to develop a wide range of behavioral problems (Cantwell, Baker, & Mattison, 1981; Cohen, Davine, & Meloche-Kelly, 1989; DuPaul, McGoey, Eckert, & VanBrakle, 2001), than are children not suffering from these symptoms. Research also cogently suggests that the comorbidity of speech and language disorders with ADHD merits routine screening of children suspected of having either type of problem, especially during their younger years. Children with concurrent ADHD and language disorders appear to have a much poorer prognosis than those with those with ADHD alone (Baker & Cantwell, 1992).

Within school settings, children with ADHD appear to be victims both of their temperaments and of their learning histories, which often involve beginning but not completing tasks. The negatively reinforcing model utilized by most educators in this circumstance tends to focus on misbehavior rather than on termination of the behavior. This may further disrupt the classroom by having a disinhibitory effect on other students. Although many years ago it was suggested that children with ADHD were intellectually less competent than their peers, it now appears more likely that weak performance on intellectual tasks results from the impact of impulsivity and inattention on test-taking behavior than from an innate lack of intelligence (Barkley, 1995). Kaplan, Crawford, Dewey, and Fisher (2000) identified a normal IQ distribution in children diagnosed with ADHD. Children with ADHD often underperform but may not underachieve during the elementary years. However, it has been reported that by high school at least 80% of these children fall behind in a basic academic subject requiring repetition and attention for competence, such as basic math knowledge, spelling, or written language (for reviews, see Barkley, 2006; Goldstein & Goldstein, 1998). Depending on diagnostic criteria, approximately 20–30% of children with ADHD also suffer from a concomitant, often language-based, learning disability (for a review, see Willcutt & Pennington, 2000). Although it has been hypothesized that ADHD may prevent a child from achieving his or her academic potential (Stott, 1981), the presence of a learning disability may make a child appear more inattentive than others (Aaron, Joshi, Palmer, Smith, & Kirby, 2002; McGee & Share, 1988).

Sociometric and play studies suggest that children with ADHD are not chosen as often by their peers to be best friends or partners in activities (Bagwell, Molina, Pelham, & Hoza, 2001; Pelham & Milich, 1984). They appear to be cognizant of their difficulties— an awareness that probably precipitates lower self-esteem for children with ADHD (Glow & Glow, 1980). Moreover, they appear to experience either high-prevalence, low-impact problems that result in poor social acceptance or low incidence, high impact problems that result in social rejection (Pelham & Milich, 1984). In addition, these children have difficulty adapting their behavior to different situational demands (Whalen, Henker, Collins, McAuliffe, & Vaux, 1979). It has been suggested that the impulsive behavioral patterns of children with ADHD are most responsible for their social difficulty; this may place those with comorbid hyperactive–impulsive problems of greater severity at even greater risk of developing social difficulties (Hodgens, Cole, & Boldizar, 2000; Pelham & Bender, 1982). ADHD has also been found to be a risk factor for a wide variety of ineffective social coping strategies as youth make the transition into adolescence (Young, Chadwick, Heptinstall, Taylor, & Sonuga-Barke, 2005). It should be noted as well that children who demonstrate satisfactory symptom and impairment reduction with medication appear to exhibit fewer chronic social impairments (Gallagher et al., 2004).

Some primary symptoms of ADHD may diminish in intensity by adolescence (Weiss & Hechtman, 1979). However, most adolescents with ADHD continue to experience significant problems (Milich & Loney, 1979; for reviews, see Barkley, 2006; Goldstein & Ellison, 2002). At least 80% of adolescents with ADHD continue to manifest symptoms consistent with ADHD. Sixty percent develop at least one additional disruptive disorder (Barkley, Fischer, Edelbrock, & Smallish, 1990). Between 20% and 60% of adolescents with ADHD are involved in antisocial behavior, whereas the usual occurrence is 3–4% (Satterfield, Hoppe, & Schell, 1982). At least 50–70% of these adolescents develop oppositional defiant disorder, often during their younger years, with a significant number progressing to conduct disorder (Barkley et al., 1990). However, the high prevalence of antisocial problems in adolescents with ADHD is likely to reflect the comorbidity of ADHD with other disruptive disorders, principally conduct disorder (Barkley, McMurray, Edelbrock, & Robbins, 1989). As Barkley (1997) succinctly points out, the preponderance of the available data suggests that while ADHD is clearly a risk factor for the development of adolescent antisocial problems, life experiences (principally factors within families) most powerfully contribute to the onset and maintenance of delinquency, conduct disorder, and subsequent young adult antisocial problems (see also Dalsgaard, Mortenson, Frydenberg, & Thomsen, 2002).

NEUROPSYCHOLOGICAL IMPAIRMENTS

The ecological validity of laboratory tests to identify the presence of ADHD symptoms and to determine their severity has been increasingly questioned (Barkley, 1991b; Barkley & Grodzinsky, 1994). Because ADHD is a disorder defined by behavior in the real world, it is not surprising that laboratory measures frequently fall short in identifying and defining symptoms of the disorder, in comparison to naturalistic observation, history, and organized report in the form of questionnaires. Nonetheless, it has been increasingly recognized that neuropsychologists take comfort in supplementing their clinical impressions with laboratory-generated, objective scores (DuPaul, Guevremont, & Barkley, 1991). It is acknowledged that these scores cannot be used alone to make the diagnosis of ADHD, but they may be helpful in the process of differential diagnosis (e.g., when is impulsivity a function of ADHD vs. other disorders?), as well as in determining severity or related prognosis in a group of individuals with ADHD (Gordon, 1995; Hall, Halperin, Schwartz, & Newcorn, 1997).

The development of a norm-referenced, psychometric assessment battery specifically designed for ADHD has been an elusive goal for researchers and clinicians. Thus, when one reviews the extensive literature attempting to hypothetically and objectively define specific neuropsychological impairments occurring consistently in children with ADHD, it is not surprising that no tried and true battery or specific pattern of impairment has come to light. As Levine (1992) has noted, ADHD symptoms appear to reflect "elusive entities and ... mistaken identities." The comorbidity issue, and many tests' lack of specificity in discriminating ADHD from other disorders, further complicate this endeavor. Compromised scores may be due to a variety of causes, leading some researchers to suggest that a profile of test scores be utilized in defining and explaining neuropsychological impairments in children with ADHD (Aylward, Verhulst, & Bell, 1993; Naglieri, 2000). Neuropsychologists should be aware that clinic or laboratory tests alone or in combination have been found to result in classification decisions that frequently disagree with a diagnosis of ADHD based on parent interview, history, and behavior rating scales (Doyle, Biederman, & Seidman, 2000; DuPaul, Anastopoulos, Shelton, Guevremont, & Metevia, 1992). Furthermore, although Szatmari, Offord, Siegel, Finlayson, and Tuff (1990) report that neuropsychological tests appear to distinguish children with ADHD from those with pure anxiety or affective (mood) disorders, they may not as efficiently distinguish ADHD from other disruptive disorders. These authors concluded that neuropsychological test scores are more strongly associated with externalizing than with internalizing diagnoses. They also appear to correlate with psychiatric symptoms at school but not at home. Moreover, scores on traditional neuropsychological instruments used to infer attention and impulse problems often do not correlate with each other (Naglieri, Goldstein, Delauder, & Schwebach, 2005). Thus it is not surprising that Barkley (1991a) suggests that when results of standardized behavior ratings, observations, and history conflict with laboratory measures, the latter should be disregarded in favor of the former, as these are considered more ecologically valid sources of data.

Cherkes-Julkowski, Stolzenberg, and Siegal (1991) suggest that perhaps performance on neuropsychological tests by children with

ADHD is a function of an inability to control focus of attention. These authors suggest that when prompts are provided during testing, children with ADHD perform significantly better. In a study evaluating children with ADHD with and without medication, compared to children with learning disabilities and a group of nondisabled controls, the greatest gains for prompts were observed in the unmedicated group with ADHD. However, neuropsychologists should be cautioned that prompts, especially on measures designed to evaluate response inhibition may actually test a child's ability to follow directions rather than to inhibit. Neuropsychologists should also keep in mind that there are data suggesting that level of reinforcement during test performance may have an impact on scores as well. Devers, Bradley-Johnson, and Johnson (1994) found that a 12-point improvement in Verbal IQ scores accrued when token reinforcers followed immediately for correct responses. The impact of praise on test performance has not been systematically evaluated. Finally, Draeger, Prior, and Sanson (1986) reported a greater deterioration in the performance of children with ADHD on a continuous-performance test than in control children's performance when the examiner left the room. These authors suggest that even an examiner's presence acts to mitigate test performance. It may well be that some children who perform poorly on test measures under these circumstances have an application deficit rather than an ability deficit.

EVALUATION

Due to the pervasive, multisetting nature of problems related to ADHD, and ADHD's high comorbidity with other childhood disorders, assessment for ADHD involves a thorough emotional, developmental, and behavioral evaluation. It should be noted, however, that the diagnosis of ADHD should be firmly based on the accepted standard, which at present is the DSM-IV-TR diagnostic criteria set. Professionals should be aware that efforts to include additional data to prove or disprove the diagnosis run the risk of introducing increasing variance (Naglieri, Goldstein, & Schwebach, 2004). The comprehensive evaluation should col-

lect data concerning the child's behavior at home, with friends, and at school; academic and intellectual functioning; medical status; and emotional development. It is suggested that professionals consider the following multistep process to accompany the evaluation of ADHD:

1. A complete history must be obtained. This is not a cursory process. Sufficient time (approximately 1½–2 hours) should be set aside to obtain a narrative of the child's development, behavior, extended family history, family relations, and current functioning. Within the context of the interview, efforts should be made to trace a developmental course that appears to fit the picture of ADHD, as well as to identify core symptoms and those related to other childhood disorders. Obtaining thorough knowledge of the diagnostic criteria for common and uncommon (e.g., high-functioning autism) childhood internalizing and externalizing disorders should be a paramount concern for the neuropsychologist, to facilitate the identification of high- as well as low-prevalence disorders.

2. Data obtained from the history should be supplemented by the completion of several standardized, factor-analyzed questionnaires concerning children's problems. At least two adults who interact with the child on a regular basis, ideally a parent and a teacher, should be requested to complete questionnaires. For general child assessment, valuable questionnaires are the Child Behavior Checklist (CBCL; Achenbach & Rescorla, 2001) and the Behavior Assessment System for Children, Second Edition (Reynolds & Kamphaus, 2004). The CBCL is a well-developed questionnaire that organizes childhood behavior on a disruptive–nondisruptive continuum. Research indicates that the Attention Problems scale in an earlier version of the CBCL correlates well with the two-factor DSM-IV ADHD diagnosis (Achenbach, 1996). The Conners 3rd Edition (Conners, 2008), the Comprehensive Teacher's Rating Scale (Ullman, Sleator, & Sprague, 1988), the Childhood Attention Problems Scale (Edelbrock, 1990), and the Academic Performance and ADHD Rating Scales (DuPaul, 1990) are also helpful. However, these questionnaires alone do not provide sufficient information for diagnosis;

they simply provide an organized report of behavior. They describe what the observer sees, but not why it is being seen.

3. From the history and questionnaires, the professional should be able to generate a consistent set of data and a series of hypotheses to explain the child's behavior across a variety of settings.

4. Requests should be made to review school records, including report cards and results of group achievement testing. If weak performance or learning disabilities are suspected, or if the child is already receiving special education services, the neuropsychologist should review all assessment data as well as the child's individualized education program. Then it is proper to decide which tests and what amount of time should be used to arrive at the most accurate evaluation of the child. Neuropsychologists should be cautioned that, as just reviewed, no specific laboratory tests to evaluate ADHD have demonstrated sufficient positive and negative predictive power to be relied on. The primary purpose of face-to-face assessment with a child should be to address issues related to the child's emotional status, self-esteem, cognitive development, and possible learning disabilities. Observation of the child's behavior during assessment may also yield clues regarding his or her interpersonal style and temperament.

5. Although a number of paper-and-pencil tasks have been used over the years in research settings to identify symptoms of ADHD, most have not lent themselves easily to clinical use. In research studies some of these tests, such as the Matching Familiar Figures Test (Kagan, 1964), have appeared to show strong positive and negative predictive power for identifying impulsive children. However, in clinical practice, such instruments have not proven reliable for confirming the diagnosis of ADHD. Computerized instruments designed to measure sustained attention and the ability to inhibit impulsive responding (Conners, 2004; Gordon, 1993; Greenberg, 1991) have become increasingly popular among neuropsychologists. However, it is important to remember that although these instruments may demonstrate strong positive predictive power (i.e., if a child fails such a task, it strongly confirms the presence of symptoms related to ADHD), they

possess poor negative predictive power (i.e., if a child passes a task, conclusions cannot be drawn one way or the other concerning the diagnosis) (McGee, Clark, & Symons, 2000). Nonetheless, many neuropsychologists rely on such instruments to provide additional data as part of the diagnostic process, rather than specifically to confirm or disconfirm the diagnosis of ADHD (Riccio, Reynolds, & Lowe, 2001). The interested reader is referred to Homack and Reynolds (2005) for a thorough review of the literature concerning computerized assessment of ADHD. Although several studies have suggested that measurement of specific intellectual processes may differentiate youth with various subtypes of ADHD (Naglieri, 1999; Paolito, 1999), data generated by instruments such as the Cognitive Assessment System (Naglieri & Das, 1997) are not necessary in making the diagnosis of ADHD but can provide useful information concerning differences in cognitive processes among diagnosed youth.

TREATMENT

Treatment of ADHD must be multidisciplinary, multimodal, and maintained over a long period (for reviews, see Goldstein & Ellison, 2002; Goldstein & Goldstein, 1998; Teeter, 1998). By far the most effective short-term interventions for ADHD are combinations of medical, behavioral, and environmental techniques.

Medication has demonstrated the ability to reduce the manipulative power of a child's behavior in eliciting certain responses from teachers, peers, and family members. An extensive literature attests to the benefits of medicine, specifically stimulants, in reducing key symptoms of ADHD and thus improving daily functioning (Klein, 1987; for reviews, see Barkley, 2006; Goldstein & Goldstein, 1998). Stimulants and other drugs principally affecting dopamine and norepinephrine (Volkow et al., 2001) have consistently have been reported to improve academic achievement and productivity, as well as accuracy of classwork (Douglas, Barr, O'Neill, & Britton, 1986); improved attention span, reading comprehension, complex problem solving, and inhibitory processes have also been noted (Balthazor, Wagner, & Pelham, 1991; Pelham, 1987). Related problems, including peer interactions, peer status, and even relationships with family members, have been reported to be improved with stimulants as well (Whalen & Henker, 1991).

Behavior management increases the salience of behaving in a way consistent with environmental expectations. The manipulation of the environment (e.g., making tasks more interesting and payoffs more valuable) reduces the risk of problems within the natural setting. Zentall (1995) suggests that students with ADHD possess an active learning style, with a demonstrated need to move, talk, respond, question, choose, debate, and even provoke. Thus, in classroom settings, children with ADHD do not fare well in sedentary situations. Interventions for managing ADHD in the classroom have included positive and negative contingent teacher attention, token economies, peer-mediated and group contingencies, time-out, home–school contingencies, reductive techniques based on reinforcement, and cognitive-behavioral strategies (Abramowitz & O'Leary, 1991). Environmental and task modifications are also critical for classroom success for the child with ADHD. However, additional research is needed, especially in the area of school-based intervention, for adolescents with ADHD.

Though they are popular, cognitive strategies (e.g., teaching a child to stop, look, and listen) as well as other nontraditional treatments (e.g., dietary manipulation, electroencephalographic biofeedback, etc.) to reduce symptoms of ADHD have not received consistent support in scientific research. The interested reader is referred to Braswell (1998) for a review of these issues. However, Shure (1994) suggests that the patient application of cognitive training over a long period of time in real-world settings can improve the self-regulatory skills of children with ADHD, and recent studies of cognitive-behavioral interventions for ADHD are beginning to yield promising results (Aberson, Shure, & Goldstein, 2007; Fabiano et al., 2009).

Regardless of the treatment modality employed, the basic underlying premise in managing problems of ADHD involves increasing the child's capacity to inhibit responding. This is consistent with the theoretical construct that the core problem for ADHD reflects an inability to take sufficient time to think or respond consistently to consequences.

SUMMARY

Professionals must be prepared to rely extensively upon history, report, and observation, and less so upon structured laboratory testing, in attempting to understand the behavior and problems of children with ADHD. This chapter has provided an overview of the current literature concerning the definition, genetic, neurobiology, evaluation, and treatment of ADHD in children.

REFERENCES

Aaron, P. G., Joshi, R. M., Palmer, H., Smith, M., & Kirby, E. (2002). Separating genuine cases of reading disability from reading deficits caused by predominantly inattentive ADHD behavior. *Journal of Learning Disabilities, 35,* 425–435.

Aberson, B., Shure, M. B., & Goldstein, S. (2007). Social problem-solving intervention can help children with ADHD. *Journal of Attention Disorders, 11,* 4–7.

Abramowitz, A. J., & O'Leary, S. G. (1991). Behavior interventions for the classroom: Implications for students with ADHD. *School Psychology Review, 20,* 220–234.

Accardo, P. J., Blondis, T. J., & Whitman, B. Y. (1990). Disorders of attention and activity level in a referral population. *Pediatrics, 85,* 426–431.

Achenbach, T. M. (1996). Subtyping ADHD: The request for suggestions about relating empirically based assessment to DSM-IV. *ADHD Report, 4,* 5–9.

Achenbach, T. M., & Rescorla, L. A. (2001). *Manual for ASEBA school-age forms and profiles.* Burlington: University of Vermont, Research Center for Children, Youth, and Families.

Altfas, J. R. (2002). Prevalence of ADHD among adults in obesity treatment. *Biomedical Psychology, 2,* 1–14.

American Psychiatric Association (APA). (1994). *Diagnostic and statistical manual of mental disorders* (4th ed., rev.). Washington, DC: Author.

American Psychiatric Association (APA). (2000). *Diagnostic and statistical manual of mental disorders* (4th ed., text rev.). Washington, DC: Author.

Anastopoulos, A. D., Barkley, R., & Shelton, T. (1994). The history and diagnosis of attention deficit/hyperactivity disorder. *Therapeutic Care and Education, 3,* 96–110.

Aylward, G. P., Verhulst, S. J., & Bell, S. (1993, September). *Inter-relationships between measures of attention deficit disorders: Same scores, different reasons.* Paper presented at the Society for Behavioral Pediatrics meeting, Providence, RI.

Bagwell, C. L., Molina, D. S., Pelham, W. E., & Hoza, B. (2001). ADHD and problems in peer relations: Predictions from childhood to adolescence. *Journal of the American Academy of Child and Adolescent Psychiatry, 40*, 1285–1299.

Baker, L., & Cantwell, D. P. (1987). A prospective psychiatric follow-up of children with speech/language disorders. *Journal of the American Academy of Child Psychiatry, 26*, 546–553.

Baker, L., & Cantwell, D. P. (1992). Attention deficit disorder and speech/language disorders. *Comprehensive Mental Health Care, 2*, 3–16.

Balthazor, M. J., Wagner, R. K., & Pelham, W. E. (1991). The specificity of the effects of stimulant medication on classroom learning-related measures of cognitive processing for attention deficit disorder children. *Journal of Abnormal Child Psychology, 19*, 35–52.

Barkley, R. A. (1991a). Attention-deficit hyperactivity disorder. *Psychiatric Annals, 21*, 725–733.

Barkley, R. A. (1991b). The ecological validity of laboratory and analogue assessment methods of ADHD symptoms. *Journal of Abnormal Child Psychology, 19*, 149–178.

Barkley, R. A. (1995). ADHD and I.Q. *ADHD Report, 3*, 1–3.

Barkley, R. A. (1997). *Defiant children: A clinician's manual for assessment and parent training* (2nd ed.). New York: Guilford Press.

Barkley, R. A. (2006). *Attention-deficit/hyperactivity disorder: A handbook for diagnosis and treatment* (3rd ed.). New York: Guilford Press.

Barkley, R. A., Fischer, M., Edelbrock, C. S., & Smallish, L. (1990). The adolescent outcome of hyperactive children diagnosed by research criteria: I. An eight year prospective follow-up study. *Journal of the American Academy of Child and Adolescent Psychiatry, 29*, 546–557.

Barkley, R. A., Fischer, M., Smallish, L., & Fletcher, K. (2004). Young adult follow-up of hyperactive children: Antisocial activities and drug use. *Journal of Child Psychology and Psychiatry, 45*, 195–207.

Barkley, R. A., & Gordon, M. (2002). Research on comorbidity, adaptive functioning and cognitive impairments in adults with ADHD: Implications for a clinical practice. In S. Goldstein & A. T. Ellison (Eds.), *Clinician's guide to adult ADHD: Assessment and intervention* (pp. 143–169). San Diego, CA: Academic Press.

Barkley, R. A., & Grodzinsky, G. M. (1994). Are tests of frontal lobe functions useful in the diagnosis of attention deficit disorder? *Clinical Neuropsychologist, 8*, 121–139.

Barkley, R. A., McMurray, M. B., Edelbrock, C. S., & Robbins, K. (1989). The response of aggressive and non-aggressive ADHD children to two doses of methylphenidate. *Journal of the American Academy of Child and Adolescent Psychiatry, 28*, 873–881.

Bastain, T. M., Lewczyk, C. M., Sharp, W. S., James, R. S., Long, R. T., Eagen, P. B., et al. (2002). Cytogenetic abnormalities in ADHD. *Journal of the American Academy of Child and Adolescent Psychiatry, 41*, 806–810.

Benjamin, J., Li, L., Patterson, C., Greenberg, B. D., Murphy, D. L., & Hamer, D. H. (1996). Population and familial association between the D4 dopamine receptor gene and measures of novelty seeking. *Nature Genetics, 12*, 81–84.

Biederman, J., Faraone, S. V., Keenan, K., Knee, D., & Tsuang, M. T. (1990). Family-genetic and psychosocial risk factors in DSM-III attention deficit disorders. *Journal of the American Academy of Child and Adolescent Psychiatry, 29*, 526–533.

Biederman, J., Faraone, S. V., Keenan, K., Benjamin, J., Krifcher, B., Moore, C., et al. (1992). Further evidence for family-genetic risk factors in attention deficit hyperactivity disorder: Patterns of comorbidity in probands and relatives in psychiatrically and paediatrically referred samples. *Archives of General Psychiatry, 49*, 728–738.

Biederman, J., Faraone, S., Mick, E., Wozniak, J., Chen, L., Ouelette, C., et al. (1996). Attention deficit hyperactivity disorder in juvenile mania: An overlooked comorbidity? *Journal of the American Academy of Child and Adolescent Psychiatry, 35*, 997–1008.

Biederman, J., Kim, J. W., Doyle, A. E., Mick, E., Fagerness, J., Smoller, J. W., et al. (2008). Sexually dimorphic effects of four genes (COMT, SLC6A2, MAOA, SLC6A4) in genetic associations of ADHD: A preliminary study. *American Journal of Medical Genetics, Part B, 147B*, 1511–1518.

Biederman, J., Mick, E., Faraone, S. V., Braaten, E., Doyle, A., Spencer, T., et al. (2002). Influence of gender on attention deficit hyperactivity disorder in children referred to a psychiatric clinic. *American Journal of Psychiatry, 159*, 36–42.

Biederman, J., Petty, C. R., Fried, R., Black, S., Faneuil, A., Doyle, A. E., et al. (2008). Discordance between psychometric testing and questionnaire-based definition of executive function deficits in individuals with ADHD. *Journal of Attention Disorders, 12*, 92–102.

Blondis, T. A., Snow, J. H., Stein, M., & Roizen, N. J. (1991). Appropriate use of measures of attention and activity for the diagnosis and management of attention deficit hyperactivity disorder. In P. J. Accardo, T. A. Blondis, & B. Y. Whitman (Eds.), *Attention deficit disorders and hyperactivity in children* (pp. 85–120). New York: Dekker.

Bloom, D. R., Levin, H. S., Ewing-Cobbs, L., Saunders, A. E., Song, J., Fletcher, J. M., et al.

(2001). Lifetime and novel psychiatric disorders after pediatric traumatic brain injury. *Journal of the American Academy of Child and Adolescent Psychiatry, 40,* 572–579.

Brand, E. F., Das-Smaal, E. A., & De Jonge, B. F. (1996). Subtypes of children with attention disabilities. *Child Neuropsychology, 2,* 109–122.

Braswell, L. (1998). Cognitive behavioral approaches as adjunctive treatments for ADHD children and their families. In S. Goldstein & M. Goldstein (Eds.), *Managing attention deficit hyperactivity disorder in children: A guide for practitioners* (2nd ed., pp. 533–544). New York: Wiley.

Cantwell, D. P., Baker, L., & Mattison, R. (1981). Prevalence, type and correlates of psychiatric disorder in 200 children with communication disorder. *Journal of Developmental and Behavioral Pediatrics, 2,* 131–136.

Cardon, L. R., Smith, S. D., Fulker, D. W., Kimberling, W. J., Pennington, B. F., & De Fries, J. C. (1994). Quantitative trait locus for reading disability in chromosome 6. *Science, 266,* 276–279.

Carey, W. B. (1970). A simplified method for measuring infant temperament. *Journal of Pediatrics, 77,* 188–194.

Carlson, C. L., & Mann, M. (2002). Sluggish cognitive tempo predicts a different pattern of impairment in the attention deficit hyperactivity disorder—predominantly inattentive type. *Journal of Clinical Child and Adolescent Psychology, 31,* 123–129.

Castellanos, F. X., Giedd, J. N., Marsh, W. L., Hamburger, S. D., Vaituzis, A. C., Dickstein, D. P., et al. (1996). Quantitative brain magnetic resonance imaging in attention-deficit hyperactivity disorder. *Archives of General Psychiatry, 53,* 607–616.

Castle, L., Aubert, R. E., Verbrugge, R. R., Khalid, M., & Epstein, R. S. (2007). Trends in Medication for ADHD. *Journal of Attention Disorders, 10,* 335–342.

Centers for Disease Control and Prevention (CDC). (2005). Mental health in the United States: Prevalence of diagnosis and medication treatment of attention deficit/hyperactivity disorder—United States, 2003. *Morbidity and Mortality Weekly Report, 54,* 842–847.

Chabildas, N., Pennington, B. F., & Willicutt, E. G. (2001). A comparison of the neuropsychological profiles of the DSM-IV subtypes of ADHD. *Journal of Abnormal Child Psychology, 29,* 529–540.

Cherkes-Julkowski, M., Stolzenberg, J., & Siegal, L. (1991). Prompted cognitive testing as a diagnostic compensation for attentional deficits: The Raven Standard Progressive Matrices and attention deficit disorder. *Learning Disabilities, 2,* 1–7.

Chess, S., & Thomas, A. (1986). *Temperament in clinical practice.* New York: Guilford Press.

Clark, C., Prior, M., & Kinsella, G. J. (2000). Do executive function deficits differentiate between adolescents with ADHD and oppositional defiant/conduct disorder: A neuropsychological study using the Six Elements Test and the Hayling Sentence Completion Test. *Journal of Abnormal Child Psychology, 28,* 403–414.

Cohen, N. J., Davine, M., & Meloche-Kelly, M. (1989). Prevalence of unsuspected language disorders in a child psychiatric population. *Journal of the American Academy of Child and Adolescent Psychiatry, 28,* 107–111.

Cohen, N. J., Sullivan, S., Minde, K. K., Novak, C. ., & Helwig, C. (1981). Evaluation of the relative effectiveness of methylphenidate and cognitive behavior modification in the treatment of kindergarten-aged hyperactive children. *Journal of Abnormal Child Psychology, 9,* 43–54.

Comings, D. E., Wu, S., & Chiu, C. (1996). Polygenic inheritance of Tourette syndrome, stuttering, attention deficit hyperactivity, conduct and oppositional defiant disorder. *American Journal of Medical Genetics, 67,* 264–288.

Conners, C. K. (2004). *Conners Continuous Performance Test II (Version 5).* North Tonawanda, NY: Multi-Health Systems.

Conners, C. K. (2008). *Conners 3rd Edition.* North Tonawanda, NY: Multi-Health Systems.

Cook, E. H., Stein, M. A., Krasowski, M. D., Cox, N. J., Olkon, D. M., Kieffer, J. E., et. al. (1995). Association of attention deficit disorder and the dopamine transporter gene. *American Journal of Human Genetics, 56,* 993–998.

Crighton, A. (1798). *An inquiry into the nature and origin of mental derangement* (2 vols.). London: Strand.

Cuffe, S. P., Moore, C. G., & McKeown, R. E. (2005). Prevalence and correlates of ADHD symptoms in the National Health Interview Survey. *Journal of Attention Disorders, 9(2),* 392–401.

Crystal, D. S., Ostrander, R., Chen, R., & August, G. J. (2001). Multi-method assessment of psychopathology among DSM-IV subtypes of children with ADHD: Self, parent and teacher reports. *Journal of Abnormal Child Psychology, 29,* 189–205.

Daigneault, S., Braun, C. M. J., & Whitaker, H. A. (1992). An empirical test of two opposing theoretical models of prefrontal function. *Brain and Cognition, 19,* 48–71.

Dalsgaard, S., Mortenson, P., Frydenberg, M., & Thomsen, P. H. (2002). Conduct problems: Gender and adult psychiatric outcome of children with ADHD. *British Journal of Psychiatry, 181,* 416–421.

De Fries, J. C., & Fulker, D. W. (1985). Multiple regression analysis of twin data. *Behavior Genetics, 15,* 467–473.

De Fries, J. C., & Fulker, D. W. (1988). Multiple regression analysis of twin data: etiology of deviant scores versus individual differences. *Acta*

Geneticae Medicae et Gemellologiae (Roma), 37, 205–216.

Devers, R., Bradley-Johnson, S., & Johnson, C. M. (1994). The effect of token reinforcement on WISC-R performance for fifth through ninth grade American Indians. *Psychological Record, 44,* 441–449.

Douglas, V. I., Barr, R. G., O'Neil, M. E., & Britton, B. G. (1986). Short-term effects of methylphenidate on the cognitive, learning, and academic performance of children with attention deficit disorder in the laboratory and classroom. *Journal of Child Psychology and Psychiatry, 27,* 191-211.

Doyle, A. E., Biederman, J., & Seidman, L. J. (2000). Diagnostic efficacy of neuropsychological test scores for discriminating boys with and without ADHD. *Journal of Consulting and Clinical Psychology, 68,* 477–488.

Draeger, S., Prior, M., & Sanson, A. (1986). Visual and auditory attention performance in hyperactive children: Competence or compliance. *Journal of Abnormal Child Psychology, 14,* 411–424.

DuPaul, G. J. (1990). *Academic Performance Rating Scale and ADHD Rating Scale.* Worcester: University of Massachusetts. Department of Psychiatry.

DuPaul, G. J., Anastopoulos, A. D., Shelton, T. L., Guevremont, D. C., & Metevia, L. (1992). Multimethod assessment of attention-deficit hyperactivity disorder: The diagnostic utility of clinic-based tests. *Journal of Clinical Child Psychology, 21,* 394–402.

DuPaul, G. J., Guevremont, D. C., & Barkley, R. A. (1991). Attention deficit hyperactivity disorder in adolescence: Critical assessment parameters. *Clinical Psychological Review, 11,* 231–245.

DuPaul, G. J., McGoey, K. E., Eckert, T. L., & Van Brakle, J. V. (2001). Preschool children with ADHD: Impairments in behavioral, social and school functioning. *Journal of the American Academy of Child and Adolescent Psychiatry, 40,* 508–515.

Eaves, L. J., Silberg, J. L., & Hewitt, J. K. (1993). Genes, personality, and psychopathology: A latent class analysis of liability to symptoms of attention deficit hyperactivity disorder in twins. In R. Plomin & G. McClean (Eds.), *Nature, nurture, and psychology* (pp. 285–303). Washington, DC: American Psychological Association.

Ebstein, E. B., Novick, O., Umansky, R., Priel, B., Osher, Y., Blaine, D., et al. (1996). Dopamine D4 receptor (D4DR) exon III polymorphism associated with the human personality trait of novelty seeking. *Nature Genetics, 12,* 78–80.

Edelbrock, C. (1990). Childhood Attention Problems (CAP) scale. In R. A. Barkley, *Attention-deficit hyperactivity disorder: A handbook for diagnosis and treatment* (pp. 320–321). New York: Guilford Press.

Edelbrock, C., Rende, R., Plomin, R., & Thompson, L. A. (1995). A twin study of competence and problem behavior in childhood and early adolescence. *Journal of Psychology and Psychiatry, 36,* 775–785.

Eiraldi, R. B., Power, T. J., & Nezu, C. M. (1997). Patterns of comorbidity associated with subtypes of attention deficit/hyperactivity disorder among six- to twelve-year-old children. *Journal of the American Academy of Child and Adolescent Psychiatry, 36,* 503–514.

Ellis, A. W. (1985). The cognitive neuropsychology of development (and acquired) dyslexia: A critical survey. *Cognitive Neuropsychology, 2,* 169–205.

Fabiano, G. A., Pelham, W. E., Coles, E. K., Gnagy, E. M., Chronis-Tuscano, A., & O'Connor, B. C. (2009). A meta-analysis of behavioral treatments for ADHD. *Clinical Psychology Review, 29*(2), 129–140.

Faraone, S. V., & Biederman, J. (2005). What is the prevalence of adult ADHD?: Results of a population screen of 966 adults. *Journal of Attention Disorders, 9*(2), 384–391.

Faraone, S. V., Biederman, J., Chen, W. J., & Krifcher, B. (1992). Segregation analyses of attention deficit hyperactivity disorder. *Psychiatric Genetics, 2,* 257–275.

Faraone, S. V., Biederman, J., & Friedman, D. (2000). Validity of DSM-IV subtypes of attention-deficit/hyperactivity disorder: A family study perspective. *Journal of the American Academy of Child and Adolescent Psychiatry, 59,* 300–307.

Faraone, S. V., Doyle, A. E., Lasky-Su, J., Sklar, P. B., D'Angelo, E., Gonzalez-Heydrich, J., et al. (2008). Linkage analysis of attention deficit hyperactivity disorder. *American Journal of Medical Genetics, Part B, 147B,* 1387–1391.

Faraone, S. V., & Khan, S. A. (2006). Candidate gene studies of attention-deficit/hyperactivity disorder. *Journal of Clinical Psychiatry, 67,* 13–20.

Faraone, S. V., Perlis, R. H., Doyle, A. E., Smoller, J. W., Goralnick, J. J., Holmgren, M. A., et al. (2005). Molecular genetics of attention-deficit/ hyperactivity disorder. *Biological Psychiatry, 57,* 1313–1323.

Fergusson, D. M., & Horwood, L. J. (1992). Attention deficit and reading achievement. *Journal of Child Psychology and Psychiatry, 33,* 375–385.

Fuster, J. M. (1989). A theory of prefrontal functions: The prefrontal cortex and the temporal organization of behavior. In J. M. Fuster (Ed.), *The prefrontal cortex: Anatomy, physiology, and neuropsychology of the frontal lobe* (pp. 123–164). New York: Raven Press.

Gadow, K. D., Sprafkin, J., & Nolan, E. (2001). DSM-IV symptoms in community and clinic preschool children. *Journal of the American Academy of Child and Adolescent Psychiatry, 40,* 1383–1392.

Gallagher, R., Fleiss, K., Etkovich, J., Cousins, L.,

Greenfield, B., Martin, D., et al. (2004). Social functioning in children with ADHD treated with long-term methylphenidate and multi-modal psychosocial treatment. *Journal of the American Academy of Child and Adolescent Psychiatry, 43*, 820–829.

Geurts, H. M., Verte, S., Oosterlaan, J., Roeyers, H., & Sergeant, J. A. (2005). ADHD subtypes: Do they differ in their executive functioning profile? *Archives of Clinical Neuropsychology, 20*, 457–477.

Gibson, E., & Radner, N. (1979). Attention: Perceiver as performer. In G. Hale & M. Lewis (Eds.), *Attention and development* (pp. 235–267). New York: Plenum Press.

Gillis, J. J., Gilger, J. W., Pennington, B. F., & De Fries, J. C. (1992). Attention deficit disorders in reading disabled twins: Evidence for a genetic etiology. *Journal of Abnormal Child Psychology, 20*, 303–315.

Glow, R. A., & Glow, P. H. (1980). Peer and self-rating: Children's perception of behavior relevant to hyperkinetic impulse disorder. *Journal of Abnormal Psychology, 8*, 471–490.

Goldstein, S., & Brooks, R. (2007). *Understanding and managing children's classroom behavior.* Hoboken, NJ: Wiley.

Goldstein, S., & Ellison, A. T. (Eds.). (2002). *Clinician's guide to adult ADHD: Assessment and intervention.* San Diego, CA: Academic Press.

Goldstein, S., & Goldstein, M. (1998). *Understanding and managing attention deficit hyperactivity disorder in children: A guide for practitioners* (2nd ed.). New York: Wiley.

Goldstein, S., & Naglieri, J. (2006). The role of intellectual processes in the DSM-V diagnosis of ADHD. *Journal of Attention Disorders, 10(1)*, 3–8.

Goldstein, S., & Schwebach, A. (2005). Attention-deficit/hyperactivity disorder. In S. Goldstein & C. R. Reynolds (Eds.), *Handbook of neurodevelopmental and genetic disorders in adults* (pp. 115–146). New York: Guilford Press.

Goodman, R., & Stevenson, J. (1989). A twin study of hyperactivity: II. The aetiological role of genes, family relationships and perinatal activity. *Journal of Child Psychology and Psychiatry, 30*, 691–709.

Gordon, M. (1993). Do computerized measures of attention have a legitimate role in ADHD evaluations? *ADHD Report, 1*, 5–6.

Gordon, M. (1995). *How to own and operate an ADHD clinic.* DeWitt, NY: Gordon Systems.

Gordon, M., Antshel, K., Faraone, S., Barkley, R., Lewandowski, L., Hudziak, J., et al. (2006). Symptoms versus impairment: The case for respecting DSM-IV's Criterion D. *Journal of Attention Disorders, 9(3)*, 465–475.

Gordon, M., & McClure, F. D. (1983). *The objective assessment of attention deficit disorders.* Paper presented at the 91st Annual Convention of the American Psychological Association, Anaheim, CA.

Greenberg, L. (1991). *Test of Variables of Attention (TOVA).* St. Paul, MN: Attention Technology.

Guevremont, D. C., DuPaul, G. J., & Barkley, R. A. (1993). Behavioral assessment of attention deficit hyperactivity disorder. In J. L. Matson (Ed.), *Handbook of hyperactivity in children* (pp. 150–168). Needham Heights, MA: Allyn & Bacon.

Haenlein, M., & Caul, W. F. (1987). Attention deficit disorder with hyperactivity: A specific hypothesis of reward dysfunction. *Journal of the American Academy of Child and Adolescent Psychiatry, 26*, 356–362.

Hagen, J. W., & Hale, G. H. (1973). The development of attention in children. *Child Psychology, 7*, 117–137.

Hagerman, R. (1991). Organic causes of ADHD. *ADD-VANCE, 3*, 4–6.

Hall, S. J., Halperin, J. M., Schwartz, S. T., & Newcorn, J. H. (1997). Behavioral and executive functions in children with attention deficit hyperactivity disorder and reading disability. *Journal of Attention Disorders, 1*, 235–247.

Halperin, J. M., Newcorn, J. H., Matier, K., Sharma, V., McKay, K. E., & Schwartz, S. (1993). Discriminant validity of attention-deficit hyperactivity disorder. *Journal of the American Academy of Child and Adolescent Psychiatry, 32*, 1038–1043.

Harrier, L. K., & DeOrnellas, K. (2005). Performance of children diagnosed with ADHD on selected planning and reconstitution tests. *Applied Neuropsychology, 12*, 106–119.

Hart, C. C., & Harter, S. L. (2001, October 31–November 3). *Measurement of right frontal lobe functioning and ADHD.* Abstract from the 21st Annual Meeting of the National Academy of Neuropsychology.

Hechtman, L. (1993). Genetic and neurobiological aspects of attention deficit hyperactivity disorder: A review. *Journal of Psychiatric Neuroscience, 9*, 193–201.

Hodgens, J., Cole, J., & Boldizar, J. (2000). Peer-based differences among boys with ADHD. *Journal of Clinical Child Psychology, 29*, 443–452.

Homack, S. R., & Reynolds, C. R. (2005). Continuous performance testing in differential diagnosis of ADHD. *ADHD Report, 13(5)*, 5–9.

Houshyar, S., & Kaufman, J. (2005). Resiliency in maltreated children. In S. Goldstein & R. Brooks (Eds.), *Handbook of resilience in children.* New York: Kluwer Academic/Plenum Press.

James, W. (1890). *The principles of psychology.* New York: Holt.

Kagan, J. (1964). *The Matching Familiar Figures Test.* Unpublished manuscript, Harvard University.

Kaplan, B. J., Crawford, S. G., Dewey, D. M., &

Fisher, G. C. (2000). The I.Q.'s of children with ADHD are normally distributed. *Journal of Learning Disabilities, 33,* 425–432.

Katz, M. (1997). *Playing a poor hand well.* New York: Norton.

Klein, R. G. (1987). Pharmacotherapy of childhood hyperactivity: An update. In H. Y. Meltzer (Ed.), *Psychopharmacology: The third generation of progress* (pp. 287–301). New York: Raven Press.

Lahey, B. B., Applegate, B., McBurnett, K., Biederman, J., Greenhill, L., Hynd, G., et al. (1994). DSM-IV field trial for attention/deficit hyperactivity disorder in children and adolescents. *American Journal of Psychiatry, 151,* 1673–1685.

Lahey, B. B., Pelham, W. E., Loney, J., Lee, S., & Willcutt, E. (2005). Instability of the DSM-IV subtypes of ADHD from preschool through elementary school. *Archives of General Psychiatry, 62,* 896–902.

LaHoste, G. J., Swanson, J. M., Wigal, S. B., Glabe, C., Wigal, T., King, N., et al. (1996). Dopamine D4 receptor gene polymorphism is associated with attention deficit hyperactivity disorder. *Molecular Psychiatry, 1,* 121–124.

Levine, M. D. (1992). Commentary: Attentional disorders: Elusive entities and their mistaken identities. *Journal of Child Neurology, 7,* 449–453.

Levy, F., Hay, D. A., McStephen, M., Wood, C., & Waldman, I. (1997). Attention-deficit hyperactivity disorder: A category or a continuum? Genetic analysis of a large-scale twin study. *Journal of the American Academy of Child and Adolescent Psychiatry, 36,* 737–744.

Lowe, N., Kirley, A., Hawi, Z., Sham, P., Wickham, H., Kratochvil, C. J., et al. (2004). Joint analysis of the DRD5 marker concludes association with ADHD confined to the predominantly inattentive and combined subtypes. *American Journal of Human Genetics, 74,* 348–356.

Luk, S. L., Leung, P. W., & Yuen, J. (1991). Clinic observations in the assessment of pervasiveness of childhood hyperactivity. *Journal of Child Psychology and Psychiatry, 32,* 833–850.

Mautner, V. F., Kluwe, L., Thakker, S. D., & Laerk, R. A. (2002). Treatment of ADHD in neurofibromatosis type 1. *Developmental Medicine and Child Neurology, 44,* 164–170.

McGee, R. A., Clark, S. E., & Symons, D. K. (2000). Does the Conners' Continuous Performance Test aid in ADHD diagnosis? *Journal of Abnormal Child Psychology, 28,* 415–424.

McGee, R., & Share, D. L. (1988). Attention deficit disorder hyperactivity and academic failure: Which comes first and what should be treated? *Journal of the American Academy of Child and Adolescent Psychiatry, 27,* 318–325.

Medco Health Solutions. (2005). *ADHD medication use growing faster among adults than children: New research.* Retrieved from *www.medco. com*

Mesulam, M. M. (1985). *Principles of behavioral neurology.* Philadelphia: Davis.

Milich, R. S., & Loney, J. (1979). The role of hyperactive and aggressive symptomatology in predicting adolescent outcome among hyperactive children. *Journal of Pediatric Psychology, 4,* 93–112.

Mirskey, A. F., Anthony, B. J., Duncan, C. C., Ahearn, M. B., & Kellam, S. G. (1991). Analysis of the elements of attention: A neuropsychological approach. *Neuropsychology Review, 2,* 109–145.

Mrug, S., Hoza, B., Gerdes, A. C., Hinshaw, S., Arnold, L. E., Hechtman, L., et al. (2009). Discriminating between children with ADHD and classmates using peer variables. *Journal of Attention Disorders, 12,* 372–380.

Murphy, K., Barkley, R., & Bush, T. (2002). Young adults with ADHD: Subtype differences in comorbidity, educational and clinical history. *Journal of Nervous and Mental Disease, 190,* 1–11.

Naglieri, J. A. (1999). *Essentials for CAS assessment.* New York: Wiley.

Naglieri, J. (2000). Can profile analysis of ability test scores work?: An illustration using the PASS theory and CAS with an unselected cohort. *School Psychology Quarterly, 15,* 419–433.

Naglieri, J. A., & Das, J. P. (1997). *Cognitive Assessment System.* Itasca, IL: Riverside.

Naglieri, J. A., & Das, J. P. (2006). Are intellectual processes important in the diagnosis and treatment of ADHD? *ADHD Report, 14*(1), 1–6.

Naglieri, J., Goldstein, S., Delauder, B., & Schwebach, A. (2005). Relationships between the WISC-III and the Cognitive Assessment System with Conners' Rating Scales and Continuous Performance Tests. *Archives of Clinical Neuropsychology, 20,* 385–401.

Naglieri, J., Goldstein, S., & Schwebach, A. (2004). Can there be reliable identification of ADHD with divergent conceptualization and inconsistent test results? *ADHD Report, 12,* 6–9.

Neale, B. M., Lasky-Su, J., Anney, R., Franke, B., Zhou, K., Maller, J. B., et al. (2008). Genome-wide association scan of attention deficit hyperactivity disorder. *American Journal of Medical Genetics, Part B, 147B,* 1337–1344.

O'Neill, M. E., & Douglas, V. I. (1996). Rehearsal strategies and recall performance with boys with and without attention deficit hyperactivity disorder. *Journal of Pediatric Psychology, 21,* 73–88.

Paolito, A. W. (1999). Clinical validation of the Cognitive Assessment System for children with ADHD. *ADHD Report, 1,* 1–5.

Pelham, W. E. (1987). What do we know about the use and effects of CNS stimulants in ADD? In J. Loney (Ed.), *The young hyperactive child: Answers to questions about diagnosis, prognosis and treatment* (pp. 99–110). New York: Haworth Press.

Pelham, W. E., & Bender, M. E. (1982). Peer relationships in hyperactive children. In K. D. Gadow & I. Bialer (Eds.), *Advances in learning and behavioral disabilities* (Vol. 1, pp. 365–436). Greenwich, CT: JAI Press.

Pelham, W. E., & Milich, R. (1984). Peer relations of children with hyperactivity/attention deficit disorder. *Journal of Learning Disabilities, 17,* 560–568.

Picano, J. J., Klusman, L. E., Hornbestel, L. K., & Moulton, J. M. (1992). Replication of three-component solution for common measures of attention in HIV seropositive males. *Archives of Clinical Neuropsychology, 7,* 271–274.

Posner, M. I. (1987). Selective attention in head injury. In H. S. Levin, J. Grafman, & H. M. Eisenberg (Eds.), *Neurobehavioral recovery from head injury* (pp. 144–157). New York: Oxford University Press.

Posner, M. I., & Snyder, C. R. (1975). Attention and cognitive control. In R. Solso (Ed.), *Information processing and cognition: The Loyola Symposium* (Vol. 2, pp. 163–187). Hillsdale, NJ: Erlbaum.

Rabiner, D. L., Anastopoulos, A. D., Costello, J., Hoyle, R. H., & Swartzwelder, H. S. (2008). Adjustment to college in students with ADHD. *Journal of Attention Disorders, 11,* 689–699.

Reynolds, C. R., & Kamphaus, R. W. (2004). *The Behavior Assessment System for Children, Second Edition.* Bloomington, MN: Pearson Assessments.

Riccio, C. A., Reynolds, C. R., & Lowe, P. A. (2001). *Clinical applications of continuous performance tests: Measuring attention and impulsive responding in children and adults.* New York: Wiley.

Robin, A. L., Tzelepis, A., & Bedway, M. (2008). A cluster analysis of personality style in adults with ADHD. *Journal of Attention Disorders, 12,* 254–263.

Rutter, M., MacDonald, H., Le Couteur, A., Harrington, R., Bolton, P., & Bailey, A. (1990). Genetic factors in child psychiatric disorders: II. Empirical findings. *Journal of Child Psychology and Psychiatry, 31,* 39–83.

Safer, D. J. (1973). A familial factor in minimal brain dysfunction. *Behavior Genetics, 3,* 175–186.

Satterfield, J. H., Hoppe, C. M., & Schell, A. M. (1982). A perspective study of delinquency in 110 adolescent boys with attention deficit disorder and 88 normal adolescent boys. *American Journal of Psychiatry, 139,* 795–798.

Seidman, L. J., Biederman, J., Faraone, S. V., Weber, W., Mennin, D., & Jones, J. (1997). A pilot study of neuropsychological functioning in girls with ADHD. *Journal of the American Academy of Child and Adolescent Psychiatry, 36,* 366–373.

Semrud-Clikeman, M., Steingard, R. J., Filipek, P., Biederman, J., Bekken, K., & Renshaw, P. F. (2000). Using MRI to examine brain–behavior relationships in males with attention deficit disorder with hyperactivity. *Journal of the American Academy of Child and Adolescent Psychiatry, 39,* 477–484.

Sherman, D. K., Iacono, W. G., & McGue, M. K. (1997). Attention-deficit hyperactivity disorder dimensions: A twin study of inattention and impulsivity–hyperactivity. *Journal of the American Academy of Child and Adolescent Psychiatry, 36,* 745–753.

Shum, D. H., MacFarland, K. A., & Bain, J. D. (1990). Construct validity of eight tests of attention: Comparison of normal and closed head injured samples. *Clinical Neuropsychologist, 4,* 151–162.

Shure, M. (1994). *Raising a thinking child.* New York: Holt.

Silverthorn, P., Frick, P. J., Kuper, K., & Ott, J. (1996). Attention deficit hyperactivity disorder and sex: A test of two etiological models to explain the male predominance. *Journal of Clinical Child Psychology, 25,* 52–59.

Skinner, B. F. (1953). *Science and human behavior.* New York: Macmillan.

Sprafkin, J., Gadow, K. D., Weiss, M. D., Schneider, J., & Nolan, E. E. (2007). Psychiatric comorbidity in ADHD symptom subtypes in clinic and community adults. *Journal of Attention Disorders, 11,* 114–124.

Stein, M. (1997). We have tried everything and nothing works: Family-centered pediatrics and clinical problem solving. *Journal of Developmental and Behavioral Pediatrics, 18,* 114–119.

Stevenson, J. (1992). Evidence for a genetic etiology in hyperactivity in children. *Behavior Genetics, 22,* 337–344.

Still, G. F. (1902). Some abnormal psychical conditions in children. *Lancet, 1,* 1008–1012, 1077–1082, 1163–1168.

Stott, D. H. (1981). Behavior disturbance and failure to learn: A study of cause and effect. *Educational Research, 23,* 163–172.

Swanson, J. M., Flodman, P., Kennedy, J., Spence, M. A., Moyzis, R., Schuck, S., et al. (2000). Dopamine genes and ADHD. *Neuroscience and Biobehavioral Reviews, 24,* 21–25.

Szatmari, P., Offord, D. R., Siegel, L. S., Finlayson, M. A., & Tuff, L. (1990). The clinical significance of neurocognitive impairments among children with psychiatric disorders: Diagnosis and situational specificity. *Journal of Child Psychology and Psychiatry, 31,* 287–299.

Tarver-Behring, S., Barkley, R. A., & Karlsson, J. (1985). The mother–child interactions of hyperactive boys and their normal siblings. *American Journal of Orthopsychiatry, 355,* 202–209.

Teeter, P. A. (1998). *Interventions for ADHD: Treatment in developmental context.* New York: Guilford Press.

Terestman, N. (1980). Mood quality and intensity in nursery school children as predictors of behavior disorder. *American Journal of Orthopsychiatry, 50*, 125–138.

Thapar, A., Hervas, A., & McGuffin, P. (1995). Childhood hyperactivity scores are highly heritable and show siblings competition effects: Twin study evidence. *Behavior Genetics, 35*, 537–544.

Thomas, A., & Chess, S. (1977). *Temperament and development.* New York: Brunner/Mazel.

Titchener, E. B. (1924). *A textbook of psychology.* New York: Macmillan.

Ullmann, R. K., Sleator, E. K., & Sprague, R. K. (1988). *ADD-H: Comprehensive Teacher's Rating Scale* (2nd ed.). Champaign, IL: MetriTech.

Vaidya, C. J., Bunge, S. A., Dudukovic, N. M., Zalecki, C. A., Elliott, G. R., & Gabrieli, J. D. (2005). Altered neurosubstraits of cognitive control and childhood ADHD: Evidence from functional magnetic resonance imaging. *American Journal of Psychiatry, 162*, 1605–1613.

Voeller, K. S. (1991). Towards a neurobiologic nosology of attention deficit hyperactivity disorder. *Journal of Child Neurology, 6*, S2–S8.

Volkow, N. D., Wang, G., Fowler, J. S., Logan, J., Gerasimov, M., Maynard, L., et al. (2001). Therapeutic doses of oral methylphenidate significantly increase extra cellular dopamine in the human brain. *Journal of Neuroscience, 21*, 1–5.

Warren, R. P., Odell, J. D., Warren, L. W., Burger, R. A., Maciulis, A., Daniels, W. W., et al. (1995). Reading disability, attention-deficit hyperactivity disorder and the immune system. *Science, 268*, 786–787.

Weiss, G., & Hechtman, L. (1979). The hyperactive child syndrome. *Science, 205*, 1348–1354.

Wender, P. H. (1975). The minimal brain dysfunction syndrome. *Annual Review of Medicine, 26*, 45–62.

Whalen, C. K., & Henker, B. (1991). Therapies for hyperactive children: Comparisons, combinations and compromises. *Journal of Consulting and Clinical Psychology, 59*, 126–137.

Whalen, C. K., Henker, B., Collins, B., McAuliffe, S., & Vaux, A. (1979). Peer interaction in a structured communication task: Comparisons of normal and hyperactive boys and of methylphenidate (Ritalin) and placebo effects. *Child Development, 50*, 388–401.

Willcutt, E. G., & Pennington, B. F. (2000). Comorbidity of reading disability and attention-deficit/hyperactivity disorder: Differences by gender and subtype. *Journal of Learning Disabilities, 33*, 179–191.

Willerman, L. (1973). Activity level and hyperactivity in twins. *Child Development, 44*, 288–293.

Winsberg, B. G., & Comings, D. E. (1999). Association of the dopamine transported gene (DAT1) with poor methylphenidate response. *Journal of the American Academy of Child and Adolescent Psychiatry, 38*, 1474–1477.

Young, S., Chadwick, O., Heptinstall, E., Taylor, E., & Sonuga-Barke, E. J. S. (2005). The adolescent outcome of hyperactive girls. *European Child and Adolescent Psychiatry, 14*, 245–254.

Zahn-Waxler, C., Schmitz, S., Fulker, D., Robinson, J., & Emde, R. (1996). Behavior problems in five-year-old monozygotic and dizygotic twins: Genetic and environmental influences, patterns of regulation, and internationalization of control. *Development and Psychopathology, 8*, 103–122.

Zametkin, A. J., & Rapoport, J. L. (1987). Neurobiology of attention deficit disorder with hyperactivity: Where have we come in 50 years? *Journal of American Academy of Child and Adolescent Psychiatry, 26*, 676–686.

Zametkin, A. J., Nordahl, T. E., & Gross, M. (1990). Cerebral glucose metabolism adults with hyperactivity in childhood onset. *Archives of General Psychiatry, 50*, 333–340.

Zentall, S. S. (1984). Context effects in the behavioral ratings of hyperactivity. *Journal of Abnormal Child Psychology 12*, 345–352.

Zentall, S. S. (1995). Modifying classroom tasks and environments. In S. Goldstein (Ed.), *Understanding and managing children's classroom behavior* (pp. 356–374). New York: Wiley.

CHAPTER 8

Oppositional, Conduct, and Aggressive Disorders

LISA L. WEYANDT
GENEVIEVE VERDI
ANTHONY SWENTOSKY

Aggression, disruptive behaviors, and acting-out behaviors are common at various stages of development. When these externalizing behaviors increase in frequency and duration, however, and cause impairment in child and family functioning, they become causes of concern for individuals, families, and society at large. The purposes of the present chapter are to provide a brief history of oppositional defiant disorder (ODD) and conduct disorder (CD), and to review the current literature concerning developmental course, genetic factors, and biological markers of the behaviors characterizing these disorders. Information is also provided concerning assessment and treatment strategies for children and adolescents with ODD and CD.

HISTORY

The nosology of ODD, CD, and aggression has evolved over the last 40 years in terms of conceptualization, research approaches, and treatment protocols. Hartup (2005) notes that three specific changes have occurred in the understanding of the development of aggression in individuals, as well as the way the subject is empirically assessed.

Although the theoretical and empirical emphasis of researchers historically centered on specific stimuli and events that elicited aggressive behaviors, contemporary research emphasizes the assessment of aggressive individuals within bioecological systems. A second change identified by Hartup (2005) is that research on aggression and antisocial behavior has converged into one field of study, whereas early explorations tended to approach the two categories of behavior as distinct and unrelated. A final major trend in the aggression literature relates to the study of aggression via a developmentally oriented paradigm. Early studies (Kuhn, Madsen, & Becker, 1967; Noble, 1973; Rosekrans & Hartup, 1967; Rule & Duker, 1973) on aggression typically assessed individuals only at one particular time point; very little attention was given to age differences. Today, however, the most informative studies of aggression are developmental in nature, often employing longitudinal designs to better identify the precursors and outcomes of aggressive behaviors in children and adolescents (Broidy et al., 2003; Tremblay et al., 2005).

Despite these methodological shifts and numerous other methodological improvements in the study of how aggression, CD, and ODD develop, many uncertainties and opportunities for improved research remain. For instance, it is difficult to determine whether children and adolescents in previous studies of CD and ODD would meet current diagnostic criteria for these disorders (Robins, 1999). As the theoretical and methodological changes concerning CD and ODD have occurred, the diagnostic criteria of these disorders have also evolved. In fact, CD and ODD were not recognized officially by the American Psychiatric Association (APA) until 1980, when the *Diagnostic and Statistical Manual of Mental Disorders* (DSM-III) was published. Since 1980, the diagnostic criteria for these disorders have become more developmentally focused and more empirically based (APA, 2000). For example, the DSM-IV-TR (APA, 2000) describe these three subtypes of CD:

1. Childhood-onset type
2. Adolescent-onset type
3. Unspecified onset (in which the age of onset of CD is unknown)

Three different subtypes were identified in DSM-III-R (APA, 1987):

1. Group type
2. Solitary aggressive type
3. Undifferentiated type

Also, in DSM-IV-TR it is explained that ODD is "often," but not always, a developmental antecedent of CD (APA, 2000, p. 101), supporting the nature of the DSM-IV-TR diagnoses of ODD and CD as based on developmentally oriented examinations of child and adolescent behavior. As illustrated in Table 8.1, the diagnostic criteria for CD have also expanded from 13 possible symptoms in DSM-III-R to 15 possible symptoms in DSM-IV-TR. Fewer criteria are included in the current symptomology for ODD; DSM-III-R lists nine possible symptoms, whereas DSM-IV-TR has only eight possible symptoms. As seen in Table 8.2, the use of swearing or obscene language is the omitted symptom. These changes in diagnostic emphasis and specific diagnostic criteria under-

TABLE 8.1. Comparing DSM-III-R and DSM-IV-TR Diagnostic Symptoms for CD

DSM-III-R	DSM-IV-TR
1. Frequent initiation of physical fights	1. Frequent initiation of physical fights
2. Use of a weapon in more than one fight	2. Use of a weapon that can cause serious injury to others (e.g., a bat, brick, gun, knife)
3. Physical cruelty to people	3. Physical cruelty to people
4. Physical cruelty to animals	4. Physical cruelty to animals
5. Stealing while confronting a victim (e.g., mugging, snatching a purse, etc.)	5. Stealing while confronting a victim
6. Forcing someone into sexual activity	6. Forcing someone into sexual activity
7. Deliberately setting fires	7. Deliberately setting fires with the intention to cause serious damage
8. Deliberately destroying others' property (other than by setting fires)	8. Deliberately destroying others' property (other than by setting fires)
9. Breaking into someone else's home, building, or car	9. Breaking into someone else's home, car, or building
10. Frequent lying (other than to avoid sexual or physical abuse)	10. Frequent lying to obtain favors or goods, or to get out of obligations
11. Stealing without confronting a victim, more than once (including forgery)	11. Stealing things of nontrivial value without confronting a victim (e.g., shoplifting, but not breaking and entering; forgery)
12. Running away from home overnight at least twice while residing in parents' or parental surrogates' home (or once without returning)	12. Running away from home overnight at least twice while residing in parents' or parental surrogates' home (or once without returning for a long period)
13. Frequent truancy from school (for older person, frequent absence from work)	13. Frequent truancy from school, beginning before 13 years of age
	14. Frequently staying out at night despite parents' prohibitions, beginning before 13 years of age
	15. Frequent bullying, threats, or intimidation of others

TABLE 8.2. Comparing DSM-III-R and DSM-IV-TR Diagnostic Symptoms for ODD

DSM-III-R	DSM-IV-TR
1. Frequent loss of temper	1. Frequent loss of temper
2. Frequent arguements with adults	2. Frequent arguements with adults
3. Frequent active defiance or refusal of adults' rules or requests (e.g., refusal to do home chores)	3. Frequent active defiance of or noncompliance with adults' rules or requests
4. Frequent deliberate acts that annoy other people (e.g., grabbing other children's belongings)	4. Frequent deliberate annoyance of other people
5. Frequent blame of others for own mistakes	5. Frequent blame of others for own mistakes or misbehavior
6. Frequent touchiness or readiness to be annoyed by others	6. Frequent touchiness or readiness to be annoyed by others
7. Frequent anger and resentment	7. Frequent anger and resentment
8. Frequent spitefulness and vindictiveness	8. Frequent spitefulness and vindictiveness
9. Frequent swearing or use of obscene language	

score the fact that a complete understanding of ODD and CD has not yet been achieved. As reflected in the changes accompanying the DSM-IV-TR diagnostic criteria for ODD and CD, an effective method for improving the understanding of these disorders is examining these disorders in reference to their developmental courses (Broidy et al., 2003; Tremblay et al., 2005).

DEVELOPMENTAL COURSES

The development of aggressive and antisocial behaviors, and of the behavioral disorders that they characterize, is a dynamic process in which multiple factors play a part (Burke, Loeber, & Birmaher, 2002). Environmental factors (Burke et al., 2002; Burt, Krueger, McGue, & Iacono, 2001), family and parental factors (Frick et al., 1992; Joussemet et al., 2008; Tremblay et al., 2005), genetic factors (Eley, Lichtenstein, & Moffitt, 2003; Rhee & Waldman, 2002), individual personal factors (Morrell & Murray, 2003), and biological factors (Beauchaine, Hong, & Marsh, 2008; Raine, 2002) have all been identified as influences in the development of these disorders. Any number of these factors may combine cumulatively or interactively to have particularly potent effects on infant and youth development (Odgers et al., 2007). To add to the complexity, the similarity of various behavioral symptoms (e.g., loss of temper, display of anger, physical fighting, violation of rules) that are representative of aggressive and antisocial behaviors, ODD, and CD (Dick, Viken, Kaprio, Pulk-

kinen, & Rose, 2005; Gelhorn, Sakai, Price, & Crowley, 2007; Maughan, Rowe, Messer, Goodman, & Meltzer, 2004) increases the difficulty in identifying and treating these behaviors and disorders separately.

The literature points to numerous relevant risk factors for aggressive behavior, ODD, and CD, providing the foundation for an understanding of the multifaceted developmental characteristics and processes that may lead to these outcomes. Moreover, identifying youth at greater risk for diagnosis may help reduce prevalence rates through prevention, intervention, and individualized treatments (Tremblay & Cote, 2005). Identifying these youth is an arduous task, however, because youth often follow multiple blurred developmental pathways that lead to outcomes of varying severity (Broidy et al., 2003; Nagin & Tremblay, 1999).

Efficiently organizing and effectively interpreting the relevant research in this area constitute a unique challenge because of the vast diversity in the methodological approaches and perspectives used to accomplish these tasks. For purposes of clarity, the developmental course of aggression, ODD, and CD are explained here from three separate perspectives: (1) childhood characteristics as predictors, (2) age differences in prevalence rates, and (3) developmental trajectories. The separation of these three different approaches is not intended to imply that the approaches are mutually exclusive or completely distinct from each other. Indeed, throughout much of the existing literature, overlap among these perspectives is the norm rather than the exception. This organizational method simply provides a structure for the organization and clarification of the current literature base (Lahey, 2008).

Childhood Characteristics

It is a truism of developmental psychology that experiences and environmental circumstances during childhood and adolescence can have lifelong effects on individuals (Afifi, Brownridge, Cox, & Sareen, 2006; Bifulco, Brown, Moran, Ball, & Campbell, 1998; Kendler, Neale, Kessler, Heath, & Eaves, 1992; Moffitt, 1993a; Reid & Patterson, 1989; Surtees et al., 2003). Although the particular mechanisms through which these effects occur are debatable, understanding the childhood experiences and characteristics that may lead to aggressive behavior, ODD, and CD will result in a better understanding of these behaviors and disorders.

Risk factors are identifiable beginning at the earliest stages of development; certain personality and cognitive characteristics of infants and toddlers have been hypothesized to increase the risk of future oppositional and conduct problems. Moffitt (1993a) has posited that neuropsychological deficits, difficult infant and child temperaments, and negative parenting behaviors and attitudes interact during infancy and early childhood to foster the development of antisocial behaviors representative of ODD and CD. Support for several components of this theory is found in the work of Lynam, Moffitt, and Stouthamer-Loeber (1993), who conducted a longitudinal study involving boys from infancy to age 13. Results indicated that 13-year-old boys who engaged in high levels of delinquency had significantly lower IQ scores than boys who engaged in lower levels of delinquent behaviors. Similarly, Piquero (2001) found that in a sample of 207 children and adolescents, Verbal and Performance scores on the Wechsler Intelligence Scale for Children had a significant effect on later engagement in violent and nonviolent offending. Furthermore, children and adolescents with higher scores on the Verbal scale of this assessment were significantly less likely than those with lower scores on the Verbal scale to participate in both violent and nonviolent offending as juveniles (Piquero, 2001). In a review of the literature on this topic, Teichner and Golden (2000) concluded that

researchers have consistently illustrated the existence of neuropsychological deficits such as verbal difficulties, inattention, and problems with cognitive flexibility, concept formation, and planning abilities in aggressive adolescents and youth with CD.

In addition to neuropsychological deficits, children who demonstrate delinquent behaviors and conduct problems often have academic difficulties, such as reading and vocabulary problems (Arnold et al., 2005; Willcutt & Pennington, 2000; Williams & McGee, 1994). Dionne, Tremblay, Boivin, Laplante, and Pérusse (2003) explored the relationship between expressive vocabulary and physical aggression in 19-month-olds, finding a significant negative correlation ($r = -.20$). Similarly, Bennett, Brown, Boyle, Racine, and Offord (2003) found after controlling for income, gender, maternal depression, family functioning, and previous CD symptoms that low reading achievement at school entry predicted conduct problems at a 30-month follow-up. Numerous additional studies have supported a relationship between poor academic performance and increased risk for aggressive behavior, ODD, and CD (Henrich, Schwab-Stone, Fanti, Jones, & Ruchkin, 2004; Loveland, Lounsbury, Welsh, & Buboltz, 2007; Swaim, Henry, & Kelly, 2006).

A "difficult" child temperament has likewise been linked to subsequent conduct problems. Lahey and colleagues (2008) found that maternal ratings of infant fussiness, positive affect, predictability, and activity level each made independent contributions to maternal ratings of conduct problems during ages 4–13. Similarly, negative emotionality at 17 months was found to be related to reactive aggression at 72 months (Vitaro, Barker, Boivin, Brendgen, & Tremblay, 2006), independently of harsh parenting practices. In addition to childhood temperament, parenting style has been correlated with child risk for aggression behaviors. Maternal attributions of internal, global, and stable causes of oppositional behavior have also been found to be predictive of oppositional behavior in children (Johnston, Hommersen, & Seipp, 2009). Controlling or power-assertive parenting has been found to be related to high rates of physical aggression in children and adolescents (Cote, Vaillancourt, Barker, Nagin, & Tremblay, 2007; Joussemet et al., 2008; Olweus, 1980). Rowe, Maughan, Pickles, Costello, and Angold (2002) found that rates of such adverse parenting practices as overintrusive parenting, inadequate supervision, and harsh discipline were higher in children and adolescents diagnosed with CD and ODD than in children and adolescents without these disorders.

Current research suggests that the relationship between child and parent characteristics may be bidirectional. Reid and Patterson (1989) postulated that the effects of difficult infant temperament, as well as other childhood risk factors, on later antisocial behavior are mediated by irritable, ineffective discipline and poor parental monitoring. Recent studies support this interpretation of the findings, further suggesting that difficult child temperament and poor parenting practices reciprocally influence each other; that is, a difficult child temperament elicits harsh parenting practices, which in turn exacerbate the difficult child temperament (Burke, Pardini, & Loeber, 2008; Lahey et al., 2008). Burke and colleagues (2008) found that boys who demonstrated more adverse child behaviors at ages 1 and 2, and whose parents could also be classified as unresponsive, were at increased risk for manifesting conduct problems at ages 3–3½. These findings indicate that even during the first years of life, the interplay between child temperament and parenting behaviors can increase the risk of behavioral problems in later childhood or adolescence.

Age Differences in Prevalence Rates

Despite the overlap in DSM-IV-TR (APA, 2000) diagnostic criteria for CD and ODD, research suggests that prevalence rates for ODD tend to decline in late childhood and early adolescence, whereas rates of CD increase steadily through midadolescence (Maughan et al., 2004). Maughan and colleagues (2004) have suggested that this decrease in overall prevalence of ODD is not due to a true decrease in oppositional behaviors, but rather to a proportional increase in CD symptoms and diagnoses. Because of the diagnostic criterion specifying that a child with ODD can no longer be diagnosed with that disorder once he or she meets diagnostic criteria for CD (APA, 2000), the increasingly intense aggressive behaviors

that may present in later childhood or adolescence render a previously diagnosed child ineligible for the ODD diagnosis. Research suggests that oppositional behaviors in children diagnosed with a behavioral disorder may not decrease in late childhood or early adolescence, but instead typically increase in number of symptoms and severity (Maughan et al., 2004). It is necessary to consider specific diagnostic criteria in interpreting the relational trends between ODD and CD.

A consistent and robust finding regarding the prevalence rates of CD is that CD is much more commonly diagnosed in males than in females (Loeber, Burke, Lahey, Winters, & Zera, 2000; Maughan et al., 2004). Findings regarding the gender difference in prevalence rates of ODD are also fairly consistent, with most studies indicating an equal gender prevalence or a slightly greater rate of occurrence among males (Loeber et al., 2000). Maughan and colleagues (2004) conducted a cross-sectional study using a nationally representative sample of 10,438 youth ages 5–15 years, finding that 0.8% of females and 2.1% of males met DSM-IV criteria for CD. The prevalence rates in the sample for ODD were 1.4% for females and 3.2% for males. Rowe and colleagues (2002) conducted a longitudinal study using a rural community sample of 4,500 children ages 9, 11, and 13 years, and obtained similar results: 1.1% of females and 3.1% of males met DSM-IV criteria for CD, whereas 1.5% of girls and 2% of boys met criteria for ODD. Although the differences between males and females in CD prevalence rates may appear minimal, they represent statistically significant differences that are consistently found across many studies (Gelhorn et al., 2007; Lahey et al., 2000; Sakai, Risk, Tanaka, & Price, 2008). Given these findings, it is not surprising that boys also demonstrate higher rates of physical aggression (Joussemet et al., 2008) and aggressive behavior in school (Thomas, Bierman, Thompson, & Powers, 2008) than girls. These gender differences are also consistent across parent and youth reports (Lahey et al., 2000).

Developmental Trajectories

Arguably the most popular approach to studying the origins of aggression, ODD, and CD involves examining the developmental trajectories of these behaviors and disorders (Broidy et al., 2003; Tremblay et al., 2005; White, Bates, & Buyske, 2001). Researchers developing trajectory models begin by examining manifestations of physical aggression among very young children. Tremblay and colleagues (2005) conducted a longitudinal study of 572 families, administering assessments of physical aggression at 17, 30, and 42 months after birth. Across this early age range, three trajectories of physical aggression were found: (1) children who displayed little or no aggression (28% of the sample), (2) children who followed a rising trajectory of modest physical aggression (58% of the sample), and (3) children following a rising trajectory of high physical aggression (14% of the sample). This study also found that children whose mothers engaged in coercive parenting had a history of antisocial behavior during their school years, smoked during pregnancy, or started childrearing early were at increased risk for following a rising modest- or high-aggression trajectory, as were children whose parents had low incomes, had problems living together, or were separated.

Numerous developmental trajectory studies have been carried out that involve older children and adolescents, and that are generally more refined and complex in terms of methodology. Some studies examine the developmental trajectories of aggressive behaviors (Brame, Nagin, & Tremblay, 2001; Murray-Close, Ostrov, & Crick, 2007; Tremblay et al., 2005), while other studies examine the trajectories of delinquent or antisocial behaviors (Connell & Frye, 2006; Hoeve et al., 2008; Landsheer & van Dijkum, 2005). Also, the number of externalizing behavior trajectories that are identified often depends on the specific sample analyzed (Broidy et al., 2003).

Moffitt (1993a) proposes a dual-taxonomy model of antisocial behaviors in which most delinquent individuals follow an adolescence-limited course, while a small group of delinquent individuals follow a life-course-persistent course of antisocial behavior. Individuals in the adolescence-limited group are hypothesized to display transient antisocial behaviors due to a biological and social maturity gap that leads to the mimicking of temporarily desirable behaviors of antisocial models. According to this theory, in-dividuals following the adolescence-limited course of antisocial behaviors are considered to be demonstrating normal adaptive behaviors. By contrast, those following the life-course-persistent trajectory are believed to have neuropsychological deficits that interact negatively with suboptimal childrearing environments and lead to a continued and increased likelihood of antisocial behaviors. Partial support for Moffitt's developmental trajectories of antisocial behavior was demonstrated in a study by White and colleagues (2001). In addition to the adolescence-limited, life-course-persistent, and no-antisocial-behavior groups, an additional, late-onset group was identified. This group consisted of adolescents who displayed very little delinquency in early adolescence, but displayed increasing delinquency from late adolescence to adulthood.

Subsequent studies examining possible developmental trajectories of aggressive, oppositional, and antisocial behaviors are characterized by considerable variability in the number and types of trajectories identified. For example, Broidy and colleagues (2003) analyzed data from six different sites located in three different countries, examining the developmental trajectories of aggressive and delinquent behavior in children and adolescents. For the male subsample, the number of developmental trajectories identified ranged from three to four, while the number of developmental trajectories identified for female participants ranged from two to four. Notably, no evidence was found for late-onset physical aggression for boys or girls.

A longitudinal study conducted by Nagin and Tremblay (1999) followed boys from 6 to 17 years of age and identified four distinct developmental trajectories for both aggressive behaviors and oppositional behaviors: a chronic-problem trajectory, a high-level near-desister trajectory, a moderate-level desister trajectory, and a no-problem trajectory. Two subtypes of the chronic-problem trajectory were found. A chronic-oppositional-behavior trajectory was associated with future covert delinquency, whereas a chronic-physical-aggression trajectory was associated with future overt delinquency and more serious delinquent acts. No evidence emerged for a subgroup displaying a late-onset or adolescent-onset trajectory of either category of externalizing behavior. A similar four-trajectory model was found for conduct problems among 2- to 8-year-old boys from low-income families. Shaw, Gilliom, Ingoldsby, and Nagin (2003) identified a persistent-problem trajectory, a high-level desister trajectory, a moderate-level desister trajectory, and a consistent low-level trajectory.

Although trajectory studies differ with regard to the specific behaviors of interest, the literature has consistently supported the notion that a particular group of children and adolescents demonstrates a chronic or life-course-persistent trajectory; that is, they display elevated levels of these problematic behaviors throughout their lives. The individuals who follow these chronic trajectories are typically at very high risk for poor developmental outcomes (e.g., continued use of physical violence, adolescent offending, health problems) (Bongers, Koot, van der Ende, & Verhulst, 2007; Broidy et al., 2003; Odgers et al., 2007).

GENETICS AND FAMILY PATTERNS

The current paradigm for understanding genetic contributions to aggressive and oppositional behaviors is based on the theory of polygenetic inheritance. It is now widely accepted that the development of these behaviors, and therefore the development of ODD and CD, does not result from one specific problematic gene (Burt & Mikolajewski, 2008; Caspi, McClay, Moffitt, Mill, & Martin, 2002; Haberstick, Smolen, & Hewitt, 2006; Pérusse & Gendreau, 2005; Plomin, Nitz, & Rowe, 1990; Schmidt, Fox, & Hamer, 2007; Schmidt, Fox, Rubin, Hu, & Hamer, 2002). Initial studies of the genetic contributions to externalizing disorders used antiquated methodologies like chromosomal analyses and single-gene approaches to examine the co-occurrence of a particular gene whose location was hypothesized to be correlated with a specific behavior or disorder (Plomin et al., 1990). In more recent years, molecular genetic studies use a candidate-gene approach, which attempts to identify and locate multiple genes that may influence the physiological systems believed to be involved in aggressive and oppositional behavior (Pérusse & Gendreau, 2005). Twin studies, adoption studies, and familial ag-

gregation studies have also endeavored to measure the overall genetic contribution to the development of aggressive and oppositional behaviors (Rhee & Waldman, 2002).

Twin and Adoption Studies

Twin and adoption studies have provided the preponderance of information to date about genetic influences on aggressive and oppositional behaviors. Eley and colleagues (2003) found strong genetic effects on childhood aggressive antisocial behavior. In adolescence, however, the strength of genetic influences has been observed to be commensurate with that of environmental influences.

Twin studies have indicated that the high comorbidity among ODD, CD, and attention-deficit/hyperactivity disorder (ADHD) can be largely explained by shared genetic influences, although the presence of each individual disorder is also attributed in part to unique genetic influences (Dick et al., 2005). In a study (Burt et al., 2001) of 11-year-old twins ($n = 1,506$), CD was primarily influenced by genetic factors, while ODD was strongly influenced by both genetic and environmental factors. In a related study of 584 adolescents from 293 same-sex twin pairs, Young and colleagues (2009) found that conduct problems in childhood were more heritable than those presenting during late adolescence. The authors suggest that in late adolescence, shared environmental influences may make a larger contribution to the emergence of conduct problems than they do during childhood.

A meta-analysis (Rhee & Waldman, 2002) of 51 twin and adoption studies operationalized aggressive and oppositional behaviors in four different ways: DSM diagnosis of antisocial personality disorder (APD) or CD; delinquency and criminality; aggressive behavior; and antisocial behavior. The combined additive and nonadditive genetic effects on these operationalizations of aggressive behavior had a heritability rate of 41%. Heritability rates were also found to differ significantly, depending on whether aggressiveness was assessed through self-reports or through reports by others, with heritability rates being significantly lower when self-reports were used. This finding suggests that heritability rates differ according to measurement method.

Further evidence supporting the hypothesis that heritability rates of aggression vary as a function of assessment method comes from studies of genetic influences on aggressive behaviors that have used laboratory observational methods of measuring such behaviors. In one of the very few studies (Plomin, Foch, & Rowe, 1981) using an observational measure of physical aggression, no hereditary influences on observed aggressive behaviors were found. In a study analyzing the genetic and environmental influences on child conduct problems and parenting behaviors, Deater-Deckard (2000) found significant genetic influences when parent reports of child conduct problems were used, but no significant genetic influence when observational measures were used. Although more studies using observational measures are desperately needed, the range of genetic influence in research to date varies from 0% when behavioral measures are used to at least 41% when self-reports and reports by others are used (Deater-Deckard, 2000; Rhee & Waldman, 2002).

Familial Aggregation and Transmission

A substantial amount of research suggests that delinquent behavior (Farrington, Joliffe, Loeber, Stouthamer-Loeber, & Kalb, 2001); APD and CD (Lahey et al., 1988); and childhood-persistent aggression and childhood-persistent antisocial behavior all tend to aggregate in families (Zoccolillo et al., 2005). Specifically, Lahey and colleagues (1988) showed that youth with childhood-onset CD were more likely to have a family history of antisocial behavior than youth with adolescent-onset CD.

Loeber and Dishion (1983) found that parental criminality was one of four primary predictors of young male delinquency. In a study of 1,517 European American and African American boys using parental reports of family delinquency and criminality, 8% of the families in the study accounted for 43% of the total reported arrests (Farrington et al., 2001). Similarly, having one relative who was arrested increased the probability that another family member would be arrested. Also, male relatives who were arrested tended to be married to females who were arrested. Although arrests of brothers, sisters, mothers, uncles, aunts, and grandparents all predicted boys' delinquency, having an arrested father was the strongest of these predictors. In a related study, Jafee, Moffitt, Caspi, and Taylor (2003) found that fathers' antisocial behavior was a significant predictor of children's antisocial behavior. Furthermore, living with fathers who frequently demonstrated antisocial behavior explained a significant amount of additional variance in children's antisocial behavior. These results indicate that children whose fathers engage in high levels of antisocial behavior are at an increased risk of engaging in their own antisocial behaviors if their fathers live in the home. Collectively, these studies provide further evidence for both genetic and environmental influences on the development of childhood antisocial behaviors.

BIOLOGICAL AND NEUROPSYCHOLOGICAL MARKERS

The body of research concerning biological and neuropsychological markers for ODD and CD has contributed few definitive answers to date, but a significant number of potentially informative hypotheses have emerged, many of which are likely to be clarified in future studies. Many researchers in this field have suggested that biological deficits in certain individuals may predispose them to engage in aggressive or antisocial behaviors.

Various specific biological markers for conduct problems have been presented in the literature (Anastassiou-Hadjicharlambous & Warden, 2008; Kruesi et al., 1992; Raine, 2002; Steiner & Dunne, 1997). These include responses to medication and irregular neurotransmitter functions, such as observed suppressed levels of central serotonin in aggressive children. Prenatal maternal behaviors have also been identified as potential contributors to an individual's development of CD through influencing the noradrenergic functioning and cholinergic receptors of the child (Raine, 2002). Depressed cortisol levels have been presented as another possible biological marker for traits of CD in both males (Loney, Butler, Lima, Counts, & Eckel, 2006; McBurnett et al., 1991) and females (Pajer, Gardner, Rubin, Perel, & Neal, 2001). Yet another possible marker of aggressive disorders in children may be levels of the thyroid hormones triiodothyronine (T3) and free thyroxine (FT4) (Ramklint, Stalenheim, von Knorring, & von Knorring, 2000). Adults with a history of CD exhibited elevated levels of both T3 and FT4.

One frequently presented biological correlate of conduct disorders in children is a depressed autonomic nervous system, with resulting insufficient physiological arousal. For example, work by Anastassiou-Hadjicharlambous and Warden (2008) found that children with a CD diagnosis who scored highly on measures of callousness and lack of emotionality were observed to display a smaller change in physiological arousal (as measured by heart rate) than peers. Ortiz and Raine (2004) conducted a meta-analysis of 40 studies (with an overall sample of 5,868 children) and found that antisocial children had significantly lower resting heart rates than either psychiatric or normal controls. Raine (2002) likewise identified low physiological arousal (as demonstrated by low resting heart rate) as a biological marker for children and adolescents exhibiting antisocial and aggressive behavior, linking the sluggish autonomic response to reduced noradrenergic functioning. A related biological marker of aggressive disorders related to temperament is low withdrawal response, often typified by low levels of fear response (Fowles, 1980, 2000; Fung et al., 2005). Low physiological arousal puts individuals at risk for CD (McBurnett, Harris, Swanson, & Pfiffner, 1993), via a hypothetical pathway characterized by low arousal both at baseline and in the presence of stimuli (Raine, 2002).

The hypothesized lack of fear response in individuals with CD has been assessed in several ways, with perhaps the most well-received research demonstrating reduced electrodermal responses to possible punishment (Fowles, 2000; Fung et al., 2005) among aggressive individuals. This biological deficit may have long-reaching implications, as children with abnormally low levels of fear may never form appropriate guilt responses to inappropriate behavior, may never develop a social conscience, and may not experience appropriate concern about possible punishment resulting from maladaptive behaviors (Kochanska, Murray, & Coy, 1997). Indeed, distinct temperamental pathways to conduct problems have therefore been defined (Frick & Morris, 2004), linked with low fear response and heightened reactivity (Nigg, 2006).

Though a dearth of research on the topic makes findings difficult to generalize, it has also been suggested that gender differences exist in various autonomic correlates with aggression. Reduced autonomic functioning has been observed in aggressive boys with conduct problems, but not necessarily in girls with conduct problems (Beauchaine et al., 2008). Striatal hyperdopaminergic functioning has also been associated with externalizing behavior disorders in boys, with research indicating that externalizing pathologies such as ADHD and CD are characterized by deficits in predicted reward processing (Beauchaine et al., 2008). These findings are noteworthy, as they suggest that associated antisocial behaviors may be extremely difficult to change in young men once they have been acquired.

More recently, researchers have begun to focus on neuroimaging studies and anatomical correlates of conduct problems. Specifically, several studies have implicated abnormalities in the prefrontal cortex as biological correlates of such problems. Berman and Siegal (1976) were among the first to suggest impaired frontal lobe functioning as a correlate of aggressive and antisocial behaviors. Both prefrontal structural and functional deficits have since been correlated with antisocial and aggressive behavior in both youth and adults. Baving, Laucht, and Schmidt (2000), for example, observed atypical patterns of frontal brain activity in school-age boys and girls with ODD. It has also been suggested that such brain differences may vary on the basis of gender. Nevertheless, an atypical activation pattern of cognitive activity has been observed in both boys and girls with ODD. Raine (2002) posits that the prefrontal cortices of youth with conduct disorders may develop more slowly than those of peers, resulting in the lack of inhibitory control over maladaptive behaviors commonly associated with the diagnosis of CD. Functional abnormalities linked specifically to inhibition have been identified processes in the brains of boys with CD (Rubia et al., 2008). Among adolescent boys diagnosed with CD, a pattern of brain atypicality has been observed in the bilateral temporoparietal region, commonly thought to be associated with self-monitoring of task performance (Rubia et al., 2008). A comparison group of boys with ADHD demonstrated a deficit in activation of the left prefrontal cortex, commonly associated with inhibitory control. These findings support the possibility that although individuals with ADHD and CD may present with a similar behavioral phenotype, unique cognitive abnormalities are contributing to the behaviors in each group of individuals. It is important to note once again that these neuroanatomical studies are correlational in nature, and do not reveal the underlying causes of the differences found. Furthermore, results across studies are highly conflicting; some studies report anatomical or functional differences between children with and without antisocial behaviors, while others do not (Weyandt, 2005).

A number of researchers (Seguin, Nagin, Assaad, & Tremblay, 2004; Teichner & Golden, 2000) have also hypothesized that individuals with CD and other aggressive disorders exhibit deficits in neuropsychological executive functions. In both genders, CD has been linked to significant impairment in cognitive ability, inhibition/set shifting, planning ability, verbal memory, and visual–spatial tasks (Olvera, Semrud-Clikeman, Pliszka, & O'Donnell, 2005). Verbal skill deficits have been repeatedly observed in individuals with CD (Olvera et al., 2005; Moffitt, 1993b). Indeed, some have hypothesized that deficits in verbal/language ability may contribute to many of the maladaptive behaviors manifested by youth with aggressive disorders; their noncompliance may in part be attributable to poor comprehension and undeveloped problem-solving skills. Other executive functioning deficits observed among individuals with CD have included problems with abstract reasoning and concept formation, sustaining attention and concentration, planning abilities, formulating goals, initiating purposive sequences of behavior, inhibiting impulsive behaviors, and self-monitoring (Moffitt, 1993b). Gaps exist in the research, however. For example, much remains to be explored regarding possible gender differences in the manifestation of aggressive disorders. Whereas some of the literature suggests that girls with CD may exhibit specific deficits in neuropsychological functioning (e.g., in overall cognitive ability and visual–spatial abilities) (Pajer et

al., 2008), other data suggest that few if any significant gender differences exist (Herba, Tranah, Rubia, & Yule, 2006). It is imperative to note, however, that executive functioning deficits are *not* unique to CD; they have been found in children and adults with a variety of disorders, such as hydrocephalus, meningitis, phenylketonuria, traumatic brain injury, autism, obsessive–compulsive disorder, Gilles de la Tourette syndrome, and ADHD (Weyandt, 2005).

Furthermore, evidence for executive dysfunction varies widely across studies. Children with comorbid attention and oppositional disorders have been observed to score significantly lower on measures of executive functioning, language comprehension, and short-term memory than their nondisordered peers (Youngwirth, Harvey, Gates, Hashim, & Friedman-Weieneth, 2007). In numerous studies, however, after ADHD is controlled for, executive function deficits in youth with conduct problems are dramatically reduced (Olvera et al., 2005; van Goozen et al., 2004; Youngwirth et al., 2007). Other research has suggested the possibility that children with ODD do not experience impaired executive functioning in terms of controlling inhibitions, but rather in relation to self-regulating their behavior under conditions of motivational inhibition (van Goozen et al., 2004). Recently, Weyandt (2009) has emphasized that executive function deficits are not unique to particular disorders (such as CD/ODD); nor are they necessary or sufficient for diagnosis. Findings are mixed in terms of what comorbid disorders are related to impaired executive functioning in children with externalizing disorders, and future research should attempt to clarify the relationship among executive function deficits, externalizing behavior type, gender, age, and severity of behavior disturbance. Additional studies suggest that adolescents with aggression and conduct issues experience impaired functioning of motor inhibition (Herba et al., 2006). Although many studies have found evidence of neuropsychological impairment in youth with CD, it is important to note that many such youth have quite normal neuropsychological functioning (Teichner & Golden, 2000). Future research should strive to discern whether specific executive function deficits are characteristic of and unique to aggressive disorders.

Although the specific biological factors that contribute to CD and other forms of aggressive behavior remain under investigation, it appears highly likely that conduct problems have a genetically heritable component, as noted earlier. For example, twin studies have found higher concordance rates of elevated levels of aggressive disorders and antisocial behaviors in monozygotic twins than in dizygotic twins (Reid, Dorr, Walker, & Bonner, 1986; Scourfield, Van den Bree, Martin, & McGuffin, 2005). More recently (Dick et al., 2004), a genome screen of individuals with CD identified regions on two chromosomes (19 and 2) that may influence whether or not an individual will develop CD. Although much related research must be done in the future to clarify the findings, the results of the genome screen indicate a probable genetic etiology for CD.

RISK FACTORS
FOR PHENOTYPIC EXPRESSION

Although a genetic and biological predisposition to conduct problems is well illustrated by the literature, it is also certain that exogenous factors contribute to the development of maladaptive behaviors consistent with ODD or CD. Several psychosocial and environmental factors are believed to increase individual risk for developing conduct problems. For example, a child born with a biological predisposition to develop CD may be exposed prenatally to substances that add to his or her risk for developing this disorder,

as research indicates that the offspring of parents with substance use disorders were at greater risk for a diagnosis of CD (Johnson, Cohen, Kasen, & Brook, 2008). Furthermore, research has found that a child who is exposed to or victimized by violence is likelier to become oppositional, as is a child whose family is unstable (in terms of geography, financial well-being, or relationships); who is frequently unsupervised; who experiences precocious exposure to substance use; or whose parents have a history of ODD, CD, or ADHD (Mayo Clinic, n.d.). Certainly, however, it is difficult to know whether a child with CD has inherited a biological basis for the behaviors or is merely modeling the aggressive and antisocial behaviors of one or both parents (Holmes, Slaughter, & Kashani, 2004).

Both dispositional and contextual risk factors for developing CD have likewise been identified. In addition to the biological factors discussed previously, dispositional risk factors include a preference for dangerous activities, high level of impulsivity, academic underachievement, and deficits in processing social information (Frick, 2004). Contextual risk factors for CD include all those for ODD, as well as parental psychopathology, peer rejection, impoverished living conditions, and association with deviant peers.

Clearly, several categories of risk factors for phenotypic expression of aggressive behaviors have been identified: individual, genetic, environmental, and familial. Table 8.3 summarizes the known risk factors for CD and ODD. Although a significant number

TABLE 8.3. Risk Factors for Developing CD or ODD

CD	ODD
• Impulse control dysfunction (as with ADHD) • Difficult temperament in early childhood • Aggression toward peers/rejection by peers • Social withdrawal/lack of social skills • Depression/anxiety • Academic underachievement • Poor parental relations: inconsistent supervision, harsh punishment, rejection, parental alcoholism • Large family size (4+ children) • Exposure to violence and neglect • Prenatal malnutrition and exposure to toxins	• Having a parent with a mood or substance use disorder • Being abused or neglected • Harsh or inconsistent discipline • Lack of supervision • Poor relationship with one or both parents • Family instability (e.g., divorce, multiple moves, or changing schools or child care providers frequently) • Parents with a history of ADHD, ODD, or conduct problems • Financial problems in the family • Exposure to violence • Substance abuse in the child or adolescent

of risk factors exist for these disorders, an equally substantial number of interventions and treatment options have been identified for implementation when such behaviors occur.

ASSESSMENT

Appropriate assessment of an individual who is displaying symptoms of ODD or CD should follow a multimethod, multi-informant, multisetting strategy (Steiner & Dunne, 1997). Data should be obtained from both the individual and his or her parents, and from other family members as appropriate. A thorough developmental and social history of the individual must be obtained, particularly in regard to relevant DSM-IV-TR criteria (APA, 2000). The evaluator should investigate the presence and quality of peer and sibling relationships, as well as school functioning. A multisetting approach is of particular importance here, as some individuals with ODD or CD encounter problems in some settings long before others; for instance, an individual who is maladaptive at home and school may be functional in some community settings. Other types of assessment that may add important information to the evaluation include a family assessment; a physical examination; and a thorough assessment of the individual's cognitive, behavioral, and social functioning (Hughes, Crothers, & Jimerson, 2007; Steiner & Dunne, 1997).

The essential diagnostic feature of CD, according to DSM-IV-TR (APA, 2000) is "a repetitive and persistent pattern of behavior in which the basic rights of others or major age-appropriate societal norms or rules are violated" (p. 98). The individual being assessed must meet at least three of the criteria listed in the right column of Table 8.1, which fall into four categories of maladaptive behaviors: aggression to people and animals (criteria 1–6 and 15 in the table), destruction of property (criteria 7–8 in the table), deceitfulness or theft (criteria 9–11 in the table), and serious violations of rules (criteria 12–14 in the table). If it is determined that an individual had met at least three of these criteria in the last 12 months (and at least one within the last 6 months), and that the behaviors in question are having a sig-

nificant negative impact on his or her social, occupational, or academic functioning, the individual may be diagnosed with CD.

As also noted earlier, three subtypes of CD have been identified: childhood-onset type, adolescent-onset type, and unspecified onset. All of these may be described as mild, moderate, or severe in nature (APA, 2000). The first two subtypes differ somewhat in terms of their manifestations in observable behaviors. The childhood-onset type of CD often presents in the form of physical aggression and poor peer relationships. The adolescent-onset type is characterized by fewer instances of aggressive behaviors, and poor social relations typically involve interactions with authority figures rather than peers. Regardless of subtype, the behavior problems associated with a CD diagnosis tend to present across settings and to impair functioning in school, home, and the community (APA, 2000). In addition to the diagnostic criteria already discussed, CD is often typified by a lack of empathy or concern for others and an absence of (appropriate) emotions of guilt or remorse (APA, 2000). Individuals with CD often exhibit precocious sexual and substance-related behaviors and are likelier than peers to engage in reckless or risk-taking acts. Common comorbid diagnoses for individuals with CD include ADHD, as well as learning, anxiety, mood, and substance-related disorders (APA, 2000).

According to APA (2000), an individual who fails to meet the diagnostic criteria for CD but demonstrates a similar pattern of maladaptive tendencies may be diagnosed with ODD. Typically, individuals with ODD do not display the same severity of behavior as those with CD; nor do their transgressions typically include violence/aggression toward others, destruction of property, or theft (APA, 2000). The essential feature of the ODD diagnosis is a pattern of "negativistic, hostile, and defiant behavior" (APA, 2000, p. 102) lasting 6 months or more; it must exist independently of a psychotic/mood disorder diagnosis, and must cause significant impairment in an individual's functioning. Four of the eight criteria listed in the right column of Table 8.2 must be displayed over the course of the 6-month period.

For individuals with ODD, related behaviors can be manifested in a number of different ways (APA, 2000). ODD-related behaviors emerge most often in the home, but can be problematic in school or social settings as well. Conflicts with authority figures (such as teachers and parents) can become commonplace for an individual with ODD, as can precocious substance use, mood lability, and a low tolerance for frustration. Children with ODD are likelier than their peers to be codiagnosed with ADHD, learning disorders, and communication disorders (APA, 2000).

Specific assessment tools have been identified as effective in determining whether or not an individual has CD or ODD. One instrument designed to assess the possible presence of CD in a child or adolescent is the Antisocial Personality Disorder Questionnaire (Myers, Stewart, & Brown, 1998), a structured interview designed to assess both CD and APD. The reliability and validity of the questionnaire have been determined by associations with more well-established assessment procedures (Brown, Gleghorn, Schuckit, Myers, & Mott, 1996). Other, more widely used comprehensive assessments of mental health have also been found to be appropriate tools for evaluating the presence of CD or ODD in children and adolescents. The National Institute of Mental Health's Diagnostic Interview Schedule for Children, Version IV (DISC-IV), for example, has been found to demonstrate reliability and validity in evaluating individuals suspected of having CD. The DISC-IV does not solely assess CD; rather, it is designed to assess a large number of psychiatric disorders in children and adolescents (Shaffer, Fisher, Luca, Dulcan, & Schwab-Stone, 2000). A subcategory of questions from the assessment specifically addresses behaviors relevant to the diagnostic criteria for CD. The Child Behavior Checklist (CBCL; Achenbach & Rescorla, 2001) includes inventories to be completed by parents, teacher, and the individual experiencing disordered behavior; earlier versions of the CBCL have been identified as reliable and valid for purposes of diagnosing both ODD (Abolt & Thyer, 2002) and CD (Lowe, 1998). As stated previously, however, it is important to note that both of these disorders are best evaluated via a multimodal approach; as such, the implications of any singular assessment should be interpreted with caution.

TREATMENT

Treating children and adolescents with disruptive behavior disorders, as well as studying the treatment of children with such disorders, is an arduous task due to the heterogeneity of risk factors (Teichner & Golden, 2000; Tremblay et al., 2005; Powell, Lochman, & Boxmeyer, 2007) and developmental pathways (Broidy et al., 2003; Moffitt, 1993a; White et al., 2001) encompassed in these disorders. In addition, as children grow older, the number of experienced risk factors inevitably increases, requiring a wider range of factors that treatments need to address. Therefore, earlier interventions are preferable because they can target children's problematic behaviors at a time when they are less complex and stable (Jensen, 2008). Many different treatment approaches are used to treat aggression, ODD, and CD. Some treatment approaches have been studied more extensively than others (Kazdin, 1997), and some have shown to be more effective than others. Evidence supporting some of the major treatment approaches is discussed below. This discussion does not provide an exhaustive explanation of all available treatments; it simply touches upon some of the most commonly used treatments for these disorders (Frick, 2001; Kazdin, 2007).

Cognitive Problem-Solving Skills Training

Among the most widely used cognitive-behavioral treatments for aggression, ODD, and CD is cognitive problem-solving skills training (CPST) or cognitive-behavioral skills training. This therapeutic approach attempts to train children and adolescents to alter the deficient cognitive processes that are believed to lead to their disruptive behaviors. The primary goals of CPST and similar treatments are to help children and adolescents improve their inhibition of impulsive and aggressive actions, recognize individual and social problems, consider alternative solutions to problems, and select and pursue the most adaptive solutions (Frick, 2001; Kazdin, 1997). Although there is an evidence base that supports the use of CPST (Dangel, Deschner, & Rasp, 1989; de Castro, Bosch, Veerman, & Koops, 2003; Frick,

2001; Kazdin, 1997), more research needs to be done to determine how CPST needs to be modified for different age groups and different cultures (Kazdin, 1997), as well as how to improve generalization of newly learned behaviors (Frick, 2001).

Parent Management Training

The most researched and most effective treatment for ODD and CD to date is parent management training (PMT; Brestan & Eyberg, 1998; Taylor & Biglan, 1998). PMT focuses on improving parent–child interactions through implementing more efficient and consistent disciplinary strategies, changing the antecedents of behaviors in order to increase the likelihood of children's prosocial behaviors, and improving parents' abilities to monitor and supervise their children appropriately (Frick, 2001). The American Psychological Association's Division 12 considers PMT an empirically validated treatment for children with oppositional behavior (American Psychological Association Task Force, 1993). Costin and Chambers (2007) showed that PMT was effective in treating primary-school-age children with ODD in a community-based setting, regardless of whether or not they had another comorbid disorder. As one might expect, one of the key limitations of PMT is that it can often be difficult to maintain parental participation throughout the entire course of treatment (Frick, 2001).

Psychopharmacological Interventions

Various types of medications have demonstrated minimal to modest levels of effectiveness for treating symptoms of aggression, ODD, and CD. Connor, Barkley, and Davis (2000) demonstrated that clonidine, an antihypertensive medication, was effective in reducing ODD and CD symptoms in children and adolescents with either ODD or CD and comorbid ADHD. Studies have shown evidence that lithium decreases aggressive behavior in children and adolescents with CD (Campbell et al., 1995; Malone, Delaney, Luebbert, Cater, & Campbell, 2000). Evidence also suggests that typical antipsychotics are superior to placebos in treating children and adolescents with ODD and CD;

however, their common side effects have led to an increased interest in atypical antipsychotics (Findling, 2008). Of the atypical antipsychotics used for aggression, ODD, and CD, risperidone has been the most extensively studied. Risperidone was found to be effective and well tolerated in reducing conduct and behavioral problems in children ages 5–12 (Aman, De Smedt, Derivan, Lyons, & Findling, 2002). Also, Buitelaar, van der Gaag, Rutger, Cohen-Kettenis, and Melman (2001) found that risperidone was effective and well tolerated in treating adolescents with extreme aggression. Although many possible psychopharmacological interventions exist for treating symptoms of ODD and CD, these medicines must be administered with caution because of the potential side effects. It is also important to note that the U.S. Food and Drug Administration has not approved any medication specifically for the treatment of CD or ODD.

Multisystemic Therapy

Because of the complexity in the risk factors, causal factors, and developmental pathways associated with aggression, ODD, and CD, it has been suggested that multiple treatment approaches originating from multiple theoretical traditions may be best for reducing the symptoms of these disorders (Jensen, 2008). Multisystemic therapy (MST) often takes a family-based approach to treatment while also including PMT, CPST, and even psychopharmacological strategies that may be most appropriate for any given child or adolescent (Kazdin, 1997). In a meta-analysis of the effectiveness of MST for treating antisocial behaviors in youth, Curtis, Ronan, and Borduin (2004) found that youth and families who received MST were offending less and functioning better afterward than 70% of the youth and families who received alternative treatments. In a review of the literature on effective treatments for delinquent youth, Kurtz (2002) states that MST significantly reduces reoffending rates, and that this success is probably due to MST's multimodal approach.

Although the approaches described above have evidence supporting their effectiveness, their effectiveness is typically limited. When selecting a treatment plan, service providers should be sure to take a comprehensive approach that takes into account the individual factors that lead to each child's disruptive behaviors (Frick, 2001).

CONCLUSION

In summary, recent advances have been made in conceptualizing and understanding factors that contribute to the development of aggressive behaviors, ODD, and CD in children and adolescents. Current research supports a role for genetic, developmental, physiological, and environmental factors, and these factors are believed to interact in complex ways that lead to the onset of antisocial behavior in children. The literature is replete with methodological problems, however, including small sample sizes, comorbidity, differences in inclusion criteria, low statistical power, herterogeneity of participants, and confounding variables. Further research is needed to clarify the similarities and differences among boys and girls with CD and ODD; the roles of genetic and familial variables; and the contribution of neurochemical and neuroanatomical factors to the development of aggressive and antisocial behaviors in children and adolescents. Advances in each of these areas will lead to more valid and reliable approaches to identifying and treating these behaviors in children and adolescents.

REFERENCES

Abolt, T., & Thyer, B. A. (2002). Social work assessment of children with oppositional defiant disorder: Reliability and validity of the Child Behavior Checklist. *Social Work in Mental Health, 1*(1), 73–84.

Achenbach, T. M., & Rescorla, L. A. (2001). *Manual for ASEBA school-age forms and profiles.*. Burlington: University of Vermont, Research Center for Children, Youth, and Families.

Afifi, T. O., Brownridge, D. A., Cox, B. J., & Sareen, J. (2006). Physical punishment, childhood abuse and psychiatric disorders. *Child Abuse and Neglect, 30*, 1093–1103.

Aman, M. G., De Smedt, G., Derivan, A., Lyons, B., & Findling, R. L. (2002). Double-blind, placebo-controlled study of risperidone for the treatment of disruptive behaviors in children with subaverage intelligence. *American Journal of Psychiatry, 159*, 1337–1346.

American Psychiatric Association (APA). (1980). *Diagnostic and statistical manual of mental disorders* (3rd ed.). Washington, DC: Author.

American Psychiatric Association (APA). (1987). *Diagnostic and statistical manual of mental disorders* (3rd ed., rev.). Washington, DC: Author.

American Psychiatric Association (APA). (2000). *Diagnostic and statistical manual of mental disorders* (4th ed., text rev.). Washington, DC: Author.

American Psychological Assocation Task Force on Promotion and Dissemination of Psychological Procedures. (1993). Washington, DC: Author.

Anastassiou-Hadjicharalambous, X., & Warden, D. (2008). Physiologically-indexed and self-perceived affective empathy in conduct-disordered children high and low on callous-unemotional traits. *Child Psychiatry and Human Development, 39*(4), 503–517.

Arnold, E., Goldston, D., Walsh, A., Reboussin, B. A., Daniel, S. S., Hickman, E., et al. (2005). Severity of emotional and behavioral problems among poor and typical readers. *Journal of Abnormal Child Psychology, 33*, 205–217.

Baving, L., Laucht, M., & Schmidt, M. H. (2000). Oppositional children differ from healthy children in frontal brain activation. *Journal of Abnormal Child Psychology, 28*(3), 267–275.

Beauchaine, T. P., Hong, J., & Marsh, P. (2008). Sex differences in autonomic correlates of conduct problems and aggression. *Journal of the American Academy of Child and Adolescent Psychiatry, 47*(7), 788–796.

Bennett, K. J., Brown, K. S., Boyle, M., Racine, Y., & Offord, D. (2003). Does low reading achievement at school entry cause conduct problems. *Social Science and Medicine, 56*, 2443–2448.

Berman, A., & Siegal, A. (1976). Adaptive and learning skills in juvenile delinquents: A neuropsychological analysis. *Journal of Learning Disabilities, 9*, 583–590.

Bifulco, A., Brown, G. W., Moran, P., Ball, C., & Campbell, C. (1998). Predicting depression in women: The role of past and present vulnerability. *Psychological Medicine, 28*, 39–50.

Bongers, I. L., Koot, H. M., van der Ende, J., & Verhulst, F. C. (2007). Predicting young adult social functioning from developmental trajectories of externalizing behavior. *Psychological Medicine, 38*, 989–999.

Brame, B., Nagin, D. S., & Tremblay, R. E. (2001). Developmental trajectories of physical aggression from school entry to late adolescence. *Journal of Child Psychology and Psychiatry, 42*, 503–512.

Brestan, E. V., & Eyberg, S. M. (1998). Effective psychosocial treatments of conduct-disordered children and adolescents: 29 years, 82 studies, and 5,272 kids. *Journal of Clinical Child Psychology, 27*(2), 180–189.

Broidy, L. M., Nagin, D. S., Tremblay, R. E., Bates,

J. E., Brame, B., & Dodge, K. A. (2003). Developmental trajectories of childhood disruptive behaviors and adolescent delinquency: A six-site, cross- national study. *Developmental Psychology, 39*(2), 222–245.

Brown, S. A., Gleghorn, A., Schuckit, M., Myers, M. G., & Mott, M. A. (1996). Conduct disorder among adolescent substance abusers. *Journal of Studies on Alcohol, 57,* 314–324.

Buitelaar, J. K., van der Gaag, R. J., Cohen-Kettenis, P., & Melman, C. T. (2001). A randomized, controlled trial of risperidone in the treatment of aggression in hospitalized adolescents with subaverage cognitive abilities. *Journal of Clinical Psychiatry, 62,* 239–248.

Burke, J. D., Loeber, R., & Birmaher, B. (2002). Oppositional defiant disorder and conduct disorder: A review of the past 10 years: II. *Journal of the American Academy of Child and Adolescent Psychiatry, 41*(11), 1275–1293.

Burke, J. D., Pardini, D. A., & Loeber, R. (2008). Reciprocal relationships between parenting behavior and disruptive psychopathology from childhood through adolescence. *Journal of Abnormal Child Psychology, 36,* 679–692.

Burt, S. A., Krueger, R. F., McGue, M., & Iacono, W. G. (2001). Sources of covariation among attention-deficit/hyperactivity disorder, oppositional defiant disorder, and conduct disorder: The importance of shared environment. *Journal of Abnormal Psychology, 110*(4), 516–525.

Burt, S. A., & Mikolajewski, A. J. (2008). Preliminary evidence that specific candidate genes are associated with adolescent-onset antisocial behavior. *Aggressive Behavior, 34,* 437–445.

Campbell, M., Adams, P. B., Small, A. M., Kafantaris, V., Silva, R. R., & Shell, J. (1995). Lithium in hospitalized aggressive children with conduct disorder: A double-blind and placebo-controlled study. *Journal of the American Academy of Child and Adolescent Psychiatry, 34,* 445–453.

Caspi, A., McClay, J., Moffitt, T. E., Mill, J., & Martin, J. (2002). Role of genotype in the cycle of violence in maltreated children. *Science, 297,* 851–854.

Connell, A. M., & Frye, A. A. (2006). Growth mixture modeling in developmental psychology: Overview and demonstration of heterogeneity in developmental trajectories of adolescent antisocial behavior. *Infant and Child Development, 15,* 609–621.

Connor, D. F., Barkley, R. A., & Davis, H. T. (2000). A pilot study of methylphenidate, clonidine, or the combination in ADHD comorbid with aggressive oppositional defiant or conduct disorder. *Clinical Pediatrics, 39,* 15–25.

Costin, J., & Chambers, S. M. (2007). Parent management training as a treatment for children with oppositional defiant disorder referred to a mental

health clinic. *Clinical Child Psychology and Psychiatry, 12,* 511–524.

Cote, S. M., Vaillancourt, T., Barker, E. D., Nagin, D., & Tremblay, R. E. (2007). The joint development of physical and indirect aggression: Predictors of continuity and change during childhood. *Development and Psychopathology, 19,* 37–55.

Curtis, N. M., Ronan, K. R., & Borduin, C. M. (2004). Multisystemic treatment: A meta-analysis of outcome studies. *Journal of Family Psychology, 18*(3), 411–419.

Dangel, R. F., Deschner, J. P., & Rasp, R. R. (1989). Anger control training for adolescents in residential treatment. *Behavior Modification, 13*(4), 447–458.

Deater-Deckard, K. (2000). Parenting and child behavioral adjustment in early childhood: A quantitative genetic approach to studying family processes. *Child Development, 71*(2), 468–484.

de Castro, B. O., Bosch, J. D., Veerman, J. W., & Koops, W. (2003). The effects of emotion regulation, attribution, and delay prompts on aggressive boys' social problem solving. *Cognitive Therapy and Research, 27*(2), 153–166.

Dick, D. M., Li, T. K., Edenberg, H. J., Hesselbrock, V., Kramer, J., Kuperman, S., et al. (2004). A genome-wide screen for genes influencing conduct disorder. *Molecular Psychiatry, 9,* 81–86.

Dick, D. M., Viken, R. J., Kaprio, J., Pulkkinen, L., & Rose, R. J. (2005). Understanding the covariation among childhood externalizing disorders: Genetic and environmental influences on conduct disorder, attention deficit hyperactivity disorder, and oppositional defiant disorder symptoms. *Journal of Abnormal Child Psychology, 33,* 219–229.

Dionne, G., Tremblay, R., Boivin, M., Laplante, D., & Pérusse, D. (2003). Physical aggression and expressive vocabulary in 19-month-old twins. *Developmental Psychology, 39*(2), 261–273.

Eley, T. C., Lichtenstein, P., & Moffitt, T. E. (2003). A longitudinal behavioral genetic analysis of the etiology of aggressive and nonaggressive antisocial behavior. *Development and Psychopathology, 15,* 383–402.

Farrington, D. P., Jolliffe, D., Loeber, R., Stouthamer-Loeber, M., & Kalb, L. M. (2001). The concentration of offenders in families, and family criminality in the prediction of boys' delinquency. *Journal of Adolescence, 24,* 579–596.

Findling, R. L. (2008). Atypical antipsychotic treatment of disruptive behavior disorders in children and adolescents. *Journal of Clinical Psychiatry, 69,* 9–14.

Fowles, D. C. (1980). The three arousal model: Implications of Gray's two-factor learning theory for heart rate, electrodermal activity, and psychopathy. *Psychophysiology, 17*(2), 87–104.

Fowles, D. C. (2000). Electrodermal hyporeactivity and antisocial behavior: Does anxiety mediate the relationship? *Journal of Affective Disorders, 61*, 177–189.

Frick, P. J. (2001). Effective interventions for children and adolescents with conduct disorder. *Canadian Journal of Psychiatry, 46*, 597–608.

Frick, P. J. (2004). Developmental pathways to conduct disorder: Implications for serving youth who show severe aggressive and antisocial behavior. *Psychology in the Schools, 41*(8), 823–834.

Frick, P. J., Lahey, B. B., Loeber, R., Stouthamer-Loeber, M., Christ, M. A., & Hanson, K. (1992). Familial risk factors to oppositional defiant disorder and conduct disorder: Parental psychopathology and maternal parenting. *Journal of Consulting and Clinical Psychology, 60*(1), 49–55.

Frick, P. J., & Morris, A. S. (2004). Temperament and developmental pathways to conduct problems. *Journal of Clinical Child and Adolescent Psychology, 33*, 54–68.

Fung, M. T., Raine, A., Loeber, R., Lynam, D. R., Steinhauer, S. R., Venables, P. H., et al. (2005). Reduced electrodermal activity in psychopathy-prone adolescents. *Journal of Abnormal Psychology, 114*, 187–196.

Gelhorn, H. L., Sakai, J. T., Price, R. K., & Crowley, T. J. (2007). DSM-IV conduct disorder criteria as predictors of antisocial personality disorder. *Comprehensive Psychiatry, 48*, 529–538.

Haberstick, B. C., Smolen, A., & Hewitt, J. K. (2006). Family-based association test of the 5HTTLPR and aggressive behavior in a general population sample of children. *Biological Psychiatry, 59*, 836–843.

Hartup, W. W. (2005). The development of aggression: Where do we stand? In R. E. Tremblay, W. W. Hartup, & J. Archer (Eds.), *Developmental origins of aggression* (pp. 3–22). New York: Guilford Press.

Henrich, C. C., Schwab-Stone, M., Fanti, K., Jones, S. M., & Ruchkin, V. (2004). The association of community violence exposure with middle-school achievement: A prospective study. *Journal of Applied Developmental Psychology, 25*, 327–348.

Herba, C. M., Tranah, T., Rubia, K., & Yule, W. (2006). Conduct problems in adolescence: Three domains of inhibition and effect of gender. *Developmental Neuropsychology, 30*(2), 659–695.

Hoeve, M., Blokland, A., Dubas, J. S., Loeber, R., Gerris, J. R. M., & van der Laan, P. H. (2008). Trajectories of delinquency and parenting styles. *Journal of Abnormal Child Psychology, 36*, 223–235.

Holmes, S. E., Slaughter, J. R., & Kashani, J. (2001). Risk factors in childhood that lead to the development of conduct disorder and antisocial personality disorder. *Child Psychiatry and Human Development, 31*(3), 183–193.

Hughes, T. L., Crothers, L. M., & Jimerson, S. R. (2007). *Assessing, identifying, and treating conduct disorder at school.* New York: Springer.

Jafee, S. R., Moffitt, T. E., Caspi, A., & Taylor, A. (2003). Life with (or without) father: The benefits of living with two biological parents depend on the father's antisocial behavior. *Child Development, 74*(1), 109–126.

Jensen, P. S. (2008). The role of psychosocial therapies in managing aggression in children and adolescents. *Journal of Clinical Psychiatry, 69*, 37–42.

Johnson, J. G., Cohen, P., Kasen, S., & Brook, J. S. (2008). Parental concordance and offspring risk for anxiety, conduct, depressive, and substance use disorders. *Psychopathology, 41*(2), 124–128.

Johnston, C., Hommersen, P., & Seipp, C. M. (2009). Maternal attributions and child oppositional behavior: A longitudinal study of boys with and without attention deficit/hyperactivity disorder. *Journal of Consulting and Clinical Psychology, 77*(1), 189–195.

Joussemet, M., Vitaro, F., Barker, E. D., Cote, S., Nagin, D. S., Zoccolillo, M., et al. (2008). Controlling parenting and physical aggression during elementary school. *Child Development, 79*(2), 411–425.

Kazdin, A. E. (1997). A model for developing effective treatments: Progression and interplay of theory, research, and practice. *Journal of Clinical Child Psychiatry, 26*, 114–129.

Kazdin, A. E. (2007). Progress in treating children referred for severe aggressive and antisocial behavior. *NYS Psychologist, 19*(5), 7–12.

Kendler, K. S., Neale, M. C., Kessler, R. C., Heath, A. C., & Eaves, L. J. (1992). Childhood parental loss and adult psychopathology in women: A twin study perspective. *Archives of General Psychiatry, 49*, 109–116.

Kochanska, G., Murray, K., & Coy, K. C. (1997). Inhibitory control as a contributor to conscience in childhood: From toddler to early school age. *Child Development, 68*, 263–277.

Kruesi, M. J. P., Hibbs, E. D., Zahn, T. P., Keysor, C. S., Hamburger, S. D., Bartko, J. J., et al. (1992). A two-year prospective follow-up study of children and adolescents with disruptive behavior disorders. *Archives of General Psychiatry, 47*, 419–426.

Kuhn, D. Z., Madsen, C. H., Jr., & Becker, W. C. (1967). Effects of exposure to an aggressive model and "frustration" on children's aggressive behavior. *Child Development, 38*, 739–745.

Kurtz, A. (2002). What works for delinquency?: The effectiveness of interventions for teenage offending behaviour. *Journal of Forensic Psychiatry, 13*(3), 671–692.

Lahey, B. B. (2008). Oppositional defiant disorder, conduct disorder, and juvenile delinquency. In T. P. Beauchaine & S. P. Hinshaw (Eds.), *Child and adolescent psychopathology* (pp. 335–369). Hoboken, NJ: Wiley.

Lahey, B. B., Piacentini, J. C., McBurnett, K., Stone, P., Hartdagen, S., & Hynd, G. (1988). Psychopathology in the parents of children with conduct disorder and hyperactivity. *Journal of the American Academy of Child and Adolescent Psychiatry, 27,* 163–170.

Lahey, B. B., Schwab-Stone, M., Goodman, S. H., Waldman, I. D., Canino, G., Rathouz, P. J., et al. (2000). Age and gender differences in oppositional behavior and conduct problems: A cross-sectional household study of middle childhood and adolescence. *Journal of Abnormal Psychology, 109*(3), 488–503.

Lahey, B. B., Van Hulle, C. A., Keenan, K., Rathouz, P. J., D'Onofrio, B. M., Rodgers, J. L., et al. (2008). Temperament and parenting during the first year of life predict future child conduct problems. *Journal of Abnormal Child Psychology, 36,* 1139–1158.

Landsheer, J. A., & van Dijkum, C. (2005). Male and female delinquency trajectories from pre- through middle adolescence and their continuation in late adolescence. *Adolescence, 40,* 729–748.

Loeber, R., Burke, J. D., Lahey, B. B., Winters, A., & Zera, M. (2000). Oppositional defiant and conduct disorder: A review of the past 10 years. II. *Journal of the American Academy of Child and Adolescent Psychiatry, 39*(12), 1468–1484.

Loeber, R., & Dishion, T. (1983). Early predictors of male delinquency: A review. *Psychological Bulletin, 94*(1), 68–99.

Loney, B. R., Butler, M. A., Lima, E. N., Counts, C. A., & Eckel, L. A. (2006). The relation between salivary cortisol, callous-unemotional traits, and conduct problems in an adolescent non-referred sample. *Journal of Child Psychology and Psychiatry, 47*(1), 30–36.

Loveland, J. M., Lounsbury, J. W., Welsh, D., & Bubultz, W. C. (2007). The validity of physical aggression in predicting adolescent academic performance. *British Journal of Educational Psychology, 77,* 167–176.

Lowe, L. A. (1998). Using the Child Behavior Checklist in assessing conduct disorder: Issues of reliability and validity. *Research on Social Work Practice, 8*(3), 286–301.

Lynam, D., Moffitt, T., & Stouthamer-Loeber, M. (1993). Explaining the relation between IQ and delinquency: Class, race, test motivation, school failure, or self-control? *Journal of Abnormal Psychology, 102*(2), 187–196.

Malone, R. P., Delaney, M. A., Luebbert, J. F., Cater, J., & Campbell, M. (2000). A double-blind placebo-controlled study of lithium in hospitalized aggressive children and adolescents with conduct disorder. *Archives of General Psychiatry, 57,* 649–654.

Maughan, B., Rowe, R., Messer, J., Goodman, R., & Meltzer, H. (2004). Conduct disorder and oppositional defiant disorder in a national sample: developmental epidemiology. *Journal of Child Psychology and Psychiatry, 45*(3), 609–621.

Mayo Clinic. (n.d.) Oppositional defiant disorder: Risk factors. Retrieved January 18, 2009, from *www.mayoclinic.com/health/oppositional-defiant-disorder/DS00630/DSECTION=risk-factors Risk factors*

McBurnett, K., Harris, S., Swanson, J. M., & Pfiffner, L. J. (1993). Neuropsychological and psychophysiological differentiation of inattention/overactivity and aggression/defiance symptom groups. *Journal of Clinical Child Psychology, 22*(2), 165–171.

McBurnett, K., Lahey, B. B., Frick, P. J., Risch, C., Loeber, R., Hart, E. L., et al. (1991). Anxiety, inhibition, and conduct disorder in children: Relation to salivary cortisol. *Journal of the American Academy of Child and Adolescent Psychiatry, 30*(2), 192–196.

Moffitt, T. E. (1993a). Adolescence-limited and life-course-persistent antisocial behavior: A developmental taxonomy. *Psychological Review, 100*(4), 674–201.

Moffitt, T. E. (1993b). The neuropsychology of conduct disorder. *Developmental Psychopathology, 5,* 135–151.

Morrell, J., & Murray, L. (2003). Parenting and the development of conduct disorder and hyperactive symptoms in childhood: A prospective longitudinal study from 2 months to 8 years. *Journal of Child Psychology and Psychiatry, 44*(4), 489–508.

Murray-Close, D., Ostrov, J., & Crick, N. (2007). A short-term longitudinal study of growth of relational aggression during middle childhood: Associations with gender, friendship intimacy, and internalizing problems. *Developmental Psychopathology, 19*(1), 187–203.

Myers, M. J., Stewart, D. G., & Brown, S. A. (1998). Progression from conduct disorder to antisocial personality disorder following treatment for adolescent substance abuse. *American Journal of Psychiatry, 155,* 479–485.

Nagin, D., & Tremblay, R. E. (1999). Trajectories of boys' physical aggression, opposition, and hyperactivity on the path to physically violent and nonviolent juvenile delinquency. *Child Development, 70*(5), 1181–1196.

Nigg, J. T. (2006). Temperament and developmental psychopathology. *Journal of Child Psychology and Psychiatry, 47*(3–4), 395–422.

Noble, G. (1973). Effects of different forms of filmed aggression on children's constructive and destructive play. *Journal of Personality and Social Psychology, 26,* 54–59.

Odgers, C. L., Caspi, A., Broadbent, J. M., Dickson,

N., Hancox, R. J., Harrington, H., et al. (2007). Prediction of differential adult health burden by conduct problem subtypes in males. *Archives of General Psychiatry, 64*, 476–484.

Olvera, R. L., Semrud-Clikeman, M., Pliszka, S. R., & O'Donnell, L. (2005). Neuropsychological deficits in adolescents with conduct disorder and comorbid bipolar disorder: A pilot study. *Bipolar Disorders, 7*(1), 57–67.

Olweus, D. (1980). Familial and temperamental determinants of aggressive behavior in adolescent boys: A causal analysis. *Developmental Psychology, 16*(6), 644–660.

Ortiz, J., & Raine, A. (2004). Heart rate level and antisocial behavior in children and adolescents: A meta-analysis. *Journal of the American Academy of Child and Adolescent Psychiatry, 43*(2), 154–162.

Pajer, K., Gardner, W., Rubin, R. T., Perel, J., & Neal, S. (2001). Decreased cortisol levels in adolescent girls with conduct disorder. *Archives of General Psychiatry, 58*(3), 297–302.

Pajer, K., Chung, J., Leininger, L., Wang, W. Gardner, W., & Yeates, K. (2008). Neuropsychological function in adolescent girls with conduct disorder. *Journal of the American Academy of Child and Adolescent Psychiatry, 47*(4), 416–425.

Pérusse, D., & Gendreau, P. L. (2005). Genetics and the development of aggression. In R. E. Tremblay, W. W. Hartup, & J. Archer (Eds.), *Developmental origins of aggression* (pp. 220–241). New York: Guilford Press.

Piquero, A. (2001). Testing Moffitt's neuropsychological variation hypothesis for the prediction of life- course persistent offending. *Psychology, Crime and Law, 7*, 193–216.

Plomin, R., Foch, T. T., & Rowe, D. C. (1981). Bobo clown aggression in childhood: Environment not genes. *Journal of Research in Personality, 15*, 331–342.

Plomin, R., Nitz, K., & Rowe, D. C. (1990). Behavioral genetics and aggressive behavior in childhood. In M. Lewis & S. M. Miller (Eds.), *Handbook of developmental psychopathology* (pp. 119–133). New York: Plenum Press.

Powell, N. R., Lochman, J. E., & Boxmeyer, C. L. (2007). The prevention of conduct problems. *International Review of Psychiatry, 19*(6), 597–605.

Raine A. (2002). Annotation: The role of prefrontal deficits, low autonomic arousal, and early health factors in the development of antisocial and aggressive behavior in children. *Journal of Child Psychology and Psychiatry, 43*(4), 417–434.

Ramklint, M., Stalenheim, E. G., von Knorring, A. L., & von Knorring, L. (2000). Triiodothyronine (T3) related to conduct disorder in a forensic psychiatric population. *European Journal of Psychiatry, 14*(1), 33–41.

Reid, J. B., & Patterson, G. R. (1989). The development of antisocial behavior patterns in childhood and adolescence. *European Journal of Personality, 3*, 107–119.

Reid, W. H., Dorr, D., Walker, J. I., & Bonner, J. W. (Eds.). (1986). *Unmasking the psychopath: Antisocial personality and related syndromes.* New York: Norton.

Rhee, S. H., & Waldman, I. D. (2002). Genetic and environmental influences on antisocial behavior: A meta-analysis of twin and adoption studies. *Psychological Bulletin, 128*(3), 490–529.

Robins, L. N. (1999). A 70-year history of conduct disorder: Variations in definition, prevalence and correlates. In P. Cohen, C. Slomkowski, & L. N. Robins (Eds.), *Historical and geographical influences on psychopathology* (pp. 37–56). Mahwah, NJ: Erlbaum.

Rosekrans, M. A., & Hartup, W. W. (1967). Imitative influences of consistent and inconsistent responses consequences to a model on aggressive behavior in children. *Journal of Personality and Social Psychology, 7*, 429–434.

Rowe, R., Maughan, B., Pickles, A., Costello, E., & Angold, A. (2002). The relationship between DSM-IV oppositional defiant disorder and conduct disorder: Findings from the Great Smoky Mountains Study. *Journal of Child Psychology and Psychiatry, 43*(3), 365–373.

Rubia, K., Halari, R., Smith, A. B., Mohammed, M., Scott, S., Giampietro, V., et al. (2008). Dissociated functional brain abnormalities of inhibition in boys with pure conduct disorder and in boys with pure attention deficit hyperactivity disorder. *American Journal of Psychiatry, 165*(7), 889–897.

Rule, B. G., & Duker, P. (1973). Effects of intentions and consequences on children's evaluations of aggressors. *Journal of Personality and Social Psychology, 27*, 184–189.

Sakai, J. T., Risk, N. K., Tanaka, C. A., & Price, R. K. (2008). Conduct disorder among Asians and Native Hawaiian/Pacific Islanders in the USA. *Psychological Medicine, 38*, 1013–1025.

Schmidt, L. A., Fox, N. A., & Hamer, D. H. (2007). Evidence for a gene–gene interaction in predicting children's behavior problems: Association of 5-HTT short and DRD4 long genotypes with internalizing and externalizing behaviors in seven year-old children. *Development and Psychopathology, 19*, 1105–1116.

Schmidt, L. A., Fox, N. A., Rubin, K. H., Hu, S., & Hamer, D. H. (2002). Molecular genetics of shyness and aggression in preschoolers. *Personality and Individual Differences, 33*, 227–238.

Scourfield, J., Van den Bree, M., Martin, N., & McGuffin, P. (2005). Conduct problems in children and adolescents: A twin study. *Archives of General Psychiatry, 61*(5), 489–496.

Seguin, J. R., Nagin, D., Assaad, J. M., & Tremblay, R. E. (2004). Cognitive-neuropsychological function in chronic physical aggression and hyperactivity. *Journal of Abnormal Psychology, 113*, 603–613.

Shaw, D. S., Gilliom, M., Ingoldsby, E. M., & Nagin, D. S. (2003). Trajectories leading to school-age conduct problems. *Developmental Psychology, 392*(2), 189–200.

Shaffer, D., Fisher, P., Lucas, C. P., Dulcan, M. K., & Schwab-Stone, M. E. (2000). NIMH Diagnostic Interview Schedule for Children, Version IV (NIMH DISC-IV): Description, differences from previous versions, and reliability of some common diagnoses. *Journal of the American Academy of Child and Adolescent Psychiatry, 39*(1), 28–38.

Steiner, H., & Dunne, J. E. (1997). Assessment summary of the practice parameters for the assessment and treatment of children and adolescents with conduct disorder. *Journal of the American Academy of Child and Adolescent Psychiatry, 36*(10), 1482–1485.

Surtees, P. G., Wainwright, N. W. J., Day, N., Brayne, C., Luben, R. L., & Khaw, K. -T. (2003). Adverse experience in childhood as a developmental risk factor for altered immune status in adulthood. *International Journal of Behavioral Medicine, 10*, 251–268.

Swaim, R. C., Henry, K. L., & Kelly, K. (2006). Predictors of aggressive behaviors among rural middle school youth. *Journal of Primary Prevention, 27*(3), 229–243.

Taylor, T. K., & Biglan, A. (1998). Behavioral family interventions for improving child-rearing: A review for clinicians and policy makers. *Clinical Child and Family Psychological Review, 1*, 41–60.

Teichner, G., & Golden, C. J. (2000). The relationship of neuropsychological impairment to conduct disorder in adolescence: A conceptual review. *Aggression and Violent Behavior, 5*(6), 509–528.

Thomas, D. E., Bierman, K. L., Thompson, C., & Powers, C. J. (2008). Double jeopardy: Child and school characteristics that predict aggressive–disruptive behavior in first grade. *School Psychology Review, 37*(4), 516–532.

Tremblay, R. E., & Cote, S. (2005). The developmental origins of aggression: Where are we going? In R. E. Tremblay, W. W. Hartup, & J. Archer (Eds.), *Developmental origins of aggression* (pp. 447–464). New York: Guilford Press.

Tremblay, R. E., Nagin, D. S., Seguin, J. R., Zoccolillo, M., Zelazo, P. D., Boivin, M., et al. (2005). Physical aggression during early childhood: Trajectories and predictors. *Canadian Child and Adolescent Psychiatry Review, 14* (1), 3–9.

van Goozen, S. H., Cohen-Kettenis, P. T., Snoek, H., Matthys, W., Swaab-Barneveld, H., & van Engeland, H. (2004). Executive functioning in children: A comparison of hospitalised ODD and ODD/ADHD children and normal controls. *Journal of Child Psychology and Psychiatry, 45*(2), 284–292.

Vitaro, F., Barker, E. D., Boivin, M., Brendgen, M., & Tremblay, R. E. (2006). Do early difficult temperament and harsh parenting differentially predict reactive and proactive aggression? *Journal of Abnormal Child Psychology, 34*, 685–695.

Weyandt, L. L. (2005). Executive function in children, adolescents, and adults with attention deficit hyperactivity disorder: Introduction to the special issue. *Developmental Neuropsychology, 27*(1), 1–10.

Weyandt, L. L. (2009). Executive functions and attention-deficit hyperactivity disorder. *ADHD Report, 17*(6), 1–7.

White, H. R., Bates, M. E., & Buyske, S. (2001). Adolescence-limited versus persistent delinquency: Extending Moffitt's hypothesis into adulthood. *Journal of Abnormal Psychology, 110*(4), 600–609.

Willcutt, E. G., & Pennington, B. F. (2000). Psychiatric comorbidity in children and adolescents with reading disability. *Journal of Child Psychology and Psychiatry, 41*, 1039–1048.

Williams, S., & McGee, R. (1994). Reading attainment and juvenile delinquency. *Journal of Child Psychology and Psychiatry, 35*, 441–459.

Young, S. E., Friedman, N. P., Miyake, A., Willcutt, E. G., Corley, R. P., Haberstick, B. C., et al. (2009). Behavioral disinhibition: Liability for externalizing spectrum disorders and its genetic and environmental relation to response inhibition across adolescence. *Journal of Abnormal Psychology, 118*(1), 117–130.

Youngwirth, S. D., Harvey, E. A., Gates, A., Hashim, R. L., & Friedman-Weieneth, J. L. (2007). Neuropsychological abilities of preschool-aged children who display hyperactivity and/or oppositional-defiant behavior problems. *Child Neuropsychology, 13*(5), 422–443.

Zoccolillo, M., Romano, E., Joubert, D., Mazzerello, T., Cote, S., Boivin, M., et al. (2005). The intergenerational transmission of aggression and antisocial behavior. In R. E. Tremblay, W. W. Hartup, & J. Archer (Eds.), *Developmental origins of aggression* (pp. 353–375). New York: Guilford Press.

CHAPTER 9

Gilles de la Tourette Syndrome

ALICIA HUGHES
BRIAN P. DALY
RONALD T. BROWN

Gilles de la Tourette syndrome (Tourette syndrome, or TS) is a genetic neuropsychiatric disorder consisting of chronic motor and verbal tics that typically persist for at least 1 year (American Psychiatric Association [APA], 2000). The disorder frequently has its origins during middle childhood, with a mean age of 7 years. Typically, motor tics precede the onset of vocal tics (Brown et al., 2008). A *tic* is a recurring, stereotypical, nonrhythmic vocalization or motor movement that may occur suddenly and without warning; it is always of short duration (APA, 2000). Individuals frequently describe their tics as irresistible, although tics can be suppressed for varying periods of time. Frequently tics are exacerbated by stress: Numerous environmental factors have been associated with fluctuation of symptoms in children and adolescents with TS (Silva, Munoz, Barickman, & Friedhoff, 1995). Such environmental stressors for children and adolescents frequently include emotional trauma and events causing anxiety (e.g., social gatherings). The frequency of tics has been observed to decrease during activities that require sustained attention and concentration, as well as during sleep. Finally, the number, frequency, severity, and type of tics may change over the course of time.

Motor and vocal tics are classified as either *simple* or *complex* (APA, 2000). Simple motor tics may include eye blinking, jerking of the neck, shrugging of the shoulders, facial grimacing, and coughing. Typical complex motor tics consist of grooming behaviors, facial gestures, touching, jumping, stomping feet, and smelling objects. Motor tics frequently involve the head and other parts of the body, including the torso and the upper and lower limbs. Simple vocal tics often include clearing of the throat, clicking, sniffing, grunting, snorting, and barking (e.g., yelps). Finally, complex vocal tics may involve the repetition of words or phrases out of context, *coprolalia* (use of obscenities or curse words), *palilalia* (repetition of one's own sounds or words), and *echolalia* (repetition of recently heard sounds, words, or phrases) (APA, 2000). The prevalence of coprolalia is actually quite low, although it is frequently mentioned in connection with TS in the mass media.

Core features of TS include multiple motor tics and one or more vocal tics. Motor and vocal tics may appear either simultaneously or separately during different periods of time (APA, 2000). To meet diagnostic criteria for TS, tics must occur many times throughout the course of the day for a period of more than 1 year. In addition, the tic symptoms must be present and not absent for a period of at least 3 consecutive months. Finally, the presence of the disorder must result in significant impairment in occupational, social, or emotional functioning.

TS is conceptualized as a clinical spectrum disorder that includes a range of functional impairments. Kurlan (1994) has observed that the mildest form of TS includes largely asymptomatic features in which only brain morphology is affected, whereas children who suffer from moderate TS evidence academic and behavioral problems and may even require special education services at school. In the most severe form of the disorder, children with TS may require pharmacotherapy so that they can function in society.

The prevalence of TS is estimated to be between 1 and 8 cases per 1,000 males and between 0.1 and 4 cases per 1,000 females (Peterson, Pine, Cohen, & Brook, 2001). Clearly, the syndrome is more prevalent in males than among females, with estimates ranging from 2:1 to 10:1 in favor of males. Variability in prevalence data has been attributed to sample populations (i.e., clinic vs. community samples), the sensitivity and specificity of the various diagnostic instruments employed, and the age distribution of the population that is sampled (Peterson et al., 2001). Those epidemiological studies that have employed a direct examination of individuals in outpatient clinics have yielded the highest prevalence estimates of TS, while surveys of community populations have yielded the lowest prevalence estimates. Because traditional structured diagnostic interviews are not sufficiently sensitive to discriminate the presence of mild tics from overt TS, it is important to note that clinic-based studies arte likely to overestimate the prevalence of TS. Thus structured diagnostic interviews are apt to yield a preponderance of false positives, whereas community-based investigations employing surveys for the identification of TS tend to underestimate the prevalence of TS due to the underreporting of symptoms (Peterson et al., 2001). It is also noteworthy that epidemiological studies of pediatric populations yield higher prevalence estimates than do studies that include their adolescent or adult counterparts. The higher prevalence of TS in pediatric populations has been attributed to a decrease in tic severity at puberty. In fact, prevalence estimates of TS in adolescents ages 16–17 years are quite similar to adult prevalence estimates (Apter et al., 1993), suggesting a rapid decrease in symptoms at adolescence.

HISTORY

Jean-Marc Itard recorded the first known report of TS in the early 19th century (Hyde & Weinberger, 1995). Itard provided a case history of a French noblewoman who displayed motor tics at the age of 7 years, and who subsequently developed involuntary vocalizations consisting of screams and strange cries. Later in her life, the woman developed coprolalia and was forced to live in seclusion until her death. Nearly 50 years later, under the supervision of the well-known neurologist Jean Martin Charcot, Gilles de la Tourette presented a series of case studies that detailed the history and symptoms of several individual patients with the same syndrome; the syndrome was subsequently named for Tourette. Early descriptions provided by Charcot included information regarding the waxing and waning of multiple motor and vocal tics, the early age of onset, and the importance of genetic influences on the disorder (Keen-Kim & Freimer, 2006).

TS is a syndrome that has been frequently misunderstood and underdiagnosed (Sprague & Newell, 1986). In the early 1940s, during the psychoanalytic movement in Europe and North America, several case studies were offered that were interpreted to support a psychodynamic interpretation of the tics (e.g., Mahler & Rangell, 1943). TS was considered a psychiatric disorder at that time, due to the patients' ability to voluntarily suppress the behaviors associated with the syndrome and the tendency of tics to be exacerbated during periods of high stress. Although the psychiatric interpretation of the symptoms associated with TS has been discounted over the past several years, the relationship of tic symptoms to important events in individuals' lives generally suggests that these factors can influence the course of TS to some extent. Nonetheless, the etiology of tic disorders is unclear: Most tics are believed to have an organic etiology, while some are believed to be exacerbated by psychogenic factors (Mansdorf, 1995). Over the past three decades, compelling evidence has been mounted to support an organic etiology of TS. Advances in the study of the human genome, coupled with significant developments in the neurosciences and specifically in neuroimaging, have resulted in the reclassification of TS as a neurological movement disorder (Peterson et al., 2001). In support of this notion, several biological markers have been linked with TS. For example, the neurotransmitter dopamine has been demonstrated either to precipitate or to exacerbate symptoms of TS (Peterson et al., 2001), although the exact nature of dopamine's effects is still being debated (see later text). Furthermore, several provocative hypotheses have been posited suggesting significant abnormal brain morphology among individuals with TS, particularly within the basal ganglia and limbic system. These burgeoning developments in the neurosciences have resulted in valuable treatment pathways for pharmacological interventions.

DEVELOPMENTAL COURSE

Although previous thinking suggested a variable and unpredictable developmental course of symptoms associated with TS, recent longitudinal studies have provided compelling evidence to indicate that TS actually follows a rather common developmental course. Specifically, in the majority of cases, tics associated with TS first appear in childhood, generally decrease in late adolescence and young adulthood, and remain at a very mild threshold or even in remission during adulthood. However, tics are described as continuing from late adolescence well into adulthood in a minority of cases. Although the developmental course has some predictability, the clinical course of TS can be fluctuating and variable. General trends in the developmental and clinical course of TS are described below.

Childhood

Data on the prevalence rate of TS indicate a 10-fold higher rate among children than among adults (Burd, Kerbeshian, Wikenheiser, & Fisher, 1986a, 1986b). Typically, tics first appear between the ages of 5 and 6 years, with tic severity peaking at about 10–12 years of age, prior to decreasing or entering full remission in most individuals by early adulthood (Pappert, Goetz, Louis, Blasucci, & Leurgans, 2003). The onset of tics is gradual, with motor tics typically preceding vocal tics, and simple tics preceding more complex tics (Leckman & Cohen, 1999). For example, at about ages 6–7 years, initial symptoms of TS include eye blinking and facial or head and neck tics. Following these simple motor tics are the development of vocal tics and a rostral–caudal progression of more complex multiple motor tics (Brown et al., 2008).

Clinically, children typically experience a waxing–waning course in which periods of tic intensity are interspersed with periods of relative symptom stability. Risk factors associated with the exacerbation of tics during childhood include periods of excitement, anxiety, stress, and fatigue. In contrast, as noted previously, tics decrease substantially during sleep. In its most severe form, TS may involve coprolalia; again, however, this is relatively rare and occurs in fewer than 10% of individuals diagnosed with TS.

Comorbid psychiatric conditions are common in children diagnosed with TS, particularly attention-deficit/hyperactivity disorder (ADHD), obsessive–compulsive disorder (OCD), anxiety, depression, and learning disabilities (Freeman et al., 2000). Whereas comorbid attention difficulties typically emerge slightly before or around the same time as the tics, obsessive–compulsive symptoms typically emerge 3–6 years after the onset of tics (Bruun & Budman, 1997). Psychosocial and learning challenges also occur in childhood, with results from a longitudinal study indicating that over one-half of children with TS demonstrate significant social or academic problems (Pappert et al., 2003).

Adolescence

Although tics may be particularly severe during early adolescence, findings from longitudinal studies indicate that approximately one-half to two-thirds of adolescents will experience a significant reduction, or complete remission, in tic expression by late adolescence or early adulthood (Pappert et al., 2003; Peterson et al., 2001). Nonetheless, adolescents with TS often experience variable and unpredictable symptoms; the fluctuations may be due to changes in hormone levels or noncompliance with medication. For adolescents who continue to present with severe tic symptoms through late adolescence, the prognosis is relatively poor (Leckman et al., 1997). That is, late adolescents with a mild presentation of symptoms will typically persist in having a mild presentation during adulthood; those still experiencing severe symptoms during the late adolescence are likely to continue having more frequent and severe tics throughout their lives.

With regard to comorbidity patterns, one investigation provided data to indicate that over 65% of late adolescents reported that learning difficulties and behavioral problems (e.g., ADHD and OCD) resulted in as much daily functional impairment as, or more than, the tics themselves (Erenberg, Cruse, & Rothner, 1987). Like adolescents with other chronic illnesses, adolescents with TS may experience psychosocial challenges that include depression, low self-esteem, and social isolation. These adolescents may be the targets of ridicule and aggression from peers; several studies have demonstrated that tic severity is inversely associated with social acceptance (Boudjouk, Woods, Miltenberger, & Long, 2000).

GENETICS AND FAMILY PATTERNS

Although the precise etiology of TS is unknown, the strongest biological evidence to date indicates a complex interaction of multiple factors: genetics, prenatal and perinatal factors, and the effects of some infections. Family and twin studies support a strong genetic component. For example, family members of individuals with TS are at increased risk for having a tic disorder or OCD (Pauls & Leckman, 1986). It is noteworthy that the majority of individuals who are genetically predisposed to TS experience few and very mild symptoms, and thus rarely present to health care providers for the management of their symptoms. However, individuals may also demonstrate tics in a milder form, such as transient tic disorder or chronic tic disorder. Furthermore, a small percentage of individuals with this genetic vulnerability present with the full phenotypic expression of the syndrome. In this section of the chapter, we review the literature pertaining to the genetics of TS, focusing specifically on family genetic and twin studies.

Family Genetic Studies

Family genetic studies have provided significant insight into the understanding of TS, with findings generally indicating that the disorder clearly aggregates in families and that the majority of cases are inherited. The prevalence of TS among first-degree relatives is approximately 10–15%, while the rate of other tics is about 15–20% (Hebebrand et al., 1997; Walkup et al., 1996). These rates are significantly higher than the rates of TS and tics in control participants with no family history of the disorder. Bilineal transmission occurs in up to one-quarter of families affected by TS (Hanna, Janjua, Contant, & Jankovic, 1999), meaning that some individuals inherit the genetic susceptibility from both parents. For example, McMahon, Carter, Fredine, and Pauls (2003) found that children with two parents affected by TS and/or OCD were three times more likely to develop tics than children with only one affected parent. In a similar familial investigation, 43% of young children who had a parent or sibling with TS developed tic disorder (Carter, Pauls, Leckman, & Cohen, 1994).

The results of segregation analyses of TS family data have revealed considerable variability, leaving the mode of inheritance for TS uncertain and still controversial among investigators. Early studies initially concluded that TS results from the inheritance of a single, dominant autosomal gene with incomplete penetrance and variable expression (Cohen & Leckman, 1994; Eapen, Pauls, & Robertson, 1993). However, more recent studies have yielded findings interpreted to suggest a more complex multifactorial/polygenic model with intermediate penetrance (Cavallini, Pasquale, Bellodi, & Smeraldi, 1999; Seuchter et al., 2000; Walkup et al., 1996), or a mixed model of genetic–environmental causes (Keen-Kim & Freimer, 2006).

According to the autosomal dominant model, TS is a disorder of incomplete penetrance because not all individuals who inherit the genetic vulnerability will manifest the symptoms. In addition, among those family members who do show symptoms, there is variability in symptom expression; that is, different manifestations occur in various family members. For example, family members with the same pattern of genetic inheritance may present with differing levels or types of symptoms: Some may be diagnosed with chronic tic disorder, while other family members are diagnosed with OCD (Pauls et al., 1990). This suggests that the expression of the gene may result in TS, a milder tic disorder, or even obsessive–compulsive symptoms with no tics at all (van de Wetering & Heutink, 1993). Data from family studies also reveal a sex-specific penetrance, accounting for the higher prevalence of TS among males; as noted earlier, estimated male-to-female ratios range between 2:1 and 10:1 (Marcus & Kurlan, 2001).

Twin Studies

Twin studies also provide strong support for a genetic component in the etiology of TS (Pauls & Leckman, 1988). Studies reveal a concordance rate of about 60% for TS in monozygotic twins, while only 10% of fraternal twins demonstrate concordance for TS (Pauls & Leckman, 1986; van de Wetering & Heutink, 1993). For chronic motor tics, monozygotic twins demonstrate approximately 77% concordance, whereas dizygotic twins demonstrate only 23% concordance (Price, Kidd, Cohen, Pauls, & Leckman, 1985).

Although researchers have examined several candidate genes in an attempt to isolate a TS gene, results have proven inconclusive or negative (Leckman, 2002; Rosa, Jankovic, & Ashizawa, 2003). Nevertheless, initial findings from genetic linkage studies suggest that several chromosome regions may contain susceptibility loci for TS (for a review, see Pauls, 2003).

BIOLOGICAL AND NEUROPSYCHOLOGICAL MARKERS

Neurobiology

At the present time, the pathogenesis of tic disorders at a molecular and cellular level is unknown (Hoekstra, Anderson, et al., 2004). In addition, the precise neurobiological abnormality of TS remains inconclusive (Singer & Minzer, 2003); however, TS is considered a neurobehavioral disorder,

with likely involvement of the basal ganglia and associated cortical circuits such as the corticostriatal–thalamocortical pathways (Hoekstra, Anderson, et al., 2004; Phelps, 2008; Singer & Minzer, 2003). Early research findings suggested that, on average, individuals with TS have reduced volume and abnormal lateralization of their basal ganglia (Peterson, 1995). Evidence for the involvement of the basal ganglia in other movement disorders (e.g., Huntington disorder) is well established, thereby lending support to the role of the basal ganglia in other movement disorders, including TS (Abbruzzese & Berardelli, 2003). Finally, evaluation of the phenomenology and natural history of tic disorders also suggests involvement of the corticostriatal–thalamocortical circuits (Mink, 2001).

Peterson and colleagues (2003) employed volumetric magnetic resonance imaging (MRI) in children and adults with TS. Results revealed significant reductions in the caudate nucleus, which represents one part of the basal ganglia. In a similar MRI study of individuals with TS, Singer (2000) reported abnormalities in the caudate or lenticular nuclei. Findings from a prospective study of children diagnosed with TS revealed significant inverse correlations between the volume of the caudate nucleus and severity of tics in early adulthood (Bloch, Leckman, Zhu, & Peterson, 2005). Specifically, the smaller the caudate nucleus in childhood, the more acute the tics were during adulthood. Interestingly, there was no association with tic severity at the time of the MRI scan. Findings were interpreted to support abnormalities of the caudate nucleus and striatal–cortical circuits in individuals with TS (Bloch et al., 2005). In their review of the literature, Hoekstra, Anderson, and colleagues (2004) report consistent findings between MRI studies and positron emission tomography [PET], single-photon emission computed tomography [SPECT], and functional MRI [fMRI] studies, thereby definitively documenting involvement of the basal ganglia in TS.

It has been suggested that dopamine receptor abnormalities are involved in TS. This contention is primarily derived from the therapeutic response to neuroleptics among individuals with TS. Specifically, the neuroleptic haloperidol, a dopamine receptor antagonist, has demonstrated success in the management of TS through reduction of tics. Indeed, pharmacological agents that block dopamine receptors are considered the most effective tic-suppressing medications (Bruggerman et al., 2001). However, findings from studies of dopamine receptors are equivocal. For example, Heinz and colleagues (1998) reported a correlation between dopamine receptor binding and tic severity, whereas findings from another investigation demonstrated no difference between individuals with TS and those receiving placebo controls (Wong et al., 1997). Another research team employed SPECT to evaluate dopamine receptor capacity in five monozygotic twin pairs with TS. Findings revealed greater dopamine receptor capacity in the caudate nucleus for the more severely affected cotwin in each pair (Wolf et al., 1996). In contrast, D2 and D3 dopamine receptor availability has remained unaltered in PET (Turjanski et al., 1994) and SPECT (George et al., 1994) studies. Taken together, these findings suggest the lack of a unified dopaminergic hypothesis in TS (Hoekstra, Anderson, et al., 2004).

Neuropsychological Characteristics

Individuals with TS do not exhibit any impairment in general intellectual ability (Como, 2001). Furthermore, neuropsychological function for the majority of children with TS has been demonstrated to be within normal limits when compared to that of age-matched peers (Yeates & Bornstein, 1996). However, some individuals with TS do exhibit impairment in neuropsychological functioning (Bornstein, 1990). What is less clear, however, is whether the impairment results from pathology associated with comorbidities (e.g., ADHD, OCD, learning disabilities) or from dysfunction in the frontostriatal area of the brain that is associated with pure TS (Osmon & Smerz, 2005). Certainly individuals with TS demonstrate high prevalence rates of comorbid learning disabilities (Burd, Freeman, Klug, & Kerbeshian, 2006), as well as ADHD and OCD (Alsobrook & Pauls, 1997; Freeman, 1997). Alternatively, some evidence suggests that impairment may be associated with neuroanatomical and neurophysiological abnormalities, such as pathology in fronto-

striatal structures (for a review, see Osmon & Smerz, 2005).

For those individuals with TS who suffer from compromised neuropsychological functioning, findings in the literature are generally consistent in implicating deficits in visual processing and psychomotor difficulties (Osmon & Smerz, 2005). Specifically, the most common deficits appear to be in visual processing, including difficulties with visual–motor and visual–spatial integration. It is noteworthy, however, that most individuals with TS do not demonstrate any difficulty with visual processing abilities (Schultz et al., 1998). Deficits in psychomotor abilities frequently include impairments in fine motor skills (Como, 2001) and speedy execution of movement (Georgiu, Bradshaw, Phillips, Bradshaw, & Chiu, 1995).

Attention and executive function problems also occur among some individuals with TS. In a study of evoked potential response, Johannes and colleagues (1997) demonstrated that individuals with TS struggled on more complex attention tasks. Nonetheless, current research on attention problems in individuals with TS suggests that these difficulties are associated with comorbidity of specific disorders and not with TS per se. Furthermore, the evidence for executive functioning deficits is equivocal. For example, whereas Harris and colleagues (1995) found evidence of deficits in executive function, another investigation that examined TS in monozygotic twins found no evidence of executive dysfunction (Randolph, Hyde, Gold, Goldberg, & Weinberger, 1993).

RISK FACTORS FOR PHENOTYPIC EXPRESSION

Because there is a less than 100% concordance rate for TS and/or tics in monozygotic twins, nongenetic influences such as environmental prenatal and postnatal factors must also play a role in TS. Research evidence further indicates that environmental factors contribute to the development and phenotypic expression of TS (e.g., Leckman et al., 1987; Pauls, 2003; Price et al., 1985). However, the role of environmental factors in TS has received far less empirical attention than the role of genetics. In this section, we briefly review findings from studies that have examined risk factors posited in the development and phenotypic expression of TS in children and adolescents.

The role of adverse pre- and perinatal events in the development and phenotypic expression of TS and tic disorders has probably received the most research attention to date. Increased risk for TS has been associated with (1) parental age (Burd et al., 1999), (2) low birthweight (Leckman et al., 1987), (3) lower Apgar scores (Burd et al., 1999), and (4) birth/obstetrical complications (Leckman et al., 1990). For example, Leckman and colleagues (1990) found that obstetrical complications were more common in individuals who developed TS than in individuals from the population at large. Obstetrical complications that cause injury to the basal ganglia and hypoxia, resulting in ischemia to vulnerable parts of the brain, have been implicated in the development of TS (Peterson, Riddle, Gore, Cohen, & Leckman, 1994). Tic severity has been associated with (1) maternal prenatal smoking (Mathews et al., 2006), (2) low birthweight (Hyde, Aaronson, Randolph, Rickler, & Weinberger, 1992; Leckman et al., 1987), and (3) birth complications (Leckman et al., 1990). In addition, maternal stress during pregnancy and severe nausea or vomiting during the first trimester of pregnancy have been found to be associated with tic severity (Leckman et al., 1990). It has been posited that environmental stressors may alter dopamine levels in the central nervous system, which may result in a teratogenic effect on the fetus (Fredhoff, 1986). With respect to comorbid disorders, maternal use of coffee, alcohol, and tobacco has been associated with OCD in patients with TS (Santangelo et al., 1994). For example, Mathews and colleagues (2006) examined the association between prenatal/perinatal adverse events and tic severity in a large sample of individuals with TS. Findings from this investigation revealed that prenatal maternal smoking was associated with increased tic severity and with the presence of OCD.

A number of other environmental risk factors, such as psychosocial stressors, use of stimulant medications, and infections, have been posited to influence the course and severity of TS. Findings from both cross-sectional and longitudinal studies have suggested that TS is sensitive to psychosocial stress (e.g., Findley et al., 2003; Hoekstra, Steenhuis, Kallenberg, & Minderaa, 2004; Silva et al., 1995). For example, data from a recent longitudinal study of children and adolescents with TS and/or OCD revealed that current levels of psychosocial stress predicted future tic severity (Lin et al., 2007).

The use of stimulant medication remains of concern as a possible risk for tics and TS (Walkup, 2001). Findings from studies examining the impact of stimulant medication suggest that there is no clear and consistent relationship between tic severity and stimulant medication in children with tics and ADHD (Gadow, Sverd, & Sprafkin, 1999; Nolan, Gadow, & Sprafkin, 1999). However, it remains unclear whether some children who take stimulant medication may be at increased risk of developing or exacerbating tics.

The association between infections, especially streptococcal infections, and TS is somewhat controversial. The term *pediatric autoimmune neuropsychiatric disorder associated with streptococcal infection* (PANDAS) was coined on the basis of findings from a retrospective study that reported the sudden onset of tics and obsessive–compulsive symptoms temporally associated with streptococcal infection in a sample of children (Swedo et al., 1998). It is hypothesized that cross-reactive antibodies induced by group A streptococcal infection bind to basal ganglia antigens and thereby result in TS symptoms and PANDAS. In such cases, TS symptoms begin suddenly following streptococcal infection, but then follow a typical course. However, findings from studies examining the association between streptococcal infections and TS have been mixed. For example, data from a recent study of children and adults indicated that individuals with TS had higher rates of group A streptococcal and anti-basal-ganglia antibodies, compared to a healthy comparison control group (Church, Dale, Lees, Giovannoni, & Robertson, 2003). However, several prospective studies have not revealed differences in antistreptococcal antibodies among children with TS (Loiselle, Wendtlandt, Rohde, & Singer, 2003; Luo et al., 2004; Perrin et al., 2004). Thus it seems unlikely from the research evidence that streptococcal infection is a specific risk factor for the development or phenotypic expression of TS, except in a few rare cases (Phelps, 2008).

PSYCHOLOGICAL FACTORS RELATED TO SYMPTOMATOLOGY AND ADJUSTMENT

The extant literature demonstrates that TS is a stress-sensitive condition (Shapiro & Shapiro, 1998). As noted earlier, findings from cross-sectional and longitudinal studies have consistently demonstrated that TS is sensitive to psychosocial stress (Findley et al., 2003; Hoekstra, Steenhuis, et al., 2004; Silva et al., 1995). In a recent prospective longitudinal study, Lin and colleagues (2007) found that current levels of stress and depression independently predicted future tic severity in children and adolescents with TS and OCD. Stressful life events such as beginning a new school year, waiting for test results, family conflict, and moving to a new residence are also associated with an increase in tic severity (Malatesta, 1990).

Research studies examining emotional distress or disorders have also found associations with tic severity (Burd et al., 2006). For example, in a study of children and adolescents with TS, anxiety was the most commonly reported factor associated with tic severity (Silva et al., 1995). In addition, findings from a recent study indicate that comorbid OCD, other anxiety disorders, mood disorders, and anger control problems are all associated with increased tic severity (Burd et al., 2006).

Several studies have indicated that severity of tics is associated with disruptive behavior problems and disorders, as well as with poorer social and academic competence (Burd et al., 2006; Zhu, Leung, Liu, Zhou, & Su, 2006). For instance, Zhu and colleagues (2006) found that delinquent behavior, thought problems, attention problems, and aggression were all positively associated with tic severity; they also found that deficits in social and school competence were positively related to severity of tic symptoms. Findings in the literature with respect to ADHD are equivocal, with some results indicating a positive relationship between ADHD and tic severity (Carter et al., 2000), while other studies have revealed no significant relationship between tic severity and a comorbid diagnosis of ADHD (Burd et al., 2006).

With respect to adjustment, research suggests that children with TS and comorbid ADHD exhibit poorer functioning compared to those with TS alone and to their normally developing counterparts (Bawden, Stokes, Camfield, Camfield, & Salisbury, 1998; Carter et al., 2000; Spitzer, Williams, Gibbon, & First, 1990). Specifically, findings indicate that children with TS who have a comorbid diagnosis of ADHD exhibit more internalizing and externalizing behavioral problems and poorer social adaptation (Carter et al., 2000), as well as more aggressive behavior problems (Bawden et al., 1998) and poorer global functioning (Spitzer et al., 1990), than children with TS alone do. Carter and colleagues (2000) found that children with TS alone were not significantly different in terms of externalizing and social problems compared to normal controls, but did exhibit a higher frequency of internalizing problems. Thus these findings may be interpreted to suggest that some social-emotional and behavior adjustment difficulties may specifically be results of ADHD symptoms as opposed to TS.

ASSESSMENT

An assessment process that includes multiple methods and perspectives is frequently promoted as the best evidence-based assessment strategy in the child and adolescent health and mental health literature. Assessment instruments available for TS include clinician-observer rating scales, self-report rating scales, parent rating scales, and video-based rating scales. We provide a brief review of some of the more widely used methods for the assessment of TS in children and adolescents. Furthermore, we discuss differential diagnosis and assessment for common comorbid conditions.

Clinician-Observer Rating Scales

Clinician-observer rating scales are used to assess for the various dimensions of tic behavior, including type, duration, frequency, intensity, location, complexity, suppression, and functional impairment. These rating scales are designed to be completed by an experienced clinician after a clinical interview. Some of the most commonly used clinician-observer rating scales are the Shapiro Tourette's Syndrome Severity Scale (STSSS; Shapiro & Shapiro, 1984), the Yale Global Tic Severity Scale (YGTSS; Leckman et al., 1989), and the Hopkins Motor and Vocal Tic Scale (HMVTS; Walkup, Rosenberg, Brown, & Singer, 1992).

The STSSS is an easy-to-use measure that consists of a composite rating scale of tic severity based on five factors: the degree to which the tics are noticeable to others; whether the tics elicit comments or curiosity; whether others consider the identified patient as unusual or bizarre; whether the tics interfere with daily functioning; and whether the identified patient is incapacitated, homebound, or hospitalized because of the tics. The clinician sums the ratings for the five factors to derive a total global severity rating. The STSSS has demonstrated adequate reliability and validity (Shapiro, Shapiro, Young, & Feinberg, 1988). The STSSS is primarily a measure of social impairment associated with TS and therefore does not provide an assessment of the tics' characteristics as experienced by the patient.

The YGTSS is a semistructured clinician-rated instrument that assesses the nature of motor and vocal tics, as well as the functional impairments associated with these tics. The nature and severity of motor and vocal tics are assessed on five separate dimensions: number, frequency, intensity, complexity, and interference. The five dimensions are each rated on a 6-point scale for motor and vocal tics, and the scores are then summed to yield a total tic score. The YGTSS also includes a separate overall impairment rating ranging from 0 (no impairment) to 50 (severe impairment). A global severity score is derived by summing the overall impairment rating and the total tic score. The YGTSS has demonstrated adequate reliably and validity (Storch et al., 2005), and has been shown to be sensitive to treatment effects (e.g., Gilbert, Batterson, Sethuraman, & Sallee, 2004). Although the YGTSS provides an assessment of the nature and functional impairment of tics and has good psychometric properties, it does not assess for other common symptoms associated with TS; it also takes more time to complete than some other clinician rating scales.

The HMVTS was created to provide a quick, simple, and accurate assessment of the nature of tics and the resulting degree of impairment. However, similar to the other two rating scales discussed here, the HMVTS does not assess for other common symptoms associated with TS in children and adolescents. The HMVTS consists of a series of linear visual analogue scales on which a caregiver/parent and a physician separately rank each tic symptom (motor and vocal), taking into consideration the tics' frequency, intensity and interference with daily functioning. Caregivers are instructed that the lines range from 0 (no tics) to 10 (most severe). The scales can be divided into four severity ranges: mild, moderate, moderately severe, and severe. Three final scores are derived for both motor and vocal tics based on the caregiver's ratings, the clinician's rating, and an overall assessment. Final scores use a 5-point rating scale ranging from 1 (no tics) to 5 (severe tics). Research reveals that the HMVTS has adequate psychometric properties (Walkup et al., 1992).

Self-Report and Parent Rating Scales

Self-report and parent rating scales are frequently used to assess TS, due to their ease of administration and scoring. Child self-report rating scales may also be helpful in obtaining a subjective impression of the symptoms (Goetz & Kompoliti, 2001). In addition, parent report rating scales are important because they provide information about how the child behaves in the home setting and how the child is observed by significant people in her or his life.

The Motor tic, Obsessions and compulsions, Vocal tic, Evaluation Survey (MOVES; Gaffney, Sieg, & Hellings, 1994) is one of the only self-report rating scales that may be employed across the developmental spectrum, since it has been developed for children, adolescents, and adults. The MOVES is a brief 16-item self-report measure of TS. Items are self-rated on a 4-point scale from 0 (never) to 3 (always). The MOVES yields five subscales: Motor Tics, Vocal Tics, Obsessions, Compulsions, and Associated Symptoms (e.g., echolalia, echopraxia, coprolalia, and copropraxia). Scores on the subscales may be combined to form a Tic subscale or an Obsessive–Compulsive subscale. The MOVES has demonstrated adequate psychometric properties (e.g., Gaffney et al., 1994).

Several parent/caregiver rating scales are commonly used to assess TS. The Tourette Syndrome Symptom List (TSSL; Cohen, Leckman, & Shaywitz, 1985) is among the most commonly employed measures to assist caregivers and parents in making daily or weekly ratings of tic behavior. The TSSL is a 29-item list of symptoms, each of which is rated on a 5-point scale from 1 (symptom not present) to 5 (symptoms almost always present); the 29 symptoms include a wide range of simple and complex tics and other behavioral symptoms associated with TS (e.g., outbursts, defiance). Although the TSSL has been used with considerable frequency, it has not undergone rigorous psychometric validation and does not address the full range of symptomatology that accompanies childhood TS (Kompoliti & Goetz, 1997).

The Tourette's Disorder Scale—Parent Rated (TODS-PR; Shytle et al., 2003) was developed to improve upon previous TS rating scales by including the assessment of other clinically relevant symptoms (e.g., tics, inattention, hyperactivity, aggression, obsessions, compulsions, and emotional disturbance) seen in children with TS. The TODS-PR is a 15-item parent-rated measure with severity ratings for each item ranging from 0 to 10 (0 = not at all and 10 = extremely). An overall total score is calculated by summing the item scores (minimum score = 0, maximum score = 150). The TODS-PR has demonstrated good internal consistency, convergent validity, and discriminant validity, and has been shown to be sensitive to treatment effects (Shytle et al., 2003; Storch et al., 2004).

Video-Based Rating Scales

Video-based rating scales can be used to assess the nature of a patient's tics via behavioral observation. This type of methodology can provide objective information about the individual's tics that can be difficult to obtain otherwise because tics are fleeting in nature and because they are sometimes suppressed in the presence of a clinician. Examples of behavioral observation tasks that can be used to assess tics include reading, sitting quietly alone or in the presence of an observer, engaging in casual conversion, or performing mathematical computations or other mental tasks. The behavioral tasks can be chosen to distract—or, more importantly, to provide a more relaxed environment for—the individual with suspected tic disorder, in order to obtain a more accurate assessment of the nature of the patient's tics (Goetz & Kompoliti, 2001). Although video-based rating scales provide an objective assessment of tics that may not always be possible to obtain by other measures, these scales can be time-consuming and difficult to implement outside a research setting, due to lack of equipment or space.

Differential Diagnosis among the Tic Disorders

TS is differentiated from the other tic disorders primarily by the requirement that the child or adolescent must exhibit *both* multiple motor tics and at least one vocal tic for more than 1 year. Chronic tic disorder requires at least one motor or vocal tic, but not *both* for 1 year. Transient tic disorder requires that the tics occur many times throughout the day for at least 4 weeks, but less than 1 year. If the tics occur for less than 4 weeks and/or do not occur for many times throughout the day, then tic disorder not otherwise specified may be the appropriate diagnosis.

Common Comorbid Conditions

As noted earlier, TS is frequently comorbid with other psychiatric disorders in children and adolescents; comorbidity estimates range as high as 90% (Robertson, 2000). Research indicates that comorbid conditions include a wide range of psychiatric disorders, such as anxiety, mood, conduct, and substance use disorders (Gaze, Kepley, & Walkup, 2006). ADHD and OCD are among the most common comorbid conditions reported. Given the high rates of comorbidity in children and adolescents with TS, a comprehensive assessment of psychiatric disorders is essential in order to minimize the impact of the comorbid condition(s) on tic severity and to provide the most appropriate treatment for both the TS and the co-occurring disorder(s).

TREATMENT

Therapies that have demonstrated empirically validated evidence for the management of TS include behavioral treatments, pharmacotherapy, and their combination.

Behavioral Treatments

Although several behavioral interventions have been examined for the management of TS, habit reversal training (HRT; Azrin & Nunn, 1973) is among the most widely recognized and has received the most rigorous empirical attention. Originally, HRT consisted of eight components. However, it has since been simplified based on a component analysis, which indicated three critical components: (1) awareness training, (2) competing-response practice, and (3) social support (Woods & Miltenberger, 1995). Awareness training has several components (i.e., response description, response detection, identifying early warning signs, and identifying high-risk situations), all of which are geared toward increasing awareness and are based on the premise that increased awareness of tics facilitates self-control. Competing response training occurs once awareness training has been mastered. This training entails teaching individuals with TS to produce any physical response that is incompatible with the tic and to tense the identified tic-opposing muscles until the urge to produce the tic subsides. Social support involves having the individual's caregivers, family, and friends provide prompting, praise, and support for the individual to use the newly learned skills outside of treatment. HRT is based on the rationale that tics are maintained by unawareness of their occurrence, excessive practice, response chaining, and social reinforcement of the tics. A task force of the American Psychological Association published criteria for empirically supported treatments (American Psychological Association Task Force, 1995), including criteria for describing treatments as "well established" and "probably efficacious." From a review of the literature, Carr and Chong (2005) conclude that HRT meets the "probably efficacious" criteria.

Exposure with response prevention (ERP) is a behavioral treatment that is most frequently used to treat OCD, but also has received empirical attention for the treatment of TS. ERP entails exposing the individual to sensations and urges that precede the tics and then preventing the tic response. The rationale for ERT in managing TS is that tic reduction occurs as a result of habituation to premonitory sensations and urges. Recent results from a study that compared ERT to HRT for the treatment of TS indicated that both treatments significantly reduced tics, but that the treatment groups did not differ from each other (Verdellen, Keijsers, Cath, & Hoogduin, 2004). Although the results from this study are preliminary, the data do suggest that the two treatments are comparable in helping to reduce tic symptoms in individuals with TS.

Pharmacological Treatments

Research evidence suggests that neuroleptic agents (both atypical and typical antipsychotics) that block postsynaptic dopamine receptors are presently the most effective medications for the treatment of tics (Gilbert, 2006; Phelps, 2008). Typical neuroleptic medications such as haloperidol (Haldol) and pimozide (Orap) have received the most rigorous empirical attention and have demonstrated efficacy in numerous double-blind placebo controlled studies (for a review, see Sandor, 2003). Atypical neuroleptics such as risperidone (Risperdal) and ziprasidone (Geodan) have also demonstrated efficacy for the management of tics (Gilbert et al., 2004; Sallee et al., 2000). For example, in a recent randomized double-blind crossover study that compared risperidone to pimozide, risperidone was associated with significantly lower tic severity scores, but greater weight gain. Although research suggests that risperidone is associated with greater weight gain, atypical neuroleptics generally tend to have fewer or less severe adverse side effects than typical neuroleptics do. Adverse side effects associated with the typical neuroleptics, such as extrapyramidal symptoms and sedation, can result in patients' discontinuing the medication. Thus the atypical neuroleptics show promise in the management of tics in children and adolescents.

Although neuroleptic medications that block postsynaptic dopamine receptors are considered the most effective medications for the treatment of tics, placebo-controlled studies provide evidence for several alternative pharmacological treatments for tics (for a review, see Gilbert et al., 2006). For example, findings from a recent double-blind study indicated that clonidine (Catapres) was as effective at reducing tics as the atypical neuroleptic risperidone (Gaffney et al., 2002). In addition, clonidine and gaunfacine (Tenex) are two psychotropic agents that have been shown to reduce both tics and impulsivity (Scahill et al., 2001; Tourette Syndrome Study Group, 2002). Thus, given that children and adolescents with TS frequently have a comorbid diagnosis of ADHD or demonstrate impulsivity, findings from research studies to date suggest that these two medications may be particularly beneficial for children with TS and comorbid ADHD. This is especially relevant, given the widespread concerns that stimulant medications typically used for the treatment of ADHD may exacerbate tics. However, findings from a study comparing clonidine, methylphenidate (Ritalin), and placebo for the treatment of ADHD in children with tics indicated that all treatments were superior to placebo with respect to reducing both ADHD and tic symptoms (Tourette Syndrome Study Group, 2002). Therefore, contrary to the popular belief that stimulant medication exacerbates tic symptoms, results from this study suggest that methylphenidate is effective at reducing tics in children and adolescents with tics and ADHD. However, tic exacerbation remains possible in some susceptible individuals, and this possibility warrants careful monitoring during stimulant treatment. Recent findings from a randomized double-blind study examining the nonstimulant medication atomoxetine (Strattera) indicated greater ADHD symptom improvement and greater reduction in tic severity compared to placebo for the treatment of ADHD in children and adolescents with TS (Spencer et al., 2008).

Many medications have been shown to be effective at treating tics in open-label studies (see Gilbert, 2006, for a review). However, due to the lack of control groups in these studies, extraneous variables may have influenced the outcome measures and led to overestimates of the treatment effects. As such, findings from these studies should be viewed with caution, and the data must be interpreted judiciously in the management of children and adolescents with TS.

SUMMARY AND CONCLUSIONS

Over the past few decades, significant advances in empirical developments have increased our understanding of the assessment and management of TS, together with the comorbidities that are frequently associated with this disorder. In particular, neuroimaging research over the past 10 years has yielded fairly compelling evidence that TS has a strong biological component. Moreover, research on the role of dopamine in both the development and the course of TS and other movement disorders has allowed for significant advances in the pharmacotherapy of these disorders. Finally, it has become particularly clear that TS has a strong familial and genetic component. The developments in human genome research that have furthered our understanding of the genetics of TS have assisted in predicting those individuals who are at greatest risk for the phenotypic expression of the disorder, and also provide promising avenues for the treatment of TS based on specific genetic markers.

Whereas much has been learned about the biology of TS over the past decade, important progress has also been made in our understanding of the environmental factors associated with the course of the disorder. Clearly, a next step in research efforts will be a greater understanding of how the interaction between biological factors (e.g., genetics, neurotransmitters) and environmental factors results in the expression of the disease, and of how both biology and environment can be manipulated for the purpose of managing TS. Although specific biological markers must clearly be present for phenotypic expression of the disease, environmental factors may mediate or moderate the phenotypic expression of the disorder. This remains an important and fruitful area for research in the years to come.

The clinical assessment of children with TS is especially complex, as this disorder is frequently comorbid with a number of psychiatric disorders, including anxiety disorders, mood disorders, ADHD, and learning disabilities. The impact of these comorbid psychiatric disorders on the symptom display and natural history of TS remains an important area for future investigation. Conversely, the impact of TS on the symptom display and natural history of the various comorbid psychiatric disorders is also an important area for further study.

Finally, behavioral treatments and pharmacotherapy are the therapies of choice in the management of TS because of their firm evidence base. Both behavioral and pharmacological approaches have been demonstrated to be efficacious in the short term, although there are no long-term studies of the efficacy and durability of these treatment approaches. Furthermore, the relative efficacy of pharmacotherapy and behavior management is an important research question that necessitates careful study. In addition, the efficacy of combined behavioral and pharmacological approaches, compared to either of these approaches employed alone, needs systematic investigation. Finally, the sequencing of these treatments and the points in time at which each treatment approach might be employed constitute still another important area for study. We anticipate that careful investigation and the continued developments of translational and clinical research will result in better identification of children and adolescents suffering from TS, as well as in enhanced quality of life for these youth and their families.

REFERENCES

Abbruzzese, G., & Berardelli, A. (2003). Sensorimotor integration in movement disorders. *Movement Disorders, 18,* 231–240.

Alsobrook, J. P., II, & Pauls, D. L. (1997). The genetics of Tourette syndrome. *Neurologic Clinics of North America, 15,* 381–393.

American Psychiatric Association (APA). *Diagnostic and statistical manual of mental disorders* (4th ed., text rev.). Washington, DC: Author.

American Psychological Association Task Force on Promotion and Dissemination of Psychological Procedures. (1995). Training in and dissemination of empirically-validated psychological treatments: Report and recommendations. *Clinical Psychologist, 48,* 3–24.

Apter, A., Pauls, D. L., Bleich, A., Zohar, A. H., Kron, S., Ratzoni, G., et al. (1993). An epidemiological study of Gilles de la Tourette's syndrome in Israel. *Archives of General Psychiatry, 50,* 734–738.

Azrin, N. H., & Nunn, R. G. (1973). Habit reversal: A method of eliminating nervous habits and tics. *Behaviour Research and Therapy, 11,* 619–628.

Bawden, H. N., Stokes, A., Camfield, C. S., Camfield, P. R., & Salisbury, S. (1998). Peer relationship problems in children with Tourette's disorder or diabetes mellitus. *Journal of Child Psychology and Psychiatry, 39,* 663–668.

Bloch, M. H., Leckman, J. F., Zhu, H., & Peterson, B. S. (2005). Caudate volumes in childhood predict symptom severity in adults with Tourette syndrome. *Neurology, 65,* 1253–1258.

Bornstein, R. A. (1990). Neuropsychological performance in children with Tourette's syndrome. *Psychiatry Research, 33,* 73–81.

Boudjouk, P. J., Woods, D. W., Miltenberger, R. G., & Long, E. S. (2000). Negative peer evaluation in adolescents: Effects of tic disorders and trichotillomania. *Child and Family Behavior Therapy, 22,* 17–28.

Brown, R. T., Antonuccio, D., DuPaul, G. J., Fristad, M., King, C. A., Leslie, L. K., et al. (2008). *Psychopharmacological, psychosocial, and combined interventions for childhood disorders: Evidence base, contextual factors, and future directions.* Washington, DC: American Psychological Association.

Bruggerman, R., van der Linden, C., Buitelaar, J. K., Gericke, G. S., Hawkridge, S. M., & Temlett, J. A. (2001). Risperidone versus pimozide in Tourette's disorder: A comparative double-blind parallel group study. *Journal of Clinical Psychiatry, 62,* 50–56.

Bruun, R. D., & Budman, C. L. (1997). The course and prognosis of Tourette syndrome. *Neurologic Clinics of North America, 15,* 291–298.

Burd, L., Freeman, R. D., Klug, M. G., & Kerbeshian, J. (2006). Variables associated with increased tic severity in 5,500 participants with Tourette syndrome. *Journal of Developmental and Physical Disabilities, 18,* 13–24.

Burd, L., Kerbeshian, J., Wikenheiser, M., & Fisher, W. (1986a). Prevalence of Gilles de la Tourette's syndrome in North Dakota adults. *American Journal of Psychiatry, 143,* 787–788.

Burd, L., Kerbeshian, J., Wikenheiser, M., & Fisher, W. (1986b). A prevalence study of Gilles de la Tourette syndrome in North Dakota school-age children. *Journal of the American Academy of Child and Adolescent Psychiatry, 25,* 552–553.

Burd, L., Severud, R., Klug, M.G., & Kerbeshian, J. (1999). Prenatal and perinatal risk factors for Tourette disorder. *Journal of Perinatal Medicine, 27,* 295–302.

Carr, J. E., & Chong, I. M. (2005). Habit reversal treatment of tic disorders: A methodological critique of the literature. *Behavior Modification, 29,* 858–875.

Carter, A. S., O'Donnell, D. A., Schultz, R. T., Scahill, L., Leckman, J. F., & Pauls, D. L. (2000). Social and emotional adjustment in children affected with Gilles de la Tourette's syndrome: Associations with ADHD and family functioning. *Journal of Child Psychology and Psychiatry, 41,* 215–223.

Carter, A. S., Pauls, D. L., Leckman, J. F., & Cohen, D. J. (1994). A prospective longitudinal study of Gilles de la Tourette's syndrome. *Journal of the American Academy of Child and Adolescent Psychiatry, 33*, 377–385.

Cavallini, M. C., Pasquale, L., Bellodi, L., & Smeraldi, E. (1999). Complex segregation analysis for obsessive compulsive disorder and related disorders. *American Journal of Medical Genetics, 88*, 38–43.

Church, A. J., Dale, R. C., Lees, A. J., Giovannoni, G., & Robertson, M. M. (2003). Tourette's syndrome: A cross sectional study to examine the PANDAS hypothesis. *Journal of Neurology, Neurosurgery and Psychiatry, 74*, 602–607.

Cohen, D. J., & Leckman, J. F. (1994). Developmental psychopathology and neurobiology of Tourette's syndrome. *Journal of the American Academy of Child and Adolescent Psychiatry, 33*, 2–15.

Cohen, D. J., Leckman, J. F., & Shaywitz, B. A. (1985). The Tourette syndrome and other tics. In D. Shaffer, A. Ehrhard, & L. Greenhill (Eds.), *The clinical guide to child psychiatry* (pp. 566–573). New York: Free Press.

Como, P. G. (2001). Neuropsychological function in Tourette syndrome. *Advances in Neurology, 85*, 103–111.

Eapen, V., Pauls, D. L., & Robertson, M. M. (1993). Evidence for autosomal dominant transmission in Tourette's syndrome: United Kingdom cohort study. *British Journal of Psychiatry, 162*, 593–596.

Erenberg, G., Cruse, R. P., & Rothner, A. D. (1987). The natural history of Tourette's syndrome: A follow-up study. *Annals of Neurology, 22*, 383–385.

Findley, D. B., Leckman, J. F., Katsovich, L., Lin, H., Zhang, H., Grantz, H., et al. (2003). Development of the Yale Children's Global Stress Index (YCGSI) and its application in children and adolescents with Tourette syndrome and obsessive–compulsive disorder. *American Journal of Child and Adolescent Psychiatry, 4*, 450–457.

Fredhoff, A. J. (1986). Insights into the pathophysiology and pathogenesis of Gilles de la Tourette syndrome. *Revue Neurologique, 142*, 860–864.

Freeman, R. D. (1997). Attention deficit hyperactivity disorder in the presence of Tourette syndrome. *Neurologic Clinics of North America, 15*, 411–420.

Freeman, R., Fast, D., Burd, L., Kerbeshian, J., Robertson, M., & Sandor, P. (2000). An international perspective on Tourette syndrome: Selected findings from 3500 individuals in 22 countries. *Developmental Medicine and Child Neurology, 42*, 436–447.

Gadow, K. D., Sverd, J., & Sprafkin, J. (1999). Stimulant medication withdrawal during long-term therapy in children with comorbid attention-deficit hyperactivity disorder and chronic multiple tic disorder. *Archives of General Psychiatry, 56*, 330–336.

Gaffney, G. R., Perry, P. J., Lund, B. C., Bever-Stille, K. A., Arndt, S., & Kuperman, S. (2002). Risperidone versus clonidine in the treatment of children and adolescents with Tourette's syndrome. *Journal of the American Academy of Child and Adolescent Psychiatry, 41*, 330–336.

Gaffney, G. R., Sieg, K., & Hellings, J. (1994). The MOVES: A self-rating scale for Tourette's syndrome. *Journal of Child and Adolescent Psychopharmacology, 4*, 269–280.

Gaze, C., Kepley, H. O., & Walkup, J. T. (2006). Co-occurring psychiatric disorders in children and adolescents with Tourette syndrome. *Journal of Child Neurology, 21*, 657–664.

George, M. S., Robertson, M. M., Costa, D. C., Ell, P. J., Trimble, M. R., Pilowsky, L., et al. (1994). Dopamine receptor availability in Tourette's syndrome. *Psychiatry Research, 55*, 193–203.

Georgiou, N., Bradshaw, J., Phillips, J., Bradshaw, J. A., & Chiu, E. (1995). Advance information and movement sequencing in Gilles de la Tourette's syndrome. *Journal of Neurology, Neurosurgery and Psychiatry, 58*, 184–191.

Gilbert, D. (2006). Treatment of children and adolescents with tics and Tourette syndrome. *Journal of Child Neurology, 21*, 690–700.

Gilbert, D. L., Batterson, J. R., Scthuraman, G., & Sallee, F. R. (2004). Tic reduction with Risperidone versus pimozide in a randomized, double-blind, cross-over trial. *Journal of the American Academy of Child and Adolescent Psychiatry, 43*, 206–214.

Goetz, C. G., & Kompoliti, K. (2001). Rating scales and quantitative assessment of tics. *Advances in Neurology, 85*, 31–42.

Hanna, P. A., Janjua, F. N., Contant, C. F., & Jankovic, J. (1999). Bilineal transmission in Tourette syndrome. *Neurology, 53*, 813–818.

Harris, E. L., Schuerholz, L. J., Singer, H. S., Reader, M. J., Brown, J. E., Cox, C., et al. (1995). Executive function in children with Tourette syndrome and/or attention deficit hyperactivity disorder. *Journal of the International Neuropsychological Society, 1*, 511–516.

Hebebrand, J., Klug, B., Fimmers, R., Seutcher, S. A., Wettke-Schafer, R., Deget, F., et al. (1997). Rates for tic disorders and obsessive compulsive symptomatology in families of children and adolescents with Gilles de la Tourette syndrome. *Journal of Psychiatric Research, 31*, 519–530.

Heinz, A., Knable, M., Wolf, S., Jones, D. W., Gorey, J. G., Hyde, T. M., et al. (1998). Tourette's syndrome beta-CIT SPECT correlates of vocal tic severity. *Neurology, 51*, 1069–1074.

Hoekstra, P. J., Anderson, G. M., Limburg, P. C., Korf, J., Kallenberg, C. G. M., & Minderaa, R. B. (2004). Neurobiology and neuroimmunology of Tourette's syndrome: An update. *Cellular and Molecular Life Sciences, 61,* 886–898.

Hoekstra, P. J., Steenhuis, M. P., Kallenberg, C. G. M., & Minderaa, R. B. (2004). Association of small life events with self reports of tic severity in pediatric and adult tic disorder patients: A prospective longitudinal study. *Journal of Clinical Psychiatry, 65,* 426–431.

Hyde, T. M., Aaronson, B. A., Randolph, C., Rickler, K. C., & Weinberger, D. R. (1992). Relationship of birth weight to the phenotypic expression of Gilles de la Tourette's syndrome in monozygotic twins. *Neurology, 42,* 652–658.

Hyde, T. M., & Weinberger, D. R. (1995). Tourette's syndrome: A model neuropsychiatric disorder. *Journal of the American Medical Association, 239,* 498–511.

Johannes, S., Weber, A., Muller-Vahl, K. R., Kolbe, H., Dengler, R., & Munte, T. F. (1997). Event-related brain potentials show changed attentional mechanisms in Gilles de la Tourette syndrome. *European Journal of Neurology, 4,* 152–161.

Keen-Kim, D., & Freimer, N. B. (2006). Genetics and epidemiology of Tourette syndrome. *Journal of Child Neurology, 21,* 665–671.

Kompoliti, K. & Goetz, C. G. (1997). Tourette's syndrome: Clinical rating and quantitative assessment of tics. *Neurologic Clinics, 15,* 239–254.

Kurlan, R. (1994). Hypothesis II: Tourette's syndrome is part of a clinical spectrum that includes normal brain development. *Archives of Neurology, 51,* 1145–1151.

Leckman, J. F. (2002). Tourette's syndrome. *Lancet, 360,* 1577–1586.

Leckman, J. F., & Cohen, D. J. (1999). *Tourette's syndrome—tics, obsessions, compulsions: Developmental psychopathology and clinical care.* New York: Wiley.

Leckman, J. F., Dolnansky, E. S., Hardin, M. T., Clubb, M., Walkup, J. T., Stevenson, J., et al. (1990). Perinatal factors in the expression of Tourette's syndrome: An exploratory study. *Journal of the American Academy of Child and Adolescent Psychiatry, 29,* 220–226.

Leckman, J. F, Peterson, B. S., Anderson, G. M., Arnsten, A. F., Pauls, D. L., & Cohen, D. J. (1997). Pathogenesis of Tourette's syndrome. *Journal of Child Psychology and Psychiatry, 38,* 119–142.

Leckman, J. F., Price, R. A., Walkup, J. T., Ort, S. I., Pauls, D. L., & Cohen, D. J. (1987). Nongenetic factors in Gilles de la Tourette syndrome. *Arches of General Psychiatry, 44,* 100.

Leckman, J. F., Riddle, M. A., Hardin, M. T., Ort, S. I., Swartz, K. L., Stevenson, J., et al. (1989). The Yale Global Tic Severity Scale: Initial testing of a clinician-rated scale of tic severity. *Journal of the American Academy of Child and Adolescent Psychiatry, 28,* 566–573.

Lin, H., Katsovich, L., Ghebremichael, M., Findley,

D. B., Grantz, H., Lombroso, P. J., et al. (2007). Psychosocial stress predicts future symptom severities in children and adolescents with Tourette syndrome and/or obsessive–compulsive disorder. *Journal of Child Psychology and Psychiatry, 48,* 157–166.

Loiselle, C. R., Wendlandt, J. T., Rohde, C. A., & Singer, H. S. (2003). Antistreptococcal, neuronal, and nuclear antibodies in Tourette syndrome. *Pediatric Neurology, 28,* 119–125.

Luo, F., Leckman, J. F., Katsovich, L., Findley, D., Grantz, H., Tucker, D. M., et al. (2004). Prospective longitudinal study of children with tic disorders and OCD: Relationship of symptom exacerbations to newly acquired streptococcal infections. *Pediatrics, 113,* 578–585.

Mahler, M. S., & Rangell, L. (1943). A psychosomatic study of maladie des tics (Gilles de la Tourette's disease). *Psychiatric Quarterly, 17,* 579.

Malatesta, V. J. (1990). Behavioral case formulation: An experimental assessment study of transient tic disorder. *Journal of Psychopathology and Behavioral Assessment, 12,* 219–232.

Mansdorf, I. J. (1995). Tic disorders. In R. T. Ammerman & M. Hersen (Eds.), *Handbook of child behavior therapy in the psychiatric setting* (pp. 323–340). New York: Wiley.

Marcus, D., & Kurlan, R. (2001). Tics and its disorders. *Neurologic Clinics, 19,* 735–758.

Mathews, C. A., Bimson, B., Lowe, T. L., Herrera, L. D., Budman, C. L., Erenberg, G., et al. (2006). Association between maternal smoking and increased symptom severity in Tourette's syndrome. *American Journal of Psychiatry, 163,* 1066–1073.

McMahon, W. M., Carter, A. S., Fredine, N., & Pauls, D. L. (2003). Children at familial risk for Tourette's disorder: Child and parent diagnoses. *American Journal of Medical Genetics, Part B (Neuropsychiatric Genetics), 121,* 105–111.

Mink, J. W. (2001). Basal ganglia dysfunction in Tourette's syndrome: A new hypothesis. *Pediatric Neurology, 25,* 190–198.

Nolan, E. E., Gadow, K. D., & Sprafkin, J. (1999). Stimulant medication withdrawal during long-term therapy in children with comorbid attention-deficit hyperactivity disorder and chronic multiple tic disorder. *Pediatrics, 103,* 730–737.

Osmon, D. C., & Smerz, J. M. (2005). Neuropsychological evaluation in the diagnosis and treatment of Tourette's syndrome. *Behavior Modification, 29,* 746–783.

Pappert, E. J., Goetz, C. G., Louis, E. D., Blasucci, L., & Leurgans, S. (2003). Objective assessments of longitudinal outcome in Gilles de la Tourette's syndrome. *Neurology, 61,* 936–940.

Pauls, D. L. (2003). An update on the genetics of Gilles de la Tourette syndrome. *Journal of Psychosomatic Research, 55,* 7–12.

Pauls, D. L., & Leckman, J. F. (1986). The inheritance of Gilles de la Tourette's syndrome and associated behaviors: Evidence for autosomal dominant transmission. *New England Journal of Medicine, 315*, 993–997.

Pauls, D. L., & Leckman, J. F. (1988). Genetics of Tourette syndrome. In D. J. Cohen, R. Bruun, & J. F. Leckman (Eds.), *Tourette syndrome and tic disorders: Clinical understanding and treatment* (pp. 91–102). New York: Wiley.

Pauls, D. L., Pakstis, A. J., Kurlan, R., Kidd, K. K., Leckman, J. F., Cohen, D. J., et al. (1990). Segregation and linkage analyses of Tourette's syndrome and related disorders. *Journal of the American Academy of Child and Adolescent Psychiatry, 29*, 195–203.

Perrin, E. M., Murphy, M. I., Casey, J. R., Pichichero, M. E., Runyan, D. K., Willer, W. C., et al. (2004). Does group A beta hemolytic streptococcal infection increase risk for behavioral and neuropsychiatric symptoms in children? *Archives of Pediatric and Adolescent Medicine, 158*, 848–856.

Peterson, B. S. (1995). Neuroimaging in child and adolescent neuropsychiatric disorders. *Archives of General Psychiatry, 34*, 1560–1576.

Peterson, B. S., Pine, D. S., Cohen, P., & Brook, J. S. (2001). Prospective, longitudinal study of tic, obsessive–compulsive, and attention-deficit/hyperactivity disorder in an epidemiological sample. *Journal of the American Academy of Child and Adolescent Psychiatry, 40*, 685–695.

Peterson, B. S., Riddle, M. A., Gore, J. C., Cohen, D. J., & Leckman, J. F. (1994). CNA T2 relaxation time asymmetries in Tourette's syndrome. *Psychiatry Research: Neuroimaging, 55*, 205–221.

Peterson, B. S., Thomas, P., Kane, M. J., Scahill, L. Zhang, H., & Bronen, R. (2003). Basal ganglia volumes in patients with Tourette's syndrome. *Archives of General Psychiatry, 60*, 415–424.

Phelps, L. (2008). Tourette's disorder: Genetic update, neurological correlates, and evidence-based interventions. *School Psychology Quarterly, 23*, 282–289.

Price, R. A., Kidd, K. K., Cohen, D. J., Pauls, D. L., & Leckman, J. F. (1985). A twin study of Tourette syndrome. *Archives of General Psychiatry, 42*, 815–820.

Randolph, C., Hyde, T. M., Gold, J. M., Goldberg, T. E., & Weinberger, D. R. (1993). Tourette's syndrome in monozygotic twins: Relationship of tic severity to neuropsychological function *Archives of Neurology, 50*, 725–728.

Robertson, M. M. (2000). Tourette syndrome, associated conditions and the complexities of treatment. *Brain, 123*, 425–462.

Rosa, A. L., Jankovic, J., & Ashizawa, T. (2003). Screening for mutations in the MECP2 (Rett syndrome) gene in Gilles de la Tourette syndrome. *Archives of Neurology, 60*, 502–503.

Sallee, F. D., Kurlan, R., Goetz, C. G., Singer, H., Scahill, L., Law, G., et al., (2000). Ziprasidone treatment of children and adolescents with Tourette's syndrome: A pilot study. *Journal of the American Academy of Child and Adolescent Psychiatry, 39*, 292–299.

Sandor, P. (2003). Pharmacological management of tics in patients with TS. *Journal of Psychosomatic Research, 55*, 41–48.

Santangelo, S. L., Pauls, D. L., Goldstein, J. M., Faraone, S. V., Tsuang, M. T., & Leckman, J. F. (1994). Tourette's syndrome: What are the influences of gender and comorbid obsessive–compulsive disorder? *Journal of the American Academy of Child and Adolescent Psychiatry; 33*, 795–804.

Scahill, L., Chappell, P. B., Kim, Y. S., Schultz, R. T., Katsovich, L., Shepard, E., et al. (2001). A placebo-controlled study of guanfacine in the treatment of children with tics and ADHD. *American Journal of Psychiatry, 158*, 1067–1074.

Schultz, R. T., Carter, A. S., Gladstone, M., Scahill, L., Leckman, J. F., Peterson, B. S., et al. (1998). Visual–motor integration functioning in children with Tourette syndrome. *Neuropsychology, 12*, 134–145.

Seuchter, S. A., Hebebrand, J., Klug, B., Knapp, M., Lemkuhl, G., Poustka, F., et al., (2000). Complex segregation analysis of families ascertained through Gilles de la Tourette syndrome. *Genetic Epidemiology, 18*, 33–47.

Shapiro, A. K., & Shapiro, E. (1984). Controlled study of pimozide vs. placebo in Tourette's syndrome. *Journal of the American Academy of Child and Adolescent Psychiatry, 23*, 161–173.

Shapiro, A. K., & Shapiro, E. S. (1998). Signs, symptoms, and clinical course. In D.J. Cohen, R.D. Bruun, & J.F. Leckman (Eds.), *Tourette's syndrome and tic disorders: Clinical understanding and treatment* (pp. 127–193). New York: Wiley.

Shapiro, A. K., Shapiro, E. S., Young, J. G., & Feinberg, T. E. (1988). Measurement in tic disorders. In A. K. Shapiro, E. S. Shapiro, & J. G. Young (Eds.), *Gilles de la Tourette syndrome* (2nd ed., pp. 451–480). New York: Raven Press.

Shytle, R. D., Silver, A. A., Sheehan, K. H., Wilkinson, B. J., Newman, M., Sanberg, P. R., et al. (2003). The Tourette's Disorder Scale (TODS): Development, reliability and validity. *Assessment, 10*, 273–287.

Silva, R. R., Munoz, D. M., Barickman, J. & Friedhoff, A. J. (1995). Environmental factors and related fluctuation of symptoms in children and adolescents with Tourette's disorder. *Journal of Child Psychology and Psychiatry, 36*, 305–312.

Singer, H. S. (2000). Current issues in Tourette syndrome. *Movement Disorders, 15*, 1051–1063.

Singer, H. S., & Minzer, K. (2003). Neurobiology of Tourette's syndrome: Concepts of neuroanatomic localization and neurochemical abnormalities. *Brain Development, 25*, S70–S84.

Spencer, T. J., Sallee, F. R., Gilbert, D. L., Dunn, D. W., McCracken, J. T., Coffey, B. J., et al. (2008). Atomoxetine treatment of ADHD in children with comorbid Tourette syndrome. *Journal of Attention Disorders, 11*, 470–481.

Spitzer, R. L., Williams, J. B. W., Gibbon, M., & First, M. B. (1990). *Structured Clinical Interview for DSM-III-R, Non-Patient Edition (SCID-NP, Version 1.0)*. Washington, DC: American Psychiatric Press.

Sprague, R. L., & Newell, K. M. (1986). *Brain and behavior relationships*. Washington, DC: American Psychological Association.

Storch, E. A., Murphy, T. K., Geffken, G. R., Soto, O., Sajid, M., Allen, P., et al. (2004). Further psychometric properties of the Tourette's Disorder Scale—Parent Rated Version (TODS-PR). *Child Psychiatry and Human Development, 35*, 107–120.

Swedo, S. E., Leonard, H. L., Garvey, M., Mittleman, B., Allen, A. J., Perlmutter, S., et al. (1998). Pediatric autoimmune neuropsychiatric disorders associated with streptococcal infections: Clinical descriptions in the first 50 cases. *American Journal of Psychiatry, 155*, 264–271.

Tourette Syndrome Study Group. (2002). Treatment of ADHD in children with tics. A randomized controlled trial. *Neurology, 58*, 527–536.

Turjanski, N., Sawle, G. V., Playford, E. D., Weeks, R., Lammertsma, A. A., Lees A. J., et al. (1994). PET studies of the presynaptic and postsynaptic dopaminergic system in Tourette's syndrome. *Journal of Neurology, Neurosurgery and Psychiatry, 57*, 688–692.

van de Wetering, B. J., & Heutink, P. (1993). The genetics of the Gilles de la Tourette syndrome: A review. *Journal of Laboratory and Clinical Medicine, 121*, 638–645.

Verdellen, C. W. J., Keijsers, G. P. J., Cath, D. C., & Hoogduin, C. A. L. (2004). Exposure with response prevention versus habit reversal in Tourettes's syndrome: A controlled study. *Behaviour Research and Therapy, 42*, 501–511.

Walkup, J. T. (2001). Epidenetic and environmental risk factors in Tourette syndrome. *Advances in Neurology, 85*, 273–279.

Walkup, J. T., LaBuda, M. C., Singer, H. S., Brown, J., Riddle, M. A., & Hurko, O. (1996). Family study and segregation analysis of Tourette syndrome: Evidence for a mixed model of inheritance. *American Journal of Human Genetics, 59*, 684–693.

Walkup, J. T., Rosenberg, L. A., Brown, J., & Singer, H. S. (1992). The validity of instruments measuring tic severity in Tourette's syndrome. *Journal of the American Academy of Child and Adolescent Psychiatry 31*, 472–477.

Wolf, S. S., Jones, D. W., Knable, M. B., Gorey, J. G., Lee, K. S., Hyde, T. M., et al. (1996). Tourette syndrome: Prediction of phenotypic variation in monozygotic twins by caudate nucleus D2 receptor binding. *Science, 273*, 1225–1227.

Wong, D., Singer, H., Brandt, J., Shaya, E., Chen, C., Brown, J., et al. (1997). D2–like dopamine receptor density in Tourette syndrome measured by PET. *Journal of Nuclear Medicine, 38*, 1243–1247.

Woods, D. W., & Miltenberger, R. G. (1995). *Tic disorders, trichotillomania, and other repetitive behavior disorders: Behavioral approaches to analysis and treatment*. Norwell, MA: Kluwer Academic.

Yeates, K. O., & Bornstein, R. A. (1996). Neuropsychological correlates of learning disability subtypes in children with Tourette's syndrome. *Journal of the International Neuropsychological Society, 2*, 375–382.

Zhu, Y., Leung, K. M. Liu, P., Zhou, M., & Su, L. (2006). Comorbid behavioural problems in Tourette's syndrome are positively correlated with the severity of tic symptoms. *Australian and New Zealand Journal of Psychiatry, 40*, 67–73.

CHAPTER 10

Anxiety Disorders

STEVEN R. PLISZKA

The last decade has seen major growth in research on child and adolescent anxiety disorders, with new data emerging from longitudinal, family/genetic, neuroimaging, and treatment studies. This has allowed investigators to develop new hypotheses about the etiology of these disorders, as well as to make evidence-based recommendations to clinicians regarding treatment approaches. It is key to begin with a definition of *anxiety*. *Fear* can be defined as a negative brain state brought on by the immediate presence of threatening stimuli (e.g., a predator or an oncoming car), whereas *anxiety* is a similar brain state "engaged when encountering sustained cues that more ambiguously predict threat" (Pine, Helfinstein, Bar-Haim, Nelson, & Fox, 2009, p. 213). Thus fear and anxiety are differentiated by the immediacy of the threat, which may be physical (e.g., an approaching hurricane) or social (e.g., an upcoming examination). Anxiety is adaptive if it causes an individual to take action against a threat (e.g., evacuating the coast or studying for the examination), but becomes symptomatic if it is so severe that the person is persistently in a negative state (i.e., always worrying) or needs to avoid situations to an extent that is self-defeating. Anxiety is generally also associated with physical symptoms of high arousal, such as muscle tension, poor sleep, internal feelings of restlessness, sweating, heart racing, or shortness of breath. When the symptoms of physical arousal are extreme and uncontrollable, a *panic attack* is said to occur.

Anxiety disorders are subdivided by the *Diagnostic and Statistical Manual of Mental Disorders*, fourth edition, text revision (American Psychiatric Association, 2000) into generalized anxiety disorder (GAD), specific phobia, agoraphobia, panic disorder, social phobia (social anxiety disorder), posttraumatic stress disorder (PTSD), acute stress disorder, and obsessive–compulsive disorder (OCD). Separation anxiety disorder (SAD) is the only anxiety disorder that is required to have an onset during childhood and is not diagnosed in adults (although children with SAD are at high risk for adult anxiety disorders, as we shall see).

TYPICAL DEVELOPMENT OF ANXIETY

Klein (1994) has reviewed the developmental course of anxiety and fear in children. In infants, fears of loud noises or loss of support predominate. Fear of strangers arises next, at about 8 months of age, with separation anxiety apparent at about 12–15 months. Fears of imaginary creatures arise during early childhood, and as children enter primary school, fears about performance, health, and personal harm become more pronounced. Silverman, La Greca, and Wasserstein (1995) extensively studied the worries of 272 elementary school children ages 7–12 years. Children were given a structured interview that assessed worries in 14 areas: school, performance, classmates, friends, war, disasters, money, health, future events, personal harm, "little things," appearance, family, and "other." The children were asked whether they worried about each broad category, and, if so, were then asked to list specific worries within that area. Children next rated the intensity of their worry and filled out a number of standardized anxiety rating forms. One-week test–retest reliability of the interview was very good, suggesting that children in this age group are reliable reporters of their worries, at least over the short term. The average child reported about 8 worries, spanning an average of 6 of the 14 areas. The most common worries were about school, health, and personal harm, with friends and appearance ranked the lowest. European American and Hispanic girls reported more worries than boys, but African American boys had as many worries as girls. The number of worries reported by a child correlated highly with the child's self-rating on anxiety scales.

Muris, Meesters, Merckelbach, Sermon, and Zwakhalen (1998) examined anxiety in 193 nonreferred children. Sixty (31%) of the sample stated that they never worried at all. The other children reported that they worried two to three times per week, with the most common worries being about school, dying, getting sick, or being teased. Girls worried more than boys. Other studies have examined anxiety in an unreferred population of children (Ialongo, Edelsohn, Werthamer-Larsson, Crockett, & Kellam, 1994). Over 1,000 first-grade children filled out the Revised Children's Manifest Anxiety Scale (RCMAS). Teacher ratings of classroom adaptive behavior, peer ratings, and achievement measures were also obtained. About 400 of these children filled out the RCMAS again 4 months later; the intraclass correlation coefficients were .64 for boys and .42 for girls, showing good stability of

the anxiety scores. Children with the highest anxiety scores showed lower achievement in mathematics and reading. Interestingly, self-ratings of anxiety did not predict peer or teacher nominations for shyness. Although none of the children in the study underwent a structured interview for psychiatric disorder, the findings with regard to achievement are not consistent with the notion that anxiety in childhood is a benign phenomenon. Also, the studies reviewed above show that children can reliably rate their anxious symptoms and articulate their worries; thus greater confidence can be placed in studies that base the diagnosis of anxiety on a child's report.

The experience of anxiety is closely related to *emotional regulation*, defined as a "voluntary and goal directed process aimed at modifying emotional state to achieve social and biological adaptation, as well as individual goals" (Hannesdottir & Ollendick, 2007, p. 276). For instance, a child may be afraid of water, but may work to consciously suppress the fear when peers are watching. Success or failure of emotional regulation may lead to an adaptive response (e.g., jumping in the pool and discovering that there is nothing to be worried about) or a maladaptive one (e.g., refusing to go to a pool party). Some children with anxiety disorders may not differ from typically developing children in terms of the fear or anxiety experienced internally, but in their ability to regulate their emotions. Deficits in emotional regulation occur with other emotional states (i.e., anger, elation) and thus are not specific to anxiety disorders. Indeed, some parents may identify general "negative affect" as anxiety in some situations, particularly in children with disruptive behavior disorders; this may complicate the interpretation of both research and treatment outcome findings (March et al., 2000).

EPIDEMIOLOGY AND COMORBIDITY

Epidemiological studies of the anxiety disorders in children and adolescents have yielded broadly similar results and are shown in Table 10.1. Anxiety disorders as a group are the most common forms of mental disorders in children and adolescents. The National Comorbidity Survey Replication Adolescent

Supplement (NCS-A) involved face-to-face interviews with nearly 10,000 adolescents ages 12–17 from 2001 to 2004; a lay interview for psychiatric disorders was used. Information from parents was also obtained (Kessler, Avenevoli, Costello, et al., 2009). The full results of the NCS-A are yet to be published at this writing, but data are available from a subsample of 347 adolescents that were administered both the lay interview and the Schedule for Affective Disorders and Schizophrenia for School-Age Children (K-SADS) (Kessler, Avenevoli, Green, et al., 2009). The lay interview showed good concordance with the K-SADS. In this subsample, the lifetime prevalence on the K-SADS for any anxiety disorders was 25%, with specific phobia being most common (12.7%), followed by social phobia (9.2%). GAD (3.3%), PTSD (4.2%), and panic disorder (2.1%) were less common. Clearly, many adolescents had more than one anxiety disorder—a finding consistent with older research. Half of children with DSM-III-R overanxious disorder were also found to have SAD, particularly younger patients (Strauss, Lease, Last, & Francis, 1988). Over a quarter of patients with SAD also have phobias (Benjamin, Costello, & Warren, 1990).

Anxiety disorders are comorbid with other mental disorders as well. In a population of 104 prepubertal children with major depressive disorder (MDD), 41% met criteria for an anxiety disorder, with SAD being the most prevalent (Kovacs, Gatsonis, Paulauskas, & Richards, 1989). In most cases, the anxiety disorder predated the first episode of MDD and persisted after the remission of the depression; this suggested that the depression and anxiety were clearly distinct from each other, rather than that the anxiety was an epiphenomenon of the depression. Angold and Costello (1993) reviewed nine epidemiological studies of childhood mental disorder where at least some of the data were obtained from the children themselves. They examined the rates of depressive comorbidity with the anxiety disorders, which ranged from a low of 6.6% to a high of 69%. In most of the studies, however, only about 10–20% of the anxious children were depressed. The overlap of depression and anxiety is thus asymmetrical: Whereas approximately a quarter of anxious children are depressed, well over half and sometimes up to 75% of children with depressive disorders have comorbid anxiety disorders.

There is also a well-studied overlap of anxiety and disruptive behavior disorders. Children with anxiety disorders have been found to have higher than expected rates of attention-deficit/hyperactivity disorder (ADHD) and oppositional defiant disorder (ODD) (Strauss et al., 1988). Chavira, Garland, Daley, and Hough (2008) examined mental disorders in a subset of 1,715 participants ages 6–18 years

TABLE 10.1. Epidemiology of Anxiety Disorders in Children and Adolescents

Study	Age group (years)	Comment	SAD	GAD[a]	Prevalences of anxiety diagnoses (%) Specific (simple) phobia	Social phobia	Any anxiety disorder
Anderson et al. (1987)	11		3.5	2.9	2.4	—	—
Bird et al. (1988)	4–16	CGAS < 61	4.7	—	2.6	—	—
		CGAS = 61–70	2.1		1.3		
Costello (1989)	7–11	CGAS < 70	4.1	4.6	9.2	1.0	—
Shaffer et al. (1996)	9–17	Parent Youth Combined[b]	1.4	1.9	0.7	2.8	5.3
			1.6	2.6	1.6	2.3	7.1
			3.9	5.7	2.6	5.4	13.0
Kessler et al. (2009b)	12–18	K-SADS	NA	3.3	12.7	9.2	25.0

Note. CGAS, Children's Global Assessment Scale; K-SADS, Schedule for Affective Disorders and Schizophrenia for School-Age Children.
[a]Includes DSM-III/DSM-III-R overanxious disorder.
[b]Used "either–or" method.

who received care in a public sector, such as child welfare or juvenile justice. They compared participants (mean age ~14 years) with anxiety disorders to those with an anxiety disorder and a physical illness to those with a physical illness alone or no physical illness. There was no control group of children not treated in the public health sector. Children with anxiety disorders had very significant rates of depressive disorders (28.4%), disruptive disorders (59.2%), and substance use disorders (21.4%). The additional comorbidity of a physical illness further increased psychiatric comorbidity. Conversely, up to 25–33% of children with ADHD or other disruptive behavior disorders will meet criteria for an anxiety disorder (Angold, Costello, & Erkanli, 1999; Pliszka, Carlson, & Swanson, 1999).

LONGITUDINAL COURSE

Of 14 prospective, long-term epidemiological follow-up studies reviewed by Hirshfeld-Becker, Micco, Simoes, and Henin (2008), 13 showed that childhood anxiety disorders are associated with an increased rate of anxiety disorders in adulthood. Table 10.2 shows selected results from several of the larger studies. Of interest, Woodward and Fergusson

(2001) found a clear dose–response relationship between the number of anxiety disorders in childhood and the likelihood of later adult anxiety disorders. It is also clear that anxiety disorders predict MDD (Gregory et al., 2007); this indicates that anxiety disorders of childhood are not benign conditions that resolve with maturity.

GENETICS AND FAMILY PATTERNS

Studies performed over the last decade have confirmed that parents with anxiety disorders have elevated rates of anxiety disorders among their children. Hirshfeld-Becker and colleagues (2008) combined results from 14 studies examining the rates of anxiety disorders in children of parents who themselves had anxiety disorders compared to control parents. These studies involved 1,371 participants; the 465 children of parents with anxiety disorders had a rate of anxiety disorders of 37%, compared with a rate of 15% among children of control parents ($p <$ .0001). In general, if a parent has a particular anxiety disorder, a child is at risk for the full range of anxiety disorders, not just the anxiety disorder afflicting the parent. Parental MDD and bipolar disorder also increase the risk for childhood anxiety disorders

TABLE 10.2. Selected Prospective Studies Examining Long-Term Outcome of Childhood Anxiety Disorders

Study	Sample	Results at follow-up
Newman et al. (1996)	961 children assessed at ages 11, 13, 15, 18, and 21	Among those with anxiety disorder at age 21, 61.5% had a childhood disorder.
Pine et al. (1998)	776 children ages 9–19 years, assessed at ages 14, 16, and 22 years	Those with an early anxiety disorder were 2.5–3.8 times more likely to have the disorder at follow-up.
Woodward and Fergusson (2001)	964 children in birth cohort, ages 15–16 years, followed for 1–5 years	Rates of anxiety disorder at follow-up: ≥3 anxiety disorders at baseline: 77% 2 anxiety disorders at baseline: 46% 1 anxiety disorder at baseline: 42% No anxiety disorder at baseline: 13%
Kim-Cohen et al. (2003)	1,037 in birth cohort, ages 11–26 years, assessed over 15 years	Anxiety disorder before age 15 predicted anxiety disorder in adulthood (odds ratio = 2.9).
Gregory et al. (2007)	963 children in birth cohort, assessed at ages 11–32 years	Adults with a variety of anxiety disorders had elevated rates of anxiety disorders in childhood, as well as higher rates of MDD. Adults with PTSD had elevated rates of disruptive behavior disorders.

(Grigoroiu-Serbanescu et al., 1989; Weissman et al., 2006). Last, Hersen, Kazdin, Orvaschel, and Perrin (1991) interviewed the first- and second-degree relatives of 94 children with anxiety disorders, as well as the relatives of 58 children with ADHD and 87 controls. There was a significantly higher rate of anxiety disorders in the relatives of the anxious children (35%), compared to the relatives of children with ADHD (24%) or normal controls (16%).

Family studies such as those reviewed above cannot tell us whether genetic or environmental factors (or a combination of both) are involved in the transmission of the disorder. There have been very few adoption studies of anxiety disorders. Twin studies have found that about 30–40% of the variability of anxiety symptoms can be attributed to genetics (i.e., heritability = 0.3–0.4) (Hettema, Neale, & Kendler, 2001; Smoller & Tsuang, 1998). Hettema, Prescott, Myers, Neale, and Kendler (2005) examined data from more than 5,000 twin pairs to look at the role of genes and environment in six different anxiety disorders. Since the different anxiety disorders were highly comorbid in the sample, Hettema and colleagues sought to determine whether there were unique or shared genes or environmental factors for each disorder. The heritability of six anxiety disorders ranged from 0.2 to 0.3, but two different genetic factors were found: one shared by GAD, panic disorder, and agoraphobia; the other by three phobic disorders (social, animal, and situational). Shared environmental factors did not exceed 0.11 for any anxiety disorder. Nonshared environment accounted for 62–79% of the variance. There was a common nonshared environmental factor for each of the six disorders, but each disorder had a specific environmental factor as well.

BIOLOGICAL MARKERS

There has been a major expansion of hypotheses about the biological nature of the genetic diathesis to anxiety disorders, fueled by the technical revolutions in genetics and neuroimaging. Despite these advances, the complex etiology of anxiety disorders remains a mystery, and there are no genetic clinical applications at this writing. More-over, as indicated above, these fascinating advances in the neurobiology of anxiety should not blind us to equally impressive work on family and environmental factors in anxiety (reviewed in the next section).

Animal Models

Serotonin (5-HT) has long been implicated in the pathophysiology of many psychiatric disorders, particularly anxiety and depressive disorders. Mice genetically engineered to lack the 5-HT1A autoreceptor show increased anxiety in a variety of tasks (Klemenhagen, Gordon, David, Hen, & Gross, 2006). If the 5-HT1A receptor is functional during the first 15 days of life, the mice do not develop levels of anxiety higher than wild-type mice, but if the 5-HT1A receptor is disabled in mice at birth, then the mice are more anxious even if the receptor is enabled after day 21 of life (Gross et al., 2002; Santarelli et al., 2003). Similar effects are found if mice have the 5-HT transporter (5-HTT) knocked out in postnatal days 4–21 (Leonardo & Hen, 2008). These models suggest that excessive 5-HT in early life may enhance anxiety; this is paradoxical, considering that specific serotonin reuptake inhibitors (SSRIs) enhance the availability of serotonin acutely, though it is highly likely that chronic effects of SSRIs are more complex and may lead to a diminution of 5-HT influence.

Recent studies in rodents have shown that epigenetic events (i.e., environmental influences on gene expression) may be key in anxious behaviors. Rat pups raised by mothers that do not engage in the normal amount of licking and grooming develop a highly reactive hypothalamic–pituitary–adrenocortical axis (HPA) with high levels of corticotropin-releasing hormone (CRH), adrenocorticotropin, and plasma cortisol in response to stress (Meaney, 2001; Ogren & Lombroso, 2008). The behavior of the maternal rats appears to be mediated through a complex process wherein tactile stimulation causes increased release of thyroid hormone. This, combined with activation of the 5-HT system, leads to activation of genes that control the expression of nerve growth factor. Tactile stimulation also leads to demethylation of the DNA that controls the transcription of glucocorticoid receptors; this allows the nerve growth factor to activate glucocorticoid receptor transcription in the hippocampus. This appears to be the step that down-regulates the HPA axis, and these effects are lifelong (Kaffman & Meaney, 2007).

Human Genetic Studies

As noted, one-third of the variance in childhood anxiety disorders can be attributed to genetics (Jang, 2005). Lesch and colleagues (1996) first identified a common functional polymorphism in the 5-HTT gene (SLC6A4). The 5-HTT-linked polymorphic region (5-HTTLPR) can have two elements: a short (s) allele consisting of a 14-base-pair repeat, and a long (l) allele consisting of a 16-base-pair repeat. The s allele has been associated with half the reuptake of 5-HT *in vitro* than the l allele, but whether this translates into more 5-HT transmission in humans carrying an s allele is unclear (Hariri & Holmes, 2006). Furthermore, the l allele exists in two forms (l_a and l_g), with the l_g allele also showing lower levels of 5-HTT (Parsey et al., 2006). A very large number of studies now show that persons carrying an s allele exhibit higher levels of anxiety, depression, and other forms of negative affect than do persons homozygous for the l allele (Lesch et al., 1996; Schinka, Busch, & Robichaux-Keene, 2004; Sen, Burmeister, & Ghosh, 2004). In children, however, the picture has been more mixed: The s allele was associated in one study with shyness (Battaglia et al., 2005); the opposite finding (l allele related to shyness) was obtained in another (Arbelle et al., 2003); and still other studies showed no relationship of the s allele to shyness, anxiety, or depression in children (Schmidt, Fox, Rubin, Hu, & Hamer, 2002; Young, Smolen, Stallings, Corley, & Hewitt, 2003). Persons carrying the s allele are more prone to depression if exposed to environmental stressors (Caspi et al., 2003; Kendler, Kuhn, Vittum, Prescott, & Riley, 2005), though it is unclear whether this relationship holds for anxiety disorders. As reviewed below, the greatest interest of 5-HTTLPR may be in relationship to neuroimaging findings (Munafo, Brown, & Hariri, 2008).

Several other genes have been studied in childhood anxiety but findings are very preliminary. Infants with at least one copy of both the 7-repeat DRD4 allele *and* the l allele of 5-HTTLPR showed less anxiety than infants with other genotypes did to approach of a novel stimulus. Infants who had the 7-repeat DRD4 allele *and* who were homozygous for the s allele showed more anxiety and resistance to a stranger's initiation of interaction (Lakatos et al., 2003). Interestingly, these two polymorphisms were not related to maternal ratings of infant temperament. Smoller and Tsuang (1998) found an association between an allele of the CRH gene and behavioral inhibition (BI) in young children, with the association being more marked in children of parents with panic disorder. The association of CRH and BI is intriguing, given the animal data reviewed above and the association of BI with the development of anxiety disorders.

Behavioral Inhibition

Kagan and colleagues (Kagan, Reznick, Clarke, & Snidman, 1984; Kagan, Reznick, & Snidman, 1988) initially described the phenomena of BI in children. Children were brought to a playroom where they interacted with an unfamiliar person or objects. About 15% of the sample showed *behavioral inhibition*, defined as a long latency to speak, play, or interact with a stranger, as well as maintenance of increased proximity to the mother. Such a pattern of behavior is highly stable over time (Reznick et al., 1986). High rates of motor activity and crying in infants as young as 4 months predict BI at ages 9 and 14 months (Kagan & Snidman, 1991). *In utero* heart rates may also be a predictor of BI (Snidman, Kagan, & Riordan, 1995). Inhibited children show increased heart rate, pupillary dilation, salivary cortisol, and urinary norepinephrine during stressful tasks, compared to uninhibited children (Kagan, Reznick, & Snidman, 1987; Kagan et al., 1988; Snidman et al., 1995). Inhibited children also show less secure attachments to their mothers as assessed by the Strange Situation, and are rated higher than uninhibited children on the Child Behavior Checklist Internalizing scale (Manassis, Bradley, Goldberg, Hood, & Swinson, 1995).

A number of studies have shown a relationship between BI and both adult and child anxiety disorders (Biederman et al., 1990; Hirshfeld et al., 1992; Rosenbaum et al., 1988, 1992). Children of parents with panic disorder and agoraphobia had significantly higher rates of BI than children of controls or children of parents with MDD (Rosenbaum et al., 1988). Conversely, children who were identified as having BI had an increased risk of anxiety disorders (Biederman et al., 1990), as did their parents (Rosenbaum et al., 1992). At a 3-year follow-up, children who showed the most consistent BI had the greatest likelihood of having an anxiety disorder; these children were also more likely to show multiple anxiety disorders (Biederman et al., 1990; Hirshfeld et al., 1992). Hirshfeld-Becker and colleagues (2008) found that 22% of preschoolers with BI showed an anxiety disorder by age 10, compared to only 8% of children without BI, even after the investigators controlled for parental diagnosis. It should be emphasized that not all children with BI go on to develop anxiety disorders; the above-cited studies found that about 40–60% of the inhibited children were free of anxiety disorders, depending on the time of follow-up.

EEG Frontal Asymmetry

Frontal lobe "power" can be assessed by quantifying the relative amounts of alpha, beta, and other wavelengths obtained from various frontal electroencephalographic (EEG) leads. Greater alpha power is associated with reduced activation and lower cerebral blood flow (Cook, O'Hara, Uijtdehaage, Mandelkern, & Leuchter, 1998; Goldman, Stern, Engel, & Cohen, 2000). Davidson (1992) first used this finding to explore the neurobiological basis of negative affect, using EEG measures of frontal lobe activation. In adults, left anterior cerebral hemisphere activation was associated with positive affect, whereas right anterior hemisphere activation was more associated with negative affect. Davidson hypothesized that the left frontal areas of the cerebrum are part of an "approach" system, whereas the right frontal areas mediate "withdrawal." Adults who consistently show left-sided activation in the resting state report more positive emotional responses to a pleasant film. In contrast, adults with greater right-sided activation report more intense negative feelings to a film with fearful or disgusting stimuli (Wheeler, Davidson, & Tomarken, 1993). Left-sided activation is more likely to be shown when individuals perform working memory tasks under reward conditions (Pizzagalli, Sherwood, Henriques, & Davidson, 2005). Infants show greater right-sided activation when a bad-tasting substance is placed on their tongues, whereas a good-tasting substance elicits left-sided EEG activation (Fox & Davidson, 1986). At age 10 months, infants watching a film of an actress crying or laughing showed right or left activation of the anterior EEG, respectively (Davidson & Fox, 1982). Left frontal activation is found when 10-month-olds observe the approach of their mothers, while right activation is noted when a stranger approaches (Fox & Davidson, 1988). Using the criteria of Kagan and colleagues (1984), Davidson (1992) classified 31-month-olds into three groups of 28 subjects: inhibited, uninhibited, and a middle group. When the children were 38 months of age, EEG recordings were obtained both at rest and during several tasks. The inhibited children showed significantly more right-sided activation in the midfrontal electrodes than did the middle or uninhibited children. Uninhibited children, in contrast, showed greater left-sided activation than either of these groups.

More recent studies have suggested that the left–right hemispheric distinction is related to the approach–withdrawal distinction rather than to a positive–negative affect discrimination. Left-sided activation has been shown to be related to anger as well as positive affect (Harmon-Jones, Lueck, Fearn, & Harmon-Jones, 2006), and deactivation of the left anterior cortex by transcortical magnetic stimulation interferes with the processing of anger (van Honk & Schutter, 2006). In this variation of Davidson's model, both anger and happiness are viewed as "approach" emotions, as anger might lead an organism to be aggressive against a potential foe. Family history complicates the interpretation of this straightforward analysis, however. Forbes and colleagues (2006) assessed frontal asymmetry in 74 children, 44 of whom had mothers with childhood-onset depression. Whereas right frontal asymmetry was associated with depression/anxiety in children of nondepressed mothers, anxiety/depression was associated with left frontal asymmetry in the children of mothers with a history of depression. Gender effects were found as well, with only boys showing a relationship of left frontal asymmetry with aggression. Gender effects were also found for frontal EEG asymmetry in an adult twin study; furthermore, EEG asymmetry was only heritable in young adults (Smit, Posthuma, Boomsma, & De Geus, 2007). This suggests that as people age, environment and experience may shape this "biological" trait.

Anxiety Sensitivity

Anxiety sensitivity is the tendency to experience any state of high arousal as harmful, unpleasant, and portending harmful physical or psychological consequences (McNally, 2002). High rates of anxiety sensitivity (assessed by questionnaire) in high school students predicts the onset of panic disorder, even after comorbid depression is controlled for (Hayward, Killen, Kraemer, & Taylor, 2000). Adolescents who rate themselves as chronically anxious are more likely to have acute anxiety attack in response to hyperventilation (Leen-Feldner, Reardon, & Zvolensky, 2007). Anxious children are more sensitive to bodily cues that anticipate negative emotions (Thompson, 2001). Thus persons at risk for anxiety disorders may experience a normal increase in physiological arousal after a stressor as intolerable, leading to avoidance of situations that are not ordinarily threatening. Consistent with this, offspring of parents with anxiety disorders show increased heart rates under stress (Battaglia et al., 1997), elevated salivary cortisol (Warren et al., 2003), and an increased startle reflex (Grillon, Dierker, & Merikangas, 1997).

RISK FACTORS FOR PHENOTYPIC EXPRESSION

Given the relatively low amount of the variance in anxiety disorders that is attributable to genetics, a substantial amount of the remaining variance must be attributed to environmental factors. For the most part, prospective studies show a relationship between health problems, divorce, abuse, and parental loss in early childhood on the one hand, and later anxiety disorders on the other (Kroes et al., 2002). As these variables may be associated with a variety of psychiatric disorders, a wide body of research has focused on specific aspects of the parent–child relationship that might be related to the development of anxiety.

Emotional Dysregulation/ Information Processing

If an emotion is experienced as overwhelming or noxious, an individual must find a way to regulate it, and there is evidence that anxious children have major difficulties in this regard (Hannesdottir & Ollendick, 2007). Anxious children have less ability than controls to hide their emotions in order to obtain an interpersonal goal (Southam-Gerow & Kendall, 2000). Like adults with anxiety, anxious children tend to give higher priority to the processing of threatening information than nonanxious subjects do (Vasey & MacLeod, 2001). Hadwin, Garner, and Perez-Olivas (2006) extensively reviewed the data on information processing in anxious children. There is good evidence to suggest that anxious children show clear attentional biases to threatening stimuli and are more likely to interpret ambiguous situations as threatening. Although adults show memory biases for negative past events, this finding is not as well replicated in children. Pine and colleagues (2009) reviewed three developmental models of information processing in anxiety disorders of childhood: (1) Such biases may emerge very early in development as a possible neurobiological factor; (2) information-processing biases are a late feature, and perhaps an actual consequence, of the anxiety disorder; and (3) these biases emerge from interactions between a child and a caretaker. With regard to the third model, it is clear that biases to threatening stimuli can be induced by training in individuals who do not have anxiety disorders.

Parenting Behaviors

McLeod, Wood, and Weisz (2007), examining how the characteristics of parental behavior are related to childhood anxiety behaviors, reviewed 47 studies involving 12,879 subjects. Overall, parenting behaviors accounted for 4% of the variance in anxiety symptoms, but the effect size was larger for diagnosed anxiety disorders (0.35). More specifically, parental rejection and parental control accounted for 4% and 6% of the variation in anxiety, respectively. Parental autonomy granting has the largest relationship with anxiety, accounting for 18% of the variance. Fisak and Grills-Taquechel (2007) reviewed studies related specifically to the role of parental modeling in the development of childhood anxiety. *Social referencing* is the process by which young children use their parents' reaction to stimuli to form their own emotional reaction to the same event. In one study, mothers of toddlers were coached to make either anxious or nonanxious responses to the appearance of a toy spider or snake (Gerull & Rapee, 2002). Toddlers who were shown their mothers reacting fearfully to a toy were more likely to avoid the toy. The effect was particularly pronounced in girls. A similar effect was found when mothers were coached to respond anxiously to a stranger in the laboratory (de Rosnay, Cooper, Tsigaras, & Murray, 2006). Thus parents with anxiety disorders may model anxious responses to events, which toddlers and young children use to determine their own emotional responses. Retrospective studies show that anxious adults report that their parents reinforced their anxious behaviors (e.g., allowing them to stay home from school) (Ehlers, 1993). Parents of anxious children have been shown to deliver a larger number of messages conveying dangerousness of the environment than parents of typically developing children do (Beidel & Turner, 1997). In summary, there is evidence to support the hypothesis that parents may transmit anxiety to children by not granting age-appropriate autonomy, modeling (social referencing), reinforcing anxious behaviors, and transferring information that the world is dangerous. Further prospective studies are needed to determine to what degree child temperament influences parenting style.

NEUROIMAGING

Some of the most exciting work in understanding the pathophysiology of anxiety in the last decade has come from the integration of genetic and neuroimaging studies, particularly functional magnetic resonance imaging (fMRI) (Munafo et al., 2008; Pine et al., 2009). Most of this work has focused on the neural processing of angry versus neutral (or happy) faces, so a brief summary of what is known about recognition of facial emotion is in order (see Vuilleumier & Pourtois, 2007, for a review). Recognition of facial features and emotion strongly involves the facial fusiform area (FFA) in the ventral temporal cortex. Visual stimuli reach this area by traveling from the retina to the lateral geniculate nucleus and then on to the primary visual areas in the occipital cortex; from there it is processed in various secondary visual areas, including the FFA. The FFA responds more strongly to faces than to other objects. This pathway is relatively "slow." There is also a direct pathway to the amygdala that bypasses the lateral geniculate; furthermore, the amygdala will respond to fairly coarse features of facial expression. The amygdala responds more strongly to angry/threatening faces than to neutral/happy faces. From an evolutionary perspective, this may allow social mammals to respond rapidly to a threat from a peer—ultimately by either withdrawing or approaching.

A now well-replicated finding is that anxious individuals have an attention bias to angry faces; that is, they take longer than controls to disengage from focusing on an angry face in order to respond to a probe (Bar-Haim, Lamy, Pergamin, Bakermans-Kranenburg, & van IJzendoorn, 2007). This task is easily adapted to an fMRI paradigm. The blood-oxygen-level-dependent signal (a measure of the flow of oxygenated blood to an active brain region) is assessed in various brain regions during the presentation of an angry face relative to a neutral face. The magnitude of this contrast can then be compared between anxious and nonanxious subjects, or it can be correlated with subjects' response on an anxiety rating scale. Monk and colleagues (2008) found that anxious adolescents showed greater activation of the amygdala than controls when the faces were presented for only 17 milliseconds; such activation was correlated with the reaction time to disengage from the faces and respond to the probe. In a second study (Monk et al., 2006), the subjects were exposed to the faces for 500 milliseconds. At the longer exposure, the controls and anxious subjects had equal activation of the amygdala; however, now the anxious subjects had greater activity in the ventrolateral prefrontal cortex (PFC).

Reaction time on the task was now correlated negatively with the degree of this activity. Pine and colleagues (2009) suggested that when a threat is briefly presented, anxious adolescents have abnormally increased acute activity of the amygdala (which may be related to arousal or physical discomfort). Once the amygdala is activated, ventrolateral PFC processing comes online to cope with the anxiety, and this secondary process is disturbed in anxious individuals.

Social interactions in humans go well beyond reading facial expression. Guyer and colleagues (2008) asked anxious adolescents and controls to look at pictures of teenagers and rate how much they would like to interact with them in an online chat session. They were told that the people in the picture would be rating them. They then viewed the pictures during the fMRI scan; anxious adolescents had greater amygdala activation than controls when viewing peers they had negatively evaluated (even though the peers were pictured smiling). A measure of ventrolateral PFC–amygdala connectivity correlated positively with baseline anxiety ratings; anxious subjects showed greater connectivity than controls. This again suggests that anxious subjects tend to have their attention captured by negatively perceived social stimuli; perhaps the aberrant frontal–amygdala connections lead to perseveration on the anxiety-provoking stimulus.

Genetic studies are increasingly being combined with neuroimaging to yield greater understanding of these brain–behavior relationships. Increased activation of the amygdala in response to fearful faces is related not only to diagnostic status, but to an individual's underlying genotype. A meta-analysis of 14 fMRI studies comparing carriers of the s allele of the 5-HTTLPR genotype to homozygous l carriers showed the s carriers to have greater activation of the amygdala to angry faces ($p < .001$), though genotype explained only 10% of the variance on the task. In adolescents, the relationship between 5-HTTLPR genotype and diagnosis has proved complex. No difference was found in 5-HTTLPR genotype distribution between adolescents with GAD or MDD and controls (Lau et al., 2009). In healthy controls, s or l_g carriers had greater amygdala activation to fearful faces than l_a

carriers had. In contrast, patients homozygous for the l_a genotype had greater activation of the amygdala than patients who were s/l_g carriers had.

As exciting as neuroimaging and genetics are, the Lau and colleagues study shows the need for caution in interpreting results. The 5-HTTLPR s/l findings may at best relate to an underlying endophenotype of emotional reactivity, rather than to anxiety/mood disorders per se (Hariri & Holmes, 2006). This endophenotype may be influenced by many other genes (most unknown at this point) and by environmental interactions. As we shall see below, neuroimaging findings can be altered by both psychosocial and psychopharmacological treatments; thus they should not be viewed as "hard-wired" into the brain.

ASSESSMENT

Despite advances in genetics and neuroimaging, diagnosis of anxiety disorders in children is based on clinical interview. The clinician should obtain data from the primary caregiver(s); from the child; and (when appropriate and possible) from other adults who interact with the child, such as teachers or day care workers. The clinician should screen for anxiety disorders regardless of the chief complaint that has brought the child to the evaluation. In the research arena, both the K-SADS (Kaufman et al., 1997) and the Diagnostic Interview Schedule for Children, Version IV (Shaffer, Fisher, Lucas, Dulcan, & Schwab-Stone, 2000) contain extensive sections covering all the DSM-IV/DSM-IV-TR anxiety disorders. In a regular clinical setting, the practitioner should ask questions covering each of these disorders. It is most convenient to begin with GAD, asking whether the child worries excessively about either past behavior or upcoming events; the clinician must be certain that the parent does not mistakenly perceive fear of punishment for misbehavior or oppositionality about future tasks as anxiety (see the caveat regarding negative affect, below). Does the child have unrealistic fears about events in the world (e.g., a tornado hitting the house, wars starting, earthquakes)? Does he or she feel stressed about an event for which the child is clearly capable and prepared? GAD also requires some physiological symptoms (e.g., insomnia, restlessness, muscle tension). From these questions, it is a logical segue into questions about social anxiety (e.g., the child's fears that people don't like him or her, avoiding parties due to fears of interacting with others). Social anxiety should be distinguished from avoidant personality disorder, as in the latter the child does not *desire* to interact with others. If a child has separation difficulties (e.g., school refusal, not sleeping alone, unable to stay with sitter or relatives), the clinician should ask about the full range of SAD symptoms, followed by questions about panic attacks. Finally, specific phobia and OCD can be covered. Parents sometimes report excessive interest in video games or other pleasurable activities as "obsessive"; therefore, the clinician should be certain to determine whether the obsessions or compulsions are repetitive, ritualistic, irrational, and generally unwanted by the child.

The clinical interview can be supplemented by a wide range of parent and child rating scales for anxiety, shown in Table 10.3. Careful attention to a child's reading level and attention span is required for the use of self-report scales; young children should not be asked to fill out ratings unsupervised. Rating scales should be used as screening tools or as part of a mental health assessment. Lack of concordance between parent and child reports of anxiety (whether symptoms are elicited by rating scale or by clinical interview) is a common problem (Bird, Gould, & Staghezza, 1992). Parents may be unaware of the child's symptoms. In contrast, if a parent reports that the child is anxious while the child denies all symptoms, careful review is needed. If a child's nonverbal behavior is highly suggestive of anxiety) (fearful facial expression, apparent muscle tension, low voice volume), or if other adults beside the parent report objective signs of anxiety (e.g., teacher reports child is afraid to go out at recess), the parent's report is validated in spite of the child's denial of anxiety.

As ADHD and depression are frequently comorbid with anxiety disorders, questioning about these diagnoses is necessary. Clini-

TABLE 10.3. Selected Rating Scales Used in the Assessment of Child and Adolescent Anxiety Disorders

Instrument	Description
Revised Children's Manifest Anxiety Scale: Second Edition (RCMAS-2)	Recently updated anxiety scale measuring the level and nature of anxiety as experienced by children, using a yes–no response format. Age-stratified norms based on a national sample of more than 2,300 children and teens. Scale has 49 items covering Physiological Anxiety, Worry, Social Anxiety, Defensiveness, and Inconsistent Responding (Reynolds & Richmond, 2008).
Screen for Child Anxiety Related Emotional Disorders (SCARED)	A 38-item scale with parent and child forms. Subject responds to each item with 0 (not true), 1 (sometimes true), or 2 (often true). Yields five factors: Somatic/Panic, General Anxiety, Separation Anxiety, Social Phobia, and School Phobia. Discriminates depressed/anxious children from those with disruptive behavior disorders; no norms as yet (Birmaher et al., 1997).
Multidimensional Anxiety Scale for Children (MASC)	A 39-item scale with four factors: Physical Symptoms, Social Anxiety, Separation Anxiety, and Harm Avoidance. Fourth-grade reading level (March, Parker, Sullivan, Stallings, & Conners, 1997).
Pediatric Anxiety Rating Scale (PARS)	A clinician-rated, 50-item symptom checklist with items grouped into the following categories: Social Interactions or Performance Situations (9 items), Separation (10 items), Generalized (8 items), Specific Phobia (4 items), Physical Signs and Symptoms (13 items), and Other (6 items). Each symptom is scored by the interviewing clinician as present or absent (yes–no) during the previous week (Research Unit on Pediatric Psychopharmacology Anxiety Study Group, 2002).

cians should not attribute hyperactivity and impulsivity to psychodynamically driven anxiety. Children with ADHD, ODD, depression, or anxiety can more broadly show excessive "negative affect" (March et al., 2000). This consists of whining, crying, stubbornness, or temper tantrums in response to stressors. It should be distinguished from anxiety per se; its presence alone should not lead to a diagnosis of anxiety disorder if the child does not also meet the criteria for one of the DSM-IV-TR anxiety disorders discussed above.

TREATMENT

Over the last two decades, both psychopharmacological and psychosocial interventions (particularly cognitive-behavioral therapy [CBT]) have been the focus of large-scale, well-designed randomized controlled trials (RCTs) in children and adolescents. These studies have extensively documented their efficacy relative to placebo or waiting-list controls, giving the modern clinician a potent armamentarium to treat these disorders.

Selective Serotonin Reuptake Inhibitors

The SSRIs fluoxetine, sertraline, fluvoxamine, and paroxetine have all been the foci of large-scale RCTs in the treatment of child and adolescent OCD (Reinblatt & Riddle, 2007). March and colleagues (1998) randomly assigned 187 children or adolescents to placebo or sertraline (mean daily dose 167 mg) and found that 53% responded to sertraline versus 37% to placebo. Fluoxetine was superior to placebo (49% vs. 25% at a mean dose of 25 mg/day) in adolescents with OCD (Geller et al., 2001). In another study, Liebowitz and colleagues (2002) found that 57% of subjects with OCD responded to fluoxetine versus 32% to placebo. Fluvoxamine (mean dose 165 mg/day) was superior to placebo (42% vs. 26%) in a 10-week RCT (Riddle et al., 2001). Paroxetine was the subject of two large RCTs (Geller et al., 2003a, 2004); both showed the superiority of the active drug to placebo. The Pediatric OCD Treatment Study (POTS) Team (2004) randomly assigned 112 subjects to CBT alone, sertraline alone, combination treatment, or placebo

for 12 weeks. The sertraline dose range was 25–200 mg, with a mean daily dose of 170 mg. The Children's Yale–Brown Obsessive–Compulsive Scale was the primary outcome measure. Results indicated a statistically significant advantage for CBT alone ($p = .003$), sertraline alone ($p = .007$), and combined treatment ($p = .001$) compared with placebo. Combined treatment also proved superior to CBT alone ($p = .008$) and to sertraline alone ($p = .006$), which did not differ from each other. The response rates for the four groups were 53.5% for the combined group, 39.3% for the CBT group, 21.4% for the sertraline group, and 3.6% for the placebo group. It is not clear why the sertraline group response rate was so much lower in the POTS study than the 53% response rate in the earlier study (March et al., 1998). It should be also noted that the placebo group response rate was substantially lower in this study than in all the others. There were site differences in terms of the CBT response rate; that is, CBT was more efficacious in some localities than in others, suggesting differences in culture or therapist characteristics that affected the outcome. A meta-analysis of 12 studies of SSRIs in OCD showed a highly significant difference between drug and placebo (Geller et al., 2003b), with no difference among the various SSRIs.

SSRIs have also been studied in non-OCD anxiety disorders, though controlled studies are less numerous than for OCD. In a large-sample study, children and adolescents with GAD were randomly assigned to either fluvoxamine or placebo for 8 weeks; the active drug was found to be markedly superior to placebo (76% vs. 29%) (Walkup et al., 2001). Birmaher and colleagues (2003) found 20 mg/day of fluoxetine superior to placebo in 74 children with a variety of non-OCD diagnoses (61% vs. 35%). Ninety percent of children and adolescents with GAD randomly assigned to sertraline responded, compared with a mere 10% in the placebo group (Rynn, Siqueland, & Rickels, 2001). Wagner and colleagues (2004) found paroxetine superior to placebo in subjects ages 8–17 years who had social phobia. Most recently, a major study randomly assigned 488 children with a variety of anxiety disorders to treatment with sertraline, CBT, combined treatment, or placebo (Walkup et al., 2008). The proportions of responders were 80.7%

for combination therapy, 59.7% for CBT, and 54.9% for sertraline, with all therapies being superior to placebo (23.7%). Combination therapy was superior to both monotherapies.

The *number needed to treat* (NNT) is the number of patients who need to be treated in order to prevent one additional bad outcome (95% chance that at least one patient has responded above the placebo rate). In the above-reviewed studies, the NNT was 2–6, indicating significant efficacy. All these studies reported side effects of agitation, insomnia, gastrointestinal upset, and suicidal ideation. In a meta-analysis examining the effects of antidepressants in both anxious and depressed children and adolescents, Bridge and colleagues (2007) found that the SSRIs had better-established efficacy in non-OCD anxiety disorders, with intermediate efficacy for OCD, whereas the efficacy for MDD was more limited. In terms of suicidal ideation, the *number needed to harm* (NNH, the opposite of NNT) was 143, clearly showing that the cost–benefit ratio is in favor of treating anxiety disorders with SSRIs. Nonetheless, in line with the Food and Drug Administration's boxed warning in the package inserts of all antidepressants, parents and patients should be warned about

the possibility of increased thoughts of self-harm before the patients are started on any antidepressant (see "Individualizing Treatment," below).

Cognitive-Behavioral Treatment

Kendall (1993) theorized that childhood anxiety is based on cognitive distortions: "Anxious children seem preoccupied with concerns about evaluations by self and others and the likelihood of severe negative consequences. They seem to misperceive characteristically the demands of the environment and routinely add stress to a variety of situations" (p. 239). CBT promotes changing negative cognitions in conjunction with using behavior therapy techniques known to decrease anxiety. Kendall's CBT approach, which requires 16–20 sessions, is summarized in Table 10.4. CBT has become the best-validated psychosocial intervention for the treatment of child and adolescent anxiety; it has been the focus of several meta-analyses and reviews in the last decade (Cartwright-Hatton, Roberts, Chitsabesan, Fothergill, & Harrington, 2004; James, Soler, & Weatherall, 2005; Munoz-Solomando, Kendall, & Whittington, 2008). In non-OCD, non-phobic anxiety, the pooled response rate

TABLE 10.4. Cognitive-Behavioral Therapy (CBT) According to Kendall's Model

Session 1	Build rapport; collect information on situations that promote anxiety and on how the child responds to the anxiety.
Session 2	Teach child to identify different types of feelings.
Session 3	Rank-order anxiety-provoking situations. Help child distinguish anxiety response from other types of emotions.
Session 4	Relaxation training; give child personalized audiocassette for use outside of sessions.
Session 5	Teach child to modify self-talk (replace negative with positive) and use self-talk to reduce anxiety.
Session 6	Emphasize coping self-talk and verbal self-redirection.
Session 7	Teach child to self-evaluate and self-reward positive, nonanxious coping responses.
Session 8	Review all of the skills above.
Session 9	Have child practice skills and watch therapist model handling anxiety; use role playing to rehearse handling anxiety-provoking situations.
Sessions 10–15	Expose child to real and imagined anxiety-provoking situations. Continue practice.
Session 16	Termination issues; discuss therapy experience; encourage the child to consider how to use new coping skills in everyday life.

to CBT was 56.5% compared to 34.8% in no-treatment controls (Cartwright-Hatton et al., 2004). Similar results (56% for CBT, 28.2% for controls) were found in a subsequent meta-analysis (James et al., 2005). Four controlled studies ($N = 222$ subjects) using CBT for treatment of OCD were included in a meta-analysis, but the POTS results reviewed earlier were viewed as the best estimate for the effect size of this modality (O'Kearney, Anstey, & von Sanden, 2006). The response rates of anxiety disorders of childhood and adolescents are comparable to those for SSRIs, and the studies reviewed above also favor the superiority of combined medication and CBT over either modality alone.

When CBT was compared to education support for youth with school refusal (separation anxiety), both treatments were equally efficacious (Last, Hansen, & Franco, 1998). Silverman and colleagues (1999) randomly assigned 81 children with phobia to an exposure-based contingency management treatment condition, an exposure-based cognitive self-control treatment condition, or an education support control condition. Whereas both exposure-based treatments were superior to education support at the end of the 10-week intervention, all the groups were equally improved at the 3-, 6-, and 12-month follow ups. This raises the issue as to whether CBT is in fact superior to other psychosocial interventions or nonspecific social support. Recently, Hudson and colleagues (2009) randomly assigned 112 children with anxiety disorders (ages 7–16 years) to either group CBT or an attention control group for 10 sessions. Parents attended the groups as well. CBT was superior to the control group in reducing anxiety at follow-up; 6 months after treatment, the children receiving CBT had a remission rate of 69% (vs. 45% of those who received the attention control), suggesting that CBT yields specific benefits over supportive therapy. CBT has also been provided in school-based and family contexts (Bernstein, Bernat, Victor, & Layne, 2008; Creswell & Cartwright-Hatton, 2007).

Individualizing Treatment

The studies reviewed above suggest that combining CBT with medication yields a success rate better than either modality alone, whereas CBT and medication alone appear to have equal efficacy (Walkup et al., 2008). Thus clinicians have a great deal of flexibility in determining a treatment plan, and family preferences can be taken into account. It is perfectly reasonable for a clinician to choose CBT alone if the family does not wish to have their child on medication. Conversely, some families and children find CBT difficult or do not have the resources to pursue it regularly, and medication alone is a good treatment option in such situations. Also, when a child has spontaneous panic attacks or separation anxiety with physiological arousal, medication treatment is sometimes necessary as a first step just to stabilize the child so that the therapist can work with him or her. If a child has not responded to 6–10 weeks of monotherapy with either CBT or an SSRI, then combined therapy should be strongly considered.

Neuroimaging Effects of Treatment

One of the more exciting recent developments has been work showing how the brain changes both anatomically and physiologically in response to either pharmacotherapy or CBT. CBT and paroxetine appear to have different effects on brain functioning in children and adolescents with OCD. Twelve weeks of paroxetine reduced glutamate/glutamine caudate concentrations as well as thalamic volume to levels seen in controls (Gilbert et al., 2000; Rosenberg, McMaster, et al., 2000)—effects not seen in a separate sample of children treated with OCD with cognitive therapy alone, despite an equally good response of symptoms (Benazon, Moore, & Rosenberg, 2003; Rosenberg, Benazon, Gilbert, Sullivan, & Moore, 2000). Thus the brain changes were associated with response in one form of treatment but not in another, suggesting different biological routes to recovery. Paroxetine has been shown to alter amygdala volume symmetry (Szeszko et al., 2004). In another study, patients with OCD had less gray matter bilaterally in the PFC at baseline than controls did, but after 6 months of paroxetine treatment, there was a trend for gray matter volume to be increased in the patient group (Lazaro et al., 2006). In the future, such studies may lead to a better understanding of why some patients do not respond to treatment.

CONCLUSION

Our understanding of the nature and treatment of anxiety disorders in children and adolescents has increased greatly in the last decade. Genetic factors account for about one-third of the variance in anxiety symptoms, but multiple genes are likely to be involved. Furthermore, these genes most likely exert their effects through endophenotypes, such as emotional dysregulation, attention bias to threatening stimuli, or BI. Thus environmental factors can exert their effects in the development of the endophenotype itself, and then again in combining with the endophenotype to bring about the full disorder. Most encouraging has been the development of evidence-based treatments such as CBT and SSRIs. Intriguingly, in children and adolescents, the evidence for the efficacy of SSRIs is stronger in anxiety disorders than in depressive disorders. Nonetheless, caution is warranted in treating anxious children and adolescents with these agents; it is necessary to discuss the risk of suicidal ideation with patients and their families. Future advances in genetics and neuroimaging may lead to even more effective pharmacological and psychosocial interventions.

REFERENCES

American Psychiatric Association. (2000). *Diagnostic and statistical manual of mental disorders* (4th ed., text rev.). Washington, DC: Author.

Anderson, J. C., Williams, S., McGee, R., & Silva, P. A. (1987). DSM-III disorders in preadolescent children: Prevalence in a large community sample. *Archives of General Psychiatry, 44*, 69–76.

Angold, A., & Costello, E. J. (1993). Depressive comorbidity in children and adolescents: Empirical, theoretical, and methodological issues. *American Journal of Psychiatry, 150*, 1779–1791.

Angold, A., Costello, E. J., & Erkanli, A. (1999). Comorbidity. *Journal of Child Psychology and Psychiatry, 40*, 57–87.

Arbelle, S., Benjamin, J., Golin, M., Kremer, I., Belmaker, R. H., & Ebstein, R. P. (2003). Relation of shyness in grade school children to the genotype for the long form of the serotonin transporter promoter region polymorphism. *American Journal of Psychiatry, 160*, 671–676.

Bar-Haim, Y., Lamy, D., Pergamin, L., Bakermans-Kranenburg, M. J., & van IJzendoorn, M. H. (2007). Threat-related attentional bias in anxious and nonanxious individuals: A meta-analytic study. *Psychological Bulletin, 133*, 1–24.

Battaglia, M., Bajo, S., Strambi, L. F., Brambilla, F., Castronovo, C., Vanni, G., et al. (1997). Physiological and behavioral responses to minor stressors in offspring of patients with panic disorder. *Journal of Psychiatric Research, 31*, 365–376.

Battaglia, M., Ogliari, A., Zanoni, A., Citterio, A., Pozzoli, U., Giorda, R., et al. (2005). Influence of the serotonin transporter promoter gene and shyness on children's cerebral responses to facial expressions. *Archives of General Psychiatry, 62*, 85–94.

Beidel, D. C., & Turner, S. M. (1997). At risk for anxiety: I. Psychopathology in the offspring of anxious parents. *Journal of the American Academy of Child and Adolescent Psychiatry, 36*, 918–924.

Benazon, N. R., Moore, G. J., & Rosenberg, D. R. (2003). Neurochemical analyses in pediatric obsessive–compulsive disorder in patients treated with cognitive-behavioral therapy. *Journal of the American Academy of Child and Adolescent Psychiatry, 42*, 1279–1285.

Benjamin, R. S., Costello, E. J., & Warren, M. (1990). Anxiety disorders in a pediatric sample. *Journal of Anxiety Disorders, 4*, 293–316.

Bernstein, G. A., Bernat, D. H., Victor, A. M., & Layne, A. E. (2008). School-based interventions for anxious children: 3-, 6-, and 12-month follow-ups. *Journal of the American Academy of Child and Adolescent Psychiatry, 47*, 1039–1047.

Biederman, J., Rosenbaum, J. F., Hirshfeld, D. R., Faraone, S. V., Bolduc, E. A., Gersten, M., et al. (1990). Psychiatric correlates of behavioral inhibition in young children of parents with and without psychiatric disorders. *Archives of General Psychiatry, 47*, 21–26.

Bird, H. R., Canino, G., & Rubio-Stipec, M. (1988). Estimates of prevalence of childhood maladjustment in a community survey in Puerto Rico. *Archives of General Psychiatry, 45*, 1120–1126.

Bird, H. R., Gould, M. S., & Staghezza, B. (1992). Aggregating data from multiple informants in child psychiatry epidemiological research. *Journal of the American Academy of Child and Adolescent Psychiatry, 31*, 78–85.

Birmaher, B., Axelson, D. A., Monk, K., Kalas, C., Clark, D. B., Ehmann, M., et al. (2003). Fluoxetine for the treatment of childhood anxiety disorders. *Journal of the American Academy of Child and Adolescent Psychiatry, 42*, 415–423.

Birmaher, B., Khetarpal, S., Brent, D., Cully, M., Balach, L., Kaufman, J., et al. (1997). The Screen for Child Anxiety Related Emotional Disorders (SCARED): Scale construction and psychometric characteristics. *Journal of the American Academy of Child and Adolescent Psychiatry, 36*, 545–553.

Bridge, J. A., Iyengar, S., Salary, C. B., Barbe, R. P., Birmaher, B., Pincus, H. A., et al. (2007). Clinical response and risk for reported suicidal ideation and suicide attempts in pediatric antidepressant treatment: A meta-analysis of randomized controlled trials. *Journal of the American Medical Association, 297,* 1683–1696.

Cartwright-Hatton, S., Roberts, C., Chitsabesan, P., Fothergill, C., & Harrington, R. (2004). Systematic review of the efficacy of cognitive behaviour therapies for childhood and adolescent anxiety disorders. *British Journal of Clinical Psychology, 43,* 421–436.

Caspi, A., Sugden, K., Moffitt, T. E., Taylor, A., Craig, I. W., Harrington, H., et al. (2003). Influence of life stress on depression: moderation by a polymorphism in the 5-HTT gene. *Science, 301,* 386–389.

Chavira, D. A., Garland, A. F., Daley, S., & Hough, R. (2008). The impact of medical comorbidity on mental health and functional health outcomes among children with anxiety disorders. *Journal of Developmental and Behavioral Pediatrics, 29,* 394–402.

Cook, I. A., O'Hara, R., Uijtdehaage, S. H., Mandelkern, M., & Leuchter, A. F. (1998). Assessing the accuracy of topographic EEG mapping for determining local brain function. *Electroencephalography and Clinical Neurophysiology, 107,* 408–414.

Costello, E. J. (1989). Child psychiatric disorders and their correlates: A primary care pediatric sample. *Journal of the American Academy of Child and Adolescent Psychiatry, 28,* 851–855.

Creswell, C., & Cartwright-Hatton, S. (2007). Family treatment of child anxiety: Outcomes, limitations and future directions. *Clinical Child and Family Psychology Review, 10,* 232–252.

Davidson, R. J. (1992). Anterior asymmetry and the nature of emotion. *Brain and Cognition, 20,* 125–151.

Davidson, R. J., & Fox, N. A. (1982). Asymmetrical brain activity discriminates between positive versus negative affective stimuli in human infants. *Science, 218,* 1235–1237.

de Rosnay, M., Cooper, P. J., Tsigaras, N., & Murray, L. (2006). Transmission of social anxiety from mother to infant: An experimental study using a social referencing paradigm. *Behaviour Research and Therapy, 44,* 1165–1175.

Ehlers, A. (1993). Somatic symptoms and panic attacks: A retrospective study of learning experiences. *Behaviour Research and Therapy, 31,* 269–278.

Fisak, B., Jr., & Grills-Taquechel, A. E. (2007). Parental modeling, reinforcement, and information transfer: Risk factors in the development of child anxiety? *Clinical Child and Family Psychology Review, 10,* 213–231.

Forbes, E. E., Shaw, D. S., Fox, N. A., Cohn, J. F., Silk, J. S., & Kovacs, M. (2006). Maternal depression, child frontal asymmetry, and child affective behavior as factors in child behavior problems. *Journal of Child Psychology and Psychiatry, 47,* 79–87.

Fox, N. A., & Davidson, R. J. (1986). Taste-elicited changes in facial signs of emotion and the asymmetry of brain electrical activity in human newborns. *Neuropsychologia, 24,* 417–422.

Fox, N. A., & Davidson, R. J. (1988). Patterns of brain electrical activity during facial signs of emotion in ten month old infants. *Developmental Psychology, 24,* 230–236.

Geller, D. A., Biederman, J., Stewart, S. E., Mullin, B., Farrell, C., Wagner, K. D., et al. (2003a). Impact of comorbidity on treatment response to paroxetine in pediatric obsessive–compulsive disorder: Is the use of exclusion criteria empirically supported in randomized clinical trials? *Journal of Child and Adolescent Psychopharmacology, 13*(Suppl. 1), S19–S29.

Geller, D. A., Biederman, J., Stewart, S. E., Mullin, B., Martin, A., Spencer, T., et al. (2003b). Which SSRI?: A meta-analysis of pharmacotherapy trials in pediatric obsessive–compulsive disorder. *American Journal of Psychiatry, 160,* 1919–1928.

Geller, D. A., Hoog, S. L., Heiligenstein, J. H., Ricardi, R. K., Tamura, R., Kluszynski, S., et al. (2001). Fluoxetine treatment for obsessive-compulsive disorder in children and adolescents: A placebo-controlled clinical trial. *Journal of the American Academy of Child and Adolescent Psychiatry, 40,* 773–779.

Geller, D. A., Wagner, K. D., Emslie, G., Murphy, T., Carpenter, D. J., Wetherhold, E., et al. (2004). Paroxetine treatment in children and adolescents with obsessive–compulsive disorder: A randomized, multicenter, double-blind, placebo-controlled trial. *Journal of the American Academy of Child and Adolescent Psychiatry, 43,* 1387–1396.

Gerull, F. C., & Rapee, R. M. (2002). Mother knows best: Effects of maternal modelling on the acquisition of fear and avoidance behaviour in toddlers. *Behaviour Research and Therapy, 40,* 279–287.

Gilbert, A. R., Moore, G. J., Keshavan, M. S., Paulson, L. A., Narula, V., MacMaster, F. P., et al. (2000). Decrease in thalamic volumes of pediatric patients with obsessive–compulsive disorder who are taking paroxetine. *Archives of General Psychiatry, 57,* 449–456.

Goldman, R. I., Stern, J. M., Engel, J., Jr., & Cohen, M. S. (2000). Acquiring simultaneous EEG and functional MRI. *Clinical Neurophysiology, 111,* 1974–1980.

Gregory, A. M., Caspi, A., Moffitt, T. E., Koenen,

K., Eley, T. C., & Poulton, R. (2007). Juvenile mental health histories of adults with anxiety disorders. *American Journal of Psychiatry, 164,* 301–308.

Grigoroiu-Serbanescu, M., Chrstodorescu, D., Jipescu, I., Totoescu, A., Marinescu, E., & Ardelean, V. (1989). Psychopathology in children aged 10–17 of bipolar parents: Psychopathology rate and correlates of the severity of the psychopathology. *Journal of Affective Disorders, 16,* 167–179.

Grillon, C., Dierker, L., & Merikangas, K. R. (1997). Startle modulation in children at risk for anxiety disorders and/or alcoholism. *Journal of the American Academy of Child and Adolescent Psychiatry, 36,* 925–932.

Gross, C., Zhuang, X., Stark, K., Ramboz, S., Oosting, R., Kirby, L., et al. (2002). Serotonin1A receptor acts during development to establish normal anxiety-like behaviour in the adult. *Nature, 416,* 396–400.

Guyer, A. E., Lau, J. Y., McClure-Tone, E. B., Parrish, J., Shiffrin, N. D., Reynolds, R. C., et al. (2008). Amygdala and ventrolateral prefrontal cortex function during anticipated peer evaluation in pediatric social anxiety. *Archives of General Psychiatry, 65,* 1303–1312.

Hadwin, J. A., Garner, M., & Perez-Olivas, G. (2006). The development of information processing biases in childhood anxiety: A review and exploration of its origins in parenting. *Clinical Psychology Review, 26,* 876–894.

Hannesdottir, D. K., & Ollendick, T. H. (2007). The role of emotion regulation in the treatment of child anxiety disorders. *Clinical Child and Family Psychology Review, 10,* 275–293.

Hariri, A. R., & Holmes, A. (2006). Genetics of emotional regulation: The role of the serotonin transporter in neural function. *Trends in Cognitive Sciences, 10,* 182–191.

Harmon-Jones, E., Lueck, L., Fearn, M., & Harmon-Jones, C. (2006). The effect of personal relevance and approach-related action expectation on relative left frontal cortical activity. *Psychological Science, 17,* 434–440.

Hayward, C., Killen, J. D., Kraemer, H. C., & Taylor, C. B. (2000). Predictors of panic attacks in adolescents. *Journal of the American Academy of Child and Adolescent Psychiatry, 39,* 207–214.

Hettema, J. M., Neale, M. C., & Kendler, K. S. (2001). A review and meta-analysis of the genetic epidemiology of anxiety disorders. *American Journal of Psychiatry, 158,* 1568–1578.

Hettema, J. M., Prescott, C. A., Myers, J. M., Neale, M. C., & Kendler, K. S. (2005). The structure of genetic and environmental risk factors for anxiety disorders in men and women. *Archives of General Psychiatry, 62,* 182–189.

Hirshfeld, D. R., Rosenbaum, J. F., Biederman, J., Bolduc, E. A., Faraone, S. V., Snidman, N., et al. (1992). Stable behavioral inhibition and its association with anxiety disorder. *Journal of the American Academy of Child and Adolescent Psychiatry, 31,* 103–111.

Hirshfeld-Becker, D. R., Micco, J. A., Simoes, N. A., & Henin, A. (2008). High risk studies and developmental antecedents of anxiety disorders. *American Journal of Medical Genetics, Part C (Seminars in Medical Genetics), 148C,* 99–117.

Hudson, J. L., Rapee, R. M., Deveney, C., Schniering, C. A., Lyneham, H. J., & Bovopoulos, N. (2009). Cognitive-behavioral treatment versus an active control for children and adolescents with anxiety disorders: A randomized trial. *Journal of the American Academy of Child and Adolescent Psychiatry, 48,* 533–544.

Ialongo, N., Edelsohn, G., Werthamer-Larsson, L., Crockett, L., & Kellam, S. (1994). The significance of self-reported anxious symptoms in first-grade children. *Journal of Abnormal Child Psychology, 22,* 441–455.

James, A., Soler, A., & Weatherall, R. (2005). Cognitive behavioural therapy for anxiety disorders in children and adolescents. *Cochrane Database of Systematic Reviews,* Issue 4 (Article No. CD004690), DOI: 10.1002/14651858.CD004690.pub2.

Jang, K. L. (2005). *The behavioral genetics of psychopathology: A clinical guide.* Mahwah, NJ: Erlbaum.

Kaffman, A., & Meaney, M. J. (2007). Neurodevelopmental sequelae of postnatal maternal care in rodents: Clinical and research implications of molecular insights. *Journal of Child Psychology and Psychiatry, 48,* 224–244.

Kagan, J., Reznick, J. S., Clarke, C., & Snidman, N. (1984). Behavioral inhibition to the unfamiliar. *Child Development, 55,* 2212–2225.

Kagan, J., Reznick, J. S., & Snidman, N. (1987). The physiology and psychology of behaviorial inhibition in children. *Child Development, 58,* 1459–1473.

Kagan, J., Reznick, J. S., & Snidman, N. (1988). Biological basis of childhood shyness. *Science, 240,* 167–171.

Kagan, J., & Snidman, N. (1991). Infant predictors of inhibited and uninhibited profiles. *Psychological Science, 2,* 40.

Kaufman, J., Birmaher, B., Brent, D., Rao, U., Flynn, C., Moreci, P., et al. (1997). Schedule for Affective Disorders and Schizophrenia for School-Age Children—Present and Lifetime Version (K-SADS-PL): Initial reliability and validity data. *Journal of the American Academy of Child and Adolescent Psychiatry, 36,* 980–988.

Kendall, P. C. (1993). Cognitive-behavioral therapies with youth: Guiding theory, current status, and emerging developments. *Journal of Consulting and Clinical Psychology, 61,* 235–247.

Kendler, K. S., Kuhn, J. W., Vittum, J., Prescott, C. A., & Riley, B. (2005). The interaction of stressful life events and a serotonin transporter polymorphism in the prediction of episodes of major depression: A replication. *Archives of General Psychiatry, 62,* 529–535.

Kessler, R. C., Avenevoli, S., Costello, E. J., Green, J. G., Gruber, M. J., Heeringa, S., et al. (2009). National Comorbidity Survey Replication Adolescent Supplement (NCS-A): II. Overview and design. *Journal of the American Academy of Child and Adolescent Psychiatry, 48,* 380–385.

Kessler, R. C., Avenevoli, S., Green, J., Gruber, M. J., Guyer, M., He, Y., et al. (2009). National Comorbidity Survey Replication Adolescent Supplement (NCS-A): III. Concordance of DSM-IV/CIDI diagnoses with clinical reassessments. *Journal of the American Academy of Child and Adolescent Psychiatry, 48,* 386–399.

Kim-Cohen, J., Caspi, A., Moffitt, T. E., Harrington, H., Milne, B. J., & Poulton, R. (2003). Prior juvenile diagnoses in adults with mental disorder: Developmental follow-back of a prospective-longitudinal cohort. *Archives of General Psychiatry, 60,* 709–717.

Klein, R. G. (1994). Anxiety disorders. In M. Rutter, E. Taylor, & L. Hersov (Eds.), *Child and adolescent psychiatry: Modern approaches* (3rd ed., pp. 351–374). Oxford, UK: Blackwell Scientific.

Klemenhagen, K. C., Gordon, J. A., David, D. J., Hen, R., & Gross, C. T. (2006). Increased fear response to contextual cues in mice lacking the 5-HT1A receptor. *Neuropsychopharmacology, 31,* 101–111.

Kovacs, M., Gatsonis, C., Paulauskas, S. L., & Richards, C. (1989). Depressive disorders in childhood: IV. A longitudinal study of comorbidity with a risk for anxiety disorders. *Archives of General Psychiatry, 46,* 776–782.

Kroes, M., Kalff, A. C., Steyaert, J., Kessels, A. G., Feron, F. J., Hendriksen, J. G., et al. (2002). A longitudinal community study: Do psychosocial risk factors and Child Behavior Checklist Scores at 5 years of age predict psychiatric diagnoses at a later age? *Journal of the American Academy of Child and Adolescent Psychiatry, 41,* 955–963.

Lakatos, K., Nemoda, Z., Birkas, E., Ronai, Z., Kovacs, E., Ney, K., et al. (2003). Association of D4 dopamine receptor gene and serotonin transporter promoter polymorphisms with infants' response to novelty. *Molecular Psychiatry, 8,* 90–97.

Last, C. G., Hansen, C., & Franco, N. (1998). Cognitive-behavioral treatment of school phobia. *Journal of the American Academy of Child and Adolescent Psychiatry, 37,* 404–411.

Last, C. G., Hersen, M., Kazdin, A., Orvaschel, H., & Perrin, S. (1991). Anxiety disorders in children and their families. *Archives of General Psychiatry, 48,* 928–934.

Lau, J. Y., Goldman, D., Buzas, B., Fromm, S. J., Guyer, A. E., Hodgkinson, C., et al. (2009). Amygdala function and 5-HTT gene variants in adolescent anxiety and major depressive disorder. *Biological Psychiatry, 65,* 349–355.

Lazaro, L., Bargallo, N., Castro-Fornieles, J., Falcon, C., Andres, S., Prieto, T., et al. (2006, October). *Brain changes in children and adolescents with obsessive compulsive disorder.* Paper presented at the 53rd Annual Meeting of the American Academy of Child and Adolescent Psychiatry, San Diego, CA.

Leen-Feldner, E. W., Reardon, L. E., & Zvolensky, M. J. (2007). Pubertal status and emotional reactivity to a voluntary hyperventilation challenge predicting panic symptoms and somatic complaints: A laboratory-based multi-informant test. *Behavior Modification, 31,* 8–31.

Leonardo, E. D., & Hen, R. (2008). Anxiety as a developmental disorder. *Neuropsychopharmacology, 33,* 134–140.

Lesch, K. P., Bengel, D., Heils, A., Sabol, S. Z., Greenberg, B. D., Petri, S., et al. (1996). Association of anxiety-related traits with a polymorphism in the serotonin transporter gene regulatory region. *Science, 274,* 1527–1531.

Liebowitz, M. R., Turner, S. M., Piacentini, J., Beidel, D. C., Clarvit, S. R., Davies, S. O., et al. (2002). Fluoxetine in children and adolescents with OCD: A placebo-controlled trial. *Journal of the American Academy of Child and Adolescent Psychiatry, 41,* 1431–1438.

Manassis, K., Bradley, S., Goldberg, S., Hood, J., & Swinson, R. P. (1995). Behavioural inhibition, attachment and anxiety in children of mothers with anxiety disorders. *Canadian Journal of Psychiatry, 40,* 87–92.

March, J. S., Biederman, J., Wolkow, R., Safferman, A., Mardekian, J., Cook, E. H., et al. (1998). Sertaline in children and adolescents with obsessive compulsive disorder: A multicenter, randomized, controlled trial. *Journal of the American Medical Association, 280,* 1752–1756.

March, J. S., Parker, J. D. A., Sullivan, K., Stallings, P., & Conners, C. K. (1997). The Multidimensional Anxiety Scale for Children (MASC): Factor structure, reliability, and validity. *Journal of the American Academy of Child and Adolescent Psychiatry, 36,* 554–565.

March, J. S., Swanson, J. M., Arnold, L. E., Hoza, B., Conners, C. K., Hinshaw, S. P., et al. (2000). Anxiety as a predictor and outcome variable in the Multimodal Treatment Study of Children with ADHD (MTA). *Journal of Abnormal Child Psychology, 28,* 527–541.

McLeod, B. D., Wood, J. J., & Weisz, J. R. (2007). Examining the association between parenting and childhood anxiety: A meta-analysis. *Clinical Psychology Review, 27,* 155–172.

McNally, R. J. (2002). Anxiety sensitivity and panic disorder. *Biological Psychiatry, 52,* 938–946.

Meaney, M. J. (2001). Maternal care, gene expression, and the transmission of individual differences in stress reactivity across generations. *Annual Review of Neuroscience, 24*, 1161–1192.

Monk, C. S., Nelson, E. E., McClure, E. B., Mogg, K., Bradley, B. P., Leibenluft, E., et al. (2006). Ventrolateral prefrontal cortex activation and attentional bias in response to angry faces in adolescents with generalized anxiety disorder. *American Journal of Psychiatry, 163*, 1091–1097.

Monk, C. S., Telzer, E. H., Mogg, K., Bradley, B. P., Mai, X., Louro, H. M., et al. (2008). Amygdala and ventrolateral prefrontal cortex activation to masked angry faces in children and adolescents with generalized anxiety disorder. *Archives of General Psychiatry, 65*, 568–576.

Munafo, M. R., Brown, S. M., & Hariri, A. R. (2008). Serotonin transporter (5-HTTLPR) genotype and amygdala activation: A meta-analysis. *Biological Psychiatry, 63*, 852–857.

Munoz-Solomando, A., Kendall, T., & Whittington, C. J. (2008). Cognitive behavioural therapy for children and adolescents. *Current Opinion in Psychiatry, 21*, 332–337.

Muris, P., Meesters, C., Merckelbach, H., Sermon, A., & Zwakhalen, S. (1998). Worry in normal children. *Journal of the American Academy of Child and Adolescent Psychiatry, 37*, 703–710.

Newman, D. L., Moffitt, T. E., Caspi, A., Magdol, L., Silva, P. A., & Stanton, W. R. (1996). Psychiatric disorder in a birth cohort of young adults: Prevalence, comorbidity, clinical significance, and new case incidence from ages 11 to 21. *Journal of Consulting and Clinical Psychology, 64*, 552–562.

O'Kearney, R. T., Anstey, K. J., & von Sanden, C. (2006). Behavioural and cognitive-behavioural therapy for obsessive–compulsive disorder in children and adolescents. *Cochrane Database of Systematic Reviews*, Issue 4 (Article No. CD004856), DOI: 10.1002/14651858.CD004856.pub2.

Ogren, M. P., & Lombroso, P. J. (2008). Epigenetics: Behavioral influences on gene function. Part I. Maternal behavior permanently affects adult behavior in offspring. *Journal of the American Academy of Child and Adolescent Psychiatry, 47*, 240–244.

Parsey, R. V., Hastings, R. S., Oquendo, M. A., Hu, X., Goldman, D., Huang, Y. Y., et al. (2006). Effect of a triallelic functional polymorphism of the serotonin-transporter-linked promoter region on expression of serotonin transporter in the human brain. *American Journal of Psychiatry, 163*, 48–51.

Pediatric OCD Treatment Study (POTS) Team (2004). Cognitive-behavior therapy, sertraline, and their combination for children and adolescents with obsessive–compulsive disorder: The Pediatric OCD Treatment Study (POTS) random-ized controlled trial. *Journal of the American Medical Association, 292*, 1969–1976.

Pine, D. S., Cohen, P., Gurley, D., Brook, J., & Ma, Y. (1998). The risk for early-adulthood anxiety and depressive disorders in adolescents with anxiety and depressive disorders. *Archives of General Psychiatry, 55*, 56–64.

Pine, D. S., Helfinstein, S. M., Bar-Haim, Y., Nelson, E., & Fox, N. A. (2009). Challenges in developing novel treatments for childhood disorders: Lessons from research on anxiety. *Neuropsychopharmacology, 34*, 213–228.

Pizzagalli, D. A., Sherwood, R. J., Henriques, J. B., & Davidson, R. J. (2005). Frontal brain asymmetry and reward responsiveness: A source-localization study. *Psychological Science, 16*, 805–813.

Pliszka, S. R., Carlson, C. L., & Swanson, J. M. (1999). *ADHD with comorbid disorders: Clinicial assessment and management*. New York: Guilford Press.

Reinblatt, S. P., & Riddle, M. A. (2007). The pharmacological management of childhood anxiety disorders: A review. *Psychopharmacology (Berlin), 191*, 67–86.

Research Unit on Pediatric Psychopharmacology Anxiety Study Group. (2002). The Pediatric Anxiety Rating Scale (PARS): Development and psychometric properties. *Journal of the American Academy of Child and Adolescent Psychiatry, 41*, 1061–1069.

Reynolds, C. R., & Richmond, B. O. (2008). *Revised Children's Manifest Anxiety Scale: Second Edition (RCMAS-2)*. Los Angeles: Western Psychological Services.

Reznick, J. S., Kagan, J., Snidman, N., Gersten, M., Baak, K., & Rosenberg, A. (1986). Inhibited and uninhibited children: A follow up study. *Child Development, 57*, 660–680.

Riddle, M. A., Reeve, E. A., Yaryura-Tobias, J. A., Yang, H. M., Claghorn, J. L., Gaffney, G., et al. (2001). Fluvoxamine for children and adolescents with obsessive–compulsive disorder: A randomized, controlled, multicenter trial. *Journal of the American Academy of Child and Adolescent Psychiatry, 40*, 222–229.

Rosenbaum, J. F., Biederman, J., Bolduc, E. A., Hirshfeld, D. R., Faraone, S. V., & Kagan, J. (1992). Comorbidity of parental anxiety disorders as risk for childhood-onset anxiety in inhibited children. *American Journal of Psychiatry, 149*, 475–481.

Rosenbaum, J. F., Biederman, J., Gersten, M., Hirshfeld, D. R., Meminger, S. R., Herman, J. B., et al. (1988). Behavioral inhibition in children of parents with panic disorder and agoraphobia: A controlled study. *Archives of General Psychiatry, 45*, 463–470.

Rosenberg, D. R., Benazon, N. R., Gilbert, A., Sullivan, A., & Moore, G. J. (2000). Thalamic volume in pediatric obsessive–compulsive disorder patients before and after cognitive behavioral therapy. *Biological Psychiatry, 48,* 294–300.

Rosenberg, D. R., MacMaster, F. P., Keshavan, M. S., Fitzgerald, K. D., Stewart, C. M., & Moore, G. J. (2000). Decrease in caudate glutamatergic concentrations in pediatric obsessive–compulsive disorder patients taking paroxetine. *Journal of the American Academy of Child and Adolescent Psychiatry, 39,* 1096–1103.

Rynn, M. A., Siqueland, L., & Rickels, K. (2001). Placebo-controlled trial of sertraline in the treatment of children with generalized anxiety disorder. *American Journal of Psychiatry, 158,* 2008–2014.

Santarelli, L., Saxe, M., Gross, C., Surget, A., Battaglia, F., Dulawa, S., et al. (2003). Requirement of hippocampal neurogenesis for the behavioral effects of antidepressants. *Science, 301,* 805–809.

Schinka, J. A., Busch, R. M., & Robichaux-Keene, N. (2004). A meta-analysis of the association between the serotonin transporter gene polymorphism (5-HTTLPR) and trait anxiety. *Molecular Psychiatry, 9,* 197–202.

Schmidt, L. A., Fox, N. A., Rubin, K. H., Hu, S., & Hamer, D. (2002). Molecular genetics of shyness and aggression in preschoolers. *Personality and Individual Differences, 33,* 227–238.

Sen, S., Burmeister, M., & Ghosh, D. (2004). Meta-analysis of the association between a serotonin transporter promoter polymorphism (5-HTTLPR) and anxiety-related personality traits. *American Journal of Medical Genetics, Part B (Neuropsychiatric Genetics), 127B,* 85–89.

Shaffer, D., Fisher, P., Dulcan, M. K., Davies, M., Piacentini, J., Schwab-Stone, M. E., et al. (1996). The NIMH Diagnostic Interview Schedule for Children Version 2.3 (DISC 2.3): Description, acceptability, prevalence rates, and performance in the MECA study. Methods for the Epidemiology of Child and Adolescent Mental Disorders. *Journal of the American Academy of Child and Adolescent Psychiatry, 35,* 865–877.

Shaffer, D., Fisher, P., Lucas, C. P., Dulcan, M. K., & Schwab-Stone, M. E. (2000). NIMH Diagnostic Interview Schedule for Children Version IV (NIMH DISC-IV): Description, differences from previous versions, and reliability of some common diagnoses. *Journal of the American Academy of Child and Adolescent Psychiatry, 39,* 28–38.

Silverman, W. K., Kurtines, W. M., Ginsburg, G. S., Weems, C. F., Rabian, B., & Serafini, L. T. (1999). Contingency management, self-control, and education support in the treatment of childhood phobic disorders: A randomized clinical trial. *Journal of Consulting and Clinical Psychology, 67,* 675–687.

Silverman, W. K., La Greca, A. M., & Wasserstein, S. (1995). What do children worry about?: Worries and their relation to anxiety. *Child Development, 66,* 671–686.

Smit, D. J., Posthuma, D., Boomsma, D. I., & De Geus, E. J. (2007). The relation between frontal EEG asymmetry and the risk for anxiety and depression. *Biological Psychology, 74,* 26–33.

Smoller, J. W., & Tsuang, M. T. (1998). Panic and phobic anxiety: Defining phenotypes for genetic studies. *American Journal of Psychiatry, 155,* 1152–1162.

Snidman, N., Kagan, J., & Riordan, L. (1995). Cardiac function and behavioral reactivity during infancy. *Psychophysiology, 32,* 199.

Southam-Gerow, M. A., & Kendall, P. C. (2000). A preliminary study of the emotion understanding of youths referred for treatment of anxiety disorders. *Journal of Clinical Child Psychology, 29,* 319–327.

Strauss, C. C., Lease, C. A., Last, C. G., & Francis, G. (1988). Overanxious disorder: An examination of developmental differences. *Journal of Abnormal Child Psychology, 16,* 433–443.

Szeszko, P. R., MacMillan, S., McMeniman, M., Lorch, E., Madden, R., Ivey, J., et al. (2004). Amygdala volume reductions in pediatric patients with obsessive–compulsive disorder treated with paroxetine: Preliminary findings. *Neuropsychopharmacology, 29,* 826–832.

Thompson, R. A. (2001). Childhood anxiety disorders from the perspective of emotion regulation and attachment. In M. W. Vasey & M. R. Dadds (Eds.), *The developmental psychopathology of anxiety* (pp. 160–182). Oxford, UK: Oxford University Press.

van Honk, J., & Schutter, D. J. (2006). From affective valence to motivational direction: The frontal asymmetry of emotion revised. *Psychological Science, 17,* 963–965.

Vasey, M. W., & MacLeod, C. (2001). Information-processing factors in childhood anxiety: A review and developmental perspective. In M. W. Vasey & M. R. Dadds (Eds.), *The developmental psychopathology of anxiety* (pp. 253–277). Oxford, UK: Oxford University Press.

Vuilleumier, P., & Pourtois, G. (2007). Distributed and interactive brain mechanisms during emotion face perception: Evidence from functional neuroimaging. *Neuropsychologia, 45,* 174–194.

Wagner, K. D., Berard, R., Stein, M. B., Wetherhold, E., Carpenter, D. J., Perera, P., et al. (2004). A multicenter, randomized, double-blind, placebo-controlled trial of paroxetine in children and adolescents with social anxiety disorder. *Archives of General Psychiatry, 61,* 1153–1162.

Walkup, J. T., Albano, A. M., Piacentini, J., Birmaher, B., Compton, S. N., Sherrill, J. T., et al. (2008). Cognitive behavioral therapy, sertraline, or a combination in childhood anxiety. *New England Journal of Medicine, 359,* 2753–2766.

Walkup, J. T., Labellarte, M. J., Riddle, M. A.,

Pine, D. S., Greenhill, L., Klein, R., et al. (2001). Fluvoxamine for the treatment of anxiety disorders in children and adolescents. *New England Journal of Medicine, 344,* 1279–1285.

Warren, S. L., Gunnar, M. R., Kagan, J., Anders, T. F., Simmens, S. J., Rones, M., et al. (2003). Maternal panic disorder: Infant temperament, neurophysiology, and parenting behaviors. *Journal of the American Academy of Child and Adolescent Psychiatry, 42,* 814–825.

Weissman, M. M., Wickramaratne, P., Nomura, Y., Warner, V., Pilowsky, D., & Verdeli, H. (2006). Offspring of depressed parents: 20 years later. *American Journal of Psychiatry, 163,* 1001–1008.

Wheeler, R. E., Davidson, R. J., & Tomarken, A. J. (1993). Frontal brain asymmetry and emotional reactivity: A biological substrate of affective style. *Psychophysiology, 30,* 82–89.

Woodward, L. J., & Fergusson, D. M. (2001). Life course outcomes of young people with anxiety disorders in adolescence. *Journal of the American Academy of Child and Adolescent Psychiatry, 40,* 1086–1093.

Young, S. E., Smolen, A., Stallings, M. C., Corley, R. P., & Hewitt, J. K. (2003). Sibling-based association analyses of the serotonin transporter polymorphism and internalizing behavior problems in children. *Journal of Child Psychology and Psychiatry, 44,* 961–967.

CHAPTER 11

Mood Disorders

SUSAN M. SWEARER
CIXIN WANG
JAMI GIVENS
BRANDI BERRY
DAWN REINEMANN

According to the *Diagnostic and Statistical Manual of Mental Disorders*, fourth edition, text revision (DSM-IV-TR; American Psychiatric Association [APA], 2000), mood disorders are predominantly characterized by disturbances in affect, including depressed and/or manic states. Depressive disorders include major depressive disorder (MDD), dysthymic disorder (DD), and depressive disorder not otherwise specified (DDNOS). These three depressive disorders differ in the number of symptoms required to meet the diagnostic criteria, as well as the severity and duration of the symptoms (APA, 2000; Reinemann & Swearer, 2005). Bipolar disorders include full-blown bipolar disorder (bipolar I) and the milder and perhaps more common forms of bipolar disorder (bipolar II, cyclothymic disorder, and bipolar disorder NOS) (Akiskal & Mallya, 1987).

BACKGROUND AND HISTORY

Diagnostic Criteria

MDD is characterized by one or more major depressive episodes (MDEs) without a history of manic, mixed, or hypomanic episodes (APA, 2000). The main features of MDEs are the presence of depressed mood or loss of interest or pleasure almost all the time, over at least 2 weeks of time. For children and adolescents, their mood can be irritable rather than depressed. Children and adolescents must also experience at least four additional symptoms to meet the criteria, including significant weight loss, insomnia or hypersomnia, psychomotor agitation or retardation, loss of energy, feelings of worthlessness or excessive guilt, inability to concentrate, and suicidal ideation. Symptoms of DD are less severe than those of MDD; however, symptoms must exist over a longer period of time (at least 1 year for children and adolescents, and 2 years for adults). DD is characterized by chronic and persistent mood disturbance, including depressed mood (or irritable mood for children and adolescents) and at least two additional depressive symptoms. For children and adolescents, any symptom-free period during the 1-year period of dysthymic symptoms should be no longer than 2 months and should be free of MDEs. When some symptoms of mood disturbance exist, but the youth does not meet the criteria for MDD or DD, a diagnosis of DDNOS may be used (APA, 2000; Stark, Sander, et al., 2006).

Bipolar disorders are characterized by the occurrence of manic or mixed episodes (bipolar I) or hypomanic episodes (bipolar II) in addition to MDEs (APA, 2000). The main features of manic episodes include persistently elevated, expansive, or irritable mood for at least a week, and three or more other symptoms, including grandiosity, pressure to talk, decreased need for sleep, flight of ideas, distractibility, increase in goal-directed behavior, and excessive involvement in pleasurable activities with high risk for painful consequences. Hypomanic erpisodes are shorter (at least 4 days) and less severe than manic episodes. If children present with hypomanic symptoms and depressive symptoms, but these are not sufficient or severe enough to meet full criteria for a manic episode or an MDE, a diagnosis of cyclothymic disorder may be given (if other criteria are also met). If children present with bipolar features but do not meet criteria for any bipolar disorder, a diagnosis of bipolar disorder NOS may be used. The diagnosis of bipolar disorders among children and adolescents is difficult because bipolar disorders in youth present in a very different way from the classic cycles of manic and depressive episodes often seen among adults (Geller & DelBello, 2003). Children and adolescents usually experience rapid mood changes (e.g., mood and energy shifts as frequent as several times within a day). As a result, most children do not meet the duration criteria (4–7 days) for bipolar I or bipolar II disorder in DSM-IV-TR (Birmaher, 2007).

PREVALENCE

The results on the prevalence rates of childhood and adolescent depression vary (see Table 11.1). Angold, Costello, and Erkanli (1999) conducted a review of 21 population-based studies published between 1987 and 1997 on children and adolescents, and found that the prevalence rate (3-month to 12-month) of depressive disorders (including MDD and DD) varied from 0.3% to 8%. Other recent studies suggest that rates of depressive disorders among adolescents range from 2.6% to 24% (Costello, Mustillo, Erkanli, Keeler, & Angold, 2003; Garber, 2000; Lewinsohn, Clarke, Seeley, & Rohde, 1994; Riolo, Nguyen, Greden, & King, 2005; Rushton, Forcier, & Schectman, 2002). The large variation in prevalence rates may be due to different assessment methods used

(Kessler, 2002); different compositions of the samples (e.g., in terms of age and ethnicity); and different time intervals examined. Studies using point prevalence and a shorter interval, such as a 3-month interval, usually show lower prevalence rates than studies using longer intervals (12 months or more) (Costello, Egger, & Angold, 2004). Studies on point prevalence of MDD have shown that the current rates of depression are usually less than 1% among children (reviewed by Merikangas & Angst, 1995), and vary from 1.2% to 6% among adolescents (reviewed by Kessler, Avenevoli, & Merikangas, 2001). The Methods for Epidemiology of Child and Adolescent Mental Disorders Study found that the current prevalence rate of major depression among youths ages 9 through 17 years was 4.8% (Lahey et al., 1996). Studies on adolescents from clinic samples usually show higher prevalence rates of depression, ranging from 13% to 61% (e.g., Hodge & Siegel, 1985; Peterson et al., 1993).

According to DSM-IV-TR (APA, 2000), the lifetime prevalence rates for bipolar disorders in the general population are as follows: from 0.4% to 1.6% for bipolar I disorder, approximately 0.5% for bipolar II disorder, and from 0.4% to 1% for cyclothymic disorder. Most epidemiological studies have focused on adults, and fewer studies have been conducted with younger populations. Most epidemiological studies also rely on youth self-reports instead of clinical interviews, which may lead to an underestimation of the prevalence of bipolar disorders (Youngstrom, Findling, Youngstrom, & Calabrese, 2005). Studies using clinical interviews among children and adolescents have shown that the prevalence of bipolar I disorder ranges from approximately 1% to 1.5% (Kashani et al., 1987; Lewinsohn, Klein, & Seeley, 1995, 2000) in community samples. The prevalence of bipolar I disorder is higher (6–22%) among clinical samples and incarcerated adolescents (Biederman et al., 1996; Pliszka, Sherman, Barrow, & Irick, 2000).

DEVELOPMENTAL COURSE

The age of onset for an initial MDE varies across studies (Merikangas & Angst, 1995). The age of onset for MDD varies from childhood to adulthood, with an average age in

TABLE 11.1 Prevalence Rates of Youth Mood and Depressive Disorders

Study	Authors (date)	Ages of youth (years)	Source	Diagnostic criteria	MDD prevalence %	DD prevalence %	Bipolar disorders prevalence %
NCS	Kessler et al. (1994)	15–18	National	DSM-III-R/ UM-CIDI[1]	14.1 lifetime		
NHANES III	Jonas et al. (2003)	17–19	National	DSM-III/ DIS	7.2 lifetime (MDE)	4.7 lifetime	
MECA	Lahey et al. (1996)	9–17	National	DSM-III-R	4.8 point		
	Whitaker et al. (1990)	14–17	High school	DSM-III, clinical interview	4.0 lifetime	4.9 lifetime	
	Lewinsohn et al. (1991)	14–18	High school	DSM-III-R, K-SADS-E	18.4 lifetime 2.9 point	3.2 lifetime	
	Lewinsohn et al. (1993)	14–18 (grades 9–12)	High school	DSM-III-R, K-SADS-E, LIFE	2.57 point 3.12 point 18.48 lifetime 24.01 lifetime	0.53 point 0.13 point 3.22 lifetime 2.98 lifetime	
	Lewinsohn et al. (1995)	14–18		DSM-III-R, K-SADS	18.49 lifetime		0.53–0.64 point; 0.94–0.95 lifetime
	Lewinsohn et al. (2000)	15–18		DSM-IV, K-SADS-PL	18.25 lifetime		1.12 lifetime

Note. The studies are selected if structured diagnostic interviews were used and if the studies were published between 1989 and 2009. NCS, National Comorbidity Survey; DSM-III-R/UM-CIDI, diagnosis based on DSM-III-R criteria and made with a modified version of the Composite International Diagnostic Interview; NHANES III, Third National Health and Nutrition Examination Survey; DSM-III/DIS, diagnosis based on DSM-III criteria and made with the Diagnostic Interview Schedule; MECA, Methods for Epidemiology of Child and Adolescent Mental Disorders Study; K-SADS-E, Schedule for Affective Disorders and Schizophrenia for School-Age Children, Epidemiologic Version (Chambers et al., 1985); K-SADS-PL, Present and Lifetime Version of the K-SADS; LIFE, Longitudinal Interval Follow-Up Evaluation (Shapiro & Keller, 1979).

the mid-20s. DD tends to have an earlier onset (APA, 2000). In general, depression is very rare during childhood, but after age 12 the prevalence rate increases (Merikangas & Angst, 1995). This is discussed further below.

Evidence has shown that bipolar disorders may first occur during childhood or adolescence. Retrospective studies show that most adults with bipolar disorders (20–65.3%) reported experiencing symptoms during childhood and adolescence. In a community sample, the mean age of onset for the first episode was 11.75 years for children with bipolar disorders (Lewinsohn et al., 1995). Some studies suggest that early onset of bi-polar disorders is related to increased frequency of mood swings, longer duration of illness (Suppes et al., 2001), and lower global functioning (Wozniak et al., 1995).

The average length of MDD among adolescents is about 8–9 months, and the length of DD ranges from 3 to 4 years (Stark, Sander, et al., 2006). Patients with untreated MDD can remain symptomatic for up to 24 months (Ingram, Miranda, & Segal, 1998). Most children and adolescents do not meet the criteria for depressive disorders after 1 or 2 years (Kendall, 1993). However, not meeting the criteria for depressive disorders does not mean the absence of depressive symptoms, and adolescents may continue to show some symptoms of depression. Research has reported that recurrence of depressive symptoms is common among adolescents (Reinemann & Swearer, 2005). In one study, adolescents with bipolar disorders had longer symptom duration and more mixed cycling episodes than adults with these disorders had (Birmaher et al., 2006). Another study showed that the duration of bipolar disorders ranged from 0.7 to 125 months, with a mean of 50 months (Lewinsohn et al., 1995). Studies show that between 37% and 70% of adolescents with bipolar disorders recover from the initial episode after 1–2 years (Birmaher et al., 2006; Geller, Craney, et al., 2001; Geller et al., 2002); however, the relapse rates are also high, ranging from approximately 23% to 80% (Birmaher et al., 2006; Geller, Craney, et al., 2001; Geller et al., 2002; Pavuluri, Birmaher, & Naylor, 2005).

Researchers suggest that the basic characteristics of depression are similar in children, adolescents, and adults (e.g., APA, 2000; Stark, Sander, et al., 2006), but that the frequency of the common depressive symptoms changes with age. Adolescents typically display more anhedonia, hopelessness, hypersomnia, and weight change; children report more somatic complaints and agitation, and present with a depressive appearance (Kendall, 1993; Nurcombe, 1992).

Studies have also shown that the prevalence rate of depressive disorders increases during adolescence (Cantwell, 1990; Costello et al., 2003; Hankin et al., 1998; Lewinsohn et al., 1994; Reinemann & Swearer, 2005). Using a structured diagnostic interview in a longitudinal study, researchers found that the lifetime prevalence of depressive disorders increased from 1.07% to 5.66% during ages 11–15, and then jumped to 20.67% at age 18. The peak (lifetime prevalence of depression and new onset of depression) occurred between ages 15 and 18 (Hankin et al., 1998), which was hypothesized to coincide with pubertal changes. Similarly, in a randomly selected sample of 1,710 high school students, researchers found that older adolescents were more likely than younger adolescents to have a diagnosis of DD (Lewinsohn, Hops, Roberts, Seeley, & Andrews, 1993).

Longitudinal studies have shown continuity in depression over time, especially in children who have early-onset depression with other comorbid disorders (see Kessler et al., 2001, for a review). However, only a small portion (9%) of those children and adolescents who experienced MDD during their early years continue to experience it as adults (Lewinsohn, Rohde, Seeley, Klein, & Gotlib, 2000).

GENETICS AND FAMILY PATTERNS

Evidence suggests that family influences, such as maternal depression, may contribute to the development of depression via genetic as well as environmental factors (Burge & Hammen, 1991). Similar findings suggest that genetic influences as well as environmental factors appear to contribute to risk for developing bipolar disorders (Du Rocher Schudlich, Youngstrom, Calabrese, & Findling, 2008). Thus, in the quest to identify factors and events that may cause or contribute to the development of mood disorders, both genetic and environmental factors must be explored.

Some identified risk factors appear to be largely environmental. Maternal stress as well as harsh parenting and discipline, for instance, were found to be risk factors for both internalizing and externalizing problems in children (Bayer, Hiscock, Ukomune, Price, & Wake, 2008). Furthermore, having a single parent and/or experiencing parental conflict also predicted children's development of internalizing problems. In addition, a review of the literature by Wells, Deykin, and Klermin (1985) concluded that parental loss through death or separation was also a salient risk factor for depression. Endrass and colleagues (2007) found that a history of problematic social behavior, such as truancy and running away from home, increased one's risk of developing bipolar II disorder—perhaps by increasing one's exposure to stressful life events such as negative consequences for those behaviors. Low parental financial status was also found to be a risk factor for the development of bipolar II disorder, increasing risk by over 90%.

Other risk factors for the development of mood disorders appear to stem predominantly from genetic factors. In one study, a family history of depression was found to be a risk factor for the development of depression (Angst, Gamma, & Endrass, 2003). In fact, following the conclusion of a literature review on depression, Wells and colleagues (1985) identified parental mental illness and/or alcoholism as the strongest risk factors for depression. In addition, parents' mood disorders have been found to be significantly related to their children's development of bipolar disorders, depression, and/or oppositional defiant disorder (Du Rocher Schudlich et al., 2008). Furthermore, family histories of bipolar disorders as well as generalized anxiety disorder were found to predict bipolar II disorder (Endrass et al., 2007).

It has been noted that familial psychopathology may be the result of genetic influences, environmental factors, or both (Althoff, Faraone, Rettew, Morley, & Hudziak, 2005). In fact, genetic factors may influence one's environment, and the environment may have an impact on physiology. Reiss (2008) has described three potential ways in which parental depression may be transmitted to children. First, the parent may pass on genes that cause or contribute to depression in the child. However, a parent's depression may also undermine his or her parenting style, thus affecting the child's environment. Finally, a depressed mother may expose her fetus to high levels of cortisol, affecting the fetus's hypothalamic–pituitary–adrenal axis. Thus stressful environmental factors may affect a mother's cortisol levels, which may then have an impact on her fetus. In addition to these three possibilities, a parent's genetic makeup may affect the way that parent behaves, which may influence the child's environment. This dynamic appeared in Du Rocher Schudlich and colleagues' (2008) study, which found that parents' mood disorders were correlated with increased conflict and impaired family functioning, which then contributed to children's development of bipolar disorders. Thus separating genetic and environmental contributors is a difficult and complicated process.

To begin teasing these factors apart, family and adoption studies have been conducted to investigate genetic as well as environmental influences of risk. As Althoff and colleagues (2005) describe, family studies may help determine whether a disorder is heritable, but they yield little information on genetic effects. Adoption studies yield clearer information on the magnitude of genetic versus environmental contributions of specific disorders. Thus, both are usually necessary to determine whether a disorder is heritable, and if so, to what extent it is being passed on via genetic versus environmental factors.

One family study interviewed probands with and without a diagnosis of DD, chronic MDD, or episodic MDD, as well as one or more relatives, across three time periods to screen for psychopathology (Klein, Shankman, Lewinsohn, Rohde, & Seeley, 2004). The relatives of probands with either type of depression exhibited significantly higher rates of MDD than did the relatives of probands without a diagnosis of a mood disorder. Relatives of probands with chronic MDD or DD were 40% more likely to exhibit MDD than were the relatives of probands with episodic MDD. Thus it appears that depression, especially chronic forms of depression, is familial.

Bipolar I disorder also appears to be familial, given one study's finding that a monozygotic twin of a proband with bipolar I disorder was 60 times more likely to develop bipolar I disorder than members of the general population were (Craddock, Khodel, Van, & Reich, 1995, as cited in Potash & DePaulo, 2000). First-degree relatives of a proband with bipolar I disorder were 7 times more likely to develop bipolar I disorder than were members of the general population. Both of these findings suggest a strong degree of family factors for bipolar I disorder. As previously discussed, however, studies on family influences yield little information on the contributions of genetic versus environmental factors; thus adoption studies are necessary to tease apart these effects more clearly.

An adoption study that explored environmental contributions to the development of adolescent depression involved administering clinical interviews to 568 adopted adolescents, 416 nonadopted adolescents, and their parents (Tully, Iacono, & McGue, 2008). These interviews assessed lifetime diagnoses of MDD. For both sets of adolescents, maternal but not paternal depression was associated with a higher risk of developing MDD and disruptive behavior disorders. Thus Tully and colleagues (2008) concluded that environmental factors elevate the risk that adolescents will develop MDD and/or disruptive behavior disorders in families with depressed mothers, whether or not the mothers are biologically related to the adolescents.

Contrary to Tully and colleagues (2008), who found powerful evidence for the contribution of environmental factors in the development of depression, Mendlewicz and Rainer (1977) found evidence suggesting that genetics play a powerful role in the transmission of bipolar disorder. In this study, biological and adoptive parents of adoptees with manic–depressive disorder, now known as bipolar disorder, were interviewed. The investigators found that the biological parents showed higher rates of psychiatric illness than the adoptive parents did. However, as Althoff and colleagues (2005) noted, there have been few adoption studies of any mood disorder, and there have been no adoption studies of pediatric bipolar disorders. Some of the studies that have been undertaken have become quite dated, while others still struggle to separate the effects of genetic versus environmental factors. Thus, more research is clearly needed to identify the extent to which genetic and environmental factors contribute to the development of mood disorders in children and adolescents.

BIOLOGICAL AND NEUROPSYCHOLOGICAL MARKERS

The etiology of mood disorders is largely unknown (Zhang, Hauser, Conty, Emrich, & Dietrich, 2007). To yield more information on potential contributors to depression, Zhang and colleagues (2007) assessed the behavioral and electrophysiological characteristics of healthy individuals with and without familial risk for depression. Those with high risk for depression due to family history showed greater accuracy but slower speed than individuals at lower risk due to lack of family history did. High-risk individuals also showed significantly reduced P3b amplitudes over left temporal areas, compared to low-risk individuals. Thus P3b, a component of event-related potentials, may be a neurocognitive marker of vulnerability for the development of depression.

Another study exploring markers of depression involved administering electroencephalograms (EEGs) and questionnaires to assess for depression and anxiety in 732 twins and nontwin siblings, in order to examine the link between frontal asymmetry of EEG alpha power (FA) and risk for the development of depression and anxiety (Smit, Posthuma, Boomsma, & De Geus, 2006). The results showed that FA was only heritable during young adulthood and was higher for females than for males. A gender difference was also found in the link between FA and depression/anxiety; that is, a significant relationship was only found for females. Thus, FA may be a valid endophenotype for females in young adulthood.

In yet another study, a genome-wide linkage scan explored chromosomes that may contain genes that contributing to the development of early-onset, recurrent MDD (Holmans et al., 2007). The results of the evidence gathered from 656 families with two or more such cases showed that regions of 8p, 15q, and 17p may contain such genes. A similar study done by Levinson and colleagues (2007) examined DNA markers on chromosomes 15q25–26 for 631 families, and found modestly positive evidence in favor of a link between genes in these chromosomal regions and susceptibility to MDD.

Similar studies have been conducted to explore biological and neuropsychological markers of bipolar disorders. Frampton, Allen, and Cross (2008) used a variety of tests to assess the neurocognitive functioning of three groups of participants: those with first-degree relatives with bipolar disorders who also had diagnoses of bipolar disorder (referred to in this study as the BP group); those with first-degree relatives with bipolar disorder who did not have the disorder themselves (who composed the FD group); and individuals without bipolar disorder or a family history of it (who made up the NC group). Though this finding was not significant, the NC group generally tended to perform better than the FD group, who in turn performed better than the BP group. Even after the investigators controlled for mood symptoms, the NC group outperformed the BP and FD groups on the visual–spatial/constructional domain, which was assessed via tests such as the Wechsler Block Design subtest and the Judgment of Line Orientation test. Furthermore, the BP group performed significantly worse than the FD and NC groups on the Wechsler Digit Symbol subtest. Thus deficits on these neuropsychological tests may be endophenotypes for bipolar disorder.

In another study, a genome-wide linkage scan was conducted to explore genes that may contribute to susceptibility to the development of bipolar disorders (Zandi et al., 2007). Participants with or without a major mood disorder were genotyped, and evidence showed that chromosomes 2q24 and 3q28 may contain such genes; however, the findings were not significant. A review of the literature led Althoff and colleagues (2005) to identify chromosomes 12p, 14q, and 15q as potentially containing genes that contribute to early-onset bipolar disorder. Althoff and colleagues concluded that an early onset of bipolar disorder may be connected with greater familial risk to relatives. Furthermore, it was hypothesized that early-onset bipolar disorder may be a more severe form or separate form of bipolar disorder.

RISK FACTORS
FOR PHENOTYPIC EXPRESSION

Gender

Research has found no gender differences in depression between boys and girls before the onset of puberty (e.g., Speier, Sherak, Hirsch, & Cantwell, 1995). However, during adolescence, more girls are diagnosed with depressive disorders than boys (Cantwell, 1990; Hankin et al., 1998; Lewinsohn et al., 1993, 1994; McGee, Feehan, Williams, & Anderson, 1992; Reinemann & Swearer, 2005). The gender difference seems to emerge between ages 13 and 15 (Ge, Conger, & Elder, 2001; Hankin et al., 1998). This gender difference continues into adulthood, with the prevalence of depression being twice as high among women as among men. For bipolar disorders, gender differences have been less studied, and no clear gender difference in the prevalence of bipolar I has been documented (APA, 2000). Bipolar II disorder may be more common in women than in men (APA, 2000); however, there is no empirical support for this difference among children and adolescents.

Ethnic, Cultural,
and Socioeconomic Differences

Recent studies have shown that the experience and interpretation of depressive symptoms are likely to be different among different cultural and ethnic groups. In certain cultures, depressive symptoms may be demonstrated in terms of somatic complaints instead of depressed mood. Depressive experiences may be expressed in terms of an "imbalance" of internal energy in Chinese and some Asian cultures, headaches in Hispanic and Mediterranean cultures, and problems of the "heart" in Middle Eastern cultures (APA, 2000). The prevalence of depressive disorders may be different among cultures as well. Some Asian cultures, such as China, Japan, and Taiwan, have been found to have lower prevalence rates of depressive disorders than those in Western cultures among adults (Bland, 1997; Hwu, Chang, Yeh, Chang, & Yeh, 1996; Simon, Von Korff, Picvinelli, Fullerton, & Ormel, 1999), as well as among adolescents (Doi, Roberts, Takeuchi, & Suzuki, 2001).

There is some evidence that adolescents from ethnic minority groups may experience more depressive symptoms than European American adolescents do (Rushton et al., 2002). Studies on mental health outcomes among children and adolescents have shown that African American youth (Brown, Meadows, & Elder, 2007; Gore & Aseltine, 2003) and Hispanic American youth reported more depressive symptoms than European Americans did (Brown et al., 2007; Gore & Aseltine, 2003; Siegal, Aneshensel, Taub, Driscoll, & Cantwell, 1998). Epidemiological studies have also shown that the prevalence of MDD is higher among African American youth (Doi et al., 2001) and Hispanic American youth (Doi et al., 2001) than among European American youth. Some researchers suggest that the ethnicity differences may be attributable to the socioeconomic differences among different ethnic groups. In one study, the significant association between adolescent depression and ethnicity disappeared after the investigators controlled for sociodemographic variables such as family income and parental education (Doi et al., 2001). However, another study showed that the ethnic difference between Hispanic Americans and European Americans still existed even after the researchers controlled for socioeconomic differences (Siegel et al., 1998). It is possible that higher depressive symptoms among minority groups reflect their greater exposure to challenging social conditions, such as ongoing stressors, above and beyond the common measure of socioeconomic status (Siegal et al., 1998). Limited epidemiological data from community samples do not support significant racial differences in the prevalence of bipolar disorders among children and adolescents (Lewinsohn et al., 1995; Lewinsohn, Klein, & Seeley, 2000).

The effects of socioeconomic factors, such as family income and parental educational level, on adolescent depression have also been documented (Doi et al., 2001; Siegal et al., 1998). Children and adolescents from low-income families are at greater risk for experiencing stressful life events, which may lead to higher rates of mood disorders (Reinherz, Giaconia, Lefkowitz, Pakiz, & Frost, 1993; Siegal et al., 1998).

ASSESSMENT

The primary purpose of assessing psychological disorders in children and adolescents is to gather sufficient information to make a diagnosis, determine prognosis, guide treatment, and monitor and evaluate treatment goals (Klein, Dougherty, & Olino, 2005). A complete assessment determines whether the level of intervention should target the individual, the environment, or both (Stark, 1990). Assessment of depression evaluates the symptoms, severity, and syndrome of depression (Chrisman, Egger, Compton, Curry, & Goldston, 2006). During the first phase of assessment, a preliminary diagnosis is made. The therapist determines whether the diagnosis of MDD or DD is met, and rules out other diagnoses (e.g., bipolar disorders, depression due to a medical condition or substance). Case conceptualization begins, and symptoms that may guide or influence treatment are evaluated (e.g., suicidal ideation, psychotic symptoms; Klein et al., 2005). The chronology and course of depressive symptoms are evaluated (Chrisman et al., 2006), as well as the prior history of depression, comorbidity with other disorders, functional impairment, and environmental stressors. When treatment for depression begins, assessment continues in order to monitor the change in depressive symptoms and determine whether the treatment needs to be continued, changed, or terminated. Assessment information should be gathered through multiple informants, including the child, parents, and teachers (Klein et al., 2005).

The assessment of pediatric bipolar disorders is less well defined. Psychology as a field has been skeptical of diagnosing children and adolescents with bipolar disorders, and this skepticism has probably decreased efforts to establish accurate assessment strategies. However, these disorders can only be correctly diagnosed through careful assessment, which will in turn decrease the risk of overdiagnosing disorders that appear to be recent "trendy" conditions. A differential diagnosis is also difficult, as few assessment strategies for the diagnosis of pediatric bipolar disorders have been designed (Youngstrom, 2007). Diagnosis is further complicated by symptom overlap between these disorders and other disorders (e.g., overlap between manic and ADHD symptoms), high rates of comorbidity, and mood changes inherent to bipolar disorders (Youngstrom et al., 2005).

Youngstrom and colleagues (2005) suggest a provisional evidence-based approach to pediatric bipolar disorder assessment. The authors suggest gathering four types of information from multiple sources. First, due to the heritability of bipolar disorders, it is important to gather detailed information regarding any family history of mood disorders. It is also suggested that clinicians assess symptoms that are specific to bipolar disorders (Youngstrom et al., 2005), such as increased energy and grandiosity (see Youngstrom, Birmaher, & Findling, 2008). Symptoms such as irritability and aggressive behaviors are certainly common in bipolar disorders; however, they are not exclusive to a bipolar diagnosis and may be found in other childhood and adolescent disorders (Youngstrom et al., 2005, 2008). Clinicians should also gather evidence regarding mood functioning changes over time, as information and documentation about mood cycling will aid in bipolar disorder diagnosis. Finally, the gathering of assessment information should be extended beyond the initial meeting, as a diagnosis of a bipolar disorder should stem from more than a single assessment period (Youngstrom et al., 2005).

Common to all psychological assessments is a multimethod evaluation, including reports from multiple informants. Such reports aid in diagnosis, as children often lack the ability to describe their emotions and experiences (Smith & Handler, 2007). Approaches used in the assessment of mood disorders include behavior checklists and rating scales, clinical interviews, and observational information.

Behavior Checklists and Rating Scales

Rating scales are standardized lists of questions based on cumulative experience with youth. Such scales rely on quantifiable information as a means of determining deviance from normative behaviors (Piacentini, 1993). A rating scale can either be administered by a clinician or completed by a youth, a parent, or a teacher. Self-report measures are more relevant for reporting the covert nature of depressive symptoms (Klein et al., 2005), but are less useful in diagnosing bipolar disorders, as youth are less likely to be knowledgeable about or even aware of their manic symptoms (Youngstrom, 2007). It is generally recommended that a combination of a clinical interview and self-report measures (see Table 11.2) be used in order to gather the information needed for diagnosis and treatment. Repeated administration of rating scales is also a useful way to monitor treatment gains (Piacentini, 1993).

Clinical Interviews

Both structured and semistructured interviews have been established to assess psychological disorders in youth. The benefits of structured interviews include their systematic, comprehensive nature and high interrater reliability (Klein et al., 2005). Although structured interviews have some limitations, including a lack of flexibility (Klein et al., 2005) and lengthy administration times, they may aid in the assessment of mood disorders in youth, as young children are often not able to provide detailed answers or respond well to open-ended questions (Stark, 1990). Some clinical interviews used to diagnose depressive and/or bipolar disorders in children and adolescents include the National Institute of Mental Health Diagnostic Interview Schedule for Children, Version IV (NIMH DISC-IV; Shaffer, Fisher, Lucas, Dulcan, & Schwab-Stone, 2000); the Schedule for Affective Disorders and Schizophrenia for School-Age Children, also referred to as the Kiddie-SADS (K-SADS; Puig-Antich & Chambers, 1978); The Washington University in St. Louis K-SADS (WASH-U-K-SADS; Geller, Zimerman, et al., 2001; the

Diagnostic Interview for Children and Adolescents (DICA: Reich, 2000); and the Child and Adolescent Psychiatric Assessment (CAPA; Angold & Costello, 1995, 2000; Angold et al., 1995).

Observation

Observational tools are capable of addressing limitations inherent in self-report data, including children's and adolescents' limited capacity for self-reflection (Rudolph & Lambert, 2007). When developing a treatment plan for depression, a therapist observes a child's behavior to determine whether this behavior is playing a role in maladaptive family interactions. Maladaptive messages and covert family rules are observed within the context of the family, in order to establish the behaviors and communications that may be maintaining the youth's depressive cognitions (Stark, 1990). Information from direct observation of the youth and caregiver during the clinical interview can be incorporated into the multimethod assessment. Observation records are also useful for monitoring mood highs and lows, allowing the clinician to differentiate between bipolar disorders and unipolar depressive disorders (Youngstrom, 2007).

TREATMENT AND PROGNOSIS

Pharmacotherapy

Although medication is typically reserved for severely impaired children and adolescents, or for use when other treatments have not been effective (Brown, Carpenter, & Simerly, 2005), the number of prescriptions written for children and adolescents in the United States is growing (Deveaugh-Geiss et al., 2006). In fact, psychopharmacological treatments are likely to be the first treatments for pediatric bipolar disorders (Feeny, Danielson, Schwartz, Youngstrom, & Findling, 2006). Unlike children with depressive disorders, children diagnosed with bipolar disorders almost always require pharmacological treatment (Brown et al., 2005). A study by Moreno, Arango, Parellada, Shaffer, and Bird (2007) examined the psychotropic medications given to youth referred to outpatient physicians for bipolar disorders from 1999 to 2003 and found that 90.6% received psychotropic medication ($N = 154$).

TABLE 11.2. Mood Disorder Rating Scales Published in the *Mental Measurements Yearbook (MMY)*

Scale name	Author(s) and *MMY* date	Original publisher and date	Ages; number of items
Adolescent Psychopathology Scale (APS)	Reynolds (2003)	Psychological Assessment Resources (1998)	Ages 12–19; 346 items
Adolescent Symptom Inventory–4 (ASI-4)	Gadow & Sprafkin (2003a)	Checkmate Plus (1998)	Ages 12–18; teacher form (106 items), parent form (120 items)
Beck Depression Inventory–II (BDI-II)	Beck et al. (2001)	Psychological Corporation (1996)	Ages 13–adult; 21 items
Children's Depression Inventory (CDI)	Kovacs (1992)	Multi-Health Systems	Ages 7–17; forms: long (21 items), short (10 items), parent (17 items), teacher (12 items)
Clinical Assessment of Depression (CAD)	Bracken & Howell (2004)	Psychological Assessment Resources (2004)	Ages 8–79; 50 items
Hilson Adolescent Profile (HAP)	Inwald et al. (1992)	Hilson Research (1992)	Ages 10–19; 310 items
Internalizing Symptoms Scale for Children (ISSC)	Merrell & Walters (2001)	PRO-ED (1998)	Ages 8–13; 48 items
Millon Clinical Multiaxial Inventory–III (MCMI-III)	Millon et al. (2001)	National Computer Systems (1997)	Ages 18–adult; 175 items
Multiscore Depression Inventory (MDI)	Berndt (1992)	Western Psychological Services (1986)	Ages 13–adult; 118 items
Multiscore Depression Inventory for Children (MDI-C)	Berndt & Kaiser (2001)	Western Psychological Services (1996)	Ages 8–17; 79 items
Reynolds Adolescent Depression Scale–2nd Edition (RADS-2)	Reynolds (2005)	Psychological Assessment Resources (2002)	Ages 11–20; 30 items
Reynolds Child Depression Scale	Reynolds (1992)	Psychological Assessment Resources (1989)	Ages 8–12; 30 items
State–Trait Depression Adjective Checklists (ST-DACL)	Lubin (1998)	Psychological Assessment Resources (1994)	Ages 14–adult; forms A–D, 108 adjectives
Weinberg Depression Scale for Children and Adolescents (WDSCA)	Weinberg et al. (2001)	PRO-ED (1998)	Fourth-grade reading level; 56 items
Youth's Inventory–4 (YI-4)	Gadow & Sprafkin (2003b)	Checkmate Plus (1999)	Ages 12–18; 118 items

Many psychopharmacological treatments for mood disorders have demonstrated effectiveness with the adult population, but the effectiveness with children is in need of future research. Four major classes of antidepressants exist, with selective serotonin reuptake inhibitors (SSRIs) being the most commonly prescribed for depressive disorders (Bennett, Teeling, & Feely, 2005; Brown et al., 2005). SSRIs prevent the reabsorption of serotonin, making more serotonin available to the brain. SSRIs have fewer side effects than the other antidepressants, but the benefits of SSRIs may take 4–8 weeks to take effect (Brown et al., 2005). Tricyclic antidepressants (TCAs) also target the neurotransmitters in the brain; however, their side effects are usually harsh, making TCAs a second or third choice for treatment in most cases. The risk of overdose is also higher, so TCAs are not typically prescribed without the assurance of prudent supervision (Brown et al., 2005; Fombonne & Zinck, 2008). Monoamine oxidase inhibitors are also rarely used in children and adolescents because of the significant dietary restrictions they require.

Psychopharmacological treatments for bipolar disorders in children and adolescents most often include lithium. In fact, lithium (also widely used for adult bipolar disorders) is the only medication for the treatment of acute mania and bipolar I disorder in adolescents that has been approved by the U.S. Food and Drug Administration (FDA) for youth 12 years and older (Hamrin & Pachler, 2007). Lithium affects neurotransmitters in the brain, including norepinephrine, dopamine, and serotonin. It has several negative side effects, however; these include nausea, vomiting, tremor, sleepiness, weight gain, and damage to the kidneys. Mood stabilizers are also prescribed for youth diagnosed with bipolar disorders. Mood stabilizers also have negative side effects, and both lithium and mood stabilizers require blood level monitoring (Brown et al., 2005). For medication treatment guidelines for children and adolescents diagnosed with bipolar disorders, see Kowatch and colleagues (2005).

Medication Use for Children and Adolescents

Much debate has risen about the use of psychotropic medications for children and adolescents. Further research is needed to determine whether the medications described above are indeed efficacious treatments for children and adolescents. Studies have been limited and methodologically flawed in some cases (Moreno, Laje, et al., 2007). However, controlled studies have indicated favorable outcomes in the treatment of depressive disorders with SSRIs (Emslie et al., 1997, 2002; Keller et al., 2001; Treatment for Adolescents with Depression Study [TADS] Team, 2004). Studies comparing medication and placebo have found both paroxetine (Keller et al., 2001) and fluoxetine (TADS Team, 2004) to be significantly more effective than placebo. The TADS Team (2007) also found that fluoxetine accelerated treatment improvements measured at 12 weeks.

The efficacy of medication use with children and adolescents diagnosed with bipolar disorders is also emerging through controlled and uncontrolled studies. Studies using open-label treatment have yielded preliminary results for the efficacy of lithium (e.g., Kafantaris, Coletti, Dicker, Padula, & Kane, 2003) and other medications, including ziprasidone (Biederman et al., 2007). Geller and colleagues (1998) conducted a randomized controlled treatment study of adolescents ($N = 25$) with comorbid bipolar I disorder and substance abuse. Adolescents assigned to the lithium group showed significantly greater improvement in both bipolar and substance abuse symptoms than those assigned to the placebo group did. It is less clear how children and adolescents respond to mood stabilizers and anticonvulsants compared to lithium; at least one study detected no significant differences between these treatments (Kowatch et al., 2000).

Black-Box Warnings

Safety concerns regarding the use of antidepressants in youth arose following a report by the Medicine and Healthcare Products Regulatory Agency in the United Kingdom in 2003 (Fombonne & Zinck, 2008). Following these concerns, the U.S. FDA conducted an investigation examining the use of SSRIs. The FDA found that SSRIs had a significant risk for youth, in that taking these medications might increase the risk of suicidal events; however, no deaths due to SSRIs were discovered (Fombonne & Zinck,

2008). The FDA has placed "black-box" label warnings on SSRIs to warn that SSRIs have been linked to depression and suicide attempts in some children. Fluoxetine is the only medication that the FDA has approved for use by children (Brown et al., 2005), as its use has proven effective in at least two studies.

Psychosocial Treatments

Cognitive-behavioral therapy (CBT) has been effective in treating unipolar depression and meets the criteria for a well-established treatment for depressive disorders (Compton et al., 2004). We briefly describe three treatment programs based on CBT and interpersonal process, with empirical support for their effectiveness in treating childhood and adolescent depression. The ACTION program (Stark, Schnoebelen, et al., 2007, Stark, Simpson, Schnoebelen, et al., 2007; Stark et al., 2008; Stark, Simpson, Yancy, & Molnar, 2007), the Adolescent Coping with Depression course (CWD-A; Lewinsohn, Clarke, Hops, & Andrews, 1990), and interpersonal psychotherapy for depressed adolescents (IPT-A; Mufson, Dorta, Moreau, & Weissman, 2004) all have evidence for their effectiveness with youth.

Compared to the literature on depression, less attention has been given to psychosocial interventions for pediatric bipolar disorders, leaving many psychologists unprepared for the rising numbers of referrals for these disorders (Youngstrom, 2007). In fact, there are no proven efficacious or effective treatments for bipolar disorders in youth (Youngstrom et al., 2005). However, psychoeducation, CBT, and family therapy have all shown promise. Preliminary effectiveness has been indicated for CBT (Feeny et al., 2006), child- and family-focused CBT (CFF-CBT; Pavuluri et al., 2004), and multifamily psychoeducation groups (Goldberg-Arnold & Fristad, 2003). The first and second of these are also briefly described.

The ACTION Program

The ACTION program (Stark et al., 2008; Stark, Schnoebelen, et al., 2007; Stark, Simpson, Schnoebelen, et al., 2007; Stark, Simpson, Yancy, et al., 2007) is a group treatment for depressed girls ages 9–13

years. This small-group CBT intervention is structured according to a therapist's manual, contains workbooks for the girls and their parents, and is conducted in the school environment. A self-control model is the basis for the treatment program, which includes affective education, coping skills training, problem-solving training, and cognitive restructuring. The girls in the group are taught to use coping skills through the cognitive-behavioral model (Stark et al., 2008). Parent training is implemented concurrently, with the aim to teach parents the same skills their children are learning and to help them reinforce and support their children's skill acquisition (Stark, Sander, Hargrave, et al., 2006). Stark, Sander, Hauser, and colleagues (2006) obtained preliminary results suggesting that 70% of girls no longer experienced depressive symptoms following the ACTION program.

Adolescent Coping with Depression Course

The CWD-A (Lewinsohn et al., 1990) is based on the assumption that depressed youth do not receive reinforcement, do not engage in pleasant activities, and behave in a way that contributes to a loss of support. This program incorporates pleasant events and reinforcement while addressing negative cognitions and deficits in interpersonal skills. The CWD-A teaches adolescents how to use coping skills and problem solving (Rohde, Lewinsohn, Clarke, Hops, & Seeley, 2005). The program also integrates a parallel parent component (Lewinsohn et al., 1990; Rohde et al., 2005). CWD-A administered either on an individual basis or with a parent has proven effective in the treatment of adolescent depression: Lewinsohn and colleagues (1990) found that participants in both these forms of active treatment had significantly improved depression scores, which were maintained 2 years after treatment.

Interpersonal Psychotherapy for Depressed Adolescents

IPT-A (Mufson, Dorta, Moreau, & Weissman, 2004) is a brief, manualized treatment that addresses common adolescent issues through focusing on decreasing depressive symptoms and increasing interpersonal functions. Mufson and colleagues developed

IPT-A with the assumption that depression is maintained in an environment involving interpersonal and social difficulties. Parents are involved in the initial session, and are asked for further involvement during treatment if a clinician and adolescent believe that this would be helpful (Mufson, Dorta, Moreau, & Weissman, 2004; Young & Mufson, 2008). IPT-A has proven to be an efficacious treatment for depression. A study by Mufson, Dorta, Wickramaratne, and colleagues (2004) found that IPT-A was superior to treatment as usual in reducing depressive symptoms and improving overall functioning. A 1994 study by Mufson and colleagues determined that following the course of IPT-A treatment, none of the 12- to 18-year-olds previously diagnosed with MDD met the diagnostic criteria.

CBT for Bipolar Disorders

There is less research on psychotherapy for children and adolescents with bipolar disorders, as noted above. However, pilot studies have indicated that CBT and psychoeducational treatments are effective at reducing and managing bipolar symptoms (Geller & DelBello, 2003). On the basis of research indicating that CBT techniques are effective for adults diagnosed with bipolar disorders, Feeny and colleagues (2006) created a manualized form of CBT for adolescents, modeled after the TADS treatment and substance abuse work. Each session followed the same format: (1) reviewing symptoms; (2) reviewing the previous session's homework; (3) setting an agenda (e.g., a fight with the family); (4) teaching a new skill (e.g., problem solving); (5) applying the new skill to the agenda item; and (6) assigning homework for the next session. After 12 sessions, adolescents in a pilot study (*N* = 16; ages 10–17 years) who received CBT (plus medication) had fewer manic and depressive symptoms as established by parent report than the control group (medication only).

Family Involvement in Therapy

For the most part, families have not been involved in the treatment of depressed youth. In fact, only 32% of treatments include parents (Sander & McCarty, 2005), despite the findings that depressed youth are involved

in disruptive family environments (Stark & Brookman, 1992). Family involvement is often implemented as a parallel process to individual treatment of depression. Parents attend therapy sessions in order to promote the acquisition of their children's newly learned skills, enhance communication, and become educated about their children's depression. For example, parallel family therapy is seen in the ACTION program (Stark et al., 2008; Stark, Schnoebelen, et al., 2007; Stark, Simpson, Schnoebelen, et al., 2007) and the CWD-A (Lewinsohn et al., 1990). Parents are included, but to a lesser extent, in IPT-A (Mufson, Dorta, Moreau, & Weissman, 2004; Young & Mufson, 2008).

Family therapy for bipolar disorders has recently been extended to the treatment of children and adolescents. CFF-CBT (Pavuluri et al., 2004) was adapted from an adult family-focused treatment (Miklowitz & Goldstein, 1997). CFF-CBT was designed to be used in conjunction with medication and to specifically address the developmental needs of children, adolescents, and their families. This technique combines CBT with interpersonal therapy techniques. Other characteristics of CFF-CBT include addressing rapid cycling through psychoeducation, mood monitoring, and affect regulation techniques. Interpersonal problem-solving strategies are implemented to address irritability as well as mixed episodes. A preliminary exploratory study using CFF-CBT found that participants' functioning significantly improved following treatment (Pavuluri et al., 2004).

SUMMARY

In this chapter, the literature on the diagnostic criteria; prevalence; developmental course; genetics and family patterns; biological and neuropsychological markers; and risk factors (with gender and ethnic/cultural/socioeconomic differences) in juvenile mood disorders has been reviewed. The importance of multimethod assessment has been described, and promising treatments for depressive and bipolar disorders in youth have been briefly reviewed. Congruent with a risk reduction model (Mrazek & Haggerty, 1994) of mental health disorders, it is important for clinicians working with youth and their families to view prevention, treatment, and maintenance strategies as interconnected aims. The combination of these preventative and treatment efforts will stand the best chance of reducing the rates of depressive and bipolar disorders among children and adolescents.

REFERENCES

Akiskal, H. S., & Mallya, G. (1987). Criteria for the "soft" bipolar spectrum: treatment implications. *Psychopharmacology Bulletin, 23*, 68–73.

Althoff, R. R., Faraone, S. V., Rettew, D. C., Morley, C. P., & Hudziak, J. J. (2005). Family, twin, adoption, and molecular genetic studies of juvenile bipolar disorder. *Bipolar Disorders, 7*, 598–609.

American Psychiatric Association (APA). (2000). *Diagnostic and statistical manual of mental disorders* (4th ed., text rev.). Washington, DC: Author.

Angold, A., & Costello, J. (1995). A test–retest reliability study of child-reported psychiatric symptoms and diagnoses using the Child and Adolescent Psychiatric Assessment (CAPA-C). *Psychological Medicine, 25*, 755–762.

Angold, A., & Costello, J. (2000). The Child and Adolescent Psychiatric Assessment (CAPA). *Journal of the American Academy of Child and Adolescent Psychiatry, 39*, 49–58.

Angold, A., Costello, J. E., & Erkanli, A. (1999). Comorbidity. *Journal of Child Psychology and Psychiatry, 40*, 57–87.

Angold, A., Prendergast, M., Cox, A., Harrington, R., Simonoff, E., & Rutter, M. (1995). The Child and Adolescent Psychiatric Assessment (CAPA). *Psychological Medicine, 25*, 739–753.

Angst, J., Gamma, A., & Endrass, J. (2003). Risk factors for the bipolar and depression spectra. *Acta Psychiatrica Scandinavica, 108*, 15–19.

Bayer, J.K., Hiscock, H., Ukomune, O.C., Price, A., & Wake, M. (2008). Early childhood aetiology of mental health problems: A longitudinal population-based study. *Journal of Child Psychology and Psychiatry, 49*, 1166–1174.

Beck, A., Steer, G., & Brown, R. (2001). Beck Depression Inventory–II. In B. S. Plake & J. C. Impara (Eds.), *The fourteenth mental measurements yearbook* [Electronic version]. Retrieved June 4, 2009, from *www.unl.edu/buros*

Bennett, K., Teeling, M., & Feely, J. (2005). Overprescribing antidepressants to children: Pharmacoepidemiological study in primary care. *British Medical Journal, 331*, 1451–1452.

Berndt, E. (1992). Test review of Multiscore Depression Inventory. In J. J. Kramer & J. C. Conoley (Eds.), *The eleventh mental measurements yearbook* [Electronic version]. Retrieved June 4, 2009, from *www.unl.edu/buros*

Berndt, S., & Kaiser, C. (2001). Multiscore Depression Inventory for Children. In B. S. Plake & J. C. Impara (Eds.), *The fourteenth mental measurements yearbook* [Electronic version]. Retrieved June 4, 2009, from *www.unl.edu/buros*

Biederman, J., Faraone, S., Mick, E., Wozniak, J., Ghen, L., Ouellette, G., et al. (1996). Attention-deficit hyperactivity disorder and juvenile mania: An overlooked comorbidity? *Journal of the American Academy of Child and Adolescent Psychiatry, 35*, 997–1008.

Biederman, J., Mick, E., Spencer, T., Dougherty, M., Aleardi, M., & Wozniak, J. (2007). A prospective open-label treatment trial of ziprasidone monotherapy in children and adolescents with bipolar disorder. *Bipolar Disorders, 9*, 888–894.

Birmaher, B. (2007). Longitudinal course of pediatric bipolar disorder. *American Journal of Psychiatry, 164*, 537–539.

Birmaher, B., Axelson, D., Strober, M., Gill, M., Valeri, S., Chiappetta, L., et al. (2006). Clinical course of children and adolescents with bipolar spectrum disorders. *Archives of General Psychiatry, 63*, 175–183.

Bland, R. C. (1997). Epidemiology of affective disorders: A review. *Canadian Journal of Psychology, 42*, 367–377.

Bracken, B., & Howell, K. (2007). Clinical Assessment of Depression. In K. F. Geisinger, R. A. Spies, J. F. Carlson, & B. S. Plake (Eds.), *The seventeenth mental measurements yearbook* [Electronic version]. Retrieved June 4, 2009, from *www.unl.edu/buros*

Brown, J., Meadows, S., & Elder, G. (2007). Race-ethnic inequality and psychological distress: Depressive symptoms from adolescence to young adulthood. *Developmental Psychology, 43*, 1295–1311.

Brown, R.T., Carpenter, L.A., & Simerly, E. (2005). *Mental health medications for children: A primer.* New York: Guilford Press.

Burge, D., & Hammen, C. (1991). Maternal communication: Predictors of outcome at follow-up in a sample of children at high and low risk for depression. *Journal of Abnormal Psychology, 100*, 174–180.

Cantwell, D. P. (1990). Depression across the early life span. In M. Lewis & S. M. Miller (Eds.), *Handbook of developmental psychopathology* (pp. 293–333). New York: Plenum Press.

Chambers, W. J., Puig-Antich, J., Hirsch, M., Paez, P., Ambrosini, P. J., Tabrizi, M. A., et al. (1985). The assessment of affective disorders in children and adolescents by semistructured interview: Test–retest reliability of the Schedule for Affective Disorders and Schizophrenia for School-Age Children, Present Episode Version. *Archives of General Psychiatry, 42*, 696–702.

Chrisman, A., Egger, H., Compton, S.N., Curry, J., & Goldston, D.B. (2006). Assessment of childhood depression. *Child and Adolescent Mental Health, 11*, 111–116.

Compton, S. N., March, J. S., Brent, D., Albano, A. M., Weersing, V. R., & Curry, J. (2004). Cognitive-behavioral psychotherapy for anxiety and depressive disorders in children and adolescents: An evidence-based medicine review. *Journal of American Academy of Child and Adolescent Psychiatry, 43*, 930–959.

Costello, E. J., Egger, H. L., & Angold, A. (2004). Developmental epidemiology of anxiety disorders. In T. H. Ollendick & J. S. March (Eds.), *Phobic and anxiety disorder in children and adolescents: A clinician's guide to effective psychosocial and pharmacological interventions* (pp. 61–91). New York: Oxford University Press.

Costello, E. J., Mustillo, S., Erkanli, A., Keeler, G., & Angold, A. (2003). Prevalence and development of psychiatric disorders in childhood and adolescence. *Archives of General Psychiatry, 60*, 837–844.

Deveaugh-Geiss, J., March, J., Shapiro, M., Andreason, P. J., Emslie, G., Ford, L. M., et al. (2006). Child and adolescent psychopharmacology in the new millennium: A workshop for academia, industry, and government. *Journal of the American Academy of Child and Adolescent Psychiatry, 45*, 261–270.

Doi, Y., Roberts, R., Takeuchi, K., & Suzuki, S. (2001). Multiethnic comparison of adolescent major depression based on the DSM-IV criteria in a U.S.–Japan study. *Journal of the American Academy of Child and Adolescent Psychiatry, 40*, 1308–1315.

Du Rocher Schudlich, T. D., Youngstrom, E. A., Calabrese, J. R., & Findling, R. L. (2008). The role of family functioning in bipolar disorder in families. *Journal of Abnormal Child Psychology, 36*, 849–863.

Emslie, G. J., Heiligenstein, J. H., Wagner, K. D., Hoog, S. L., Ernest, D. E., & Brown, E. (2002). Fluoxetine for acute treatment of depression in children and adolescents: A placebo-controlled, randomized clinical trial. *Journal of the American Academy of Child and Adolescent Psychiatry, 41*, 1205–1215.

Emslie, G. J., Rush, J., Weinberg, W. A., Kowatch, R. A., Hughes, C. W., Carmody, T., et al. (1997). A double-blind, randomized, placebo-controlled trial of fluoxetine in children and adolescents with depression. *Archives of General Psychiatry, 54*, 1031–1037.

Endrass, J., Vetter, S., Gamma, A. Gallo, W., Rossegger, A., Urbaniok, F., et al. (2007). Are behavioral problems in childhood and adolescence associated with bipolar disorder in early adulthood? *European Archives of Psychiatry and Clinical Neuroscience, 257*, 217–221.

Feeny, N. C., Danielson, C. K., Schwartz, L., Youngstrom, E. A., & Findling, R. L. (2006). Cognitive-behavioral therapy for bipolar disorders in adolescents: A pilot study. *Bipolar Disorders, 8*, 508–515.

Fombonne, E., & Zinck, S. (2008). Psychopharmacological treatment of depression. In J. R. Z. Abela & B. L. Hankin (Eds.), *Handbook of depression in children and adolescents* (pp. 207–223). New York: Guilford Press.

Frampton, L.V., Allen, D. N., & Cross, C. L. (2008). Neurocognitive endophenotypes for bipolar disorder. *Bipolar Disorders, 10*, 387–399.

Gadow, K., & Sprafkin, J. (2003a). Test review of Adolescent Symptom Inventory–4. In B. S. Plake, J. C. Impara, & R. A. Spies (Eds.), *The fifteenth mental measurements yearbook* [Electronic version]. Retrieved June 4, 2009, from *www.unl.edu/buros*

Gadow, K., & Sprafkin, J. (2003b). Test review of Youth's Inventory–4. In B. S. Plake, J. C. Impara, & R. A. Spies (Eds.), *The fifteenth mental measurements yearbook* [Electronic version]. Retrieved June 4, 2009 from *www.unl.edu/buros*

Garber, J. (2000). Development and depression. *Handbook of developmental psychopathology* (2nd ed., pp. 467–490). Dordrecht, The Netherlands: Kluwer Academic.

Ge, X., Conger, R. D., & Elder, G. H. (2001). Pubertal transition, stressful life events, and the emergence of gender differences in adolescent depressive symptoms. *Developmental Psychology, 37*, 404–417.

Geller, B., Craney, J., Bolhofner, K., DelBello, M., Williams, M., & Zimerman, B. (2001). One-year recovery and relapse rates of children with prepubertal and early adolescent bipolar disorder phenotype. *American Journal of Psychiatry, 158*, 303–305.

Geller, B., Craney, J., Bolhofner, K., Nickelsburg, M., Williams, M., & Zimerman, B. (2002). Two-year prospective follow-up of children with a prepubertal and early adolescent bipolar phenotype. *American Journal of Psychiatry, 159*, 927–933.

Geller, B., & DelBello, M. P. (Eds.). (2003). *Bipolar disorder in childhood and early adolescence.* New York: Guilford Press.

Geller, B., Williams, M., Zimerman, B., Frazier, J., Beringer, L., & Warner, K. (1998). Prepubertal and early adolescent bipolarity differentiate from ADHD by manic symptoms, grandiose delusions, ultra-rapid or ultradian cycling. *Journal of Affective Disorders, 51*, 81–91.

Geller, B., Zimerman, B., Williams, M., Bolhofner, K., Craney, J. L., DelBello, M. P., et al. (2001). Reliability of the Washington University in St. Louis Kiddie Schedule for Affective Disorders and Schizophrenia (WASH-U-K-SADS) mania and rapid cycling sections. *Journal of the Ameri-*

can Academy of Child and Adolescent Psychiatry, 40, 450–455.

Goldberg-Arnold, J. S., & Fristad, M. A. (2003). Psychotherapy for children with bipolar disorder. In B. Geller & M. P. DelBello (Eds.), Bipolar disorder in childhood and early adolescence (pp. 272–294). New York: Guilford Press.

Gore, S., & Aseltine, R. H., Jr. (2003). Race and ethnic differences in depressed mood following the transition from high school. Journal of Health and Social Behavior, 44, 370–389.

Hamrin, V., & Pachler, M. (2007). Pediatric bipolar disorder: Evidence-based psychopharmacological treatments. Journal of Child and Adolescent Psychiatric Nursing, 20, 40–58.

Hankin, B., Abramson, L., Moffitt, T., Silva, P., McGee, R., & Angell, K. (1998). Development of depression from preadolescence to young adulthood: Emerging gender differences in a 10-year longitudinal study. Journal of Abnormal Psychology, 107, 128–140.

Hodge, D. R., & Siegel, L. J. (1985). Depression in children and adolescents. In E. E. Beckham & W. R. Leber (Eds.), Handbook of depression: Treatment, assessment, and research (pp. 517–555). Homewood, IL: Dorsey Press.

Holmans, P., Weissman, M., Zubenko, G., Scheftner, W., Crowe, R., DePaulo, J., Jr., et al. (2007). Genetics of recurrent early-onset major depression (GenRED): Final genome scan report. American Journal of Psychiatry, 164, 248–258.

Hwu, H. G., Chang, I. H., Yeh, E. K., Chang, C. J., & Yeh, L. L. (1996). Major depressive disorder in Taiwan defined by the Chinese Diagnostic Interview Schedule. Journal of Nervous and Mental Disease, 184, 497–502.

Ingram, R. E., Miranda, J., & Segal, Z. V. (1998). Cognitive vulnerability to depression. New York: Guilford Press.

Inwald, R., Brobst, K., & Morrissey, R. (1992). Test review of Hilson Adolescent Profile. In J. J. Kramer & J. C. Conoley (Eds.), The eleventh mental measurements yearbook [Electronic version]. Retrieved June 4, 2009, from www.unl.edu/buros

Jonas, B. S., Brody, D., Roper, M., & Narrow, W. (2003). Prevalence of mood disorders in a national sample of young American adults. Social Psychiatry and Psychiatric Epidemiology, 38, 618–624.

Kafantaris, V., Coletti, D., Dicker, R., Padula, G., & Kane, J. (2003). Lithium treatment of acute mania in adolescents: A large open trial. Journal of the American Academy of Child and Adolescent Psychiatry, 42, 1038–1045.

Kashani, H., Beck, N., Hoeper, E., Fallahi, C., Corcoran, C., McAllister, J., et al. (1987). Psychiatric disorders in a community sample of adolescents. American Journal of Psychiatry, 144(8), 584–589.

Keller, M., Ryan, N., Strober, M., Klein, R., Kutcher, S., Birmaher, B., et al. (2001). Efficacy of paroxetine in the treatment of adolescent major depression: A randomized, controlled trial. Journal of the American Academy of Child and Adolescent Psychiatry, 40, 762–772.

Kendall, P. C. (1993). Cognitive-behavioral therapies with youth: Guiding theory, current status, and emerging developments. Journal of Consulting and Clinical Psychology, 61, 235–247

Kessler, R. C. (2002). Epidemiology of depression. In I. H. Gotlib & C. L. Hammen (Eds.), Handbook of depression (pp. 23–42). New York: Guilford Press.

Kessler, R. C., Avenevoli, S., & Merikangas, S. K. (2001). Mood disorders in children and adolescents: An epidemiological perspective. Biological Psychiatry, 49, 1002–1014.

Kessler, R. C., McGonagle, K., Zhao, S., & Nelson, C. (1994). Lifetime and 12-month prevalence of DSM-III-R psychiatric disorders in the United States: Results from the National Comorbidity Study. Archives of General Psychiatry, 51(1), 8–19.

Kessler, R. C., McGonagle, K. A., Zhao, S., Nelson, C. B., Hughes, M., Eshleman, S., et al. (2001). Lifetime and 12-month prevalence of DSM-III-R psychiatric disorders in the United States: Results from the National Comorbidity Survey. Archives of General Psychiatry, 51, 8–19.

Klein, D. N., Dougherty, L. R., & Olino, T. M. (2005). Towards guidelines for evidence-based assessment of depression in children and adolescents. Journal of Clinical Child and Adolescent Psychology, 34, 412–432.

Klein, D. N., Shankman, S., Lewinsohn, P., Rohde, P., & Seeley, J. (2004). Family study of chronic depression in a community sample of young adults. American Journal of Psychiatry, 161, 646–653.

Kovacs, M. (2007). Children's Depression Inventory [2003 Update]. In K. F. Geisinger, R. A. Spies, J. F. Carlson, & B. S. Plake (Eds.), The seventeenth mental measurements yearbook [Electronic version]. Retrieved June 4, 2009, from www.unl.edu/buros

Kowatch, R. A., Suppes, T., Carmody, T. J., Bucci, J. P., Hume, J. H., Kromelis, M., et al. (2000). Effect size of lithium divalproex sodium and carbamazepine in children and adolescents with bipolar disorder. Journal of the American Academy of Child and Adolescent Psychiatry, 39, 713–720.

Kowatch, R.A., Fristad, M., Birmaher, B., Wagner, K.D., Findling, R.L., Hellander, M., et al. (2005). Treatment guidelines for children and adolescents with bipolar disorder: Child Psychiatric Workgroup on Bipolar Disorder. Journal of the American Academy of Child and Adolescent Psychiatry, 44, 213–235.

Lahey, B., Flagg, E., Bird, H., Schwab-Stone, M., Canino, G., Dulcan, M., et al. (1996). The

NIMH methods for the Epidemiology of Child and Adolescent Mental Disorders (MECA) Study: Background and methodology. *Journal of the American Academy of Child and Adolescent Psychiatry, 35,* 855–864.

Levinson, D., Oleg, V., Knowles, J., Potash, J., Weissman, M., Scheftner, W., et al. (2007). Genetics of recurrent early-onset major depression (GenRED): Significant linkage on chromosome 15q25–26 after fine mapping with single nucleotide polymorphism markers. *American Journal of Psychiatry, 164,* 259–264.

Lewinsohn, P. M., Clarke, G. N., Hops, H., & Andrews, J. A. (1990). Cognitive-behavioral treatment for depressed adolescents. *Behavior Therapy, 21,* 385–401.

Lewinsohn, P. M., Clarke, G. N., Seeley, J. R., & Rohde, P. (1994). Major depression in community adolescents: Age at onset, episode duration and time to recurrence. *Journal of American Academy of Child and Adolescence Psychiatry, 33,* 809–818.

Lewinsohn, P. M., Hops, H., Roberts, R. E., Seeley, J. R., & Andrews, J. A. (1993). Adolescent psychopathology: I. Prevalence and incidence of depression and other DSM-III-R disorders in high school students. *Journal of Abnormal Psychology, 102,* 133–144.

Lewinsohn, P. M., Klein, D. N., & Seeley, J. R. (1995). Bipolar disorders in a community sample of older adolescents: Prevalence, phenomenology, comorbidity, and course. *Journal of the American Academy of Child and Adolescent Psychiatry, 34,* 454–463.

Lewinsohn, P. M., Klein, D. N., & Seeley, J. R. (2000). Bipolar disorder during adolescence and young adulthood in a community sample. *Bipolar Disorder, 2,* 281–293.

Lewinsohn, P. M., Rohde, P., Seeley, J. R., & Hope, H. (1991). Comorbidity of unipolar depression: I. Major depression with dysthymia. *Journal of Abnormal Psychology, 100,* 205–213.

Lewinsohn, P. M., Rohde, P., Seeley, J. R., Klein, D. N., & Gotlib, I. H. (2000). Natural course of adolescent major depressive disorder in community sample: Predictors of recurrence in young adults. *American Journal of Psychiatry, 157,* 1584–1591.

Lubin, B. (1998). State–Trait Depression Adjective Checklists. In J. C. Impara & B. S. Plake (Eds.), *The thirteenth mental measurements yearbook* [Electronic version]. Retrieved June 4, 2009, from *www.unl.edu/buros*

McGee, R., Feehan, M., Williams, S., & Anderson, J. (1992). DSM-III disorders from age 11 to age 15 years. *Journal of American Academy of Child and Adolescent Psychiatry, 31,* 50–59.

Mendlewicz, J., & Rainer, J. (1977). Adoption study supporting genetic transmission in manic–depressive illness. *Nature, 268,* 327–329.

Merikangas, K. R., & Angst, J. (1995). The challenge of depressive disorders in adolescence. In M. Rutter (Ed.), *Psychosocial disturbances in young people: Challenges for prevention* (pp. 131–165). Cambridge, UK: Cambridge University Press.

Merrell, K., & Walters, A. (2001). Internalizing Symptoms Scale for Children. In B. S. Plake & J. C. Impara (Eds.), *The fourteenth mental measurements yearbook* [Electronic version]. Retrieved June 4, 2009, from *www.unl.edu/buros*

Miklowitz, D., & Goldstein, M. (1997). *Bipolar disorder: A family-focused treatment approach.* New York: Guilford Press.

Millon, T., Davis, R., & Millon, C. (2001). Millon Clinical Multiaxial Inventory–III. In B. S. Plake & J. C. Impara (Eds.), *The fourteenth mental measurements yearbook* [Electronic version]. Retrieved June 4, 2009, from *www.unl.edu/buros*

Moreno, C., Arango, C., Parellada, M., Shaffer, D., & Bird, H. (2007). Antidepressants in child and adolescent depression: Where are the bugs? *Acta Psychiatrica Scandinavica, 115,* 184–195.

Moreno, C., Laje, G., Blanco, C., Jiang, H., Schmidt, A., & Olfson, M. (2007). National trends in the outpatient diagnosis and treatment of bipolar disorder in youth. *Archives of General Psychiatry, 64,* 1032–1039.

Mrazek, P. J., & Haggerty, R. J. (1994). *Reducing risks for mental disorders: Frontiers for preventive intervention research.* Washington, DC: National Academy Press.

Mufson, L., Dorta, K. P., Wickramaratne, P., Normura, Y., Oflson, M., & Weissman, M. M. (2004). A randomized effectiveness trial of interpersonal psychotherapy for depressed adolescents. *Archives of General Psychiatry, 63,* 577–584.

Mufson, L., Dorta, K. P., Moreau, D., & Weissman, M. M. (2004). *Interpersonal psychotherapy for depressed adolescents* (2nd ed.). New York: Guilford Press.

Mufson, L., Moreau, D., Weissman, M. M., Wickramaratne, P., Martin, J., & Samoilov, A. (1994). The modification of interpersonal psychotherapy with depressed adolescents IPT-A: Phase I and Phase II studies. *Journal of the American Academy of Child and Adolescent Psychiatry, 33,* 695–705.

Nurcombe, B. (1992). The evolution and validity of the diagnosis of major depression in childhood and adolescence. In D. Cicchetti & S. T. Toth (Eds.), *Rochester Symposium on Developmental Psychopathology: Vol. 4. Developmental perspectives on depression* (pp. 1–27). Rochester, NY: University of Rochester Press.

Pavuluri, M. N., Birmaher, B., & Naylor, M. (2005). Pediatric bipolar disorder: A review of the past ten years. *Journal of American Academy of Child and Adolescent Psychiatry, 44,* 846–871.

Pavuluri, M. N., Graczyk, P. A., Henry, D. B., Carbray, J. A., Heidenreich, J., & Miklowitz, D. J.

(2004). Child- and family-focused cognitive-behavioral therapy for pediatric bipolar disorder: Development and preliminary results. *Journal of the American Academy of Child and Adolescent Psychiatry, 43,* 529–537.

Peterson, A. C., Compas, B. E., Brooks-Gunn, J., Stemmler, M., Ey, S., & Grant, K. E. (1993). Depression in adolescence. *American Psychologist, 48,* 155–168.

Piacentini, J. (1993). Checklists and rating scales. In T.H. Ollendick & M. Hersen (Eds.), *Handbook of child and adolescent assessment* (pp. 82–97). Boston: Allyn & Bacon.

Pliszka, S. R., Sherman, J. O., Barrow, M. V., & Irick, S. (2000). Affective disorder in juvenile offenders: A preliminary study. *American Journal of Psychiatry, 157,* 130–132.

Potash, J. B., & DePaulo, J. R., Jr. (2000). Searching high and low: A review of the genetics of bipolar disorder. *Bipolar Disorders, 2,* 8–26.

Puig-Antich, J., & Chambers, W. (1978). *The Schedule for Affective Disorders and Schizophrenia for School-Age Children (Kiddie-SADS).* New York: New York State Psychiatric Institute.

Reich, W. (2000). Diagnostic Interview for Children and Adolescents (DICA). *Journal of the American Academy of Child and Adolescent Psychiatry, 39,* 59–66.

Reinemann, D. H. S., & Swearer, S. M. (2005). Depressive disorders. In S. Goldstein & C. R. Reynolds (Eds.), *Handbook of neurodevelopmental and genetic disorders in adults* (pp. 195–224). New York: Guilford Press.

Reinherz, H. Z., Giaconia, R. M., Lefkowitz, E. S., Pakiz, B., & Frost, A. K. (1993). Prevalence of psychiatric disorders in a community population of older adolescents. *Journal of the American Academy of Child and Adolescent Psychiatry, 32,* 369–377.

Reiss, D. (2008). Transmission and treatment of depression. *American Journal of Psychiatry, 165,* 1083–1085.

Reynolds, C. (1992). Reynolds Child Depression Scale. From J. J. Kramer & J. C. Conoley (Eds.). *The eleventh mental measurements yearbook* [Electronic version]. Retrieved June 4, 2009, from *www.unl.edu/buros*

Reynolds, C. (2003). Adolescent Psychopathology Scale. From B. S. Plake, J. C. Impara, & R. A. Spies (Eds.), *The fifteenth mental measurements yearbook* [Electronic version]. Retrieved June 4, 2009, from *www.unl.edu/buros*

Reynolds, C. (2005). Reynolds Adolescent Depression Scale–2nd Edition. In R. A. Spies & B. S. Plake (Eds.), *The sixteenth mental measurements yearbook* [Electronic version]. Retrieved June 4, 2009, from *www.unl.edu/buros*

Riolo, S., Nguyen, T., Greden, J., & King, C. (2005). Prevalence of depression by race/ethnicity: Findings from the National Health and Nutrition Ex-amination Survey III. *American Journal of Public Health, 95,* 998–1000.

Rohde, P., Lewinsohn, P. M., Clarke, G. N., Hops, H., & Seeley, J. R. (2005). The Adolescent Coping with Depression course: A cognitive-behavioral approach to the treatment of adolescent depression. In E. D. Hibbs & P. S. Jensen (Eds.), *Psychosocial treatments for child and adolescent disorders: Empirically based strategies for clinical practice* (2nd ed., pp. 219–237). Washington, DC: American Psychological Association.

Rudolph, K. D., & Lambert, S. F. (2007). Child and adolescent depression. In E. J. Mash & R. A. Barkley (Eds.), *Assessment of childhood disorders* (4th ed., pp. 213–252). New York: Guilford Press.

Rushton, J. L., Forcier, M., & Schectman, R. M. (2002). Epidemiology of depressive symptoms in the National Longitudinal Study of Adolescent Health. *Journal of the American Academy of Child and Adolescent Psychiatry, 41,* 199–205.

Sander, J.B., & McCarty, C.A. (2005). Youth depression in the family context: Familial risk factors and models of treatment. *Clinical Child and Family Psychology Review, 8*(3), 203–219.

Shaffer, D., Fisher, P., Lucas, C., Dulcan, M., & Schwab-Stone, M. (2000). NIMH Diagnostic Interview Schedule for Children Version IV (NIMH DISC-IV): Description, differences from previous versions, and reliability of some common diagnoses. *Journal of the American Academy of Child and Adolescent Psychiatry, 39,* 28–38.

Shapiro, R., & Keller, M. (1979). *Longitudinal Interval Follow-Up Evaluation (LIFE).* Unpublished manuscript.

Siegal, J. M., Aneshensel, C. S., Taub, B., Driscoll, A. K., & Cantwell, D. P. (1998). Adolescent depressed mood in a multiethnic sample. The entity from which ERIC acquires the content, including journal, organization, and conference names, or by means of online submission from the author. *Journal of Youth and Adolescence, 27,* 413–427.

Simon, G. E., Von Korff, M., Picvinelli, M., Fullerton, C., & Ormel, J. (1999). An international study of the relation between somatic symptoms and depression. *New England Journal of Medicine, 341,* 1329–1335.

Smit, D., Posthuma, D., Boomsma, D., & De Geus, E. (2006). The relation between frontal EEG asymmetry and the risk for anxiety and depression. *Biological Psychology, 74,* 26–33.

Smith, S. R., & Handler, L. (2007). The clinical practice of child and adolescent assessment. In S. R. Smith & L. Handler (Eds.), *The clinical assessment of children and adolescents: A practitioner's handbook* (pp. 1–15). New York: Routledge.

Speier, P. L., Sherak, D. L., Hirsch, S., & Cantwell, D. P. (1995). Depression in children and adolescents. In E. E. Beckham & W. R. Leber (Eds.), *Handbook of depression* (2nd ed., pp. 467–481). New York: Guilford Press.

Stark, K. D. (1990). *Childhood depression: School-based intervention.* New York: Guilford Press.

Stark, K. D., & Brookman, C. S. (1992). Childhood depression: Theory and family–school intervention. In M. J. Fine & C. Carlson (Eds.), *The handbook of family–school intervention: A systems perspective* (pp. 247–271). Needham Heights, MA: Allyn & Bacon.

Stark, K. D., Hargrave, J., Hersh, B., Greenberg, M., Herren, J., & Fisher, M. (2008). Treatment of childhood depression: The ACTION treatment program. In J. R. Z. Abela & B. L. Hankin (Eds.), *Handbook of depression in children and adolescents* (pp. 224–249). New York: Guilford Press.

Stark, K. D., Sander, J. B., Hargrave, J., Schnoebelen, S., Simpson, J., & Molnar, J. (2006). Treatment of depression in children and adolescence: Cognitive-behavioral procedures for the individual and family. In P. C. Kendall (Ed.), *Child and adolescent therapy: Cognitive-behavioral procedures* (3rd ed., pp. 169–216). New York: Guilford Press.

Stark, K. D., Sander, J., Hauser, M., Simpson, J., Schnoebelen, S., Glenn, R., et al. (2006). Depressive disorders during childhood and adolescence. In E. J. Mash & R. A. Barkley (Eds.), *Treatment of childhood disorders* (pp. 336–407). New York: Guilford Press.

Stark, K. D., Schnoebelen, S., Simpson, J., Hargrave, J., Glenn, R., & Molnar, J. (2007). *Children's workbook for ACTION.* Broadmore, PA: Workbook.

Stark, K. D., Simpson, J., Schnoebelen, S., Hargrave, J., Glenn, R., & Molnar, J. (2007). *Therapist's manual for ACTION.* Broadmore, PA: Workbook.

Stark, K. D., Simpson, J., Yancy, M., & Molnar, J. (2007). *Parent training manual for ACTION.* Broadmore, PA: Workbook.

Suppes, T., Leverich, F., Keck, P., Nolen, W., Denicoff, K., Altshuler, L., et al. (2001). The Stanley Foundation Bipolar Treatment Outcome Network II: Demographics and illness characteristics of the first 261 patients. *Journal of Affective Disorders, 67,* 45–59.

Treatment for Adolescents with Depression Study (TADS) Team. (2004). Fluoxetine, cognitive-behavioral therapy, and their combination for adolescents with depression. *Journal of the American Medical Association, 292,* 807–820.

Treatment for Adolescents with Depression Study (TADS) Team. (2007). The Treatment for Adolescents with Depression Study (TADS): Long-term effectiveness and safety outcomes. *Archives of General Psychiatry, 64,* 1132–1144.

Tully, E., Iacono, W., & McGue, M. (2008). An adoption study of parental depression as an environmental liability for adolescent depression and childhood disruptive disorders. *American Journal of Psychiatry, 165,* 1148–1154.

Weinberg, W., Harper, C., & Emslie, G. (2001). Weinberg Depression Scale for Children and Adolescents. In B. S. Plake & J. C. Impara (Eds.), *The fourteenth mental measurements yearbook* [Electronic version]. Retrieved June 4, 2009, from *www.unl.edu/buros*

Wells, V. E., Deykin, E. Y., & Klerman, G. L. (1985). Risk factors for depression in adolescence. *Psychiatric Development, 3,* 83–108.

Whitaker, A., Johnson, J., Shaffer, D., Rapoport, J. L., Kalikow, K., Walsh, B. T., et al. (1990). Uncommon troubles in young people: Prevalence estimates of selected psychiatric disorders in a nonreferred population. *Archives of General Psychiatry, 47,* 487–496.

Wozniak, J., Biederman, J., Kiely, K., Ablon, J., Faraone, S., Mundy, E., et al. (1995). Manic-like symptoms suggestive of childhood-onset bipolar disorder in clinically referred children. *Journal of the American Academy of Child and Adolescent Psychiatry, 34,* 867–876.

Young, J. F., & Mufson, L. (2008). Interpersonal psychotherapy for treatment and prevention of adolescent depression. In J. R. Z. Abela & B. L. Hankin (Eds.), *Handbook of depression in children and adolescents* (pp. 288–306). New York: Guilford Press.

Youngstrom, E. A. (2007). Pediatric bipolar disorder. In E. J. Mash & R. A. Barkley (Eds.), *Assessment of childhood disorders* (4th ed., pp. 253–304). New York: Guilford Press.

Youngstrom, E. A., Birmaher, B., & Findling, R. L. (2008). Pediatric bipolar disorder: Validity, phenomenology, and recommendations for diagnosis. *Bipolar Disorders, 10,* 194–214.

Youngstrom, E. A., Findling, R. L., Youngstrom, J. K., & Calabrese, J. R. (2005). Toward an evidence-based assessment of pediatric bipolar disorder. *Journal of Clinical Child and Adolescent Psychology, 34*(3), 433–448.

Zandi, P., Badner, J., Steele, J., Wilour, V., Miao, K., MacKinnon, D., et al. (2007). Genome-wide linkage scan of 98 bipolar pedigrees and analysis of clinical covariates. *Molecular Psychiatry, 12,* 630–639.

Zhang, Y., Hauser, U., Conty, C., Emrich, H., & Dietrich, D. (2007). Familial risk for depression and P3b component as a possible neurocognitive vulnerability marker. *Neuropsychobiology, 55,* 14–20.

CHAPTER 12

Autism Spectrum Disorders

BLYTHE CORBETT
JOAN GUNTHER

Although it does not represent an official diagnostic category, the term *autism spectrum disorders* (ASDs) has become an increasingly familiar label for the pervasive developmental disorders (PDDs) found in the *Diagnostic and Statistical Manual of Mental Disorders*, fourth edition, text revision (DSM-IV-TR; American Psychiatric Association [APA], 2000). The ASDs include autistic disorder, Asperger's disorder (Asperger syndrome), and PDD not otherwise specified (PDD-NOS); two rare PDDs, Retts disorder (Rett syndrome) and childhood disintegrative disorder, are also included (APA, 2000). In this chapter, we first provide a brief historical framework, and then highlight some of the most recent conceptualizations and findings related to these complex disorders.

The term *autistic*, first used in 1911 by a Swiss psychiatrist named Bleuler, originated from the Greek word meaning "self." Bleuler used it to depict the tendency observed in individuals with schizophrenia to isolate themselves socially and focus their attention on their "inner life" (Parnas, Bovet, & Zahavi, 2002). Leo Kanner is credited with the original account of the disorder of autism. His keen observations led to his description of common features among 11 children seen in his Baltimore, Maryland clinic in 1943. Making use of Bleuler's word *autistic*, Kanner (1943) identified *early infantile autism* as consisting of symptoms including social deficits, language peculiarities, and insistence on sameness.

At almost the same time a physician in Vienna, Austria, named Hans Asperger made use of Bleuler's term in a paper he titled "Autistic Psychopathy in Childhood" (Asperger, 1991). The paper, originally published in 1944, portrayed a group of children Asperger described as possessing such characteristics as abnormal nonverbal behaviors, emotional peculiarities, social challenges, and circumscribed interests (Hippler & Klicpera, 2003). Although Kanner's and Asperger's observed symptoms still constitute many of the basic criteria for the ASDs, ideas about their diagnoses, prevalence, theory, and treatment approaches have evolved throughout the years.

Various behaviors associated with autism may be observed in infancy; however, impairments in one of the three core domains (reciprocal social interaction, language used as social communication, and symbolic/imaginative play) must be apparent before 3 years of age (Filipek et al., 2000). Autistic disorder, often referred to as *classic autism*, is marked by impairment across all three areas: deficits in social functioning; impaired verbal and nonverbal communication; and a repertoire of repetitive, restricted, and stereotyped behaviors (APA, 2000). PDD-NOS, also known as *atypical autism*, is a condition in which impairment in all three domains exists, but the full diagnostic criteria for a specific PDD are not met. Asperger syndrome is characterized by social impairments and stereotyped patterns of behavior, interests, or activities; however, there is no cognitive impairment or clinically significant delay in language development (APA, 1994). Rett syndrome is a genetic malady that primarily affects girls and is characterized by a decline in functioning across several domains after a period of normal functioning. Deficits include problems with social interaction, motor coordination, and receptive and expressive language development. In addition, purposeful hand movements are replaced with nonpurposeful movements resembling hand washing or hand wringing. (For a complete discussion of Rett syndrome, see R. T. Brown & McMillan, Chapter 22, this volume.) Similarly, childhood disintegrative disorder is distinguished by significant behavioral, cognitive, and language regression following at least 2 years of typical development. Significant impairment is noted in at least two of the following domains: receptive or expressive language, social skills, adaptive skills, bowel or bladder control, play skills, or motor skills (APA, 2000).

Subgroups of individuals with autism are frequently categorized as "low-functioning" or "high-functioning." Not only are these labels unofficial diagnoses, but they lack agreed-upon definitions. Some research refers to individuals with autism of normal intelligence as "high-functioning" (Allik, Larsson, & Smedje, 2006); therefore, individuals referred to as "low-functioning" possess below-average intelligence. It is currently estimated that nearly 70% of individuals with autism have IQs in the range of mental retardation/intellectual disability (Shattuck et al., 2007). An extensive review of 215 articles published between 1937 and 2003 indicates that the prevalence rates of mental retardation in autism were not empirically derived and did not consider the impact of autism on the assessment measure scores. Consideration of such evidence suggests that the prevalence rates of intellectual disability may actually fall somewhere between 40% and 55% (Edelson, 2006).

A subgroup of roughly 30% of individuals with autism have a developmental profile known as *autistic regression*, which is characterized by a period of typical development or mild autistic traits followed by deterioration, usually between the ages of 2 and 3 years (Davidovitch, Glick, Holtzman, Tirosh, & Safir, 2000). The lost skills most commonly include language ability, but losses in social behavior, motor skills, and play may also occur, along with the onset of repetitive and stereotyped behavior. Autistic regression differs from childhood disintegrative disorder in that children with the latter disorder demonstrate typical development until at least the age of 2, followed by a sharp decline in skills before the age of 10 (APA, 2000).

Although screening instruments such as the Social Communication Questionnaire (SCQ) (Berument, Rutter, Lord, Pickles, & Bailey, 1999) may indicate a need for further evaluation, a diagnosis of an ASD requires a comprehensive evaluation, including cognitive and language testing. A thorough diagnostic evaluation frequently includes instruments designed exclusively for supporting the diagnosis of autism, such as the Autism Diagnostic Observation Schedule (ADOS—Gotham, Risi, Pickles, & Lord, 2007; Lord, Rutter, DiLavore, & Risi, 1999), the Autism Diagnostic Interview—Revised (ADI-R—Le Couteur, Rutter, Lord, & Rios, 1989; Lord, Rutter, & Le Couteur, 1994), or the Childhood Autism Rating Scale (CARS—Schopler, Reichler, DeVellis, & Daly, 1980). An inclusive evaluation also often incorporates neurological and genetic assessments (Filipek et al., 2000).

Research conducted in the United States determined that although parents noticed symptoms of autism in children as young as 6 months of age, diagnoses were not made until 3 or 4 years of age (Planche, Lazartigues, & Lemonnier, 2004). A United Kingdom study estimated the average age at an ASD diagnosis as 6 years, although most families noted some characteristics of autism as early as 18 months of age (Howlin & Moore, 1997). Some studies have distinguished the average ages of diagnosis for different ASDs. For instance, Mandell, Novak, and Zubritsky (2005) indicated that the average ages of diagnosis for autism, PDD-NOS, and Asperger syndrome were 3.1 years, 3.9 years, and 7.2 years, respectively.

GENDER RATIOS, PREVALENCE, AND INCIDENCE

Numerous researchers have published data estimating the occurrence of autism based on demographic factors, such as gender and intelligence. It is generally believed that the ratio of males to females with an ASD is approximately 4:1 (Gillberg & Wing, 1999; Tidmarsh & Volkmar, 2003; Wing & Gould, 1979). Although this gender proportion holds true for persons of average IQ, the proportion significantly changes to a male–female ratio of approximately 2:1 for those with intellectual disability (Ehlers & Gillberg, 1993: Wing & Gould, 1979). A large U.S. study showed that the male–female ratio decreased as the level of intellectual impairment reciprocally increased from mild to profound (Yeargin-Allsopp et al., 2003).

The *prevalence* of autism refers to the proportion of individuals in a population that have autism at any stated time, whereas the *incidence* refers to the number of new diagnoses in a population throughout a period of time. The Centers for Disease Control and Prevention's 2009 Surveillance Summaries detailed the 2006 reporting period of 11 sites in the United States and determined that approximately 1 in 110 children age 8 in the United States were characterized as having an ASD. In an excellent review, Fombonne (2005) summarizes several studies finding the prevalence of classic autism to be approximately 13 per 10,000 individuals, that of PDD-NOS to be 20.8 per 10,000 individuals, and that of Asperger syndrome to be 2.6 per 10,000. Taken together, the estimated prevalence for all PDDs was at least 36.4 per 10,000 individuals. Although a genuine increase in the number of children developing ASD cannot be ruled out, the incidence and prevalence of autism may be partially due to broadened criteria, health care providers' increased familiarity with ASD symptoms, greater public awareness, and improved case finding (Fombonne, 2005; Gernsbacher, Dawson, & Goldsmith, 2005).

ETIOLOGY

The causes of autism are referred to as either *idiopathic* or *secondary*. Secondary autism, accounting for approximately 15% of individuals with autism, refers to cases in which an environmental toxin or genetic abnormality can be identified. Idiopathic autism, or autism with unknown etiology, makes up the remaining 85% of cases. Of these individuals, approximately 30% have *complex autism*, which is delineated by dysmorphic features or other structural or brain abnormalities (*www.genome.gov*). The other 70% or so of these individuals have *essential autism*, which is demarcated by a lack of physical abnormalities (*www.genome.gov*; Miles et al., 2005).

Psychoanalytic Theory

Numerous theories regarding the etiology of autism have been presented over the last several decades. Kanner (1943) maintained that the autistic characteristics of the children he studied might have been attributable to their parents' lack of warmth and affection. This view continued into the 1960s with the "refrigerator mother" hypothesis of autism, suggesting that "cold" styles of mothering led to a child's autism. Genetic, biological, and neuroanatomical findings since then have provided compelling evidence to refute these early notions.

Genetics

The first strong evidence for a genetic role in the etiology of autism emerged from a twin study published in the 1970s in England (Folstein & Rutter, 1977b). It is now well accepted that ASDs have a strong genetic component: The concordance rate in monozygotic twins (60% autism, 90% broader phenotype) is much higher than that in dizygotic twins (3%), and the sibling recurrence risk ratio is 5–10 times that for the general population (Bailey, Phillips, & Rutter, 1996; Folstein & Rutter, 1977a, 1977b; Skaar et al., 2005). In general, it is thought that genetic and chromosomal abnormalities account for approximately 90% of ASDs (Freitag, 2007).

Since a single gene or group of genes has not been unequivocally linked to autism, it has been suggested that the broad ASD phenotypes are likely to be polygenetic, with upwards of 15 interacting genes (Risch et al., 1999). Studies have located various genetic loci related to autism; however, only a few of these regions have been confirmed. A number of methods are used to identify possible relevant genome regions.

Linkage Studies

Linkage studies attempt to identify particular genes or sequences of genes that are passed from parent to child. Autism linkage studies have met with minimal success. However, regions on 17q11–21, 7q, and 2q24–31 have been sufficiently replicated and are now considered suggestive of linkage (Cantor et al., 2005; Kumar & Christian, 2009).

Cytogenetic Studies

Cytogenetic studies attempt to identify inherited chromosomal abnormalities. These studies initially identify relatively large chromosomal regions, with identification of particular genes requiring further analysis. For example, it is estimated that abnormalities in the region 15q11–13 account for approximately 1–2% of cases of autism (Cook, Lindgren, et al., 1997; Matsuura et al., 1997; Peters, Beaudet, Madduri, & Bacino, 2004). Studies of this region indicate deficiencies of the UBE3 (Samaco, Hogart, & LaSalle, 2005) and GABRB3 (Fatemi, Reutiman, Folsom, & Thuras, 2009) genes in ASDs. The UBE3A gene directs the production of the enzyme ubiquitin protein ligase E3A, which helps to regulate neuronal activity by breaking down proteins within the cell (Sutcliffe, 2008), and has been implicated in both autism and Angelman syndrome (Samaco et al., 2005). The GABRB3 gene is a receptor for gamma-aminobutyric acid (GABA), the major inhibitory transmitter of the central nervous system (CNS). It is approximated that all cytogenetic abnormalities account for 6–7% of ASD cases in which there is no dysmorphia or intellectual disability, with higher percentages in the populations that have these characteristics (Marshall et al., 2008).

Association Studies

Association studies attempt to identify specific variations in the human DNA to evaluate candidate genes and pathways believed to be associated with particular conditions. These investigations have led to the compilation of a list of possible genes associated with autism. For a recent comprehensive review, see Abrahams and Geschwind (2008).

Findings from Related Genetic Syndromes and Medical Disorders

Autism candidate genes have also been identified through the study of genetic syndromes with a co-occurring ASD. Examples include Rett syndrome, which is the only ASD currently shown to have a genetic cause. Rett syndrome is most commonly caused by de novo mutations or deletions of the methyl-CpG-binding protein 2 (MECP2) gene (Amir et al., 1999). Additional syndromes of interest include tuberous sclerosis (e.g., Smalley, 1998), Angelman syndrome (e.g., Peters et al., 2004; Trillingsgaard & Østergaard, 2004), 22q deletion (Manning et al., 2004), Joubert syndrome (Holroyd, Reiss, & Bryan, 1991; Ozonoff, Williams, Gale, & Miller, 1999), Potocki–Lupski syndrome (Potocki et al., 2007), Smith–Lemili–Opitz syndrome (Bukelis, Porter, Zimmerman, & Tierney, 2007), Timothy syndrome (Barrett & Tsien, 2008), and fragile X syndrome (Hagerman et al., 1986; Rogers, Wehner, & Hagerman, 2001). Significant knowledge can be gained by studying these related syndromes.

Studies of fragile X and Rett syndromes implicate synaptic dysfunction as an etiological factor for autism, whereas studies of tuberous sclerosis implicate common pathways ostensibly giving rise to ASDs. The autism presentation found in fragile X often meets full diagnostic criteria; therefore, the fragile X FMR1 gene mutation may be considered a cause of autism (Hagerman, Rivera, & Hagerman, 2008). Even so, it is estimated that only 2% of children with autism have a full mutation of the fragile X mental retardation protein (FMR1) (Reddy, 2005). Due to the high male preponderance in ASDs and the association with fragile X syndrome, one might be inclined to conclude that autism is an X-linked disorder. However, because of male-to-male transmissions (Hallmayer et al., 1996) and chromosomal abnormalities resulting from maternal transmission (Simic & Turk, 2004), it is unlikely that autism is a prominently X-linked disorder.

Known medical disorders give rise to etiological hypotheses as well. For example, epilepsy is associated with autism in an estimated 30% of cases (Gubbay, Lobascher, & Kingerlee, 1970). Therefore, some forms of ASD may be associated with aberrant neural conduction and transmission. Nevertheless, even when taken together, the syndromes and known medical disorders are thought to account for fewer than 10% of ASD cases (Chakrabarti & Fombonne, 2005; Hertz-Picciotto et al., 2006).

Advanced Technology Findings

Higher-resolution technologies, including microarray analysis, have dramatically increased detection of promising genetic leads. Again, Abrahams and Gechwind's (2008) exemplary review cites microarray studies that reveal approximately 900 genes (many found on the 15q chromosome) and numerous pathways appearing to be dysregulated in ASDs. In addition, copy number variations (CNVs) have recently been found. A CNV is a segment of DNA wherein differences in copy numbers are found when the genomes of different individuals are compared. A repeatedly occurring de novo deletion was found on approximately 30 genes on chromosomal region 16p11 (Kumar et al., 2008). CNV research suggests that the incidence of autism ascribed to the structural variation of chromosomes may be much higher than the 6–7% that were identified by traditional cytogenetic approaches. Clearly, much knowledge can be gained from determining the function of the individual genes, as well as from understanding the repeated duplications. For comprehensive reviews, see Abrahams and Geschwind (2008) and Muhle, Trentacoste, and Rapin (2004). The tremendous advances in genetic technology, and the still unanswered questions regarding the causes of ASDs, draw attention to the complexity of the ASDs and the need for larger sample sizes.

Proteomics

The search for potential biomarkers in ASDs is a critical pursuit that has led to novel methods of molecular profiling for systematic and unbiased biomarker discovery. *Proteomics* uses separation and mass spectrometry methods that support ongoing genetic approaches by identifying aberrant proteins and by-products that may be related to genetic alterations associated with autism and other genetic disorders (Junaid & Pullarkat, 2001). A proteomic approach was used to quantify 6,348 peptides in a comprehensive investigation of serum from young children with high-functioning ($n = 35$) and low-functioning ($n = 34$) autism, matched in gender and age to a cohort of typically developing ($n = 35$) children (Corbett et al., 2007). Corbett and colleagues used statistical and protein-matching methods to identify four known proteins (which included apolipoproteins and complement proteins) that differentiated the children with autism from the neurotypical children. Such findings contribute to a growing body of evidence that immune factors may be implicated in the neuropathology of ASDs in a subset of children (see below).

Environmental Factors

The increasing incidence rates of ASDs have directed attention toward possible contributory factors in the environment. Suspected environmental factors are numerous and include prenatal infections, perinatal insults, viral infections, heavy metals, mercury, pesticides, polychlorinated biphenyls, and childhood vaccines containing thimerosal (Fatemi, 2008b; Muhle et al., 2004; Szpir, 2006). The vaccine controversy is discussed later in this chapter (see "Controversial Topics," below).

A breakthrough study (Nelson et al., 2001) analyzed the blood of newborns collected via heel stick; it revealed that several neuropeptides, such as vasoactive intestinal peptide (VIP) and brain-derived neurotropic factor (BDNF), were elevated in children who were later diagnosed with autism or mental retardation. Importantly, the identified peptides were not elevated in children with cerebral palsy or with typical development. These findings suggest detectable differences in peripheral neonatal blood at the time of birth between the children with autism and mental retardation and those without such disorders.

A number of studies indicate that several well-known teratogens may be related to autism, including maternal rubella infection, ethanol, valproic acid, and thalidomide. A large study by Chess (1977) found an increased rate of autism in children who were prenatally exposed to rubella. Another study reported a cohort of children exposed to ethanol before birth that were identified as exhibiting not only the dysmorphic facial features of fetal alcohol syndrome (FAS), but also the behavioral symptoms of autism (Nanson, 1992). Additional studies have reported similarities between children exposed to valproic acid and those with autism, including posterior rotation of the ears (Christianson, Chesler, & Kromberg, 1994; Williams & Hersh, 1997). Finally, various reports have shown an association with autism in cases of thalidomide embryopathy (Miller, 1991; Stromland & Miller, 1993), specifically suggesting exposure between the 20th and 24th days of gestation.

Immunological Considerations

An increase in the frequency of autoimmune disorders has been reported in the families of persons with autism (Comi, Zimmerman, Frye, Law, & Peeden, 1999; Croen, Grether, Yoshida, Odouli, & Van de Water, 2005). It is interesting to note that several genes in autism relate to immune regulation and function; these include genes for human leukocyte antigen (HLA) presentation molecules and various components of the complement protein system (e.g., Ferrante et al., 2000; Odell et al., 2005; Purcell, Jeon, Zimmerman, Blue, & Pevsner, 2001; Torres, Maciulis, & Odell, 2001; Torres, Maciulis, Stubbs, Cutler, & Odell, 2002; van Gent, Heijnen, & Treffers, 1997; Warren et al., 1996). Abnormalities of various cytokines and chemokines have been reported, including interleukin-12 (IL-12), IL-10, tumor necrosis factor-alpha (TNF-α), TNF receptor II, and interferon-gamma (IFN-γ). It has been suggested that alterations in cytokine levels may be associated with different clinical phenotypes within autism (e.g., Ashwood & Van de Water, 2004; De-Felice et al., 2003; Jyonouchi, Geng, Ruby, Reddy, & Zimmerman-Bier, 2005; Molloy et al., 2006; Singh, 1996; Zimmerman et al., 2005). Additional alterations linked to the immune system include autoantibodies in the blood, which have been speculated to be directed to CNS or brain antigens (e.g., Ashwood & Van de Water, 2004; Croen, Braunschweig, et al., 2008; Pessah et al., 2008; Silva et al., 2004; Singer et al., 2008; Singh

& Rivas, 2004; Vargas, Nascimbene, Krishnan, Zimmerman, & Pardo, 2005; Wills et al., 2009; Zimmerman et al., 2007). The presence of inflammation within the brain and cerebrospinal fluid (CSF) of individuals with autism, indicating innate neuroimmune system activation, provides compelling evidence of immunopathogenic mechanisms in at least a subset of these individuals (Vargas et al., 2005).

A growing body of research supports the hypothesis that aberrant maternal immune response may be associated with the pathogenesis of some cases of autism (e.g., Croen Matevia, Yoshida, & Grether, 2008; Lee et al., 2006; Nelson et al., 2006; Zimmerman et al., 2007). In a relatively recent investigation, neonatal blood from children later diagnosed with autism was compared to blood from children with Down syndrome and with neurotypical development; the comparison revealed distinct developmental trajectories and concentrations across the groups. The findings suggest that intrauterine inflammation may be an etiological pathogenic mechanism in autism (Nelson et al., 2006). Other investigations using various animal models and analyzing the serum of mothers have provided evidence for prenatal maternal immune responses and autoantibodies in some cases (Croen, Braunschweig, et al., 2008; Martin et al., 2008; Singer et al., 2008; Zimmerman et al., 2007). Despite a lack of consistent findings, the preponderance of evidence from cellular to neuroanatomical findings strongly supports a prenatal or very early postnatal etiology in autism, underscoring the need to continue to pursue the influential role of maternal immunological factors in the heterogeneous ASDs. There is also evidence that developmental parental factors, such as age, play into the complexity of prenatal effects in autism (Durkin et al., 2008; Saha et al., 2009; Tsuchiya et al., 2008).

NEURAL MECHANISMS

In recent years, considerable efforts have been made to identify the neural substrates of autism by using a variety of neuroscientific methods, such as human pathology, animal models, positron emission tomography (PET), magnetic resonance imaging (MRI), functional MRI (fMRI), and electroen-cephalography (EEG). Some of the notable advances in these areas are briefly outlined below. We focus on the brain regions and structures most consistently implicated in the neuropathology of autism.

Cerebrum and Total Cerebral Volume

Postmortem investigations allow the careful study of neurobiological substrates that may be related to gross or functional brain ab-normalities. To date, fewer than 100 cases of individuals with autism have been investi-gated via neuropathological techniques, and many of these cases have been potentially confounded by comorbid conditions such as mental retardation or seizures (Amaral, Schumann, & Nordahl, 2008). Bauman and Kemper were among the first to utilize pathological techniques through a series of influential qualitative studies on six brains of individuals with autism (Bauman & Kem-per, 1985; Kemper & Bauman, 1993). The primary cortical features that distinguished these brains were described as small neu-ronal cell size and increased cell-packing density in the anterior cingulate (Kemper & Bauman, 1993). Subsequently, Bailey and colleagues (1998) examined six cases of au-tism revealing different patterns of pathol-ogy, including megalenencephaly, cortical dysgenesis, and increased neuronal density.

A relatively consistent neuroanatomical finding, based on retrospective and longitudi-nal head circumference (a proxy for cerebral volume) and MRI data, has been an enlarged total cerebral volume in children with autism (Aylward, Minshew, Field, Sparks, & Singh, 2002; Courchesne, Carper, & Akshoomoff, 2003; Courchesne et al., 2001; Hazlett et al., 2005; Sparks et al., 2002). Specifically, enlarged cortical gray and cerebellar and cerebral white matter volumes have been re-ported at 2–3 years of age, but not in older children with autism (Aylward et al., 2002). Courchesne and colleagues (2001) hypothe-sized that abnormal brain growth regulation results in premature overgrowth resulting in brain enlargement, followed by a period of protracted growth. In addition to develop-mental factors, distinctions based on gender have been demonstrated, with males but not females with autism showing increased total brain volume (Piven, Arndt, Bailey, &

Andreasen, 1996). It may be reasoned that some of the inconsistencies across studies are attributable to differences in methodol-ogy, inclusion criteria, and developmental factors. Although the precise time trajectory may be argued, a convergence of data im-plicates a period of aberrant brain growth as a neural precursor for the anatomical and biobehavioral manifestation of autism.

Minicolumns

Another leading theory involves atypical development of the neuronal architecture, specifically the minicolumnar structure. Minicolumns have been described as a self-contained system of afferent, efferent, and interneuronal connections (Casanova, Bux-hoeveden, & Gomez, 2003). Cassanova and colleagues investigated the notion of in-creased cell-packing density to explain cere-bral enlargement in the brains of individuals (5–28 years of age) diagnosed with autism, compared to the brains of control subjects. The investigations revealed that within the group with autism there was altered organi-zation, resulting in an increase in the number of minicolumns and reduced cells within the columns in the frontal and temporal lobes (Casanova, Buxhoeveden, Switala, & Roy, 2002a, 2002b). Subsequent investigations supported and extended the findings to re-veal that minicolumnopathy consisting of a greater number of minicolumns contributed to plausible differences in brain size, distinc-tions in the gray and white matter ratios, and interareal connectivity in persons with autism (e.g., Casanova, 2006; Casanova et al., 2006).

Amygdala

Individuals with autism often exhibit dif-ficulty with emotion and face processing (e.g., Adolphs, Sears, & Piven, 2001; Ash-win, Wheelwright, & Baron-Cohen, 2006; Baron-Cohen et al., 1999; Critchley et al., 2000; Macdonald et al., 1989; Schultz et al., 2000) and increased stress and anxiety (Amaral & Corbett, 2003; Corbett, Men-doza, Abdullah, Wegelin, & Levine, 2006; Muris, Steerneman, Merckelbach, Hol-drinet, & Meesters, 1998) as part of their symptom profile. Thus the amygdala, which is involved in these processes, has been im-plicated in the neuropathology of autism.

Baron-Cohen and colleagues (2000) speculated that early dysfunction of this key brain structure may be largely responsible for impaired social and emotional functioning, in the often-referred-to "amygdala theory of autism."

Early neuropathological case series revealed clusters of small, tightly packed neurons in the medial nuclei of the amygdaloid complex of persons with autism (Bauman & Kemper, 1985; Kemper & Bauman, 1998). More recently, a quantitative investigation using stereological analysis showed fewer neurons in the amygdala overall and in the lateral nucleus, despite a lack of difference in overall volume of the amygdala, individual subdivisions, or cell size (Schumann & Amaral, 2006). Volumetric studies using MRI have revealed increased (Abell et al., 1999; Howard et al., 2000), decreased (Aylward et al., 1999; Pierce & Courchesne, 2000), or inconclusive amygdala differences in subjects with autism (Corbett, Carmean, et al., 2009; Palmen, Durston, Nederveen, & Van Engeland, 2006). The discrepancies across these studies may be the results of differences in developmental factors (Corbett, Carmean, et al., 2009; Schumann et al., 2004; Sparks et al., 2002), level of social impairment (Munson et al., 2006; Nacewicz et al., 2006), comorbid features such as anxiety (Corbett, Carmean, et al., 2009), or restricted/repetitive behavior (Dziobek, Fleck, Rogers, Wolf, & Convit, 2006)—all of which ostensibly play pivotal roles in the structure (and presumably the function) of the amygdala.

In addition, suggestive evidence for a role of the amygdala in autism comes from a variety of functional imaging studies (e.g., Ashwin, Baron-Cohen, Wheelwright, O'Riordan, & Bullmore, 2007; Baron-Cohen et al., 1999). In general, individuals with ASDs show reduced or differential activation of the amygdala and the "social brain" network, amidst increased activity and greater reliance on other brain regions (e.g., superior temporal cortex and anterior cingulate cortex) (Ashwin et al., 2006; Baron-Cohen et al., 1999; Corbett, Carmean, et al., 2009; Critchley et al., 2000; Schultz et al., 2003; Wang, Dapretto, Hariri, Sigman, & Bookheimer, 2004). However, it is important to note that other factors, such as the familiarity of the stimulus (Pierce, Haist, Sedaghat, & Courchesne, 2004) and

whether or not the participant is looking in the eyes, may help determine whether or not the amygdala is recruited (Dalton et al., 2005; Spezio, Huang, Castelli, & Adolphs, 2007). Also, as noted above, the level of social impairment (Nacewicz et al., 2006) anxiety (Corbett, Carmean, et al., 2009; Juranek et al., 2006) or of restricted/repetitive behavior (Dziobek et al., 2006) appears to play a role in the structure and function of the amygdala.

Hippocampus

Another part of the limbic system, the hippocampus—located in the medial temporal lobe of the brain, and critical in the formation of long-term memory—has been shown to be enlarged in children and adolescents with autism as compared to neurotypical peers (Schumann et al., 2004). This brain structure was also shown in early pathological reports to contain smaller neurons and increased cell-packing density (Kemper & Bauman, 1993). However, this finding is not consistently observed (Bailey et al., 1998). Differences in the shape of the hippocampus have also been recently reported (Dager et al., 2007; Nicolson et al., 2006), and such alterations may be associated with the severity of cognitive and neuropsychological impairment (Dager et al., 2007).

Cerebellum

Still another key brain region showing abnormalities associated with autism at both the microscopic and macroscopic levels is the cerebellum, a brain structure often referred to as "the little brain." It is located at the base of the brain and is involved in motor coordination/control and integration of sensory perception. Research in autism has revealed reduced size and number of Purkinje neurons located in the vermis and cerebral hemisphere, as well as atypical cerebellar volumes (Bailey et al., 1998; Bauman & Kemper, 1985; Ritvo et al., 1986). The speed of growth has been shown to be more rapid, and both hypoplasia and hyperplasia have been reported, ostensibly dependent on the age of the cases and the region studied (Courchesne et al., 1994; Hardan, Minshew, Harenski, & Keshavan, 2001; Hashimoto et al., 1995). Since the cerebellum is involved in many brain processes, such as motor planning, language processing, sequencing, and imagery, abnormalities in structure and function of the cerebellum may affect many areas of functioning related to some of the core deficits in ASDs (Bauman & Kemper, 2003).

Neural Networks

It is apparent that early brain overgrowth and differences in neuronal architecture set the stage for a cascade of atypical biological events and connections contributing to broad limitations in perceptual and cognitive processes. Complementing this idea, one of the current leading hypotheses conceptualizes ASDs as resulting from developmental disconnection between key highly evolved neural structures (Frith, 2004; Geschwind & Levitt, 2007). Converging evidence from widespread disturbances in circuitry, cytoarchitecture, brain structure, and function suggest that higher-order association areas are disturbed (e.g., Bauman & Kemper, 2005; Carper & Courchesne, 2005; Just, Cherkassky, Keller, Kana, & Minshew, 2007; Koshino et al., 2008), and that such disturbances are likely to be results of early disruption in distributed networks. It is apparent that combining neuroscientific approaches in hypothesis-driven theoretical ways may provide complementary information and significantly advance our understanding of ASDs.

Mirror Neurons

In addition, the synthesis of single-cell investigations and animal studies may hold the key to aberrant neural substrates important in perspective taking, imitation, and empathy in ASDs. In the early 1990s, several Italian scientists led by Giacomo Rizzolatti were using single-cell recording to study the neurons involved in grasping when they observed that the same nerve fired when a monkey reached to pick up an object or when the monkey simply viewed a human picking up the object (Fogassi et al., 1992). The discovery of these so-called "mirror neurons" provides a simple mechanism for understanding the actions of others by experiencing the action passively in one's mind. In humans, fMRI studies have localized a mirror neuron system to the inferior frontal cortex and the superior parietal lobe (Iacoboni et al., 1999). Human mirror neurons not only allow us to understand and imitate actions; they also appear to be involved in understanding the intentions of others (Iacoboni et al., 2005). Moreover, mirror neurons allow us to experience the emotions of others, thus serving as the foundation of empathy and intentionality (Gallese, 2003; Gallese, Keysers, & Rizzolatti, 2004).

In a study using fMRI, children with ASDs showed a lack of mirror neuron activity in the pars opercularis of the inferior frontal gyrus, which was negatively correlated with social impairment (Dapretto et al., 2006). Similar findings have been reported in studies using event-related potentials, thereby supporting the hypothesis that the mirror neuron system may be dysfunctional in autism (Oberman et al., 2005). Furthermore, reduction in gray matter in the mirror neuron region has been reported in individuals with ASDs (Hadjikhani, Joseph, Snyder, & Tager-Flusberg, 2006), as have atypical activation patterns associated with face processing (Hadjikhani, Joseph, Snyder, & Tager-Flusberg, 2007).

NEUROBIOLOGY

Many neurochemical investigations of autism have been conducted. The identification of biological markers has the potential to facilitate the early and accurate diagnosis of ASDs, to provide direction for biologically based treatments, and to facilitate the identification of subgroups or phenotypes within the spectrum. The more promising pursuits involve serotonin (5-HT), oxytocin (OT), acetylcholine, cortisol, glutamate, and GABA; research on these is briefly reviewed. Studies of dopamine, norepinephrine, and endogenous opioids have been less fruitful.

Serotonin

5-HT is arguably the most studied neurobiological candidate. 5-HT is derived from the fatty acid tryptophan. Serotonergic neuron cell bodies are primarily distributed in clusters in the raphe nuclei of the medulla, pons, and midbrain. The behavioral effects of 5-HT are vast and complex; they include the regulation of mood, arousal, hormone release, pain sensitivity, eating, sexual behavior, and temperature. One of the more consistent early biological findings in autism relates to hyperserotonemia, which occurs in approximately one-third of individuals with autism (e.g., Anderson et al., 1987; McBride et al., 1998; Ritvo et al., 1970; Schain & Freedman, 1961) as well as family members, suggesting a genetic susceptibility (Cook, Leventhal, & Freedman, 1988; Cook et al., 1990; Leventhal, Cook, Morford, Ravitz, & Freedman, 1990). It has since been determined that the majority of whole-blood 5-HT resides in the platelets, which is the factor contributing to the elevated levels of 5-HT in autism (Anderson et al., 1987; Cook et al., 1988). However, research has shown that the prevalence of hyperserotonemia within autism is influenced by pubertal status (lower 5-HT in postpubertal youth) and race (European American youth show lower 5-HT than Hispanic or African American youth), emphasizing the importance of controlling for these potential confounds in neurobiological research (McBride et al., 1998). In addition, the measurement of peripheral 5-HT makes it challenging to form assumptions about central effects. Thus the primary metabolite of 5-HT, 5-hydroxyindoleacetic acid (5-HIAA), investigated via CSF, PET, and treatment studies, has led to the notion that developmental regulation of 5-HT synthesis is dysregulated in autism (Whitaker-Azmitia, 2005). In fact, two polymorphisms have been reported for the serotonin transporter gene (SLC6A4) (e.g., Cook, Courchesne, et al., 1997; Tordjman et al., 2001; Yirmiya et al., 2001). The aforementioned literature of a plausible "serotonin hypothesis" of autism has contributed to the pursuit of pharmaceutical treatment. Importantly, selective serotonin reuptake inhibitors (SSRIs) are among the most frequently prescribed psychotropic medications for individuals with autism (Langworthy-Lam, Aman, & Van Bourgondien, 2002).

The Limbic–Hypothalamic–Pituitary–Adrenal Axis and Cortisol

In addition to being a key regulatory system of stress, the limbic–hypothalamic–pituitary–adrenocortical (LHPA) axis is a major part of the neuroendocrine system. As its name indicates, it involves a network of interactions among the hypothalamus, the pituitary gland, and the adrenal glands. The LHPA axis is involved in the regulation of many biological processes involving mood and emotions, energy metabolism, digestion, immune functioning, and sexual behavior. The responsiveness of the LHPA axis is affected by specific psychological and social factors, which can enhance or diminish the stress response (e.g., Levine, 2000; Levine & Mody, 2003).

A growing body of research has focused on the functioning of the LHPA axis in terms of the diurnal regulation, stress responsiveness, and feedback mechanisms of key regulatory hormones. Some early studies reported dysfunction of the tonic regulation of the LHPA axis in autism (Nir et al., 1995; Yamazaki, Saito, Okada, Fujieda, & Yamashita, 1975) as well as alterations in the normal circadian rhythm (Aihara & Hashimoto, 1989; Hill, Wagner, Shedlarski, & Sears, 1977; Hoshino et al., 1984), which appeared more prominent in low-functioning children with autism. Nevertheless, other investigations have failed to replicate such findings (Richdale & Prior, 1992; Tordjman et al., 1997), instead suggesting that amidst normal temporal placement of the diurnal rhythm, elevations in cortisol during the day may reflect enhanced stress (Richdale & Prior, 1992). Differences in concentration of adrenocorticotropic hormone have also been reported (Curin et al., 2003). An important confounding factor in some of the the earlier studies relates to the potential stressful effects of venipuncture; this confound has been minimized with the advent of salivary cortisol as a valid and reliable index of the unbound hormone in blood (Kirschbaum & Hellhammer, 1994). Thus the majority of recent investigations evaluate cortisol, one of the primary glucocorticoid hormones in humans. Cortisol follows a circadian rhythm: high concentrations in the morning, a decline throughout the day, and the lowest levels in the evening. Response to stress in salivary cortisol can be detected approximately 20 minutes after presentation of a stressor.

Recent work has shown that children with high-functioning autism demonstrate notable variability in diurnal rhythmicity, higher evening cortisol, and alterations in morning cortisol over time (Corbett et al., 2006; Corbett, Mendoza, Wegelin, Carmean, & Levine, 2008). Importantly, the variability in the cortisol rhythm of persons with autism may be related to such factors as sensory sensitivity and cumulative stress associated with changes in routine throughout the day (Corbett, Schupp, Levine, & Mendoza, 2009). In addition, several studies have shown an exaggerated stress response to various medical and environmental events (Corbett et al., 2006; Maher, Harper, Macleay, & King, 1975; Richdale & Prior, 1992; Tordjman et al., 1997), although individual and group differences exist (Corbett, Mendoza, et al., 2008). These findings emphasize the notable heterogeneity in ASDs not only in behavioral profile, but in underlying biological presentation.

Oxytocin

OT is a hypothalamic peptide synthesized in the paraventricular nucleus and the supraoptic nucleus. Receptors for OT are located throughout the brain, including the limbic system. OT is crucial to the formation of social bonds (Carter, 1998; Insel, 1997; Insel et al., 1993; Winslow, Noble, Lyons, Sterk, & Insel, 2003; Winslow, Shapiro, Carter, & Insel, 1993). Research with both animal models (e.g., Bales, Kim, Lewis-Reese, & Sue Carter, 2004; Carter, 1998; Insel, O'Brien, & Leckman, 1999; Winslow et al., 2003; Young, Wang, & Insel, 1998) and humans (Kirsch, et al., 2005; Kosfeld, Heinrichs, Zak, Fischbacher, & Fehr, 2005) provides compelling evidence for the involvement of OT in mediating complex social behavior. Furthermore, it appears that OT is an important moderator of stress (Carter, 1998; Kirsch et al., 2005; Kosfeld et al., 2005; Neumann, 2002; Neumann, Kromer, Toschi, & Ebner, 2000).

Due to its important role in social behavior, OT has been proposed as a plausible neurobiological substrate in autism (Insel, 1997). Previously it was reported that individuals with autism exhibit impaired OT processing, resulting in higher levels of plasma OT-X (a precursor to the normal adult form of OT) and lower levels of OT itself (Green et al., 2001; Modahl et al., 1998). Furthermore, higher levels of OT have been found in autistic children characterized as aloof (Modahl et al., 1998). Although treatments have only recently been explored,

early reports suggest that administration of OT may improve the ability of adults with ASDs to determine the emotional significance of speech (Hollander et al., 2007) and may reduce repetitive behaviors (Hollander et al., 2003). Most recently, genetic associations have been reported between the OT receptor gene (OXTR) and autism (Jacob et al., 2007; Wu et al., 2005; Ylisaukko-oja et al., 2006).

Melatonin

The sleep patterns of individuals with ASDs have been reported to be disturbed to varying degrees (Goodlin-Jones, Tang, Liu, & Anders, 2008; Johnson & Malow, 2008; Krakowiak, Goodlin-Jones, Hertz-Picciotto, Croen, & Hansen, 2008; Malow, McGrew, Harvey, Henderson, & Stone, 2006). Melatonin (also known chemically as N-acetyl-5-methoxytryptamine), a naturally occurring hormone produced by the pineal gland, is considered a key regulator of circadian and seasonal rhythms and is important for human cognition. Low and abnormal patterns of melatonin (Nir et al., 1995; Tordjman, Anderson, Pichard, Charbuy, & Touitou, 2005), which ostensibly contribute to reported sleep disturbances, have been noted in individuals with ASDs. Recently, evidence for a link between low melatonin level and the ASMT gene (which encodes the last enzyme of melatonin synthesis) has been reported; this is hypothesized to be a risk factor for ASDs (Melke et al., 2008). Such neurobiological and genetic findings provide support for a role of synaptic and clock genes as susceptibility risk factors in ASDs (Bourgeron, 2007). Moreover, recent investigations showing the beneficial effects of melatonin in the treatment of ASDs and sleep disturbances has been promising (Andersen, Kaczmarska, McGrew, & Malow, 2008; Garstang & Wallis, 2006; Giannotti, Cortesi, Cerquiglini, & Bernabei, 2006)

Glutamate and GABA

Glutamate and GABA are two essential neurotransmitters in the CNS; they are principally responsible for excitatory and inhibitory communication throughout the brain, respectively. Since many brain regions have been implicated in the neuropathology of autism, research on the functioning of these neurotransmitters would seem to be a promising area, but they have received comparatively limited consideration. The majority of the findings suggest that the GABAergic system in autism is suppressed and therefore results in enhanced glutamate activity (Fatemi, 2008a; Fatemi et al., 2002; Hussman, 2001). As noted, approximately 30% of persons with autism have comorbid seizures (Volkmar & Nelson, 1990). GABA(B) receptors play a critical role in maintaining the excitatory–inhibitory balance in the CNS, such that imbalance in these regulatory receptors can result in seizures. Recently, Fatemi and colleagues (2009) investigated four GABA(B) receptor subunits in the cerebellum, Brodmann area 9 (BA 9), and BA 40, showing reductions in the levels of at least two of the GABA subunits. Interestingly, the presence of seizures did not significantly alter GABA expression. The findings provide strong evidence for pervasive GABAergic dysfunction in the brains of persons with autism.

TREATMENT

Even when individuals with ASDs share behavioral and genetic profiles, it is important to keep their unique strengths, challenges, and needs in mind when choosing among available treatment options. Individualized treatments may include consultations with and services from a number of professionals and paraprofessionals, including medical doctors, psychiatrists, geneticists, psychologists, teachers, classroom support services, speech and language therapists, occupational therapists, and physical therapists. Moreover, it has been strongly suggested that care providers and educators receive specialized training in ASDs to be most effective. Intervention models that utilize more intensive and interactive training, including hands-on activities, modeling, practice, and feedback, appear most effective (Swiezy, Stuart, & Korzekwa, 2008). Consistency is critical not only in a child's behavioral and education programming, but also in service delivery across medical, home, educational, and community settings (Swiezy et al., 2008). Regardless of treatment choice, it is well established that early diagnosis and inter-

vention offer the best opportunity for the optimal development and outcome of children with ASDs (Birnbrauer & Leach, 1993; Harris, Handleman, Gordon, Kristoff, & Fuentes, 1991; Lovaas, Newsom, & Hickman, 1987). The impact of experience on the developing brain is particularly strong for the acquisition of certain skills (Knudsen, 2004), such as language and social skills (Wetherby, Watt, Morgan, & Shumway, 2007). Outcome predictors include age at time of admission, level of IQ, language functioning, and diagnostic severity (e.g., Smith, Groen, & Wynn, 2000). It is believed that the success of early intervention may be due to brain plasticity (Dawson & Zanolli, 2003).

Behavioral Approaches

Applied Behavior Analysis

Applied behavior analysis (ABA) is based on scientifically derived theories of learning and behavior. ABA breaks down complex behaviors into individual teachable skills through a process referred to as *task analysis*. These skills are then taught in a systematic, step-by-step format as part of an individualized, comprehensive behavioral program. This use of intensive, structured behavioral methods was introduced by Lovaas (e.g., Lovaas, 1987; Lovaas, Koegel, & Schreibman, 1979). In Lovaas's approach, a trainer gives an instruction or presents a stimulus, requires a behaviorally defined response from the child, and presents a consequence that either rewards an appropriate response or marks an inappropriate one. The systematic presentation of a stimulus, including the child's response or nonresponse, is commonly known as a trial. Consequently, ABA is sometimes referred to as *discrete-trial training*. Although the two terms have become virtually interchangeable, ABA is intended to refer to the science of behavior analysis (Kates-McElrath & Axelrod, 2006).

Not only do successful ABA programs teach skills; they also utilize functional behavior analysis to reduce maladaptive behaviors that impede the effectiveness of educational and intervention programs (Matson & Rivet, 2008; Murphy et al., 2005). Maladaptive behaviors in autism can range from stereotypical actions that are odd but harmless, such as rocking or hand flapping, to self-injury, such as biting or head banging. In addition, some individuals with autism may exhibit impulsive behaviors (e.g., running into traffic) or aggressive behaviors (e.g., hitting others) (Joosten, Bundy, & Einfeld, 2009; Matson & Rivet, 2008). The ABA approach takes great care to ensure that behavioral improvements are the direct results of the employed technique (e.g., Steege, Mace, Perry, & Longenecker, 2007). Despite procedural concerns regarding Lovaas's initial research (Gresham & Macmillan, 1997; Mundy, 1993; Schopler, Short, & Mesibov, 1989), it is well established that early intervention based on ABA can result in significant, comprehensive, and lasting improvements for children with autism (e.g., Birnbrauer & Leach, 1993; Eikeseth, Smith, Jahr, & Eldevik, 2002; Lovaas, 1987; Lovaas et al., 1979; Lovaas & Smith, 1989; McEachin, Smith, & Lovaas, 1993; Smith et al., 2000).

Verbal Behavior Intervention

Verbal behavior intervention is sometimes used along with ABA; it is based on B. F. Skinner's work proposing that language, just like any other behavior, is based on operant principles (Sundberg & Michael, 2001). Skinner considered a functional analysis of language to consist primarily of *mands* (requests), *tacts* (words that are under the control of the nonverbal environment, including nouns, verbs, adjectives, etc.), *echoics* (vocal imitation), and *intraverbals* (conversational language).

Pivotal Response Training

Although based on the principles of ABA, pivotal response training (PRT) targets behavioral change in a different manner. Whereas ABA targets individual behaviors and teaches specific skills (e.g., putting a shirt on), PRT focuses on increasing children's motivation by focusing on their interests and responding to their initiations. Pivotal skills such as communication, social exchanges, and self-management are targeted. Research indicates that PRT is successful at increasing language ability in children with autism (Koegel, O'Dell, & Koegel, 1987; Laski, Charlop, & Schreibman, 1988), symbolic play (Stahmer, 1995), and social behaviors (Pierce & Schreibman, 1997).

Developmental Approaches

Developmental treatments for autism focus on a child's inherent strengths to increase social, emotional, and cognitive skills.

Developmental, Individual-Difference, Relationship-Based/Floortime Model

The floortime model assumes that a child's actions are purposeful. Within this framework, the caregiver is encouraged to build a relationship by following the child's lead (Wieder & Greenspan, 2003). It is believed that social and communication skills will follow. Independent, peer-reviewed studies on this method are lacking.

Relationship Development Interaction

Relationship development interaction (RDI) attempts to address the social deficits of autism by fostering positive interactions. Proponents believe that the experience of positive social interactions will encourage a child to value interpersonal relationships, and thus will promote the acquisition of language and social skills. Some research indicates that this may be an effective treatment to enhance the social-emotional functioning of children with ASDs (Mahoney & Perales, 2003).

Educational Approaches

A number of public school systems utilize Treatment and Education of Autistic and related Communication-Handicapped Children (TEACCH) procedures. In the TEACH model, a variety of approaches are used to address an individual's deficits while encouraging independence. A TEACCH classroom has well-defined work stations for separate tasks and relies on visual supports (written or picture schedules). Several studies have demonstrated the effectiveness of the TEACCH model in regard to learning, communication, socialization, self-care, and behavior improvements (Panerai, Ferrante, & Caputo, 1997; Schopler, 2000; Schopler, Brehm, Kinsbourne, & Reichler, 1971).

Visual Approaches

Video Modeling

Video modeling is a well-validated behavioral intervention that relies on visual–auditory technology for the active presentation of material on a television or computer screen. Targeted behaviors are presented to the learner in short scenes that are viewed, imitated, and practiced. Video modeling has been shown to be particularly helpful for children with autism, as a result of reducing the field of view, providing the opportunity for repeated viewing of the targeted behavior, and presenting the material in a highly reinforcing format (Corbett & Abdullah, 2005). Such modeling has been used to target a variety of behaviors, including language, social skills, perspective taking, play, academics, and adaptive skills (Charlop-Christy, Le, & Freeman, 2000; Charlop & Milstein, 1989; Corbett, 2003; LeBlanc et al., 2003).

Picture Exchange Communication System

The Picture Exchange Communication System (PECS) is an augmented communication system that utilizes pictures to help children with autism functionally communicate (Bondy & Frost, 1994; Siegel, 1999). Communicating with pictures is especially helpful for those with motor planning difficulties who have trouble engaging in sign language. A study evaluating the efficacy of this system found that children with autism demonstrated improvements in social communication and a decrease in maladaptive behaviors (Charlop-Christy, Carpenter, Le, LeBlanc, & Kellet, 2002).

Specific Treatments

Depending on a child's individual needs, it may also be important to include other therapies in a tailored treatment approach.

Speech Therapy

Speech therapy is used not only to habilitate articulation errors, but also to enhance social and communication skills through the development of pragmatic language. Pragmatic language training assists those who misuse language or misunderstand the meaning or intent of others' communications. Speech and language therapy includes the teaching of nonverbal communication and augmentative communication skills.

Occupational Therapy

Occupational therapy remediates fine and gross motor skills, as well as sensory processing deficits. Many people with autism are hypersensitive or hyposensitive to touch, light, or noise. Sensory integration techniques used to address such concerns may include sensory brushing, swinging bouncing, or deep pressure. Although anecdotal reports indicate improvement in regulation and focus (Iarocci & McDonald, 2006; Kane, Luiselli, Dearborn, & Young, 2004), there is a lack of empirically driven research to support the efficacy of these approaches (Baranek, 2002; Dawson & Watling, 2000; Kane et al., 2004).

Social Skills Training

Difficulties in relating to people and engaging in reciprocal conversation are core features of ASDs. Although reciprocal conversation skills are typically learned through common day-to-day events of a child's life, it is often necessary to teach these skills directly and specifically to a child with an ASD. Basic skills include eye contact, listening, joint attention, imitation, and turn taking. Successful social interactions also require the sophisticated integration of nonverbal communication (e.g., facial expression, body language, communicative gestures), verbal communication (e.g., tone of voice, prosody), perspective taking, emotion processing, and many other social signals. Many types of social skill interventions have been developed, such as trained-peer interactions, social skills groups, cartoon stories, social scripts, video modeling (see above), and drama therapy. Specific approaches include Michelle Garcia Winner's Social Thinking Curriculum (*www.socialthinking. com*) and Carol Gray's Social Stories (*www. thegraycenter.org*).

Well-designed studies have shown several of these strategies to be effective. For example, a 20-week curriculum was designed to address the social-emotional functioning of 18 boys ages 8–12 years who were diagnosed with autism, Asperger syndrome, or PDD-

NOS (Solomon, Goodlin-Jones, & Anders, 2004). Specific targeted skills included basic conversation, facial recognition, emotional understanding, and individual and group problem solving. While the boys attended the 90-minute social skills sessions, their parents participated in semistructured psychoeducational training. The study showed statistically significant improvements in emotion recognition and problem-solving ability, and a reduction in inappropriate behaviors. In addition, decreases on depression scores were found for older and more cognitively impaired boys and for mothers (Solomon et al., 2004). (For excellent reviews of other social skill interventions, see Rao, Beidel, & Murray, 2008; Rogers, 2000; and Stichter, Randolph, Gage, & Schmidt, 2007.)

Pharmaceutical Approaches

As noted throughout this chapter, the behavior problems of individuals with ASDs may hinder their ability to function in the world. Psychopharmacological treatments are frequently considered when behavioral or educational approaches do not adequately manage problematic behaviors. Although few medications have been approved for the treatment of ASDs by the U.S. Food and Drug Administration (FDA) (*www.fda.gov/bbs/topics/news/2006*), a number of medications for ASDs are prescribed "off-label"; that is, they are prescribed to individuals or for symptoms outside the scope approved by the FDA (Moussavand & Findling, 2007).

It appears that a large percentage of individuals on the autism spectrum take some form of medication. Two surveys found that approximately half of subjects with PDDs were taking prescription medications (Aman, Lam, & Van Bourgondien, 2005; Hanson et al., 2007). One of these surveys (Aman et al., 2005) found that 16.5% of participants were prescribed an antipsychotic drug. Antipsychotic medications have been used for some time to treat severe behavior problems, presumably by reducing the activity of dopamine in the brain (Posey, Stigler, Erickson, & McDougle, 2008). The typical antipsychotic haloperidol (Haldol) has been used to treat autism-related hyperactivity, aggression, withdrawal, and stereotypic behavior (McCracken et al., 2002). However, Haldol has been associated with the development of drug-related dyskinesias (abnormal involuntary movements); thus other medications, such as atypical antipsychotics, are often considered (Campbell et al., 1997). Atypical antipsychotics, such as risperidone, not only affect dopamine but also reduce 5-HT (Posey et al., 2008). A number of studies have determined the effectiveness of risperidone for behaviors associated with autism. For example, a double-blind, placebo-controlled study of adults with autism found that risperidone was effective for the reduction of repetitive and aggressive behaviors (McDougle et al., 1998). In addition, the Research Units on Pediatric Psychopharmacology (RUPP) Autism Network completed an 8-week, double-blind, placebo-controlled study of risperidone for children and adolescents with autism. A 57% reduction in rate of irritability was noted in the individuals treated with risperidone, as compared with a 14% reduction in the placebo group (McCracken et al., 2002). These, among other studies, led to the FDA's 2006 approval of risperidone for the treatment of irritability, aggression, self-injury, and temper tantrums in children and adolescents with autism (*www.fda.gov/bbs/topics/news/2006*). Other atypical antipsychotics have been considered to treat autistic symptoms, including olanzapine (Zyprexa) (Potenza, Holmes, Kanes, & McDougle, 1999) and ziprasidone (Geodon) (Malone, Delaney, Hyman, & Cater, 2007).

Although SSRIs are usually prescribed for symptoms of anxiety, depression, and obsessive–compulsive disorder, a number of studies (e.g., DeLong, Teague, & McSwain Kamran, 1998) have found decreased repetitive behaviors, along with improvement in language, and social behaviors. Children with autism have also been treated with anticonvulsants (Aman, Van Bourgondien, Wolford, & Sarphare, 1995), such as topriamate (Topomax) and valproic acid (Depokote), as well as stimulant medications (Ritalin) to decrease impulsivity and hyperactivity (Quintana et al., 1995).

CONTROVERSIAL TOPICS

Autism has long been plagued by a plethora of controversial theories and treatments spawned from anecdotal reports, parental urgency, and sensationalized media reports.

Most of these have not been subjected to rigorous clinical research. It is easy to understand how parents looking for solutions will eagerly consider alternative ideas and treatments; however, pursuing ineffective interventions, even if they are not actively harmful, wastes valuable time and resources that might be applied to more meaningful and productive endeavors (Baranek, 2002).

Complementary and Alternative Medicine

Complementary and alternative medicine (CAM) treatments are often selected by parents because they ostensibly target the causes of autism, as opposed to the symptoms. Levy and Hyman (2005) have categorized CAM approaches based on the proposed mechanisms underlying the symptoms: immune modulation, gastrointestinal functioning, neurotransmitter functioning, or nonbiological mechanisms. The use of CAM approaches is widespread, as shown in a large chart review study from one leading U.S. children's hospital revealing that such approaches had been used for 30% of children with autism; in 9% of these cases, the methods were considered potentially dangerous (Levy, Mandell, Merhar, Ittenbach, & Pinto-Martin, 2003). Several CAM treatments that have captivated certain sectors of the autism community; some of these are described below.

Secretin

A highly publicized patient series reported the incidental findings of improved social and language skills in three children with ASDs following the administration of secretin, a peptide hormone (Horvath et al., 1998). Despite the absence of empirical evidence regarding the amelioration of symptoms, parents eagerly sought secretin treatment. As a result, dozens of experimental trials were initiated to investigate the effect of single and repeated doses of intravenous porcine secretin; many of these were well-designed, double-blind, placebo-controlled crossover trials. The results consistently showed secretin's lack of efficacy for the treatment of autistic disorder (e.g., Corbett et al., 2001; Levy, Souders, et al., 2003; Owley et al., 2001; Sandler et al., 1999).

Tomatis and Related Methods

The Tomatis method, which has often been compared to auditory integration therapy (Berard, 1993), is another controversial treatment showing limited if any benefit for children with autism (for a review, see Baranek, 2002). Both the Tomatis method and auditory integration therapy are forms of sound therapy that use high- and low-frequency-filtered music designed to modulate the acoustical signal. Anecdotal reports of Tomatis claim that using modified music stimulates connections between the ear and the CNS, resulting in improved communication and behavior in children with autism (Thompson & Andrews, 2000). However, in a recent double-blind, placebo-controlled, crossover study, no treatment effects were observed (Corbett, Shickman, & Ferrer, 2008).

Other methods lacking empirical support, to name a few, include the Rapid Prompting Method and the Son-Rise Program. The Rapid Prompting Method incorporates nearly continuous interaction and prompting, paired with an alphabet board for responses (*www.halo-soma.org*). The Son-Rise Program emphasizes building a non-force-based, nonjudgmental relationship with a child (*www.autismtreatmentcenter.org*).

Biomedical Treatments

Finally, biomedical treatments for ASDs are based on the idea that specific *in utero* or postbirth environmental insults may contribute to the onset of these disorders. Biomedical theories contend that interactions between genes and environment have the potential to trigger an ASD. Environmental insults are thought to include toxic chemicals (e.g., heavy metals, medications, antibiotics, pesticides, preservatives), as well as reductions in nutrients presumably due to modern food preparation, cooking, and diet (Taylor & Rogers, 2005). Although biomedical concerns encompass all major systems of the body, the most widely publicized biomedical treatments have been associated with the gastrointestinal and immune systems.

Gastrointestinal concerns have included the so-called "leaky gut syndrome," which purportedly leads to increased permeability of the intestines, resulting in an inability to break down proteins from dairy (casein) and grains (gluten). Gluten–casein elimination diets have been designed to target this problem (Cornish, 2002; Knivsberg, Reichelt, Hoien, & Nodland, 2002). It is further theorized that gastrointestinal problems and poor absorption of nutrients may result in nutritional imbalances or deficiencies, as well as a buildup of toxins in the system. Proponents have subsequently recommended supplemental enzymes, vitamins, and minerals to address nutritional deficiencies. Detoxification with vitamin B12 and chelation therapy have both been used to diminish the alleged buildup of heavy metals in body tissue (Martineau, Barthelemy, Cheliakine, & Lelord, 1988). Other measures have included the use of intravenous immune globulin in which antibodies extracted from plasma are administered to treat the immune system and are alleged to address core symptoms of autism. For more information, see the Autism Research Institute website (*www.autism.com*).

It is important to note that most CAM approaches are not generally accepted by the mainstream medical community, as they are often based on anecdotal reports and limited scientific evidence or theory. Levy and colleagues have methodically reviewed many CAM practices, providing the rationale to refute the use of several, while presenting emerging evidence for some that are promising (Levy & Hyman, 2005, 2008; Levy, Mandell, et al., 2003).

The Vaccine Controversy

More than a decade of confusion ensued after a leading medical journal, *Lancet*, published Andrew Wakefield's 1998 article contending that ASDs and the measles/mumps/rubella vaccine were linked. In February 2010, *Lancet* retracted the entire study from published record after the General Medical Council of the United Kingdom found Wakefield's findings to be false. The association between ASDs and vaccines appears to be essentially a temporal link, due to the fact that symptoms often begin between 18 and 24 months of age—a period that often coincides with immunizations. It was also suggested that thimerosol, a mercury-based preservative for many vaccines, had toxic

effects contributing to the onset of autism (e.g., Bernard, Enayati, Redwood, Roger, & Binstock, 2001; Hornig, Chian, & Lipkin, 2004). Although the point is still being contended by some, the Immunization Safety Review (2004) refuted a causal link between autism and vaccines containing thimerosal. The potentially dangerous aftermath of such poorly investigated claims is demonstrated through the unfortunate reoccurrence of measles. Measles was thought to be eradicated in the United States; however, 64 new confirmed cases were reported to the Centers for Disease Control and Prevention in 2008. It is thought that this increase was at least partially due to the unsupported links between immunizations and ASDs.

COMORBIDITY AND PHENOTYPES

Comorbid symptoms, such as anxiety, depression, and attention-deficit/hyperactivity disorder (ADHD), contribute to the heterogeneous ASD profile. Children and adolescents with ASDs experience significantly greater mood disturbance and anxiety than peers do (Gillott, Furniss, & Walter, 2001; Kim, Szatmari, Bryson, Steiner, & Wilson, 2000). It has also been shown that more severe cases of autism are often distinguished by the presence of anxiety (Rescorla, 1988). It has been suggested that social skills and physiological arousal may provide protective and predisposing factors, respectively, in adolescents with ASDs (Bellini, 2006).

Despite the frequent report of co-occurring ADHD symptoms, the current diagnostic manual (APA, 2000) prevents the practice of diagnosing ADHD along with a PDD. Nevertheless, neuropsychological models are emerging to elucidate the co-occurrence of ASDs and ADHD, and to support the high preponderance of comorbid features (e.g., Corbett & Constantine, 2006; Corbett, Constantine, Hendren, Rocke, & Ozonoff, 2009; Geurts, Verte, Oosterlaan, Roeyers, & Sergeant, 2004; Goldberg et al., 2005; Goldstein & Schwebach, 2004; Landa & Goldberg, 2005). An additive or interactive effect stemming from dysfunction in various neural networks may contribute to the heterogeneous profile (e.g., Castellanos, Sonuga-Barke, Milham, & Tannock, 2006; Nigg, Willcutt, Doyle, & Sonuga-Barke,

2005; Sergeant, Geurts, Huijbregts, Scheres, & Oosterlaan, 2003; Sonuga-Barke, 2005). It has been proposed that children with both sets of symptoms are more functionally impaired and may respond differently to treatment (Arnold et al., 2006; Goldstein & Schwebach, 2004; Kadesjo & Gillberg, 2001; Posey, et al., 2006).

ADULT CARE AND TREATMENT

Most ASD research focuses on the assessment and treatment of children, whereas comparatively little is known about adults with ASDs (Eaves & Ho, 2008). Investigations to determine the particular concerns of both young adults and elderly persons with ASDs are clearly needed. Limited research in sexuality reveals that adults with autism demonstrate both appropriate and inappropriate sexual desires, understanding, and behaviors (Hellemans, Colson, Verbraeken, Vermeiren, & Deboutte, 2007; Stokes, Newton, & Kaur, 2007). A 5-year longitudinal follow-up study measured the lifestyle outcomes of 140 males with ASDs; occupation, living situation, interpersonal relationships, and participation in leisure activities were assessed (Cederlund, Hagberg, Billstedt, Gillberg, & Gillberg, 2008). In general, individuals with Asperger syndrome fared better than those with autism. Twenty-seven percent of those with Asperger syndrome demonstrated good outcomes, whereas the remainder reported fair to poor outcomes. Of the individuals with autism, none reported good outcomes, and the majority reported very poor outcomes. Not surprisingly, lower IQ was associated with poorer outcomes for both groups (Cederlund et al., 2008). Regarding emotional status, relatively high rates of depression, anxiety, and suicidal ideation have been described in adults with ASDs (Shtayermman, 2007). Currently, a few successful interventions are directed at teaching adults with autism. For example, the TEACCH approach has been successfully adapted to work with adults (Van Bourgondien & Schopler, 1996). In addition, a 10-session, 2- to 3-hour program designed to teach self-determination has shown promise (Fullterton, 1999). Importantly, challenging behaviors must be considered when designing programs for adults, just as

they are for children with ASDs (Matson & Rivet, 2008).

CONCLUSIONS

It is important to note that this brief review of some key findings about ASDs is not exhaustive and cannot begin to capture the depth and breadth of this ever-expanding field. It is apparent that in order to make sense of this complex spectrum of neurodevelopmental disorders, many approaches, ranging from cellular to behavioral, need to be employed and synthesized. However, equally important are multidisciplinary efforts to bring together discrepant findings and to create models that may ultimately lead to workable theories. For example, identifying the similarities and differences in neuroanatomy and comparing these with clinical presentations will permit expanded insight into underlying neurobiology (Bauman & Kemper, 2003). Although the field has accumulated significant data, such findings are infrequently integrated into systematic theories or translated into new hypothesis-driven treatments. Currently, the ASD field is poised to usher in a new era grounded in the scientific method—an era that "moves beyond the descriptive phase of observations to form hypotheses, collect data systematically, define the evidence, and establish testable theories" (Zimmerman, 2008, p. vi).

There is a tendency in the field to leap quickly from data to theory, without the necessary systematic replication and validation steps in between. This is especially critical in the study of a population with such a heterogeneous presentation. To this end, there has been a concerted effort in the field to use consistent diagnostic tools to improve the selection, identification, and characterization of persons with ASDs. Furthermore, larger studies using comparable methodologies are needed to replicate and extend promising findings from smaller pilot studies. The expanded awareness of ASDs has also resulted in exponential growth of a broad array of approaches and interpretations. Amidst the greater insight, however, the ASD field has been plagued by a number of isolated and unusual findings that have resulted in public debate and unfounded theories. This state of affairs has detoured scientific inquiry and funding. Thus, in the years to come, it will be important to allow rigorous scientific findings to guide the field, rather than public opinion or anecdotal reports in the mass media. In the process, meaningful isolated findings will have an opportunity to emerge and be integrated into system-based approaches that can be explored in sound theoretical frameworks.

REFERENCES

Abell, F., Krams, M., Ashburner, J., Passingham, R., Friston, K., Frackowiak, R., et al. (1999). The neuroanatomy of autism: A voxel-based whole brain analysis of structural scans. *NeuroReport, 10*(8), 1647–1651.

Abrahams, B. S., & Geschwind, D. H. (2008). Advances in autism genetics: On the threshold of a new neurobiology. *Nature Reviews Genetics, 9*(5), 341–355.

Adolphs, R., Sears, L., & Piven, J. (2001). Abnormal processing of social information from faces in autism. *Journal of Cognitive Neuroscience, 13*(2), 232–240.

Aihara, R., & Hashimoto, T. (1989). [Neuroendocrinologic studies on autism]. *No To Hattatsu, 21*(2), 154–162.

Allik, H., Larsson, J. O., & Smedje, H. (2006). Insomnia in school-age children with Asperger syndrome or high-functioning autism. *BMC Psychiatry, 6*, 18.

Aman, M. G., Lam, K. S., & Van Bourgondien, M. E. (2005). Medication patterns in patients with autism: Temporal, regional, and demographic influences. *Journal of Child Adolescent Psychopharmacology, 15*(1), 116–126.

Aman, M. G., Van Bourgondien, M. E., Wolford, P. L., & Sarphare, G. (1995). Psychotropic and anticonvulsant drugs in subjects with autism: Prevalence and patterns of use. *Journal of American Academy of Child and Adolescent Psychiatry, 34*(12), 1672–1681.

Amaral, D. G., & Corbett, B. A. (2003). The amygdala, autism and anxiety. *Novartis Foundation Symposium, 251*, 177–187 (discussion 187–197, 281–297).

Amaral, D. G., Schumann, C. M., & Nordahl, C. W. (2008). Neuroanatomy of autism. *Trends in Neurosciences, 31*(3), 137–145.

American Psychiatric Association (APA). (2000). *Diagnostic and statistical manual of mental disorders* (4th ed., text rev.). Washington, DC: Author.

Amir, R. E., Van den Veyver, I. B., Wan, M., Tran, C. Q., Francke, U., & Zoghbi, H. Y. (1999). Rett syndrome is caused by mutations in X-linked MECP2, encoding methyl-CpG-binding protein 2. *Nature Genetics, 23*(2), 185–188.

Andersen, I. M., Kaczmarska, J., McGrew, S. G., & Malow, B. A. (2008). Melatonin for insomnia in children with autism spectrum disorders. *Journal of Child Neurology, 23*(5), 482–485.

Anderson, G. M., Freedman, D. X., Cohen, D. J., Volkmar, F. R., Hoder, E. L., McPhedran, P., et al. (1987). Whole blood serotonin in autistic and normal subjects. *Journal of Child Psychology and Psychiatry, 28*(6), 885–900.

Arnold, L. E., Aman, M. G., Cook, A. M., Witwer, A. N., Hall, K. L., Thompson, S., et al. (2006). Atomoxetine for hyperactivity in autism spectrum disorders: Placebo-controlled crossover pilot trial. *Journal of American Academy of Child and Adolescent Psychiatry, 45*(10), 1196–1205.

Ashwin, C., Baron-Cohen, S., Wheelwright, S., O'Riordan, M., & Bullmore, E. T. (2007). Differential activation of the amygdala and the 'social brain' during fearful face-processing in Asperger syndrome. *Neuropsychologia, 45*(1), 2–14.

Ashwin, C., Wheelwright, S., & Baron-Cohen, S. (2006). Finding a face in the crowd: Testing the anger superiority effect in Asperger syndrome. *Brain and Cognition, 61*(1), 78–95.

Ashwood, P., & Van de Water, J. (2004). A review of autism and the immune response. *Clinical and Developmental Immunology, 11*(2), 165–174.

Asperger, H. (1991). Autistic psychopathy in childhood. In U. Frith (Ed.), *Autism and Asperger syndrome* (pp. 37–92). Cambridge, UK: Cambridge University Press.

Aylward, E. H., Minshew, N. J., Field, K., Sparks, B. F., & Singh, N. (2002). Effects of age on brain volume and head circumference in autism. *Neurology, 59*(2), 175–183.

Aylward, E. H., Minshew, N. J., Goldstein, G., Honeycutt, N. A., Augustine, A. M., Yates, K. O., et al. (1999). MRI volumes of amygdala and hippocampus in non-mentally retarded autistic adolescents and adults. *Neurology, 53*(9), 2145–2150.

Bailey, A., Luthert, P., Dean, A., Harding, B., Janota, I., Montgomery, M., et al. (1998). A clinicopathological study of autism. *Brain, 121*(Pt. 5), 889–905.

Bailey, A., Phillips, W., & Rutter, M. (1996). Autism: Towards an integration of clinical, genetic, neuropsychological, and neurobiological perspectives. *Journal of Child Psychology and Psychiatry, 37*(1), 89–126.

Bales, K. L., Kim, A. J., Lewis-Reese, A. D., & Sue Carter, C. (2004). Both oxytocin and vasopressin may influence alloparental behavior in male prairie voles. *Hormones and Behavior, 45*(5), 354–361.

Baranek, G. T. (2002). Efficacy of sensory and motor interventions for children with autism. *Journal of Autism and Developmental Disorders, 32*(5), 397–422.

Baron-Cohen, S., Ring, H. A., Bullmore, E. T.,

Wheelwright, S., Ashwin, C., & Williams, S. C. (2000). The amygdala theory of autism. *Neuroscience and Biobehavioral Reviews, 24*(3), 355–364.

Baron-Cohen, S., Ring, H. A., Wheelwright, S., Bullmore, E. T., Brammer, M. J., Simmons, A., et al. (1999). Social intelligence in the normal and autistic brain: An fMRI study. *European Journal of Neuroscience, 11*(6), 1891–1898.

Barrett, C. F., & Tsien, R. W. (2008). The Timothy syndrome mutation differentially affects voltage- and calcium-dependent inactivation of CaV1.2 L-type calcium channels. *Proceedings of the National Academy of Sciences, USA, 105*(6), 2157–2162.

Bauman, M. L., & Kemper, T. L. (1985). Histoanatomic observations of the brain in early infantile autism. *Neurology, 35*(6), 866–874.

Bauman, M. L., & Kemper, T. L. (2003). The neuropathology of the autism spectrum disorders: What have we learned? *Novartis Foundation Symposium, 251,* 112–122 (discussion 122–118, 281–297).

Bauman, M. L., & Kemper, T. L. (2005). Neuroanatomic observations of the brain in autism: A review and future directions. *International Journal of Developmental Neuroscience, 23*(2–3), 183–187.

Bellini, S. (2006). The development of social anxiety in adolescents with autism spectrum disorders. *Focus on Autism and Other Developmental Disabilities, 21*(3), 138–145.

Berard, G. (1993). *Hearing equals behavior.* New Canaan, CT: Keats.

Bernard, S., Enayati, A., Redwood, L., Roger, H., & Binstock, T. (2001). Autism: A novel form of mercury poisoning. *Medical Hypotheses, 56*(4), 462–471.

Berument, S. K., Rutter, M., Lord, C., Pickles, A., & Bailey, A. (1999). Autism screening questionnaire: Diagnostic validity. *British Journal of Psychiatry, 175,* 444–451.

Birnbrauer, J. S., & Leach, D. J. (1993). The Murdock early intervention program after 2 years. *Behavior Change, 10,* 63–74.

Bondy, A., & Frost, L. (1994). The Picture Exchange Communication System. *Focus on Autistic Behavior, 9,* 1–19.

Bourgeron, T. (2007). The possible interplay of synaptic and clock genes in autism spectrum disorders. *Cold Spring Harbor Symposium on Quantitative Biology, 72,* 645–654.

Bukelis, I., Porter, F. D., Zimmerman, A. W., & Tierney, E. (2007). Smith–Lemli–Opitz syndrome and autism spectrum disorder. *American Journal of Psychiatry, 164*(11), 1655–1661.

Campbell, M., Armenteros, J. L., Malone, R. P., Adams, P. B., Eisenberg, Z. W., & Overall, J. E. (1997). Neuroleptic-related dyskinesias in autistic children: A prospective, longitudinal study. *Journal of the American Academy of Child and Adolescent Psychiatry, 36*(6), 835–843.

Cantor, R. M., Kono, N., Duvall, J. A., Alvarez-Retuerto, A., Stone, J. L., Alarcon, M., et al. (2005). Replication of autism linkage: fine-mapping peak at 17q21. *American Journal of Human Genetics, 76*(6), 1050–1056.

Carper, R. A., & Courchesne, E. (2005). Localized enlargement of the frontal cortex in early autism. *Biological Psychiatry, 57*(2), 126–133.

Carter, C. S. (1998). Neuroendocrine perspectives on social attachment and love. *Psychoneuroendocrinology, 23*(8), 779–818.

Casanova, M. F. (2006). Neuropathological and genetic findings in autism: The significance of a putative minicolumnopathy. *Neuroscientist, 12*(5), 435–441.

Casanova, M. F., Buxhoeveden, D., & Gomez, J. (2003). Disruption in the inhibitory architecture of the cell minicolumn: Implications for autisim. *Neuroscientist, 9*(6), 496–507.

Casanova, M. F., Buxhoeveden, D. P., Switala, A. E., & Roy, E. (2002a). Minicolumnar pathology in autism. *Neurology, 58*(3), 428–432.

Casanova, M. F., Buxhoeveden, D. P., Switala, A. E., & Roy, E. (2002b). Neuronal density and architecture (Gray Level Index) in the brains of autistic patients. *Journal of Child Neurology, 17*(7), 515–521.

Casanova, M. F., van Kooten, I. A., Switala, A. E., van Engeland, H., Heinsen, H., Steinbusch, H. W., et al. (2006). Minicolumnar abnormalities in autism. *Acta Neuropathologica, 112*(3), 287–303.

Castellanos, F. X., Sonuga-Barke, E. J., Milham, M. P., & Tannock, R. (2006). Characterizing cognition in ADHD: Beyond executive dysfunction. *Trends in Cognitive Sciences, 10*(3), 117–123.

Cederlund, M., Hagberg, B., Billstedt, E., Gillberg, I. C., & Gillberg, C. (2008). Asperger syndrome and autism: A comparative longitudinal follow-up study more than 5 years after original diagnosis. *Journal of Autism and Developmental Disorders, 38*(1), 72–85.

Centers for Disease Control and Prevention. (2008). Measles—United States, January 1–April 25, 2008. Retrieved from *www.cdc.gov/mmwr/preview/mmwrhtml.mm57e501a1.htm*

Centers for Disease Control and Prevention. (2009). Prevalence of autism spectrum disorders—Autism and Developmental Disabilities Monitoring Network, United States, 2006. *MMWR Surveillance, 58*(10), 1–20.

Chakrabarti, S., & Fombonne, E. (2005). Pervasive developmental disorders in preschool children: Confirmation of high prevalence. *American Journal of Psychiatry, 162*(6), 1133–1141.

Charlop-Christy, M. H., Carpenter, M., Le, L., LeBlanc, L. A., & Kellet, K. (2002). Using the Picture Exchange Communication System (PECS) with children with autism: Assessment of PECS acquisition, speech, social-communicative behavior, and problem behavior. *Journal of Applied Behavior Analysis, 35*(3), 213–231.

Charlop-Christy, M. H., Le, L., & Freeman, K. A. (2000). A comparison of video modeling with *in vivo* modeling for teaching children with autism. *Journal of Autism and Developmental Disorders, 30*(6), 537–552.

Charlop, M. H., & Milstein, J. P. (1989). Teaching autistic children conversational speech using video modeling. *Journal of Applied Behavior Analysis, 22*(3), 275–285.

Chess, S. (1977). Follow-up report on autism in congenital rubella. *Journal of Autism and Childhood Schizophrenia, 7*(1), 69–81.

Christianson, A. L., Chesler, N., & Kromberg, J. G. (1994). Fetal valproate syndrome: clinical and neuro-developmental features in two sibling pairs. *Developmental Medicine and Child Neurology, 36*(4), 361–369.

Comi, A. M., Zimmerman, A. W., Frye, V. H., Law, P. A., & Peeden, J. N. (1999). Familial clustering of autoimmune disorders and evaluation of medical risk factors in autism. *Journal of Child Neurology, 14*(6), 388–394.

Cook, E. H., Jr., Courchesne, R., Lord, C., Cox, N. J., Yan, S., Lincoln, A., et al. (1997). Evidence of linkage between the serotonin transporter and autistic disorder. *Molecular Psychiatry, 2*(3), 247–250.

Cook, E. H., Jr., Leventhal, B. L., & Freedman, D. X. (1988). Free serotonin in plasma: Autistic children and their first-degree relatives. *Biological Psychiatry, 24*(4), 488–491.

Cook, E. H., Jr., Leventhal, B. L., Heller, W., Metz, J., Wainwright, M., & Freedman, D. X. (1990). Autistic children and their first-degree relatives: Relationships between serotonin and norepinephrine levels and intelligence. *Journal of Neuropsychiatry and Clinical Neurosciences, 2*(3), 268–274.

Cook, E. H., Jr., Lindgren, V., Leventhal, B. L., Courchesne, R., Lincoln, A., Shulman, C., et al. (1997). Autism or atypical autism in maternally but not paternally derived proximal 15q duplication. *American Journal of Human Genetics, 60*(4), 928–934.

Corbett, B. A. (2003). Video modeling: A window into the world of autism. *Behavior Analyst Today, 4*(3), 367–377.

Corbett, B. A., & Abdullah, M. (2005). Video modeling: Why does it work for children with autism? *Journal of Early and Intensive Behavior Intervention, 2*(1), 2–8.

Corbett, B. A., Carmean, V., Ravizza, S., Wendelken, C., Henry, M. L., Carter, C., et al. (2009). A functional and structural study of emotion and face processing in children with autism. *Psychiatry Research, 173*(3), 196–205.

Corbett, B. A., & Constantine, L. J. (2006). Autism and attention deficit hyperactivity disorder: Assessing attention and response control with the integrated visual and auditory continuous performance test. *Child Neuropsychology, 12*(4–5), 335–348.

Corbett, B. A., Constantine, L. J., Hendren, R., Rocke, D., & Ozonoff, S. (2009). Examining executive functioning in children with autism spectrum disorder, attention deficit hyperactivity disorder and typical development. *Psychiatry Research, 166*(2–3), 210–222.

Corbett, B. A., Kantor, A. B., Schulman, H., Walker, W. L., Lit, L., Ashwood, P., et al. (2007). A proteomic study of serum from children with autism showing differential expression of apolipoproteins and complement proteins. *Molecular Psychiatry, 12*(3), 292–306.

Corbett, B. A., Khan, K., Czapansky-Beilman, D., Brady, N., Dropik, P., Goldman, D. Z., et al. (2001). A double-blind, placebo-controlled crossover study investigating the effect of porcine secretin in children with autism. *Clinical Pediatrics (Philadelphia), 40*(6), 327–331.

Corbett, B. A., Mendoza, S., Abdullah, M., Wegelin, J. A., & Levine, S. (2006). Cortisol circadian rhythms and response to stress in children with autism. *Psychoneuroendocrinology, 31*(1), 59–68.

Corbett, B. A., Mendoza, S., Wegelin, J. A., Carmean, V., & Levine, S. (2008). Variable cortisol circadian rhythms in children with autism and anticipatory stress. *Journal of Psychiatry and Neuroscience, 33*(3), 227–234.

Corbett, B. A., Shickman, K., & Ferrer, E. (2008). Brief report: The effects of Tomatis sound therapy on language in children with autism. *Journal of Autism and Developmental Disorders, 38*(3), 562–566.

Corbett, B. A., Schupp, C. W., Levine, S., & Mendoza, S. (2009). Comparing cortisol, stress and sensory sensitivity in children with autism. *Autism Research, 2*, 32–39.

Cornish, E. (2002). Gluten and casein free diets in autism: A study of the effects on food choice and nutrition. *Journal of Human Nutrition and Dietetics, 15*(4), 261–269.

Courchesne, E., Carper, R., & Akshoomoff, N. (2003). Evidence of brain overgrowth in the first year of life in autism. *Journal of the American Medical Association, 290*(3), 337–344.

Courchesne, E., Karns, C. M., Davis, H. R., Ziccardi, R., Carper, R. A., Tigue, Z. D., et al. (2001). Unusual brain growth patterns in early life in patients with autistic disorder: An MRI study. *Neurology, 57*(2), 245–254.

Courchesne, E., Saitoh, O., Townsend, J. P., Yeung-Courchesne, R., Press, G. A., Lincoln, A. J., et al. (1994). Cerebellar hypoplasia and hyperplasia in infantile autism. *Lancet, 343*, 63–64.

Critchley, H. D., Daly, E. M., Bullmore, E. T., Williams, S. C., Van Amelsvoort, T., Robertson, D. M., et al. (2000). The functional neuroanatomy of social behaviour: Changes in cerebral blood flow when people with autistic disorder process facial expressions. *Brain, 123*(Pt. 11), 2203–2212.

Croen, L. A., Braunschweig, D., Haapanen, L., Yoshida, C. K., Fireman, B., Grether, J. K., et al. (2008). Maternal mid-pregnancy autoantibodies to fetal brain protein: The Early Markers for Autism Study. *Biological Psychiatry, 64*(7), 583–588.

Croen, L. A., Grether, J. K., Yoshida, C. K., Odouli, R., & Van de Water, J. (2005). Maternal autoimmune diseases, asthma and allergies, and childhood autism spectrum disorders: A case–control study. *Archives of Pediatrics and Adolescent Medicine, 159*(2), 151–157.

Croen, L. A., Matevia, M., Yoshida, C. K., & Grether, J. K. (2008). Maternal Rh D status, anti-D immune globulin exposure during pregnancy, and risk of autism spectrum disorders. *American Journal of Obstetrics and Gynecology, 199*(3), 234. e1–e6.

Curin, J. M., Terzic, J., Petkovic, Z. B., Zekan, L., Terzic, I. M., & Susnjara, I. M. (2003). Lower cortisol and higher ACTH levels in individuals with autism. *Journal of Autism and Developmental Disorders, 33*(4), 443–448.

Dager, S. R., Wang, L., Friedman, S. D., Shaw, D. W., Constantino, J. N., Artru, A. A., et al. (2007). Shape mapping of the hippocampus in young children with autism spectrum disorder. *American Journal of Neuroradiology, 28*(4), 672–677.

Dalton, K. M., Nacewicz, B. M., Johnstone, T., Schaefer, H. S., Gernsbacher, M. A., Goldsmith, H. H., et al. (2005). Gaze fixation and the neural circuitry of face processing in autism. *Nature Neuroscience, 8*(4), 519–526.

Dapretto, M., Davies, M. S., Pfeifer, J. H., Scott, A. A., Sigman, M., Bookheimer, S. Y., et al. (2006). Understanding emotions in others: Mirror neuron dysfunction in children with autism spectrum disorders. *Nature Neuroscience, 9*(1), 28–30.

Davidovitch, M., Glick, L., Holtzman, G., Tirosh, E., & Safir, M. P. (2000). Developmental regression in autism: Maternal perception. *Journal of Autism and Developmental Disorders, 30*(2), 113–119.

Dawson, G., & Watling, R. (2000). Interventions to facilitate auditory, visual, and motor integration in autism: a review of the evidence. *Journal of Autism and Developmental Disorders, 30*(5), 415–421.

Dawson, G., & Zanolli, K. (2003). Early intervention and brain plasticity in autism. *Novartis Foundation Symposium, 251*, 266–274 (discussion, 274–280, 281–297).

DeFelice, M. L., Ruchelli, E. D., Markowitz, J. E., Strogatz, M., Reddy, K. P., Kadivar, K., et al. (2003). Intestinal cytokines in children with pervasive developmental disorders. *American Journal of Gastroenterology, 98*(8), 1777–1782.

DeLong, G. R., Teague, L. A., & McSwain Kamran, M. (1998). Effects of fluoxetine treatment in young children with idiopathic autism. *Developmental Medicine and Child Neurology, 40*(8), 551–562.

Durkin, M. S., Maenner, M. J., Newschaffer, C. J., Lee, L. C., Cunniff, C. M., Daniels, J. L., et al. (2008). Advanced parental age and the risk of autism spectrum disorder. *American Journal of Epidemiology, 168*(11), 1268–1276.

Dziobek, I., Fleck, S., Rogers, K., Wolf, O. T., & Convit, A. (2006). The "amygdala theory of autism" revisited: Linking structure to behavior. *Neuropsychologia, 44*(10), 1891–1899.

Eaves, L. C., & Ho, H. H. (2008). Young adult outcome of autism spectrum disorders. *Journal of Autism and Developmental Disorders, 38*(4), 739–747.

Edelson, M. G. (2006). Are the majority of children with autism mentally retarded?: A systematic evaluation of the data. *Focus on Autism and Other Developmental Disabilities, 21*, 66–83.

Ehlers, S., & Gillberg, C. (1993). The epidemiology of Asperger syndrome. A total population study. *Journal of Child Psychology and Psychiatry, 34*(8), 1327–1350.

Eikeseth, S., Smith, T., Jahr, E., & Eldevik, S. (2002). Intensive behavioral treatment at school for 4- to 7-year-old children with autism. A 1-year comparison controlled study. *Behavior Modification, 26*(1), 49–68.

Fatemi, S. H. (2008a). The hyperglutamatergic hypothesis of autism [Letter]. *Progress in Neuro-Psychopharmacology and Biological Psychiatry, 32*(3), 911 (author reply, 912–913).

Fatemi, S. H. (2008b). The role of neurodevelopmental genes in infectious etiology of autism. *American Journal of Biochemistry and Biotechnology, 4*, 177–182.

Fatemi, S. H., Halt, A. R., Stary, J. M., Kanodia, R., Schulz, S. C., & Realmuto, G. R. (2002). Glutamic acid decarboxylase 65 and 67 kDa proteins are reduced in autistic parietal and cerebellar cortices. *Biological Psychiatry, 52*(8), 805–810.

Fatemi, S. H., Reutiman, T. J., Folsom, T. D., & Thuras, P. D. (2009). GABA(A) receptor downregulation in brains of subjects with autism. *Journal of Autism and Developmental Disorders, 39*(2), 223–230.

Ferrante, R. J., Andreassen, O. A., Jenkins, B. G., Dedeoglu, A., Kuemmerle, S., Kubilus, J. K., et al. (2000). Neuroprotective effects of creatine in a transgenic mouse model of Huntington's disease. *Journal of Neuroscience, 20*(12), 4389–4397.

Filipek, P. A., Accardo, P. J., Ashwal, S., Baranek, G. T., Cook, E. H., Jr., Dawson, G., et al. (2000).

Practice parameter: Screening and diagnosis of autism. Report of the Quality Standards Subcommittee of the American Academy of Neurology and the Child Neurology Society. *Neurology, 55*(4), 468–479.

Fogassi, L., Gallese, V., di Pellegrino, G., Fadiga, L., Gentilucci, M., Luppino, G., et al. (1992). Space coding by premotor cortex. *Experimental Brain Research, 89*(3), 686–690.

Folstein, S., & Rutter, M. (1977a). Genetic influences and infantile autism. *Nature, 265,* 726–728.

Folstein, S., & Rutter, M. (1977b). Infantile autism: A genetic study of 21 twin pairs. *Journal of Child Psychology and Psychiatry, 18*(4), 297–321.

Fombonne, E. (2005). Epidemiology of autistic disorder and other pervasive developmental disorders. *Journal of Clinical Psychiatry, 66*(Suppl. 10), 3–8.

Freitag, C. M. (2007). The genetics of autistic disorders and its clinical relevance: a review of the literature. *Molecular Psychiatry, 12*(1), 2–22.

Frith, C. (2004). Is autism a disconnection disorder? *Lancet Neurology, 3*(10), 577.

Fullerton, A. C. P. (1999). Developing skills and concepts for self-determination in young adults with autism. *Focus on Autism and Other Developmental Disabilities, 14*(1), 42–63.

Gallese, V. (2003). The roots of empathy: The shared manifold hypothesis and the neural basis of intersubjectivity. *Psychopathology, 36*(4), 171–180.

Gallese, V., Keysers, C., & Rizzolatti, G. (2004). A unifying view of the basis of social cognition. *Trends in Cognitive Sciences, 8*(9), 396–403.

Garstang, J., & Wallis, M. (2006). Randomized controlled trial of melatonin for children with autistic spectrum disorders and sleep problems. *Child: Care, Health, and Development, 32*(5), 585–589.

Gernsbacher, M. A., Dawson, M., & Goldsmith, H. H. (2005). Three reasons not to believe in an autism epidemic. *Current Directions in Psychological Science, 14*(2), 55–58.

Geschwind, D. H., & Levitt, P. (2007). Autism spectrum disorders: Developmental disconnection syndromes. *Current Opinion in Neurobiology, 17*(1), 103–111.

Geurts, H. M., Verte, S., Oosterlaan, J., Roeyers, H., & Sergeant, J. A. (2004). How specific are executive functioning deficits in attention deficit hyperactivity disorder and autism? *Journal of Child Psychology and Psychiatry, 45*(4), 836–854.

Giannotti, F., Cortesi, F., Cerquiglini, A., & Bernabei, P. (2006). An open-label study of controlled-release melatonin in treatment of sleep disorders in children with autism. *Journal of Autism and Developmental Disorders, 36*(6), 741–752.

Gillberg, C., & Wing, L. (1999). Autism: Not an extremely rare disorder. *Acta Psychiatrica Scandinavica, 99*(6), 399–406.

Gillott, A., Furniss, F., & Walter, A. (2001). Anxiety in high-functioning children with autism. *Autism, 5*(3), 277–286.

Goldberg, M. C., Mostofsky, S. H., Cutting, L. E., Mahone, E. M., Astor, B. C., Denckla, M. B., et al. (2005). Subtle executive impairment in children with autism and children with ADHD. *Journal of Autism and Developmental Disorders, 35*(3), 279–293.

Goldstein, S., & Schwebach, A. J. (2004). The comorbidity of pervasive developmental disorder and attention deficit hyperactivity disorder: Results of a retrospective chart review. *Journal of Autism and Developmental Disorders, 34*(3), 329–339.

Goodlin-Jones, B. L., Tang, K., Liu, J., & Anders, T. F. (2008). Sleep patterns in preschool-age children with autism, developmental delay, and typical development. *Journal of the American Academy of Child and Adolescent Psychiatry, 47*(8), 930–938.

Gotham, K., Risi, S., Pickles, A., & Lord, C. (2007). The Autism Diagnostic Observation Schedule: Revised algorithms for improved diagnostic validity. *Journal of Autism and Developmental Disorders, 37*(4), 613–627.

Green, L., Fein, D., Modahl, C., Feinstein, C., Waterhouse, L., & Morris, M. (2001). Oxytocin and autistic disorder: Alterations in peptide forms. *Biological Psychiatry, 50*(8), 609–613.

Gresham, F. M., & Macmillan, D. L. (1997). Autistic recovery?: An analysis and critique of the empirical evidence on the Early Intervention Project. *Behavioral Disorders, 22,* 185–201.

Gubbay, S. S., Lobascher, M., & Kingerlee, P. (1970). A neurological appraisal of autistic children: Results of a Western Australian survey. *Developmental Medicine and Child Neurology, 12*(4), 422–429.

Hadjikhani, N., Joseph, R. M., Snyder, J., & Tager-Flusberg, H. (2006). Anatomical differences in the mirror neuron system and social cognition network in autism. *Cerebral Cortex, 16*(9), 1276–1282.

Hadjikhani, N., Joseph, R. M., Snyder, J., & Tager-Flusberg, H. (2007). Abnormal activation of the social brain during face perception in autism. *Human Brain Mapping, 28*(5), 441–449.

Hagerman, R. J., Chudley, A. E., Knoll, J. H., Jackson, A. W., III, Kemper, M., & Ahmad, R. (1986). Autism in fragile X females. *American Journal of Medical Genetics, 23*(1–2), 375–380.

Hagerman, R. J., Rivera, S. M., & Hagerman, P. (2008). The fragile X family of disorders: A model for autism and targeted treatments. *Current Pediatric Reviews, 4,* 40–52.

Hallmayer, J., Spiker, D., Lotspeich, L., McMahon, W. M., Petersen, P. B., Nicholas, P., et al. (1996). Male-to-male transmission in extended pedigrees with multiple cases of autism. *American Journal of Medical Genetics, 67*(1), 13–18.

Hanson, E., Kalish, L. A., Bunce, E., Curtis, C., McDaniel, S., Ware, J., et al. (2007). Use of complementary and alternative medicine among children diagnosed with autism spectrum disorder. *Journal of Autism and Developmental Disorders, 37*(4), 628–636.

Hardan, A. Y., Minshew, N. J., Harenski, K., & Keshavan, M. S. (2001). Posterior fossa magnetic resonance imaging in autism. *Journal of the American Acad of Child and Adolescent Psychiatry, 40*(6), 666–672.

Harris, S. L., Handleman, J. S., Gordon, R., Kristoff, B., & Fuentes, F. (1991). Changes in cognitive and language functioning of preschool children with autism. *Journal of Autism and Developmental Disorders, 21*(3), 281–290.

Hashimoto, T., Tayama, M., Murakawa, K., Yoshimoto, T., Miyazaki, M., Harada, M., et al. (1995). Development of the brainstem and cerebellum in autistic patients. *Journal of Autism and Developmental Disorders, 25*(1), 1–18.

Hazlett, H. C., Poe, M., Gerig, G., Smith, R. G., Provenzale, J., Ross, A., et al. (2005). Magnetic resonance imaging and head circumference study of brain size in autism: Birth through age 2 years. *Archives of General Psychiatry, 62*(12), 1366–1376.

Hellemans, H., Colson, K., Verbraeken, C., Vermeiren, R., & Deboutte, D. (2007). Sexual behavior in high-functioning male adolescents and young adults with autism spectrum disorder. *Journal of Autism and Developmental Disorders, 37*(2), 260–269.

Hertz-Picciotto, I., Croen, L. A., Hansen, R., Jones, C. R., van de Water, J., & Pessah, I. N. (2006). The CHARGE study: An epidemiologic investigation of genetic and environmental factors contributing to autism. *Environmental Health Perspectives, 114*(7), 1119–1125.

Hill, S. D., Wagner, E. A., Shedlarski, J. G., Jr., & Sears, S. P. (1977). Diurnal cortisol and temperature variation of normal and autistic children. *Developmental Psychobiology, 10*(6), 579–583.

Hippler, K., & Klicpera, C. (2003). A retrospective analysis of the clinical case records of 'autistic psychopaths' diagnosed by Hans Asperger and his team at the University Children's Hospital, Vienna. *Philosophical Transactions of the Royal Society of London, Series B, 358*, 291–301.

Hollander, E., Bartz, J., Chaplin, W., Phillips, A., Sumner, J., Soorya, L., et al. (2007). Oxytocin increases retention of social cognition in autism. *Biological Psychiatry, 61*(4), 498–503.

Hollander, E., Novotny, S., Hanratty, M., Yaffe, R., DeCaria, C. M., Aronowitz, B. R., et al. (2003). Oxytocin infusion reduces repetitive behaviors in adults with autistic and Asperger's disorders. *Neuropsychopharmacology, 28*(1), 193–198.

Holroyd, S., Reiss, A. L., & Bryan, R. N. (1991). Autistic features in Joubert syndrome: A genetic disorder with agenesis of the cerebellar vermis. *Biological Psychiatry, 29*(3), 287–294.

Hornig, M., Chian, D., & Lipkin, W. I. (2004). Neurotoxic effects of postnatal thimerosal are mouse strain dependent. *Molecular Psychiatry, 9*(9), 833–845.

Horvath, K., Stefanatos, G., Sokolski, K. N., Wachtel, R., Nabors, L., & Tildon, J. T. (1998). Improved social and language skills after secretin administration in patients with autistic spectrum disorders. *Journal of the Association for Academic Minority Physicians, 9*(1), 9–15.

Hoshino, Y., Ohno, Y., Murata, S., Yokoyama, F., Kaneko, M., & Kumashiro, H. (1984). Dexamethasone suppression test in autistic children. *Folia Psychiatrica Neurologica Japonica, 38*(4), 445–449.

Howard, M. A., Cowell, P. E., Boucher, J., Broks, P., Mayes, A., Farrant, A., et al. (2000). Convergent neuroanatomical and behavioural evidence of an amygdala hypothesis of autism. *NeuroReport, 11*(13), 2931–2935.

Howlin, P., & Moore, A. (1997). Diagnosis in autism. A survey of over 1200 patients in the UK. *Autism, 1*, 135–162.

Hussman, J. P. (2001). Suppressed GABAergic inhibition as a common factor in suspected etiologies of autism. *Journal of Autism and Developmental Disorders, 31*(2), 247–248.

Iacoboni, M., Molnar-Szakacs, I., Gallese, V., Buccino, G., Mazziotta, J. C., & Rizzolatti, G. (2005). Grasping the intentions of others with one's own mirror neuron system. *PLoS Biology, 3*(3), e79.

Iacoboni, M., Woods, R. P., Brass, M., Bekkering, H., Mazziotta, J. C., & Rizzolatti, G. (1999). Cortical mechanisms of human imitation. *Science, 286*, 2526–2528.

Iarocci, G., & McDonald, J. (2006). Sensory integration and the perceptual experience of persons with autism. *Journal of Autism and Developmental Disorders, 36*(1), 77–90.

Immunization Society Review. (2004). Vaccines and autism (Executive Summary). Retrieved from *books.nap.edu/openbook.php?record_id=10997&page=1.*

Insel, T. R. (1997). A neurobiological basis of social attachment. *American Journal of Psychiatry, 154*(6), 726–735.

Insel, T. R., O'Brien, D. J., & Leckman, J. F. (1999). Oxytocin, vasopressin, and autism: Is there a connection? *Biological Psychiatry, 45*(2), 145–157.

Insel, T. R., Winslow, J. T., Williams, J. R., Hastings, N., Shapiro, L. E., & Carter, C. S. (1993). The role of neurohypophyseal peptides in the central mediation of complex social processes: Evidence from comparative studies. *Regulatory Peptides, 45*(1–2), 127–131.

Jacob, S., Brune, C. W., Carter, C. S., Leventhal, B. L., Lord, C., & Cook, E. H., Jr. (2007). Association of the oxytocin receptor gene (OXTR) in Caucasian children and adolescents with autism. *Neuroscience Letters, 417*(1), 6–9.

Johnson, K. P., & Malow, B. A. (2008). Sleep in children with autism spectrum disorders. *Current Neurology and Neuroscience Reports, 8*(2), 155–161.

Joosten, A. V., Bundy, A. C., & Einfeld, S. L. (2009). Intrinsic and extrinsic motivation for stereotypic and repetitive behavior. *Journal of Autism and Developmental Disorders, 39*(3), 521–531.

Junaid, M. A., & Pullarkat, R. K. (2001). Proteomic approach for the elucidation of biological defects in autism. *Journal of Autism and Developmental Disorders., 31*(6), 557–560.

Juranek, J., Filipek, P. A., Berenji, G. R., Modahl, C., Osann, K., & Spence, M. A. (2006). Association between amygdala volume and anxiety level: Magnetic resonance imaging (MRI) study in autistic children. *Journal of Child Neurology, 21*(12), 1051–1058.

Just, M. A., Cherkassky, V. L., Keller, T. A., Kana, R. K., & Minshew, N. J. (2007). Functional and anatomical cortical underconnectivity in autism: Evidence from an FMRI study of an executive function task and corpus callosum morphometry. *Cerebral Cortex, 17*(4), 951–961.

Jyonouchi, H., Geng, L., Ruby, A., Reddy, C., & Zimmerman-Bier, B. (2005). Evaluation of an association between gastrointestinal symptoms and cytokine production against common dietary proteins in children with autism spectrum disorders. *Journal of Pediatriacs, 146*(5), 605–610.

Kadesjo, B., & Gillberg, C. (2001). The comorbidity of ADHD in the general population of Swedish school-age children. *Journal of Child Psychology and Psychiatry, 42*(4), 487–492.

Kane, A., Luiselli, J.K., Dearborn, S., & Young, N. (2004). Wearing a weighted vest as intervention for children with autism/pervasive developmental disorder. *Scientific Review of Mental Health Practice, 3*(2), 19–24.

Kanner, L. (1943). Autistic disturbances of affective contact. *Nervous Child, 2*, 217–250.

Kates-McElrath, K. A., & Axelrod, S. (2006). Behavioral intervention for autism: A distinction between two behavior analytic approaches. *Behavior Analyst Today, 7*, 242–252.

Kemper, T. L., & Bauman, M. L. (1993). The contribution of neuropathologic studies to the understanding of autism. *Neurologic Clinics, 11*(1), 175–187.

Kemper, T. L., & Bauman, M. L. (1998). Neuropathology of infantile autism. *Journal of Neuropathology and Experimental Neurology, 57*(7), 645–652.

Kim, J. A., Szatmari, P., Bryson, S. E., Steiner, D. L., & Wilson, F. J. (2000). The prevalence of anxiety and mood problems among children with autism and Asperger syndrome. *Autism, 4*(2), 117–132.

Kirsch, P., Esslinger, C., Chen, Q., Mier, D., Lis, S.,

Siddhanti, S., et al. (2005). Oxytocin modulates neural circuitry for social cognition and fear in humans. *Journal of Neuroscience, 25*, 11489–11493.

Kirschbaum, C., & Hellhammer, D. H. (1994). Salivary cortisol in psychoneuroendocrine research: Recent developments and applications. *Psychoneuroendocrinology, 19*(4), 313–333.

Knivsberg, A. M., Reichelt, K. L., Hoien, T., & Nodland, M. (2002). A randomised, controlled study of dietary intervention in autistic syndromes. *Nutritional Neuroscience, 5*(4), 251–261.

Knudsen, E. I. (2004). Sensitive periods in the development of the brain and behavior. *Journal of Cognitive Neuroscience, 16*(8), 1412–1425.

Koegel, R. L., O'Dell, M. C., & Koegel, L. K. (1987). A natural language teaching paradigm for nonverbal autistic children. *Journal of Autism and Developmental Disorders, 17*(2), 187–200.

Kosfeld, M., Heinrichs, M., Zak, P. J., Fischbacher, U., & Fehr, E. (2005). Oxytocin increases trust in humans. *Nature, 435*, 673–676.

Koshino, H., Kana, R. K., Keller, T. A., Cherkassky, V. L., Minshew, N. J., & Just, M. A. (2008). fMRI investigation of working memory for faces in autism: Visual coding and underconnectivity with frontal areas. *Cerebral Cortex, 18*(2), 289–300.

Krakowiak, P., Goodlin-Jones, B., Hertz-Picciotto, I., Croen, L. A., & Hansen, R. L. (2008). Sleep problems in children with autism spectrum disorders, developmental delays, and typical development: A population-based study. *Journal of Sleep Research, 17*(2), 197–206.

Kumar, R. A., & Christian, S. L. (2009). Genetics of autism spectrum disorders. *Current Neurology and Neuroscience Reports, 9*(3), 188–197.

Kumar, R. A., KaraMohamed, S., Sudi, J., Conrad, D. F., Brune, C., Badner, J. A., et al. (2008). Recurrent 16p11.2 microdeletions in autism. *Human Molecular Genetics, 17*(4), 628–638.

Lancet. (2010). Retraction–Ileal-lymphoid-nodular hyperplasia, non-specific colitis, and pervasive developmental disorder in children. *Lancet, 375*, 445.

Landa, R. J., & Goldberg, M. C. (2005). Language, social, and executive functions in high functioning autism: A continuum of performance. *Journal of Autism and Developmental Disorders, 35*(5), 557–573.

Langworthy-Lam, K. S., Aman, M. G., & Van Bourgondien, M. E. (2002). Prevalence and patterns of use of psychoactive medicines in individuals with autism in the Autism Society of North Carolina. *Journal of Child and Adolescent Psychopharmacol, 12*(4), 311–321.

Laski, K. E., Charlop, M. H., & Schreibman, L. (1988). Training parents to use the natural language paradigm to increase their autistic children's speech. *Journal of Applied Behavior Analysis, 21*(4), 391–400.

LeBlanc, L. A., Coates, A. M., Daneshvar, S.,

Charlop-Christy, M. H., Morris, C., & Lancaster, B. M. (2003). Using video modeling and reinforcement to teach perspective-taking skills to children with autism. *Journal of Applied Behavior Analysis, 36*(2), 253–257.

Lee, L. C., Zachary, A. A., Leffell, M. S., Newschaffer, C. J., Matteson, K. J., Tyler, J. D., et al. (2006). HLA-DR4 in families with autism. *Pediatric Neurology, 35*(5), 303–307.

Leventhal, B. L., Cook, E. H., Jr., Morford, M., Ravitz, A., & Freedman, D. X. (1990). Relationships of whole blood serotonin and plasma norepinephrine within families. *Journal of Autism and Developmental Disorders, 20*(4), 499–511.

Levine, S. (2000). Influence of psychological variables on the activity of the hypothalamic–pituitary–adrenal axis. *European Journal of Pharmacology, 405*(1–3), 149–160.

Levine, S., & Mody, T. (2003). The long-term psychobiological consequences of intermittent postnatal separation in the squirrel monkey. *Neuroscience and Biobehavioral Reviews, 27*(1–2), 83–89.

Levy, S. E., & Hyman, S. L. (2005). Novel treatments for autistic spectrum disorders. *Mental Retardation and Developmental Disabilies Research Reviews, 11*(2), 131–142.

Levy, S. E., & Hyman, S. L. (2008). Complementary and alternative medicine treatments for children with autism spectrum disorders. *Child and Adolescent Psychiatric Clinics of North America, 17*(4), 803–820.

Levy, S. E., Mandell, D. S., Merhar, S., Ittenbach, R. F., & Pinto-Martin, J. A. (2003). Use of complementary and alternative medicine among children recently diagnosed with autistic spectrum disorder. *Journal of Developmental and Behavioral Pediatrics, 24*(6), 418–423.

Levy, S. E., Souders, M. C., Wray, J., Jawad, A. F., Gallagher, P. R., Coplan, J., et al. (2003). Children with autistic spectrum disorders: I. Comparison of placebo and single dose of human synthetic secretin. *Archives of Disease in Childhood, 88*(8), 731–736.

Lord, C., Rutter, M., DiLavore, P., & Risi, S. (1999). *Autism Diagnostic Observation Schedule—WPS.* Los Angeles: Western Psychological Services.

Lord, C., Rutter, M., & Le Couteur, A. (1994). Autism Diagnostic Interview—Revised: A revised version of a diagnostic interview for caregivers of individuals with possible pervasive developmental disorders. *Journal of Autism and Developmental Disorders, 24*, 659–685.

Lovaas, O. I. (1987). Behavioral treatment and normal educational and intellectual functioning in young autistic children. *Journal of Consulting and Clinical Psychology, 55*(1), 3–9.

Lovaas, O. I., Koegel, R. L., & Schreibman, L. (1979). Stimulus overselectivity in autism: A review of research. *Psychological Bulletin, 86*(6), 1236–1254.

Lovaas, O. I., Newsom, C., & Hickman, C. (1987). Self-stimulatory behavior and perceptual reinforcement. *Journal of Applied Behavior Analysis, 20*(1), 45–68.

Lovaas, O. I., & Smith, T. (1989). A comprehensive behavioral theory of autistic children: Paradigm for research and treatment. *Journal of Behavior Therapy and Experimental Psychiatry, 20*(1), 17–29.

Macdonald, H., Rutter, M., Howlin, P., Rios, P., Le Conteur, A., Evered, C., et al. (1989). Recognition and expression of emotional cues by autistic and normal adults. *Journal of Child Psychology and Psychiatry, 30*(6), 865–877.

Maher, K. R., Harper, J. F., Macleay, A., & King, M. G. (1975). Peculiarities in the endocrine response to insulin stress in early infantile autism. *Journal of Nervous and Mental Disease, 161*(3), 180–184.

Mahoney, G. P., & Perales, F. (2003). Using relationship focused intervention to enhance the social-emotional functioning of young children with autism spectrum disorders. *Topics in Early Childhood Special Education, 23*(2), 77–90.

Malone, R. P., Delaney, M. A., Hyman, S. B., & Cater, J. R. (2007). Ziprasidone in adolescents with autism: An open-label pilot study. *Journal of Adolescent Psychopharmacology, 17*(6), 779–790.

Malow, B. A., McGrew, S. G., Harvey, M., Henderson, L. M., & Stone, W. L. (2006). Impact of treating sleep apnea in a child with autism spectrum disorder. *Pediatric Neurology, 34*(4), 325–328.

Mandell, D. S., Novak, M. M., & Zubritsky, C. D. (2005). Factors associated with age of diagnosis among children with autism spectrum disorders. *Pediatrics, 116*(6), 1480–1486.

Manning, M. A., Cassidy, S. B., Clericuzio, C., Cherry, A. M., Schwartz, S., Hudgins, L., et al. (2004). Terminal 22q deletion syndrome: A newly recognized cause of speech and language disability in the autism spectrum. *Pediatrics, 114*(2), 451–457.

Marshall, C. R., Noor, A., Vincent, J. B., Lionel, A. C., Feuk, L., Skaug, J., et al. (2008). Structural variation of chromosomes in autism spectrum disorder. *American Journal of Human Genetics, 82*(2), 477–488.

Martin, L. A., Ashwood, P., Braunschweig, D., Cabanlit, M., Van de Water, J., & Amaral, D. G. (2008). Stereotypies and hyperactivity in rhesus monkeys exposed to IgG from mothers of children with autism. *Brain, Behavior, and Immunity, 22*(6), 806–816.

Martineau, J., Barthelemy, C., Cheliakine, C., & Lelord, G. (1988). Brief report: An open middle-term study of combined vitamin B6–magnesium in a subgroup of autistic children selected on their sensitivity to this treatment. *Journal of Autism and Developmental Disorders, 18*(3), 435–447.

Matson, J. L., & Rivet, T. T. (2008). Characteristics of challenging behaviours in adults with autistic disorder, PDD-NOS, and intellectual disability. *Journal of Intellectual and Developmental Disabilities, 33*(4), 323–329.

Matsuura, T., Sutcliffe, J. S., Fang, P., Galjaard, R. J., Jiang, Y. H., Benton, C. S., et al. (1997). De novo truncating mutations in E6–AP ubiquitin-protein ligase gene (UBE3A) in Angelman syndrome. *Nature Genetics, 15*(1), 74–77.

McBride, P. A., Anderson, G. M., Hertzig, M. E., Snow, M. E., Thompson, S. M., Khait, V. D., et al. (1998). Effects of diagnosis, race, and puberty on platelet serotonin levels in autism and mental retardation. *Journal of the American Academy of Child and Adolescent Psychiatry, 37*(7), 767–776.

McCracken, J. T., McGough, J., Shah, B., Cronin, P., Hong, D., Aman, M. G., et al. (2002). Risperidone in children with autism and serious behavioral problems. *New England Journal of Medicine, 347*(5), 314–321.

McDougle, C. J., Holmes, J. P., Carlson, D. C., Pelton, G. H., Cohen, D. J., & Price, L. H. (1998). A double-blind, placebo-controlled study of risperidone in adults with autistic disorder and other pervasive developmental disorders. *Archives of General Psychiatry, 55*(7), 633–641.

McEachin, J. J., Smith, T., & Lovaas, O. I. (1993). Long-term outcome for children with autism who received early intensive behavioral treatment. *American Journal of Mental Retardation, 97*(4), 359–372 (discussion, 373–391).

Melke, J., Goubran Botros, H., Chaste, P., Betancur, C., Nygren, G., Anckarsater, H., et al. (2008). Abnormal melatonin synthesis in autism spectrum disorders. *Molecular Psychiatry, 13*(1), 90–98.

Miles, J. H., Takahashi, T. N., Bagby, S., Sahota, P. K., Vaslow, D. F., Wang, C. H., et al. (2005). Essential versus complex autism: Definition of fundamental prognostic subtypes. *American Journal of Medical Genetics, Part A, 135*(2), 171–180.

Miller, M. T. (1991). Thalidomide embryopathy: A model for the study of congenital incomitant horizontal strabismus. *Transactions of the American Ophthalmological Society, 89*, 623–674.

Modahl, C., Green, L., Fein, D., Morris, M., Waterhouse, L., Feinstein, C., et al. (1998). Plasma oxytocin levels in autistic children. *Biological Psychiatry, 43*(4), 270–277.

Molloy, C. A., Morrow, A. L., Meinzen-Derr, J., Schleifer, K., Dienger, K., Manning-Courtney, P., et al. (2006). Elevated cytokine levels in children with autism spectrum disorder. *Journal of Neuroimmunology, 172*, 198–205.

Moussavand, S. F., & Findling, R. L. (2007). Recent advances in the pharmacological treatment of pervasive developmental disorders. *Current Pediatric Reviews, 3*(1), 79–91.

Muhle, R., Trentacoste, S. V., & Rapin, I. (2004). The genetics of autism. *Pediatrics, 113*(5), e-72–e486.

Mundy, P. (1993). Normal versus high-functioning status in children with autism. *American Journal on Mental Retardation, 97*, 381–384.

Munson, J., Dawson, G., Abbott, R., Faja, S., Webb, S. J., Friedman, S. D., et al. (2006). Amygdalar volume and behavioral development in autism. *Archives of General Psychiatry, 63*(6), 686–693.

Muris, P., Steerneman, P., Merckelbach, H., Holdrinet, I., & Meesters, C. (1998). Comorbid anxiety symptoms in children with pervasive developmental disorders. *Journal of Anxiety Disorders, 12*(4), 387–393.

Murphy, G. H., Beadle-Brown, J., Wing, L., Gould, J., Shah, A., & Holmes, N. (2005). Chronicity of challenging behaviours in people with severe intellectual disabilities and/or autism: A total population sample. *Journal of Autism and Developmental Disorders, 35*(4), 405–418.

Nacewicz, B. M., Dalton, K. M., Johnstone, T., Long, M. T., McAuliff, E. M., Oakes, T. R., et al. (2006). Amygdala volume and nonverbal social impairment in adolescent and adult males with autism. *Archives of General Psychiatry, 63*(12), 1417–1428.

Nanson, J. L. (1992). Autism in fetal alcohol syndrome: A report of six cases. *Alcoholism: Clinical and Experimental Research, 16*(3), 558–565.

Nelson, K. B., Grether, J. K., Croen, L. A., Dambrosia, J. M., Dickens, B. F., Jelliffe, L. L., et al. (2001). Neuropeptides and neurotrophins in neonatal blood of children with autism or mental retardation. *Annals of Neurology, 49*(5), 597–606.

Nelson, P. G., Kuddo, T., Song, E. Y., Dambrosia, J. M., Kohler, S., Satyanarayana, G., et al. (2006). Selected neurotrophins, neuropeptides, and cytokines: Developmental trajectory and concentrations in neonatal blood of children with autism or Down syndrome. *International Journal of Developmental Neuroscience, 24*(1), 73–80.

Neumann, I. D. (2002). Involvement of the brain oxytocin system in stress coping: Interactions with the hypothalamo–pituitary–adrenal axis. *Progress in Brain Research, 139*, 147–162.

Neumann, I. D., Kromer, S. A., Toschi, N., & Ebner, K. (2000). Brain oxytocin inhibits the (re)activity of the hypothalamo–pituitary–adrenal axis in male rats: Involvement of hypothalamic and limbic brain regions. *Regulatory Peptides, 96*(1–2), 31–38.

Nicolson, R., DeVito, T. J., Vidal, C. N., Sui, Y., Hayashi, K. M., Drost, D. J., et al. (2006). Detection and mapping of hippocampal abnormalities in autism. *Psychiatry Research, 148*(1), 11–21.

Nigg, J. T., Willcutt, E. G., Doyle, A. E., & Sonuga-Barke, E. J. (2005). Causal heterogeneity in attention-deficit/hyperactivity disorder: Do we need neuropsychologically impaired subtypes? *Biological Psychiatry, 57*(11), 1224–1230.

Nir, I., Meir, D., Zilber, N., Knobler, H., Hadjez, J., & Lerner, Y. (1995). Brief report: Circadian melatonin, thyroid-stimulating hormone, prolactin, and cortisol levels in serum of young adults with autism. *Journal of Autism and Developmental Disorders, 25*(6), 641–654.

Oberman, L. M., Hubbard, E. M., McCleery, J. P., Altschuler, E. L., Ramachandran, V. S., & Pineda, J. A. (2005). EEG evidence for mirror neuron dysfunction in autism spectrum disorders. *Brain Research: Cognitive Brain Research, 24*(2), 190–198.

Odell, D., Maciulis, A., Cutler, A., Warren, L., McMahon, W. M., Coon, H., et al. (2005). Confirmation of the association of the C4B null allelle in autism. *Human Immunology, 66*(2), 140–145.

Owley, T., McMahon, W., Cook, E. H., Laulhere, T., South, M., Mays, L. Z., et al. (2001). Multisite, double-blind, placebo-controlled trial of porcine secretin in autism. *Journal of the American Academy of Child and Adolescent Psychiatry, 40*(11), 1293–1299.

Ozonoff, S., Williams, B. J., Gale, S., & Miller, J. N. (1999). Autism and autistic behavior in Joubert syndrome. *Journal of Child Neurology, 14*(10), 636–641.

Palmen, S. J., Durston, S., Nederveen, H., & Van Engeland, H. (2006). No evidence for preferential involvement of medial temporal lobe structures in high-functioning autism. *Psychological Medicine, 36*(6), 827–834.

Panerai, S., Ferrante, L., & Caputo, V. (1997). The TEACCH strategy in mentally retarded children with autism: A multidimensional assessment. Pilot study. Treatment and Education of Autistic and Communication Handicapped children. *Journal of Autism and Developmental Disorders, 27*(3), 345–347.

Parnas, J., Bovet, P., & Zahavi, D. (2002). Schizophrenic autism: Clinical phenomenology and pathogenetic implications. *World Psychiatry, 1*(3), 131–136.

Pessah, I. N., Seegal, R. F., Lein, P. J., LaSalle, J., Yee, B. K., Van De Water, J., et al. (2008). Immunologic and neurodevelopmental susceptibilities of autism. *Neurotoxicology, 29*(3), 532–545.

Peters, S. U., Beaudet, A. L., Madduri, N., & Bacino, C. A. (2004). Autism in Angelman syndrome: Implications for autism research. *Clinical Genetics, 66*(6), 530–536.

Pierce, K., & Courchesne, E. (2000). Exploring the neurofunctional organization of face processing in autism. *Archives of General Psychiatry, 57*(4), 344–346.

Pierce, K., Haist, F., Sedaghat, F., & Courchesne, E. (2004). The brain response to personally familiar faces in autism: Findings of fusiform activity and beyond. *Brain, 127*(Pt. 12), 2703–2716.

Pierce, K., & Schreibman, L. (1997). Multiple peer use of pivotal response training to increase social behaviors of classmates with autism: results from trained and untrained peers. *Journal of Applied Behavior Analysis, 30*(1), 157–160.

Piven, J., Arndt, S., Bailey, J., & Andreasen, N. (1996). Regional brain enlargement in autism: A magnetic resonance imaging study. *Journal of the American Academy of Child and Adolescent Psychiatry, 35*(4), 530–536.

Planche, P., Lazartigues, A., Lemonnier, E. (2004). Identification of the early signs of autism spectrum disorder: Age at detection and conjectures about development. In O. T. Ryaskin (Ed.), *Focus on autism research* (pp. 103–123). New York: Nova Biomedical Books.

Posey, D. J., Stigler, K. A., Erickson, C. A., & McDougle, C. J. (2008). Antipsychotics in the treatment of autism. *Journal of Clinical Investigation, 118*(1), 6–14.

Posey, D. J., Wiegand, R. E., Wilkerson, J., Maynard, M., Stigler, K. A., & McDougle, C. J. (2006). Open-label atomoxetine for attention-deficit/ hyperactivity disorder symptoms associated with high-functioning pervasive developmental disorders. *Journal of Child and Adolescent Psychopharmacology, 16*(5), 599–610.

Potenza, M. N., Holmes, J. P., Kanes, S. J., & McDougle, C. J. (1999). Olanzapine treatment of children, adolescents, and adults with pervasive developmental disorders: An open-label pilot study. *Journal of Clinical Psychopharmacology, 19*(1), 37–44.

Potocki, L., Bi, W., Treadwell-Deering, D., Carvalho, C. M., Eifert, A., Friedman, E. M., et al. (2007). Characterization of Potocki–Lupski syndrome (dup(17)(p11.2p11.2)) and delineation of a dosage-sensitive critical interval that can convey an autism phenotype. *American Journal of Human Genetics, 80*(4), 633–649.

Purcell, A. E., Jeon, O. H., Zimmerman, A. W., Blue, M. E., & Pevsner, J. (2001). Postmortem brain abnormalities of the glutamate neurotransmitter system in autism. *Neurology, 57*(9), 1618–1628.

Quintana, H., Birmaher, B., Stedge, D., Lennon, S., Freed, J., Bridge, J., et al. (1995). Use of methylphenidate in the treatment of children with autistic disorder. *Journal of Autism and Developmental Disorders, 25*(3), 283–294.

Rao, P. A., Beidel, D. C., & Murray, M. J. (2008). Social skills interventions for children with Asperger's syndrome or high-functioning autism: A review and recommendations. *Journal of Autism and Developmental Disorders, 38*(2), 353–361.

Reddy, K. S. (2005). Cytogenetic abnormalities and fragile-X syndrome in autism spectrum disorder. *BMC Medical Genetics, 6*, 3.

Rescorla, L. (1988). Cluster analytic identification

of autistic preschoolers. *Journal of Autism and Developmental Disorders, 18*(4), 475–492.

Richdale, A. L., & Prior, M. R. (1992). Urinary cortisol circadian rhythm in a group of high-functioning children with autism. *Journal of Autism and Developmental Disorders, 22*(3), 433–447.

Risch, N., Spiker, D., Lotspeich, L., Nouri, N., Hinds, D., Hallmayer, J., et al. (1999). A genomic screen of autism: Evidence for a multilocus etiology. *American Journal of Human Genetics, 65*(2), 493–507.

Ritvo, E. R., Freeman, B. J., Scheibel, A. B., Duong, T., Robinson, H., Guthrie, D., et al. (1986). Lower Purkinje cell counts in the cerebella of four autistic subjects: Initial findings of the UCLA–NSAC Autopsy Research Report. *American Journal of Psychiatry, 143*(7), 862–866.

Ritvo, E. R., Yuwiler, A., Geller, E., Ornitz, E. M., Saeger, K., & Plotkin, S. (1970). Increased blood serotonin and platelets in early infantile autism. *Archives of General Psychiatry, 23*(6), 566–572.

Rogers, S. J. (2000). Interventions that facilitate socialization in children with autism. *Journal of Autism and Developmental Disorders, 30*(5), 399–409.

Rogers, S. J., Wehner, D. E., & Hagerman, R. (2001). The behavioral phenotype in fragile X: Symptoms of autism in very young children with fragile X syndrome, idiopathic autism, and other developmental disorders. *Journal of Developmental and Behavioral Pediatrics, 22*(6), 409–417.

Saha, S., Barnett, A. G., Foldi, C., Burne, T. H., Eyles, D. W., Buka, S. L., et al. (2009). Advanced paternal age is associated with impaired neurocognitive outcomes during infancy and childhood. *PLoS Medicine, 6*(3), e40.

Samaco, R. C., Hogart, A., & LaSalle, J. M. (2005). Epigenetic overlap in autism-spectrum neurodevelopmental disorders: MECP2 deficiency causes reduced expression of UBE3A and GABRB3. *Human Molecular Genetics, 14*(4), 483–492.

Sandler, A. D., Sutton, K. A., DeWeese, J., Girardi, M. A., Sheppard, V., & Bodfish, J. W. (1999). Lack of benefit of a single dose of synthetic human secretin in the treatment of autism and pervasive developmental disorder. *New England Journal of Medicine, 341*(24), 1801–1806.

Schain, R. J., & Freedman, D. X. (1961). Studies on 5–hydroxyindole metabolism in autistic and other mentally retarded children. *Journal of Pediatrics, 58*, 315–320.

Schopler, E. (2000). International priorities for developing autism services via the TEACCH Model-1. *International Journal of Mental Health, 29*, 3–97.

Schopler, E., Brehm, S. S., Kinsbourne, M., & Reichler, R. J. (1971). Effect of treatment structure on development in autistic children. *Archives of General Psychiatry, 24*(5), 415–421.

Schopler, E., Reichler, R. J., DeVellis, R. F., & Daly, K. (1980). Toward objective classification of childhood autism: Childhood Autism Rating Scale (CARS). *Journal of Autism and Developmental Disorders, 10*(1), 91–103.

Schopler, E., Short, A., & Mesibov, G. (1989). Relation of behavioral treatment to "normal functioning": Comment on Lovaas. *Journal of Consulting and Clinical Psychology, 57*(1), 162–164.

Schultz, R. T., Gauthier, I., Klin, A., Fulbright, R. K., Anderson, A. W., Volkmar, F., et al. (2000). Abnormal ventral temporal cortical activity during face discrimination among individuals with autism and Asperger syndrome. *Archives of General Psychiatry, 57*(4), 331–340.

Schultz, R. T., Grelotti, D. J., Klin, A., Kleinman, J., Van der Gaag, C., Marois, R., et al. (2003). The role of the fusiform face area in social cognition: Implications for the pathobiology of autism. *Philosophical Transactions of the Royal Society of London, Series B, 358*, 415–427.

Schumann, C. M., & Amaral, D. G. (2006). Stereological analysis of amygdala neuron number in autism. *Journal of Neuroscience, 26*, 7674–7679.

Schumann, C. M., Hamstra, J., Goodlin-Jones, B. L., Lotspeich, L. J., Kwon, H., Buonocore, M. H., et al. (2004). The amygdala is enlarged in children but not adolescents with autism; the hippocampus is enlarged at all ages. *Journal of Neuroscience, 24*, 6392–6401.

Sergeant, J. A., Geurts, H., Huijbregts, S., Scheres, A., & Oosterlaan, J. (2003). The top and the bottom of ADHD: A neuropsychological perspective. *Neuroscience and Biobehavioral Reviews, 27*(7), 583–592.

Shattuck, P. T., Seltzer, M. M., Greenberg, J. S., Orsmond, G. I., Bolt, D., Kring, S., et al. (2007). Change in autism symptoms and maladaptive behaviors in adolescents and adults with an autism spectrum disorder. *Journal of Autism and Developmental Disorders, 37*(9), 1735–1747.

Shtayermman, O. (2007). Peer victimization in adolescents and young adults diagnosed with Asperger's syndrome: A link to depressive symptomatology, anxiety symptomatology and suicidal ideation. *Issues in Comprehensive Pediatric Nursing, 30*(3), 87–107.

Siegel, B. (1999). Autistic learning disabilities and individualizing treatment for autistic spectrum disorders. *Infants and Young Children: An Interdisciplinary Journal of Special Care Practices, 12*(2), 27–35.

Silva, S. C., Correia, C., Fesel, C., Barreto, M., Coutinho, A. M., Marques, C., et al. (2004). Autoantibody repertoires to brain tissue in autism nuclear families. *Journal of Neuroimmunology, 152*(1–2), 176–182.

Simic, M., & Turk, J. (2004). Autistic spectrum disorder associated with partial duplication of chromosome 15: Three case reports. *European Child and Adolescent Psychiatry, 13*(6), 389–393.

Singer, H. S., Morris, C. M., Gause, C. D., Gillin, P. K., Crawford, S., & Zimmerman, A. W. (2008). Antibodies against fetal brain in sera of mothers with autistic children. *Journal of Neuroimmunology, 194*(1–2), 165–172.

Singh, V. K. (1996). Plasma increase of interleukin-12 and interferon-gamma. Pathological significance in autism. *Journal of Neuroimmunology, 66*(1–2), 143–145.

Singh, V. K., & Rivas, W. H. (2004). Detection of antinuclear and antilaminin antibodies in autistic children who received thimerosal-containing vaccines. *Journal of Biomedical Science, 11*(5), 607–610.

Skaar, D. A., Shao, Y., Haines, J. L., Stenger, J. E., Jaworski, J., Martin, E. R., et al. (2005). Analysis of the RELN gene as a genetic risk factor for autism. *Molecular Psychiatry, 10*(6), 563–571.

Smalley, S. L. (1998). Autism and tuberous sclerosis. *Journal of Autism and Developmental Disorders, 28*(5), 407–414.

Smith, T., Groen, A. D., & Wynn, J. W. (2000). Randomized trial of intensive early intervention for children with pervasive developmental disorder. *American Journal of Mental Retardation, 105*(4), 269–285.

Solomon, M., Goodlin-Jones, B. L., & Anders, T. F. (2004). A social adjustment enhancement intervention for high functioning autism, Asperger's syndrome, and pervasive developmental disorder NOS. *Journal of Autism and Developmental Disorders, 34*(6), 649–668.

Sonuga-Barke, E. J. (2005). Causal models of attention-deficit/hyperactivity disorder: From common simple deficits to multiple developmental pathways. *Biological Psychiatry, 57*(11), 1231–1238.

Sparks, B. F., Friedman, S. D., Shaw, D. W., Aylward, E. H., Echelard, D., Artru, A. A., et al. (2002). Brain structural abnormalities in young children with autism spectrum disorder. *Neurology, 59*(2), 184–192.

Spezio, M. L., Huang, P. Y., Castelli, F., & Adolphs, R. (2007). Amygdala damage impairs eye contact during conversations with real people. *Journal of Neuroscience, 27*, 3994–3997.

Stahmer, A. C. (1995). Teaching symbolic play skills to children with autism using pivotal response training. *Journal of Autism and Developmental Disorders, 25*(2), 123–141.

Steege, M. W., Mace, C., Perry, L., & Longenecker, H. (2007). Applied behavior analysis: Beyond discrete trial teaching. *Psychology in the Schools, 44*(1), 91–99.

Stichter, J. P., Randolph, J., Gage, N., & Schmidt, C. (2007). A review of recommended social competency programs for students with autism spectrum disorders. *Exceptionality, 15*(4), 219–232.

Stokes, M., Newton, N., & Kaur, A. (2007). Stalking, and social and romantic functioning among adolescents and adults with autism spectrum disorder. *Journal of Autism and Developmental Disorders, 37*(10), 1969–1986.

Stromland, K., & Miller, M. T. (1993). Thalidomide embryopathy: Revisited 27 years later. *Acta Ophthalmologica (Copenhagen), 71*(2), 238–245.

Sundberg, M. L., & Michael, J. (2001). The benefits of Skinner's analysis of verbal behavior for children with autism. *Behavior Modification, 25*(5), 698–724.

Sutcliffe, J. S. (2008). Genetics: Insights into the pathogenesis of autism. *Science, 321*, 208–209.

Swiezy, N., Stuart, M., & Korzekwa, P. (2008). Bridging for success in autism: Training and collaboration across medical, educational, and community systems. *Child and Adolescent Psychiatric Clinics of North America, 17*(4), 907–922.

Szpir, M. (2006). New thinking on neurodevelopment. *Environmental Health Perspectives, 114*(2), A100–A107.

Taylor, E., & Rogers, J. W. (2005). Practitioner review: Early adversity and developmental disorders. *Journal of Child Psychology and Psychiatry, 46*(5), 451–467.

Thompson, B. M., & Andrews, S. R. (2000). An historical commentary on the physiological effects of music: Tomatis, Mozart and neuropsychology. *Integrative Physiological and Behavioral Science, 35*(3), 174–188.

Tidmarsh, L., & Volkmar, F. R. (2003). Diagnosis and epidemiology of autism spectrum disorders. *Canadian Journal of Psychiatry, 48*(8), 517–525.

Tordjman, S., Anderson, G. M., McBride, P. A., Hertzig, M. E., Snow, M. E., Hall, L. M., et al. (1997). Plasma beta-endorphin, adrenocorticotropin hormone, and cortisol in autism. *Journal of Child Psychology and Psychiatry, 38*(6), 705–715.

Tordjman, S., Anderson, G. M., Pichard, N., Charbuy, H., & Touitou, Y. (2005). Nocturnal excretion of 6–sulphatoxymelatonin in children and adolescents with autistic disorder. *Biological Psychiatry, 57*(2), 134–138.

Tordjman, S., Gutknecht, L., Carlier, M., Spitz, E., Antoine, C., Slama, F., et al. (2001). Role of the serotonin transporter gene in the behavioral expression of autism. *Molecular Psychiatry, 6*(4), 434–439.

Torres, A. R., Maciulis, A., & Odell, D. (2001). The association of MHC genes with autism. *Frontiers in Bioscience, 6*, D936–D943.

Torres, A. R., Maciulis, A., Stubbs, E. G., Cutler, A., & Odell, D. (2002). The transmission disequilibrium test suggests that HLA-DR4 and DR13 are linked to autism spectrum disorder. *Human Immunology, 63*(4), 311–316.

Trillingsgaard, A., & Østergaard, J. R. (2004). Autism in Angelman syndrome: An exploration of comorbidity. *Autism, 8*(2), 163–174.

Tsuchiya, K. J., Matsumoto, K., Miyachi, T., Tsujii, M., Nakamura, K., Takagai, S., et al. (2008). Paternal age at birth and high-functioning autistic-spectrum disorder in offspring. *British Journal of Psychiatry, 193*(4), 316–321.

Van Bourgondien, M. E., & Schopler, E. (1996). Intervention for adults with autism. *Journal of Rehabilitation, 62*(1), 65–72.

van Gent T., Heijnen, C. J., & Treffers, P. D. (1997). Autism and the immune system. *Journal of Child Psychology and Psychiatry, 38*(3), 337–349.

Vargas, D. L., Nascimbene, C., Krishnan, C., Zimmerman, A. W., & Pardo, C. A. (2005). Neuroglial activation and neuroinflammation in the brain of patients with autism. *Annals of Neurology, 57*(1), 67–81.

Volkmar, F. R., & Nelson, D. S. (1990). Seizure disorders in autism. *Journal of the American Academy of Child and Adolescent Psychiatry, 29*(1), 127–129.

Wakefield, A. J., Murch, S. H., Anthony, A., Linnell, J., Casson, D. M., Malik, M., et al. (1998). Illeal-lymphoid-nodular hyperplasia, non-specific colitis, and pervasive developmental disorder in children. *Lancet, 351*, 637–641.

Wang, A. T., Dapretto, M., Hariri, A. R., Sigman, M., & Bookheimer, S. Y. (2004). Neural correlates of facial affect processing in children and adolescents with autism spectrum disorder. *Journal of the American Academy of Child and Adolescent Psychiatry, 43*(4), 481–490.

Warren, R. P., Odell, J. D., Warren, W. L., Burger, R. A., Maciulis, A., Daniels, W. W., et al. (1996). Strong association of the third hypervariable region of HLA-DR beta 1 with autism. *Journal of Neuroimmunology, 67*(2), 97–102.

Wetherby, A. M., Watt, N., Morgan, L., & Shumway, S. (2007). Social communication profiles of children with autism spectrum disorders late in the second year of life. *Journal of Autism and Developmental Disorders, 37*(5), 960–975.

Whitaker-Azmitia, P. M. (2005). Behavioral and cellular consequences of increasing serotonergic activity during brain development: A role in autism? *International Journal of Developmental Neuroscience, 23*(1), 75–83.

Wieder, S., & Greenspan, S. I. (2003). Climbing the symbolic ladder in the DIR model through floor time/interactive play. *Autism, 7*(4), 425–435.

Williams, P. G., & Hersh, J. H. (1997). A male with fetal valproate syndrome and autism. *Developmental Medicine and Child Neurology, 39*(9), 632–634.

Wills, S., Cabanlit, M., Bennett, J., Ashwood, P., Amaral, D. G., & Van de Water, J. (2009). Detection of autoantibodies to neural cells of the cerebellum in the plasma of subjects with autism spectrum disorders. *Brain Behavior Immunity, 23*(1), 64–74.

Wing, L., & Gould, J. (1979). Severe impairments of social interaction and associated abnormalities in children: Epidemiology and classification. *Journal of Autism and Developmental Disorders, 9*(1), 11–29.

Winslow, J. T., Noble, P. L., Lyons, C. K., Sterk, S. M., & Insel, T. R. (2003). Rearing effects on cerebrospinal fluid oxytocin concentration and social buffering in rhesus monkeys. *Neuropsychopharmacology, 28*(5), 910–918.

Winslow, J. T., Shapiro, L., Carter, C. S., & Insel, T. R. (1993). Oxytocin and complex social behavior: species comparisons. *Psychopharmacology Bulletin, 29*(3), 409–414.

Wu, S., Jia, M., Ruan, Y., Liu, J., Guo, Y., Shuang, M., et al. (2005). Positive association of the oxytocin receptor gene (OXTR) with autism in the Chinese Han population. *Biological Psychiatry, 58*(1), 74–77.

Yamazaki, K., Saito, Y., Okada, F., Fujieda, T., & Yamashita, I. (1975). An application of neuroendocrinological studies in autistic children and Heller's syndrome. *Journal of Autism and Child Schizophrenia, 5*(4), 323–332.

Yeargin-Allsopp, M., Rice, C., Karapurkar, T., Doernberg, N., Boyle, C., & Murphy, C. (2003). Prevalence of autism in a US metropolitan area. *Journal of the American Medical Association, 289*(1), 49–55.

Yirmiya, N., Pilowsky, T., Nemanov, L., Arbelle, S., Feinsilver, T., Fried, I., et al. (2001). Evidence for an association with the serotonin transporter promoter region polymorphism and autism. *American Journal of Medical Genetics, 105*(4), 381–386.

Ylisaukko-oja, T., Alarcon, M., Cantor, R. M., Auranen, M., Vanhala, R., Kempas, E., et al. (2006). Search for autism loci by combined analysis of Autism Genetic Resource Exchange and Finnish families. *Annals of Neurology, 59*(1), 145–155.

Young, L. J., Wang, Z., & Insel, T. R. (1998). Neuroendocrine bases of monogamy. *Trends in Neurosciences, 21*(2), 71–75.

Zimmerman, A. W. (Ed.). (2008). *Current clinical neurology.* Totowa, NJ: Humana Press.

Zimmerman, A. W., Connors, S. L., Matteson, K. J., Lee, L. C., Singer, H. S., Castaneda, J. A., et al. (2007). Maternal antibrain antibodies in autism. *Brain, Behavior, and Immunity, 21*(3), 351–357.

Zimmerman, A. W., Jyonouchi, H., Comi, A. M., Connors, S. L., Milstien, S., Varsou, A., et al. (2005). Cerebrospinal fluid and serum markers of inflammation in autism. *Pediatric Neurology, 33*(3), 195–201.

CHAPTER 13

Turner Syndrome

M. PAIGE POWELL
TIMOTHY SCHULTE

Turner syndrome (TS) is one of the most widely known and examined chromosomal abnormalities in females (White, 1994). The syndrome—which is characterized by extremely short stature; a lack of spontaneous development of secondary sexual characteristics, with accompanying infertility; a broad chest; webbed neck; and a myriad of skeletal, renal, and cardiac abnormalities—was first identified in 1938 by Henry H. Turner. In 1959, Ford, Jones, Polani, de Almeida, and Briggs were able to identify the genetic abnormality associated with the syndrome: They linked it with a loss of or an abnormality in one of the two X chromosomes present in females. This defect of the X chromosome can lead to a large number of physical, neuropsychological, and emotional sequelae.

ETIOLOGY

TS occurs in approximately 1 out of every 2,000–3,000 live births of female children (Jones, 1988; Orten, 1990; Orten & Orten, 1992; Ross, 1990). However, the actual conception rate for TS is much higher (about 2%). It is estimated that only 1% of pregnancies with female fetuses with TS chromosomal abnormalities actually result

in live births; the other 99% of the fetuses are spontaneously aborted (Hassold, 1986; Hook & Warburton, 1983; Jones, 1988; Temple & Carney, 1993). TS is found across all racial and ethnic groups (Rovet, 1995).

A number of chromosomal abnormalities can result in TS. The first identified and most common form of TS is referred to in the literature as "pure" TS (Jones, 1988; Temple & Carney, 1993). This form is referred to as 45,X0, indicating that there is an absence of one of the X chromosomes that the fetus should have received from a parent, usually the paternal chromosome (Jacobs et al., 1990; Jones, 1988). Females with this form of TS have only one X chromosome. Approximately 50% of cases of TS have this genotype. The second most common form of TS is *mosaicism*, which occurs in 30–40% of cases. In mosaicism, the cell division that replicates the chromosomes fails to replicate the genetic material completely, and some cells contain a slightly different set of chromosomal material. Mosaicism can occur in females with 45,X0 or in females with the normal chromosomal pattern of 46,XX. Other types of abnormalities occur less frequently; these include a partial deletion of one arm of the X chromosome (46,X,del[Xp] or 46,X,del[Xq]), isochromosomes (46,X,i[Xq]), and rings (46,X,r[X]) (Jones, 1988; Ross, Roeltgen, Kushner, Wei, & Zinn, 2000; Ross, Zinn, & McCauley, 2000; Temple & Carney, 1993). The chromosomal abnormality is thought to occur during the division of the sex cell of the parent, and there does not appear to be a significant maternal age factor (Jones, 1988).

CLINICAL PRESENTATION

Physical Manifestations

There are many physical abnormalities present with TS. These physical problems not only vary across patients, but vary depending on which chromosomal abnormality is present. The most obvious and common physical characteristics of TS include extremely short stature, often between 4 feet, 6 inches and 4 feet, 10 inches (Jones, 1988); a short, webbed neck; a broad chest with broadly spaced nipples; cubitus valgus (i.e., an unusual carrying angle for the elbows); a short fourth or fifth metacarpal or metatarsal; and a lack of development of secondary sexual characteristics, such as enlarged breasts and pubic hair. The lack of development of secondary sexual characteristics occurs due to ovarian (gonadal) dysgenesis. During the fetal stage of development and after birth, there is a massive loss of oocytes or egg cells (ovarian dysgenesis), which results in a lack of development of the ovaries. This results not only in a failure to develop secondary sexual characteristics, but, for the vast majority of women with TS, in infertility (Jones, 1988).

Girls and women with TS have a wide variety of other skeletal and facial abnormalities, including scoliosis (curvature of the spine), a narrow and high-arched palate, ptosis (drooping eyelids), strabismus, a low posterior hairline, low and rotated ears, and inner-ear defects resulting in recurrent ear infections and hearing problems. Other observable symptoms include hypoplastic or underdeveloped nails, increase in pigmented moles, and lymphedema (swelling of the hands and feet). Finally, serious medical problems can be found: heart defects, such as coarctation (narrowing) of the aorta, and kidney problems (e.g., horseshoe kidney, double or cleft renal pelvis). Further medical complications can include high blood pressure, obesity, diabetes mellitus, Hashimoto thyroiditis, cataracts, and arthritis (Jones,

1988). There is evidence that people with the "pure" form of TS, the 45,X0 type, are likely to have more malformations than people with the mosaic or other forms of TS (Jones, 1988).

In the past, for most girls and women with TS, diagnosis of TS typically occurred during late adolescence. The referral for a genetic evaluation was usually precipitated by the fact that a young woman had failed to begin puberty (Rovet, 1993). Because of the late diagnosis, many children and adults with TS did not receive the appropriate medical, psychological, or educational intervention (Rovet, 1993). However, the diagnosis of TS is beginning to occur earlier, during infancy and early childhood (Mathiesen, Reilly, & Skuse, 1992), allowing children to receive appropriate intervention at an earlier age. Prenatal detection of TS may occur during routine chorionic villous sampling or amniocentesis. In addition, ultrasound findings such as cardiac anomalies, renal anomalies, poly- or ogliohydramnios, or fetal growth retardation may trigger chromosomal studies for the fetus (Saenger et al., 2001).

Neuropsychological and Psychoeducational Manifestations

Neuropsychological Manifestations

For many years after the discovery of the syndrome, it was widely believed that women with TS also had mental retardation/intellectual disability. This occasionally continued to be reported until relatively recently (Orten & Orten, 1992). Research has shown that this is not the case, and that girls and women with TS have Verbal IQ (VIQ) score distributions similar to those of the general population (Bender, Puck, Salbenblatt, & Robinson, 1984; Garron, 1977; Lewandowski, Costenbader, & Richman, 1984; McCauley, Ito, & Kay, 1986; McCauley, Kay, Ito, & Treder, 1987; Money, 1963; Money & Alexander, 1966; Rovet, 1990, 2004; Rovet & Netley, 1982; Shaffer, 1962; Waber, 1979). However, the Performance IQ (PIQ) scores tend to be somewhat lower than VIQ scores in people with TS, and these lower-than-expected PIQ scores may result in lower global IQ scores (Rovet, 1995). The lower PIQ scores on the Wechsler scales are thought to be due to difficulties in tasks that require visual–spatial processing.

Shaffer (1962) was the first researcher to suggest the presence of a specific cognitive profile for TS. His study documented that women with TS had an average PIQ that was approximately 19 points lower than their average VIQ. The pattern of VIQ scores higher than PIQ scores has been consistently documented in the literature, with the actual difference or degree of difference varying from study to study (ranging between 8 and 21 points on average) (Bender et al., 1984; Buckley, 1971; Downey et al., 1991; Garron, 1977; Lewandowski, 1985; Lewandowski et al., 1984; McCauley et al., 1986, 1987; McGlone, 1985; Money, 1963; Money & Alexander, 1966; Netley & Rovet, 1982; Pennington et al., 1985; Rovet, 1990; Rovet & Netley, 1982; Shaffer, 1962; Waber, 1979). Despite the consistent finding that PIQ is lower than VIQ in most girls and women with TS, a homogeneous cognitive profile has not been documented for females with TS (Rovet, 1990). However, several deficits on specific subtests of intelligence scales have been reported.

In the first study to examine the specific deficits in TS (Shaffer, 1962), Verbal Comprehension on the Wechsler scales was found to be high, with poorer scores on Performance subtests requiring perceptual organization (Block Design and Object Assembly) and freedom from distractibility (Arithmetic and Digit Span). These findings have also been confirmed across the literature. Specific Wechsler Performance subtest deficits found in women and girls with TS, compared to control subjects, include the following: Arithmetic, Digit Span, Object Assembly, Block Design, and Digit Symbol (Dellantonio, Lis, Saviolo, Rigon, & Tenconi, 1984; Downey et al., 1991; Lewandowski et al., 1984; Money, 1963, 1964; Shucard, Shucard, Clopper, & Schachter, 1992; Temple & Carney, 1995).

Although the literature has been clear and consistent regarding the findings of deficiencies in nonverbal, visual–spatial areas in TS, it has been less clear about the exact nature and cause of the deficits. Across studies, a wide variety of deficits have been noted. The most widely reported deficits are visual–spatial processing deficits (Downey et al., 1991; Money, 1993; Robinson et al., 1986; Rovet, 1993; Rovet & Netley, 1982; Temple & Carney, 1995). Other specific deficits that have been reported include problems with visual memory (Alexander & Money,

1966; Downey et al., 1991; Lewandowski, 1985; Lewandowski et al., 1984, Ross, Roeltgen, & Cutler, 1995), deficits in visual-constructional skills (Downey et al., 1991; McCauley et al., 1987; Murphy et al., 1994; Robinson et al., 1986; Temple & Carney, 1995), difficulties with visual discrimination and part–whole perception (Silbert, Wolff, & Lilienthal, 1977), and problems with visual–motor integration (Lewandowski et al., 1984).

In addition, deficits have been identified in attention, executive functioning, memory, face processing, and motor skills. In the area of attention, difficulties with inhibitory control and auditory attention have been found, whereas difficulties with sustained attention and focusing have not been identified as problematic for people with TS (Romans, Roeltgen, Kushner, & Ross, 1997; Ross, Zinn, & McCauley, 2000). In addition, the research has found that difficulties with distraction, planning, and production in a fluent manner have been identified as executive functioning concerns for individuals with TS (Romans et al., 1997; Temple et al., 1996), but not difficulty with set shifting. For the area of memory, deficits in short-term recall and poor visual working memory have been identified (Buchanan, Pavlovic, & Rovet, 1998). Deficits in overall working memory have also been identified (Berch, 1996; Buchanan et al., 1998).

Recent studies have focused on face-processing abilities, which may underlie difficulties with social interaction. Girls with TS were found to have more difficulties with general face recognition, emotion processing, and recognition of familiar faces in both upright and inverted positions (Elgar, Campbell, & Skuse, 2002; Lawrence, Kuntsi, Coleman, Campbell, & Skuse, 2003) than control subjects had. Finally, motor clumsiness and decreased movement speed have also been identified as deficits for girls and women with TS (Ross, Roeltgen, Feuillan, Kushner, & Cutler, 1998; Ross, Kushner, & Roeltgen, 1996; Ross, Roeltgen, et al., 2000). Research completed by Nijhuis-van der Sanden, Smits-Englesman, and Eling (2000) and Nijhuis-van der Sanden, Eling, Van Asseldonk, and Van Galen (2004) has found that girls with TS have the same accuracy in motor tasks as their typical peers, but that movement speed is much lower, regardless of task demands. Difficulties with planning movements have also been reported (Nijhuis-van der Sanden et al., 2004). The various cognitive deficits that have been identified in TS do appear to continue across the lifespan (Downey et al., 1991; Garron, 1977; Ross, Zinn, & McCauley, 2000). However, some skills do appear to improve with age, including motor planning skills (Romans, Stephanatos, Roeltgen, Kushner, & Ross, 1998).

Neurological Findings

Many studies have attempted to identify the actual area(s) of dysfunction within the brain associated with the typical cognitive deficits seen in TS. Currently there are two theories with some empirical support. Both of these theories revolve around the issue of lateralization of the brain. The human brain has two hemispheres, left and right, each of which is responsible for certain cognitive tasks (i.e., the brain is lateralized). The left hemisphere is thought to be responsible for language and symbolic operations. The right hemisphere is thought to be responsible for nonverbal information processing (Watson, 1981). The first theory regarding dysfunction within the brain and lateralization in TS is that women and girls with TS have generalized, diffuse right-hemispheric dysfunction (Dellantonio et al., 1984; Kolb & Heaton, 1975; Rovet, 1990, 1995; Rovet & Netley, 1981; Shucard et al., 1992; Silbert et al., 1977). This makes intuitive sense, in view of the findings that women and girls with TS tend to have intact verbal skills (left hemisphere) and difficulties with nonverbal, visual–spatial tasks (right hemisphere).

The second theory suggests that there is a lack of, or failure in, development of normal lateralization of the brain in people with TS (or global hemispheric dysfunction). Several researchers have found an apparent lack of lateralization in the brains of girls and women with TS (Bender, Linden, & Robinson, 1994; Bender et al., 1984; McGlone, 1985; Netley & Rovet, 1982; Nijhuis-van der Sanden et al., 2000; Pennington et al., 1985; Rovet, 1990).

Research with neuroimaging and other techniques has supported the idea that specific brain areas are dysfunctional in girls and women with TS. Tamm, Menon, and Reiss (2003) found dysfunction in the pre-

frontal cortex regions involving inhibition, attention and working memory. Cutter and colleagues (2006) found reduced white matter in the cerebellar hemispheres, parieto-occipital regions, and the splenium of the corpus callosum. They also found increased white matter in the temporal and orbitofrontal lobes and genui of the corpus callosum, as well as lower concentrations of N-acetyl aspirate in the parietal lobe and high choline levels in the hippocampus. Finally, they found that the origin of the X chromosome (maternal or paternal) had an impact on the volume of right amygdala–hippocampal areas, gray matter volume in the caudate nucleu and thalamus, and bilateral white matter in the temporal lobes: The presence of the maternal X chromosome led to a poorer outcome. Hart, Davenport, Hooper, and Belger (2006) found that women with TS has less activation of frontoparietal araes of the brain during visual–spatial working memory tasks than did controls. Finally, research by Rezaie and colleagues (2008) found that women with TS had increased leftward brain asymmetry restricted to the posterior of the brain and the superior temporal and parieto-occipital association cortex. Clark, Klonoff, and Hayden (1990) also found differences in the occipital cortex.

Psychoeducational Manifestations

Given the various neuropsychological deficits found with TS—specifically, difficulties with visual–spatial, visual–motor, and memory tasks—it is not surprising that educational difficulties are also associated with TS. The most common learning problem for girls with TS is in the area of mathematics. Many authors have reported that TS is associated with poorer performance on the Arithmetic subtests of the Wechsler scales (Downey et al., 1991; Garron, 1977; Money & Alexander, 1966; Shaffer, 1962). In addition, girls with TS have been found to have low achievement in mathematics (Mazzocco, 1998; Rovet, 1995; Siegel, Clopper, & Stabler, 1998). Rovet (1995) reported that the mathematics problems appear to be more related to the conceptual/factual area than to the actual computational area. She also reported that older girls are more likely to have a mathematics disability than younger girls, probably due to the fact that math becomes more conceptual and relies more on memory skills as children progress through school. Mazzocco and her colleagues (Mazzocco, 1998, 2001; Mazzocco, Bhatia, & Lesniak-Karpiak, 2006; Murphy & Mazzocco, 2008) have done more specific assessment of the mathematical difficulties of girls with TS. These studies have found that mathematics deficits are evident as early as kindergarten. It appears that girls with TS have no difficulty understanding and applying math concepts; they appear to have more difficulty with processing speed and completing timed tasks. The visual–spatial aspects and verbal and working memory aspects of mathematics may also contribute to the difficulty girls with TS have in math.

Although reading has generally been found to be a well-developed skill for girls with TS (Mazzocco, 2001; Temple, Carney, & Mullarkey, 1996), Rovet (1995) reported that some girls may experience difficulty with reading decoding skills, but not comprehension skills. Spelling and reading skills appear to remain intact. Rovet (1993) noted that reading disabilities at times coexist with the mathematics disabilities in TS, but that they have not been found to occur alone.

A growing body of literature has begun to compare children with TS to children who have nonverbal learning disabilities (NLD) (Rovet, 1995; Williams, Richman, & Yarbrough, 1992). Children with NLD are a subgroup of children with learning disabilities who have particular difficulty with visual-perceptual skills. These skill deficits result in difficulties with mathematics, nonverbal reasoning, and socialization (Strang & Rourke, 1983). There is also a VIQ-PIQ discrepancy in NLD, with VIQ being higher than PIQ. Manifestations of NLD are most common in children who have identifiable brain disorders such as neurofibromatosis, head injuries, or loss or absence of brain tissue, as well as in children who have undergone radiation treatment for cancer (Rourke, 1985).

Correlations between Phenotype and Neuropsychological and Educational Deficits

As in the physical features associated with TS, there appears to be extensive heterogeneity in the neuropsychological deficits as-

sociated with TS. Several studies have examined the impact of phenotype (i.e., 45,X0 vs. mosaicism) on these deficits. As a rule, it has been found that TS subjects with the mosaic form of TS tend to have fewer cognitive and visual–spatial difficulties than girls with the "pure" form of TS have (Bender et al., 1994; El Abd, Turk, & Hill, 1995; Rovet & Ireland, 1994; Temple & Carney, 1993). More recent literature has focused on the parental origin of the X chromosome loss (Kesler et al., 2003; Loesch et al., 2005; Skuse et al., 1997), but has not been conclusive as to whether the origin of the loss has an impact on cognitive or behavioral phenotype.

Psychosocial Aspects

Over the past 20 years, an increasing amount of attention has been given to the psychosocial aspects of TS. Overall, research has found that girls and women with TS tend to have fewer severe mental disorders than those found in the general population of females. Women with TS are less likely to experience the "positive" symptomatology of psychopathology, such as acting-out behaviors, suicidal ideation, and alcohol/drug use. However, they do appear to experience more of the "negative" symptomatology of psychopathology, such as a lack of emotional reactivity and few or poor relationships with peers and other intimates (Downey, Ehrhardt, Gruen, Bell, & Morishima, 1989). Other personality characteristics that have been commonly associated with TS have included high stress tolerance, unassertiveness, overcompliance, and a lack of emotional maturity (Baekgaard, Nyborg, & Nielsen, 1978; Downey et al., 1989; Higurashi et al., 1986; McCauley et al., 1986; McCauley, Ross, Kushner, & Culter, 1995; McCauley, Sybert, & Ehrhardt, 1986; Nielsen, Nyborg, & Dahl, 1977).

Issues in Childhood and Adolescence

The three major psychosocial areas of concern for girls with TS are the areas of self-esteem, peer relationships, and social isolation—areas that appear to be highly interrelated. Across studies, girls with TS have been found to have low self-esteem (McCauley et al., 1986, 1995; Perheentupa et al., 1974). Among the major sources contributing to a child's sense of self-worth are the child's interactions with others, especially peers and family members. Major differences in appearance, such as short stature and the other physical anomalies associated with TS, can have a lasting impact on a developing child's sense of self and self-worth. Short children are often teased and bullied by peers at school, which may adversely affect their self-esteem (Skuse, 1987), and this appears to be a major problem for girls with TS (McCauley et al., 1986). A child with TS, who may be less assertive than her peers (Skuse, 1987), may have greater difficulty in handling the teasing in a proactive manner. In addition, because children are often treated according to the age they appear to be rather than their actual chronological age, a child or adolescent with TS may experience the added burden of being treated like a much younger child and not having the behavioral expectations that would correspond to her chronological age (Alley, 1983). This again will set her apart from her peers and have an impact upon self-esteem. Furthermore, it has been found that for girls with TS, the greater the number of physical anomalies, the lower the self-esteem (El Abd et al., 1995). Finally, difficulties with motor coordination and hearing difficulties due to inner-ear abnormalities may affect self-esteem as well (El Abd et al., 1995).

Academic difficulties can also result in lowered self-esteem in children. There is a vast literature base examining the impact of learning disabilities on the development of a child's self-esteem and feelings of self-worth (Taylor, 1989). The psychosocial problems that are evident in children with learning disabilities, such as poor task motivation, poor social skills, externalizing behaviors, depression, and somatic complaints, may continue into adulthood (Jorm, Share, Matthews, & Maclean, 1986).

As girls with TS grow older, the delay in the onset of puberty may further decrease their self-esteem during adolescence (Skuse, 1987). There has been some evidence to suggest that girls with TS have average self-esteem until puberty, at which time they begin to fall behind their peers both physically and socially, and their self-esteem decreases. As they fall behind, they begin to withdraw and are viewed as socially immature (Perheentupa et al., 1974). Problems with social isolation and poor peer relations are reported across the literature (Nielsen et al., 1977; Rovet, 1993; Skuse, 1987). As girls are teased for their physical abnormalities, including short stature, they may withdraw from peer interactions. Poor peer relations may also be due to hormonal deficits. As puberty is delayed, children with TS fail to go through the hormonal changes of adolescence and may be seen as emotionally immature as well as physically immature (Skuse, 1987). They may prefer to be with children younger than themselves (McCauley et al., 1995; Rovet & Ireland, 1994). Social difficulties may also be related to the visual–spatial processing problems associated with TS because children with these difficulties, including girls with TS, often have problems with understanding the social cues and facial expressions of others (affective discrimination) (McCauley et al., 1987; Waber, 1979).

Other psychosocial difficulties that have been associated with TS are behavior problems. Skuse, Cave, O'Herlihy, and South (1998) found that a large number of the adolescent girls in their study exhibited adjustment problems in such areas as somatic symptoms, anxiety, and social immaturity. Sonis and colleagues (1983) found that parents of girls with TS reported more behavior problems for their daughters than did parents of girls in a non-TS control group. The parents of the girls with TS reported that their daughters were experiencing poor peer relationships, immaturity, and poor attention skills. In an effort to rule out short stature as the cause for the problems that girls with TS experience, McCauley and colleagues (1986) compared girls who had TS with girls who had short stature but not TS. The results of that study indicated that the girls with TS had more behavior problems and poorer peer relationships than their constitutionally short counterparts. The girls with TS were reported by parents and teachers to be socially immature and to have many problems associated with externalizing behavior, such as impulsivity, overactivity, and poor attention span. Rovet (1995) also found more "hyperactivity" among girls with TS. Rovet and Ireland (1994) found that girls with TS tended to score lower on measures of social competence and higher on measures of general behavior problems. These behavior problems were most noticeable in the areas of social relationships, attention problems, immaturity, hyperactivity, and anxiety. In addition, girls with TS were found to experience more problems in school. These problems do appear to increase across childhood (Skuse, 1987).

Finally, there have also been reports of a connection between the occurrence of anorexia nervosa in adolescents and adults with TS and the advent of hormone therapy (Kron, Katz, Gorzynski, & Weiner, 1977; Muhs & Lieberz, 1993; Taipale, Niittyma- ki, & Nevalainen, 1982). This appears to be related to the onset of sexual development and to anxiety caused by the new sexual feelings that occur. It is believed that the development of anorexia nervosa in girls with TS who have begun hormonal treatment has an etiology similar to that in typically developing girls (Muhs & Lieberz, 1993; Taipale et al., 1982). It has also been attributed to a distorted body image caused by a combination of the "stocky" body build usually associated with TS and the perceptual deficits that exist with TS (Darby, Garfinkel, Vale, Kirwan, & Brown, 1981).

Issues in Adulthood

Like the cognitive aspects of TS, many of the psychosocial difficulties reported in children with TS continue into adulthood. Women with TS have also been found to experience difficulties with self-esteem (McCauley et al., 1986; Pavlidis, McCauley, & Sybert, 1995). The impaired development of secondary sexual characteristics and the subsequent infertility often contribute to low self-esteem in adults with TS (El Abd et al., 1995; Pavlidis et al., 1995; Skuse, 1987). In addition, women with TS may continue to be less emotionally mature and continue to experience poor, or a low number of, peer relationships (Nielsen et al., 1977).

As reported above, children with TS may tend to be more hyperactive than their same-age peers (McCauley et al., 1986; Rovet, 1995; Rovet & Ireland, 1994; Sonis et al, 1983); however, adults with TS may have lower levels of activity than expected (Downey et al., 1989; Higurashi et al., 1986; Money & Mittenthal, 1970; Pavlidis et al., 1995; Rovet, 1995). The reason for this difference is not readily discernible. In addition, adult women with TS may be likely to

experience mild depressive symptomatology. However, there does not appear to be a consistent pattern of psychological problems; nor does there seem to be an increase in the frequency of psychological problems over that seen in the general population (Money & Mittenthal, 1970; Shaffer, 1962). In addition, Orten and Orten (1992) found that women with TS reported that they were satisfied with their lives and happy. Women with TS do appear to be less independent of their parents and less likely to marry or live with partners than the general population (Nielsen et al., 1977; Nielsen & Stradiot, 1987; Orten & Orten, 1992).

Given the reported perceptual and educational problems associated with TS, another area of potential concern is the educational and occupational achievement of adults with TS. Despite the findings that the perceptual and educational difficulties found in childhood continue into adulthood (Garron, 1977; Nielsen & Stradiot, 1987), women with TS have been found to perform at an average or above-average level academically and to be gainfully employed in a wide variety of occupations (Nielsen et al., 1977; Nielsen & Stradiot, 1987; Orten & Orten, 1992).

Despite the delay in or lack of development of secondary sexual characteristics, it does appear that women with TS have a strong female gender identity (Ehrhardt, Greenberg, & Money, 1970; Money & Mittenthal, 1970). However, women with TS may be less sexually active than average (Pavlidis et al., 1995). They also report less interest in sexual relationships (Downey et al., 1989). Even with this lack of sexual activity, and maybe because of the lack of interest in sexual relationships, women with TS report moderate to high levels of sexual satisfaction (Pavlidis et al., 1995). However, higher sexual satisfaction was associated with higher frequency of sexual intercourse and a higher health status. Raboch, Kobilkòva, Horejsi, Starka, and Raboch (1987) have hypothesized that the lower levels of interest in sex may be related to lower levels of sexual hormones. They also found that once women with TS were in stable, good relationships, any differences in interest and participation in sexual relationships disappeared. Health status appears to be significantly related to a number of psychosocial issues for adults with TS. Pavlidis and colleagues (1995) found that health status was associated with higher self-esteem and greater sexual satisfaction.

Correlations between Phenotype and Psychosocial Problems

Again, as with physical manifestations and neuropsychological manifestations, there is a wide heterogeneity in psychosocial difficulties. These also appear to be related to phenotype. Children and adults with the mosaicism phenotype appear to have fewer behavioral difficulties than those with other forms of TS (Pasaro Mendez, Fernandez, Goyanes, & Mendez, 1994; Rovet & Ireland, 1994; Temple & Carney, 1993).

ASSESSMENT

Given the wide variety of difficulties that may be associated with TS, every child with this syndrome must be provided with a thorough neuropsychological evaluation. It is critical that neuropsychological and education problems be identified and treated early in a child's academic career (Rovet, 1993). In order to assess for all of the possible sequelae of TS, it is important to develop a comprehensive battery. This battery should include, at a minimum, measures of intelligence, achievement (including instruments designed for intense assessment of mathematics and reading), nonverbal (visual-perceptual) skills, executive function, memory, and personality/behavior.

Assessment for deficits associated with the cognitive phenotype of TS should start with the use of a well-standardized comprehensive assessment instrument that explores several facets of cognitive functioning, verbal and nonverbal. Academic achievement is another critical area for assessment in TS. It is critical for learning disabilities to be diagnosed so that appropriate interventions can be implemented. Given the likelihood of academic problems, especially in the area of mathematics, it is very important to obtain a thorough educational evaluation.

In addition to broad achievement measures, more specialized instruments may also be of use in diagnosing learning disabilities and designing intervention strategies. Because people with TS may exhibit a variety of visual-perceptual problems, it is important to obtain a broad range of assessment in this area. Visual-perceptual instruments can be divided into a number of areas, including measures of visual-perceptual or gestalt integration, spatial relations and visual matching, and visual-constructional skills. In addition, it can be helpful to assess the processing of aural and visual stimuli, sequencing, and recall. Executive functioning is an area that can be critical to assess for girls and women with TS, given the broad range of effects that deficits in this area can contribute to. Memory (both visual and auditory), attention, and concentration should be assessed as well.

Finally, assessment of psychological adjustment is very important in evaluating people with TS. Personality measures can be divided into three general categories: parent/teacher reports, child self-reports, and projective measures. In each of these categories, it is essential to assess psychological symptomatology, self-esteem, and social skills that may require clinical attention. Assessment of psychological symptomatology should include instruments designed to assess for more general psychopathology, as well as instruments designed to assess depression, anxiety, social anxiety, and self-esteem more specifically. Assessment of information processing and coping styles can also be helpful for planning intervention for people with TS.

INTERVENTIONS

Intervention for children and adults with TS is critical for a positive life outcome. A girl or woman with TS is at risk for developing a wide range of sequelae. The clinical needs of patients with TS fall across four areas: medical, social, academic, and sexual issues (Mullins, Lynch, Orten, & Youll, 1991).

Medical Interventions

Because a wide variety of medical problems can occur with TS, it is critical that regular medical care be obtained (Mullins et al, 1991; Orten, 1990; Orten & Orten, 1994; Rovet, 1995). It is also critical that every girl or woman with TS and her family receive accurate and sensitive medical information (Orten, 1990). In 2000 there was a consensus workshop at the Fifth International Symposium on Turner Syndrome, which resulted in a set of comprehensive recommendations for the diagnosis and management of TS (Saenger et al., 2001). This set of guidelines suggested a multidisciplinary approach to treatment and management. Early in life, assessment of cardiac and renal complications associated with TS is recommended. In addition, assessment of hypertension is recommended. Due to ear malformations and a high prevalence of otitis media, assessment of hearing is recommended, as well as assessment of potential speech problems. Other areas to address include the eyes, orthopedic concerns (e.g., scoliosis), orthodontic concerns (due to small mandibles), weight, lymphedema, and glucose intolerance.

Management of short stature is also recommended, given the impact that this can have on socialization and academic achievement. This includes growth hormone therapy to stimulate growth and thus to increase adult height. The management of puberty through the use of estrogen replacement therapy to stimulate the development of secondary sexual characteristics and healthy bones and tissue is also encouraged. With early and timely use of estrogen and growth hormone, most girls with TS can be brought to normal height (Rosenfeld et al., 1992). This can have a critical impact on the development of self-esteem in these children. If the teasing that begins when a child with TS begins to lag behind her peers can be avoided by helping the child reach her developmental/physical milestones on time, self-esteem may be spared (Orten, 1990; Orten & Orten, 1994; Perheentupa et al., 1974). Interestingly, research exploring the impact of the use of estrogen on memory in girls with TS has suggested improvements in both verbal and nonverbal memory (Ross, Roeltgen, et al., 2000).

During adulthood, continued treatment for medical conditions is critical, and there is an increased emphasis on fertility issues. With recent advances in fertility interventions, such as *in vitro* fertilization with a donor egg, pregnancy is now a possibility for some women with TS and their partners. For women with functional ovaries, the timing of pregnancy can be critical, given the risk of premature ovarian failure. The cryptopreservation of ovarian tissue and immature oocytes is a current line of research designed to allow women with TS to become pregnant with their own eggs.

Psychosocial Interventions

As the review above has shown, girls and women with TS can experience a wide variety of psychosocial problems. For our purposes here, these difficulties are divided into two categories. The first area for attention is the treatment of issues of concern associated with the diagnosis of TS. The second area is the treatment of specific symptomatology.

Issues of Concern Related to the Diagnosis

One of the first issues that people diagnosed with TS have to cope with is the diagnosis of a chronic syndrome with wide-ranging ramifications. Persons who are diagnosed with a chronic, lifelong illness must adapt to both the physical and psychological sequelae of the illness, as well as the fact that their lives and potentially their views of self have been altered. Russo (1986) and Varni and Wallander (1988) discuss the need for people with chronic illnesses to address the specific stressors that affect their lives and to develop positive coping strategies to deal with these stressors. Positive adjustments lead to resilience, and poor adjustment leads to vulnerability to stressors (Varni & Wallander, 1988). Self-esteem issues are often involved in this adjustment. Both a person with TS and her family members will have many emotional reactions at the time of diagnosis, and these reactions are similar to those experienced when any major medical condition is diagnosed (Orten & Orten, 1994). According to Orten and Orten, these reactions can fall into four categories.

The first category of adjustment is the need to resolve "the personal meaning of TS" (Orten & Orten, 1994, p. 241). The age at diagnosis will have an impact on the initial issues involved in obtaining personal meaning. For younger children, the main issues may revolve around medical aspects of the syndrome and potential medical interventions (treatments, hospitalizations, and the like). During the teenage years, issues may include "being different" from others and the physical anomalies the patients may have. For late adolescents and adults, issues surrounding fertility and parenthood may arise. Coming to terms with these issues may be complicated by the severity of the medical problems that a girl or woman faces. The impact of the diagnosis can also be mediated by the parents' reactions to the diagnosis (Orten & Orten, 1994).

A second category of adjustment is coping with the reactions of others, especially reactions to the patients' short stature. Teasing about short stature often begins during the elementary school years. If growth hormone therapy is initiated at the appropriate times, this problem may be avoided. However, girls with TS may also be teased about other physical abnormalities. For adult women, short stature and youthful appearance can cause difficulties in the workplace. Teaching ways to cope and deal with teasing and potential discrimination in a positive and helpful manner is a critical part of intervention for girls and women with TS (Orten & Orten, 1994).

Deciding whether and, if so, when to tell others about the diagnosis is another issue of particular concern for girls and women with TS. For children, one form this question may take is whether or not to inform the school about the diagnosis. As with any medical or psychological problem, informing the school can lead to positive outcomes, such as greater understanding of and more accommodations to the special needs of the child; however, it can also result in the child's being stigmatized and treated differently in a negative way. The decision to inform or not to inform the school is one that needs to be made jointly by the treatment team, the parents, and the child if she is mature enough to participate in the decision (Orten & Orten, 1994).

Whether or not to tell dating partners or potential intimate relationships about TS is a question that is often faced in adulthood. Issues surrounding fertility and parenthood again become critical. These issues can have an impact on a partner as well as a woman with TS.

A final area that girls and women have to deal with when coming to terms with TS are the physical problems and their impact on lifestyle and quality of life. Often this involves grieving for lost abilities. It is important for girls and women to understand the potential medical and cognitive implications of TS, and to deal with these on a day-to-day basis.

One of the major mediating factors in coping with stress is perceived social support (Varni, Rubinfeld, Talbot, & Setoguchi, 1989). Because of this, a support group model for intervention may be very appropriate. Support groups, with members who face similar issues, can provide reassurance, information, and advice. Psychoeducational models often meet the needs and desires of participants in TS support groups (Mullins et al., 1991). Attention to family members and to their coping with the diagnosis and sequelae of TS is also important because families can be a major source of support for some girls and women (Mullins et al., 1991; Orten & Orten, 1994). A survey by Orten and Orten (1992) found that a large number of parents were provided with incomplete and pessimistic medical explanations at the time of diagnosis, and that the parents were very dissatisfied (and at times angry) with the explanations that they were given. Thus one of the first areas of intervention with families is to assure that they receive accurate and adequate medical, psychological, and developmental information regarding TS (Orten, 1990).

Good information for women with TS and families of girls with TS can be found in a number of places. One is the Turner Syndrome Society of the United States (*www.turnersyndrome.org*). This is a nonprofit organization with the following missions: to increase public awareness, to increase understanding of the people who are affected by TS, to provide a forum for those affected by TS to become acquainted with one another, and to provide an opportunity for interaction between health care professionals and those affected by TS. The society sponsors a conference each year and offers a number of publications on TS. Other web resources include the MedlinePlus Medical Encyclopedia and the Mayo Clinic website. In addition, good family communication is important in helping girls and women with TS cope with issues surrounding it. Finally, individual therapy may be important for some girls and women at various stages of their lives.

Other Specific Psychosocial Symptomatology

As mentioned above, there are several areas of potential psychosocial symptomatology for girls and women with TS. Unfortunately, little empirical research has been conducted on psychosocial interventions for people with TS. The first is the area of social skills. Most interventions in this area have been cognitive-behavioral in nature. Target behaviors have included increasing the rate of social interaction, enhancing prosocial skills, and decreasing antisocial or aggressive behaviors. Interventions have included social problem-solving training, anger coping training, coaching, and behavioral rehearsal. These interventions can take place in individual therapy or groups (Smith, Barkley, & Shapiro, 2006). The second major area of concern is the symptomatology of hyperactivity and inattention in some girls with TS. The most common treatment approaches for these problems are cognitive-behavioral and psychopharmacological or a combination of the two (Smith et al., 2006). The National Cooperation Growth Study supported the need for a combination of educational, behavioral, and medical treatment (Siegel et al., 1998).

Academic Interventions

Early intervention is critical in helping children with learning disabilities. The first issue of concern when implementing academic interventions are the individual needs of each child. Some children will require placement in a special education program, while others may benefit from tutoring alone. It is also important to make sure that the expectations for each child are developmentally appropriate and follow a developmental sequence. In addition, interventions work best when parents and the school work as a team with the child to deal with the special needs of the child. Finally, it is very helpful to utilize areas of strength to remediate or circumvent areas of weakness. This is one of the reasons why a thorough educational assessment is important. Although there are a wide variety of intervention models for working with children with special academic needs, it is most critical that the intervention "fit" a child with TS and her personal strengths and weaknesses.

The only formal study that has examined an academic intervention with girls with TS was conducted by Williams and colleagues (1992). In that study, the girls with TS were compared to children with NLD, and an intervention commonly used for youth with NLD—cognitive behavior modification or strategy training (Meichenbaum, 1985)—was also utilized with the girls with TS. The intervention included the use of verbal mediation skills for planning and executing a learning task. This allowed the girls with TS to use a well-developed skill area, their verbal skills, to help them learn ways of performing a nonverbal task. The results of this study showed a significant improvement in spatial task performance in both groups following the cognitive behavior modification training. This suggests that girls with TS may be responsive to remediation of their educational deficits.

SUMMARY AND CONCLUSIONS

Turner syndrome, a chromosomal abnormality that affects only females, can result in myriad lifelong physical/medical, psychosocial, and educational problems. The type and severity of the problems may vary widely across patients. However, there are some hallmark symptoms associated with the syndrome; these include short stature, failure to develop secondary sexual characteristics at puberty, infertility, visual-perceptual difficulties, executive functioning and memory, academic problems with mathematics, and social skill difficulties. Many of the physical/medical problems can be dealt with through supportive therapy, including hormone replacement therapy. Special attention should be given to the psychosocial sequelae of the syndrome, and appropriate therapeutic interventions should be undertaken. Finally, early and appropriate intervention is critical for continued academic success. With the proper support, encouragement, and interventions, girls and women with TS can live long, productive, and happy lives.

REFERENCES

Alexander, D., & Money, J. (1966). Turner's syndrome and Gerstmann's syndrome: Neuropsychological comparisons. *Neuropsychologica, 4,* 265–273.

Alley, T. R. (1983). Growth produced changes in body shape and size as determinants of perceived age and adult caregiving. *Child Development, 54,* 241–248.

Baekgaard, W., Nyborg, H., & Nielsen, J. (1978). Neuroticism and extroversion in Turner's syndrome. *Journal of Abnormal Psychology, 87,* 583–586.

Bender, B. G., Linden, M. G., & Robinson, A. (1994). Neurocognitive and psychosocial phenotypes associated with Turner syndrome. In S. H. Broman & J. Grafman (Eds.), *Atypical cognitive deficits in developmental disorders* (pp. 197–216). Hillsdale, NJ: Erlbaum.

Bender, B. G., Puck, M., Salbenblatt, J., & Robinson, A. (1984). Cognitive development of unselected girls with complete and partial X monosomy. *Pediatrics, 73,* 175–182.

Berch, D. B. (1996). Memory. In J. Rovet (Ed.), *Turner syndrome across the lifespan* (pp. 140–145). Toronto: Klein Graphics.

Buchanan, L., Pavlovic, J., & Rovet, J. (1998). A reexamination of the visuospatial definition of Turner syndrome: Contributions of working memory. *Developmental Psychology, 14,* 341–367.

Buckley, F. (1971). Preliminary report on intelligence quotient scores of patients with Turner's syndrome: A replication study. *British Journal of Psychiatry, 119,* 513–514.

Clark, C., Klonoff, H., & Hayden, M. (1990). Regional cerebral glucose metabolism in Turner syndrome. *Canadian Journal of Neurological Science, 17,* 140–144.

Cutter, W. J., Daly, E. M., Robertson, D. M., Chitnis, X. A., van Amelsvoort, T. A., Simmons, A., et al. (2006). Influence of X chromosome and hormones on human brain development: A magnetic resonance imaging and proton magnetic resonance spectroscopy study of Turner syndrome. *Biological Psychiatry, 59,* 272–282.

Darby, P. L., Garfinkel, P. E., Vale, J. M., Kirwan, P. J., & Brown, G. M. (1981). Anorexia nervosa and "Turner syndrome": Cause or coincidence? *Psychological Medicine, 11,* 141–145.

Dellantonio, A., Lis, A., Saviolo, N., Rigon, F., & Tenconi, R. (1984). Spatial performance and hemispheric specialization in the Turner syndrome. *Acta Medica Auxologica, 16,* 193–203.

Downey, J., Ehrhardt, A., Gruen, R., Bell, J., & Morishima, A. (1989). Psychopathology and social functioning in women with Turner syndrome. *Journal of Nervous and Mental Disease, 177,* 191–200.

Downey, J., Elkin, E. J., Ehrhardt, A. A., Meyer-Bahlburg, H. F., Ball, J. J., & Morishima, A. (1991). Cognitive ability and everyday functioning in women with Turner syndrome. *Journal of Learning Disabilities, 24,* 32–39.

Ehrhardt, A. A., Greenberg, N., & Money, J. (1970). Female gender identity and absence of fetal hormones: Turner's syndrome. *Johns Hopkins Medical Journal, 126,* 142–155.

El Abd, S., Turk, J., & Hill, P. (1995). Annotation: Psychological characteristics of Turner syndrome. *Journal of Child Psychology and Psychiatry, 36,* 1109–1125.

Elgar, K., Campbell, R., & Skuse, D. (2002). Are you looking at me?: Accuracy in processing line-of-sight in Turner syndrome. *Proceedings of the Royal Society of London, Series B, 269*(1508), 2415–2422.

Ford, C. E., Jones, K. W., Polani, P. E., de Almeida, J. C., & Briggs, J. H. (1959). A sex chromosome anomaly in a case of gonadal dysgenesis (Turner's syndrome). *Lancet, i,* 711–713.

Garron, D. C. (1977). Intelligence among persons with Turner's syndrome. *Behavior Genetics, 7,* 105–127.

Hart, S. J., Davenport, M. L., Hooper, S. R., & Belger, A. (2006). Visuospatial executive function in Turner Syndrome: Functional MRI and neurocognitive findings. *Brain, 129,* 1125–1136.

Hassold, T. J. (1986). Chromosome abnormalities in human reproductive wastage. *Trends in Genetics, 2,* 105–110.

Higurashi, M., Kawai, H., Segawa, M., Iijima, K., Ikeda, Y., Tanaka, F., et al. (1986). Growth, psychological characteristics, and sleep wakefulness cycle of children with sex chromosome abnormalities. *March of Dimes Birth Defects Foundation: Original Article Series, 22,* 251–275.

Hook, E. B., & Warburton, D. (1983). The distribution of chromosomal genotypes associated with Turner's syndrome, live birth prevalence rates and evidence of diminished fetal mortality and severity in genotypes associated with structural X abnormalities or mosaicism. *Human Genetics, 64,* 24–27.

Jacobs, P. A., Betts, P. R., Cockwell, A. E., Crolla, J. A., Mackenzie, M. J., Robinson, D. O., et al. (1990). A cytogenic and molecular reappraisal of a series of patients with Turner's syndrome. *Annals of Human Genetics, 54,* 209–223.

Jones, K. L. (1988). X0 syndrome (Turner syndrome). In K. L. Jones (Ed.), *Smith's recognizable patterns of human malformation* (pp. 74–79). Philadelphia: Saunders.

Jorm, A. F., Share, D. L., Matthews, R., & Maclean, R. (1986). Behavior problems in specific reading retarded and general reading backward children: A longitudinal study. *Journal of Child Psychology and Psychiatry, 27,* 33–43.

Kesler, S. R., Blasey, C. M., Brown, W. E., Yankowitz, J., Zeng, S. M., Bender, B. G., et al. (2003). Effects of X-monosomy and X-linked imprinting on superior temporal gyrus morphology in Turner syndrome. *Biological Psychiatry, 54,* 636–646.

Kolb, J. E., & Heaton, R. K. (1975). Lateralized neurologic deficits and psychopathology in a Turner syndrome patient. *Archives of General Psychiatry, 32,* 1198–1200.

Kron, L., Katz, J. L., Gorzynski, G., & Weiner, H.

(1977). Anorexia nervosa and gonadal dysgenesis. *Archives of General Psychiatry, 34,* 332–335.

Lawrence, K., Kuntsi, J., Coleman, M., Campbell, R., & Skuse, D. (2003). Face and emotion recognition deficits in Turner syndrome: A possible role for X-linked genes in amygdala development. *Neuropsychology, 17,* 39–49.

Lewandowski, L. J. (1985). Clinical syndromes among the learning disabled. *Journal of Learning Disabilities, 18,* 177–178.

Lewandowski, L. J., Costenbader, V., & Richman, R. (1984). Neuropsychological aspects of Turner syndrome. *International Journal of Clinical Neuropsychology, 7,* 144–147.

Loesch, D. Z., Bui, Q. M., Kelso, W., Huggins, R. M., Slater, H., Warne, G., et al. (2005). Effect of Turner's syndrome and X-linked imprinting of cognitive status: Analysis based on pedigree data. *Brain and Development, 27,* 494–503.

Mathiesen, B., Reilly, S., & Skuse, D. (1992). Oral–motor dysfunction and feeding disorders in infants with Turner syndrome. *Developmental Medicine and Child Neurology, 34,* 141–149.

Mazzocco, M. M. (1998). A process approach to describing mathematics difficulties in girls with Turner syndrome. *Pediatrics, 102,* 492–494.

Mazzocco, M. M. M. (2001). Math learning disability and math LD subtypes: Evidence from studies of Turner syndrome, fragile X, and neurofibromatosis type 1. *Journal of Learning Disabilities, 34,* 520–533.

Mazzocco, M. M., Bhatia, N. S., & Lesniak-Karpiak, K. (2006). Visuospatial skills and their association with math performance in girls with fragile X or Turner syndrome. *Child Neuropsychology, 12,* 87–110.

McCauley, E., Ito, J., & Kay, T. (1986). Psychosocial functioning in girls with the Turner syndrome and short stature. *Journal of the American Academy of Child Psychiatry, 25,* 105–112.

McCauley, E., Kay, T., Ito, J., & Treder, R. (1987). The Turner syndrome: Cognitive deficits, affective discrimination, and behavior problems. *Child Development, 58,* 464–473.

McCauley, E., Ross, R., Kushner, H., & Culter, G. (1995). Self-esteem and behavior in girls with Turner syndrome. *Journal of Developmental and Behavioral Pediatrics, 16,* 82–88.

McCauley, E., Sybert, V. P., & Ehrhardt, A. A. (1986). Psychosocial adjustment of adult women with Turner syndrome. *Clinical Genetics, 29,* 284–290.

McGlone, J. (1985). Can spatial deficits in Turner's syndrome be explained by focal CNS dysfunction or atypical speech lateralization? *Journal of Clinical and Experimental Neuropsychology, 7,* 375–394.

Meichenbaum, D. (1985). Teaching thinking: A cognitive-behavioral perspective. In S. F. Chipman, J. W. Segal, & R. Glaser (Eds.), *Thinking and learning skills: Vol. 2. Research and open questions* (pp. 407–426). Hillsdale, NJ: Erlbaum.

Money, J. (1963). Cytogenetic and psychosexual incongruities with a note on space–form blindness. *American Journal of Psychiatry, 119,* 820–827.

Money, J. (1964). Two cytogenetic syndromes: Psychologic comparisons. I. Intelligence and specific factor quotients. *Journal of Psychiatric Research, 2,* 223–231.

Money, J. (1993). Specific neurocognitive impairments associated with Turner (45,X) and Klinefelter (47,XXY) syndromes: A review. *Social Biology, 40,* 147–151.

Money, J., & Alexander, D. (1966). Turner's syndrome: Further demonstration of the presence of specific cognitional deficiencies. *Journal of Medical Genetics, 3,* 47–48.

Money, J., & Mittenthal, S. (1970). Lack of personality pathology in Turner's syndrome: Relations to cytogenetics, hormones, and physique. *Behavior Genetics, 1,* 43–56.

Muhs, A., & Lieberz, K. (1993). Anorexia nervosa and Turner's syndrome. *Psychopathology, 26,* 29–40.

Mullins, L. L., Lynch, J., Orten, J., & Youll, L. K. (1991). Developing a program to assist Turner's syndrome patients and families. *Social Work in Health Care, 16,* 69–79.

Murphy, D., Allen, G., Haxby, J., Largay, K. A., Daly, E., White, B. J., et al. (1994). X-chromosome effects on female brain: A magnetic resonance imaging study of Turner's syndrome. *Lancet, 342,* 1197–2000.

Murphy, M. M., & Mazzocco, M. M. M. (2008). Mathematics learning disabilities in girls with fragile X or Turner syndrome during late elementary school. *Journal of Learning Disabilities, 41,* 29–46.

Netley, C., & Rovet, J. (1982). Atypical hemispheric lateralization in Turner syndrome subjects. *Cortex, 18,* 377–384.

Nielsen, J., Nyborg, H., & Dahl, G. (1977). Turner's syndrome: A psychiatric-psychological study of 45 women with Turner's syndrome. *Acta Jutlandica, 45*(Monograph).

Nielsen, J., & Stradiot, M. (1987). Transcultural study of Turner's syndrome. *Clinical Genetics, 32,* 260–270.

Nijhuis-van der Sanden, M. W., Eling, P. A., Van Asseldonk, E. H., & Van Galen, G. P. (2004). Decreased movement speed in girls with Turner syndrome: A problem in motor planning or muscle initiation? *Journal of Clinical and Experimental Neuropsychology, 26,* 795–816.

Nijhuis-van der Sanden, R. W., Smits-Engelsman, B. C., & Eling, P. A. (2000). Motor performance in girls with Turner syndrome. *Developmental Medicine and Child Neurology, 42,* 685–690.

Orten, J. L. (1990). Coming up short: The physical, cognitive and social effects of Turner's syndrome. *Health and Social Work, 7,* 100–106.

Orten, J. D., & Orten, J. L. (1992). Achievement among women with Turner's syndrome. *Families in Society: The Journal of Contemporary Human Services, 73,* 424–431.

Orten, J. L., & Orten, J. D. (1994). Women with Turner's syndrome: Helping them reach their full potential. *Disability and Society, 9,* 239–248.

Pasaro Mendez, E. J., Fernandez, R. M., Goyanes, V., & Mendez, J. (1994). Turner's syndrome: A behavioral and cytogenetic study. *Journal of Genetic Psychology, 154,* 433–447.

Pavlidis, K., McCauley, E., & Sybert, V. P. (1995). Psychosocial and sexual functioning in women with Turner syndrome. *Clinical Genetics, 47,* 85–89.

Pennington, B. F., Heaton, R. K., Karzmark, P., Pendleton, M. G., Lehman, R., & Shucard, D. W. (1985). The neuropsychological phenotype in Turner syndrome. *Cortex, 21,* 391–404.

Perheentupa, J., Lenko, H. L., Nevalainen, I., Nittymaki, M., Soderheim, A., & Taipale, V. (1974). Hormone therapy in Turner's syndrome: Growth and psychological aspects. *Growth and Developmental Endocrinology, 5,* 121–127.

Raboch, J., Kobilkova, J., Horejsi, J., Starka, L., & Raboch, J. (1987). Sexual development and life of women with gonadal dysgenesis. *Journal of Sex and Marital Therapy, 13,* 117–126.

Rezaie, R., Dalyy, E. M., Cutter, W. J., Murphy, D. G. M., Robertson, D. M. W., DeLisi, L. E., et al. (2008). The influence of sex chromosome aneuploidy on brain asymmetry. *American Journal of Medical Genetics, Part B, 150B,* 74–85.

Robinson, A., Bender, B., Borelli, J., Puck, M., Salbenblatt, J., & Winter, J. (1986). Sex chromosomal aneuploidy: Prospective and longitudinal studies. In S. Ratliffe & N. Paul (Eds.), *Prospective studies on children with sex chromosome aneuploidy* (pp. 23–73). New York: Liss.

Romans, S. M., Roeltgen, D., Kushner, H., & Ross, J. L. (1997). Executive function in girls with Turner's syndrome. *Developmental Neuropsychology, 13,* 23–40.

Rosenfeld, R., Franke, J., Artie, K., Brase, J. A., Bursteen, S., Cara, J., et al. (1992). Six year results of a randomized prospective trial of human growth hormone and oxandrolone in Turner's syndrome. *Journal of Pediatrics, 121,* 49–55.

Ross, J. L. (1990). Disorders of the sex chromosomes: Medical overview. In C. S. Holmes (Ed.), *Psychoneuroendocrinology: Brain, behavior and hormonal interactions* (pp. 127–137). New York: Springer-Verlag.

Ross, J. L., Kushner, H., & Roeltgen, D. P. (1996). Developmental changes in motor function in girls with Turner syndrome. *Pediatric Neurology, 15,* 317–322.

Ross, J. L., Roeltgen, D., & Cutler, G. B. (1995). The neurodevelopmental transition between childhood and adolescence in girls with Turner syndrome. In K. A. Albertsson-Wikland & M. B. Ranke (Eds.), *Turner syndrome in a life span perspective: Research and clinical aspects* (pp. 296–308). Amsterdam: Elsevier.

Ross, J. L., Roeltgen, D., Feuillan, P., Kushner, H., & Cutler, G. B., Jr. (1998). Effects of estrogen on nonverbal processing speed and motor function in girls with Turner's syndrome. *Journal of Clinical Endocrinology and Metabolism, 83,* 3198–3204.

Ross, J. L., Roeltgen, D., Kushner, H., Wei, F., & Zinn, A. R. (2000). The Turner syndrome: Associated neurocognitive phenotype maps to distal Xp. *American Journal of Human Genetics, 67,* 672–681.

Ross, J. L., Zinn, A. R., & McCauley, E. (2000). Neurodevelopmental and psychosocial aspects of Turner syndrome. *Mental Retardation and Developmental Disabilities Research Review, 6,* 135–141.

Rourke, B. P. (Ed.). (1985). *Neuropsychology of learning disabilities: Essentials of subtype analysis.* New York: Guilford Press.

Rovet, J. (1990). The cognitive and neuropsychological characteristics of children with Turner syndrome. In D. Berch & B. Bender (Eds.), *Sex chromosome abnormalities and human behavior: Psychological studies* (pp. 38–77). Boulder, CO: Westview Press.

Rovet, J. (1993). The psychoeducational characteristics of children with Turner syndrome. *Journal of Learning Disabilities, 26,* 333–341.

Rovet, J. (1995). Turner syndrome. In B. P. Rourke (Ed.), *Syndrome of nonverbal learning disabilities: Neurodevelopmental manifestations* (pp. 351–371). New York: Guilford Press.

Rovet, J. (2004). A review of genetic and hormonal influences on neuropsychological functioning. *Child Neuropsychology, 10*(4), 262–279.

Rovet, J., & Ireland, L. (1994). The behavioral phenotype of children with Turner syndrome. *Journal of Pediatric Psychology, 19,* 779–790.

Rovet, J., & Netley, C. (1981). Turner syndrome in a pair of dizygotic twins: A single case study. *Behavior Genetics, 11,* 65–72.

Rovet, J., & Netley, C. (1982). Processing deficits in Turner's syndrome. *Developmental Psychology, 18,* 77–94.

Russo, D. C. (1986). Chronicity and normalcy as the psychological basis for research and treatment in chronic disease in children. In N. A. Krasnegor, J. D. Arasteh, & M. F. Cataldo (Eds.), *Child health behavior: A behavioral pediatrics approach* (pp. 521–536). New York: Wiley.

Saenger, P., Albertsson Wikland, K., Conway, G. S., Davenport, M., Gravholt, C. H., Hintz, R., et al. (2001). Recommendations for the diagnosis and management of Turner syndrome. *Journal of Clinical Endocrinology and Metabolism, 86,* 3061–3069.

Shaffer, J. (1962). A specific cognitive deficit observed in gonadal aplasia (Turner's syndrome). *Journal of Clinical Psychology, 18,* 403–406.

Shucard, D. W., Shucard, J. L., Clopper, R. R., & Schachter, M. (1992). Electrophysiological and neuropsychological indices of cognitive processing deficits in Turner syndrome. *Developmental Neuropsychology, 8,* 299–323.

Siegel, P. T., Clopper, R., & Stabler, B. (1998). The psychological consequences of Turner syndrome and review of the National Cooperative Growth Study psychological substudy. *Pediatrics, 102,* 488–491.

Silbert, A., Wolff, P., & Lilienthal, J. (1977). Spatial and temporal processing in patients with Turner's syndrome. *Behavior Genetics, 7,* 11–21.

Skuse, D. (1987). Annotation: The psychological consequences of being small. *Journal of Child Psychology and Psychiatry, 28,* 641–650.

Skuse, D. H., Cave, S., O'Herlihy, A., & South, R. (1998). Quality of life in children with Turner syndrome: Parent, teacher, and individual perspectives. In D. Drotar (Ed.), *Measuring health related quality of life in children and adolescents: Implications for research and practice* (pp. 313–328). Mahwah, NJ: Erlbaum.

Skuse, D. H., James, R. S., Bishop, D. V. M., Coppin, B., Dalton, P., Aamodt-Leeper, G., et al. (1997). Evidence from Turner's syndrome of an imprinted X-linked locus affecting cognitive function. *Nature, 387,* 705–708.

Smith, B. H., Barkley, R. A., & Shapiro, C. J. (2006). Attention-deficit/hyperactivity disorder. In E. J. Mash & R. A. Barkley (Eds.), *Treatment of childhood disorders* (3rd ed., pp. 65–136). New York: Guilford Press.

Sonis, W. A., Levine-Ross, J., Blue, J., Cutler, G. B., Loriaux, P. L., & Klein, R. P. (1983). *Hyperactivity and Turner's syndrome.* Paper presented at the American Academy of Child Psychiatry Meetings, San Francisco.

Strang, J. D., & Rourke, B. P. (1983). Concept formation of non-verbal reasoning abilities of children who exhibit specific academic problems with arithmetic. *Journal of Clinical Child Psychology, 12,* 33–39.

Taipale, V., Niittymaki, M., & Nevalainen, I. (1982). Turner's syndrome and anorexia nervosa symptoms. *Acta Paedopsychiatrica, 48,* 231–238.

Tamm, L., Menon, V., & Reiss, A. L. (2003). Abnormal prefrontal cortex function during response inhibition in Turner syndrome: Functional magnetic resonance imaging evidence. *Biological Psychiatry, 53,* 107–111.

Taylor, H. G. (1989). Learning disabilities. In E. J. Mash & R. A. Barkley (Eds.), *Treatment of childhood disorders* (pp. 437–480). New York: Guilford Press.

Temple, C. M., & Carney, R. A. (1993). Intellectual functioning of children with Turner syndrome: A comparison of behavioural phenotypes. *Developmental Medicine and Child Neurology, 35,* 691–698.

Temple, C. M., & Carney, R. A. (1995). Patterns of spatial functioning in Turner's syndrome. *Cortex, 31,* 109–118.

Temple, C. M., Carney, R. A., & Mullarkey, S. (1996). Frontal lobe function and executive skills in children with Turner's syndrome. *Developmental Neuropsychology, 12,* 343–363.

Turner, H. H. (1938). A syndrome of infantilism, congenital webbed neck, and cubitus valgus. *Endocrinology, 23,* 566–574.

Varni, J. W., Rubinfeld, L. A., Talbot, D., & Setoguchi, Y. (1989). Stress, social support, and depressive symptomatology in children with congenital/acquired limb deficiencies. *Journal of Developmental and Behavioral Pediatrics, 10,* 13–16.

Varni, J. W., & Wallander, J. C. (1988). Pediatric chronic disabilities: Hemophilia and spina bifida as examples. In D. K. Routh (Ed.), *Handbook of pediatric psychology* (pp. 190–221). New York: Guilford Press.

Waber, D. (1979). Neuropsychological aspects of Turner syndrome. *Developmental Medicine and Child Neurology, 21,* 58–70.

Watson, W. C. (1981). *Physiological psychology: An introduction.* Boston: Houghton Mifflin.

White, B. J. (1994). The Turner syndrome: Origin, cytogenetic variants, and factors influencing the phenotype. In S. H. Broman & J. Grafman (Eds.), *Atypical cognitive deficits in developmental disorders* (pp. 183–195). Hillsdale, NJ: Erlbaum.

Williams, J. K., Richman, L. C., & Yarbrough, D. B. (1992). Comparison of visual–spatial performance strategy training in children with Turner syndrome and learning disabilities. *Journal of Learning Disabilities, 25,* 658–663.

CHAPTER 14

Fragile X Syndrome and Fragile X–Associated Disorders

RANDI J. HAGERMAN

Fragile X syndrome (FXS) and fragile X–associated disorders (FXDs) include a broad spectrum of problems, including intellectual disability (ID) and learning disabilities; emotional problems; fragile X–associated primary ovarian insufficiency (FXPOI); and an aging syndrome associated with tremor, ataxia, and dementia, called the fragile X–associated tremor/ataxia syndrome (FXTAS). These disorders are caused by genetic mutations in the fragile X mental retardation 1 (FMR1) gene, which was discovered in 1991 (Verkerk et al., 1991). Those with FXS have a full mutation (>200 cytosine–guanine–guanine [CGG] repeats) on the front end of FMR1 leading to silencing or methylation of the gene, such that little or no FMR1 messenger RNA (mRNA) is transcribed, and subsequently little or no FMR1 protein (FMRP) is translated. It is the lack or deficiency of FMRP that leads to the physical, behavioral and cognitive deficits of FXS. In carriers with a premutation (55–200 CGG repeats), there is too much mRNA produced, two to eight times the normal level. This extra level of mRNA causes a gain of function in carriers. The resulting phenotypes include neurodevelopmental problems in some boys, such as attention-deficit/hyperactivity disorder (ADHD) and autism spectrum disorders

(ASDs); FXPOI in 20% of adult females; and FXTAS in 10% of older females and 40% of older males.

Significant advances over the last decade concerning the neurobiology of FXS have led to new treatments for FXS (Hagerman et al., 2009). FMRP, which is missing in FXS, is an RNA transport protein inhibiting the translation of many other mRNAs that occur in the neuron and are important for synaptic plasticity and learning (Bassell & Warren, 2008). In FXS there is enhanced translation of many proteins throughout the brain (Qin, Kang, Burlin, Jiang, & Smith, 2005), and one of the consequences is upregulation of the metabotropic glutamate receptor 5 (mGluR5) pathway, leading to weakening or long-term depression (LTD) of synaptic connections (Bear, Huber, & Warren, 2004). This finding has led to new treatments for FXS, specifically mGluR5 antagonists that have been shown to reverse the LTD and weak synaptic connections in the animal models for FXS (de Vrij et al., 2008; McBride et al., 2005; Yan, Rammal, Tranfaglia, & Bauchwitz, 2005). The new trials of mGluR5 antagonists in humans with FXS have included use of fenobam, which even in a single dose appeared to be promising in the treatment of adults with FXS (Berry-Kravis et al., 2009). FXS is the most common inherited form of ID and the most common single gene associated with ASDs. It is now leading the way for new targeted treatments for neurodevelopmental disorders (Hagerman et al., 2009). The mGluR5 antagonists are likely to be helpful for other causes of ASDs besides FXS.

PREVALENCE

Numerous studies have been done to determine the prevalence of both the premutation and the full mutation in the general population (Song, Barton, Sleightholme, Yao, & Fry-Smith, 2003). The premutation is more common, and it occurs in approximately 1 in 130–250 women and 1 in 250–810 males (Dombrowski et al., 2002; Fernandez-Carvajal et al., 2009; P. J. Hagerman, 2008). The full-mutation allele occurs in approximately 1 in 2,500 in the general population (P. J. Hagerman, 2008), but FXS is only recognized in 1 in 3,600 (Crawford et al., 2002). Some individuals with FXS are high-functioning and present with only learning problems or emotional problems and not ID, particularly females with the full mutation (Angkustsiri, Wirojanan, Deprey, Gane, & Hagerman, 2008). Approximately 2–3% of males with ID of unknown etiology have FXS (Slaney et al., 1995). In addition, 2–6% of individuals with ASDs have FXS (Hagerman, Rivera, & Hagerman, 2008b), so fragile X DNA testing should be carried out in all children or adults who present with ID or ASDs of unknown etiology.

FXS occurs in all racial and ethnic groups that have been studied (Sherman, 2002). A relatively high prevalence of both the premutation and the full mutation occurs in Finland, Israel, and Tunisia, suggesting a *founder effect*—that is, the presence of a carrier in the original founding population for these areas (Eichler & Nelson, 1996; Pesso et al., 2000; Song et al., 2003; Zhong et al., 1996).

INHERITANCE

The expansion from a premutation to a full mutation only occurs when the FMR1 gene is passed on to the next generation through a female. When the gene passes from a male with the premutation, he will pass on the premutation to all of his daughters because the sperm in males with FXS has only the premutation (Reyniers et al., 1993). Therefore, whether a male has a full mutation, a mosaic pattern (premutation in some cells and full mutation in others), or a premutation, he will only pass the premutation on to all of his daughters. A female, however, can pass either the premutation or the full mutation on to her children. The greater the CGG repeat number in a carrier female, the greater the chance of expansion to a full mutation in the next generation (Nolin et al., 2003). If a female has more than 100 CGG repeats, and she passes the X chromosome with the mutation on to her child, it will expand to a full mutation 100% of the time in the next generation. Since females have two X chromosomes, the risk of passing the mutation on to the next generation is 50% with each pregnancy. A carrier mother can therefore have affected daughters with FXS, daughters with the premutation, affected sons with FXS, sons with the premutation, and/or normal children without the fragile X mutation (McConkie-Rosell et al., 2007).

In contrast, a male will pass on the premutation to only his daughters but none of his sons. His sons will receive the Y chromosome and therefore will be unaffected by FXS or by the carrier state. Daughters who receive the mutation from their fathers have a high risk of producing children with FXS in the next generation. Therefore, once the diagnosis of FXS or the premutation is made, it is essential to have genetic counseling (McConkie-Rosell et al., 2007). All individuals in the family who are at risk to have the premutation or the full mutation should have fragile X DNA testing, which can be ordered by any physician and is usually covered by insurance.

It is imperative for affected families to understand the inheritance pattern of FXS. Family members should be well informed of the dynamics of inheritance, so that relatives will understand their risk for involvement from either the premutation or the full mutation. Figure 14.1 shows a family pedigree that demonstrates the change in CGG repeats through four generations and the types of clinical features in each generation

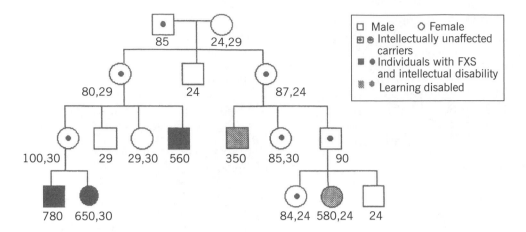

FIGURE 14.1. A pedigree of a family affected by FXS. The numbers represent the CGG repeat numbers at *FMR1* in each X chromosome. Note that the male with 350 repeats has an unmethylated full mutation; he does not have intellectual disability (ID), but does have learning disabilities. The female with 650 repeats has a full mutation and has ID, whereas the female with 580 repeats also has a full mutation, but has learning disabilities rather than ID.

that can be related to the premutation and the full mutation. Involvement in individuals with the full mutation is covered in detail below, followed by a briefer description of premutation involvement.

PHYSICAL, BEHAVIORAL, AND COGNITIVE PHENOTYPES OF FULL-MUTATION INVOLVEMENT

Physical Phenotype

Young children with FXS usually present with language and motor delays, hypotonia, and hyperactivity. The typical physical features of FXS may not be present in early childhood, so it is important not to dismiss a diagnosis of FXS solely because of a lack of these physical features (see Figure 14.2). Physical features of FXS include prominent ears, long face, hyperextensible finger joints, double-jointed thumbs, flat feet, soft skin, and a high-arched palate (Hagerman, 2002b). Most of these features can be seen in the general population, and children with FXS do not typically look dysmorphic or unusual. On occasion, ears can be dramatically prominent, with cupping in the upper part of the pinnae. Females with the full mutation are less likely than males to present with typical physical features of FXS. For males, macroorchidism (large testicles) is

also part of the physical phenotype, but it is usually not present until adolescence (Lachiewicz & Dawson, 1994). In adolescence or adulthood, the testicular volume may be two to three times normal size, although this is also not always recognized in a physical examination (Hagerman, 2002b). The degree of physical involvement and cognitive involvement in FXS correlates with the level of FMRP that is present in the blood (Loesch et al., 2004). Typical physical features of FXS are outlined in Table 14.1.

Many of the physical features in FXS are considered part of a connective tissue dysplasia (Hagerman, 2002b). The high frequency of otitis media difficulties in early childhood is probably related to the connective tissue problems, in that the eustachian tube is easily collapsible, trapping fluid in the middle ear. The connective tissue problems on occasion lead to other medical complications, such as hernias, scoliosis, and mitral valve prolapse (Hagerman, 2002b).

Growth abnormalities also may occur in FXS. Young patients often have a large head circumference, and those with FXS and autism have larger heads in early childhood than those with FXS but no autism do (Chiu et al., 2007). In puberty, however, the growth velocity may be slowed, and short stature is not uncommon in adulthood (Loesch, Huggins, & Hoang, 1995).

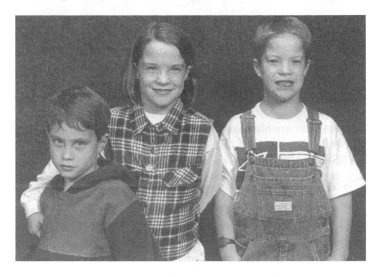

FIGURE 14.2. These siblings all have the full mutation of FXS. Although they do not display typical physical features of FXS, they do present with characteristic behavioral features of FXS (see text). Photograph used by permission of the children's parents.

TABLE 14.1. Typical Physical and Behavioral Features of FXS

Physical features	Behavioral features
Long ears	Poor eye contact
Prominent ears	Tactile defensiveness
Long face	Hand flapping
Single palmar crease	Hand biting
Cardiac murmur or click	Perseveration
	Hyperactivity
Hand calluses	Diagnosis of attention-deficit/hyperactivity disorder (ADHD)
Flat feet	
Hyperextensible finger joints	Verbal or physical outbursts
Double-jointed thumbs	Tantrums
High-arched palate	Shyness or social anxiety

Behavioral Phenotype

Behavioral features of FXS include an extremely short attention span, impulsivity, and hyperactivity, as well as hypersensitivity to visual, auditory, tactile, and olfactory stimuli (Miller et al., 1999; Roberts et al., 2001). Children with FXS often have difficulty in crowds and with loud noises because their hypersensitivity and hyperarousal often lead to tantrums or aggression. They may also overreact to some smells with a gagging or vomiting response. In addition, children with FXS may experience tactile defensiveness to such an extent that they pull away from light touch. Tags in clothes or firm textures of materials can be irritating to them. The extra stimuli associated with transitions—even going from the car into the house—can lead to behavior outbursts for children with FXS. Behavioral interventions and therapy, as described below, can be helpful in alleviating or calming the intensity of some of these behaviors.

Perseveration is a typical communicative and behavioral feature in children with FXS. Children may repeat a certain activity (e.g., stacking toys, spinning objects, flushing the toilet, or watching the same video) over and over again. Perseveration is also present in speech—not only in repeating the same phrase, but in talking about the same subject continually. Mumbling, echolalia, cluttered speech, and self-talk (i.e., carrying on a conversation with oneself, often using different vocal tones) are all commonly seen in individuals with FXS (Abbeduto & Hagerman, 1997; Hagerman, 2002b).

Autistic-like features are also common in children with FXS, including hand flapping, hand biting, toe walking, poor eye contact, tactile sensitivity, shyness, and social anxiety. Full autism—that is, autistic disorder as defined by the *Diagnostic and Statistical Manual of Mental Disorders*, fourth edition, text revision (DSM-IV-TR) and documented by standardized autism diagnostic measures such as the Autism Diagnostic Observation Schedule (ADOS)—occurs in 30% of boys with FXS, and DSM-IV-TR defined pervasive developmental disorder not otherwise specified (PDD-NOS) occurs in an additional 30% (Harris et al., 2008). Those with autism and FXS together have lower IQs than those with FXS without autism, but the severity of autism does not correlate with the level of FMRP once the IQ is controlled (Loesch et al., 2007). Autism is common in FXS, and it should be assessed in the evaluation of children with FXS because if it is present appropriate educational interventions should be carried out (including applied behavior analysis interventions, such as the Denver model or pivotal response training (Rogers & Vismara, 2008). Children with FXS are at high risk for autism because the absence or deficiency of FMRP leads to dysregulation of many proteins that are known to be associated with autism through their action in synaptic plasticity, or through dysregulation of the gamma-aminobutyric acid (GABA) and glutamate systems in the brain (Belmonte & Bourgeron, 2006). This dysregulation leads to an imbalance of inhibitory and stimulatory systems, problems with connectivity in the brain, weak synaptic connections, and growth abnormalities; some of these are related to protein tyrosine phosphatase (PTEN) dysregulation, which occurs in the absence of FMRP (Belmonte & Bourgeron, 2006; Chonchaiya et al., 2009; Hagerman, Rivera, & Hagerman, 2008).

Cognitive and Neuroanatomical Phenotypes

The majority of males with FXS have ID, with IQs lower than 70 (Bennetto & Pennington, 2002); females are less affected by FXS because they have two X chromosomes, and although the full mutation may be present on one of the X chromosomes, the other is normal and is producing FMRP. All females inactivate one of their X chromosomes, and an activation ratio, which can be calculated from the DNA studies, represents the percentage of cells with the normal X chromosome as the active chromosome. The activation ratio correlates with IQ in females and with the level of FMRP (Tassone et al., 1999). Approximately 50–70% of females with the full mutation have intellectual deficits in the

borderline or mild-ID range (de Vries et al., 1996). Females with normal IQs but with the full mutation usually demonstrate learning disabilities, including attentional and organizational problems and math difficulties. Approximately 70% of women with the full mutation who do not have an IQ deficit have problems in executive functioning, which relate to their difficulty with organization and attention (Cornish, Turk, & Hagerman, 2008). Their behavior is often impulsive, and they can be tangential in their speech, as well as mood-labile. Young girls and boys with the full mutation usually demonstrate significant shyness and social anxiety, which often interferes with social interactions and can predispose them to ASDs (Cordiero et al., unpublished raw data). On occasion the social withdrawal and anxiety may lead to quieter language and even selective mutism in school, but usually not at home (Hagerman, Hills, Scharfenaker, & Lewis, 1999).

Studies of neuroanatomical changes in FXS have helped to increase our understanding of the neurobehavioral phenotype of FXS (Reiss & Dant, 2003). In general, certain parts of the brain are generally larger in patients with FXS than in age- and IQ-matched controls. These areas include the caudate and the thalamus, although the amygdala is not enlarged, at least in younger boys with FXS (Hazlett et al., 2009). The brains of young children with idiopathic autism without FXS have a very different neuroanatomical structure from the brains of those with FXS either with or without autism. Boys with autism have a larger amygdala and a smaller caudate than boys with FXS (Hazlett et al., 2009). These findings demonstrate that the genetic etiology for autism is more important for determining brain structure than the behavioral phenotype of autism. The enlarged caudate in FXS may relate to the problems with executive functioning and ADHD that are common in these children.

PHENOTYPIC ILLUSTRATIONS

Case 1

Case 1, a boy age 4 years, 3 months, was diagnosed with FXS by FMR1 DNA testing. He has a full mutation that is fully methylated. He was born after a normal pregnancy, and his birthweight was 8 pounds, 14 ounces.

He did well in the newborn period, although his suck was poor, he was hypotonic, and his developmental milestones were mildly delayed. He sat at 10 months and walked at 15 months. At present he does not yet speak in phrases, but can use approximately 10–15 words. He began to hand-flap and bite his hands in his first year. His father called him "little butterfly" because of his hand flapping. He also chews excessively on things such as his shirt collar, has poor eye contact, and has problems with perseveration. He is easily overstimulated and has a high activity level, as well as impulsivity and distractibility. In addition, tantrums are a problem for him, although he is not physically aggressive. He has difficulty with transitions and becomes easily overwhelmed on a daily basis.

Like many children with FXS, this boy has had recurrent otitis media infections. Pressure-equalizing (PE) tubes were used to help alleviate this problem. His height is at the 75th percentile for his age, and both his weight and head circumference are at the 95th percentile for his age. He has visually prominent ears as well as ear cupping, but his face is not long. He has a high-arched palate, along with hyperextensible joints and double-jointed thumbs. In addition, his hands display a single palmar crease. His cardiac examination is normal, with no click or murmur, and he has flat feet.

His cognitive abilities were assessed several years ago with the Bayley Scales of Infant Development and the Vineland Adaptive Behavior Scales. On the Bayley, he is performing at a developmental level between 23 and 25 months. His mother describes him as difficult to motivate; she notes that he mainly enjoys watching videos and/or eating. On the Vineland, his Adaptive Behavior Composite score is 51, which is typical of a child 21–22 months of age. His other Vineland scores are as follows: Communication, 52; Daily Living Skills, 55; Socialization, 66; and Motor Skills, 49. He has not yet been able to complete the Kaufman Assessment Battery for Children (K-ABC) because of significant attention and concentration problems in addition to language deficits.

Case 2

Case 2 is a boy age 4 years, 6 months who has FXS and autism. DNA testing demon-strates a full mutation that is fully methylated, and he has no detectable FMRP in peripheral blood. His mother had a normal pregnancy, and she was delivered by cesarean section; his birthweight was 9 pounds, 5 ounces. He sat at 7 months, crawled at 11 months, walked at 21 months, and began speaking in two-word phrases at 3 years. He had significant reflux in the newborn period and was a very colicky baby. His parents noticed that his behavior was unusual even in the first year. He would frequently arch his back and focus on ceiling fans; he displayed hand flapping and poor eye contact, as well as tactile defensiveness. When he was diagnosed with autism, he was qualified to receive appropriate autism preschool services, as well as speech–language and occupational therapy. It was not until he was older than 3 years, well after his autism diagnosis was made, that he was found to also have FXS.

This boy is hyperactive with a very short attention span; he has tantrums, but these are not aggressive episodes. He has difficulty with transitions and anxiety on a daily basis. Although some of his autistic behavior has improved with therapy, he continues to seek self-stimulatory input and perseverates in spinning and twirling objects. In the past on the Vineland Adaptive Behavior Scales, his Adaptive Behavior Composite score is 54, with an age equivalent of 24 months. His other scores are as follows: Communication, 65; Daily Living Skills, 54; Socialization, 65; and Motor Skills, 51. His total score on the ADOS is 15, which is well into the autism range.

As noted above, he is already receiving special education and various therapies. He also spends part of the school day integrated into a regular kindergarten, where he is assisted by an aide. Mainstreaming him into the normal classroom is beneficial for him because he can learn from and imitate other children who are performing at a typical level. He has outgrown some of his autistic tendencies, and his interest in others and socialization skills have improved over time. However, he continues to be anxious, easily overwhelmed, and overstimulated, and he utilizes approach withdrawal behavior in most of his social interactions.

His medical history includes a history of sinusitis and recurrent otitis media infections, with more than 20 infections beginning at 6 months of age. He has not had hernias or joint dislocations, and his only surgery was for PE tubes because of the recurrent otitis media infections. He originally had a history of staring spells occurring a couple of times a week, and he was unresponsive to his name during these spells. An electroencephalogram was carried out and he was found to have spike wave discharges in the frontal and parietal areas, although no seizures were documented. Once he was started on valproic acid, his staring spells stopped, and he became more socially responsive.

His physical examination demonstrates a height at the 50th percentile, weight at the 75th percentile, and head circumference at the 98th percentile for his age. His forehead and ears are prominent, but his face is not long. He has a high-arched palate, hyperextensible joints, and flat feet, but does not have double-jointed thumbs, a single palmar crease, or hand calluses. Cardiac exam shows a normal rhythm, without murmur or click. His testicular volume is 3 ml bilaterally, which is normal for his age.

MOLECULAR–CLINICAL CORRELATIONS AND ADULT OUTCOME

As described earlier, the majority of males with FXS present with ID, although approximately 13% have IQs above 70 (Bennetto & Pennington, 2002; Hagerman, Hull, et al., 1994). This number may increase when younger children are examined. Freund, Peebles, Aylward, and Reiss (1995) found that approximately 50% of preschool boys with FXS had intellectual functioning in the typical or borderline range. Children with FXS may present with normal or near-normal expressive vocabulary abilities, and they also do well on visual matching tasks, so their initial IQ may look fairly good. However, IQ usually declines with age as more demands are made in reasoning. Significant IQ decline typically occurs in the majority of males and in about 30% of females with the full mutation (Bennetto & Pennington, 2002; Wright-Talamante et al., 1996). A few males are able to maintain IQs in the normal or borderline range in adolescence and adulthood. These individuals usually have variant DNA patterns and are producing a significant level of FMRP. For high-functioning males, a typical

pattern is a full mutation that is completely or almost completely unmethylated (Loesch, Huggins, & Hagerman, 2004). In addition, individuals with a mosaic pattern (i.e., some cells with the premutation and other cells with the full mutation) may also be high-functioning, particularly if a high percentage of cells demonstrate the premutation (Tassone et al., 1999). The higher the FMRP level, the more likely the patient is to maintain an IQ in the borderline or normal range. Studies have shown that the average IQ in adulthood for a male with the full mutation that is fully methylated is 41; the average IQ for a mosaic male is 60; and the average IQ for patients with a lack of methylation, or at least 50% of the mutation unmethylated, is 88 (Merenstein et al., 1996). Therefore, it appears that the level of FMRP produced by the gene correlates with an improved prognosis in adulthood (Tassone et al., 1999).

PREMUTATION INVOLVEMENT

Individuals with the premutation typically have IQs in the average range, and they were previously thought to be completely unaffected by the premutation. However, some children with the premutation were found to have cognitive deficits or autism, particularly boys; these findings led to further investigation of the molecular findings in those with the premutation who had problems (Tassone, Hagerman, Taylor, Mills, et al., 2000). Some of these individuals were found to have lower levels of FMRP, but the most striking and unexpected finding was elevation of the FMR1 mRNA level from two to eight times normal (Tassone, Hagerman, Taylor, Gane, et al., 2000). At the same time of this discovery, several grandfathers with the premutation were found to have a similar phenotype of tremor with action and ataxia leading to frequent falls (Hagerman et al., 2001). Further studies demonstrated that this phenotype of tremor and ataxia was seen in approximately 40% of male carriers who were older than 50 years, and that the prevalence increased with age (Jacquemont et al., 2004). This condition was found to be associated with the premutation and a toxicity to the neurons, leading to the formation of intranuclear inclusions in neurons and astrocytes, in addition to brain atrophy and white matter disease in the periventricular and subcortical regions and in the middle cerebellar peduncles (Adams et al., 2007; Jacquemont et al., 2003). This condition has been named the fragile X–associated tremor/ataxia syndrome (FXTAS), but it also includes executive function deficits, cognitive decline in all, dementia in some, and a neuropathy in most. The inclusions appear to be caused by the RNA toxicity of the premutation, but their formation may be a protective mechanism of the cell to handle the protein dysregulation that occurs in cells with the premutation (Greco et al., 2006). Various proteins become dysregulated with the toxicity of the premutation, including lamin A/C, alpha B crystallin, heat shock proteins, and ubiquitin, and they all are also sequestered in the inclusions of FXTAS (Arocena et al., 2005). Inclusions also occur in the peripheral nervous system, including autonomic ganglia throughout the body, such as pericardial ganglia, periadrenal ganglia, and myenteric plexus ganglia in the gastrointestinal system (Gokden, Al-Hinti, & Harik, 2009). This suggests that RNA toxicity affects the peripheral nervous system, leading to various types of autonomic dysfunction: impotence (which is common even before the onset of tremor and ataxia), orthostatic hypotension, hypertension, and even cardiac arrhythmias (Coffey et al., 2008; Jacquemont et al., 2003). Inclusions can also occur in the thyroid gland and in the Leidig cells of the testicles, which make testosterone (Greco et al., 2007; Louis, Moskowitz, Friez, Amaya, & Vonsattel, 2006). Testosterone deficiency is common in men with FXTAS, and thyroid dysfunction is also common, particularly in women with FXTAS (Coffey et al., 2008).

FXTAS can also occur in about 10% of women with the premutation who are older than 50 years, but dementia is rare because women are relatively protected by the second X chromosome (Coffey et al., 2008; Rodriguez-Revenga et al., 2009). Women with the premutation, however, have a higher rate of autoimmune problems (including fibromyalgia and thyroid disease) than age-matched controls without the premutation have (Coffey et al., 2008; Rodriguez-Revenga et al., 2009). In addition, about 3–4% of women with the premutation may also suffer from multiple sclerosis, and sometimes this can occur together with FXTAS (Greco et al., 2008).

An additional unique phenotype seen only in the premutation and not in the full mutation is primary ovarian insufficiency or FXPOI. Approximately 20% of women with the premutation will experience cessation of their menses before age 40, although a small percentage may become pregnant later (Sullivan et al., 2005). This is thought to relate to RNA toxicity in the ovum or in the cells that support the ovum, and it is more common with higher CGG repeat numbers in the premutation range (Sullivan et al., 2005; Wittenberger et al., 2007). In addition, women with the premutation have higher rates of depression and anxiety than the general population (Roberts et al., 2009). In individuals with FXTAS, inclusions occur throughout the limbic system, so it is likely that emotional problems in carriers are related to RNA toxicity in the limbic system.

Within the last decade, several children with the premutation have been found to have learning deficits; emotional problems such as anxiety; social deficits and ASDs; or even ID (Aziz et al., 2003; Farzin et al., 2006; Tassone, Hagerman, Taylor, Mills, et al., 2000). Although this finding led to the identification of elevated FMR1 mRNA in premutation carriers, the focus has been on the aging problems in carriers and FXTAS (P. J. Hagerman & Hagerman, 2004). However, now we know that the premutation can also cause neurodevelopmental problems, particularly in males with the premutation, because they only have one X chromosome and are not protected by the second X. Although most individuals with the premutation usually have IQs in the average range, ADHD and ASDs are not uncommon in males (Clifford et al., 2007; Farzin et al., 2006).

Case 3

Case 3 is a 12-year-old boy who was diagnosed as carrying the premutation at 8 years of age, when DNA testing demonstrated a CGG repeat number of 79. His mother had a normal pregnancy; she delivered at full term; and the birthweight was 6 pounds, 4 ounces. He did well in the newborn period and exhibited normal developmental milestones, including sitting at 6 months, walking at 11 months, riding a tricycle at 3 years of age, and riding a bicycle by 7 years of age. His coordination has been quite good, and he has played soccer and other sports, but he has had mild difficulty with handwriting and drawing. In the language area, he said words in the first year and sentences by 2 years of age. However, he was noted to be hyperactive as a toddler, and this persisted into his school years; his significant attentional problems and impulsivity led to a diagnosis of ADHD. He has also suffered from tantrums, which began at 3 years of age but became worse at age 9 and into adolescence. His mother is a premutation carrier with 70 repeats; her father (the boy's grandfather) suffers from tremor and ataxia in addition to mild dementia, and he has been recently diagnosed with FXTAS. He lives in an apartment attached to the main house, and Case 3's mother is stressed with the caretaking needs of her father.

As treatment for his ADHD, Case 3 was started on Concerta at 27 mg a day at age 8. He is now on 36 mg a day with a good response and normal growth parameters. His behavior has not included hand flapping or hand biting, but he had approximately one tantrum per week in middle childhood, and he has shown more significant problems with aggressive behavior both at home and at school within the last year. His mother has remarried during the last year, and he dislikes his stepfather. A more detailed psychological evaluation was recently carried out because of his history of both verbal and physical aggression. His emotional assessment demonstrated severe problems with anger, anxiety, mood instability, and dysthymia. It also revealed obsessive thinking focused on violent ideation. His aggressive ideation toward his stepfather was severe, and intensive counseling was initiated, in addition to a positive behavioral program in school.

Cognitive testing at age 8 years, 10 months with the K-ABC yielded an overall Mental Processing Composite score of 100, a Sequential Processing score of 108, and a Simultaneous Processing score of 95. Cognitive testing at 12 years of age with the third edition of the Wechsler Intelligence Scale for Children yielded a Full Scale IQ of 103, a Verbal IQ of 99, and a Performance IQ of 107.

Because Case 3's recent evaluation revealed not only severe ADHD but aggression and violent ideation, he was started on aripiprazole (Abilify—2 mg at bedtime, with a gradual increase to 4 mg), an atypical antipsychotic. This medication has helped to stabilize his mood, reduce his anxiety, further improve his ADHD symptoms, and decrease his aggression. He was also started in weekly counseling to help his aggression, anxiety, and dysthymia. Sertraline was subsequently started after the positive effects of the aripiprazole were noted, and it has further improved his mood, anxiety, and obsessive ideation.

Recent molecular testing for Case 3 demonstrated the presence of a premutation at 66 repeats that was completely unmethylated in 85% of his cells. However, it also showed an additional light smear in the full-mutation range with 230 repeats, and this was present in 15% of his cells and was methylated. Subsequent FMRP levels demonstrated that 70% of his lymphocytes stained positive for FMRP (Tassone et al., 1999). Case 3 is therefore a mosaic male with FXS; his cognitive abilities are in the average range, but he has significant emotional and behavioral problems, including ADHD, violent ideation, mood instability, and dysthymia. In addition, his FMR1 RNA level is 3.8 times normal, so he is also at risk for RNA toxicity. In essence, he has a "double hit"— that is, a mild decrease in FMRP levels that gives him some features of FXS, as well as elevated mRNA levels that may add to his psychopathology and perhaps to his ADHD and his social problems. My colleagues and I have never seen a patient with FXS develop FXTAS, and it is likely that the lowered level of FMRP can protect individuals from FXTAS.

ASSESSMENT ISSUES: WHO REQUIRES FMR1 DNA TESTING?

Children and adults with FXS or premutation involvement may often present with other diagnoses. These may include an ASD, such as PDD-NOS, autism, or Asperger syndrome; schizotypal personality disorder; or other diagnoses with specific etiologies, such as Tourette syndrome, Pierre Robin sequence, Soto syndrome, or even

Prader–Willi syndrome. Tics are seen in approximately 20% of patients with FXS, and abrupt mood swings and ADHD are common in those with the full mutation and in those affected by the premutation, as they are in Tourette syndrome. Children with Tourette syndrome do not usually demonstrate the cognitive deficits that are present in FXS, however. The large head circumference in childhood frequently causes FXS to be confused with Soto syndrome or cerebral gigantism. Approximately 5% of patients with FXS can have a cleft palate, which can be confused with other clefting syndromes, including Pierre Robin sequence. As previously discussed, autism and other ASDs also overlap with FXS. Obsessive–compulsive behavior is often seen in FXS, and occasionally the obsessive behavior may focus on eating, which can lead to obesity and a phenotype similar to Prader–Willi syndrome. This is called the Prader–Willi phenotype (PWP) in FXS, and it is associated with obesity, hyperphagia, delayed puberty, and often a small phallus. This PWP is not associated with a 15q deletion that is causal to Prader–Willi syndrome. However, recently a downregulation of cytoplasmic FMR1-interacting protein (CYFIP1), a sister protein that binds to FMRP and whose gene is located at the 15q region, was documented in individuals with the PWP compared to controls (Nowicki et al., 2007). The CYFIP1 level in individuals with the PWP was much lower than that of controls, and the level was also much lower than that seen in individuals with FXS without the PWP (Nowicki et al., 2007). Why CYFIP1 is down-regulated in the PWP is not known, but those with the PWP also have a higher ASD rate than is seen in FXS without the PWP (Nowicki et al., 2007).

It is important to consider fragile X testing in all individuals who have ID or ASDs, when the etiology for these problems is unknown. In addition, if there is a family history of ID, the chance that this could be due to FXS increases dramatically. As noted earlier, FXS causes 30% of X-linked ID, and in general FXS is the most common inherited form of ID or ASD known.

Not all children with hyperactivity should be tested for FXS. However, if a hyperactive child has cognitive deficits or typical physical features associated with FXS, has a family history consistent with FXDs, or

exhibits autistic-like features (e.g., hand flapping, hand biting, or poor eye contact), then the diagnosis of FXS or premutation involvement should be strongly considered, and DNA testing should be carried out. Similarly, not all children with learning disabilities need to be tested for FXS. However, if a learning disability involves math deficits (particularly in a female), and it is combined with shyness, social anxiety, or physical features related to FXS and/or with a family history of ID or consistent with an FXD, then this child should be tested for fragile X mutations. In addition, patients who have selective mutism or schizotypal personality disorder and other features consistent with FXS or FXDs should be tested.

An FXS or FXD diagnosis is important from two perspectives. First, it allows genetic counseling to be given to multiple family members who may be carriers of fragile X or affected by FXS. In addition, a diagnosis of FXS or FXD helps in the development of treatment programs, including the various interventions described below.

TREATMENT

There is no cure for FXS or FXDs, but various interventions and treatments are helpful for affected children and adults. For FXS the treatment team should include multiple professionals, including a special education teacher, a speech–language pathologist, an occupational therapist, a physician, and a psychologist (Braden, 2000; Hagerman, 2002a; Hagerman et al., 2009; Scharfenaker, O'Connor, Stackhouse, & Noble, 2002).

Medical Follow-Up and Psychopharmacology

The medical treatment of FXS includes vigorous intervention for recurrent otitis media infections, which can further exacerbate the language delays in FXS (Hagerman, Altshul-Stark, & McBogg, 1987). In addition, approximately 20% of patients have seizures; these can further interfere with normal development and academic progress, and they require treatment (Hagerman, 2002a; Hagerman et al., 2009). Other medical problems associated with loose connective tissue include rare hernias, rare joint dislocations, mitral valve prolapse, sinus infections, and gastroesophageal reflux. Medical interventions for these problems have been discussed elsewhere (Hagerman, 2002a).

Medical interventions can be most helpful for the behavior problems that are usually present in FXS. For the preschool child, tantrums and hyperarousal are common difficulties, in addition to a short attention span. Stimulant medications (see below) may benefit some preschool children, but may exacerbate behavioral problems in others (Berry-Kravis & Potanos, 2004; Hagerman et al., 2009; Hagerman, Murphy, & Wittenberger, 1988). Additional medications, including clonidine (Catapres), guanfacine (Tenex), and aripiprazole (Abilify), can also help ADHD symptoms (Hagerman et al., 2009). Abilify is an atypical antipsychotic that appears to be helpful in low doses for the majority of children and adults with FXS, not only for improving attention but also for stabilizing mood and improving anxiety and aggression (Hagerman et al., 2009). Currently a controlled trial is taking place in Indiana to test the efficacy of Abilify in the treatment of FXS.

For the treatment of moodiness, aggression, anxiety and obsessive–compulsive behavior, the selective serotonin reuptake inhibitors (SSRIs) have been remarkably helpful in FXS (Berry-Kravis & Potanos, 2004; Hagerman, Fulton, et al., 1994, 2009). The SSRIs include fluoxetine (Prozac), sertraline (Zoloft), paroxetine (Paxil), citalopram (Celexa), escitalpram (Lexapro), and fluvoxamine (Luvox). They are relatively safe and easy to monitor because they do not require regular blood work or electrocardiograms. The side effects include diarrhea, agitation, hyperactivity, sleep disturbances, abdominal pain, and the rare occurrence of mania. They are commonly used in adolescence and adulthood, and limited experience is available regarding their use in childhood. Controlled studies are needed to document their efficacy, specifically in FXS.

The most exciting aspect of treatment in FXS is the development of targeted treatments that can reverse the neurobiological abnormalities documented over the last few years. As noted at the beginning of this chapter, the absence or deficiency of FMRP leads to up-regulation downstream in the mGluR5 pathway. This pathway normally leads to LTD of synaptic plasticity, so that synaptic connections are weakened. FMRP is the inhibitor of this pathway; therefore, in the absence of FMRP there is enhanced LTD, which is thought to lead to the ID in FXS (Bear et al., 2004). Therefore, the use of mGluR5 antagonists should block this effect, and this has been proven in the mouse and *Drosophila* models of FXS (de Vrij et al., 2008; Dolen & Bear, 2008; McBride et al., 2005). Now treatment with mGluR5 antagonists has begun to be studied in patients with FXS, and preliminary positive responses have been seen in a single-dose trial of fenobam (Berry-Kravis et al., 2009). Lithium also down-regulates the mGluR5 system, and an open trial of lithium in individuals with FXS demonstrated positive behavioral effects, with some signs of improved cognition as well (Berry-Kravis et al., 2008).

Another new targeted treatment in FXS is minocycline, which lowers the level of matrix metalloproteinase (MMP9), one of a family of proteins important for synaptic plasticity. MMP9 levels are high in the absence of FMRP, and treatment of the knockout mouse model of FXS with 1 month of minocycline at birth improved synaptic connections and also improved behavior and cognition (Bilousova et al., 2009). Therefore, human trials are being initiated in children with FXS, although in children younger than 8 years minocycline can lead to the graying of teeth. Long-term minocycline treatment can lead to graying or darkening of other tissues, including skin, at any age. In addition, pseudotumor cerebri or increased intracranial pressure, as well as drug-induced lupus, can occur as a rare side effect of minocycline treatment. Further studies, including a controlled trial, are needed before minocycline can be broadly recommended for treatment of children with FXS. This new age of targeted treatments in FXS should lead to exciting benefits from treatment in cognition and behavior. It should also encourage more widespread screening efforts, including newborn screening.

Treatment of premutation involvement includes treatment of ADHD with stimulants, and treatment of the emotional problems (including anxiety and depression) with SSRIs (Bourgeois et al., 2009; Hagerman, Hall, et al., 2008). Treatment of FXPOI may include the use of hormone replacement therapy

(Wittenberger et al., 2007). Treatment of the tremor, the ataxia, and the pain problems associated with neuropathy in patients with FXTAS is more complicated; a recent review has been published on this topic (Hagerman et al., 2008a).

Speech–Language and Occupational Therapy

All children who are significantly affected by FXS can benefit from speech–language therapy and occupational therapy (Scharfenaker et al., 2002; Schopmeyer & Lowe, 1992). Speech and language deficits in FXS include auditory processing problems, cluttering, mumbling, poor pragmatics, motor dyspraxia, and difficulties with abstract reasoning. Speech–language therapy can focus on each of these deficits. Even in a child without ID, deficits in higher linguistic skills and pragmatics may exist. Strengths in the language area include memory and imitation skills, a fine sense of humor, and empathy in social interactions if there is no ASD. The memory strengths and the imitation skills can be well utilized in a therapy intervention program (Scharfenaker et al., 2002).

Sensory integration occupational therapy can also be helpful for children with FXS. Physical calming techniques, such as brushing of the arms and legs, joint compression, and deep back rubs, can be helpful in decreasing hyperarousal behavior or aggression. In addition to sensory integration therapy, a focus on fine and gross motor coordination and on motor planning is helpful in therapy. Hypotonia also improves with time and with intervention.

Additional techniques can be used to improve oral strength and verbalizations. PROMPT therapy has been studied in young children with ASDs but without FXS (Rogers et al., 2006), and anecdotal information suggests that it is also beneficial for children with FXS. For jaw and mouth strength, several approaches are suggested. For instance, introducing a variety of textured foods can help decrease oral sensitivity. Bagels, fruit leather, and chewy candy are excellent at improving oral function. Simple games, such as playing tug of war with a wet washcloth during bathtime, can also promote increased jaw strength (Scharfenaker et al., 2002). Other methods can be used for stimulat-

ing verbal expression, including the use of rhythm, movement, dancing, and singing. The combination of speech–language therapy with occupational therapy can be helpful, particularly for less verbal children with FXS (Scharfenaker et al., 2002). Therapies can be even more effective when they are implemented at home as well as in school.

The use of augmentative and alternative communication can be successful for children with FXS who are nonverbal. Many different methods of communication can be used to augment a child's speech production or provide an alternative to speech (Beukelman & Mirenda, 1992; Greiss-Hess et al., 2009), and an evaluation can determine which of these may be useful. For instance, some children may use signs and gestures to communicate with others. Pointing to pictures, or using the Picture Exchange Communication System, can also be a useful form of communication and choice making. Parents and teachers can create picture books or cards to help a child communicate his or her needs (e.g., the child can point to a picture of a glass of water when he or she is thirsty). For choice making, the child can choose between pictures of two things or activities (e.g., pictures of going outside or of playing in the house). More complicated picture boards can also be successful in generating expressive language. For instance, the child can select pictures that represent the words "I," "want," and "hug," to generate the sentence "I want [a] hug." Finally, speech output devices may be used to help a child communicate his or her needs through synthesized or digitized speech (Hagerman, 1999).

Computer-Based Interventions

Computer technology is a useful adjunct to the educational experience for children with FXS. They usually enjoy working on computers, and they show talent in this area. Computers can be utilized to enhance attention and build vocabulary skills, in addition to improving written language output. Adaptive peripherals, such as an expanded keyboard or IntelliKeys, can be useful in helping children with FXS to use a computer (IntelliTools, Inc., 1996).

The use of both visual and auditory feedback computer technology is most beneficial for children with FXS. Computers can help sustain attention in some children with FXS who are otherwise easily distracted in standard learning environments. There is such a wide variety of software available in different topics of learning that it is important to evaluate a child's cognitive level and visual–spatial, memory, motor, and language skills, in order to match a beneficial program to the child (Braden, 2002; Greiss-Hess et al., 2009; Scharfenaker et al., 2002). Some helpful programs include IntelliTalk from IntelliTools, which is a talking word processor that can speak letters, words, sentences, and a combination of all three (IntelliTools, Inc., 1996); and Co-Writer from Don Johnston, Inc., which is a combination of a dictionary and software that uses artificial intelligence to predict what a person wants to say (Greiss-Hess et al., 2009). Programs such as Co-Writer were initially established to aid people with physical limitations, but children with learning and cognitive disabilities have also benefited tremendously from these programs.

Behavioral and Educational Interventions

The use of behavioral intervention techniques, including structure and positive behavioral reinforcement, is beneficial for children with FXS. Several references outline behavioral interventions for children with FXS (Braden, 2000; Chonchaiya et al., 2009; Hills-Epstein, Riley, & Sobesky, 2002). A controlled trial of a sleep intervention in children with FXS was also beneficial (Weiskop, Richdale, & Matthews, 2005).

Children with FXS can be often educated in an inclusion setting in the regular classroom (Spiridigliozzi et al., 1994). If cognitive deficits or behavioral problems are significant, then an aide or paraprofessional can be utilized in the classroom to modify assignments or to give extra explanation to the child with FXS (and perhaps others who need it). An inclusion setting helps to improve social skills, since the child imitates the typical and appropriate behavior of the other children. Education in a segregated program exclusively with children who have special needs can be problematic, particularly if all of the other children are lower-functioning, since the child with FXS will imitate the behaviors and language of the lower-functioning children. Therefore, an inclusion setting is recommended for a child with FXS whenever possible, so that the other children in the class can model appropriate behavior for the child with FXS.

An emerging area of intervention in those with FXS is in the first year of life, as newborn screening becomes more widespread. Rogers and Vismara (2008) have reviewed early intervention efforts for young children with autism, and such interventions, including the Early Start Denver model, can be utilized in toddlers with FXS (Vismara & Rogers, 2008). As targeted treatments are shown to be safe in young children, they should also be combined with intensive early interventions to correct the central nervous system deficits in FXS and guide more normal development.

CONCLUSIONS

The broad spectrum of involvement in FXS requires a variety of interventions specific to each individual. Although there are similar physical, cognitive, and behavioral characteristics among children with FXS and FXDs, there is no set curriculum that will be effective for every child. For instance, some children who are premutation carriers may not require medical or educational intervention, whereas others may benefit from medication to help with anxiety or ADHD, or from tutoring to help with school difficulties. Children who are affected by FXS usually benefit from special education support, speech–language and occupational therapy, and medication; however, there is no set formula as to the extent of therapy or the specific medications that will be most helpful for each individual child. For this reason, it is essential for every child with FXS to be seen by a physician and a team of professionals who are familiar with FXS and can create an appropriate program for the child. A list of Fragile X clinical and research centers from throughout the United States and Canada is now expanding internationally and can be found on the website for the National Fragile X Foundation (*www.fragilex.org*). Once a family knows of the FXS or FXD diagnosis, it is helpful for the family to contact the National Fragile X Foundation, which has a network of parent support groups and resource centers around the country and internationally. The toll-free phone number of the National Fragile X Foundation is 800-688-8765. The National Fragile X Foundation can also provide educational information in papers, books, videos, and conferences for both parents and professionals.

ACKNOWLEDGMENTS

This work was partially supported by grants from the National Institute of Child Health and Human Development (Nos. HD036071 and HD 02274); Grant Nos. NIA AG032115, NCRR RR024146, and NIDCR DE019583 from the National Institute on Aging; and Grant No. 90DD0596 from the Health and Human Services Administration of Developmental Disabilities.

REFERENCES

Abbeduto, L., & Hagerman, R. J. (1997). Language and communication in fragile X syndrome. *Mental Retardation and Developmental Disabilities Research Reviews, 3*(4), 313–322.

Adams, J. S., Adams, P. E., Nguyen, D., Brunberg, J. A., Tassone, F., Zhang, W., et al. (2007). Volumetric brain changes in females with fragile X–associated tremor/ataxia syndrome (FXTAS). *Neurology, 69*(9), 851–859.

Angkustsiri, K., Wirojanan, J., Deprey, L. J., Gane, L. W., & Hagerman, R. J. (2008). Fragile X syndrome with anxiety disorder and exceptional verbal intelligence. *American Journal of Medical Genetics, Part A, 146*(3), 376–379.

Arocena, D. G., Iwahashi, C. K., Won, N., Beilina, A., Ludwig, A. L., Tassone, F., et al. (2005). Induction of inclusion formation and disruption of lamin A/C structure by premutation CGG-repeat RNA in human cultured neural cells. *Human Molecular Genetics, 14*(23), 3661–3671.

Aziz, M., Stathopulu, E., Callias, M., Taylor, C., Turk, J., Oostra, B., et al. (2003). Clinical features of boys with fragile X premutations and intermediate alleles. *American Journal of Medical Genetics, 121B*(1), 119–127.

Bassell, G. J., & Warren, S. T. (2008). Fragile X syndrome: Loss of local mRNA regulation alters synaptic development and function. *Neuron, 60*(2), 201–214.

Bear, M. F., Huber, K. M., & Warren, S. T. (2004). The mGluR theory of fragile X mental retardation. *Trends in Neurosciences, 27*(7), 370–377.

Belmonte, M. K., & Bourgeron, T. (2006). Fragile X syndrome and autism at the intersection of genetic and neural networks. *Nature Neuroscience, 9*(10), 1221–1225.

Bennetto, L., & Pennington, B. F. (2002). Neuropsychology. In R. J. Hagerman & P. J. Hagerman (Eds.), *Fragile X syndrome: Diagnosis, treatment, and research* (3rd ed., pp. 206–248). Baltimore: Johns Hopkins University Press.

Berry-Kravis, E., & Potanos, K. (2004). Psychopharmacology in fragile X syndrome—present and future. *Mental Retardation and Developmental Disabilities Research Reviews, 10*(1), 42–48.

Berry-Kravis, E., Sumis, A., Hervey, C., Nelson, M., Porges, S. W., Weng, N., et al. (2008). Open-label treatment trial of lithium to target the underlying defect in fragile X syndrome. *Journal of Developmental and Behavioral Pediatrics, 29*(4), 293–302.

Berry-Kravis, E., Hessl, D., Coffey, S., Hervey, C., Schneider, A., Yuhas, J., et al. (2009). A pilot open-label single-dose trial of fenobam in adults with fragile X syndrome. *Journal of Medical Genetics, 46*(4), 266–271.

Beukelman, D. R., & Mirenda, P. (1992). *Augmentative and alternative communication management of severe communication disorders in children and adults.* Baltimore: Brookes.

Bilousova, T. V., Dansie, L., Ngo, M., Aye, J., Charles, J. R., Ethell, D. W., et al. (2009). Minocycline promotes dendritic spine maturation and improves behavioural performance in the fragile X mouse model. *Journal of Medical Genetics, 46*(2), 94–102.

Bourgeois, J., Coffey, S., Rivera, S., Hessl, D., Gane, L., Tassone, F., et al. (2009). A review of fragile X premutation disorders: Expanding the psychiatric perspective. *Journal of Clinical Psychiatry, 70*(6), 852–862.

Braden, M. (2000). *Fragile, handle with care.* Silverthorne, CO: Spectra.

Braden, M. (2002). Academic interventions in fragile X. In R. J. Hagerman & P. J. Hagerman (Eds.), *Fragile X syndrome: Diagnosis, treatment and research* (3rd ed., pp. 428–464). Baltimore: Johns Hopkins University Press.

Chiu, S., Wegelin, J. A., Blank, J., Jenkins, M., Day, J., Hessl, D., et al. (2007). Early acceleration of head circumference in children with fragile X syndrome and autism. *Journal of Developmental and Behavioral Pediatrics, 28*(1), 31–35.

Chonchaiya, W., Schneider, A., & Hagerman, R. (2009). Fragile X: A family of disorders. *Advances in Pediatrics, 56*, 165–186.

Clifford, S., Dissanayake, C., Bui, Q., Huggins, R., Taylor, A., & Loesch, D. (2007). Autism spectrum phenotype in males and females with fragile X full mutation and premutation. *Journal of Autism and Developmental Disorders, 37*(4), 738–747.

Coffey, S. M., Cook, K., Tartaglia, N., Tassone, F., Nguyen, D. V., Pan, R., et al. (2008). Expanded clinical phenotype of women with the FMR1 premutation. *American Journal of Medical Genetics, Part A, 146A*(8), 1009–1016.

Cornish, K., Turk, J., & Hagerman, R. (2008). The fragile X continuum: New advances and perspectives. *Journal of Intellectual Disability Research, 52*(Pt. 6), 469–482.

Crawford, D. C., Meadows, K. L., Newman, J. L., Taft, L. F., Scott, E., Leslie, M., et al. (2002). Prevalence of the fragile X syndrome in African-Americans. *American Journal of Medical Genetics, 110*(3), 226–233.

de Vries, B. B., Wiegers, A. M., Smits, A. P., Mohkamsing, S., Duivenvoorden, H. J., Fryns, J. P., et al. (1996). Mental status of females with an FMR1 gene full mutation. *American Journal of Human Genetics, 58*(5), 1025–1032.

de Vrij, F. M. S., Levenga, J., van der Linde, H. C., Koekkoek, S. K., De Zeeuw, C. I., Nelson, D. L., et al. (2008). Rescue of behavioral phenotype and neuronal protrusion morphology in Fmr1 KO mice. *Neurobiology of Disease, 31*(1), 127–132.

Dolen, G., & Bear, M. F. (2008). Role for metabotropic glutamate receptor 5 (mGluR5) in the pathogenesis of fragile X syndrome. *Journal of Physiology, 586*(6), 1503–1508.

Dombrowski, C., Levesque, M. L., Morel, M. L., Rouillard, P., Morgan, K., & Rousseau, F. (2002). Premutation and intermediate-size FMR1 alleles in 10,572 males from the general population: Loss of an AGG interruption is a late event in the generation of fragile X syndrome alleles. *Human Molecular Genetics, 11*(4), 371–378.

Eichler, E. E., & Nelson, D. L. (1996). Genetic variation and evolutionary stability of the FMR1 CGG repeat in six closed human populations. *American Journal of Medical Genetics, 64*(1), 220–225.

Farzin, F., Perry, H., Hessl, D., Loesch, D., Cohen, J., Bacalman, S., et al. (2006). Autism spectrum disorders and attention-deficit/hyperactivity disorder in boys with the fragile X premutation. *Journal of Developmental and Behavioral Pediatrics, 27*(2 Suppl.), S137–S144.

Fernandez-Carvajal, I., Walichiewicz, P., Xiaosen, X., Pan, R., Hagerman, P. J., & Tassone, F. (2009). Screening for expanded alleles of the FMR1 gene in blood spots from newborn males in a Spanish population. *Journal of Molecular Diagnosis, 11*(4), 324–329.

Freund, L., Peebles, C. A., Aylward, E., & Reiss, A. L. (1995). Preliminary report on cognitive and adaptive behaviors of preschool-aged males with fragile X. *Developmental Brain Dysfunction, 8*, 242–261.

Gokden, M., Al-Hinti, J. T., & Harik, S. I. (2009). Peripheral nervous system pathology in fragile X tremor/ataxia syndrome (FXTAS). *Neuropathology, 29*(3), 280–284.

Greco, C., Tassone, F., Garcia-Arocena, D., Tartaglia, N., Coffey, S., Vartanian, T., et al. (2008). Clinical and neuropathologic findings in a woman with the FMR1 premutation and multiple sclerosis. *Archives of Neurology, 65*(8), 1114–1116.

Greco, C, Berman, R. F., Martin, R. M., Tassone, F., Schwartz, P. H., Chang, A., et al. (2006). Neuropathology of fragile X-associated tremor/ataxia syndrome (FXTAS). *Brain, 129*(Pt. 1), 243–255.

Greco, C., Soontrapornchai, K., Wirojanan, J., Gould, J. E., Hagerman, P. J., & Hagerman, R. J. (2007). Testicular and pituitary inclusion formation in fragile X associated tremor/ataxia syndrome. *Journal of Urology, 177*(4), 1434–1437.

Greiss-Hess, L., Lemons-Chitwood, K., Harris, S., Borodyanskaya, M., Hagerman, R. J., Bodine, C., et al. (2009). Assistive technology use by persons with fragile X syndrome: Three case reports. *AOTA: Special Interest Section Quarterly: Technology, 19*(1), 1–4.

Hagerman, P. J. (2008). The fragile X prevalence paradox. *Journal of Medical Genetics, 45*(8), 498–499.

Hagerman, P. J., & Hagerman, R. J. (2004). Fragile X-associated tremor/ataxia syndrome (FXTAS). *Mental Retardation and Developmental Disabilities Research Reviews, 10*(1), 25–30.

Hagerman, R. J. (1999). *Neurodevelopmental disorders: Diagnosis and treatment.* New York: Oxford University Press.

Hagerman, R. J. (2002a). Medical follow-up and pharmacotherapy. In R. J. Hagerman & P. J. Hagerman (Eds.), *Fragile X syndrome: Diagnosis, treatment, and research* (3rd ed., pp. 287–338). Baltimore: Johns Hopkins University Press.

Hagerman, R. J. (2002b). Physical and behavioral phenotype. In R. J. Hagerman & P. J. Hagerman (Eds.), *Fragile X syndrome: Diagnosis, treatment, and research* (3rd ed., pp. 3–109). Baltimore: Johns Hopkins University Press.

Hagerman, R. J., Altshul Stark, D., & McBogg, P. (1987). Recurrent otitis media in boys with the fragile X syndrome. *American Journal of Diseases of Children, 141*, 184–187.

Hagerman, R. J., Berry-Kravis, E., Kaufmann, W. E., Ono, M. Y., Tartaglia, N., Lachiewicz, A., et al. (2009). Advances in the treatment of fragile X syndrome. *Pediatrics, 123*(1), 378–390.

Hagerman, R. J., Fulton, M. J., Leaman, A., Riddle, J., Hagerman, K., & Sobesky, W. (1994). A survey of fluoxetine therapy in fragile X syndrome. *Developmental Brain Dysfunction, 7*, 155–164.

Hagerman, R. J., Hall, D. A., Coffey, S., Leehey, M., Bourgeois, J., Gould, J., et al. (2008). Treatment of fragile X-associated tremor ataxia syndrome (FXTAS) and related neurological problems. *Clinical Interventions in Aging, 3*(2), 251–262.

Hagerman, R. J., Hills, J., Scharfenaker, S., & Lewis, H. (1999). Fragile X syndrome and selective mutism. *American Journal of Medical Genetics, 83*(4), 313–317.

Hagerman, R. J., Hull, C. E., Safanda, J. F., Carpenter, I., Staley, L. W., O'Connor, R. A., et al. (1994). High functioning fragile X males: Demonstration of an unmethylated fully expanded

FMR-1 mutation associated with protein expression. *American Journal of Medical Genetics, 51*(4), 298–308.

Hagerman, R. J., Leehey, M., Heinrichs, W., Tassone, F., Wilson, R., Hills, J., et al. (2001). Intention tremor, parkinsonism, and generalized brain atrophy in male carriers of fragile X. *Neurology, 57*, 127–130.

Hagerman, R. J., Murphy, M. A., & Wittenberger, M. D. (1988). A controlled trial of stimulant medication in children with the fragile X syndrome. *American Journal of Medical Genetics, 30*(1–2), 377–392.

Hagerman, R. J., Rivera, S. M., & Hagerman, P. J. (2008). The fragile X family of disorders: A model for autism and targeted treatments. *Current Pediatric Reviews, 4*, 40–52.

Harris, S. W., Goodlin-Jones, B., Nowicki, S. T., Hessl, D., Tassone, F., Barabato, I., et al. (2008). Autism profiles of young males with fragile X syndrome. *American Journal of Mental Retardation, 113*, 427–438.

Hazlett, H., Poe, M., Lightbody, A. A., Gerig, G., MacFall, J., Ross, A., et al. (2009). Teasing apart the heterogeneity of autism: Same behavior, different brains in toddlers with fragile X syndrome and autism. *Journal of Neurodevelopmental Disorders, 1*, 81–90.

Hills-Epstein, J., Riley, K., & Sobesky, W. (2002). The treatment of emotional and behavioral problems. In R. J. Hagerman & P. J. Hagerman (Eds.), *Fragile X syndrome: Diagnosis, treatment, and research* (3rd ed., pp. 339–362). Baltimore: Johns Hopkins University Press

IntelliTools, Inc. (1996). *IntelliTools: Access to learning through technology.* Novato, CA: Author.

Jacquemont, S., Hagerman, R. J., Leehey, M., Grigsby, J., Zhang, L., Brunberg, J. A., et al. (2003). Fragile X premutation tremor/ataxia syndrome: Molecular, clinical, and neuroimaging correlates. *American Journal of Human Genetics, 72*, 869–878.

Jacquemont, S., Hagerman, R. J., Leehey, M. A., Hall, D. A., Levine, R. A., Brunberg, J. A., et al. (2004). Penetrance of the fragile X-associated tremor/ataxia syndrome in a premutation carrier population. *Journal of the American Medical Association, 291*(4), 460–469.

Lachiewicz, A. M., & Dawson, D. V. (1994). Do young boys with fragile X syndrome have macroorchidism? *Pediatrics, 93*(6, Pt. 1), 992–995.

Loesch, D. Z., Bui, Q. M., Dissanayake, C., Clifford, S., Gould, E., Bulhak-Paterson, D., et al. (2007). Molecular and cognitive predictors of the continuum of autistic behaviours in fragile X. *Neuroscience and Biobehavioral Reviews, 31*, 315–326.

Loesch, D. Z., Huggins, R. M., & Hagerman, R. J. (2004). Phenotypic variation and FMRP levels in fragile X. *Mental Retardation and Developmental Disabilities Research Reviews, 10*(1), 31–41.

Loesch, D. Z., Huggins, R. M., & Hoang, N. H. (1995). Growth in stature in fragile X families: A mixed longitudinal study. *American Journal of Medical Genetics, 58*(3), 249–256.

Louis, E., Moskowitz, C., Friez, M., Amaya, M., & Vonsattel, J. P. (2006). Parkinsonism, dysautonomia, and intranuclear inclusions in a fragile X carrier: A clinical-pathological study. *Movement Disorders, 21*(3), 420–425.

McBride, S. M., Choi, C. H., Wang, Y., Liebelt, D., Braunstein, E., Ferreiro, D., et al. (2005). Pharmacological rescue of synaptic plasticity, courtship behavior, and mushroom body defects in a *Drosophila* model of fragile X syndrome. *Neuron, 45*(5), 753–764.

McConkie-Rosell, A., Abrams, L., Finucane, B., Cronister, A., Gane, L. W., Coffey, S. M., et al. (2007). Recommendations from multi-disciplinary focus groups on cascade testing and genetic counseling for fragile X-associated disorders. *Journal of Genetic Counseling, 16*(5), 593–606.

Merenstein, S. A., Sobesky, W. E., Taylor, A. K., Riddle, J. E., Tran, H. X., & Hagerman, R. J. (1996). Molecular-clinical correlations in males with an expanded FMR1 mutation. *American Journal of Medical Genetics, 64*(2), 388–394.

Miller, L. J., McIntosh, D. N., McGrath, J., Shyu, V., Lampe, M., Taylor, A. K., et al. (1999). Electrodermal responses to sensory stimuli in individuals with fragile X syndrome: A preliminary report. *American Journal of Medical Genetics, 83*, 268–279.

Nolin, S. L., Brown, W. T., Glicksman, A., Houck, G. E., Gargano, A. D., Sullivan, A., et al. (2003). Expansion of the fragile X CGG repeat in females with premutation or intermediate alleles. *American Journal of Human Genetics, 72*, 454–464.

Nowicki, S. T., Tassone, F., Ono, M. Y., Ferranti, J., Croquette, M. F., Goodlin-Jones, B., et al. (2007). The Prader–Willi phenotype of fragile X syndrome. *Journal of Developmental and Behavioral Pediatrics, 28*(2), 133–138.

Pesso, R., Berkenstadt, M., Cuckle, H., Gak, E., Peleg, L., Frydman, M., et al. (2000). Screening for fragile X syndrome in women of reproductive age. *Prenatal Diagnosis, 20*(8), 611–614.

Qin, M., Kang, J., Burlin, T. V., Jiang, C., & Smith, C. B. (2005). Postadolescent changes in regional cerebral protein synthesis: An *in vivo* study in the FMR1 null mouse. *Journal of Neuroscience, 25*(20), 5087–5095.

Reiss, A. L., & Dant, C. C. (2003). The behavioral neurogenetics of fragile X syndrome: Analyzing gene–brain–behavior relationships in child developmental psychopathologies. *Development and Psychopathology, 15*(4), 927–968.

Reyniers, E., Vits, L., De Boulle, K., Van Roy, B., Van Velzen, D., de Graaff, E., et al. (1993). The full mutation in the FMR-1 gene of male fragile X patients is absent in their sperm [see comments]. *Nature Genetics, 4*(2), 143–146.

Roberts, J., Bailey D., Jr., Mankowski, J., Ford, A., Sideris, J., Weisenfeld, L., et al. (2009). Mood and anxiety disorders in females with the FMR1 premutation. *American Journal of Medical Genetics, Part B, Neuropsychiatric Genetics, 150B*(1), 130–139.

Roberts, J. E., Boccia, M. L., Bailey, D. B., Hatton, D., & Skinner, M. (2001). Cardiovascular indices of physiological arousal in boys with fragile X syndrome. *Developmental Psychobiology, 39*(2), 107–123.

Rodriguez-Revenga, L., Madrigal, I., Pagonabarraga, J., Xuncla, M., Badenas, C., Kulisevsky, J., et al. (2009). Penetrance of FMR1 premutation associated pathologies in fragile X syndrome families. *European Journal of Human Genetics, 17*(10), 1359–1362.

Rogers, S. J., Hayden, D., Hepburn, S., Charlifne-Smith, R., Hall, T., & Hayes, A. (2006). Teaching young nonverbal children with autism useful speech: A pilot of the Denver Model and PROMPT interventions. *Journal of Autism and Developmental Disorders, 36*(8), 1007–1024.

Rogers, S. J., & Vismara, L. A. (2008). Evidence-based comprehensive treatments for early autism. *Journal of Clinical Child and Adolescent Psychology, 37*(1), 8–38.

Scharfenaker, S., O'Connor, R., Stackhouse, T., & Noble, L. (2002). An integrated approach to intervention. In R. J. Hagerman & P. J. Hagerman (Eds.), *Fragile X syndrome: Diagnosis, treatment, and research* (3rd ed., pp. 363–427). Baltimore: Johns Hopkins University Press.

Schopmeyer, B. B., & Lowe, F. (1992). *The fragile X child.* San Diego, CA: Singular.

Sherman, S. (2002). Epidemiology. In R. J. Hagerman & P. J. Hagerman (Eds.), *Fragile X syndrome: Diagnosis, treatment, and research* (3rd ed., pp. 136–168). Baltimore: Johns Hopkins University Press.

Slaney, S. F., Wilkie, A. O., Hirst, M. C., Charlton, R., McKinley, M., Pointon, J., et al. (1995). DNA testing for fragile X syndrome in schools for learning difficulties. *Archives of Disease in Childhood, 72*(1), 33–37.

Song, F. J., Barton, P., Sleightholme, V., Yao, G. L., & Fry-Smith, A. (2003). Screening for fragile X syndrome: A literature review and modelling study. *Health Technology Assessment, 7*(16), 1–106.

Spiridigliozzi, G., Lachiewicz, A., MacMordo, C., Vizoso, A., O'Donnell, C., McConkie-Rosell, A., et al. (1994). *Educating boys with fragile X syndrome: A guide for parents and professionals.* Durham, NC: Duke University Medical Center.

Sullivan, A. K., Marcus, M., Epstein, M. P., Allen, E. G., Anido, A. E., Paquin, J. J., et al. (2005). Association of FMR1 repeat size with ovarian dysfunction. *Human Reproduction, 20*(2), 402–412.

Tassone, F., Hagerman, R. J., Iklé, D. N., Dyer, P. N., Lampe, M., Willemsen, R., et al. (1999). FMRP expression as a potential prognostic indicator in fragile X syndrome. *American Journal of Medical Genetics, 84*(3), 250–261.

Tassone, F., Hagerman, R. J., Taylor, A. K., Gane, L. W., Godfrey, T. E., & Hagerman, P. J. (2000). Elevated levels of *FMR1* mRNA in carrier males: A new mechanism of involvement in fragile X syndrome. *American Journal of Human Genetics, 66*, 6–15.

Tassone, F., Hagerman, R. J., Taylor, A. K., Mills, J. B., Harris, S. W., Gane, L. W., et al. (2000). Clinical involvement and protein expression in individuals with the *FMR1* premutation. *American Journal of Medical Genetics, 91*, 144–152.

Verkerk, A. J., Pieretti, M., Sutcliffe, J. S., Fu, Y. H., Kuhl, D. P., Pizzuti, A., et al. (1991). Identification of a gene (FMR-1) containing a CGG repeat coincident with a breakpoint cluster region exhibiting length variation in fragile X syndrome. *Cell, 65*(5), 905–914.

Vismara, L. A., & Rogers, A. (2008). The Early Start Denver model: A case study of an innovative practice. *Journal of Early Intervention, 31*(1), 91–108.

Weiskop, S., Richdale, A., & Matthews, J. (2005). Behavioural treatment to reduce sleep problems in children with autism or fragile X syndrome. *Developmental Medicine and Child Neurology, 47*(2), 94–104.

Wittenberger, M. D., Hagerman, R. J., Sherman, S. L., McConkie-Rosell, A., Welt, C. K., Rebar, R. W., et al. (2007). The FMR1 premutation and reproduction. *Fertility and Sterility, 87*(3), 456–465.

Wright-Talamante, C., Cheema, A., Riddle, J. E., Luckey, D. W., Taylor, A. K., & Hagerman, R. J. (1996). A controlled study of longitudinal IQ changes in females and males with fragile X syndrome. *American Journal of Medical Genetics, 64*(2), 350–355.

Yan, Q. J., Rammal, M., Tranfaglia, M., & Bauchwitz, R. P. (2005). Suppression of two major fragile X syndrome mouse model phenotypes by the mGluR5 antagonist MPEP. *Neuropharmacology, 49*(7), 1053–1066.

Zhong, N., Kajanoja, E., Smits, B., Pietrofesa, J., Curley, D., Wang, D., et al. (1996). Fragile X founder effects and new mutations in Finland. *American Journal of Medical Genetics, 64*(1), 226–233.

CHAPTER 15

The Mucopolysaccharidoses

MICHAEL B. BROWN

The mucopolysaccharidoses (MPS disorders) are a group of progressive, hereditary diseases that result from abnormalities of glycosaminoglycan (acid mucopolysaccharide) metabolism (Spranger, 2007). There are six types of MPS disorders, several of which have a number of subtypes (see Table 15.1). The estimated prevalence of these disorders is as follows: Hurler syndrome (MPS IH), 1 in 76,000 to 1 in 144,000 live births;

TABLE 15.1. Classification of the MPS Disorders

MPS IH	Hurler syndrome
MPS IS	Scheie syndrome
MPS IHS	Hurler–Scheie syndrome
MPS II	Hunter syndrome
MPS IIIA	Sanfilippo syndrome, Type A
MPS IIIB	Sanfilippo syndrome, Type B
MPS IIIC	Sanfilippo syndrome, Type C
MPS HID	Sanfilippo syndrome, Type D
MPS IVA	Morquio syndrome, Type A
MPS IVB	Morquio syndrome, Type B
MPS IVC	Morquio syndrome, Type C
MPS VI	Maroteaux–Lamy syndrome
MPS VII	Sly syndrome

Scheie syndrome (MPS IS), 1 in 840,000 to 1 in 1,300,000 live births; Hurler–Scheie syndrome (MPS HIS), 1 in 280,000 live births; Hunter syndrome (MPS II), 1 in 100,000 to 150,000 live births; Sanfilippo syndrome (MPS III), 1 in 24,000 to 1 in 200,000 live births; Morquio syndrome (MPS IV), 1 in 75,000 to 1 in 1,000,000 live births; and Maroteaux–Lamy syndrome (MPS VI), 1 in 100,000 to 1 in 1,300,000 live births (Chen, 2006). Very few cases of Sly syndrome (MPS VI) have been reported worldwide (Neufeld & Muenzer, 2001).

ETIOLOGY, FEATURES, AND COURSE

Pathophysiology

The MPS disorders are the largest group of lysosomal storage disorders (Herring, 2008). Lysosomes are intracellular structures containing enzymes that can break down or metabolize complex molecules. The complex molecules are brought into the lysosomes for metabolism in the course of normal physiological processes. In the MPS disorders, there is a failure of specific genes to produce a sufficient level of active enzymes necessary to break down the mucopolysaccharides. As a result, large quantities of the incom-

TABLE 15.2. Enzyme Deficiencies in MPS Disorders

Type of disorder		Enzyme deficiency
MPS IH	Hurler syndrome	Alpha-L-iduronidase
MPS IS	Scheie syndrome	Alpha-L-iduronidase
MPS IHS	Hurler–Scheie syndrome	Alpha-L-iduronidase
MPS II	Hunter syndrome	Iduronate sulfatases
MPS IIIA	Sanfilippo syndrome, Type A	Heparan-N-sulfatase
MPS IIIB	Sanfilippo syndrome, Type B	Alpha-N-acetylglucosaminidase
MPS IIIC	Sanfilippo syndrome, Type C	Acetyl CoA-alpha-glucosaminide-acetyltransferase
MPS HID	Sanfilippo syndrome, Type D	N-Acetylglucosamine-6-sulfatase
MPS IVA	Morquio syndrome, Type A	Galactose-6-sulfatase
MPS IVB	Morquio syndrome, Type B	Beta-galactosidase
MPS VI	Maroteaux–Lamy syndrome	N-Acetylgalactosamine-4-sulfatase
MPS VII	Sly syndrome	Beta-glucuronidase

pletely metabolized material accumulate in the lysosomes. The abnormal accumulation produces the symptoms and complications of these disorders. There are several enzymes required for the degradation of mucopolysaccharides, and the MPS disorders are classified according to the specific enzyme deficiencies that cause them (Bach, 2004; Herring, 2008; see Table 15.2).

Genetics

Each of the MPS disorders, with the exception of Hunter syndrome, is an autosomal recessive disorder (Chen, 2006). In an autosomal recessive disorder, each parent must be a carrier of the abnormal gene for a child to develop the disorder. Both males and females are affected by the autosomal recessive MPS disorders. The variation in the severity of clinical manifestations of the disorders in different individuals is a result of allelic mutations and the level of residual enzyme activity (Spranger, 2007).

Hunter syndrome is a recessive, sex-linked disorder (Chen, 2006). The affected gene site is located on the X chromosome, and as a result females carry the recessive gene for the disorder. The disorder consequently occurs almost exclusively in males, as males receive only one X chromosome; therefore, there is no second X chromosome to provide a dominant (normal) version of the gene to override the effect of the recessive (impaired) gene. Females can be affected if there has been an inactivation of the normal X chromosome (Spranger, 2007).

Major Features

The abnormal accumulation of incompletely metabolized mucopolysaccharides produces a number of characteristic clinical features, the most striking of which are skeletal effects. The complete range of skeletal features occurs in Hurler syndrome; these features occur to varying degrees in each of the other MPS disorders. Excessive lysosomal storage also affects other organ systems, most notably the cardiovascular, respiratory, and nervous systems. Neurological involvement results in progressive dementia in many of the MPS disorders.

MPS I (Hurler Syndrome, Scheie Syndrome, and Hurler–Scheie Syndrome)

Children with Hurler syndrome have characteristic skeletal effects known as *dysostosis multiplex* (Alman & Goldberg, 2005; Neufeld & Muenzer, 2001). Specific features include (1) widened collarbone and ribs; (2) progressive curvature of the lower spine (lumbar kyphoscoliosis); (3) significant shortening of stature; (4) shortened neck; (5) stubby, claw-shaped hands; (6) contractions of the joints; (7) enlarged head; (8) flattening of the bridge of the nose, wide nostrils, thick lips, and large and protruding tongue with open mouth; and (9) thick hair and excessive body hair. Hurler syndrome is the most severe of the three syndromes; Scheie and Hurler–Scheie syndromes both have less severe skeletal expressions. Rapidly progressing cognitive impairment is the rule in Hurler syndrome, whereas cognitive functioning is generally spared in Scheie and Hurler–Scheie syndromes.

MPS II (Hunter Syndrome)

The features of Hunter syndrome include (1) a depressed nasal bridge and distortion of facial bones; (2) enlarged head; (3) a distinctive posture of hunched shoulders, with the joints of the limbs held in partial flexion; (4) joint stiffness and a claw-like hand deformity; (5) very short stature or dwarfism; and (6) a thickening and overgrowth of hair on the body (Young, Harper, Newcombe, & Archer, 1982b).

MPS III (Sanfilippo Syndrome)

The presentation of Sanfilippo syndrome is dominated by severe neurodegenerative disturbance (Cleary & Wraith, 1993). Progressive intellectual disability occurs rapidly, accompanied by serious behavior disturbances that include hyperactive behavior, physical aggression, noncompliance, and self-stimulatory behaviors (Nidiffer & Kelly, 1983). There is usually only mild somatic involvement of the sort typical of the other MPS disorders until late in the course of the disorder (Spranger, 2007). Stature is near normal, and the facial features common to the other MPS disorders are usually not present. Joint stiffness is mild and rarely causes mobility problems.

MPS IV (Morquio Syndrome)

The primary features of Morquio syndrome are skeletal deformities, with secondary effects on the nervous and cardiovascular systems. The characteristic features include (1) shortened trunk, neck, legs, and arms; (2) short stature or dwarfism, depending on the severity of the disorder; (3) unstable knee joints; (4) enlarged elbows and wrists; (5) flattened vertebrae, with underdevelopment of a portion of the cervical vertebrae; (6) expanded thoracic rib cage, with marked inward curvature of the lumbar

spine (kyphoscoliosis); (7) waddling gait and inward-turned knees; (8) finger and joint stiffness, and early arthritis in hips and knees; (9) depressed nasal bridge and protruding lower jaw; (10) broad mouth, with the appearance of a permanent grin; and (11) dental abnormalities, including thin and pitted enamel, widely spaced conical teeth, and excessive tooth wear (Alman & Goldberg, 2005; Cervantes & Lifshitz, 1990; Nelson & Kinirons, 1988). Persons with this disorder have normal or near-normal intelligence (Cervantes & Lifschitz, 1990).

MPS VI (Maroteaux–Lamy Syndrome)

Children with Maroteaux–Lamy syndrome have dysostosis multiplex, the same characteristic skeletal effects as in Hurler syndrome. Children with this syndrome may exhibit variations in the severity of the skeletal manifestations. Intellectual functioning remains in the normal range (Bach, 2004). Both severe and milder versions of the disorder have been identified.

MPS VII (Sly Syndrome)

Sly syndrome is characterized by skeletal manifestations similar to those of Hurler syndrome but often with slower progression (Spranger, 2007). Unusual facial appearance, hepatosplenomegaly, and short stature are common. Both mild and severe forms of the disorder have been reported, along with a form of the disorder that is present at birth (Neufeld & Muenzer, 2001).

Developmental Course

The features of the MPS disorders generally become apparent in early childhood, though some of these disorders may first be diagnosed as late as adolescence. Each of the disorders has a typical developmental course that includes the age of onset of symptoms and the progression of impairment.

MPS I (Hurler, Scheie, and Hurler–Scheie Syndromes)

Children with Hurler syndrome appear normal at birth and grow rapidly during their first year (Nelson & Crocker, 1999). A deceleration of growth occurs at some point between 6 and 18 months of age (Neufeld & Muenzer, 2001). Learning peaks in the second or third year of life, and afterward developmental regression occurs, with a loss of previously learned skills. Progressive intellectual disability results, and language facility is gradually lost. The ability to walk is gradually lost, and most children with MPS IH remain incontinent (Bax & Coville, 1995). Many children have difficulty feeding themselves because of poor coordination and swallowing difficulties. The children also become less interested in the environment. Maximum functional age is usually between 2 and 4 years. Death frequently occurs by age 10 (Neufeld & Muenzer, 2001), typically as a result of cardiovascular disorders, respiratory problems, or complications of neurological damage (Nelson & Crocker, 1999).

The symptoms of Hurler–Scheie syndrome usually begin between 3 and 8 years of age (Spranger, 2007). Children develop mild facial deformities, shortened stature, and stiffened joints. Hepatosplenomegaly (enlargement of the liver and spleen) and hernia are frequent complications (Neufeld & Muenzer, 2001). Visual losses may occur due to corneal clouding or glaucoma. Intellectual development is typically normal or only mildly impaired. Hydrocephaly is common. Deafness and heart valve disorders are typical. Persons with this syndrome usually survive into adulthood.

Scheie syndrome is at the milder end of the clinical spectrum of these disorders (Spranger, 2007). This disorder is characterized by joint stiffness, deformity of the hands, and corneal clouding. Stature is usually normal, as is intellectual functioning. The diagnosis is usually made in the teens, and life expectancy is generally not affected.

MPS II (Hunter Syndrome)

Two forms of Hunter syndrome, mild and severe, have been identified based on onset, complications, and course of the disorder (Young, Harper, Newcombe, & Archer, 1982a, 1982b). Within each form, however, considerable individual variation can exist (Bach, 2004). The mild or late-onset form has an average age of onset of 4.3 years and an average age at death of 21.7 years (Young

& Harper, 1982). Physical development is typically normal at first, with the abnormal facial configuration and growth defects becoming evident by early childhood (Avery & First, 1994). Intellectual performance is also typically relatively normal. Survival is possible into the fourth decade and beyond, and persons with the disorder may continue their education, marry, and have children. Death is usually caused by cardiac or pulmonary complications (Young & Harper, 1982).

The severe or early-onset form of Hunter syndrome has an average age of onset of 2.5 years, with an average age at death of 11.8 years (Young & Harper, 1983). This form of the disorder is marked by progressive neurological involvement, which results in a plateau of learning and developmental skills at some point between ages 2 and 6. The plateau is followed by a regression in cognitive skills and behavior. Intellectual disability has an insidious onset and becomes profound. Seizure disorder is common, especially past age 10. The children become emaciated, and there is significant wasting of body mass (neurodevelopmental cachexia). Ninety percent of those affected are bedridden by age 10. Death usually results from pulmonary complications of the cachexic state (Young & Harper, 1983).

MPS III (Sanfilippo Syndrome)

Children with Sanfilippo syndrome (MPS III) are typically first diagnosed at about age 5 (Cleary & Wraith, 1993; Neufeld & Muenzer, 2001; Nidiffer & Kelly, 1983). The features of the disorder begin to appear between 2 and 6 years of age. The rate of achievement of developmental milestones is normal up to this time, although delay or loss of language and memory may be the most notable early symptoms. The presenting symptoms include hyperactivity, developmental delay, hirsutism, and poor sleep. Some children develop episodes of intractable diarrhea. There may also be increasingly severe temper tantrums and aggressive behavior. Some children have panic-like symptoms in unfamiliar places. Cognitive decline continues with progressive dementia. The skeletal features common to the MPS disorders are usually less severe in Sanfilippo syndrome and tend to become obvious only in the later stages of the disorder.

After age 10, the behavioral symptoms often become less severe. Typical problems include falls caused by lack of coordination, and difficulty with feeding as a result of impaired swallowing. Joint stiffness and spasticity interfere with mobility and may necessitate the use of a wheelchair. Seizures are not uncommon. Most individuals with Sanfilippo syndrome survive into their teens, although some persons live into their second or third decade.

There are four forms of Sanfilippo syndrome, designated as IIIA, IIIB, IIIC, and IIID, each associated with a different enzyme abnormality (see Table 15.2). The clinical presentation of each type appears similar, although there are reports of persons whose behavior was not problematic until their late teens (Kim, Berger, Bunner, & Carey, 1996) and of others who were still mobile into their 20s (Cleary & Wraith, 1993).

MPS IV (Morquio Syndrome)

Individuals with Morquio syndrome (MPS IV) appear normal at birth, and the characteristics of the disorder develop during infancy or childhood. There have traditionally been two widely recognized forms of this disorder, designated as MPS IVA and MPS IVB, which differ in the severity of symptoms and the age at detection (Neufeld & Muenzer, 2001). A more recent typology (Alman & Goldberg, 2005) includes a third variant of Morquio syndrome, MPS IVC. This mild variant of the disorder results in much less severe clinical manifestations. Stature is nearly normal, with only mild skeletal abnormalities. This form is usually first diagnosed in adolescence.

Persons with MPS IVA (the severe form of the disorder) appear normal at birth, but shortened stature appears by about 1 year of age. Final height is usually less than 50 inches. Younger children have difficulty with continence, although most children over 10 are continent (Bax & Coville, 1995). The diagnosis of the severe form of the disorder is usually made between 1 and 3 years of age. Individuals with the severe variant of the disorder usually live until their third or fourth decade (Bach, 2004). Children with MPS IVB (the intermediate form of the disorder) have the classic characteristics in a less severe form. They have a final height greater than 50 inches and usually have normal-appearing dentition. The diagnosis of this form is usually made during the childhood years.

MPS VI (Maroteaux–Lamy Syndrome)

The severe form of Maroteaux–Lamy syndrome includes pronounced skeletal deformities with intact intellectual functioning (Neufeld & Muenzer, 2001; Spranger, 2007). The head is usually large, with a short neck, broad flat nose, and wide nostrils. The skin and hair are thick and course. Liver enlargement is common, and the abdomen may protrude. The spine may be curved, and joint mobility may be limited. Stature is significantly shortened and is noticeable between 2 and 3 years of age. There is wide variation in the presentation of the disorder, including a mild version of the disorder that results in less severe skeletal involvement.

MPS VII (Sly Syndrome)

Individuals with Sly syndrome may vary in the expression of symptoms (Neufeld & Muenzer, 2001). The more severe, early-onset type of this disorder begins by age 3. Skeletal abnormalities are moderately severe and result in shortened stature. Intellectual disability is frequently moderate, but not progressive. The later-onset form of the disorder occurs after age 4. Skeletal involvement may be mild or severe. Intelligence is usually normal. A severe neonatal form of the disorder can be present and has caused infant death.

MEDICAL, PSYCHOLOGICAL, AND SOCIAL COMPLICATIONS

Any MPS disorder is a developmental disorder with significant impact on an individual's physical, psychological, and social development. Many of the complications, especially the physical and cognitive complications, are results of the accumulation of mucopolysaccharides in the tissues. The social impact is secondary to the child's level of physical disability, difficulties in communication and understanding as a result of cognitive limitations, and the presence of difficult behaviors characteristic of several MPS disorders.

Medical Complications

Complications of MPS disorders occur in many organ systems (Alman & Goldberg, 2005; Avery & First, 1994; Neufeld & Muenzer, 2001). The enlargement of the liver and spleen (hepatosplenomegaly) results in a protuberant abdomen, and hernia occurs frequently. Chronic, intractable diarrhea is frequently found in Hunter and Sanfilippo syndromes. Carpal tunnel syndrome (entrapment of nerves in the wrist) can result in further impairment in the use of the hands and arms.

Cardiovascular problems, especially valvular disorders, are usually evident in older children and adolescents with MPS disorders. Respiratory disorders are common, including increased rates of respiratory infections, airway obstruction, and pulmonary hypertension. Sleep apnea may result from obstructions in the respiratory system. Deafness, due to both progressive thickening of the skull (conduction loss) and sensory impairment, is likely in the severest forms of the disorders (Herring, 2008). Glaucoma and retinitis pigmentosa can occur, which, along with corneal clouding, often affects vision.

Dentition is frequently affected in the MPS disorders, especially in Morquio and Maroteaux–Lamy syndromes (Nelson & Kinirons, 1988; Smith, Hallett, Hall, Wardrop, & Firth, 1995). Delayed tooth eruption and weaknesses in enamel can occur. Abnormalities of tooth morphology, such as wide spacing and a sharp, conical shape, are common. Excessive wear on the tooth surface may result.

The abnormal formation of the cervical vertebrae, especially in Morquio syndrome, may lead to misalignment of these vertebrae (atlantoaxial subluxation). This can cause spinal cord compression, leading to paralysis and death (Ashraf, Crockard, Ransford, & Stevens, 1991; Neufeld & Muenzer, 2001). Spinal misalignment and narrowing of the airway also create potentially serious problems with establishing an airway and providing anesthesia if surgery is necessary.

Neuropsychological Complications

Little is known about the specific neuropsychological aspects of the MPS disorders because formal neuropsychological study of children with these disorders has rarely been undertaken (Shapiro & Klein, 1994). Children with the MPS disorders are not routinely referred for neuropsychological assessment; reasons have included the lack of treatment available for the disorders, as well as the advanced stage of the disorders by the time diagnoses are usually made. The excessive storage of mucopolysaccharides in the tissues does affect both the gray and white matter of the brain.

The primary neuropsychological complication of the MPS disorders is progressive dementia. Dementia differs from intellectual disability in that intellectual disability is a slowing in the attainment of developmental milestones, whereas dementia is a reduction in the previously attained level of functioning. In those MPS disorders that result in dementia, there is an initial slowing of development, followed by a plateau in level of functioning. Skills that have been developed are subsequently lost. Language delays occur in the severe form of Hunter syndrome and in Sanfilippo syndrome (Shapiro, Lockman, Balthazar, & Krivit, 1995). All patients with Hurler syndrome in one study who had been treated with bone marrow transplantation (BMT) had residual learning problems, although none had severe mental retardation (Guffon, Souillet, Maire, Straczek, & Guibaud, 1998).

Hydrocephaly (an accumulation of cerebrospinal fluid surrounding the brain) is common, especially in Hurler and Hunter syndromes. Children with Sanfilippo syndrome and the severe form of Hunter syndrome often have seizures (Cleary & Wraith, 1993; Young et al., 1982a). Neurological symptoms may also be caused by spinal cord compression due to the buildup of extradural soft tissue (Alman & Goldberg, 2005).

Behavioral Complications

Children with MPS disorders have a high prevalence of certain behavior problems (Bax & Colville, 1995). Parents of children with Hurler syndrome describe their children as anxious or fearful. Many are considered to be restless, with little aggressive behavior. Sleep problems are seen in some children, but these are reflections of their medical problems rather than of a behavior problem. Overactivity is common in children with Hunter syndrome up to age 10. There is a high rate of aggressive/destructive behavior in children under 5. Excessive fearfulness occurs in most and is especially likely in younger children. Problems with sleep, such as difficulty settling and going to sleep, occur frequently. Behavior problems (overactivity, aggression, and defiance) tend to arise early in the course of Hunter syndrome in children with the severe form of the disorder. In the milder form of Hunter syndrome, behavioral problems are more likely to occur in adolescence, presumably because of the adjustment problems posed by the adolescents' unusual appearance and their knowledge of their prognosis (Young et al., 1982a).

Sanfilippo syndrome causes the most dramatic behavioral symptoms of all the MPS disorders (Bax & Coville, 1995; Nidiffer & Kelly, 1983). Restlessness is a common feature in children with MPS III, and children commonly wander around home and school; they also mouth clothing and other objects. Parents often describe their children as unpredictable, with frequent aggressive and destructive behaviors, including hitting others. These behaviors seem unprovoked and do not appear to be accompanied by anger. Difficult behavior at night is also common, including staying up during the nighttime hours, wandering, and restlessness. Many families have had to use secure sleeping arrangements or resort to having a child sleep in a parent's room so as to provide supervision over night.

Children with Morquio syndrome have a relatively low level of behavioral problems, compared to those with the other MPS disorders. Sleep problems are present, especially in the 5- to 9-year-old group. Many children between ages 10 and 14 are described by their parents as fearful (Bax & Colville, 1995).

Psychosocial Complications

Family stress often occurs because of the multiple demands of the MPS disorders (Bax & Coville, 1995; Nidiffer & Kelly, 1983).

Parents are unlikely to have regular outside help in managing the day-to-day care of a child with such a disorder. They often feel uncomfortable leaving their child with other caregivers, sometimes because of the fear that the child may die while the parents are gone. In addition, parents often face increased pressures caused by repeated medical procedures, associated behavior problems, and the financial demands of having a child with a major chronic disorder. Relatively few families receive any type of assistance from a mental health care provider.

Parents are very concerned and frequently worried about their child's prognosis. Many are frustrated by the lack of information available to parents and professionals at the local level. There is often a lack of adequate community support and assistance. Parents frequently feel helpless (Nidiffer & Kelly, 1983) and isolated (Bax & Coville, 1995).

Parents feel a great deal of distress when their child becomes so impaired that they are unable to communicate with him or her (Bax & Coville, 1995). They are also concerned about the effect of the child with MPS on siblings (Nidiffer & Kelly, 1983). Sibling relationships may be affected by jealousy because of the extra parental attention to the needs of the child with MPS, or the burden of providing extra care for an ill sibling. Siblings may also be concerned that their own acceptance by their peers will be affected by the presence of a sibling with such significant problems.

IDENTIFICATION, TREATMENT, AND INTERVENTION

Because the MPS disorders occur so rarely, parents, school personnel, and local health care providers are likely to have little first-hand experience with these disorders. Early identification is important to allow for early treatment and intervention. A number of medical, educational, and allied health care specialists are required for optimal care, especially for those children with more severe forms of the disorders (see Table 15.3). Close communication and collaboration among parents, educators, and health care providers are vital to create an atmosphere of trust and support, which is necessary in dealing with these disorders.

TABLE 15.3. Treatment Providers Involved in Comprehensive Care for MPS Disorders

Physicians	Educational specialists	Health care providers
Anesthesiologist	Early intervention specialist	Pediatric dentist
Cardiologist	Special education teacher	Occupational therapist
Child psychiatrist	Instructional assistant	Physical therapist
Neurologist	School psychologist	Psychologist
Neurosurgeon	School nurse	Rehabilitation counselor
Ophthalmologist	School social worker	Speech–language clinician
Orthopedic surgeon		
Pulmonologist		

Diagnosis

Children with MPS disorders usually present for diagnosis as a result of developmental delay or the development of characteristic skeletal features. Early diagnosis is important because intervention (especially the newer therapies) is more effective in children who have not yet suffered neurological injury due to accumulation of mucopolysaccharides (Herring, 2008). Mucopolysaccharides are excreted through the urine, and analysis of mucopolysaccharide levels in the urine can be measured for an initial diagnosis. The outcome of urinary screening is sometimes inaccurate, and its utility varies with the different types of MPS disorders. More definitive diagnosis requires an enzyme assay of cultured fibroblasts or leukocytes (white blood cells). In this procedure, cell samples are taken and grown in a culture medium. The cells are then subjected to tests for the presence of the enzyme in question.

The differential diagnosis for MPS disorders includes other diseases that produce dysostosis multiplex and physical appearance typical of the MPSs (Matalan, 1996; see Table 15.4). The hyperactivity and tantrum

TABLE 15.4. Genetic Diseases Considered in the Differential Diagnosis of the MPS Disorders

GM$_1$ gangliosidosis	Mucolipidosis III
Mannosidosis	Mucolipidosis IV
Fucosidosis	Multiple sulfatase deficiency
Aspartylglucosaminuria	
Mucolipidosis I	Kneist syndrome
Mucolipidosis II (I-cell disease)	Spondyloepiphyseal dysplasias

behaviors present in Sanfilippo syndrome may be misdiagnosed as attention-deficit/hyperactivity disorder. This underscores the importance of a medical workup on all children with developmental difficulties as part of an evaluation of behavioral problems.

Prenatal diagnosis is possible and is routinely conducted when there is a known risk that the fetus will be affected by one of the disorders (Bach, 2004; Neufeld & Muenzer, 2001). Fetal fibroblasts circulating in the amniotic fluid can be obtained through amniocentesis from the 13th to the 16th week of gestation. These cells can then be cultured and assayed for activity of the relevant enzyme. Chorionic villus sampling obtains small pieces of the placenta through needle biopsy from the 10th or 11th week of gestation (Bach, 2004). These cells are then analyzed for enzyme activity or mutation analysis.

Medical Issues and Interventions

Children with MPS disorders have many characteristic medical problems that are the targets of medical interventions. There has generally been no definitive treatment for the MPS disorders, and supportive treatments are beneficial for improving children's quality of life (Rudolph, Rudolph, Hostetter, Lister, & Siegel, 2002). A number of recent efforts to develop definitive treatments have shown promise for some of the MPS disorders, however.

Supportive Treatment

Supportive treatments focus on alleviating the manifestations and complications of the MPS disorders (Neufeld & Muenzer, 2001).

Children commonly need supportive interventions for cardiovascular complications and respiratory difficulties. Upper-airway obstruction and sleep apnea may require surgical interventions, and respiratory infections and middle-ear infections need prompt and aggressive treatment. Because of the difficulties of maintaining an airway, persons with MPS disorders who need general anesthesia must be cared for in a setting that has experience in providing anesthesia services for this group (Neufeld & Muenzer, 2001).

Interventions for hearing loss are frequently necessary, and children with MPS disorders should receive regular evaluation for sensory and conductive hearing loss (Alpern, 1992). Hearing aids can be helpful for many children with these disorders who have hearing loss. Auditory training, such as instruction in making use of residual hearing and lip reading, may be useful for some children. Alternative communication skills may be necessary for higher-functioning children and adults who have tracheotomies because of airway obstruction, or who have total hearing loss.

Regular dental care is important to prevent or address potential dental problems, which are especially common for children with Morquio syndrome (Nelson & Kinirons, 1988). Surgical treatment of impacted teeth may be necessary. The possibility of endocarditis is increased by the presence of cardiovalvular disease, which is commonly present in the MPS disorders. Prophylactic treatment is indicated to prevent the occurrence of infective endocarditis secondary to dental procedures.

Skeletal and mobility difficulties are common problems for children with MPS disorders (Neufeld & Muenzer, 2001). Both surgical and nonsurgical interventions are used in the management of the orthopedic problems associated with these disorders (Herring, 2008). Surgery may be necessary to correct spinal deformity and to stabilize cervical instability in those situations where the instability may lead to neurological impairment. Surgical treatment is also indicated to reduce median nerve compression in carpal tunnel syndrome. Nonsurgical treatments include physical therapy to minimize joint contractures and the use of splints or braces. Some children will need to use a wheelchair for mobility.

Definitive Treatment

A number of efforts have been made to develop definitive biological treatments to correct the basic defects that cause the MPS disorders or to provide adequate levels of enzymes in the body. These treatments have shown promise for some of the MPS disorders. The optimal results of these definitive treatments will come from early intervention prior to the tissue and organ damage caused by accumulation of mucopolysaccharides (Muenzer & Fisher, 2004).

Two types of transplantation procedures have been used for treating MPS disorders. BMT is a form of treatment that replaces abnormal cells and supplements the genetic production of the enzyme. Hematopoietic stem cell transplantation replaces abnormal cells using infusions of umbilical cord blood. Both BMT and hematopoietic transplantation have had similar effects for MPS IH (Hurler syndrome). Improvements have been noted in improved neurological, hepatic, and cardiac functioning, along with improvements in the airway, joint movement, and hearing (Muenzer & Fisher, 2004). BMT has not had a noticeable effect on the progression of skeletal disease, however, and there is no evidence yet of the effect on skeletal disease of cord blood transplantation. BMT has been effective on the non-neuropsychological symptoms of Hunter syndrome (Guffon, Bertrand, Forest, Foulhoux, & Froissart, 2009). BMT has improved motor function for one child with Maroteaux–Lamy syndrome on long-term follow-up (Wang, Hwu, & Lin, 2008).

Shapiro and colleagues (1995) found that BMT prior to age 2 resulted in stabilization of intellectual functioning for children with Hurler syndrome who had IQs above 70 prior to the procedure. BMT did not alter the progressive course in any children with Sanfilippo syndrome. No children with Hunter syndrome received BMT prior to the age of 2, and all but one of the children failed to show an alteration in the course of the disease. This may demonstrate that the severity of the disease and the age at onset are important factors in successful outcomes of BMT. BMT, like any organ transplantation, remains an expensive procedure with significant mortality and morbidity rates (Batshaw & Tuchman, 2007).

Enzyme replacement therapy has been used successfully to reduce some of the manifestations of MPS I and MPS VI. Treatment over 26 weeks with a human recombinant form of alpha-L-iduronidase has produced reduction in urinary glycosaminoglycan excretion, improvement in liver volume, and enhanced physical endurance in children with MPS IS (Scheie) and MPS HS (Hurler–Scheie) disorders (Miebach, 2005). Because the enzyme does not cross the brain–blood barrier, it is likely not to affect the neurological manifestations of the disorder. Treatments over 24–48 weeks with N-acetylgalactosamine-4-sulfatase reduced lysosomal storage and improved physical endurance and joint function in children with Maroteaux–Lamy syndrome (MPS VI; Harmatz et al., 2004). Enzyme replacement therapy has ameliorated the non-neurological manifestations of Hunter Syndrome (Rudolph et al., 2002). Enzyme replacement therapy may also be advantageous for some children with MPS IH (Hurler syndrome) because it offers fewer risks than BMT and improves somatic symptoms (Muenzer & Fisher, 2004).

Psychosocial Issues

Like all children, children with MPS disorders have a wide range of personality traits and habits. Their feelings and behaviors are affected by many factors, including their family, the extent of their physical problems, and their level of cognitive functioning. Family and friends generally have positive feelings and relationships with their family member with an MPS disorder, and the affected child is treated by others in many ways as any child would be treated. Many have few or no issues with negative behaviors, and when such behaviors are present, they are similar to those of children experiencing problems with similar cognitive and physical effects.

Some children with MPS disorders, especially children with MPS III subtypes, may exhibit significant behavioral issues. Unfortunately, psychological services are rarely provided in the ongoing management of children with these disorders (Bax & Colville, 1995). Clinical experience with MPS disorders suggests that the difficult behaviors (such as the aggressive outbursts of children with Sanfilippo syndrome) may not respond well to behavioral intervention strategies (Nidiffer & Kelly, 1983). Behavioral interventions have been successful in decreasing the sleep problems of children with Sanfilippo syndrome (Coville, Watters, Yule, & Bax, 1996). It is important to remember that discomfort, changes in routine, and the level of environmental stimulation may lead to or exacerbate difficult behavior. A thorough assessment of behavioral problems should include an assessment of the physical environment, behavioral antecedents, and consequences of the problems, as well as an evaluation of the child's characteristics (Jacob-Timm & Daniels, 1998).

Few studies have examined psychopharmacological interventions for the behavioral difficulties of children with MPS disorders. Such interventions have produced variable responses (Cleary & Wraith, 1993). Methylphenidate has not been useful in reducing the hyperactivity of children with Sanfilippo syndrome (Jacob-Timm & Daniels, 1998). Thioridazine and haloperidol do reduce the hyperactivity, although these drugs also have potential side effects that create additional problems (Wraith, 1995). Wraith (1995) also found that benzodiazepines and chloral hydrate are effective sleep medications for children with Sanfilippo syndrome. Carbamazepine has been successfully used to reduce overactivity, aggressive outbursts, and labile mood in an adolescent with Sanfilippo syndrome (Kim et al., 1996).

Family Issues

Parents of children with MPS report that they have joys and pleasures in raising their children similar to those experienced by parents of nondisabled children. The diagnosis of a severe disorder, however, has a powerful effect on parents, who must deal not only with their own feelings but with a complex array of medical and educational providers (Chen & Miles, 2007). For parents whose children have MPS disorders, the latter dealings are often complicated by most health care and educational providers' lack of familiarity with the disorders. The path from first concerns to a definitive diagnosis is often long. Parents may be overwhelmed by the many stressors that result from having a child with a progressive genetic disorder (Perszyk & Perszyk, 2004). This is compounded by the fact that life expectancy is reduced for most children with MPS disorders.

Providing information and helping parents locate support groups (see Table 15.5) can be of great benefit to parents overwhelmed by the challenges of a child with an MPS disorder. Parents can receive enormous support from talking with other parents who can understand their situation and provide not only empathy, but good information on resources and strategies that are not otherwise widely accessible. The National MPS Society, for example, provides many invaluable programs, information and support for parents. These include an annual parent conference, regional social events, small grants for the purchase of special equipment, and a number of parent volunteers who can talk with parents whose children are newly diagnosed. Perszyk and Perszyk (2004) provide a useful description of the needs of families with children with genetic disorders over the course of these disorders. A very useful approach to working with families of children

TABLE 15.5. Information and Support Resources for Parents and Professionals

Alliance of Genetic Support Groups
    4301 Connecticut Avenue NW, Suite 404
    Washington, DC 20008-2369
    202-966-5557
    www.geneticalliance.org
    Information on a wide range of support groups in local communities.

Canadian Society for Mucopolysaccharide and Related Disease
    P.O. Box 30034
    RPO Parkgate
    North Vancouver, British Columbia, Canada
      V7H 2Y8
    800-667-1846
    www.mpssociety.ca
    An information and advocacy organization for persons with MPSs and their families.

National MPS Society
    P.O. Box 14686
    Durham, NC 27709-4686
    877-MPS-1001
    www.mpssociety.org
    A support and advocacy organization for MPS disorders. Information, names of specialists who treat these disorders, and ways to contact other families of children with these disorders are available.

with severe disabilities can be found in Chen and Miles (2007).

Empathy and emotional support are very helpful responses from treatment providers. Training parents in behavior management techniques, or providing referrals for parent counseling and/or psychopharmacological interventions, may help parents cope with their child's behavior problems. Parents may also need assistance in accessing the necessary medical care for the complications of an MPS disorder. Since the need for medical care is likely to be complex and ongoing, then parents may need assistance with insurance, government benefits, or access to community groups that could provide material assistance for the family. Parents of children with MPS III disorder face especially difficult challenges because of the combination of sleep and behavior problems (Rudolph et al., 2002). Environmental modification is necessary, and the provision of regular respite care can help families take some time for themselves.

Family members of a child with an MPS disorder may experience grief at a number of times, beginning with the diagnosis of the disorder and, for a child whose disorder is fatal, extending to the child's death (and beyond). Deterioration in the child's condition is likely to cause a renewal of the feelings of loss, grief, and helplessness that occurred when the initial diagnosis was made. Providing anticipatory guidance in advance of a child's death will increase the family members' ability to deal with bereavement (Davies et al., 2004). In a case where the disorder is likely to cause death during childhood, the family members may benefit from support and counseling to help them deal with issues of grief and loss. Referrals to resources that can assist with grief support and in-home care in the later stages of the disorder (such as a hospice or a community bereavement support group) will be useful for some families.

Genetic Counseling

Genetic counseling services can be useful for families with a history of an MPS disorder. The geneticist or genetic counselor will take a detailed history of the family to help determine the risk of the specific disorder in future children (Schonberg & Tifft, 2007).

The geneticist can also discuss the risks and benefits of prenatal diagnostic tests after pregnancy occurs. The genetic counselor can assist the parents in considering their reproductive options (such as artificial insemination with donor sperm or eggs) if the parents are found to be genetic carriers. Parents may also feel guilt because of the inherited nature of these disorders, which may affect their marital relationships or attitudes toward having more children in the future (Perszyk & Perszyk, 2004). Further counseling may be necessary to assist with difficulties related to these feelings of guilt.

Persons who are carriers of a genetic disease can be identified before they have children who may develop the disorder. Widespread population screening for MPS disorders does not occur at this time (Gahl, 1999). Screening of the mother's family is warranted for known cases of Hunter syndrome, which is an X-linked disorder. Attention to future pregnancies is prudent for the other MPS disorders, which are autosomal recessive disorders; testing will permit the identification of risk for future children who may be born with an MPS disorder. A significant problem for parents of children with Sanfilippo syndrome is that this diagnosis is usually made relatively late, making effective genetic counseling more difficult. It is not uncommon for parents to have additional children with Sanfilippo syndrome prior to having a diagnosis made for their first child (Nidiffer & Kelly, 1983).

Educational Issues and Interventions

Most children with MPS disorders are likely to need assistance in school through special education services. Students can qualify for special education services under the "multiple disabilities" or "other health-impaired" categories. Parents of children with disabilities have worked tirelessly through national support groups (e.g., in the case of MPS disorders, the National MPS Society) to help local, state, and federal decision makers understand the difficulties that they have endured in obtaining appropriate services for their children.

The fact that these disorders are degenerative or progressive is an important factor in planning for school services. Difficulties with behavior management, socialization, and medical/health care will need to be addressed. No research has addressed interventions for the specific educational and psychosocial problems posed by the MPS disorders. Adaptation of methods and technologies currently used for children with multiple disabilities is a sound approach.

Psychoeducational Assessment

Any child with an MPS disorder should receive careful evaluation of psychosocial adjustment, cognitive functioning, and behavior. Psychological testing serves several useful functions (Shapiro & Klein, 1994). Tests can document deterioration of functioning over time, allowing the clinician to determine the progression of the disease. Improvement or stability of functioning as determined by psychological testing can also provide outcome data for evaluating treatment. This may be especially useful for when working with children who are going to be or have been treated with BMT.

Psychoeducational assessment may also be useful in determining the appropriate curriculum and school placement for children with MPS disorders. Documentation of deterioration may help teachers adjust their expectations and strategies for those children who have progressive dementia. The documentation of normal intellectual functioning may also help teachers and parents have appropriately high academic and vocational expectations for children with MPS disorders that result in alterations of physical appearance without intellectual impairment.

Shapiro and Klein (1994) have described several issues relevant to the assessment of individuals with the MPS disorders, particularly the more severe variants of these disorders. Sensory deficits, including hearing loss and vision impairment (due to corneal clouding and cataracts), complicate the assessment of cognitive abilities. The behavioral problems that are characteristic of Sanfilippo syndrome, including restlessness, hyperactivity, limited attention span, disruptive behavior, and tantrums, pose serious obstacles to testing. Attention deficits, distractibility, and hyperactivity are noted in children with Hurler syndrome in early childhood. Hearing loss, vision impairment, and movement difficulties also affect the selection of psychoeducational tests. Strategies for selecting and administering tests for children with these problems and disabilities are available elsewhere (McLean, Wolery, & Bailey, 2003; Sattler, 2006, 2008; Shapiro & Klein, 1994; Teeter & Semrud-Clikeman, 2007; Vess & Douglas, 1996).

Early Intervention

Early intervention programs (formerly referred to as infant stimulation programs) are available in virtually all communities (Guralnick & Conlon, 2007). These programs include a variety of supports, interventions, and coordination services for children with developmental problems and their families. Infants and very young children with Hurler syndrome (Nelson & Crocker, 1999), and children with the other MPS disorders, may obtain substantial benefit from an early intervention/stimulation program. It is important to obtain maximum intellectual gain prior to the inevitable deterioration of cognitive skills characteristic of several variants of these disorders. The resulting gains in cognitive, language, self-help, and motor skills will be especially important before the early plateaus in learning are reached. Enrollment in a preschool early intervention program as soon as a diagnosis is made is warranted. Coordination of educational and support services during the transition from an infant/toddler program to the school setting is an essential area for professional attention.

Educational Planning and Programming

The degenerative nature of these disorders is one of the most important yet difficult factors to take into account for children's individualized education programs (IEPs). Because of the rather rapid regression in skills and behavior experienced in the severe forms of the MPS disorders, frequent monitoring is required so that changes in an IEP can quickly be made to support a child whose skills are deteriorating. Educational strategies should encourage appropriate participation, new learning, or the preservation of established skills. Alterations in the learning environment and in methods of instruction are frequently necessary to adapt to a child's cognitive, mobility, or behavior problems. The IEP should include rapidly increasing

support and assistance as regression in behavior and cognitive skills occurs. Many of the strategies that are useful for all children with severe or multiple disabilities (Best, Heller, & Bigge, 2005; Downing, 1996) will be useful for children with MPS disorders.

Planning and goal development may be difficult for educational personnel who do not have experience with children whose disorders are progressive, since the traditional focus is on improvement in skills and lessened support as improvement occurs. Plans should be based on short-term goals. Teachers frequently need additional support to accept a child's limited skills and deteriorating course. The use of specific and observable goals for maintaining cognitive and social skills will be helpful for developing educational strategies.

The ability of children with progressive disorders to maintain mobility and related physical skills is directly related to receiving a free and appropriate education. Many children with MPS disorders benefit greatly from early and regular adaptive physical activity to maintain and improve mobility, coordination, and other physical skills. The provision of adaptive physical education will also be beneficial in maintaining and/or improving social and cognitive skills.

The rapid loss of communication skills experienced by many children with MPS disorders creates significant challenges to their participation in educational activities. Speech therapy services tailored to maintaining communication skills for the longest possible time will contribute to an enhanced education experience for children with these disorders. Because hearing loss is a common consequence of the progression of MPS disorders (Alpern, 1992), special attention is required to identify and monitor hearing loss and to maintain communication in the classroom. Assistive technology services can make a significant contribution to an effective educational program. One framework for assessment, intervention, and program planning for children with hearing loss can be found elsewhere (Vess & Douglas, 1996).

Powell-Smith, Stoner, Bilter, and Sansosti (2008) provide a practical perspective on building a supportive educational environment for students with severe disabilities. Educational personnel should emphasize the development and maintenance of functional life skills and should utilize activity-based learning whenever possible. The principle of normalization helps to prevent undue restriction in the educational program or opportunities for students who have severe disabilities, such as those found in many forms of MPS disorders. Additional information on educational strategies and issues can be found in Brown and Trivette (1998) and in the National MPS Society's (2008) *Education Strategies and Resources* booklet.

Behavioral Issues

Some children with MPS disorders (especially children with MPS III) may exhibit difficult behaviors in the school setting (especially problems with overactivity, restlessness, and fearfulness). It is not uncommon for educational personnel either to fail to set limits because of a child's physical impairment, or to treat a problem behavior as a discipline issue rather than a complication of the child's medical condition. Teachers and administrators frequently need additional assistance in managing the behavior problems that may occur in children with these syndromes.

Positive behavior support principles should be used whenever possible to improve behavior, with an emphasis on use of reinforcements (Cataldo et al., 2007; Powell-Smith et al., 2008). The focus of these interventions is on improving both functioning and quality of life for a student with MPS. Positive behavior support strategies involve changes in the educational environment, as well as strategies that assist the student to function effectively within this environment. These alterations to the learning environment and instructional methods are often helpful in decreasing problem behavior. Appropriate psychopharmacological intervention may be necessary as an adjunct to behavioral and educational interventions.

Socialization

School attendance and socialization are to be encouraged and fostered through classroom integration and specific social skills interventions. Students' independence should be supported in all areas. Teachers can do much to improve the acceptance of a child through instructional activities, such as cooperative learning and encouraging support for all children in the classroom.

Socialization is an important factor in the decision about classroom placement for students with MPS disorders. Parents may have some concerns about inclusion or mainstreaming, but in general it is a positive step to keep students in classrooms with nondisabled children. Since MPS disorders are progressive, however, the grade level at which a child with an MPS disorder should be placed may not be clear and may become less so as time passes. From the perspective of socialization and participation, it is generally best for students with MPS disorders to remain in a mainstreamed classroom with children to whom they are most similar in terms of cognitive behavior and level of socialization. This may trigger some resistance from school personnel, and often requires some level of compromise with grade placement as a child grows physically larger. Suggestions for assessing the success of an inclusive educational setting for a child with MPS disorders can be found in the National MPS Society's (2008) *Education Strategies and Resources* booklet.

Adolescents with Morquio, Maroteaux–Lamy, Scheie, and Hurler–Scheie syndromes and with the mild form of Hunter syndrome have some of the same psychosocial needs as do other adolescents. During this time, sexuality and physical appearance become especially important. Additional support and education are necessary during this time, and educational personnel should work closely with parents to help address the complications that an MPS disorder may create for adolescents. Support programs for young adults are often available through national organizations such as the National MPS Society.

Academic and Career Expectations

Although there are many similarities in the manifestations of MPS disorders, children with these disorders exhibit a wide range of impairment. Teachers and parents should not assume from the outward skeletal manifestations of the disorders that intellectual development is significantly delayed. For example, children with Scheie syndrome, Hurler–Scheie syndrome, Morquio syndrome, Maroteaux-Lamy syndrome, and the less severe variant of Hunter syndrome are likely to have normal or only mildly delayed intellectual development. Appropriately high expectations of academic achievement will foster realistic self-appraisal and enhanced academic achievement.

Vocational maturity in adolescents with chronic health concerns is largely contingent on the attitudes and efforts of parents, teachers, and counselors (Brolin, 1980). Academic and vocational programming should foster independence and autonomy. Vocational goals should be set realistically high. Planning for transition from school to postsecondary education or the world of work should focus on helping students pursue vocations in a manner similar to that of their peers (Davis, Anderson, Linkowski, Berger, & Feinstein, 1991).

Developing Support Systems

Teachers and peers should be educated about the condition, abilities, and special needs of a child with an MPS disorder. Teachers may be unsure of their ability to teach children with these disorders. Their competence should be supported, as they will find that many of the skills they use in teaching nonimpaired children are the skills that will enable them to work well with children who have these syndromes.

The use of peers in the regular education classroom has been helpful to students with MPS disorders, their teachers, and their classmates. Classmates have participated in activities to promote inclusion of students with MPS disorders into the classroom milieu. Using team-based learning, for example, allows a student with MPS to participate in learning activities at his or her appropriate level. Downing and Eichinger (1996) discuss how to select, train, and utilize peers in inclusive classrooms with students who have serious disabilities.

Teachers and peers will need support in dealing with their feelings of loss in a case where the child's condition worsens and the child either leaves school or dies. The course of MPS disorders is typically chronic, so there is time to plan and prepare for this eventuality. School mental health professionals can be involved in working with the parents and the teacher in designing infor-

mation sessions about loss for students in the classroom. Frequently the local hospice has programs or outreach services that can be useful at this time.

Health Services in the School

Children with MPS disorders may have a wide range of medical problems that affect their school program. The most frequently encountered include problems with mobility, respiratory difficulties, and cardiovascular issues for which care is necessary in the school setting. Some students may have sleep apnea, which may present as daytime sleepiness. Sometimes students may have medical conditions that call for specialized medical interventions for which training is necessary. Medication may be prescribed for associated medical or behavioral issues, and teachers will need to monitor the student or perhaps administer medication. Educational and medical personnel must work together with parents to develop a health care plan to ensure that a student with an MPS disorder receive proper care while in the school setting; Heller (2004) discusses many useful suggestions for integrating health and educational programs.

SUMMARY

The MPS disorders are progressive genetic disorders that result from genetic mutations affecting the metabolism of glycosaminoglycans (acid mucopolysaccharides). Incompletely metabolized mucopolysaccharides are deposited in the lysosomes of the connective tissues, bone, and major organs. The disorders are characterized by varying degrees of physical, sensory, cognitive, and behavioral impairments secondary to accumulation of metabolites in the body. Children with some of the MPS disorders have been found to have higher rates of behavior problems, including overactivity, aggressiveness, restlessness, and fearfulness.

Supportive medical and psychosocial treatments have been most commonly provided because for many children there is no successful direct treatment for the MPS disorders. Supportive treatments focus on alleviating the manifestations and complications of the disorders. More recently, however, BMT, cord blood transplantation, and enzyme replacement therapy have had varying degrees of success for some of the disorders. Children with MPS disorders are likely to need assistance in school through special education services, where difficulties with behavior management, socialization, and medical/health care will need to be addressed.

Although MPS disorders are difficult disorders, it is important to remember that despite the stressors, parents of children with MPS report that their joys and pleasures in raising their children are similar to those experienced by parents of nondisabled children. Nevertheless, family stress levels are often high due to the multiple demands of these chronic disorders. A multidisciplinary approach to assessment and intervention is necessary, and local care providers are unlikely to have experience with these disorders. Information and evaluation from regional or national specialists may be required. Involvement of parents and professionals associated with national support groups (such as the National MPS Society) provides critical information and support for caregivers and families. Close communication and collaboration among parents, educators, and health care providers are essential to assist children with these disorders and their families.

REFERENCES

Alpern, C. S. (1992). Hunter's syndrome and its management in a public school setting. *Language, Speech, and Hearing Services in Schools, 23*, 102–106.

Alman, B. A., & Goldberg, M. J. (2005). Syndromes of orthopaedic importance. In R. T. Morrissy & S. L. Weinstein (Eds.), *Lovell and Winter's pediatric orthopaedics* (pp. 251–314). Philadelphia: Lippincott-Raven.

Ashraf, J., Crockard, H. A., Ransford, A. O., & Stevens, J. M. (1991). Transoral decompression and posterior stabilisation in Morquio's disease. *Archives of Disease in Childhood, 66*, 1318–1321.

Avery, M. E., & First, L. R. (1994). *Pediatric medicine*. Baltimore: Williams & Wilkins.

Bach, G. (2004). Prenatal diagnosis of disorders of mucopolysaccharide metabolism. In A. Milunsky (Ed.), *Genetic disorders and the fetus* (pp. 503–513). New York: Plenum Press.

Batshaw, M. L., & Tuchman, M. (2007). Inborn errors of metabolism. In M. L. Batshaw, L. Pel-

ligrino, & N. J. Roizen, (Eds.), *Children with disabilities* (pp. 285–297). Baltimore: Brookes.

Bax, M. C., & Colville, G. A. (1995). Behaviour in mucopolysaccharide disorders. *Archives of Disease in Childhood, 73*, 77–81.

Best, S. J., Heller, K. W., & Bigge, J. L. (2005). *Teaching individuals with physical or multiple disabilities*. Upper Saddle River, NJ: Pearson Education.

Brolin, D. E. (1980). *Vocational preparation of persons with handicaps*. Columbus, OH: Merrill.

Brown, M. B., & Trivette, P. S. (1998). Mucopolysaccharide disorders. In L. Phelps (Ed.), *Health related disorders in children and adolescents* (pp. 442–452). Washington, DC: American Psychological Association.

Cataldo, M. F., Kahng, S., DeLeon, I. G., Martens, B. K., Friman, P. C., & Cataldo, M. (2007). Behavioral principles, assessment, and therapy. In M. L. Batshaw, L. Pelligrino, & N. J. Roizen (Eds.), *Children with disabilities* (pp. 539–556). Baltimore: Brookes.

Cervantes, C. D., & Lifshitz, F. (1990). Skeletal dysplasias with primary abnormalities in carbohydrate, lipid, and amino acid metabolism. In S. Castells & L. Finberg (Eds.), *Metabolic bone disease in children*. New York: Dekker.

Chen, H. (2006). *Atlas of genetic diagnosis and counseling*. Totowa, NJ: Humana Press.

Chen, D., & Miles, C. (2007). Working with families. In F. P. Orelove, D. Sobsey, & R. K. Silberman (Eds.), *Educating children with multiple disabilities: A collaborative approach* (pp. 31–65). Baltimore: Brookes.

Cleary, M. A., & Wraith, J. E. (1993). Management of mucopolysaccharidosis type III. *Archives of Disease in Childhood, 69*, 403–406.

Coville, G. A., Watters, J. P., Yule, W., & Bax, M. (1996). Sleep problems in children with Sanfilippo syndrome. *Developmental Medicine and Child Neurology, 38*, 538–544.

Davies, B., Worden, J. W., Orloff, S. F., Gudmundsdottir, M., Toce, S., & Sumner, L. (2004). Bereavement. In B. S. Carter & M. Levetown (Eds.), *Pallative care for infants, children, and adolescents* (pp. 196–219). Baltimore: Johns Hopkins University Press.

Davis, S. E., Anderson, C., Linkowski, D. C., Berger, K., & Feinstein, C. F. (1991). Developmental tasks and transitions of adolescents with chronic illnesses and disabilities. In R. P. Marinelli & A. E. Dell Orto (Eds.), *The psychological and social impact of disability*. New York: Springer.

Downing, J. E. (1996). *Including students with severe and multiple disabilities in typical classrooms*. Baltimore: Brookes.

Downing, J. E., & Eichinger, J. (1996). The important role of peers in the inclusion process. In J. E. Downing (Ed.), *Including students with severe* and multiple disabilities in typical classrooms (pp. 129–146). Baltimore: Brookes.

Gahl, W. A. (1999). Lysosomal storage diseases. In F. D. Burg, J. R. Ingelfinger, E. R. Wald, & R. A. Polin (Eds.), *Gellis and Kagan's current pediatric therapy*. Philadelphia: Saunders.

Guffon, N., Bertrand, Y., Forest, I., Foulhoux, A., & Froissart, R. (2009). Bone marrow transplantation in children with Hunter syndrome: Outcome after 7 to 17 years. *Journal of Pediatrics, 154,* 733–737.

Guffon, N., Souillet, G., Maire, I., Straczek, J., & Guibaud, P. (1998). Follow-up of nine patients with Hurler syndrome after bone marrow transplantation. *Journal of Pediatrics, 133,* 119–125.

Guralnick, M. J., & Conlon, C. J. (2007). Early intervention. In M. L. Batshaw, L. Pelligrino, & N. J. Roizen (Eds.), *Children with disabilities* (pp. 511–521). Baltimore: Brookes.

Harmatz, P., Whitley, C. B., Waber, L., Pais, R., Steiner, R., Plecko, B., et al. (2004). Enzyme replacement therapy in mucopolysaccharidosis VI (Maroteaux–Lamy syndrome). *Journal of Pediatrics, 144,* 574–580.

Heller, K. W. (2004). Integrating health care and educational programs. In F. P. Orelove, D. Sobsey, & R. K. Silberman (Eds.), *Educating children with multiple disabilities: A collaborative approach* (pp. 379–424). Baltimore: Brookes.

Herring, J. A. (Ed.). (2008). *Tachdjian's pediatric orthopaedics* (4th ed.). Philadelphia: Saunders/ Elsevier.

Jacob-Timm, S., & Daniels, J. A. (1998). Sanfilippo syndrome. In L. Phelps (Ed.), *Health related disorders in children and adolescents* (pp. 571–577). Washington, DC: American Psychological Association.

Kim, W. J., Berger, P., Bunner, S., & Carey, M. P. (1996). Behavioral manifestations of genetic disorders. *Journal of the American Academy of Child and Adolescent Psychiatry, 35,* 976–977.

Matalan, R. K. (1996). Disorders of mucopolysaccharide metabolism. In R. E. Behrman, R. M. Kliegman, W. E. Nelson, & V. C. Vaughan (Eds.), *Nelson textbook of pediatrics* (15th ed.). Philadelphia: Saunders.

McLean, M., Wolery, M., & Bailey, D. B. (2003). *Assessing infants and preschoolers with special needs*. Englewood Cliffs, NJ: Prentice-Hall.

Miebach, E. (2005). Enzyme replacement therapy in mucopolysaccharidosis type I. *Acta Paediatrica, 94*(Suppl. 447), 58–60.

Muenzer, J., & Fisher, A. (2004). Advances in the treatment of mucopolysaccharidosis type I. *New England Journal of Medicine, 350,* 1932–1934.

National MPS Society. (2008). *Education strategies and resources*. Durham, NC: Author.

Nelson, J., & Kinirons, M. (1988). Clinical findings in 12 patients with MPS IV A (Morquio's disease): Further evidence for heterogeneity. Part II: Dental findings. *Clinical Genetics, 33,* 121–125.

Nelson, R. P., & Crocker, A. C. (1999). The child with multiple disabilities. In M. R. Levine, W. B. Carey, & A. C. Crocker (Eds.), *Developmental–behavioral pediatrics* (3rd ed.). Philadelphia: Saunders.

Neufeld, E. F., & Muenzer, J. (2001). The mucopolysaccharidoses. In C. R. Scriver, A. L. Beaudet, W. S. Sly, & D. Valle (Eds.), *The metabolic and molecular bases of inherited disease* (pp. 3421–3452). New York: McGraw-Hill.

Nidiffer, F. D., & Kelly, T. E. (1983). Developmental and degenerative patterns associated with cognitive, behavioural and motor difficulties in the Sanfilippo syndrome: An epidemiological study. *Journal of Mental Deficiency Research, 27,* 185–203.

Perszyk, S., & Perszyk, A. (2004). The child with a genetic condition. In B. S. Carter & M. Levetown (Eds.), *Palliative care for infants, children and adolescents* (pp. 196–219). Baltimore: Johns Hopkins University Press.

Powell-Smith, K. A., Stoner, G., Bilter, K. J., & Sansosti, F. J. (2008). Best practices in supporting the education of students with severe and low incidence disabilities. In A. Thomas & J. Grimes (Eds.), *Best practices in school psychology* (pp. 1233–1248). Washington, DC: National Association of School Psychologists.

Rudolph, C., Rudolph, A., Hostetter, M., Lister, S., & Siegel, N. (2002). *Rudolph's pediatrics*. New York: McGraw-Hill.

Sattler, J. M. (2006). *Assessment of children: Behavioral, social and clinical foundations*. San Diego, CA: Jerome M. Sattler.

Sattler, J. M. (2008). *Assessment of children: Cognitive foundations*. San Diego, CA: Jerome M. Sattler.

Schonberg, R. L., & Tifft, C. J. (2007). Birth defects and prenatal diagnosis. In M. L. Batshaw, L. Pelligrino, & N. J. Roizen (Eds.), *Children with disabilities* (pp. 83–96). Baltimore: Brookes.

Shapiro, E. G., & Klein, K. A. (1994). Childhood dementia: neuropsychological assessment with application to the natural history and treatment of degenerative storage diseases. In M. Tramontano & S. Hooper (Eds.), *Advances in child neuropsychology* (Vol. 2). New York: Springer-Verlag.

Shapiro, E. G., Lockman, L. A., Balthazar, M., & Krivit, W. (1995). Neuropsychological outcomes of several storage diseases with and without bone marrow transplantation. *Journal of Inherited Metabolic Diseases, 18,* 413–429.

Smith, K. S., Hallett, K. B., Hall, R. K., Wardrop, R. W., & Firth, N. (1995). Mucopolysacchariosis: MPS VI and associated delayed tooth eruption. *International Journal of Oral and Maxillofacial Surgery, 24,* 176–180.

Spranger, J. (2007). Mucopolysaccharidoses. In R. M. Kliegman, R. E. Behrman, H. B. Jenson, & B. M. D. Stanton (Eds.), *Nelson textbook of pediatrics* (18th ed.). Philadelphia: Saunders.

Teeter, P. A., & Semrud-Clikeman, M. (2007). *Child neuropsychology: Assessment and interventions for neurodevelopmental disorders*. New York: Springer.

Vess, S., & Douglas, L. (1996). Best practices in program planning for children who are deaf or severely hard of hearing. In A. Thomas & J. Grimes (Eds.), *Best practices in school psychology* (pp. 1123–1133). Washington, DC: National Association of School Psychologists.

Wang, C. C., Hwu, W. L., & Lin, K. H. (2008). Long-term follow-up of a girl with Maroteaux–Lamy syndrome after bone marrow transplantation. *World Journal of Pediatrics, 4,* 152–154.

Wraith, J. E. (1995). Behavior management, mobility, and medication. *The Canadian Connection,* pp. 32–37.

Young, I. D., & Harper, P. S. (1982). Mild form of Hunter's syndrome: Clinical delineation based on 31 cases. *Archives of Disease in Childhood, 57,* 828–836.

Young, I. D., & Harper, P. S. (1983). The natural history of the severe form of Hunter's syndrome: A study based on 52 cases. *Developmental Medicine and Child Neurology, 25,* 481–489.

Young, I. D., Harper, P. S., Newcombe, R. G., & Archer, I. M. (1982a). A clinical and genetic study of Hunter's syndrome: I. Heterogeneity. *Journal of Medical Genetics, 19,* 401–407.

Young, I. D., Harper, P. S., Newcombe, R. G., & Archer, I. M. (1982b). A clinical and genetic study of Hunter's syndrome: II. Differences between mild and severe forms. *Journal of Medical Genetics, 19,* 408–411.

CHAPTER 16

Noonan Syndrome

PHYLLIS ANNE TEETER ELLISON

Biogenetic disorders of childhood are of interest to pediatric neuropsychologists because they frequently interfere with children's neuropsychological, cognitive, psychosocial, and academic development. Medical complications accompany many biogenetic disorders, and these place added psychological and financial stress on family members. These interrelated variables have been systematically investigated for some syndromes (e.g., Tourette syndrome), but other genetic disorders are less well understood. Clinicians have long been interested in how genetic disorders affect development, interfere with neuropsychological and cognitive functioning, and affect overall psychological adjustment across environments—home, school, and community. In order to provide ecologically valid assessment and intervention planning, pediatric neuropsychologists should consider the impact of biogenetic disorders on these various dimensions, and should provide meaningful interventions to address these needs. Noonan syndrome (NS) is discussed in this chapter, with a focus on clinical presentation, common characteristics and associated medical and neuropsychological complications, assessment issues, and intervention planning.

NS is accompanied by multiple congenital anomalies with variable expressivity across individuals, and may be hard to detect in mildly affected individuals (Johannes, Garcia, De Vaan, & Weening, 1995; van der Burgt, 2007). It is characterized by craniofacial anomalies including ptosis, hypertelorism, and epicanthus; downslanting palpebral fissures; low-set, posteriorly angulated ears; a deeply grooved philtrum with high, wide peaks of the vermilion border of the upper lip; a high, arched palate; and micrognathia. In addition to these features, the syndrome is often accompanied by congenital heart disease (pulmonary valve stenosis), skeletal abnormalities (short stature, webbed neck, and thorax abnormalities), genital malformations, and cognitive impairments (Johannes et al., 1995, p. 571; Limal et al., 2006; van der Burgt, 2007). Risk for juvenile myelomonocytic leukemia (JMML) has also been reported in individuals with NS (Jongmans et al., 2005).

In 1883, Kobylinski reported a case of a 20-year-old male who presented with unusual features (for a review of this and other early studies, see Noonan, 1994). The patient's characteristics included small stature, low-set ears, webbed neck, micrognathia (i.e., unusual smallness of the jaw), and other symptoms overlapping with those of several present-day syndromes, including NS (Noonan, 1994, 2005). In 1930, Ullrich published case studies of children with physical anomalies resembling those of Kobylinski's patient (e.g., webbed neck and short stature) and sexual infantilism (i.e., small testes). In 1938, Turner described female children who had similar physical characteristics (e.g., webbed neck, short stature, and sexual infantilism) and whose underlying disorder was later identified as a sex chromosome abnormality. *Ullrich–Turner syndrome* (UTS) or *Turner syndrome,* as this disorder came to be called, thus was defined as a complete or partial absence of, or other anomaly in, the X chromosome in some or all body cells (Wiederman, Kunze, & Dibbem, 1992).

Ullrich expanded his interests in rat research conducted by Bonnevie, who produced mice with webbed necks and swollen limbs through genetic mutations (Noonan, 1994). Europeans adopted the term *Ullrich–Bonnevie syndrome* to describe children who are now considered to have NS. Noonan and Ehmke (1963) published reports of nine patients (six males and three females) who were believed to exhibit a distinct syndrome. These children had small stature and various facial abnormalities, including hypertelorism (i.e., abnormally large distance between eyes), ptosis (i.e., drooping of the eyelid), and low-set ears. Some of the males had undescended testes. Other abnormalities included chest deformities, and all the patients had vascular pulmonary stenosis (Noonan, 1994). Opitz and Weaver (1985) confirmed that this indeed was a separate syndrome, and suggested the name *Noonan syndrome.* Although the term *Turner phenotype* remained in use for a number of years, NS became more prevalent in the literature in about 1968; it was also soon dissociated from sex-linked abnormalities, as it was found in both males and females (Allanson, 2007; Noonan, 1994). "Soon it was realized that some female patients with normal chromosomes previously diagnosed as having the UTS were in fact females with the 'male Turner syndrome,' i.e., the same syndrome described by Noonan" (Mendez & Opitz, 1985, p. 494).

"Many pediatricians have only a limited knowledge of this condition" (Noonan, 1994, p. 548) due to a lack of research on NS. Although not sex-linked, NS is considered to be an autosomal dominant inherited condition that typically involves congenital heart disease (50–80%), with other associated physical characteristics including below-average height, facial abnormalities, and chest deformity (Limal et al., 2006; Noonan, 1994, 2005; Noonan, Raaijmakers, & Hall, 2003).

PREVALENCE RATES

Estimates of prevalence rates for NS vary from 1 per 1,000 births to 1 per 2,500 (Nora, Nora, & Sinka, 1974; van der Burgt, 2007). Some studies suggest higher rates, ranging from 1 per 1,000 for severe symptoms (Mendez & Opitz, 1985) to 1 per 100 for milder expressions (Noonan, 1994). Although not sex-linked, NS affects males and females at a 2:1 ratio (Tartaglia, Corrdeddu, Chang, & Shaw, 2004). There appear to be no racial differences in the occurrence of NS, and the syndrome has been found in countries all over the world. NS is the most common genetic disorder in children with congenital heart disease (it is found in 1.4% of children with cardiac defects), and its rate of occurrence is even higher for children undergoing surgery for pulmonary stenosis (17%; Noonan, 1994, 2005).

GENETIC FACTORS, FAMILIAL TRANSMISSION, AND PATHOGENESIS

Although symptoms of NS have a superficial resemblance to the symptoms of Turner syndrome (which involves an absent or defective chromosome), research has not verified sex-linked inheritance, in that NS occurs in both males and females (van der Burgt, 2007). A number of patients with NS also have von Recklinghausen neurofibromatosis (NFvR), so speculations that chromosome 17 (which is abnormal in patients with NFvR) was involved in NS were also investigated, without positive findings (Sharland, Taylor, Patton, & Jeffrey, 1992). While the exact genetic anomaly for NS has not been found (Noonan, 1994, 2005), there have been some advances in identifying four major genes that are associated with NS: PTPN11, KRAS, SOS1, and RAF1 (Allanson, 2005, 2007). Sequence analysis of the PTPN11 gene shows "missense" mutations in up to 50–60% of patients with NS (Jongmans, Otten, Noordam, & van der Burgt, 2004; Tartaglia et al., 2001, 2002); 10–13% show "missense" mutations in SOS1 exons 1–23 (Schubbert et al., 2006); KRAS mutations are found in fewer than 5% of patients (Schubbert et al., 2006); and "missense" mutations in RAF1 exons 1–17 are seen in 3–17% of patients (Pandit et al., 2007).

Mother-to-child inheritance seems likely, as many males have cryptorchidism (i.e., undescended testes), and some are infertile (Noonan, 1994, 2005). Approximately 30–75% of cases result from parent-to-child transmission (Allanson, 2007). Parents with many symptoms are more likely to transmit the disorder (risk is 50%), whereas those with mild symptoms have lower risks (<1%; Allanson, 2007). Although NS appears to have strong genetic transmission (i.e., a child inherits a copy of the affected gene from a parent), there is also evidence that some mutations appear spontaneously (Allanson, 2007; Mayo Clinic, 2009).

The variable expressivity of NS makes detection of mild cases difficult, so individuals may carry the gene but may not be aware of it. The phenotypic changes over the lifespan from birth to adulthood may be misleading, because a parent may not look like a child, but pictures of the parent as an infant will show similarities. Consequently, a careful review of family pictures at various ages on both maternal and paternal sides of the family may reveal whether a particular case is sporadic or familial in nature (Noonan, 1994, 2005). The risk that subsequent offspring will have NS is reduced if it is a sporadic case; however, if it runs in families, there is a 50% risk that an offspring will also have the disorder (Noonan, 1994, 2005).

Others suggest that in the developing brain, growth factors directly influence a number of proteins that generate neuronal development. Genetic mutations are thought to inhibit basal neurogenesis in favor of astrogenesis or atrocytic growth (see Gauthier et al., 2007). This variation in neuronal growth may contribute to the cognitive features of NS.

DEVELOPMENTAL CONSIDERATIONS

Prenatal Period and Early Infancy

Individuals with NS generally have an unremarkable prenatal history. About one-third of NS pregnancies do have complications caused by polyhydramnios (excess of amniotic fluid). Cystic hygromas (fetal edema) have also been found with ultrasound technology (van der Burgt, 2007), and excessive weight loss in the first week of life has been reported as well (Noonan, 1994). It has been suggested that fetuses with polyhydramnios, pleural infusions, and edema should be tested for NS (van der Burgt, 2007).

Feeding problems are relatively common; 39% of babies with NS have moderate difficulties, and 24% show severe problems that require tube feeding (Sharland, Burch, McKenna, & Patton, 1992). Projectile vomiting may also be present (Gilbert, 1996). Failure to thrive has been reported in infants with NS (Allanson, 2007), and lethargy, poor feeding, and vomiting may lead to hospitalization, according to Noonan (1994). The feeding difficulties do resolve themselves in later infancy, although repeated concerns about failure to thrive may be part of the early developmental picture.

Childhood and Early Adolescence

Both physical and cognitive/intellectual delays have been found in a relatively large number of children diagnosed with NS. Short stature is found in the majority of children (80%), and a 2-year gap between bone age and chronological age is common (Gilbert, 1996). Hypotonia may also be present (Noonan, 1994, 2005), and motor delays are common (van der Burgt, 2007). Delayed puberty has been reported; undescended testes are frequently observed; and small testicular size and infertility often occur in later stages (Gilbert, 1996; Mendez & Opitz, 1985; van der Burgt, 2007).

Thomas and Stanhope (1993) suggest that patients who are below the 3rd percentile for height before puberty should be considered as candidates for growth hormone (GH) treatment. Initial benefits in height have been found in children treated with GH (Ahmed et al., 1991; Limal et al., 2006; Osio, Dahlgren, Wikland, & Westphal, 2005). Despite promising findings, Limal and colleagues (2006) report that individuals with mutations in the PTPN11 gene are less responsive to GH treatment.

Adulthood

Although signs and symptoms of NS may lessen with age (van der Burgt, 2007), the mean height of adults with NS may be up to two standard deviations below the norm (Noonan, 1994, 2005). While 30% of adults with NS reach normal height, below-average height growth rates in adults have been documented: Up to 50% of females and 40% of males have height growth rates below the 3rd percentile (Noonan et al., 2003). Ultimate adult height is affected by parental size, and wide variations have been found, but most females reach 5 feet and males reach 5 feet, 5 inches.

PSYCHOSOCIAL COMPROMISE

The psychosocial features of NS are not well documented. Lee, Portnoy, Hill, Gillberg, and Patton (2005) have not found specific behavioral or psychopathology in children with NS, but social interactions may be compromised as a result of other complications. First, children with NS often have poor muscle tone, which tends to affect their athletic ability (Gilbert, 1996), and early milestones are often delayed (Allanson, 2007). Children with NS are thus frequently poor at sports, and this fact may reduce their natural opportunities for play and socialization. Because they also tend to mature late, they often prefer to play with younger children (Gilbert, 1996). The social consequences of chronic medical complications (cardiac, orthopedic, etc.) need further study in patients with NS. However, Lee and colleagues (2005) indicate that for the most part, children with NS show self-esteem comparable to that of age-matched peers.

Although it is important to note that there is no evidence of consistent psychiatric or behavioral disorders in patients with NS, adults with NS appear to have some psychosocial problems (Allanson, 2007). They have been found to have relatively high rates of depression (20%; Noonan, 2005). Other emotional problems include anxiety, panic attacks, problems with self-awareness, and difficulties identifying and expressing emotions (Verhoeven, Wingbermühle, Egger, van der Burgt, & Tuiner, 2008).

NEUROLOGICAL COMPROMISE

Various neurological problems in patients with NS have been described. Sharland, Burch, and colleagues (1992) reported that recurrent seizures are a problem for 13% of these patients. Infrequent peripheral neuropathy has also been reported. For example, Noonan (1994) found mild myelomeningocele (protrusion of the cord and meninges from a defect in the vertebral column) in a patient with recurring tethered cord. "Other neurologic complications have included spina bifida occulta, subarachnoid hemorrhage from aneurysm, and syringomyelia," as well as optic glioma and medulloblastoma (Noonan, 1994, p. 552). Malignant schwannoma was reported by Kaplan, Opitz, and Gosset (1968), while Noonan (1994) also found a number of benign schwannomas.

As noted earlier, Noonan (1994, 2005) and van der Burgt (2007) indicate that hypertonia is common, and it can be associated with poor coordination. The interaction of hypertonia with visual problems may account for the coordination difficulties.

MEDICAL RISKS
Congenital Heart Disease

A number of congenital heart diseases are associated with NS and are identifiable at birth (Gilbert, 1996; van der Burgt, 2007). Pulmonary stenosis, in which the valve in the pulmonary artery is misshapen (narrowed) or not adequately formed, is the most common cardiac problem (50–65%); atrial septal defect, in which the wall dividing the right and left upper heart chambers is improperly formed, is not uncommon (10%); ventricular septal hypertrophy, where there is an increase in the wall separating the right and left lower heart chambers, is also found (10%); and ventricular septal defects, where there is a hole between the right and left lower chambers, are found in approximately 5% of patients with NS (Allanson, 2007; Noonan, 1994, 2005; Shaw, Kalidas,

Crosby, Jeffery, & Patton, 2007). Noonan (1994) indicates that virtually every type of cardiac defect has been found in individuals with NS. Hypertrophic cardiomyopathy, including both the obstructive and the nonobstructive types, occurs in 20–30% of patients (Shaw et al., 2007). Cardiomyopathy frequently involves both the right and the left ventricles, is noticeable at birth or develops in later infancy or childhood, and involves muscle disarray and thick walls in the coronary arteries.

Other cardiac problems include dysplastic pulmonary valve and mitral valve prolapse. Various congenital defects may require surgery or medications, while others may not need further treatment (Gilbert, 1996; Shaw et al., 2007). Electrocardiograms are used to identify abnormal defects (e.g., left-axis deviation or dominant S wave over the precordium) and sometimes can be helpful or confirmatory in the diagnosis of NS (Noonan, 1994). Noonan (1994) suggests that all patients with NS should undergo cardiac evaluations as soon after birth as possible, as well as frequent, periodic checkups, because not all cardiac problems present at birth.

Thrombocytopenia

Some patients with NS have shown decreased numbers of blood platelets (Mendez & Opitz, 1985). In addition, various bleeding abnormalities have been reported, including factor IX deficiency and von Willebrand disease (Mendez & Opitz, 1985). Flick, Sing, Kizer, and Lazarchick (1991) estimate that as many as 20% of patients with NS have clinically significant blood coagulation abnormalities. In a case study, Flick and colleagues (1991) found that a 23-year-old patient with chronic idiopathic thrombocytopenic purpura also had cyclooxygenase deficiency, which was thought to be the primary mechanism for the patient's platelet defect. Tofil, Winkler, Watts, and Noonan (2005) caution that life-threatening bleeding may occur in patients with NS undergoing surgery.

Lymphatic System Difficulties

Although it is not pathognomonic for NS, lymphatic involvement has been found in patients with NS (Allanson, 2007; Mendez & Opitz, 1985; van der Burgt, 2007). Lymphatic dysplasia (abnormal or obstructed drainage of the lymphatic system) has produced various complications, including edema and protein-losing enteropathy. Lymphatic conditions can also create complications after surgery.

Leukemia

Persons with NS appear to have an increased risk for childhood leukemia, particularly those with a germline mutation in PTPN11 (Allanson, 2007). Jongmans and colleagues (2005) also indicate a risk for juvenile myelomonocyctic leukemia JMML in individuals with mutations in PTPN11.

Genitourinary Problems

The fact that the majority of males with NS have undescended testes (cryptorchidism), often bilaterally, may result in deficient spermatogenesis and infertility (van der Burgt, 2007). Male puberty may be delayed for as much as 2 years, which appears related to bone age (Noonan, 1994, 2005); moreover, secondary sexual characteristics may not be adequately developed (Allanson, 2007). Females are not typically infertile, and they may have either normal or delayed puberty (van der Burgt, 2007). Maternal transmission of NS is three times greater than paternal transmission, which appears likely to be due to male infertility resulting from cryptorchidism. Noonan (1994) also reports that patients with NS may have renal abnormalities (10%), but that most of these have little serious medical impact on the affected individuals.

Orthopedic Problems

A number of different orthopedic problems have been found in individuals with NS, with as many as 90% of patients showing chest deformity such as prominent-pectus cariatum or hollowed-pectus excavatum (van der Burgt, 2007). Other orthopedic problems have been reported, including scoliosis (10–15%), talipes equinovarus (a deformity of the foot in which the heel is turned inward and is plantar-flexed—typical clubfoot; 10–15%), radioulnar synostosis, cervical spine fusion, or contractures of the joints (Lee et al., 2001;

Noonan, 1994, 2005). Lee and colleagues (2001) suggest that scoliosis with thoracic lordosis may develop early in life and can be severe. Early detection and treatment are important. The hypotonia that is common may improve with age. Other anomalies include abnormal angle of the elbow, curved fifth finger, blunt and squared fingertips, shield-like chest, and widely spaced nipples (Noonan, 1994, 2005).

NEUROPSYCHOLOGICAL IMPAIRMENTS

Most of the research on NS to date has been directed at documenting the physical characteristics of NS; limited information is available about the central nervous system or neuropsychological features (intellectual, speech, or hearing problems) of the disorder (Hopkins-Acos & Bunker, 1979). A few isolated studies or single-subject designs have investigated specific neuropsychological deficits, but these investigations should be considered preliminary. Research suggests that hypotonia is common, and poor coordination is also reported (Fakouri & Fakouri, 1998; Lee et al., 2001; Noonan, 1994, 2005; van der Burgt, 2007).

Attention and Concentration

Although there are no large-scale studies documenting attention and concentration difficulties in patients with NS, attention deficits have been reported in some cases (van der Burgt, 2007).

Intellectual and Academic Development

The intellectual functioning of individuals with NS can range from mild cognitive deficiency (Lee et al., 2005; Noonan, 1994, 2005; van der Burgt, 2007) to superior abilities (Finnegan & Hughes, 1988; Money & Kalus, 1979). Mendez and Opitz (1985) reviewed 63 papers reporting the intellectual functioning of individuals with NS and found that 24% of these individuals had cognitive impairments. In a study of 100 students with NS, 5% attended schools for physically disabled students, 11% were in programs for slow learners, and 84% attended regular education classrooms and had

good school performance (Sharland, Burch, et al., 1992). Others report ranges of cognitive impairment between 15% and 35% of patients with NS (van der Burgt, 2007).

A Full Scale IQ (e.g., on the third edition of the Wechsler Intelligence Scale for Children) may mask specific abilities when there are significant Verbal–Performance discrepancies. In a small-scale study of children with NS, profile analysis showed that individuals varied in their pattern of verbal and nonverbal strengths. In one case, a patient did show a specific deficit in verbal reasoning skills; however, in four cases, praxic or nonverbal abilities were compromised (Money & Kalus, 1979). Specifically, the latter cases showed difficulty with the visual-constructional aspects of the Wechsler scales. These authors hypothesized that the visual-constructional disabilities found in patients with NS "as well as [patients with] Turner's syndrome, despite the disparity of the two syndromes cytogenetically, puts constraints on what importance may be attributed to the missing chromosome of 45,X Turner's syndrome in formulating theories regarding the X and Y chromosome as determinants of sex difference in hemispheric dominance and verbal–praxic disparity in 'normal girls' and boys" (Money & Kalus, 1979, p. 850). Further study is needed to confirm this hypothesis and to delineate more clearly any differences between verbal and nonverbal abilities in patients with NS.

Sensory, Motor, and Visual Perceptual Skills

There is ample evidence to suggest that motor, visual-perceptual, and sensory deficits are associated with NS (Hopkins-Acos & Bunker, 1979; Noonan, 1994, 2005; van der Burgt, 2007). Motor difficulties that may be secondary to hypertonia and poor muscle tone appear early in life (e.g., poor sucking in infancy) and often continue into early childhood (Gilbert, 1996). Children with NS are often described as clumsy, are frequently poor in sports, and have a tendency to "knock into objects" (Gilbert, 1996, p. 216). Visual-perceptual difficulties have also been reported, and squinting and myopia (nearsightedness) may be problems as well (Gilbert, 1996; van der Burgt, 2007).

Language Skills

Delays in language acquisition are quite common (25–75%) in children with NS, and a majority of children show articulation problems (Allanson, 2007; van der Burgt, 2007). Speech and hearing deficits have also been reported in a case study of a child with NS (Hopkins-Acos & Bunker, 1979). In this young child, "slightly depressed pure-tone thresholds" were reported with a "slight downward shift for both ears on the typano-grams," which were consistent with a "mild conductive loss" (Hopkins-Acos & Bunker, 1979, p. 497). Further speech–language evaluation showed that the child was functioning significantly below expected age levels on measures of language comprehension, with more pronounced difficulties in verbal expressive skills. A functional assessment of his communication intentions and behaviors, via systematic, structured observations of the child in his home interacting with his mother, his brother, and the clinician, also yielded signs of significant delays.

Hopkins-Acos and Bunker (1979) suggested a relationship among the child's congenital heart problems, reduced sensory–motor exploration experiences, and speech–language delays. The child did show improvement with an early intervention program designed to treat speech–language delays. When he was later placed in a normal kindergarten classroom, he made improvements in language comprehension, including three-part commands, same–different, and other verbal concepts; reading through visual recognition of letters; writing his name; social interactions; and independent and group activities. He continued to show below-average abilities in the perceptual–motor area and had difficulty catching and throwing a ball, balancing on one foot, and working with pencils or crayons. Delays were most significant in visual-perceptual, motor, and phonological development (Hopkins-Acos & Bunker, 1979). Remediation efforts focused on increasing functional skills to facilitate communication by combining non-verbal signs with appropriate verbalizations that encouraged the "reciprocal nature of social-linguistic behavior" (Hopkins-Acos & Bunker, 1979, p. 503).

The extent to which other children with NS evidence speech–language delays warrants further investigation. Consideration of the effects of early cardiac problems and restriction of sensory–motor experiences is also of interest. The extent to which children respond to early intervention is of primary concern. In addition, van der Burgt (2007) suggests that the possibility of hearing problems should be investigated early. Later studies show that hearing loss resulting from otitis media may be common in patients with NS (15–40%) (van der Burgt, 2007). Sensory–neural damage may also result in loss of hearing in the low-frequency (10%) and high-frequency (25%) ranges.

Organization, Sequencing, Learning, Memory, and Executive Functions

An extensive review of MEDLINE and PsycINFO indicated that research to date has not explored problems with organization, sequencing, learning, memory, or executive functions in individuals with NS. Gilbert (1996) does indicate that children with NS may have specific difficulties in learning to speak and may be slow to mature. The extent to which individuals with NS have compromised intellectual abilities may also predict difficulties in these areas as well, but research and clinical case reports are needed to verify this hypothesis.

In conclusion, as Hopkins-Acos and Bunker (1979) commented, most research to date has focused on the physical characteristics associated with NS, with less emphasis on neuropsychological abilities. Thus it is difficult to predict which individuals will display select deficits, apart from generalized difficulties associated with low intellectual functioning.

ASSESSMENT AND DIAGNOSTIC ISSUES

Clinical Findings That Aid in Diagnosis

The diagnosis of NS is often made from clinical findings (Noonan, 1994, 2005; van der Burgt, 2007). Typically the facial features are helpful for making a diagnosis, although these are difficult to discern in newborns. Noonan (1994) and van der Burgt (2007) indicate that the following features are typically present: (1) sloping forehead; (2) thick ears, which may be posteriorly positioned; (3) hypertelorism, with down-slanting of the palpebral fissures (folds protecting eyes), a deep-set philtrum (groove of the upper lip), and sometimes retrognathia (jaw positioned in the back of the frontal plane); (4) marked edema of the neck, with excess nuchal skin (skin on the back of the neck); (5) relatively enlarged head from infancy through age 2 years; (6) flat cheekbones with prominent, round eyes; (7) depressed nasal bridge; (8) stocky body, with chest deformities that become more prominent with age; and (9) short neck. These features do change in childhood, and the face becomes more coarse, triangular, and sharper in adolescence and adulthood. A low hairline in back may obscure web-like features on the neck. Adults tend to have obvious nasolabial folds, with a high hairline in front, and transparent, wrinkled skin (Noonan, 1994, 2005; van der Burgt, 2007).

Although a scoring system for clinicians was devised by Duncan, Fowler, and Farkas (1981), the diagnosis of NS is still relatively subjective (Noonan, 1994, 2005). However, it is important to determine the maternal use of alcohol or other teratogens (e.g., anticonvulsants) and to identify other chromosomal abnormalities, to rule out competing diagnoses. Others suggest that laboratory studies, including chromosome analysis and DNA analysis (PTPN11, KRAS), may be appropriate (van der Burgt, 2007). Extensive cardiological examination, including echocardiography, is also recommended.

Several cases of individuals with NS have shown fetal edema (Bowie & Black, 1986; van der Burgt, 2007) and cystic hygroma (i.e., a watery tumor on the neck; Donnefeld, Nazir, Sindoni, & Libviggi, 1991) *in utero*. Graham (1996) suggests that diagnosis for mildly affected individuals can be made after a careful cardiac evaluation and consideration of the adult expression of the disorder.

Key Issues in Regard to Differential Diagnosis

A number of other syndromes should be excluded when one is making a diagnosis of NS, including Turner syndrome, NFvR, and Aarskog syndrome. These syndromes are briefly reviewed in order to highlight the major features and characteristics that distinguish NS.

Turner Syndrome

Turner syndrome (see Powell & Schulte, Chapter 13, this volume, for a full discussion) is characterized by the following: short stature, webbed neck, redundant skinfolds or edema of the neck, lymphedema of the feet and hands, ptosis of the eyelids, micrognathia, renal anomalies, cardiac defects (e.g., coarctation of the aorta), poor development of secondary sexual characteristics, and primary amenorrhea. A child with Turner syndrome may not be diagnosed at birth. Despite physical features (e.g., webbed neck, ptosis, short stature) and medical problems (e.g., cardiac defects) similar to those of NS, Turner syndrome can be reliably differentiated through genetic tests.

von Recklinghausen Neurofibromatosis

NFvR (also known as NF1) is characterized by multiple *café au lait* spots and skin tumors, with skeletal (i.e., clubfoot, dislocation of the hips) and neurological signs (Wiederman et al., 1992; see Payne & North, Chapter 17, this volume, for a full discussion). NFvR is thought to be an autosomal dominant disorder with variable expressivity, and chromosome 17 has been implicated. Children may show classic signs of NFvR with NS, and are generally diagnosed as having "neurofibromatosis–Noonan syndrome" (NFNS; Wiederman et al., 1992). In some cases, the NS signs may be subtle but nonetheless clinically evident (Opitz & Weaver, 1985). Opitz and Weaver (1985) suggest that NFNS is nosologically discrete, not an unusual form of either syndrome; that it is as common as NFvR; and that it has an unknown pathogenesis, although males have different manifestations of the syndrome (fusiform swelling of nerve strands) compared to females (classic cutaneous neurofibromas and a propensity to develop retroperitoneal/visceral neurofibromas. Allanson, Hall, and Van Allen (1985) have also reported patients with NFNS, and likewise suggest that this is a single disorder distinct from the separate syndromes.

Aarskog Syndrome

Although Aarskog syndrome is considered an X-linked recessively inherited syndrome, there is some evidence that it can be partially manifested in females (i.e., short stature with facial and hand features), so there may be an autosomal recessive inheritance linkage as well (Wiederman et al., 1992). Features of Aarskog syndrome that resemble those of NS include short stature and unusual facial features (hypertelorism, downslant of the palpebral fissures, ptosis). Aarskog syndrome and NS can be differentiated, however, as NS "does not include the penoscrotal anomaly, but includes pulmonary stenosis, pterygium, [and] mental retardation" (Wiederman et al., 1992, p. 194).

TREATMENT AND
INTERVENTION PLANNING

Medical Treatment

Cardiac surgery may or may not be warranted, depending on the severity and symptoms of the heart disease (Noonan, 1994, 2005; van der Burgt, 2007). Although balloon valvuloplasty has been used to treat pulmonary stenosis, difficulties have been noted when the valve is dysplastic (i.e., abnormal in size or shape; Marantz et al., 1988). In these instances, if balloon valvuloplasty is not successful, then surgery is an alternative. Noonan (1994) also notes that in some cases the valve may need to be resected to relieve obstructions. Other surgical procedures may be needed to treat the various cardiac problems associated with NS. In rare cases, children with NS and cardiomyopathy have undergone heart transplants, but the general course and prognosis for cardiomyopathy are not well known.

Bleeding problems and easy bruising may also need attention; in such cases, platelet counts should be tracked, and aspirin products should be avoided (Noonan, 1994). Some report that these problems may resolve by adulthood (see van der Burgt, 2007). As noted earlier, cases of ALL have been reported in children with NS, although it is not known whether NS places a child at higher risk for other malignancies. Obviously, medical screening and follow-up treatment are important in these cases.

Initial research investigating GH treatment to increase height has shown promise (Limal et al., 2006; van der Burgt, 2007). There have been reports of improved growth velocity in prepubertal and pubertal children with NS. Gilbert (1996) suggests that in some cases, surgery may be warranted to treat undescended testes. Surgical intervention prior to school age may increase fertility and may decrease other malignant complications.

Psychosocial, Educational, and Emotional Interventions

Although specific treatment plans have not been investigated, techniques for addressing cognitive, speech–language, visual-perceptual, and academic difficulties may prove helpful. Access to educational services may be appropriate under the special education category of "other health-impaired." It is apparent that some children with NS may require psychological support for other issues associated with coping with a chronic medical disease. Further long-term follow-up is needed to determine whether children with NS have a predictable developmental course (particularly when cognitive difficulties are present), or whether the syndrome is so heterogeneous that its progression remains highly individual. Vocational training or preparation for the work force may be particularly challenging for individuals with associated cognitive difficulties or more serious medical problems.

Parents may benefit from counseling and realistic planning for a child's future. Family education and support are also recommended, as families may not be well informed about the disorder. Further research is needed to more clearly establish effective practices for children and adolescents with NS and their families.

CONCLUSIONS

A multidisciplinary approach is recommended for an individual with NS, so that medical follow-up, psychoeducational interventions, vocational training, and parental support can be coordinated. These interventions should be monitored regularly so that the child will have the best possible adult outcome. For children with NS, a neuropsychologist needs to move beyond being a diagnostician into playing the role of advocate and counselor. Section 504 of the Rehabilitation Act of 1973 (a civil rights law banning discrimination on the basis of disabilities) and the Individuals with Disabilities Education Improvement Act of 2004 empower children, adolescents, and adults with medical and genetic disorders to gain the vocational and educational training needed for life success. The extent to which we can foster this kind of ecologically valid intervention may optimize the potential for individuals with NS to become self-reliant, self-sufficient, and/or completely independent.

ACKNOWLEDGMENT

I would like to extend my thanks to Jane Walczak, the librarian at Children's Hospital in Milwaukee, Wisconsin, for her assistance in accessing many of the references for my research on NS.

REFERENCES

Ahmed, M. L., Foot, A. B. M., Edge, J. A., Lamkin, V. A., Savage, M. O., & Dunger, D.B. (1991). Noonan's syndrome: Abnormalities of the growth hormone/IGF-I axis and the response to treatment with human biosynthetic growth hormone. *Acta Paediatrica Scandinavica, 80,* 446-450.

Allanson, J. E. (2005). Noonan syndrome. In S. B. Cassidy & J. E. Allanson (Eds.), *Management of genetic syndromes* (pp. 402–404). New York: Wiley-Liss.

Allanson, J. E. (2007). Noonan syndrome. *American Journal of Medical Genetics, 145C,* 274–279.

Allanson, J. E., Hall, J. G., Hughes, H. E., Preus, M., & Witt, R. D. (1985). Noonan syndrome: The changing phenotype. *American Journal of Medical Genetics, 21,* 507–514.

Allanson, J. E., Hall, J.G., & Van Allen, M. I. (1985). Noonan phenotype associated with neurofibromatosis. *American Journal of Medical Genetics, 21,* 457–462.

Bowie, E. V., & Black, V. (1986). Non-immune hydrops fetalis in Noonan's syndrome. *American Journal of Diseases of Children, 140,* 758–760.

Donnefeld, A. E., Nazir, M. A., Sindoni, F., & Libviggi, R. J. (1991). Prenatal sonographic documentation of cystic hygroma regression to Noonan syndrome. *American Journal of Medical Genetics, 39,* 461–465.

Duncan, W. J., Fowler, R. S., & Farkas, L. G., (1981). A comprehensive scoring system for evaluating Noonan syndrome. *American Journal of Medical Genetics, 10,* 37–50.

Fakouri, C., & Fakouri, E. (1998). Noonan syndrome. In L. Phelps (Ed.), *A guidebook for understanding and educating health-related disorders in children and adolescents* (pp. 474–479). Washington, DC: American Psychological Association.

Finnegan, J. A., & Hughes, H. E. (1988). Very superior intelligence in a child with Noonan syndrome. *American Journal of Medical Genetics, 31,* 385–389.

Flick, J. T., Sing, A. K., Kizer, J., & Lazarchick, J. (1991). Platelet dysfunction in Noonan's syndrome: A case with a platelet cyclooxygenase-like deficiency and chronic idiopathic thrombocytopenic purpura. *American Journal of Clinical Pathology, 95,* 739–742.

Gauthier, A., Furstoss, O., Araki, T., Chan, R., Neel, B., Kaplan, D., et al. (2007). Control of CNS cell-fate decisions by SHP-2 and its dysregulation in Noonan syndrome. *Neuron, 54*(2), 245-262.

Ghaziuddin, M., Bolyard, B., & Alessi, A. (1994). Autistic disorder in Noonan syndrome. *Journal of Intellectual Disability Research, 38,* 67–72.

Gilbert, P. (1996). *The A–Z reference book of syndromes and inherited disorders.* San Diego, CA: Singular.

Govaert, P., Leroy, J. G., Pauwels, R., Vanhaesebrouck, P., De Praeter, C. Van Kets, H., et al. (1992). Perinatal manifestations of maternal yellow nail syndrome. *Pediatrics, 89,* 1016–1018.

Hopkins-Acos, P., & Bunker, K. (1979). A child with Noonan syndrome. *Journal of Speech and Hearing Disorders, 44,* 494–503.

Johannes, J. M., Garcia, E. R., De Vaan, G. A. M., & Weening, R. S. (1995). Noonan's syndrome in association with acute leukemia. *Pediatric Hematology and Oncology, 12,* 571–575.

Jongmans, M., Otten, B., Noordam, K., & van der Burgt, I. (2004). Genetics and variation in phenotype in Noonan syndrome. *Hormone Research, 62*(Suppl. 3), 56–59.

Jongmans, M., Sistermans, E. A., Rikken, A., Nillesen, W. M., Tamminga, R., Patton, M., et al. (2005). Genetic and phenotypic characterization of Noonan syndrome: New data and review of the literature. *American Journal of Medical Genetics, 134A*(2), 117–231.

Kaplan, M. S., Opitz, J. M., & Gosset, F. R. (1968). Noonan's syndrome: A case with elevated serum alkaline phosphatase levels and malignant schwannoma of the left forearm. *American Journal of Diseases of Children, 116,* 359–366.

Krishan, E. U., Wegner, K., & Garg, S. K. (1978). Congenital hypoplastic anemia terminating in acute promyelitic leukemia. *Pediatrics, 61,* 898–901.

Lee, C. K., Chang, B. S., Hong, Y. M., Yang, S. W., Lee, C. S., & Seo, J. B. (2001). Spinal deformities in Noonan syndrome: A clinical review of sixty cases. *Journal of Bone and Joint Surgery (American), 83,* 1495–1502.

Lee, D. A., Portnoy, S., Hill, P., Gillberg, C., & Patton, M. A. (2005). Psychological profile of children with Noonan syndrome. *Developmental Medicine and Child Neurology, 47*(1), 35–38.

Limal, J.M., Parfait, B., Carbol, S., Bonnet, D., Leheup, B., Lyonnet, S., et al. (2006). Noonan syndrome: relationships between genotype, growth, and growth factors. *Journal of Clinical Endocrinology and Metabolism, 91,* 300–306.

Marantz, P. M., Huta, J. C., Mullins, C. E., Murphy, D. J., Jr., Nihill, M. R., Ludomirsky, A., et al. (1988). Results of balloon valvuloplasty in typical and dysplastic pulmonary valve stenosis: Doppler echocardiographic follow-up. *Journal of the American College of Cardiology, 12,* 476-479.

Mayo Clinic. (2009). Noonan syndrome. Retrieved from *mayoclinic.com/health/noonan-syndrome/DS00857.*

Mendez, H. M. M., & Opitz, J. M. (1985). Noonan syndrome: A review. *American Journal of Medical Genetics, 21,* 493–506.

Money, J., & Kalus, M. (1979). Noonan's syndrome: IQ and specific disabilities. *American Journal of Diseases of Children, 133,* 846–850.

Noonan, J. A. (1994, September). Noonan syndrome: An update and review for the primary physician. *Clinical Pediatrics,* 548–555.

Noonan, J. A. (2005). Noonan syndrome. In S. Goldstein & C. R. Reynolds (Eds.), *Handbook of neurodevelopmental and genetic disorders in adults* (pp. 308–333). New York: Guilford Press.

Noonan, J. A., & Ehmke, D. A. (1963). Associated noncardiac malformations in children with congenital heart disease. *Journal of Pediatrics, 63,* 468–469.

Noonan, J. A., Raaijmakers, R., & Hall, B. D. (2003). Adult height in Noonan syndrome. *American Journal of Medical Genetics, Part A, 123,* 68–71.

Opitz, J. M., & Weaver, D. D. (1985). Editorial comments: The neurofibromatosis–Noonan syndrome. *American Journal of Medical Genetics, 21,* 477–490.

Osio, D., Dahlgren, J., Wikland, K. A., & Westphal, O. (2005). Improved final height with long-term growth hormone treatment in Noonan syndrome. *Acta Paediatrica, 94,* 1232–1237.

Pandit, B., Sarkozy, A., Pennacchio, L. A., Carta, C., Oishi, K., Martinelli, S., et al. (2007). Gain-of-function RAF1 mutations cause Noonan and LEOPARD syndromes with hypertrophic cardiomyopathy. *Nature Genetics, 39,* 1007–1012.

Schubbert, S., Zenker, M., Rowe, S. L., Böll, S., Klein, C., Bollag, G., et al. (2006). Germline KRAS mutations cause Noonan syndrome. *Nature Genetics, 38,* 331–336.

Sharland, M., Burch, M., McKenna, W. M., & Patton, M. A. (1992). A clinical study of Noonan syndrome. *Archives of Disease in Childhood, 61,* 178–183.

Sharland, M., Taylor, R., Patton, M. A., & Jeffrey, S. (1992). Absence of linkage of Noonan syndrome to the neurofibromatosis type I locus. *Journal of Medical Genetics, 29,* 188–190.

Shaw, A. C., Kalidas, K., Crosby, A. H., Jeffery, S., & Patton, M. A. (2007). The natural history of Noonan syndrome: A long-term follow-up study. *Archives of Disease in Childhood, 92,* 128–132.

Tartaglia, M., Cordeddu, V., Chang, H., & Shaw, A. (2004). Paternal germline origin and sex-ratio distortion in transmission of PTPN11 mutations in Noonan syndrome. *American Journal of Human Genetics, 75,* 492–497.

Tartaglia, M., Kalidas, K., Shaw, A., Song, X., Musat, D. L., van der Burgt, I., et al. (2002). PTPN11 mutations in Noonan syndrome: Molecular spectrum, genotype–phenotype correlation, and phenotypic heterogeneity. *American Journal of Human Genetics, 70,* 1555–1563.

Tartaglia, M., Mehler, E. L., Goldberg, R., Zampino, G., Brunner, H. G., Kremer, H., et al. (2001). Mutations in PTPN11, encoding the protein tyrosine phosphatase SHP-2, cause Noonan syndrome. *Nature Genetics, 29,* 465–468.

Thomas, B. C., & Stanhope, R. (1993). Long-term treatment with growth hormone in Noonan's syndrome. *Acta Paediatrica, 82,* 853–855.

Tofil, N. M., Winkler, M. K., Watts, R. G., & Noonan, J. (2005). The use of recombinant factor VIIa in a patient with Noonan syndrome and life-threatening bleeding. *Pediatric Critical Care Medicine, 6*(3), 352–354.

van der Burgt, I (2007). Noonan syndrome. *Orphanet Journal of Rare Diseases, 2,* 1–6.

Verhoeven, W., Wingbermühle, E., Egger, J., van der Burgt, I., & Tuinier, S. (2008). Noonan syndrome: Psychological and psychiatric aspects. *American Journal of Medical Genetics, 146,* 191–196.

Wiederman, H. R., Kunze, J., & Dibbem, H. (1992). *Atlas of clinical syndromes: A visual aid to diagnosis for clinicians and practicing physicians.* St. Louis, MO: Mosby/Year Book.

CHAPTER 17

Neurofibromatosis Type 1

JONATHAN M. PAYNE
KATHRYN N. NORTH

Neurofibromatosis type 1 (NF1) is an autosomal dominant genetic disorder with a prevalence of approximately 1 in 3,500 (Huson & Hughes, 1994). The hallmark features of NF1 are cell proliferation and the development of nerve sheath tumors known as *neurofibromas*. Although the diagnosis of NF1 is based on the presence of distinctive cutaneous manifestations, such as *café au lait* spots, axillary freckling, cutaneous neurofibromas, and Lisch nodules (iris hamartomas), the most common complication of NF1 in childhood is cognitive dysfunction. Although the cognitive phenotype of NF1 is quite variable, approximately 80% of children with NF1 experience moderate to severe impairment in one or more areas of cognitive functioning (Hyman, Shores, & North, 2005). The cognitive domains commonly affected include attention, executive function, language, and visual perception (Hyman et al., 2005). It is not surprising to find that cognitive deficits often undermine performance in the academic environment, and some form of learning disability (LD) is estimated to be present in up to 70% of children (Brewer, Moore, & Hiscock, 1997). In this chapter, we discuss the clinical and genetic features of NF1, the neuropsychology of the disorder, the pathogenesis underlying cognitive and learning difficulties, and the theoretical basis for future clinical trials.

HISTORICAL PERSPECTIVE

Numerous antique illustrations of patients with multiple dermal tumors, and a likely diagnosis of NF1, appeared throughout the 17th and 18th centuries (e.g., *Monstrorum Historia*, 1642, reported by Madigan & Masello, 1989; see also Zanca & Zanca, 1980). One of the earliest descriptions, discovered amongst the documents of the Bolognese physician and naturalist Ulisse Aldrovandi (1522–1605), concerns the patient "Homuncio"—a man presenting with short stature and large, flabby masses of flesh less than 2 inches thick, hanging from the left side of his head and trunk. "Buffon's girl" of 1749 shows a little girl represented with several cutaneous anomalies, including dark leaf-shaped areas of hyperpigmentation on the limbs and trunk, a large raised lesion with the appearance of "pigskin" encircling the trunk, and "life jacket"–shaped lesions with a diffuse plexiform neurofibroma (reported by Ruggieri & Polizzi, 2003). One of the most complete early accounts of the disorder dates from a case described by von Tilesius in 1793. Referred to as "Wart Man," the patient was described as having "countless growths on his skin [fibrous tumors], a few spots of irregular color on his legs [café au lait spots], a stocky large head [macrocephaly], and a somewhat high shoulder on one side [scoliosis]." It wasn't until 1882, however, that Friedrich von Recklinghausen provided the first systematic description of the clinical and pathological features of NF1, which later became known as Recklinghausen disease. He published two case reports in a monograph entitled *On Multiple Neurofibromas of the Skin and Their Relationship to Multiple Neuromas.* von Recklinghausen correctly identified the pathology of the cutaneous and subcutaneous tumors—"These skin and nerve tissues represent minglings of both neural elements and connective tissue"—and created the term *neurofibroma.*

At the turn of the 20th century, Thomson (1900) identified the genetic nature of the disorder, demonstrating that the disease was familial in 30 of 77 cases. At about this time, numerous case reports of NF1 appeared in the medical literature, often overestimating disease complications and focusing on more severe cases. Preiser and Davenport proposed autosomal dominant inheritance in 1918; however, it was not until the 1950s that the first large, reasonably accurate surveys of the disease appeared (Borberg, 1951; Crowe, Schull, & Neel, 1956).

Detailed research into the various clinical manifestations and complications of NF1 has increased markedly since the early 1980s, beginning with the landmark work of Riccardi (e.g., 1981). In 1987, definitive diagnostic criteria for NF1 and NF2 were proposed (National Institutes of Health [NIH] Consensus Development Conference, 1988), enabling accurate and uniform clinical diagnoses of the two disorders. The NF1 gene was cloned in 1990, and its gene product, neurofibromin, was identified (Wallace et al., 1990). A few years later, the NF2 gene was cloned, with merlin (also known as schwannomin) identified as its gene product (Rouleau et al., 1993). Although NF2 is also an autosomal dominant disorder, NF1 and NF2 are caused by different genes, and their clinical manifestations are quite distinct. Both are characterized by neural tumors; however, in NF2 the predominant tumors

are schwannomas of the eighth cranial (auditory) nerve, meningiomas, and peripheral nerve schwannomas (Yohay, 2006).

CLINICAL ASPECTS AND COMPLICATIONS

Prevalence

NF1 is one of the most common single-gene disorders to affect the human nervous system with a frequency of approximately 1 in 3,500 (Huson & Hughes, 1994; Riccardi, 1992; Upadhyaya & Cooper, 1998). Population-based prevalence rates range from 1 in 960 in 374,440 patients in Israel (Garty, Laor, & Danon, 1994) to 1 in 6,711 in 2,375,304 patients in Italy (Clementi, Barbujani, Turolla, & Teconi, 1990). NF1 has been identified in all ethnic groups; it occurs with equal frequency in males and females; and an estimated 2–3 million individuals are affected worldwide (Seizinger, 1993).

Diagnostic Criteria

Although von Recklinghausen described NF1 as a clinical entity in 1882, it wasn't until 1987 that accepted diagnostic criteria were established, as noted above. According to these criteria (NIH Concensus Development Conference, 1988), NF1 is present in a patient who has two or more of the following signs: (1) six or more *café au lait* macules (5 mm or larger in prepubertal individuals, 15 mm or larger in postpubertal individuals); (2) two or more neurofibromas of any type, or one or more plexiform neurofibromas; (3) freckling in the axilla or inguinal regions; (4) an optic pathway tumor (optic glioma); (5) two or more Lisch nodules (benign iris hamartomas); (6) a distinctive osseous lesion such as sphenoid wing dysplasia or thinning of the cortex of the long bones, with or without pseudoarthrosis; or (7) a first-degree relative with NF1 according to the preceding criteria. These diagnostic criteria are suitable for both adult and pediatric populations, and nearly all patients with NF1 meet the criteria by 20 years of age (DeBella, Szudek, & Friedman, 2000). The number of clinical features included in the NIH diagnostic criteria increases with age, however, making a clinical diagnosis can be difficult within the first year of life. Indeed, approximately 46% of children sporadically affected by NF1 will fail to meet NIH diagnostic criteria within the first year of life, as they typically display just one cardinal clinical feature, usually multiple *café au lait* spots (DeBella, Szudek, & Friedman, 2000). Most children with an affected parent, however, can be identified within the first year of life because the diagnosis requires just one sign in addition to a positive family history. Whereas some diagnostic features (e.g., Lisch nodules, cutaneous and subcutaneous neurofibromas) are less common in young children and do not reach maximum frequencies until adulthood, others increase rapidly during childhood. As such, the reliability of the NIH diagnostic criteria improves every year as a child grows older, and by 8 years of age, 97% of all patients with NF1 meet the criteria. Although some have suggested including NF1-specific features— such as T2-weighted hyperintensities (T2H) seen on head magnetic resonance imaging (MRI)—to provide a more reliable diagnosis for young children, results show that they do not significantly increase the sensitivity of the NIH diagnostic criteria (DeBella, Poskitt, Szudek, & Friedman, 2000).

Clinical Manifestations and Their Frequencies

The clinical complications of NF1 and their frequencies have been reviewed in several centers around the world (Friedman & Birch, 1997; Huson, Harper, & Compston, 1988; Riccardi, 1992; Young, Hyman, & North, 2002; Table 17.1).

Café au Lait *Macules*

The most common feature of NF1 is the presence of *café au lait* macules—ovoid, dark-pigmented areas of skin that can range from several millimeters in size to covering a sub-

TABLE 17.1. Prevalence of Clinical Manifestations of NF1 in Four Major Studies

Feature	Young et al. (2002) (n = 495)	Friedman & Birch (1997) (n = 1,728)	Riccardi (1992) (n = 953)	Huson et al. (1988) (n = 135)
Café au lait macules (6+)	95%	90%	100%	84%
Skinfold freckling	80%	85%	—	67%
Discrete neurofibromas	50%	54%	—	—
One plexiform neurofibroma	27%	24%	40%	32%
2+ plexiform neurofibromas	5%	5%	—	—
Internal neurofibromas	6%	—	—	—
Lisch nodules	94%	59%	84%	96%
Asymptomatic optic gliomas	4%	—	—	—
Symptomatic optic gliomas	6%	4%	—	2%
Seizures	5%	6%	6%	7%
Hydrocephalus	3%	4%	—	—
Congenital heart disease	4%	2%	—	—
Hypertension	4%	4%	—	—
Endocrine abnormalities	6%	—	—	—
Short stature	18%	—	—	34%
Precocious puberty	5%	4%	—	—
Scoliosis	23%	26%	25%	10%
Pseudoarthrosis	3%	2%	1%	4%
Sphenoid wing displasia	7%	11%	—	—
Other bone abnormalities	11%	—	—	—
Macrocephaly	38%	—	—	45%
Noonan phenotype	9%	4%	—	—
Total neoplasms	5%	5	—	—
CNS neoplasms	3%	2%	—	—

stantial portion of the body (Ward & Gutmann, 2005). The early appearance of these macules is often the first feature of NF1; if they are not present at birth, they tend to become visible within the first 2 years of life. The presence of one or more *café au lait* macules is common in the general population, but the presence of six or more macules indicates a strong likelihood of NF1.

Skinfold Freckling

A common feature of NF1 is intertriginous freckling. Up to 80% of children with NF1 display freckling within regions that are not typically exposed to sunlight (De Schepper, Boucneau, Lambert, Messiaen, & Naeyaert, 2004). Freckling is typically observed in axillary and inguinal regions, but can also be present around the base of the neck, and underneath the breasts in women (Korf, 2002). This characteristic pattern typically emerges between 3 and 5 years of age.

Neurofibromas

As noted earlier, neurofibromas are benign tumors of the nerve sheath. Although differing classification systems exist for the various forms of neurofibromas (see Rosser & Packer, 2002b, for discussion), the main types of neurofibromas are *cutaneous* and *plexiform*. Cutaneous neurofibromas tend to be discrete nodular growths that involve the dermal (and, in some cases, subcutaneous) tissue. These nodular growths typically range from 1 to 2 centimeters in size and may protrude above the skin (Korf, 2002; Rosser & Packer, 2002b). Cutaneous neurofibromas generally begin to appear at about puberty and continue to increase in number throughout adulthood, with peak plexiform growth periods during times of hormone change, such as adolescence and pregnancy. These small neurofibromas are present in almost all adults with NF1. Cutaneous neurofibromas tend to be slow-growing and are not malignant; although they do not usually cause any pain or discomfort, they may be associated with significant cosmetic burden for some individuals (Young et al., 2002).

On the other hand, plexiform neurofibromas tend to grow along the length of larger nerves and arise from multiple nerve fascicles

(Korf, 2002; Ward & Gutmann, 2005). Unlike cutaneous neurofibromas, some plexiform neurofibromas are congenital in origin, and it is these tumors that are more likely to cause significant cosmetic disfigurement and subsequent psychosocial distress (North, 1998; Rosser & Packer, 2002c). Plexiform neurofibromas may be present superficially, or may infiltrate muscle, bone, and viscera, which can cause significant pain (Rosser & Packer, 2002c; Ward & Gutmann, 2005). Superficial neurofibromas are easier to identify and tend to be visible within the first 2 years of life (Rosser & Packer, 2002c). As many plexiform neurofibromas may be silent and not identified until later in life, it is difficult to determine accurate prevalence rates; however, estimates suggest that approximately one-quarter to one-third of individuals with NF1 develop plexiform neurofibromas (Korf, 1999). Plexiform neurofibromas carry an increased potential for transformation into malignant peripheral nerve sheath tumors (Arun & Gutmann, 2004). The latter are particularly aggressive and generally have a poor response to treatment. The lifetime risk of malignant peripheral nerve sheath tumors in NF1 is approximately 8–13% (Evans et al., 2002).

Lisch Nodules

Lisch nodules are harmless iris hamartomas that do not compromise vision. Seen through a slit lamp, they are rare in children under 6 years of age, commonly appear in children between the ages of 6 and 10 years, and are present in over 98% of adults with NF1 (Lubs, Bauer, Formas, & Djokic, 1991). Lisch nodules are pathognomonic of NF1 and are an extremely useful diagnostic tool; they are also frequently used for screening parents of affected children.

Optic Pathway Gliomas

Optic pathway gliomas (OPGs) are the most common central nervous system tumors in patients with NF1, with the majority of cases involving the anterior visual pathway (see Listernick, Louis, Packer, & Gutmann, 1997, for a review). They are usually detected prior to age 6 years, with the mean age of diagnosis approximately 4 years (Gutmann, 2002; Ward & Gutmann, 2005). OPGs tend to be slow-growing and in some cases can resolve spontaneously (Rosser & Packer, 2002a). Although present in 15–20% of patients on cranial imaging, only 30–50% of OPGs become symptomatic, with common sequelae including reduced visual acuity, visual field defects, afferent pupillary defects, optic nerve atrophy, proptosis, and strabismus (Rosser & Packer, 2002a; Singhal, Birch, Kerr, Lashford, & Evans, 2002; Thiagalingam, Flaherty, Billson, & North, 2004). Precocious puberty may also occur in children with OPGs, usually as a result of hypothalamic infiltration (Listernick, Charrow, Greenwald, & Mets, 1994). The first line of treatment for symptomatic OPGs is chemotherapy; it is preferable to defer any necessary radiotherapy until after the age of 5 years, due to the cognitive sequelae associated with radiotherapy (Rosser & Packer, 2002a; Young et al., 2002). Although it is common clinical practice for patients to undergo annual ophthalmological examinations throughout their first 10 years of life, routine MRI surveillance is usually not recommended for patients with NF1 (Ward & Gutmann, 2005).

Orthopedic Abnormalities

NF1 is also associated with skeletal system abnormalities, including scoliosis, sphenoid wing dysplasia, and pseudoarthrosis, at prevalence rates of up to 20%. Most NF1-related scoliosis is mild and does not require intervention. Less common, however, is a severe, rapidly progressive dysplastic scoliosis that requires surgical correction (~5% of patients). When associated with paravertebral neurofibromas, dysplastic scoliosis can produce abrupt angle curvature, spinal cord compression, and consequent acute or chronic neurological complications.

Sphenoid wing dysplasia is generally unilateral and may or may not be associated with a local neurofibroma. Although it is usually of little clinical significance, in some instances it can progress and affect the integrity of the bony orbit. In addition, cortical thinning and bowing of the long bones, particularly the tibia, can lead to repeated fractures with incomplete healing; this can result in the appearance of a false joint, known as *pseudoarthrosis* (Stevenson et al., 1999).

GENETICS AND FAMILY PATTERNS

NF1 results from a mutation in the NF1 gene on the long arm of chromosome 17. Mutations can occur virtually anywhere within the NF1 gene and can consist of deletions, insertions, nonsense mutations, missense mutations, and intronic mutations (Yohay, 2006). NF1 is inherited in an autosomal dominant fashion, with 50% risk of transmission to offspring. Despite almost complete penetrance by adulthood, the phenotypic expression of NF1 varies dramatically among affected individuals and even within families (Viskochil, 2002). There are poor correlations between the specific mutation and disease phenotype, except in patients with entire gene deletion (~5% of patients). These individuals display a more severe phenotype, including earlier onset, large load of neurofibromas, severe and generalized cognitive impairment, dysmorphic facial features, and increased risk of malignancy. This genetic variability suggests that additional genetic and environmental factors play a role in determining the phenotypic expression of the gene; these pose a challenge to the prediction of the future course of the disorder for an affected individual (Ward & Gutmann, 2005). The NF1 gene has a high mutation rate, with > 50% of cases the result of sporadic mutations. Given the frequency of NF1, this represents one of the highest single-locus mutation rates known in humans.

The NF1 gene was first identified and successfully cloned in 1990, and encodes a 220- to 250-kDa protein called neurofibromin (Wallace et al., 1990). Neurofibromin is primarily expressed in neurons, astrocytes, oligodendrocytes, and Schwann cells, and shares high sequence homology with guanosine triphosphatase (GTPase) activator proteins (Gutmann, 2002; Ward & Gutmann, 2005). An important feature of these proteins is their involvement in the regulation of cell proliferation and differentiation, leading to the hypothesis that NF1 is a "tumor suppressor gene." In this regard, neurofibromin normally limits cell growth, and its absence or reduced expression results in increased cell growth. Like other GTPase activator proteins, neurofibromin interacts with ras, a key intracellular signaling protein that is important for regulating cell growth and survival. Ras is a GTP-binding protein that is active in the GTP-bound state and inactive in the guanosine diphosphate (GDP)–bound state. Neurofibromin inhibits the activity of ras GTPase proteins by catalyzing the hydrolysis of active GTP-bound ras to inactive GDP-bound ras. Loss of neurofibromin results in elevated levels of active GTP-bound ras, stimulating cell proliferation and tumorigenesis (Williams et al., 2009).

COGNITIVE PROFILE

One of the most common complications of NF1 in childhood is cognitive dysfunction. As noted earlier, approximately 80% of children with NF1 experience significant impairment in one or more areas of cognitive functioning (Hyman et al., 2005). Since the early 1990s, the common aim of many cognitive studies has been to determine the "cognitive profile" of children with NF1—that is, to arrive at a general consensus about the type and severity of cognitive impairments specifically related to the disorder. Although the literature indicates some common trends, there are a number of inconsistent findings, which make a clear profile difficult to define. This is likely to be a result of the variable phenotypic expression seen in NF1, but also in part to methodological differences across studies. For example, in studies attempting to investigate the impact of an NF1 gene mutation on cognition, children with NF1 have been compared to unaffected siblings in a pairwise design, to unaffected controls from the general population, or to a norm-referenced group.

General Intellectual Functioning

Historically, reports of intellectual functioning in patients with NF1 overestimated the prevalence of mental retardation, with some studies suggesting rates of 30% (Samuelsson & Axelsson, 1981). These early studies often obtained their subjects from mental institutions and hospitals, resulting in a biased sample skewed toward severe NF1-related manifestations, with mildly affected cases clearly underrepresented (Cole & Myers, 1978; Crowe et al., 1956). These studies also tended to rely on crude measures of intelligence, such as the number of years of schooling, personal history, and parental reports, rather than on standardized measures of intelligence. It is now accepted that mental retardation (IQ < 70) is not a typical manifestation of NF1, and estimates vary between 4% and 8% (Hyman et al., 2005; North et al., 1997). Although this is approximately two to three times the rate seen in the general population, it is relatively low compared to the rates for other genetic disorders affecting the central nervous system (Hyman et al., 2005; Ozonoff, 1999).

One of the most robust findings of studies examining the cognitive profile in NF1 is a distinct downward shift in the bell curve, compared with both the general population and unaffected siblings. The mean Full Scale IQ tends to cluster around the high 80s to low 90s (Hyman et al., 2005; Levine, Materek, Abel, O'Donnell, & Cutting, 2006). In the past, there has been a suggestion of a bimodal distribution of IQ scores in NF1, with a peak around 85 and another at 100 (North, Joy, Yuille, Cocks, & Hutchins, 1995; Ozonoff, 1999); however, this has proven difficult to replicate across studies. The observed lowering of IQ scores has raised discussion of whether this reflects a true downward shift, or whether a small subset of children who perform poorly on measures of intellectual functioning lower the overall group mean (North, 2000). Although a subset of children will always perform poorly on testing, the majority of studies examining IQ in NF1 find cohort scores to be normally distributed, but with the characteristic downward shift. As such, it appears that the observed lowering of IQ scores reflects a true downward shift in IQ, rather than a subset of individuals skewing the mean. This is further supported by evidence from a relatively large cohort study reporting that 61% of children with NF1 (*n* = 81) obtained Full Scale IQs at least 10 points lower than those of their siblings without NF1 (Hyman et al., 2005). Although a few studies have reported that children with NF1 display significantly lower Performance than Verbal IQs (Eliason, 1986; Legius, Descheemaeker, Spaepen, Casaer, & Fryns, 1994), the majority have not replicated this finding (e.g., Ferner, Hughes, & Weinman, 1996; Hyman et al., 2005; Moore, Slopis, Jackson, De Winter, & Leeds, 2000; North et al., 1995).

Visual–Spatial and Perceptual Skills

Visual–spatial deficits are among the most common and severe impairments associated with NF1 and constitute a core feature of the NF1 cognitive phenotype. Characterized by a difficulty organizing and accurately interpreting visual information, poor performance on the Judgment of Line Orientation (JLO) test is a consistent feature across all studies of the NF1 cognitive phenotype (e.g., Hyman et al., 2005; Moore et al., 2000; Ozonoff, 1999; Schrimsher, Billingsley, Slopis, & Moore, 2003). For example, Hyman and colleagues (2005) reported that 56% of children with NF1 performed at least one standard deviation below the mean on JLO. Others have reported mean scores for NF1 cohorts to fall more than two standard deviations below their unaffected siblings (Hofman, Harris, Bryan, & Denckla, 1994; Joy, Roberts, North, & de Silva, 1995). As JLO does not involve fine motor coordination or a timed response, it is thought to be particularly sensitive to the visual–spatial difficulties in NF1. The point has been raised that JLO relies on elements of executive functioning (an area also believed to be commonly impaired in NF1; see below), such as using visual working memory and visual tracking skills to encode a line of one orientation and compare it to an array of orientations (Cutting, Clements, Lightman, Yerby-Hammack, & Denckla, 2004; Levine et al., 2006). The specific cluster of deficits observed across multiple visual–spatial and perceptual tasks, however, provides strong evidence of a true visual–spatial deficit. The evidence for visual–spatial deficits has been further strengthened by studies demonstrating impaired performance on the JLO task after controlling for IQ and performance on fine motor tasks (Hyman et al., 2005). Apart from JLO, other common measures of visual–spatial and perceptual functioning sensitive to these deficits in children with NF1 include the Block Design subtest of the Wechsler intelligence scales, the Beery–Buktenica Visual–Motor Integration test, and the Rey–Osterrieth Complex Figure Test (Hyman et al., 2005; Kayl & Moore, 2000; Legius et al., 1994; Mazzocco et al., 1995; Schrimsher et al., 2003).

Language

Early studies in NF1 focused much effort on understanding nonverbal aspects of the disorder, giving little attention to verbal-based abilities. Mazzocco and colleagues (1995) were among the first researchers to undertake a detailed examination of language skills in children with NF1. They compared 19 children with NF1 to their siblings on a number of language tasks. The children with NF1 obtained significantly lower scores on tests of vocabulary, picture naming, written vocabulary, receptive language, and verbal reasoning than their unaffected siblings did. A deficit in phonological processing, particularly phoneme segmentation, was also identified in the NF1 group; this is an important finding, given that phonological skills are a recognized precursor of literacy skills. Dilts and colleagues (1996) compared 19 children with NF1 to their siblings on the Clinical Evaluation of Language Fundamentals—Revised test. They reported that 58% of children with NF1 failed this screening test, compared to a failure rate of 16% in the control group. Combined expressive and receptive language deficits were identified in 26% of the sample with NF1, while 32% displayed pure expressive language impairment. Pure receptive language deficits were not identified in the cohort with NF1.

These earlier findings have since been replicated across a large number of studies (e.g., Billingsley, Slopis, Swank, Jackson, & Moore, 2003; Hyman et al., 2005). Given the wide range of language skills implicated, a global language deficit has been widely accepted as a key feature of the NF1 cognitive phenotype. It is important to note, however, that NF1-related language deficits rarely occur in isolation (Ozonoff, 1999). A majority of children with NF1 who experience language difficulties are more likely to have concurrent difficulties in other cognitive domains, such as visual–spatial impairment (North, 2000).

Executive Function and Attention

An area of increasing interest and recognition is the presence of executive impairments in children with NF1. *Executive function* refers to a collection of interrelated cognitive and behavioral skills that are responsible for goal-oriented activity, such as planning, attention, inhibition, cognitive flexibility, organization, and self-monitoring (Lezak, 1995). It is well established that the frontal lobes, and in particular the prefrontal cortex, play an important role in cognitive aspects of executive function. It is generally recognized that children with NF1 experience executive impairments; complex attention, working memory, spatial planning, and organization are typically implicated. Early studies highlighted a depressed Freedom from Distractibility Index on the Wechsler intelligence scales, which incorporates aspects of attention, sequencing, and verbal working memory (e.g., Eliason, 1986). North and colleagues (1995) described their cohort as having poor problem-solving skills and poor learning of material presented in an unstructured manner. One study suggested that 60% of their patient sample displayed features of executive dysfunction, including deficits in the ability to copy a complex figure in an organized manner (Chapman, Waber, Bassett, Urion, & Korf, 1996). A further study reported that although executive deficits were highly correlated with IQ, spatial planning impairments were greater than predicted by IQ (Hyman et al., 2005).

It has been suggested that poor inhibition, complex attention, planning, and organization in children with NF1 contributes to a profile resembling attention-deficit/hyperactivity disorder (ADHD) (Levine et al., 2006; North et al., 1995; Ozonoff, 1999; Ward & Gutmann, 2005). Approximately 40% of children with NF1 meet *Diagnostic and Statistical Manual of Mental Disorders*, fourth edition, text revision (DSM-IV-TR) criteria for ADHD (Hyman et al., 2005; Koth, Cutting, & Denckla, 2000). ADHD is characterized by developmentally inappropriate levels of hyperactivity, impulsivity, and inattention. This triad of symptoms forms the basis for the three main subtypes of ADHD (inattentive, hyperactive–impulsive, and combined). The most commonly reported problem areas in NF1 are inattention and impulsivity (North et al., 1995). Indeed, Hyman and colleagues (2005) reported that out of 31 children with NF1 who met DSM-IV-TR criteria for ADHD (39% of the total sample), 65% were classified with the com-

bined subtype, 32% with the predominantly inattentive subtype, and only 3% with the predominantly hyperactive–impulsive subtype. These proportions mirror those reported for the general population with ADHD, suggesting that the underlying processes associated with attention difficulties in NF1 may be similar to those associated with ADHD and that analogous treatment strategies may thus be applied to children with comorbid NF1 and ADHD (e.g., Mautner, Kluwe, Thakker, & Leark, 2002).

Memory

Although the presence of memory deficits in children with NF1 remains an area of controversy, memory in general is thought to be spared in children with NF1 (e.g., Hofman et al., 1994; Hyman et al., 2005; Joy et al., 1995). Indeed, the memory problems that have been reported may more accurately reflect primary language or visual–spatial impairments than memory deficits per se. Furthermore, because of the significant overlap between executive function and memory, particularly working memory, future studies will need to separate the interrelationships among language, executive function, and memory (Levine et al., 2006).

Social Cognition

Concerns regarding social skills and peer interaction have often been reported in the NF1 literature. Common descriptions in this literature include "shy," "loner," "awkward around peers," and "having difficulty forming relationships with peers." However, very few studies have explored these issues in detail. Parent and teacher questionnaires exploring behavior and social skills consistently reveal that children with NF1 experience greater levels of anxiety, withdrawal, depression, and somatic complaints; are subjected to more teasing; and have poorer overall social skills (Barton & North, 2004; Johnson, Saal, Lovell, & Schorry, 1999; Prinzie et al., 2003). A handful of studies have also investigated self-concept in children with NF1 (Barton & North, 2007; Counterman, Saylor, & Pai, 1996; Dilts et al., 1996). The most recent of these found that although children with NF1 experience a poor self-concept for physical/sporting abilities, they report an inflated self-perception of their academic abilities, suggesting a lack of metacognition (i.e., skills to evaluate their own abilities) in this area (Barton & North, 2007). The impact of executive impairments on self-concept (and social cognition in general) remains unclear and needs to be addressed in future studies.

Academic Achievement and LD

Given the breadth and severity of NF1-related cognitive impairment, it is not surprising that children with the disorder are at significant risk of academic underachievement, with the reported frequency of LD estimated to fall between 20% and 70% (Brewer et al., 1997; Hyman, Shores & North, 2006). The breadth of this range is due to the lack of a standard definition of LD. The term *learning disability* typically refers to scores on tests of academic achievement that are "substantially below" those expected for children of similar age, level of schooling, and level of intelligence. However, the application of this definition varies from study to study. Whereas some report absolute levels of performance, others diagnose LD based on a discrepancy between IQ and academic achievement (e.g., Hyman et al., 2005). Hyman and colleagues (2006) made the distinction between *specific learning disability* (SLD), or academic difficulties in the presence of normal IQ, and *general learning disability* (GLD), associated with low IQ and delayed academic achievement (more than one standard deviation below the normative mean). The authors reported that 20% of their NF1 cohort (*n* = 81) exhibited SLD, 32% GLD, and 48% typical academic achievement. Of note, there was a highly significant gender effect in the group with SLD (15 out of 16 were males). Thus males with NF1 appear to have a much greater risk for SLD, whereas females with NF1 are at no greater risk of SLD than those in the general population (Hyman et al., 2006).

As early studies into the cognitive profile of children with NF1 focused primarily on the nature of visual–spatial and perceptual impairments, it had been proposed that children with NF1 could be primarily characterized as having *nonverbal learning disability* (NLD)—a syndrome consisting of impaired mathematics, visual–spatial skills, complex psychomotor abilities, and social skills in the presence of intact verbal skills (Rourke, 1988). NLD is thought to emerge in children with disordered right-hemisphere networks (from deterioration or destruction of white matter), or with a lack of access to such systems (e.g., callosal agenesis; Rourke, 1988). Although children with NF1 display certain aspects of the NLD syndrome, there has been a trend away from this conceptualization with a greater recognition of language impairment in NF1. In fact, current understanding suggests that NF1 is not related to SLD; impairments are evident in mathematics, single-word reading, reading comprehension, and spelling when children with NF1 are compared to unaffected siblings and children from the general population (e.g., Cutting, Koth, & Denckla, 2000; Hyman et al., 2005; Watt, Shores, & North, 2008).

In order to appropriately treat LD in NF1, it is important to understand the cognitive and language impairments that underlie various types of LD. Although very little is known about the relationship between cognitive impairment and mathematical LD in NF1, a handful of studies have attempted to understand the underlying cause of reading disability (Cutting et al., 2000; Mazzocco et al., 1995; Watt et al., 2008). Those that have typically report deficits in measures correlated with reading achievement. For example, Cutting and colleagues (2000) reported that rapid naming and phoneme segmentation were delayed. Similarly, Mazzocco and colleagues (1995) also reported deficits in basic linguistic abilities of phonological memory and phoneme segmentation. A recent study by Watt and colleagues (2008) demonstrated that despite average levels of general intellectual functioning, 50% of children in their cohort (15 of 30) met the diagnostic criteria for specific phonological dyslexia; that is, they demonstrated impaired nonword reading (e.g., *ganten*), but reading of irregular words (words that do not follow spelling-to-sound rules; e.g., *island*) fell within the normal range. These findings suggest that a significant proportion of children with NF1 experience a specific difficulty in employing spelling-to-sound rules to assemble a pronunciation when reading, possibly as a result of difficulties in phonological awareness.

As no studies have examined the efficacy of interventions on cognitive impairments or

LD in NF1, the next logical step is to validate remediation techniques in this group. From a clinical perspective, there is currently no suggestion that the management of NF1-related LD needs to differ from techniques employed in the general population who experience similar deficits (North et al., 1995). As such, tools for the remediation and management of ADHD and LD that have been effective in general paediatric populations may also benefit children with NF1. It is critical that future research not only focus on the categorization and subtyping of children with NF1, but also address ways of minimizing the impact of specific cognitive difficulties on learning, and examine the potential benefits of standard remediation practices for children with NF1.

DEVELOPMENTAL CONSIDERATIONS

In studies that have investigated the cognitive functioning of children with NF1, most have focused on children ages 6–16 years. Thus little is currently known about cognitive development in very young children with NF1. To the best of our knowledge, only two studies have reported specifically on the functioning of children under 6 years of age. Legius and colleagues (1994) grouped children with NF1 into three age ranges: 17 months to 4 years ($n = 7$), 4 years to 6 years ($n = 7$), and 6 years to 16 years ($n = 31$). In the youngest age range, 6 of 7 children demonstrated a delay in language and motor skills, and 4 of 7 children exhibited mild developmental delay. For children ages 4–6 years, their general intellectual functioning was in the average range, with significantly better verbal than nonverbal abilities. Three of these children were receiving remedial teaching; two had speech disorders; and attention difficulties were also identified. In the second study, Samango-Sprouse and colleagues (1994) assessed 90 infants and toddlers with NF1. Young children were reported to have depressed cognitive abilities, as well as abnormal neuromotor and perceptual motor development. Problem-solving skills were described as monochromatic (i.e., one strategy was used excessively), and a more passive interaction style was also reported. Taken together, the results of these two studies suggest that NF1-related cognitive impairments

are expressed early in life, and that they appear to mirror the difficulties identified in school-age children (i.e., attention, motor, and language difficulties).

Although these two cross-sectional studies highlight the presence of developmental delays in young children with NF1, the trajectory of the observed difficulties is unclear. We are currently conducting a longitudinal study of a cohort of very young children with NF1 (ages 5–40 months) to ascertain how delays identified in very young children develop over time, and also to identify early predictors of future academic failure. Early identification will not only enable appropriate assessment and intervention as early as possible, but will also be the key to targeting patients for specific and preventative therapies as they become available, ultimately improving the long-term outcomes of children with NF1.

Only a handful of studies have examined cognitive functioning in adults with NF1. Although early cross-sectional data suggested an improvement in cognitive performance from childhood to adulthood (Riccardi & Eichner, 1986), most subsequent evidence indicates a stable profile. In the only longitudinal study bridging childhood and adulthood, Hyman and colleagues (2003) prospectively followed 32 patients with NF1 and 11 unaffected sibling controls. Both groups underwent baseline neuropsychological assessments in childhood (mean age 12.6 years) and were reassessed after an 8-year period (mean age 20.1 years). There was no improvement in cognitive ability as the children with NF1 developed into adulthood.

PATHOGENESIS OF COGNITIVE DEFICITS

The presence of cognitive deficits in NF1 has led to an interest in understanding the neurobiological basis of the NF1 cognitive phenotype. Investigations have consistently found little or no relationship between clinical variables and the degree of cognitive impairments of NF1. For example, factors such as gender, presence of macrocephaly, clinical severity, or mode of inheritance (familial or sporadic) do not correlate with or predict cognitive dysfunction (e.g., Hyman et al., 2005; North et al., 1995). Current research, however, provides strong evidence for a relationship between cognitive dysfunction and (1) structural brain anomalies and (2) altered biochemical pathways as a direct result of a loss of neurofibromin. Below, we discuss evidence for both.

Abnormal Brain Structure

Consistent findings in the neuroimaging literature are now providing insight into brain–behavior relationships in NF1. One of the most robust findings in the literature is that children with NF1 have larger brains than their typically developing peers do (Greenwood et al., 2005; Moore, Slopis, Schomer, & Jackson, 1996; Said et al., 1996). Although this enlargement appears to be primarily localized to increases in white matter volumes, there is suggestion of increased gray matter volume in posterior regions (Greenwood et al., 2005). A number of studies have found correlations between gray matter properties and cognitive function; however, due to the diverse nature of the research questions, firm conclusions concerning the role of gray matter and cognitive impairment cannot be drawn (Greenwood et al., 2005; Moore et al., 2000; Said et al., 1996).

Other studies have targeted the influence of more specific NF1-related neuroanatomical abnormalities on cognition. A relationship has been established between corpus callosum volume and cognition. Specifically, larger corpus callosum volumes have been associated with greater severity of visual–spatial impairment and LD (Moore et al., 2000), whereas smaller volumes have been associated with more severe attention problems in children with NF1 and ADHD (Kayl, Moore, Slopis, Jackson, & Leeds, 2000). Billingsley and colleagues (2003) examined the neural correlates of language and reading dysfunction in NF1. They found that children with NF1 displayed greater symmetry of the planum temporale—a structure located on the on the superior surface of the temporal lobe within the sylvian fissure, which is thought to play a role in mapping auditory phonemes onto visual graphemes. This mirrors structural abnormalities observed in dyslexic children from the general population.

Focal areas of high intensity observed on T2-weighted MRI (T2H) are considered a hallmark feature of NF1. T2H commonly occur in the basal ganglia, cerebellum, brainstem, thalamus, and subcortical white matter, and are currently thought to represent areas of increased water content within the myelin or dysplastic areas of white matter formation. As such, T2H may be a radiological marker of more extensive white matter abnormality in individuals with NF1 (DiMario & Ramsby, 1998; North et al., 1995). T2H are estimated to be present in 55–90% of children with NF1; however, it has been predicted that with increasingly sensitive imaging techniques, the prevalence is likely to approach 100% (Gill, Hyman, Steinberg, & North, 2006). Although they are not associated with any mass effect, focal neurological deficits, or macrocephaly, there has been much debate over their relative contribution to cognitive impairment. A number of large studies using clinic-based samples and quantitative neuropsychological measures found a significant association between a lowering of IQ and the presence of T2H (e.g., Denckla et al., 1996; North et al., 1994). However, others have not (Bawden et al., 1996; Legius et al., 1995). The reasons for these contradictory findings are most likely to be differences in inclusion criteria, small sample sizes, age variations of cohorts, differences in subject populations (e.g., age variations of cohorts), and differing methods of quantifying T2H.

Of the three studies that have reported on *location* of T2H, all consistently found that thalamic T2H were associated with significantly lower IQ (Goh, Khong, Leung, & Wong, 2004; Hyman, Gill, Shores, Steinberg, & North, 2007; Moore et al., 1996). Hyman and colleagues (2007) reported that although the presence and number of T2H were not associated with IQ, discrete T2H located in the thalamus were associated with severe and generalized cognitive impairment. Thus the specific locations of T2H may be more precisely linked to the lowering of IQ and other specific cognitive functions than to their number or presence. The apparent relationship between thalamic T2H and cognitive impairment is not surprising, given that infarction, tumor, and trauma studies have demonstrated clear links between thalamic lesions and impairments in memory, executive and visual–spatial function, language, and attention.

Animal Models and Abnormal Ras Functioning

The NF1 gene encodes the protein neurofibromin, which has several known biochemical functions, including activation of the ras GTPase. Thus partial or complete loss of neurofibromin results in the up-regulation of ras signaling, which has been proposed to underlie many of the phenotypes associated with NF1. Defective ras signaling has been suggested to affect neural development, migration, and apoptosis, resulting in abnormal cortical and white matter structure (Billingsley et al., 2003; North, 2000; North et al., 1997). This hypothesis may explain the absence of focal neurological signs in the presence of high-frequency cognitive dysfunction. It also provides sound theoretical explanation for decrements in performance on neuropsychological measures with increased task complexity.

An important experimental model to examine the cognitive corollary of a partial or complete loss of neurofibromin is the $Nf1$ +/– mouse model. Importantly, human and mouse forms of neurofibromin are highly homologous (98% sequence similarity), as are the promoter sequences of the gene, suggesting that both the biochemistry of the protein and the transcriptional regulation of the gene are conserved across species. Mice heterozygous for a mutation in the $NF1$ gene ($Nf1$ +/– mice) demonstrate cognitive and behavioral abnormalities that resemble the impairments observed in humans. These cognitive impairments are not related to an increase in tumor predisposition and do not appear to be associated with any structural abnormalities in the brain. Compared to their unaffected littermates, $Nf1$ +/– mice experience difficulties on hippocampal-dependent tasks, such as the Morris water maze, and also on tasks of attention and motor coordination.

Notwithstanding the clear differences between mice and humans, there are distinct cross-species similarities in the learning deficits caused by $NF1$ mutations. $NF1$ mutations seem to affect some brain functions more than others. For example, whereas visual-spatial learning, attention, and motor coordination are impaired, other forms of learning, such as classical conditioning, appear to be intact (Silva et al., 1997). The phenotypic expression is also variable: 40–60% of $Nf1$ +/– mice exhibit cognitive impairments, but the other carriers display normal cognitive performance. Furthermore, remedial training of impaired mice on the water maze task can alleviate the learning deficit.

Although these experiments suggest that an increase in active ras could be responsible for the $Nf1$ +/– mouse cognitive phenotype, this assertion has been reinforced by studies that manipulated levels of active ras. Costa and colleagues (2002) bred $Nf1$ +/– mice to mice deficient in active ras (K-ras +/– mice) and tested both groups on a hidden water maze task. Genetic manipulation to reduce ras resulted in equivalent performance between the wild-type mice and $Nf1$ +/– /K-ras +/– mice, suggesting that learning impairments in $Nf1$ +/– mice may be caused by excessive ras activity.

Active ras has also been inhibited in $Nf1$ +/– mice via pharmacological manipulation. To achieve this, $Nf1$ +/– mice were given lovastatin, an agent commonly used to treat hyperlipidemia in children and adults, which has been shown to cross the blood–brain barrier and decrease p21ras isoprenylation and activity in the brain. Li and colleagues (2005) tested whether lovastatin could reverse cognitive and behavioral deficits in $Nf1$ +/– mice compared with a placebo control group. After several days of treatment, the $Nf1$ +/– mice treated with lovastatin demonstrated improved performance relative to the placebo group on tasks of visual–spatial learning and attention. Not only did lovastatin result in a functional improvement, but slice preparations indicated that lovastatin also rescued defects in long-term potentiation, an increase in synaptic strength between two neurons contributing to a cellular mechanism of learning and memory (Cooke & Bliss, 2006). These results provide further evidence that ras modulation by neurofibromin is essential for learning and memory in Nf1 mice, and they are potentially very significant for the development of treatments for NF1 in humans.

AREAS FOR FURTHER RESEARCH

Over the past 15 years, we in this field have achieved a much greater understanding of the NF1 cognitive phenotype and identified possible radiological markers for cognitive impairments. Many important issues, however, remain to be addressed. For example, we need a better understanding of specific neuropsychological impairments of memory, language, and executive function. Given the relatively heterogeneous nature of the NF1 phenotype, it is essential that future studies address specific hypotheses in well-defined subsamples and use multiple control groups when appropriate. Careful refinement of the cognitive profile of these patients needs to be undertaken, so that future intervention studies can be specifically targeted. As areas of cognition continue to be investigated, it is also critical for neuro-anatomical phenomena (T2H and volumetric/structural) and particularly functional brain imaging techniques to be incorporated into future studies. Not only do these methods hold promise to uncovering the neural basis of NF1-related cognitive impairment, but they may also provide a method for monitoring the effectiveness of therapy by demonstrating normalization of cognitive networks. The natural history of cognitive impairments (particularly in young children with NF1) also needs to be explored, so that appropriate assessment and intervention can be implemented as early as possible.

The ultimate goal of research into cognitive deficits in NF1 is the development of successful remediation programs to prevent the pattern of school failure that is common in children with NF1. Despite the major impact of cognitive deficits upon quality of life, current therapeutic intervention typically relies on symptomatic educational intervention, most of which is not evidence-based. With current understanding of the important role of neurofibromin in the pathogenesis of cognitive impairment, we can now move toward the development of pharmacological treatments in humans with NF1. Currently there are clinical trials underway (at about the midway point) to determine the efficacy of lovastatin for treating visual–spatial memory and attention impairments in children with NF1.

REFERENCES

Arun, D., & Gutmann, D. H. (2004). Recent advances in neurofibromatosis type 1. *Current Opinion in Neurology, 17*, 101–105.

Barton, B., & North, K. (2004). Social skills of children with neurofibromatosis type 1. *Developmental Medicine and Child Neurology, 46*, 553–563.

Barton, B., & North, K. (2007). The self-concept of children and adolescents with neurofibromatosis type 1. *Child: Care, Health, and Development, 33*, 401–408.

Bawden, H., Dooley, J., Buckley, D., Camfield, P., Gordon, K., Riding, M., et al. (1996). MRI and nonverbal cognitive deficits in children with neurofibromatosis 1. *Journal of Clinical and Experimental Neuropsychology, 18*, 784–792.

Billingsley, R. L., Slopis, J. M., Swank, P. R., Jackson, E. F., & Moore, B. D. (2003). Cortical morphology associated with language function in neurofibromatosis type I. *Brain and Language, 85*, 125–139.

Borberg, A. (1951). Clinical and genetic investigations into tuberous sclerosis and Recklinghausen's neurofibromatosis: Contribution to elucidation of inter-relationship and eugenics of syndromes. *Acta Psychiatrica et Neurologica Scandinavica, S71*, 1–239.

Brewer, V. R., Moore, B. D., & Hiscock, M. (1997). Learning disability subtypes in children with neurofibromatosis. *Journal of Learning Disabilities, 30*, 521–533.

Chapman, C. A., Waber, D. P., Bassett, N., Urion, D. K., & Korf, B. R. (1996). Neurobehavioral profiles of children with neurofibromatosis 1 referred for learning disabilities are sex-specific. *American Journal of Medical Genetics, 67*, 127–132.

Clementi, M., Barbujani, G., Turolla, L., & Teconi, R. (1990). Neurofibromatosis-1: A maximum likelihood estimation of mutation rate. *Human Genetics, 84*, 116–118.

Cole, W. G., & Myers, N. A. (1978). Neurofibromatosis in childhood. *Australian and New Zealand Journal of Surgery, 48*, 360–365.

Cooke, S. F., & Bliss, T. V. P. (2006). Plasticity in the human central nervous system. *Brain, 129*, 1659–1673.

Costa, R. M., Federov, N. B., Kogan, J. H., Murphy, G. G., Stern, J., Ohno, M., et al. (2002). Mechanism for the learning deficits in a mouse model of neurofibromatosis type 1. *Nature, 415*, 526–530.

Counterman, A. P., Saylor, C. F., & Pai, S. (1996). Psychological adjustment of children and adolescents with neurofibromatosis. *Children's Health Care, 24*, 223–234.

Crowe, F. W., Schull, W. J., & Neel, J. V. (1956). *A clinical pathological and genetic study of multiple neurofibromatosis*. Springfield, IL: Thomas.

Cutting, L. E., Clements, A. M., Lightman, A. D., Yerby-Hammack, P. D., & Denckla, M. B. (2004). Cognitive profile of neurofibromatosis type 1: Rethinking nonverbal learning disabilities. *Learning Disabilities Research and Practice, 19*, 155–165.

Cutting, L. E., Koth, C. W., & Denckla, M. B. (2000). How children with neurofibromatosis type 1 differ from "typical" learning disabled clinic attenders: Nonverbal learning disabilities revisited. *Developmental Neuropsychology, 17,* 29–47.

DeBella, K., Poskitt, K., Szudek, J., & Friedman, J. M. (2000). Use of "unidentified bright objects" on MRI for diagnosis of neurofibromatosis 1 in children. *Neurology, 54,* 1646–1651.

DeBella, K., Szudek, J., & Friedman, J. M. (2000). Use of the National Institutes of Health criteria for diagnosis of neurofibromatosis 1 in children. *Pediatrics, 105,* 608–614.

Denckla, M. B., Hofman, K., Mazzocco, M. M., Melhem, E., Reiss, A. L., Bryan, R. N., et al. (1996). Relationship between T2–weighted hyperintensities (unidentified bright objects) and lower IQs in children with neurofibromatosis-1. *American Journal of Medical Genetics, 67,* 98–102.

De Schepper, S., Boucneau, J., Lambert, J., Messiaen, L., & Naeyaert, J.-M. (2004). Pigment cell-related manifestations in neurofibromatosis type 1: An overview. *Pigment Cell Research, 18,* 13–24.

Dilts, C. V., Carey, J. C., Kircher, J. C., Hoffman, R. O., Creel, D., Ward, K., et al. (1996). Children and adolescents with neurofibromatosis 1: A behavioral phenotype. *Journal of Developmental and Behavioral Pediatrics, 17,* 229–239.

Di Mario, F. J., & Ramsby, G. (1998). Magnetic resonance imaging lesion analysis in neurofibromatosis type 1. *Archives of Neurology, 55,* 500–505.

Eliason, M. (1986). Neurofibromatosis: Implications for learning and behavior. *Journal of Developmental and Behavioral Pediatrics, 7,* 175–179.

Evans, D., G., R., Baser, M., E., McGaughran, J., Sharif, S., Howard, E., & Moran, A. (2002). Malignant peripheral nerve sheath tumours in neurofibromatosis 1. *Journal of Medical Genetics, 39,* 311–314.

Ferner, R. E., Hughes, R. A., & Weinman, J. (1996). Intellectual impairment in neurofibromatosis 1. *Journal of the Neurological Sciences, 138,* 125–133.

Friedman, J. M., & Birch, P. H. (1997). Neurofibromatosis: A descriptive analysis of the disorder in 1728 patients. *American Journal of Medical Genetics, 70,* 138–143.

Garty, B. Z., Laor, A., & Danon, Y. L. (1994). Neurofibromatosis type 1 in Israel: Survey of young adults. *Journal of Medical Genetics, 31,* 853–857.

Gill, D. S., Hyman, S. L., Steinberg, A., & North, K. N. (2006). Age-related findings on MRI in neurofibromatosis type 1. *Pediatric Radiology, 36,* 1048–1056.

Goh, W. H. S., Khong, P.-L, Leung, C. S. Y., &

Wong, V. C. N. (2004). T2–weighted hyperintensities (unidentified bright objects) in children with neurofibromatosis 1: Their impact on cognitive function. *Journal of Child Neurology, 19,* 853–858.

Greenwood, R. S., Tupler, L. A., Whitt, J. K., Buu, A., Dombeck, C. B., Harp, A. G., et al. (2005). Brain morphometry, T2–weighted hypertensities, and IQ in children with neurofibromatosis type 1. *Archives of Neurology, 62,* 1904–1908.

Gutmann, D. H. (2002). Neurofibromin in the brain. *Journal of Child Neurology, 17,* 592–601.

Hofman, K. J., Harris, E. L., Bryan, R. N., & Denckla, M. B. (1994). Neurofibromatosis type 1: the cognitive phenotype. *Journal of Pediatrics, 124,* S1–S8.

Huson, S. M., Harper, P. S., & Compston, D. A. S. (1988). Von Recklinghausen neurofibromatosis: A clinic and population study in south-east Wales. *Brain, 111,* 1355–1381.

Huson, S. M., & Hughes, R. A. C. (1994). *The neurofibromatoses: A pathogenetic and clinical overview.* London: Chapman & Hall.

Hyman, S. L., Gill, D. S., Shores, E. A., Steinberg, A., Joy, P., Gibikote, S. V., et al (2003). Natural history of cognitive deficits and their relationship to MRI-T2-hyperintensities in NF1. *Neurology, 60,* 1139–1145.

Hyman, S. L., Gill, D. S., Shores, E. A., Steinberg, A., & North, K. N. (2007). T2–hyperintensities in children with neurofibromatosis type 1 and their relationship to cognitive functioning. *Journal of Neurology, Neurosurgery and Psychiatry, 78,* 1088–1091.

Hyman, S. L., Shores, E. A., & North, K. N. (2005). The nature and frequency of cognitive deficits in children with neurofibromatosis type 1. *Neurology, 65,* 1037–1044.

Hyman, S. L., Shores, E. A., & North, K. N. (2006). Learning disabilities in children which neurofibromatosis type 1: Subtypes, cognitive profile, and attention-deficit-hyperactivity disorder. *Developmental Medicine and Child Neurology, 48,* 973–977.

Johnson, N. S., Saal, H. M., Lovell, A. M., & Schorry, E. K. (1999). Social and emotional problems in children with neurofibromatosis type 1: Evidence and proposed interventions. *Journal of Pediatrics, 134,* 767–772.

Joy, P., Roberts, C., North, K., & de Silva, M. (1995). Neuropsychological function and MRI abnormalities in neurofibromatosis type 1. *Developmental Medicine and Child Neurology, 37,* 906–914.

Kayl, A. E., & Moore, B. D. (2000). Behavioral phenotype of neurofibromatosis, type 1. *Mental Retardation and Developmental Disabilities Research Reviews, 6,* 117–124.

Kayl, A. E., Moore, B. D., Slopis, J. M., Jackson, E. F., & Leeds, N. E. (2000). Quantitative morphology of the corpus callosum in children with neurofibromatosis and attention-deficit hyperactivity disorder. *Journal of Child Neurology, 15,* 90–96.

Korf, B. R. (1999). Plexiform neurofibromas. *American Journal of Medical Genetics, 89,* 31–37.

Korf, B. R. (2002). Clinical features and pathobiology of neurofibromatosis 1. *Journal of Child Neurology, 17,* 573–578.

Koth, C. W., Cutting, L. E., & Denckla, M. B. (2000). The association of neurofibromatosis type 1 and attention deficit hyperactivity disorder. *Child Neuropsychology, 6,* 185–194.

Legius, E., Descheemaeker, M. J., Spaepen, A., Casaer, P., & Fryns, J. P. (1994). Neurofibromatosis type 1 in childhood: A study of the neuropsychological profile in 45 children. *Genetic Counseling, 5,* 51–60.

Legius, E., Descheemaeker, M. J., Steyaert, J., Spaepen, A., Vlietinck, R., Casaer, P., et al. (1995). Neurofibromatosis type 1 in childhood: Correlation of MRI findings with intelligence. *Journal of Neurology, Neurosurgery and Psychiatry, 59,* 638–640.

Levine, T. M., Materek, A., Abel, J., O'Donnell, M., & Cutting, L. E. (2006). Cognitive profile of neurofibromatosis type 1. *Seminars in Pediatric Neurology, 13,* 8–20.

Lezak, M. D. (1995). *Neuropsychological assessment* (3rd ed.). New York: Oxford University Press.

Li, W., Cui, Y., Kushner, S. A., Brown, R. A. M., Jentsch, J. D., Frankland, P. W. et al. (2005). The HMG-CoA reductase inhibitor lovastatin reverses the learning and attention deficits in a mouse model of neurofibromatosis type 1. *Current Biology, 15,* 1961–1967.

Listernick, R., Charrow, J., Greenwald, M., & Mets, M. (1994). Natural history of optic pathway tumors in children with neurofibromatosis type 1: A longitudinal study. *Journal of Pediatrics, 125,* 63–66.

Listernick, R., Louis, D. N., Packer, R. J., & Gutmann, D. H. (1997). Optic pathway gliomas in children with neurofibromatosis 1: Consensus statement from the NF1 Optic Pathway Glioma Task Force. *Annals of Neurology, 41,* 143–149.

Lubs, M.-L., E., Bauer, M. S., Formas, M. E., & Djokic, B. (1991). Lisch nodules in neurofibromatosis type 1. *New England Journal of Medicine, 324,* 1264–1266.

Madigan, P., & Masello, M. J. (1989). Report of neurofibromatosis-like case: *Monstrorum Historia,* 1642. *Neurofibromatosis, 2,* 53–56.

Mautner, V. F., Kluwe, L., Thakker, S. D., & Leark, R. A. (2002). Treatment of ADHD in neurofibromatosis type 1. *Developmental Medicine and Child Neurology, 44,* 164–170.

Mazzocco, M. M. M., Turner, J. E., Denckla, M. B., Hofman, K. J., Scalon, D. C., & Vellutino, F. R. (1995). Language and reading deficits associated with neurofibromatosis type 1: Evidence for a not-so-nonverbal learning disability. *Developmental Neuropsychology, 11,* 503–522.

Moore, B. D., Slopis, J. M., Jackson, E. F., De Winter, A. E., & Leeds, N. E. (2000). Brain volume in children with neurofibromatosis type 1: Relationship to neuropsychological status. *Neurology, 54,* 914–920.

Moore, B. D., Slopis, J. M., Schomer, D., & Jackson, E. F. (1996). Neuropsychological significance of areas of high signal intensity on brain MRIs of children with neurofibomatosis. *Neurology, 46,* 1660–1668.

National Institutes of Health (NIH) Consensus Development Conference. (1988). Neurofibromatosis: Conference statement. *Archives of Neurology, 45,* 575–578.

North, K. (1998). Neurofibromatosis 1 in childhood. *Seminars in Pediatric Neurology, 5,* 231–242.

North, K. (2000). Neurofibromatosis type 1. *American Journal of Medical Genetics, 97,* 119–127.

North, K., Joy, P., Yuille, D., Cocks, N., & Hutchins, P. (1995). Cognitive function and academic performance in children with neurofibromatosis type 1. *Developmental Medicine and Child Neurology, 37,* 427–436.

North, K., Joy, P., Yuille, D., Cocks, N., Mobbs, E., Hutchins, P., et al. (1994). Learning difficulties in neurofibromatosis 1: The significance of MRI abnormalities. *Neurology, 44,* 878–883.

North, K., Riccardi, V., Samango-Sprouse, C., Ferner, R., Moore, B., Legius, E., et al. (1997). Cognitive function and academic performance in neurofibromatosis 1: Consensus statement from the NF1 Cognitive Disorders Task Force. *Neurology, 48,* 1121–1127.

Ozonoff, S. (1999). Cognitive impairment in neurofibromatosis type 1. *American Journal of Medical Genetics, 89,* 45–52.

Preiser, S. A., & Davenport, C. B. (1918). Multiple neurofibromatosis (von Recklinghausen's disease) and its inheritance; with description of a case. *American Journal of the Medical Sciences, 156,* 507–540.

Prinzie, P., Descheemaeker, M. J., Vogels, A., Cleymans, T., Haselager, G. J., Curfs, L. M., et al. (2003). Personality profiles of children and adolescents with neurofibromatosis type 1. *American Journal of Medical Genetics, 118,* 1–7.

Riccardi, V. M. (1981). Von Recklinghausen neurofibromatosis. *New England Journal of Medicine, 305,* 1617–1627.

Riccardi, V. M. (1992). *Neurofibromatosis: Phenotype, natural history, and pathogenesis* (2nd ed.). Baltimore: John Hopkins University Press.

Riccardi, V. M., & Eichner, J.E. (1986). *Neurofibromatosis. Phenotype, natural history and pathogenesis.* Baltimore: John Hopkins University Press.

Rosser, T. L., & Packer, R. J. (2002a). Intracranial neoplasms in children with neurofibromatosis 1. *Journal of Child Neurology, 17,* 630–637.

Rosser, T. L., & Packer, R. J. (2002b). Neurofibromas in children with neurofibromatosis 1. *Journal of Child Neurology, 17,* 585–591.

Rosser, T. L., & Packer, R. J. (2002c). Therapy for plexiform neurofibromas in children with neurofibromatosis 1: An overview. *Journal of Child Neurology, 17,* 638–641.

Rouleau, G. A., Merel, P., Lutchman, M., Sanson, M., Zucman, J., Marineau, C., et al. (1993). Alteration in a new gene encoding a putative membrane-organizing protein causes neurofibromatosis type 2. *Nature, 363,* 515–521.

Rourke, B. P. (1988). The syndrome of nonverbal learning disabilities: Developmental manifestations in neurological disease, disorder, and dysfunction. *Clinical Neuropsychologist, 2,* 293–330.

Ruggieri, M., & Polizzi, A. (2003). From Aldrovandi's "Homuncio" (1592) to Buffon's girl (1749) and the "Wart Man" of Tilesius (1793): Antique illustrations of mosaicism in neurofibromatosis? *Journal of Medical Genetics, 40,* 227–232.

Said, S. M., Yeh, T. L., Greenwood, R. S., Whitt, J. K., Tupler, L. A., & Krishnan, K. R. (1996). MRI morphometric analysis and neuropsychological function in patients with neurofibromatosis. *NeuroReport, 7,* 1941–1944.

Samango-Sprouse, C., Cohen, M. S., Mott, S. H., Custer, D. A., Vaught, D. R., Stein, H. J., et al. (1994). The effect of familial vs. sporadic inheritance in the neurodevelopmental profile of young children with neurofibromatosis type 1. *American Journal of Human Genetics, 55,* 21.

Samuelsson, B., & Axelsson, R. (1981). Neurofibromatosis: A clinical and genetic study of 96 cases in Gothenburg, Sweden. *Acta Dermato-Venereologica, 95,* S67–S71.

Schrimsher, G. W., Billingsley, R. L., Slopis, J. M., & Moore, B. D. (2003). Visual–spatial performance deficits in children with neurofibromatosis type-1. *American Journal of Medical Genetics, 120A,* 326–330.

Seizinger, B. R. (1993). NF1: A prevalent cause of tumorigenesis in human cancers? *Nature Genetics, 3,* 97–99.

Silva, A. J., Frankland, P. W., Marowitz, Z., Friedman, E., Laszlo, G.S., Cioffi, D., et al. (1997). A mouse model for the learning deficits associated with neurofibromatosis type 1. *Nature Genetics, 15,* 281–284.

Singhal, S., Birch, J. M., Kerr, B., Lashford, L., & Evans, D. G. R. (2002). Neurofibromatosis type 1 and sporadic optic gliomas. *Archives of Diseases in Childhood, 87,* 65–70.

Stevenson, D. A., Birch, P. H., Friedman, J. M., Viskochil, D. H., Balestrazzi, P., Boni, S., et al. (1999). Descriptive analysis of tibial pseudarthrosis in patients with neurofibromatosis 1. *American Journal of Medical Genetics, 84,* 413–419.

Thiagalingam, S., Flaherty, M., Billson, F., & North, K. (2004). Neurofibromatosis type 1 and optic pathway gliomas: Follow-up of 54 patients. *Ophthalmology, 111,* 568–577.

Thomson, A. (1900). *On neuroma and neurofibromatosis.* Edinburgh, UK: Turnbull & Spears.

Upadhyaya, M., & Cooper, D. N. (Eds.). (1998). *Neurofibromatosis type 1: From genotype to phenotype.* Oxford, UK: BIOS Scientific.

Viskochil, D. (2002). Genetics of neurofibromatosis 1 and the NF1 gene. *Journal of Child Neurology, 17,* 562–570.

von Recklinghausen, F. (1882). *Ueber die multiplen fibrome der haut und ihre beziehung zur den multiplen neuromen.* Berlin: Hirshwald.

von Tilesius, W.G. (1793). *Historia pathologica singularis cutis turpitudinis.* Leipzig: Crudis.

Wallace, M. R., Marchuk, D. A., Andersen, L. B., Letcher, R., Odeh, H. M., Saulino, A. M., et al. (1990). Type 1 neurofibromatosis gene: Identification of a large transcript disrupted in three NF1 patients. *Science, 249,* 181–186.

Ward, B. A., & Gutmann, D. H. (2005). Neurofibromatosis 1: From lab bench to clinic. *Pediatric Neurology, 32,* 221–228.

Watt, S. E., Shores, E. A., & North, K. N. (2008). An examination of lexical and sublexical reading skills in children with neurofibromatosis type 1. *Child Neuropsychology, 14,* 401–418.

Williams, V. C., Lucas, J., Babcock, M. A., Gutmann, D. H., Korf, B., & Maria, B. L. (2009). Neurofibromatosis type 1 revisited. *Pediatrics, 123,* 124–133.

Yohay, K. H. (2006). The genetic and molecular pathogenesis of NF1 and NF2. *Seminars in Pediatric Neurology, 13,* 21–26.

Young, H., Hyman, S. L., & North, K. (2002). Neurofibromatosis 1: Clinical review and exceptions to the rules. *Journal of Child Neurology, 17,* 613–621.

Zanca, A., & Zanca, A. (1980). Antique illustrations of neurofibromatosis. *International Journal of Dermatology, 19,* 55–58.

CHAPTER 18

Sickle Cell Disease

JULIEN T. SMITH
DAVID A. BAKER

The term *sickle cell disease* (SCD) refers to a broad category of chronic hematological disorders that includes sickle cell anemia (SCA), as well as other specific genetic presentations of the disease. SCD is an autosomal recessive genetic pathology of the hemoglobin (the oxygen-binding molecules of the blood), which affects approximately 72,000 people of African, Mediterranean, Caribbean, South and Central American, Arab, and East Indian descent in the United States alone and is the most prevalent genetic hematological disorder worldwide (Ashley-Koch, Yang, & Olney, 2000; National Heart, Lung, and Blood Institute, 1996). In the United States, the disease affects approximately 1 in 350–700 African American and 1 in 1,000–1,400 Hispanic American newborns annually (National Heart, Lung, and Blood Institute, 1996; Wang, 2007). The most severe form of SCD is SCA, which presents when two copies of the hemoglobin variant (HbSS) compose the beta-globin gene. The beta-globin locus is a group of genes on the short arm of chromosome 11, responsible for hemoglobin protein synthesis. When only one copy of the hemoglobin variant (HbS) combines with a copy of another beta-globin gene variant, a heterozygous condition of SCD is present. Several heterozygous forms exist, with sickle hemoglobin C disease (HbSC), sickle beta-plus thalassemia (HbS/ß+), and sickle beta-zero thalassemia (HbS/ß°) being the most common variants. However, approximately 65% of individuals affected by SCD possess the homozygous state (HbSS), the most severe genotype; several heterozygous conditions account for the rest of the SCD population (Wang, 2007). Moreover, those who inherit the "sickle cell trait" have one normal beta-globin gene and one sickle beta-globin gene (HbS), making them trait carriers (HbAS) but generally asymptomatic, except in rare and extreme circumstances (Ashley-Koch et al., 2000). Infants with SCD are protected from abnormal hemoglobin effects by the presence of fetal hemoglobin through about 3 months of age. Adult hemoglobin completely replaces fetal hemoglobin within the first 3–6 months after birth. In individuals with SCD, the adult hemoglobin is obviously impaired, and the negative effects of the disease take hold in early childhood. Evidence suggests that children who exhibit more acute symptoms earlier in life display a more clinically severe disease course (Miller et al., 2001).

PATHOPHYSIOLOGY

The rigidity and dysfunction of erythrocytes (red blood cells) are central to the pathophysiology of SCD. In an individual with SCD, HbS allows crystal formation on the erythrocytes after releasing oxygen, leaving them less stable, unable to bond oxygen properly, more rigid, and with a shorter lifespan (10–20 days). During the deoxygenation process in the vasculature, the presence of abundant HbS molecules causes the collapse and *sickling* of the red blood cells (i.e., they become sickle-shaped). Because sickled cells are rigid, they are unable to pass through the vasculature properly, and interfere with the blood flow by clumping together and becoming lodged in the vessels. The collection of many of these trapped sickled cells can cause vaso-occlusion by blocking blood flow and preventing the oxygenation of cells. Accumulations of sickled cells lead to increased viscosity or slowed movement of blood, referred to as *sludging,* as the healthy, oxygenated blood cells cannot pass around the rigid cells or effectively move through the viscous fluid. Moreover, red blood cells in SCD also appear to have an increased binding affinity for the vascular endothelium, with stronger affinity evident in more severe clinical cases (Ballas & Mohandas, 1996; Lonergan, Cline, & Abbondanzo, 2001).

Another complication of SCD is the reduced oxygen-carrying capacity of erythrocytes that occurs when HbS polymerizes into the collapsed state. Low oxygenation can lead to acidosis and ischemis necrosis. Certain tissues are particularly susceptible to the negative effects of low oxygen and blockage, including organs such as the lungs, spleen, kidneys, and liver, as well as the central nervous system (CNS).

Given the extensive vasculature in the brain and the resulting neuropathology related to SCD, several theoretical models of the processes causing neurological damage have been proposed. For instance, Hillery and Panepinto (2004) have proposed that neuropathology in SCD is caused by several cascading and interrelated events, including increased red cell adhesion, damage to the vessel wall, inflammation, abnormal vasomotor tone/control, and increased activation of the coagulation system. Therefore, both large and small vessels are commonly implicated in the CNS complications related to SCD (Prengler, Pavlakis, Prohovnik, & Adams, 2002).

CEREBROVASCULAR ACCIDENTS: OVERT AND SILENT STROKES

Cerebrovascular accidents (CVA), or stroke, is the most broadly documented form of neurological injury in patients with SCD (Schatz & Puffer, 2006, 2007). According to the Cooperative Study of Sickle Cell Disease (CSSCD), a longitudinal, multicenter study involving over 4,000 patients, the likelihood that a child with SCA will have a stroke is 11% before age 20. Furthermore, of all patients with SCD, 6–11% will experience a stroke prior to age 15, with peak incidence occurring between 2 and 5 years of age (Ohene-Frempong et al., 1998). Silent stroke (see below) appears even more prominent in this population, with prevalence rates ranging from 15% to 27% (Balkaran et al., 1992; Schatz & Puffer, 2007); variations in imaging techniques account for such a wide range of rates (Schatz & Puffer, 2007). Approximately two-thirds of children who have one stroke have another stroke, 80% of which occur within 36 months without therapeutic intervention. Seventy-five percent of the children who experience a CVA have a cerebral infarction, while 20% have an intracerebral hemorrhage. For uncertain reasons, children are more likely to experience infarct, whereas adults are more likely to experience hemorrhage (Ohene-Frempong et al., 1998; Pavlakis, Prohovnik, Piomelli, & Devivo, 1989; Ris & Gruenich, 2000). The Stroke Prevention Trial in Sickle Cell Anemia performed in the 1990s, as well as more recent studies, have shown that children with abnormal transcranial Doppler ultrasonography (TCD) velocities who receive regular blood transfusions have a 90% lower risk of stroke (Adams et al., 1998; Lee et al., 2006). Red blood cell transfusion therapy clearly reduces the risk of recurrent stroke, but this therapy is accompanied by its own risks and uncertainties, as well as questions of whether and when it can be safely stopped (Lee et al., 2006; Pegelow, 2001).

Strokes can occur either overtly or covertly, with obvious or subtler CNS injury that may not be easily identified through standard neurological exam (Fowler et al., 1988; Mercuri et al., 1995; Swift et al., 1989). Overt strokes are defined as having an acute onset of motor symptoms that persist for at least 24 hours, as well as clear evidence of neurological injury in neuroimaging. During childhood, the majority of overt hemorrhagic strokes result from large-artery vasculopathy (Pegelow, 2001). Overt strokes commonly occur in the frontal and parietal lobes, which are supplied by the internal carotid artery and middle or anterior cerebral arteries. Overt stroke typically involves more than 40 cubic centimeters of brain tissue, whereas smaller volumes are usually associated with silent stroke (Schatz & Puffer, 2007).

Silent cerebral infarct (SCI) or silent stroke is defined as brain lesions that are detectable on magnetic resonance imaging (MRI), but without evidence of overt neurological impairment upon physical examination (Pegelow et al., 2002). With rapid improvements in neuroimaging techniques, SCI has been found to be the most prevalent mechanism of neurological injury in children with SCA, occurring in as few as 15% and as many as 35% of cases (Bernaudin et al., 2000; Buchanan, DeBaun, Quinn, & Steinberg, 2004; Pegelow et al., 2002; Steen, Emudianughe, et al., 2003; Switzer, Hess, Nichols, & Adams, 2006). Furthermore, Wang and colleagues (2001) found that approximately 10% of a sample of children under age 6 had evidence of previous SCI. Using more sensitive MRI technology (thin-slice T1- and T2-weighted sequences and fluid attenuated inversion recovery sequence), Steen, Emudianughe, and colleagues (2003) found a 35% prevalence of silent stroke, particularly in the parenchyma of the brain (supportive tissue consisting of nerve and glial cells).

With improved radiological technology, the processes and subtleties of CNS injury in patients with SCD are now better understood. Using MRI, magnetic resonance angiography (MRA), TCD, and in some instances computerized tomography, researchers have found that damage can occur in minute veins, arterioles, and surrounding tissue (Adams et al., 1988, 1992; Armstrong et al., 1996; National Institutes of Health, 1986; Pavlakis et al., 1988; Ris et al., 1996; Wiznitzer et al., 1990). Arterial border zones (so-called "watershed regions") are most susceptible to cerebral hypoperfusion and subsequent damage, especially between the anterior and middle cerebral arteries (Pavlakis et al., 1988; Wang, 2007). Reduced pressure from large-vessel disease (lesions of the intima [inner lining] in major arteries) causes slower flow rates of blood between small vessels in watershed regions and increases risk of hypoperfusion. The chronic anemia and hemodynamic insufficiency of SCD lead to vulnerability and "inadequate perfusion in border zone regions presenting a mechanism for cerebral infarction" (Pavlakis et al., 1988, p.128). The most common sites of CVA or stroke are the internal carotid artery, the anterior and middle cerebral arteries, and their boundary zones (Craft, Schatz, Glauser, Lee, &c DeBaun, 1993); these serve the middle and superior frontal gyri, as well as the temporal and parietal cortex, all common sites of stroke (Schatz & Puffer, 2007). Whereas overt stroke is associated with worse cognitive outcomes, the milder extent of neurological injury in silent stroke is offset by the higher prevalence rate and associated risk factor for future overt stroke (Schatz & McClellan, 2006). Ongoing, subtle neurological deficits caused by silent strokes, ischemia, and hypoxia are most frequently identified in the territory of penetrating arteries, the deep white matter, and striatum. Subtle cerebral impairment resulting from silent stroke may be evident only as mild sensory deficits, soft signs, or higher-order cognitive deficits. Several studies, including the CSSCD, have found neuropsychological differences between children with SCD who have had overt stroke, silent stroke, and no known stroke (see the more extensive neuropsychological discussion below). Overall, the clinical impact of SCI is not as subtle as was once believed. Children with silent strokes have an increased risk for future overt strokes or new MRI lesions (Miller et al., 2000; Pegelow et al., 2001). Risk factors for SCI include low pain rate, a history of seizures, and a leukocyte count over $11.8 \times 109/L$ (Kinney et al., 1999). In addition to these risk factors, there appears to be a genetic predisposition to stroke in individuals with SCD, as sibling studies have found that a disproportionate number of siblings without SCD experience stroke (Driscoll et al., 2003).

NONSTROKE-RELATED CAUSES OF NEUROLOGICAL COMPROMISE

In the past 10 years, improvements in imaging technology have enhanced understanding related to potential disease-related causes of cognitive challenges in SCD. Clearly, children who have experienced obvious physiological complications are at increased risk; however, children who are experiencing silent strokes, metabolic insufficiencies, and chronic oxygen deprivation are also at increased risk for reduced neurocognitive functioning. There are indicators that children with SCD who have no significant MRI abnormalities still display lower scores on tests of intellectual functioning, although these differences in many cases are not statistically significant (Schatz, Finke, Kellet, & Kramer, 2002; Steen et al., 2005; Steen, Miles, et al., 2003). Furthermore, cognitive impairment has been identified in children without evidence of stroke in clinical history or neuroimaging (Schatz, Finke, et al., 2002; Steen et al., 2005); this may be associated with severity of anemia (Bernaudin et al., 2000; Schatz, Craft, et al., 2004) or inadequate perfusion (Kirkham et al., 2001; Oguz et al., 2003). Most supportive are the findings that severe anemia seems to be associated with cognitive challenges including deficits in intellectual ability, verbal skills, attention, and working memory (Bernaudin et al., 2000; Brown et al., 1993; Schatz, Finke, & Roberts, 2004; Steen, Xiong, Mulhern, Langston, & Wang, 1999; Steen, Miles, et al., 2003). There is also evidence that higher blood flow velocity in the midcerebral artery is associated with lower verbal functioning, as well as with weaker sustained attention and executive skills (Kral et al., 2003). Schatz and Puffer (2007) conclude from these data that for children without stroke, disease severity (marked by abnormal TCD and severe anemia) is associated with cognitive dysfunction.

Furthermore, functional imaging studies also support findings that diffuse brain injury occurs within SCD without evidence of stroke. Kennan, Suzuka, Nagel, and Fabry (2004) found evidence that the brains of animal models with SCD are less protected from the effects of oxygen deprivation, resulting in diffuse and chronic CNS oxygen short-

age. Hogan, Pit-ten Cate, Vargha-Khadem, Prengler, and Kirkcham (2006) found a significant association among decreased oxygen saturation, increased cerebral blood flow velocity, and lower Full Scale IQ in an adolescent sample with SCD. Furthermore, differences in the composition of gray matter on T1-weighted MRI have been identified in the thalamus, caudate, and cortex of children with SCD (Steen et al., 1998, 1999, 2004; Steen, Eminudianughe, et al., 2003) and were presumed to represent diffuse injury secondary to hypoxia from chronic anemia. Moreover, decreased corpus callosum size was found in a small sample of children with SCD who had no visible infarcts (Schatz & Buzan, 2006).

The early literature suggested that local impairments in glucose metabolism and perfusion may also be culprits in the nonstroke-related neurocognitive effects of SCD (Rodgers et al., 1988), and more contemporary research has supported this. Glucose metabolism studies using positron emission tomography (PET) or perfusion MRI have supported the earlier hypothesis, showing that such impairments are associated with lower intellectual scores (Kirkham et al., 2001; Powars et al., 1999; Reed, Jagust, Al-Mateen, & Vichinsky, 1999), although the impact on particular neurocognitive functions is less clear.

DEVELOPMENTAL CONSIDERATIONS

Although most of the clinical manifestations of SCD are not apparent until early childhood, Wang and colleagues (1998), using MRI and MRA, found mild CNS abnormalities in a sample of very young children (ages 7–48 months) with SCA and developmental delays and MRI and MRA abnormalities. This has drastic ramifications for the ensuing development of children with SCD.

The first 2 years of life are a critical period of brain development, during which glial proliferation, myelination, dendritic branching, and development of synaptic connections are abundant, and vulnerability to neurological compromise is profound. Neurological insult during this period may have long-term cognitive and behavioral consequences because optimal brain activity is interrupted during an imperative growth period. Medical and educational professionals often overlook this debilitation, as compensatory strategies develop with physical recovery and time, and these can obscure underlying deficits temporarily or in specific situations. Neurological injury is often viewed as an acute illness that ends at about the time of discharge from the hospital, and long-term sequelae are not linked to the original injury. Early injury, however can lead to a globally compromised CNS that has been forced to reconstruct the interactive neuronal network. Theories of neurological maturation suggest that the developing brain is *plastic,* or malleable to alterations in functional area. The concept of plasticity implies that the functions of a damaged area of the brain can be "reassigned" to another, undamaged area. Although this is immediately effective in enabling an individual to regain a certain level of skill, it can lead to longer-term problems when the area of the brain that has taken over a specific ability is called upon to perform its original function. According to Teuber's so-called "crowding principle" (Woods & Teuber, 1973), recovery by reassignment occurs at the expense of other abilities. When functions are shifted in an attempt to compensate, areas become congested and less efficient. Early injury therefore jeopardizes long-term developmental progress, although this may not be immediately evident.

Further clarification of the impact of SCD on brain development is provided by research in early nutritional issues. Multiple or severe hypoglycemic episodes, or severe malnutrition in early development, can compromise brain growth (Swift et al., 1989). Iron deficiency anemia in the critical CNS growth period can clearly compromise long-term cognitive development; the effects include reduced attention, fatigue, behavioral problems, and poor academic achievement. Iron deficiency anemia can also lead to neurological soft signs, such as poor coordination and balance. Given the probability of early neurological involvement, a neurodevelopmental perspective appears essential when it comes to conceptualizing the impact of SCD on a child (Schatz & McClellan, 2006). A neurodevelopmental approach is useful in integrating how SCD expresses itself over the course of a child's development, and how

several social and environmental factors interact with the neurological condition.

SPECIFIC NEUROPSYCHOLOGICAL IMPAIRMENTS

Attention, Impulse Control, and Processing Speed

It is critical to understand the complicated labyrinth of the attention system and its relationships to neurological dysfunction. Because of the variable nature of stroke and chronic hypoxia in children with SCD, any one level or multiple levels of attention skill can be compromised. Dissecting attention skill levels and identifying specific deficits are vital to selecting the most efficacious interventions.

Both attention and impulse control appear particularly vulnerable to the neurocognitive impacts of SCD, and deficits in these are often associated with frontal lobe abnormality. Early studies of attention skills in children with SCD that did not examine physiological findings found notable attention and behavioral problems (Burlew, Evans, & Oler, 1989; Hurtig & Park, 1989; Hurtig & White, 1986). In a study using a visual orienting task (Craft, Schatz, Glauser, Lee, & DeBaun, 1994) in children with SCD who had experienced stroke, those with bifrontal injury showed more impulsivity than children with diffuse lesions, who had increased reaction time; both groups were more impaired than children with SCD without stroke and sibling controls. More recent studies have repeatedly documented problems in attention and concentration skills in pediatric patients with SCD compared to peers and/or sibling controls (Brandling-Bennett, White, Armstrong, Christ, & DeBaun, 2003; Brown et al., 1993, 2000; Craft et al., 1993; Fowler et al., 1988; Kral et al., 2003; Schatz, Brown, Pascual, Hsu, & DeBaun, 2001; Schatz, Craft, Koby, & DeBaun, 2004). Patients with histories of both overt and silent stroke have often been found to evidence the most attention challenges (Schatz & Puffer, 2007). Noll and colleagues (2001), found significantly lower scores in specific measures of attention (mental processing, working memory, rapid novel learning, verbal repetition, and error-prone behavior) in children with SCD than in matched controls. However, findings of disease-specific attention impairments have not always been supported (Craft et al., 1993; Nabors & Freymuth, 2002; Tarazi, Grant, Ely, & Barakat, 2007). Multiple dimensions of the illness, including its socioeconomic, psychosocial, and neuropsychological aspects, are likely to contribute to challenges in attention function.

Many studies have identified physiological correlates of attention and self-regulatory difficulties in SCD. Craft and colleagues (1993) found higher levels of impulsivity/intrusive errors and reduced self-regulation in subjects with anterior lesions than in a healthy sibling control group. The severity and persistence of chronic hypoxia (anemia, sleep hypoxia, reduced pulmonary function) in SCD seems to be associated with impairments of attention and working memory (Bernaudin et al., 2000; Brown et al., 1993; Noll et al., 2001; Schatz, Finke, & Roberts, 2004; Steen et al., 1999; Steen, Miles, et al., 2003). Patients with increased frontal lobe involvement, regardless of pathophysiology, may be more likely to evidence attention and self-regulatory impairments that interfere with multitasking skills (Berkelhammer et al., 2007). Damage to the anterior forebrain is a common finding; it has a negative impact on broad aspects of attention, memory, and other executive skills, as well as on specific functions of selective attention, vigilance, shifting set, planning, organization of thought/behavior, and error monitoring (Brown et al., 2000; Craft et al., 1993; DeBaun et al., 1998; Schatz et al., 1999; Schatz & Puffer, 2007). There is also evidence that higher blood flow velocity in the midcerebral artery is associated with lower verbal functioning, and specifically with weaker auditory working memory (Kral et al., 2003), which can interfere with auditory attention and processing.

Strokes, like many other neurological injuries, commonly result in difficulties with attention and concentration (DeBaun et al., 1998; Schatz et al., 1999). Interestingly, attention seems to be affected regardless of the volume of injury from stroke (Schatz et al., 1999), and is thus apparently a highly vulnerable neurocognitive construct in the pathophysiology of SCD. Whereas some research has identified stroke-associated impairments in visual processing speed (Nabors & Freymuth, 2002), others have concluded that slower response speed is not a core feature of SCD (Schatz, Finke, & Roberts, 2004). The rate at which a child processes input can have a strong impact on attention, as slower speeds are likely to lead to the appearance of inattentiveness, failure to fully process all available input, and inaccurate working memory. Slower processing thus has a negative impact on academic performance as well as social success.

Deficits in impulsivity and self-regulation, as well as in intellectual functioning (see below), are likely to be associated with increased externalizing behavioral challenges (Schatz & McClellan, 2006; Thompson et al., 2003). Children with poor self-regulatory control and limited problem-solving abilities are likely to have greater difficulties in navigating the academic and social environments, with weaker coping skills and frustration tolerance than their peers. Deficits in vigilance and impulse control have other strong academic implications (Nabors & Freymuth, 2002): They may affect learning, referral for resources, and teacher–student relationships.

Even in the absence of identifiable tissue injury, deficits in verbal working memory and processing speed have been identified (Bernaudin et al., 2000; Schatz, Finke, et al., 2002; Steen et al., 2003). Deficits in auditory processing (Schatz & Roberts, 2005) are likely to impair initial attention and subsequent encoding of verbal information, interfering with immediate and sustained attention to verbal input as well as with social information processing. An early report from the CSSCD (Wang et al., 2001) found significantly lower performance on measures of working memory and new learning in children with HbSS who had experienced silent infarcts, compared to those without abnormal imaging.

The prevalence of identified attention difficulties in neuropsychological testing and behavioral reports suggests the importance of screening for these issues, beginning quite early in life. There are presently few reliable measures to assess specific attention function in very young children, but constructs such as response latency or duration of visual focus might be targeted and measurements developed. DeBaun and colleagues (1998) found patient performance on the Test of Variables of Attention (McCarney

& Greenberg, 1990) to be highly sensitive to identification of previously unidentified silent stroke, suggesting that this may be an important screening tool for identifying attention challenges and potential silent stroke in this population.

General Intellectual and Neurocognitive Development

Many early studies compared the intellectual status of patients with SCD and healthy peers; however, discrepancies were commonly confounded by racial, economic, disease-state-related, or cohort issues. For this reason, research began to turn toward comparing patients with SCD to their healthy siblings, to control for these threats to internal validity. Even with such controls, subsequent studies continued to find lower overall scores in intellectual development in children with SCD who had experienced stroke (Fowler et al., 1988; Gold, Johnson, Treadwell, Hans, & Vichinsky, 2008; Kramer, Rooks, & Pearson, 1978; Listianingsih, Hariman, Griffith, Hurtig, & Keehn, 1991; McCormack et al., 1975), as well as those who had not (Schatz, Finke, et al., 2002; Steen et al., 2005, Steen, Miles, et al., 2003).

Early researchers knew that CNS pathology was associated with SCD. As previously stated, hypothesized mechanisms leading to neurocognitive impairment in children with SCD included microinfarction, anemia and related ischemia, and nutritional deficiencies (Brown, Armstrong, & Eckman, 1993; Powars, Wilson, Imbus, Pegelow, & Allen, 1978). But they also understood that other factors were affecting cognitive performance, such as recurrent school absence, socioeconomic status, the impact of a chronic illness on family functioning, and illness-related psychological issues (mood, adjustment, coping skills, etc.) (Hurtig & Park, 1989; Hurtig & White, 1986). Understanding which mechanisms place children with SCD at what type of neurocognitive risk is persistently evolving, but still not fully realized. Schatz and colleagues (1999) even suggested that specific cognitive profiles might be associated with various CNS lesion sites. The general neurocognitive impact of stroke in patients with SCD appears well accepted and understood, but understanding of the impact of silent stroke

or other less obvious pathophysiological aspects of SCD is still developing. Recent developments in MRI technology have shown greater sensitivity in identifying subtle focal brain injury, although comprehension of the neurocognitive correlates to particular lesion sites or types has not completely caught up. Conclusions in this area are additionally complicated by a young brain's ability to reorganize function.

To best understand the causal factors of cognitive challenges in SCD, identifying the developmental pattern of onset as well as the most vulnerable patient subgroup(s) or time period(s) is critical. It is also essential to early identification and specified intervention that might ameliorate the negative impact. Thus far, evidence related to the developmental impact of SCD has been inconsistent. There were some earlier findings that the neurocognitive impact of SCD becomes amplified with age (Brown et al., 1993; Fowler et al., 1988; Wang et al., 2001), but research attempting to identify specific age-related dynamics did not come to any firm conclusions (Noll et al., 2001; Steen et al., 1999; Swift et al., 1989; Wasserman, Wilimas, Fairclough, Mulhern, & Wang, 1991). More recent studies have begun to elucidate age-related factors in the intellectual functioning of children with SCD. Evidence of silent stroke or arterial stenosis has been identified in the MRIs of even very young children (4 years and under) (Wang et al., 1998), and declines in cognitive performance have been recognized in the youngest patients with SCD, including preschool-age children (Tarazi et al., 2007), toddlers (Thompson, Gustafson, Bonner, & Ware, 2002), and infants (Hogan et al., 2005). The magnitude of IQ difference from peers increases from toddlerhood to preschool age (Schatz & Roberts, 2007; Thompson et al., 2002), as well as from late childhood into early adolescence (Hogan et al., 2006; Schatz, Finke, et al., 2002; Wang et al., 2001). Researchers have increasingly recognized that subtle physiological consequences of the illness, along with the psychosocial impact of SCD (living with a chronic illness, painful crises, school absence, socioeconomic status, financial burdens, etc.), jointly lay the foundation of compromised neurocognition that appears to begin quite early in life.

Early concerns that the pathological sickle cell hemoglobin might be related in and of itself to lower intellectual status have received various levels of support in research findings. It was known early that the gene for abnormal hemoglobin had less of an impact on patients who had heterogeneous states of SCD or who were carriers of the trait, and a logical presumption seemed to follow that they were also less neurocognitively compromised than those with the homogeneous genotype. However, as mentioned previously, some trait carriers are susceptible to health complications in rare instances, which leads to this question: Are there neurocognitive deficits associated with being an SCD trait carrier? Wasserman and colleagues (1991) matched patients with SCD to sibling controls on intellectual, academic, and neuropsychological measures. Siblings with sickle cell trait (HbAS) performed no differently from normal-hemoglobin siblings (HbAA); this supported the findings of previous researchers (Kramer et al., 1978; McCormack et al., 1975), who had hypothesized that the abnormal hemoglobin found in SCD and sickle cell trait was not the primary factor in lower intellectual and academic performance. However, later research again suggested that sickle cell trait might predispose carriers to an increased risk of vascular abnormalities and stroke (Steen, Emudianughe, et al., 2003).

In one of the landmark studies examining the impact of silent stroke on neurocognitive functioning, Armstrong and colleagues (1996) found that children with SCD and a history of overt stroke had significantly lower neuropsychological scores than children with silent strokes or children without MRI abnormality. However, children with silent strokes had significantly lower scores than children without MRI abnormality in arithmetic, vocabulary, visual–motor speed, and coordination. Such findings were among the first to bring to light the possibility that children without overt stroke remained at risk for neurocognitive deficits, and that neuropsychological testing might identify the weaknesses even in the absence of positive neuroimaging findings. Steen and colleagues (1998) used quantitative MRI to identify encephalomalacia in the cortical gray matter of patients with SCD who had normal clinical exams and normal conventional MRI scans.

Intellectual testing also revealed significantly lower Full Scale IQ scores (borderline range) than in sibling controls (low-average range) in children with normal conventional MRI as well as quantitative MRI. Further supporting these findings was a study by Powars and colleagues (1999), who compared groups of children who had either no neurological symptoms or only soft neurological signs, using MRI and PET scans along with neurocognitive assessment. Children with normal MRI and abnormal PET scans had IQ scores that fell in the low-average range (one standard deviation below the population norm), whereas the children with normal MRI and PET scans had IQs within the average range. Additional neuropsychological deficits were identified in school achievement and psychomotor speed.

This recognition of the risk of subtle neurological impact and consequent neurocognitive sequelae began to spur significantly more research in the subsequent decade. Gold and colleagues (2008) found that 82% of their sample of patients with SCD and evidence of stroke had Full Scale IQs one or more standard deviations below the mean, whereas 50% of those with silent stroke scored one or more standard deviations below the mean for Verbal IQ, and 62.5% of those with silent stroke scored one or more standard deviations below the mean for Performance IQ. However, for children with SCD and no evidence of infarct, 45% still scored one or more standard deviations below the mean for Verbal IQ, and 35% scored one or more standard deviations below the mean for Performance IQ (compared to 16% in the general population). An increasing amount of research has thus examined the prevalence and potentially subtle neurocognitive impact of understated pathophysiology in a high percentage of patients with SCD by early adolescence (Bernaudin et al., 2000; Brown et al., 2000; Wang et al., 2001). One study (Knight, Singhal, Thomas, & Serjeant, 1995) found significantly lower IQ in adolescents with HbSS, which was attributed to the effects of early nutritional deficits on physical growth and cognitive development. Unfortunately, there has been little subsequent research on how micronutrient deficiencies in SCD may be related to neurocognitive development.

In a large prospective study, Bernaudin and colleagues (2000), found significantly impaired Full Scale and Performance IQs in a combined sample of patients with SCD and a history of overt stroke, and language-specific IQ deficits in those with silent strokes. A more unexpected finding was that the Verbal, Performance, and Full Scale IQs were also impaired in patients who had severe chronic anemia or thrombocytosis. Given this finding, the authors questioned the potential impact of early use of hydroxyurea (a medication that increases blood concentrations of fetal hemoglobin, which reduces erythrocyte sickling) on the long-term intellectual scores of SCD patients. Indeed, Puffer, Schatz, and Roberts (2007) found significantly higher scores on tests of verbal comprehension, fluid reasoning, and general cognitive ability in children with SCD who were taking hydroxyurea than in those who were not. Test performance was presumed to be associated with improved CNS oxygenation and reduced fatigue or episodes of pain. As the recognition of the early neurocognitive impact of SCD has increased, early identification and intervention are being advocated. The use of chronic transfusion therapy not only clearly reduces risk of subsequent stroke, but may also interrupt the developmental neurocognitive regression noted in many patients with SCD (Kral et al., 2006). Early identification of neurocognitive issues has been advocated and even recommended by numerous researchers to identify patients who are at risk of or already evidencing early signs of neurocognitive compromise (Armstrong et al., 1996; Gold et al., 2008).

Studies examining the intellectual functioning of patients with SCD have not consistently used neuroimaging as a criterion for subject selection, and have sometimes relied only on information from medical records to determine stroke history. Because children with unidentified silent strokes may have been included in such studies, there have been concerns that their findings might overestimate the true negative neuropsychological impact of SCD. However, in a meta-analysis, Schatz, Craft, and colleagues (2002) found the effect size of inclusion of patients with unidentified silent strokes to be small and probably noncontributory to group differences. Nevertheless, recent studies have begun to define subject populations with more caution, while additionally using

sensitive neuroimaging in an attempt to directly evaluate the specific pathophysiology of SCD outside of stroke.

Early neurological injury is commonly associated with neurodevelopmental challenges, particularly a failure to maintain a developmental pace similar to that of peers. The concept of plasticity suggests that cognitive impairment resulting from injuries that occur early has greater opportunities for recovery over time and can benefit from compensatory effects, although at the expense of other skills (Woods, 1980; Woods & Teuber, 1973). However, neuronal proliferation and differentiation are active processes in children under the age of 2, and injury occurring during these phases is commonly associated with poorer neurodevelopmental outcome than injury occurring during the synaptic pruning phases (ages 2–7) (Schatz & McClellan, 2006). Early damage to neuronal structure and organization has a long-term negative impact on neurocognitive operation, leading to greater functional cognitive and behavioral impairment over time. Impairments in the cognitive skills that are not expected early in development can be difficult to identify or discriminate at first; however, these deficits become greater liabilities as the comparative peer group naturally acquires the integrative capacities that come with myelination and learning.

The cumulative impact of the pathophysiology of SCD must be considered along with development. Undoubtedly, stroke has an immediate and long-term negative impact on neurocognitive functioning. However, repeated neurological insults of any type are typically associated with increasing cognitive, learning, and behavioral difficulties. Children who have experienced at least one stroke have an average subsequent reduction in IQ scores of 10–15 points (Schatz et al., 2001; Schatz & McClellan, 2006; Schatz & Puffer, 2007; Wang et al., 2001), and those with larger lesions have more significant IQ decrements than those with minimal encephalopathy do (Schatz, White, Moinuddin, Armstrong, & DeBaun, 2002). Such changes in intellectual functioning are likely to affect academic, social, and occupational access, performance, and attainment. Unfortunately, SCD is a disease of recurrent risk and injury. Just as the effects of repeated traumatic brain injury are diffuse in nature, recurrent silent infarcts seem to be associated with declines in general intellectual functioning over time, which probably result from more specified neurocognitive impairments (Kral et al., 2003, 2006; Schatz et al., 1999). In addition, the relationship between the extent or recurrence of neurological damage and cognitive impairment is proportional. The impact of repeated silent stroke and non-stroke-related neurological impairment may relate both to its diffuse nature and to the level of cumulative impairment (Armstrong et al., 1996; Bernaudin et al., 2000; Wang et al., 2001).

Thompson and colleagues (2003) documented reduced cognitive functioning over the period of 6 months to 3 years of age in children with SCD. Schatz and Roberts (2007) also identified age-related decline from 12 to 40 months of age in language and motor skills in patients with SCD. Furthermore, declining IQ scores with age have been extensively documented in the SCD literature (Kral et al., 2003; Steen et al., 2005; Wang et al., 2001). With the goal of determining the meaning, rather than only the presence, of SCD's effects on cognitive functioning, Schatz, Finke, and colleagues (2002) conducted a large meta-analysis of studies that examined cognitive performance over time in children with SCD. They found a reliable consistency in multiple studies identifying a decrement (4–5 standard score points) in intellectual test scores in the absence of cerebral infarct—findings that have been; subsequently confirmed (Steen et al., 2005, Steen, Miles, et al., 2003). The authors concluded that reductions over time were related to the pathophysiological impact of SCD as well as the impact of chronic illness on neurocognitive development. Kral and colleagues (2006) additionally found evidence that children without a history of overt stroke are at risk of cognitive decline with age not only in global intellectual functioning, but also in specific skills (e.g., verbal memory, sustained attention, cognitive flexibility, and visual–motor integration). Confirming the findings of developmental regression in children with SCD, Schatz and Buzan (2006) also found that age had a negative correlation with intellectual test scores in children with SCD compared to those without.

Unidentified neurological injury in patients with SCD who have normal neuroimaging may contribute to changes in intellectual performance. Using voxel-based morphometry, Baldeweg and colleagues (2005) identified deep anterior and posterior white matter arterial border zone abnormalities in children both with and without identifiable silent infarct. In addition, these children were found to have lower IQ scores, regardless of the presence of visible lesions. Using data from the CSSCD, Wang and colleagues (2001) found that over 10 years of data collection, there was a progressive decline in IQ scores for children with SCD even when their MRI findings were normal. Gold and colleagues (2008) also found that children without evidence of infarct evidenced more intellectual challenges than the normal population. Findings of lower IQ in children without abnormal neuroimaging has raised questions regarding other pathophysiological factors inherent in SCD that might have an impact on neurocognitive development. Chronic hypoxia to the brain has been repeatedly implicated as a subtle cause of reductions in neurocognitive performance over the course of development. Hogan and colleagues (2006) found that lowered IQ was a function of abnormal oxygen delivery to the brain (resulting from reduced oxyhemoglobin saturation and increased cerebral blood flow velocity), although the relationship between cerebral blood flow velocity and IQ was significant only for Verbal IQ scores. Recently, Hogan and colleagues (2006) found that children with SCD as young as 3–9 months of age evidenced higher indicators of neurocognitive dysfunction that were correlated with hematocrit, suggesting an early onset of neuropsychological impairments from that pathophysiology of SCD. Excluding subjects with silent infarcts by use of MRI, Bernaudin and colleagues (2000) and Steen and colleagues (1999) still found a notable relationship between hematocrit and cognitive functioning. Higher values of cerebral blood flow velocity, as measured by TCD, have been found to be associated with lower scores in verbal intelligence and executive abilities (Kral et al., 2003).

The increased level of neurocognitive variability (rather than only performance deficits) in children who have experienced silent stroke, have larger volumes of tissue involvement, or have abnormal MRI abnormalities is an important finding of studies examining intellectual functioning (Grueneich et al., 2004; Ris, Grueneich, & Kalinyak, 1995; Schatz et al., 1999). In children with SCD who have no evidence of overt CNS disease, the same level of variability has not been identified (Noll et al., 2001). Clearly the presence of CNS pathology, even if unidentified, is related to some level of global dysfunction. In any neurologically based cognitive dysfunction, it is often the variability that is the fundamental disability. Children with SCD have subtler, but broader and less predictable, neurocognitive profiles that are not promptly identified by grades, classroom performance, or criterion-based test scores. This variability and lack of predictably can unfortunately prolong identification of deficits and delay intervention because subtle impairments are missed or misattributed to another factor (e.g., immaturity, gender, school absence). Such a risk emphasizes the importance of early and thorough neuropsychological assessment of individual strengths and weaknesses, to inform and guide cognitive and academic intervention. Variability in cognitive development may also be partially explained by the economic hardship that many children with SCD experience. A disproportionate number of children with SCD come from families in lower socioeconomic brackets, and poverty has a well-documented impact on neurocognition in general and on developmental regression with age in particular (Brown et al., 1993; Gustafson, Bonner, Hardy, & Thompson, 2006). The psychosocial impact of poverty has yet to be clearly discriminated from the neurological impact of SCD.

Importantly, researchers have begun to raise the issue that relying solely on IQ tests as broad measures of the cognitive challenges present in SCD is not very likely to be sensitive to specific neurocognitive dysfunction (Grueneich et al., 2004; Schatz et al., 1999). Global IQ measures are also not as sensitive to age-related changes as are measures of specific abilities, particularly memory and executive functions (Steen, Miles, et al., 2003; Steen et al., 2005). Recognizing that intellectual measures may provide a weak assessment of specific cognitive deficits, Schatz and colleagues (1999), used more specific neuropsychological measures to assess four constructs of neurocognitive performance: attention/executive, spatial, language, and memory functions. Their findings indicated a specific relationship between frontal lobe compromise and attention and other executive impairments, as well as between diffuse injury and visual–spatial and language impairments.

Academic Achievement

There is a historically strong link between school attendance and academic achievement in the general population. Children with chronic illness overall have lower levels of academic achievement than their peers without such illness, even in the absence of learning disabilities (Martinez & Ercikan, 2009); this is often attributed to days of illness and number of absences. Many students with SCD will miss a considerable number of school days or have SCD-related difficulties within the classroom environment (Cant-Peterson, Palermo, Swift, Bebee, & Drotar, 2005). However, some research specifically on SCD has indicated that factors other than school absence seem to contribute to reduced academic achievement. The number of missed school days has been associated with lower scores on intellectual tests in children with SCD (Wasserman et al., 1991); however, even prior to beginning school, children with SCD evidence lower performance in kindergarten readiness and academically relevant skills, with or without a history of stroke (Chua-Lim, Moore, McCleary, Shah, & Mankad, 1993; Steen et al., 2002). Schatz (2004) reviewed the academic attainment (which he defined as grade promotion and need for remedial services) of a population of children with SCD who had no neurological documentation of stroke; he found that, compared to peers, children with SCD had increased levels of grade repetition, and their achievement was significantly lower than their cognitive performance. Cognitive ability and days of illness were predictors of attainment problems. Psychosocial and disease-related factors (e.g., pain management, medical appointments, self-esteem, delayed puberty and growth, medication regimens, and fatigue) can also affect not only attendance, but even attention and social and cognitive performance in school (Bonner, Gustafson, Shumacher, & Thompson, 1999). Thus, although attendance is a key factor in achievement, the neurocognitive and psychosocial factors within SCD potentially play a large role in the educational success (and probably in the subsequent occupational attainment) of this population.

It is not difficult to draw a connection between the pathophysiology of SCD and potential academic difficulties. Studies have indeed often found that children with SCD are more likely to be receiving some form of academic intervention, from special education services to grade retention (Kral et al., 2003; Schatz et al., 2001). Some studies examining neuroimaging results and academic functioning have identified a relationship between abnormal findings and academic difficulties (Armstrong et al., 1996; Kral et al., 2003; Schatz et al., 2001), though others have not (Brown et al., 2000; Gruenich et al., 2004). Overt stroke appears to have a greater impact on academic achievement than on intellectual functioning, particularly in mathematics (Armstrong et al., 1996; Schatz & Puffer, 2007; Wang et al., 2001). Wang and colleagues (2001) found that children with silent infarct scored lower than those without evidence of infarct on academic measures, but also found an average decline of 0.9 points per year in children with SCD and no evidence of infarct.

Certainly neurocognitive impairment does not occur in every student with SCD, but for those who do have these effects, awareness, accommodation, and intervention are critical to long-term educational success. Children with various forms of SCD—across all age groups and those with and without a history of stroke—have high rates of learning difficulties; these reflect the direct influence of neurocognitive challenges, as well as the incidental effects of chronic illness and recurrent school absences. Regardless of the source of their learning challenges, these children must be identified, as they have increased needs for academic accommodation. Measures of academic achievement have been used in students with SCD to determine severity, CNS impact, and functional outcome of the disease. However, measuring achievement along with academic attainment as defined above provides a more inclusive appraisal of the educational impact of SCD (Schatz, 2004).

The causes of academic difficulties are unquestionably multifactorial, stemming from neurocognitive to psychosocial factors. Missed school days, physiological needs (temperature regulation, adequate hydration, fatigue, etc.) and learning difficulties can impair academic performance on a daily basis, and ultimately can decrease overall achievement and attainment. Stroke-associated impairments have indeed been identified in reading, math, and spelling achievement, compared to that of peers (Nabors & Freymuth, 2006; Schatz et al., 2001). Wang and colleagues (2001) found that patients with HbSS and silent infarcts had significantly lower academic scores in math and reading, as well as lower Verbal, Performance, and Full Scale IQs, than patients without MRI abnormalities over a 5-year span. Both stroke-related and non-stroke-related neurocognitive impairment are likely to impair long-term academic performance, psychosocial success, occupational attainment, and psychological functioning well into adulthood. The significant reduction in IQ scores for children who have experienced stroke affects their academic attainment in 80% of cases (Schatz et al., 2001; Schatz & McClellan, 2006; Wang et al., 2001); however, a large proportion of children with SCD and no history of stroke also have neurocognitive challenges that create academic needs, and these children may not be identified as in need of intervention (Cant-Peterson et al., 2005).

The impairments in attention and memory that are among the most commonly reported neurocognitive consequences of neurological injury may be associated with lower general academic performance in SCD (Schatz & Puffer, 2007). In particular, new learning and organizational challenges are noted and compromise both acquisition as well as access to previously learned information. Lower skills in auditory discrimination have been identified in students with SCD screened for kindergarten readiness, and these deficits may be associated with difficulties in auditory attention, working memory, and language processing within the classroom (Schatz, 2004; Steen et al., 2002). The persistence of these impairments can lead to progressive changes in academic achievement over time, particularly in comparison to peers. As peers progress through developmental refinement of learning techniques and independent organization, and develop increased capacity for focal and sustained attention, children with neurological compromise who are impaired in achieving such developmental milestones fall further and further behind their peers.

The effects of SCD on reading acquisition and achievement have been the cause of some concern. Deficits in reading have been repeatedly identified in children with SCD compared to matched peers (Brown et al., 1993; Fowler et al., 1988; Nabors & Freymuth, 2002; Noll et al., 2001; Sanders et al., 1997; Swift et al., 1989), and children with SCD who have had silent infarct have been found to have lower reading achievement than those without (Armstrong et al., 1996; Gold et al., 2008). Specifically (and predictably), a history of left-hemisphere stroke has been associated with lower reading comprehension and spelling achievement scores in children with SCD (Cohen, Branch, McKie, & Adams, 1994). Gold and colleagues (2008) found lower single-word reading and reading comprehension scores in children with overt and silent stroke than in those without evidence of infarct. A weaker core vocabulary has been frequently identified, and certainly may contribute to reduced reading skill (Noll et al., 2001; Schatz, 2004; Schatz, Craft, et al., 2004; Wang et al., 2001). Auditory processing (discrimination of phonemes) and reduced attention may also contribute to reductions in early acquisition of reading skills (Schatz, 2004; Steen et al., 2001). Cognitive difficulty alone cannot be held responsible for the lower reading acquisition and performance of children with SCD; environmental and family factors also must be considered. Reading skills require conjoint development of phonemic awareness, fluency, and listening comprehension skills that are applied to written text in the framework of frequent practice. Consequently, such factors as family literacy skills, access to books, and parent–child interaction will have an impact on readiness to read and long-term reading proficiency; these may be areas of vulnerability in this population because of its disproportional level of lower socioeconomic status.

Math difficulties have also been commonly identified in studies examining the academic impact of SCD. Armstrong and colleagues (1996) found that children with SCD with overt stroke had significantly lower mental calculation, written calculation, and applied math scores than those with silent infarct. Children with silent infarcts consistently had lower math scores than those with normal MRI scans, although differences were not always significant. Noll and colleagues (2001) found significantly lower written calculation scores in children with SCD than in controls. Many studies have included only screening of written calculation, rather than more comprehensive assessments of full mathematical abilities (mental and written computation, word problems, applied math, sequential problem solving, etc.), so identifying specific contributors to arithmetic challenges will contribute to understanding these deficits more specifically. Cohen and colleagues (1994) found that children with SCA who had experienced right-hemisphere stroke had difficulties in arithmetic skills, but that those with left-hemisphere stroke had difficulties specifically in math calculation. Nabors and Freymuth (2002) also found that written calculation was consistently the lowest academic score (along with reading and spelling) in children with SCD, either with or without stroke. Although the differences were deemed not statistically significant, the authors did not discuss the clinical significance of the findings that all children with SCD scored lower in mental and written calculation than sibling controls did. Many other studies have found low math scores in patients with SCD, although these have not always been significantly discrepant from those of controls (Fowler et al., 1988; Kral et al., 2003; Ogunfowara, Olanrewaju, & Akenzua, 2005; Wasserman et al., 1991). Schatz (2004) found in his meta-analysis that mean math scores on screening measures (typically involving only written calculation) were most often lower, but that the effect size was nonsignificant. Studies assessing both written calculation and applied math problems might provide more information regarding these common difficulties. Swift and colleagues (1989) found a clinically significant discrepancy in both calculation and applied math scores between children with SCD and controls. Wang and colleagues (2001) found that scores in broad math skills were lower than in broad reading, that children with stroke scored significantly lower on math tasks than those with silent stroke did, and that both groups scored significantly lower than those with normal MRI.

Similar to intellectual functioning over time, there appears to be a risk of decline in math achievement over time in patients with SCD (Wang et al., 2001); again, this may be associated with challenges in school attendance, but also with neurocognitive issues in attention, problem solving, and psychomotor speed. However, prevention of stroke and intervention after stroke may serve a protective factor. Kral and colleagues (2006) found that performance on math and visual–motor integration tasks was stronger in patients who were receiving chronic transfusion therapy after stroke than in those who were not.

Among educators, there may be inadequate awareness of the academic risks associated with chronic illness generally, and certainly SCD specifically. Consequently, resource allocation may be lacking (Day & Chismark, 2006). If the number of days outside the classroom is correlated with weak attainment, individualized academic interventions in multiple environments may be quite critical to optimal academic achievement. Children with SCD who miss school due to illness may benefit from increased individual interventions either while hospitalized, while homebound, or on their return to the classroom, to minimize the negative impact of absence combined with learning challenges.

School districts in geographic areas that have high populations of children with SCD are more familiar with these children's problems of pain crises, decreased stamina, need for medically based accommodations, and school absences. However, less ethnically diverse school districts may not be as informed or experienced. In addition, educational definitions or state laws may not reflect current scientific and medical knowledge about the direct impact of SCD on brain function. The fact that the pathophysiology of SCD is associated with neurological injury may not be known to school personnel, and consequently some of these children may be served under Section 504 accommodation plans as students with health issues, rather than under individualized education programs as children with academically relevant disabilities and health concerns. Parents and medical providers may need to shoulder the responsibility of sharing this information with school personnel, particularly school psychologists, special educators, and school nurses, who can advocate for these children's needs within the school and classroom. In fact, it would best benefit the broad population with SCD to be screened for specific neuropsychological functioning, in order for those in need to access state-funded early intervention services prior to the age of 3, and have access to special education services after age 3 according to the 2004 Individuals with Disabilities Education Improvement Act (Armstrong, 2005). The routine use of screening measures throughout school may help to identify students with SCD who would benefit from intervention at a younger age, and this in turn may decrease academic and behavioral issues that are usually exacerbated with age. However, many families of children with SCD may not have access to, or may not have the knowledge to seek out, neuropsychological assessment either privately or through their local schools (Cant-Peterson et al., 2005). Preventative measures (e.g., parent education about the neurocognitive and academic issues and risks in SCD, as well as school- and family-based intervention programs to minimize environmental risks and maximize academic achievement) have begun, but more are needed. Koontz, Short, Kalinyak, and Noll (2004) successfully pilot-tested a school-based intervention program intended to educate peers and teachers about SCD. The intervention resulted in increased knowledge and perceived comfort in peers and teachers, as well as fewer school absences in the students with SCD.

Sensory, Motor, Visual–Spatial, and Visual-Perceptual Skills

An increased presence of fine motor, tactile, visual-perceptual, and visual–motor integration impairments has been found in children with SCD, although the data are variable and sometimes have not isolated the construct of fine motor skills from those of spatial and perceptual abilities for comparison. Visual–spatial deficits do appear to occur more frequently than language deficits, regardless of age at injury (Armstrong et al., 1996; Bernaudin et al., 2000; Schatz et al., 1999; Wang et al., 2001). Several studies have also noted that children with SCD have significantly poorer performance on measures of visual–motor integration and attention (Schatz, Finke, et al., 2002; Wasserman et al., 1991). Schatz, Craft, Koby, and De-Baun (2000) found that patients with SCD who had silent infarcts but no evidence of overt infarct obtained lower visual–spatial and visual–motor scores than sibling controls, who evidenced no abnormalities.

Spatial organization and processing deficits have also been found to be more likely in children with SCD who have a history of diffuse injury (Craft et al., 1993; Schatz et al., 1999). Language skills are associated with left-hemisphere control in the majority of the population, whereas visual–spatial functions are subsumed under multiple integrative brain regions. Visual–spatial functions are consequently often considered "more vulnerable" to any neurological injury. Although larger lesions are clearly associated with identifiable impairment, many children may have subtle deficits that negatively affect their abilities to attend to, organize, and sequence visual information, and to understand relationships, directionality, dimensionality, and orientation; these deficits can subsequently impair their ability to understand charts, copy from the board, or line up math problems. Overt stroke, even regardless of specific location, appears to have a greater impact on Performance IQ than on Verbal IQ (Armstrong et al., 1996; Bernaudin et al., 2000; Wang et al., 2001). Craft and colleagues (1993) found that children with silent diffuse stroke showed significantly more impairment on spatial measures than did either children with anterior lesions or healthy siblings. Understandably, injury in the posterior parietotemporal regions, as well as the total volume of the stroke, has been associated with the severity of subsequent visual spatial impairments (Craft et al., 1993; Schatz et al., 1999).

Language Skills

Although Verbal IQ deficits have frequently been reported for school-age children with SCD, a more specific profile of language abilities in SCD has become clearer within the past decade. Available studies suggest that both lesion volume and location are associated with specific language deficits (Berkelhammer et al., 2006). As expected, Cohen and colleagues (1994) found that patients with left-hemisphere stroke had a

global impairment in verbal abilities (expressive language, verbal and auditory memory, oral reading) consistent with aphasia. [PC6] On the other hand, children with specific right-hemisphere stroke have been found to evidence relative sparing of verbal functions (Schatz, Kraft, et al., 2004).

Although this and other studies have found impaired language function in children with SCD, not all are specifically related to left-sided cerebral injury. Hariman, Kirkham, Hurtig, and Keehn (1991) identified low-average to impaired levels of language functioning in children with a history of nondefined stroke, and concluded that there were more psychosocial than physical consequences. Poststroke reductions in Full Scale IQ, reading, spelling, and written language all clearly suggests an underlying language weakness. Listianingsih and colleagues (1991) found reduced language functions in children with SCD who did not have a documented history of stroke, suggesting the possibility of either inherent neuropathology or the occurrence of silent stroke. Wasserman and colleagues (1991) also found language difficulties on the Luria–Nebraska, but did not find supportive evidence of language compromise on the Wechsler Intelligence Scale for Children—Third Edition. Cohen and colleagues (1994) found significantly lower verbal function in a combined SCD group with stroke than in either a sibling control group or an age-referenced normative group. Children with abnormal MRI findings have been found to make more errors during rapid naming (Brown et al., 2000), although the role of processing speed, impulsivity, poor inhibition, and poor self-monitoring in such a task should also be considered.

Interestingly, in a survey of parents of infants and preschoolers with SCD, there was more reported concern about physical development than about language development (Gentry, Hall, & Danier, 1997). However, language developmental milestones at younger ages may not be generally understood by nonprofessionals, and may thus be underreported. Because academic skills are highly dependent on receptive and expressive abilities, language-based impairments that may be present at the beginning of formal schooling are likely to have a negative impact on acquisition of reading, spelling, and writing skills as well as social-interactive abilities.

More subtle language-based impairments may not be apparent until later years, when both academic and social demands increase and become more complex. Schatz and Roberts (2007) found that a disease-related impact on language factors was not statistically supported, although the authors did find that younger groups showed higher language functioning than older groups, indicative of age-related language decline. The authors determined that although detailed language factors at toddler and preschool ages may be too subtle to detect with current measurements, indications of language issues may be present at these early ages. At the time of kindergarten entry, children with SCD already evidence significantly lower skills in auditory discrimination—a skill that is critical to developing the foundational phonic abilities for reading and spelling, as well as receptive language and attention (Steen et al., 2002). Given the high rates of attention and other executive impairments in SCD, language-based difficulties may be associated with difficulties in verbal working memory and auditory processing (Bernaudin et al., 2000; Schatz, Finke, et al., 2002; Schatz & Roberts, 2005; Steen, Miles, et al., 2003). Schatz, Puffer, Sanchez, Stancil, and Roberts (2009) compared language-processing skills (semantic, syntactic, and phonological processing) of 5- to 7-year-old children with SCD at high or low neurological risk to the skills of peers without SCD. Children at high risk evidenced deficits in all language-processing domains, whereas those at low risk did not evidence any language deficits. This brings into question the possibility of disease-related factors that may affect language development, as well as highlighting the early-onset negative impacts that can occur in SCD. Multiple studies have reported findings of developmental regression in language-based skills over time in patients with SCD (Schatz & Roberts, 2003; Thompson et al., 2002; Wang et al., 2001); however, these findings have also been associated with psychosocial and environmental risk factors, rather than with disease severity alone.

Severe anemia has been implicated in reduced verbal skills, attention, and working memory in children with SCD (Bernaudin et al., 2000; Brown et al., 1993; Schatz, Finke, & Roberts, 2004; Steen et al., 1999; Steen, Miles, et al., 2003). There is also evidence

that higher blood flow velocity in the mid-cerebral artery is associated with lower verbal functioning, as well as with weaker sustained attention and other executive skills (Kral et al., 2003).

Organization, Sequencing, Learning, and Memory

The evidence of weaker attention in children with diffuse and anterior stroke suggests that the process of acknowledging, acquiring, organizing, retaining, and recalling information is likely to be compromised. The ability to learn and access knowledge from memory requires a sequence of attending, organizing, planning, and storing information in an efficient and accessible style. If a child cannot attend efficiently, then impairments in learning and memory are likely to result, but these may or may not reflect specific memory deficits. Weak organization and sequencing can subsequently interfere with efficient learning and memory. Memory impairments are sometimes presumed when another underlying deficit occurs in a related neuropsychological function. True memory deficits should be isolated from other impairments that lead to reduced learning efficiency, as the interventions are likely to be different.

Frontal regions play a major role in memory and learning, including skills of organization, planning/strategy development, and mental manipulation of information that facilitate encoding and access from long-term storage. Consequently, the association of memory and executive skills is quite important in general neurocognitive function. Frontal lobe injury in SCD may have a specific impact on learning and memory, which would have broad neurodevelopmental implications. Anterior forebrain lesions have been specifically associated with commonly identified deficits in memory, attention, and executive skills in general (Schatz & Puffer, 2007).

In particular, verbal working memory has been repeatedly found to be particularly impaired in patients with SCD. White, Salorio, Schatz, and DeBaun (2000) found that working memory deficits were specific to the type and location of infarct in SCD. For children with SCD and diffuse infarcts, verbal working memory span was reduced in comparison to that of controls with SCD and without infarct. For those with anterior or posterior infarcts, the ability to rehearse longer segments of verbal information was negatively affected in comparison to controls. Reed and colleagues (1999) demonstrated verbal memory deficits in each of their subjects, who were also found to have white matter lesions on PET scans. Reduced efficiency in rehearsing verbal information during initial learning, and poor retrieval of verbal information, have both been identified; these would clearly have an impact academic achievement and progress (Brandling-Bennett et al., 2003; White, Saloria, Schatz, & DeBaun, 2000). Frontal lobe injury in SCD has also been related to difficulties with manipulating verbal information in working memory and to poorer retrieval of verbal information on memory recall trials (Brandling-Bennett et al., 2003; White et al., 2000). Kral and colleagues (2003) found that abnormal TCD measures were predictive of weaker auditory working memory. Noll and colleagues (2001) compared children with SCD and no evidence of stroke with peers without a chronic illness, finding significantly reduced working memory, speed of novel learning, and both verbal and visually based short-term recall in the group with SCD. Specific strategic memory processing deficits have also been found in children with SCD who had frontal lobe infarct (Brandling-Bennett et al., 2003). Poorer long-term episodic memory, novel verbal learning, short-term independent recall of verbal information, and working memory were found in children with SCD who had frontal infarct, compared to those without evidence of infarct. Recognition and cued recall were consistent between groups, highlighting the negative impact of SCD-related impairment on new learning. Whereas the group with SCD–frontal infarct and the controls had similar strategy development during new learning, the former group did not subsequently use these strategies during independent recall and were dependent on cued recall strategies to access knowledge. Children receiving chronic transfusion therapy who also had higher TCD values performed better on verbal memory tasks (Kral et al., 2006), which is consistent with the presumed role of oxygenation in learning and memory.

Other Executive Functions

Executive functions are those operations that direct and regulate thought and behavior, including obvious social pragmatics and behavior, as well as subtle cognitive processes and integration and management of various skills. Young children are not expected to have adequate self-regulation, as their managerial/self-monitoring skills are under development. Inappropriate executive skills are often viewed as immaturity, attention-deficit/hyperactivity disorder, or delayed social development, and children with such problems are expected to "catch up" with time. Children who have experienced early CNS injury often recover acutely and appear to perform adequately or to have only subtle deficits in preschool and primary grades. Families and medical personnel often focus on the apparent recovery from acute injury and unintentionally downplay subtle impairments in comparison to the original trauma. Some children are seen as awkward or different, but not "impaired," and consequently do not receive interventions during a critical period of development. It is not until later grades, when the executive functions are socially and academically demanded, that the impairments become more obvious and less tolerable to peers, parents, and teachers. Increasing social, behavioral, and academic problems, unregulated by an impaired executive system, pose greater threats to successful development.

As noted earlier, notable evidence of frontal lobe abnormalities has been found in patients with SCD and stroke (Brown et al., 2000; Gold et al., 2008). Reports regarding the number of patients who have sustained frontal lobe damage are remarkable: Schatz and colleagues (1999) identified 86% of their subjects with stroke as having sustained frontal injury; Brown and colleagues (2000) reported that 96% of children with overt and silent stroke had sustained frontal lobe damage; and a more recent study found that 59% of patients diagnosed with infarct had sustained cortical frontal lobe damage (Gold et al., 2008). Examining cortical thickness at various age levels, Kirk and colleagues (2009) found notable thinning in multiple cortical areas, particularly in the adolescent group. The precuneus and posterior cingulate gyrus were most affected.

Although neuropsychological data were not collected, the authors presumed that cortical and subcortical connections between the parietal and frontal lobes might be at the foundation of many executive impairments in SCD. The precuneus region of the parietal lobe has high connectivity and has been implicated in such higher-order cognitive tasks as visual representation, episodic memory retrieval, perspective taking, and internal representation of self (Cavanna & Trimble, 2006), all of which involve executive skills. Schatz and Buzan (2006) found that anterior corpus callosum volume in patients with SCD did relate to deficits in attention and executive skills (particularly motor control). Higher blood flow velocity in the area of the midcerebral artery has also been associated with weaker sustained attention and executive skills (Kral et al., 2003).

Although the findings have been variable, deficits in specific executive skills such as selective attention, problem solving, planning, decision making, judgment, and set shifting have been recurrently identified (Gold et al., 2008; Schatz et al., 2001; Schatz, Finke, et al., 2002). Higher levels of deficits in executive functions are also consistently found after stroke in patients with SCD (Cohen et al., 1994). Schatz and Roberts (2007) used response delay as a measure of executive function in toddlers and preschool-age children with high- and low-neurological-risk SCD. The younger age group and lower-risk SCD group made fewer errors, indicating better working memory; they also evidenced better self-regulation and "low-intensity pleasure" (soothability and self-entertainment ability) than the older and higher-risk groups did. Such findings are indicative of early-onset self-regulatory difficulties that could play a role in the development, learning, and behavior of children with SCD.

Neurobehavioral and Psychosocial Functioning

Perspective taking and other social and emotional processes have received less attention than other neurocognitive challenges in SCD. Social-cognitive deficits in SCD might be presumed from the neurocognitive impairments identified in attention, working memory, language, and processing speed, as well as the more psychosocial impairments

resulting from days of illness, academic attainment issues, and frequency of school absence. Deficits in facial recognition and in auditory and visual processing of emotions (vocal prosody, facial expressions) have been identified in children with overt stroke (Boni, Brown, Davis, Hsu, & Hopkins, 2001). Children who experienced overt stroke were found to have more difficulty in interpreting ambiguous verbal and nonverbal cues, which would probably negatively affect their responses to the increasingly socially complex situations that occur with development. In addition, children with SCD and stroke had more difficulty reading facial expressions and decoding emotional tone from voices than those with SCD and normal MRI findings had (Boni et al., 2001). Furthermore, as mentioned previously, deficits in processing speed can also impair social skill development in this particular population.

Identified neurocognitive challenges in SCD are presumably associated with subsequent neurobehavioral difficulties. In fact, lower intellectual abilities can result in poor coping skill development. On the other hand, higher levels of intellectual functioning have been associated with lower reported levels of externalizing behavior problems (Schatz & McClellan, 2006; Thompson et al., 2003). Moreover, language deficits are often associated with children's difficulties in understanding verbal expectations and responding to directions, as well as properly expressing themselves. Children with attention impairments have difficulties in self-regulation and motivation that can also affect behavioral compliance and response to intervention. Lastly, the broad area of executive deficits (see earlier discussions) can interfere with behavioral compliance and frustration tolerance.

As noted throughout this chapter, general neuropsychological functioning in SCD has been found to be associated with socioeconomic status (Brown et al., 1993; Schatz & Roberts, 2007; Thompson et al., 2002; Wang et al., 2001). It is critical to consider the combined impact of disease state, biomedical risk factors and psychosocial risk factors because research has yet to identify a predictable and consistent relationship. Psychosocial factors have sometimes been found to be better predictors of neuropsychological performance than disease severity for preschool-age children (Tarazi et al., 2007), whereas Schatz, Finke, and colleagues (2002) found that disease severity was a predictor of cognitive functioning for children in a low-socioeconomic status group. According to a review by Schatz and Puffer (2007), there are more notable neurocognitive and academic challenges resulting from stroke related to SCD than there are behavioral difficulties. Previous assessments of behavioral issues in SCD have relied heavily on maternal report and have used measures that may be less sensitive to the unique factors associated with neurological compromise. The presence of behavioral challenges may actually be higher than is currently discussed in the literature. Given the high rates of academic difficulties/attainment problems, economic disadvantage, stressors of living with chronic illness, and other neuropsychological limitations, the absence of behavioral challenges would be unexpected and quite different from other populations with similar stressors.

Although many children with chronic illness have been found to have adjustment and mood difficulties, rates of depression have been found to be comparatively highest in children with SCD (Key, Brown, & Marsh, 2001). More specifically, these children have also been reported to have increased rates of feelings of hopelessness. However, Yang, Cepeda, Price, Shah, and Mankad (1994) noted years ago that fatigue and physical complaints may lead to higher false-positive rates of depression in children with SCD. Depressive and anxiety disorders are more widespread among medically involved children and teenagers than among their peers, and comorbidity may have a negative impact on medical outcomes and quality of life (Benton, Ifeagwu, & Smith-Whitley, 2007). Nonetheless, assessing emotional status in children and adolescents with SCD is extremely important in the overall conceptualization of their neuropsychological profile.

FUTURE DIRECTIONS IN NEUROPSYCHOLOGICAL RESEARCH

The understanding of the developmental and neurocognitive impact of SCD has advanced significantly in the past decade. SCD is now better conceptualized as a chronic illness and a neurodevelopmental disorder; researchers, clinicians, educators, and families are all improving their grasp of the risks posed by SCD, as well as the interventions needed to optimize development. Clearly, however, there is much more to understand.

With the acknowledgment that the neurocognitive effects of SCD can begin as early as 6 months of age, there need to be more routine cognitive assessments of patients with SCD in the clinics in which they are managed, within their pediatricians' care, or even in the educational setting. Routine assessment for early neurocognitive challenges would open the doors for earlier intervention, potentially decreasing the negative impact of the disease on functional cognitive skills, and thus improving the developmental trajectory. Because days out of school are so highly correlated with academic achievement, there is an obvious need for educational adaptations and accommodations to be provided within the context of the variables inherent in chronic illness. Provision of adapted academic tutoring within the hospital and home settings might minimize or alleviate the impact of missed instructional time. Improved education of academic personnel and students has already been shown to have a positive impact on the functional daily status of children with SCD; such efforts require further investigation and implementation, as well as expansion into the broad range of care providers, including families.

There has been a notable expansion of knowledge about the neuropsychological impact of SCD in recent years. However, the complexities of the brain–illness relationship are great, and will be best understood by continuing this intensive pace of investigation. Neurologically based deficits that lead to specific areas of neurocognitive function need to be better elucidated and perhaps predicted. The impact of early identification of neurocognitive impairment on cognitive rehabilitation and its outcomes is also as yet unknown in SCD. In addition, the role of early treatment interventions in optimizing neurocognitive development, particularly therapies such as hydroxyurea, needs to be more fully investigated.

The cultural implications of how patients with SCD are managed, educated, and supported in the community require more investigation as well. The mere fact that the population of patients with SCD has such a high rate of economic disadvantage explorations, so that our understanding of how to interact most effectively with these families will be improved. How this population is supported and managed reveals much about our culture.

REFERENCES

Adams, R., McKie, V., Hsu, L., Files, B., Vichinsky, E. Pegelow, C., et al. (1998). Prevention of a first stroke by transfusions in children with sickle cell anemia and abnormal results on transcranial Doppler ultrasonography. *New England Journal of Medicine, 339*(1), 5–11.

Adams, R. J., McKie, V., Nichols, F., Carl, E., Zhang, D., McKie, K., et al. (1992). The use of transcranial ultrasonography to predict stroke in sickle cell disease. *New England Journal of Medicine, 326*(9), 605–610.

Adams, R. J., Nichols, F. T, McKie, V., McKie, K., Milner, P., & Gammel, G. T. (1988). Cerebral infarction in sickle cell anemia: Mechanisms based on CT and MRI. *Neurology, 38*, 1012–1017.

Armstrong, F. D. (2005). Thalassemia and learning: Neurocognitive functioning in children. *Annals of the New York Academy Of Sciences, 1054*, 183–189.

Armstrong, F., Thompson, R., Wang, W., Zimmerman, R., Pegelow, C., Miller, S., et al. (1996). Cognitive functioning and brain magnetic resonance imaging in children with sickle cell disease. *Neuropsychology, 97*(6), 864–870.

Ashley-Koch, A., Yang, Q., & Olney, R. S. (2000). Sickle hemoglobin (HbS) allele and sickle cell disease: A HuGE review. *American Journal of Epidemiology, 151*(9), 839–845.

Baldeweg, T., Hogan, A., Saunders, D., Telfer, P., Gadian, D. G., Vargha-Khadem, F., et al. (2005). Detecting white matter injury in sickle cell disease using voxel based morphometry. *Annals of Neurology, 59*, 662–672.

Balkaran, B., Char, G., Morris, J. S., Thomas, P. W., Serjeant, B. E., & Serjeant, J. R. (1992). Stroke in a cohort of patients with homozygous sickle cell disease. *Journal of Pediatrics, 120*, 360–366.

Ballas, S. K., & Mohandas, N. (1996). Pathophysiology of vaso-occlusion. *Hematology/Oncology Clinics of North America*, 10, 1221–1239.

Benton, T. D., Ifeagwu, J. A., & Smith-Whitley, K. (2007). Anxiety and depression in children and adolescents with sickle cell disease. *Current Psychiatry Reports, 9*(2), 127–144.

Berkelhammer, L. D., Williamson, A. L., Sanford, S. D., Dirksen, C. L., Sharp, W. G., Margulies, A. S., et al. (2007). Neurocognitive sequelae of pediatric sickle cell disease: A review of the literature. *Child Neuropsychology, 13*(2), 120–131.

Bernaudin, F., Verlhac, S., Freard, F., Roudot-Thoraval, F., Benkerrou, M., Thuret, I., et al. (2000). Multicenter prospective study of children with sickle cell disease: Radiographic and psychometric correlation. *Journal of Child Neurology, 15*, 333–343.

Boni, L. C., Brown, R. T., Davis, P., Hsu, L., & Hopkins, K. (2001). Social information processing and magnetic resonance imaging in children with sickle cell disease. *Journal of Pediatric Psychology, 26*, 309–319.

Bonner, M. J., Gustafson, K. E., Shumacher, E., & Thompson, R. J. (1999). The impact of sickle cell disease on cognitive functioning and learning. *School Psychology Review, 28*, 182–193.

Brandling-Bennett, E. M., White, D. A., Armstrong, M. M., Christ, S. E., & DeBaun, M. R. (2003). Patterns of verbal long term and working memory performance reveal deficits in strategic processing in children with frontal infarcts related to sickle cell disease. *Developmental Neuropsychology, 24*, 423–434.

Brown, R., Armstrong, F., & Eckman, J. (1993). Neurocognitive aspects of pediatric sickle cell disease. *Journal of Learning Disabilities, 26*(1), 33–45.

Brown, R. T., Buchanan, I., Doepke, K., Eckman, J., Baldwin K., Goonan, B., et al. (1993). Cognitive and academic functioning in children with sickle cell disease. *Journal of Clinical Child Psychology, 22*, 207–218.

Brown, R. T., Davis, P. C., Lambert, R., Hsu, L., Hopkins, K., & Eckman, J. (2000). Neurocognitive functioning and magnetic resonance imaging in children with sickle cell disease. *Journal of Pediatric Psychology, 25*, 503–513.

Buchanan, G. R., DeBaun, M. R., Quinn, C. T., & Steinberg, M. H. (2004). Sickle cell disease. *American Society of Hematology: Education Program Book*, pp. 35–47

Burlew, A. K., Evans, R., & Oler, C. (1989). The impact of a child with sickle cell disease on family dynamics. *Annals of the New York Academy of Sciences, 565*, 161–171.

Cant-Peterson, C., Palermo, T. M., Swift, E., Bebee, A., & Drotar, D. (2005). Assessment of psychoeducational needs in a clinical sample of children with sickle cell disease. *Children's Health Care, 34*(2), 133–148.

Cavanna, A. E., & Trimble, M. R. (2006). The precuneus: A review of its functional anatomy and behavioural correlates. *Brain, 129*(3), 569–583.

Chua-Lim, C., Moore, R. B., McCleary, G., Shah, A., & Mankad, V. N. (1993). Deficiencies in school readiness skills of children with sickle cell anemia: A preliminary report. *Southern Medical Journal, 86*(4), 397–402.

Cohen, M. J., Branch, W. B., McKie, V. C., & Adams, R. J. (1994). Neuropsychological impairment in children with sickle cell anemia and cerebrovascular accidents. *Clinical Pediatrics, 33*(9), 517–524.

Craft, S., Schatz, J., Glauser, T. A., Lee, B., & De-Baun, M. R. (1993). Neuropsychological effects of stroke in children with sickle cell anemia. *Journal of Pediatrics, 123*(5), 712–717.

Craft, S., Schatz, J., Glauser, T. A., Lee, B., & DeBaun, M. R. (1994). The effects of bifrontal stroke during childhood on visual attention: Evidence from children with sickle cell anemia. *Developmental Neuropsychology, 10*(3), 285–297.

Day, S., & Chismark, E. (2006). The cognitive and academic impact of sickle cell disease. *Journal of School Nursing, 22*(6), 330–335.

DeBaun, M. R. Schatz, J., Siegel, M. J., Koby, M., Craft, S., Resar, L., et al. (1998). Cognitive screening examination for screening for silent cerebral infarcts in sickle cell disease. *Neurology, 50*, 1678–1682.

Driscoll, M. C., Hurlet, A., Styles, L., McKie, V., Files, B., Olivieri, N., et al. (2003). Stroke risk in siblings with sickle cell anemia. *Blood, 101*, 2401–2404.

Fowler, M. G., Whitt, J. K., Redding-Lallinger, A. R., Nash, K. B., Atkinson, S. S., Wells, R. J., et al. (1988). Neuropsychologic and academic functioning of children with sickle cell anemia. *Journal of Developmental and Behavioral Pediatrics, 9*, 213–220.

Gentry, B., Hall, L., & Danier, J. (1997). A parental survey of speech, language and physical development of infants and toddlers with sickle cell disease. *Perceptual and Motor Skills, 83*(3), 1105–1106.

Gold, J. I., Johnson, C. B., Treadwell, M. J., Hans, N., & Vichinsky, E. (2008). Detection and assessment of stroke in patients with sickle cell disease: Neuropsychological functioning and magnetic resonance imaging. *Pediatric Hematology and Oncology, 25*(5), 409–421.

Grueneich, R., Ris, M. D., Ball, W., Kalinyak, K. A., Noll, R., Vanatta, K., et al. (2004). Relationship of structural magnetic resonance imaging, magnetic resonance perfusion, and other disease factors to neuropsychological outcome in sickle cell disease. *Journal of Pediatric Psychology, 29*, 83–92.

Gustafson, K. E., Bonner, M. J., Hardy, K. K., & Thompson, R. J. (2006). Biopsychosocial and developmental issues in sickle cell disease. In R. Brown (Ed.), *Comprehensive handbook of childhood cancer and sickle cell disease* (pp. 431–448). New York: Oxford University Press.

Hariman, L. M., Kirkham, F. J., Hurtig, A. L., & Keehn, M. T. (1991). Functional outcomes of children with sickle cell disease affected by stroke. *Archives of Physical Medicine and Rehabilitation, 72*, 498–502.

Hillery, C. A., & Panepinto, J. A. (2004). Pathophysiology of stroke in sickle cell disease. *Microcirculation, 11*, 195–208.

Hogan, A. M., Kirkham, F. J., Prengler, M., Telfer, P., Lane, R., Vargha-Khadem, F., & et al. (2005). An exploratory study of physiological correlates of neurodevelopmental delay in infants with sickle cell disease. *British Journal of Haematology, 132*, 99–107.

Hogan, A. M., Pit-ten Cate, I. M., Vargha-Khadem, F., Prengler, M., & Kirkham, F. J. (2006). Physiological correlates of intellectual function in children with sickle cell disease: Hypoxaemia, hyperaemia and brain infarction. *Developmental Science, 9*(4), 379–387.

Hurtig, A. L., & Park, K. B. (1989). Adjustment and coping in adolescents with sickle cell disease. *Annals of the New York Academy of Sciences, 565*, 172–182.

Hurtig, A. L., & White, L. S. (1986). Psychosocial adjustment in children and adolescents with sickle cell disease. *Journal of Pediatric Psychology, 11*(3), 411–427.

Kennan, R. P., Suzaka, S. M., Nagel, R. L., & Fabry, M. E. (2004). Decreased cerebral perfusion correlates with increased BOLD hyperoxia response in transgenic models of sickle cell disease. *Magnetic Resonance in Medicine, 51*, 525–532.

Key, J. D., Brown, R. T., & Marsh, L. D. (2001). Depressive symptoms in adolescents with a chronic illness. *Children's Health Care, 30*, 283–292.

Kinney, T., Sleeper, L., Wang, W., Zimmerman, R., Pegelow, C., Ohene-Frempong, K., et al. (1999). Silent cerebral infarcts in sickle cell anemia: A risk factor analysis. *Pediatrics, 103*(3), 640.

Kirk, G. R., Haynes, M. R., Palasis, S., Brown, C., Burns, T. G., McCormick, M., et al. (2009). Regionally specific cortical thinning in children with sickle cell disease. *Cerebral Cortex, 19*(7), 1549–1556.

Kirkham, F. J., Hewes, D. K., Prengler, M., Wade, A., Lane, R., & Evans, J. P. (2001). Nocturnal hypoxaemia and central nervous system events in sickle cell disease. *Lancet, 357*, 1656–1659.

Knight, S., Singhal, A., Thomas, P., & Serjeant, G. (1995). Factors associated with lowered intelligence in homozygous sickle cell disease. *Archives of Disease in Childhood, 73*(4), 316–320.

Koontz, K., Short, A. D., Kalinyak, K., & Noll, R. B. (2004). A randomized, controlled pilot trial of a school intervention for children with sickle cell anemia. *Journal of Pediatric Psychology, 29*, 7–17.

Kral, M. C., Brown, R. T., Connelly, M., Curé, J. K., Besenski, N., Jackson, S. M., et al. (2006). Radiographic predictors of neurocognitive functioning in pediatric sickle cell disease. *Journal of Child Neurology, 21*(1), 37–44.

Kral, M. C., Brown, R. T., Neitert, P. J., Abboud, M. R., Jackson, S. M., & Hynd, G. W. (2003). Transcranial doppler ultrasonography and neurocognitive functioning in children with sickle cell disease. *Pediatrics, 112*, 324–331.

Kramer, M. S., Rooks, Y., & Pearson, H. A. (1978). Growth and development in children with sickle cell trait. *New England Journal of Medicine, 299*, 686–489.

Lee, E. J., Phoenix, D., Brown, W., & Jackson, B. S. (1997). A comparison of children with sickle cell disease and their non-diseased siblings on hopelessness, depression, and perceived competence. *Journal of Advanced Nursing, 25*, 79–86.

Lee, M. T., Piomelli, S., Granger, S., Miller, S. T., Harkness, S., Brambilla, D. J., et al. (2006). Stroke prevention trial in sickle cell anemia (STOP): Extended follow-up and final results. *Blood, 108*(3), 847–852.

Listianingsih, M. F., Hariman, M. D., Griffith, E. R., Hurtig, A. L., & Keehn, M. T. (1991). Functional outcomes of children with sickle-cell disease affected by stroke. *Archives of Physical Medicine and Rehabilitation, 72*, 498–502.

Lonergan, G., Cline, D., & Abbondanzo, S. (2001). Sickle cell anemia. *Radiographics, 21*(4), 971–994.

McCarney, D., & Greenberg, L. M. (1990). *Test of Variables of Attention*. Minneapolis, MN: Attention Technology.

McCormack, M. K., Scarr-Salapatek, S., Polesky, H., Thompson, W., Katz, S. H., & Barker, W. B. (1975). A comparison of the physical and intellectual development of black children with and without sickle-cell trait. *Pediatrics, 56*, 1021–1025.

Mercuri, E., Faundez, J., Roberts, I., Flora, S., Bouza, H., Cowan, F., et al. (1995). Neurological 'soft' signs may identify children with sickle cell disease who are at risk for stroke. *European Journal of Pediatrics, 154*, 150–156.

Miller, S. T., Macklin, E. A., Pegelow, C. H., Kinney, T. R., Sleeper, L. A., Bello, J. A., et al. (2001). Silent infarction as a risk factor for overt stroke in children with sickle cell anemia: A report from the Cooperative Study of Sickle Cell Disease. *Journal of Pediatrics, 139*, 385–390.

Miller, S. T., Sleeper, L. A., Pegelow, C. H., Enos, L. E., Wang, W. C., Weiner, S. J., et al. (2000). Prediction of adverse outcomes in children with sickle cell disease. *New England Journal of Medicine, 342*, 83–89.

Nabors, N. A., & Freymuth, A. K. (2002). Attention deficit in children with sickle cell disease. *Perceptual and Motor Skills, 95*(1), 57–67.

National Heart, Lung, and Blood Institute. (1996). *Sickle cell anemia* (NIH Publication No. 96–4057). Washington, DC: U.S. Government Printing Office.

National Institutes of Health. (1986). PET scans pinpoint brain metabolism changes in sickle cell disease. *Journal of the American Medical Association, 256*(13), 1692.

Noll, R. B., Stith, L., Gartstein, M. A., Ris, M. D., Grueneich, R., Vannatta, K., et al. (2001). Neuropsychological functioning of youths with sickle cell disease: Comparison with non-chronically ill peers. *Journal of Pediatric Psychology, 26*(2), 69–78.

Ogunfowora, O. B., Olanrewaju, D. M., & Akenzua, G. I. (2005). A comparative study of academic achievement of children with sickle cell disease and their healthy siblings. *Journal of the National Medical Association, 97*(3), 405–408.

Oguz, K. K., Golay, X., Pizzini, F. B., Freer, C. A., Winrow, N., Ichord, R., et al. (2003). Sickle cell disease: continuous arterial spin-labeling perfusion MR imaging in children. *Radiology, 227*, 567–574.

Ohene-Frempong, K., Weiner, S. J., Sleeper, L. A., Miller, S. T., Embury, S., Moohr, J. W., et al. (1998). Cerebrovascular accidents in sickle cell disease: Rates and risk factors. *Blood, 91*, 288–294.

Pavlakis, S. G., Bello, J., Prohovnik, I., Sutton, M., Ince, C., Mohr, J. P., et al. (1988). Brain infarction in sickle cell anemia: Magnetic resonance imagery correlates. *Annals of Neurology, 23*(2), 125–130.

Pavlakis, S. G., Prohovnik, I., Piomelli, S., & Devivo, D. C. (1989). Neurologic complications of sickle cell disease. *Advances in Pediatrics, 36*, 247–276.

Pegelow, C. H. (2001). Stroke in children with sickle cell anaemia: Aetiology and treatment. *Paediatric Drugs, 3*(6), 421–432.

Pegelow, C. H., Macklin, E. A., Moser, F. G., Wang, W. C., Bello, J. A., Miller, S. T., et al. (2002). Longitudinal changes in brain magnetic resonance imaging findings in children with sickle cell disease. *Blood, 99*, 3014–3018.

Pegelow, C. H., Wang, W., Granger, S., Hsu, L. L., Vichinsky, E., Moser, F. G., et al. (2001). Silent infarcts in children with sickle cell anemia and abnormal cerebral artery velocity. *Archives of Neurology, 58*, 2017–2021.

Powars, D. R., Conti, P. S., Wong, W. Y., Groncy, P., Hyman, C., Smith, E., et al. (1999). Cerebral vasculopathy in sickle cell anemia: Diagnostic contribution of positron emission tomography. *Blood, 93*, 71–79.

Powars, D. R., Wilson, B., Imbus, C., Pegelow, C. H., & Allen, J. (1978). The natural history of stroke in sickle cell disease. *American Journal of Medicine, 65*, 461–469.

Prengler, M., Pavlakis, S. G., Prohovnik, I., & Adams, R. J. (2002). Sickle cell disease: The neurological complications. *Annals of Neurology, 51*, 543–552.

Puffer, E., Schatz, J., & Roberts, C. W. (2007). The association of oral hydroxyurea therapy with improved cognitive functioning in sickle cell disease. *Child Neuropsychology, 13*(2), 142–154.

Reed, W., Jagust, W., Al-Mateen, M., & Vichinsky, E. (1999). Role of positron emission tomography in determining the extent of CNS ischemia in patients with sickle cell disease. *American Journal of Hematology, 60,* 268–272.

Ris, D., & Gruenich, R. (2000). Sickle cell disease. In K. O. Yeates, M. D. Ris, & H. G. Taylor (Eds.), *Pediatric neuropsychology* (pp. 320–335). New York: Guilford Press.

Ris, M. D., Gruenich, R., & Kalinyak, K. A. (1995). Neuropsychological risk in children with sickle cell disease. *Journal of the International Neuropsychological Society, 1,* 360.

Ris, M. D., Kalinyak, K. A., Ball, W. S., Noll, R. B., Wells, R. J., & Rucknagel, D. (1996). Pre- and post-stroke MRI and neuropsychological studies in sickle cell disease: A case study. *Archives of Clinical Neurology, 11*(6), 481–490.

Rodgers, G., Clark, C., Larson, S., Rapport, S., Nienhuis, A., & Schechter, A. (1988). Brain glucose metabolism in neurologically normal patients with sickle cell disease. *Archives of Neurology, 45,* 78–82.

Sanders, C., Gentry, B., Davis, P., Jackson, J., Saccente, S., & Dancer, J. (1997). Reading, writing, and vocabulary skills of children with strokes due to sickle cell disease. *Perceptual and Motor Skills, 85*(2), 477–478.

Schatz, J. (2004). Brief report: Academic attainment in children with sickle cell disease. *Journal of Pediatric Psychology, 29*(8), 627–633.

Schatz, J., Brown, R. T., Pascual, J. M., Hsu, L., & DeBaun, M. R. (2001). Poor school and cognitive functioning in children with silent cerebral infarcts and sickle cell disease. *Neurology, 56,* 1109–1111.

Schatz, J., & Buzan, R. F. (2006). Decreased corpus callosum size in sickle cell disease: Relationship with cerebral infarcts and cognitive functioning. *Journal of the International Neuropsychological Society, 12,* 17–23.

Schatz, J., Craft, S., Koby, M., & DeBaun, M. (2000). A lesion analysis of visual orienting performance in children with cerebral vascular injury. *Developmental Neuropsychology, 17*(1), 49–61.

Schatz, J., Craft, S., Koby, M., & DeBaun, M. R. (2004). Asymmetries in visual–spatial processing following childhood stroke. *Neuropsychology, 18*(2), 340–352.

Schatz, J., Craft, S., Koby, M., Seigal, M. J., Resar, L., Lee, R. R., et al. (1999). Neuropsychological deficits in children with sickle cell disease and cerebral infarction: The role of lesion location and volume. *Child Neuropsychology, 5,* 92–103.

Schatz, J., Finke, R. L., Kellet, J. M., & Kramer, J. H. (2002). Cognitive functioning in children with sickle cell disease: A meta-analysis. *Journal of Pediatric Psychology, 8,* 739–748.

Schatz, J., Finke, R. L., & Roberts, C. W. (2004). Interactions among biomedical and environmental factors in cognitive development: A preliminary study of sickle cell disease. *Journal of Developmental and Behavioral Pediatrics, 25,* 303–310.

Schatz, J., & McClellan, C. B. (2006). Sickle cell disease as a neurodevelopmental disorder. *Mental Retardation and Developmental Disabilities Research Reviews, 12,* 200–207.

Schatz, J., & Puffer, E. (2006). Neuropsychological aspects of sickle cell disease. In R. T. Brown (Ed.), *Comprehensive handbook of childhood cancer and sickle cell disease* (pp. 449–470). New York: Oxford University Press.

Schatz, J., & Puffer, E. S. (2007). Neuropsychological aspects of sickle cell disease. *Child Neuropsychology, 13,* 449–470.

Schatz, J., Puffer, E. S., Sanchez, C., Stancil, M., & Roberts, C. W. (2009). Language processing deficits in sickle cell disease in young school-age children. *Developmental Neuropsychology, 34*(1), 122–136.

Schatz, J., & Roberts, C. W. (2005). Short term memory in children with sickle cell disease: Executive versus modality specific processing deficits. *Archives of Clinical Neuropsychology, 20,* 1073–1085.

Schatz, J., & Roberts, C. W. (2007). Neurobehavioral impact of sickle cell disease in early childhood. *Journal of the International Neuropsychological Society, 13,* 933–943.

Schatz, J., White, D. A., Moinuddin, A., Armstrong, M., & DeBaun, M. R. (2002). Lesion burden and cognitive morbidity in children with sickle cell disease. *Child Neurology, 17*(12), 890–894.

Steen, R. G., Emudianughe, T., Hankins, G. M., Wynn, L. W., Wang, W. C., Xiong, X., et al. (2003). Brain imaging findings in patients with sickle cell disease. *Radiology, 228,* 216–225.

Steen, R. G., Fineberg-Buchner, C., Hankins, G., Weiss, L., Prifitera, A., & Mulhern, R. (2005). Cognitive deficits in children with sickle cell disease. *Journal of Child Neurology, 20*(2), 102–107.

Steen, R. G., Hankins, G., Xiong, X., Wang, W. C., Beil, K., Langston, J. W. (2003). Prospective brain imaging evaluation of children with sickle cell trait: Initial observations. *Radiology, 228,* 208–215.

Steen, R. G., Hu, X. J., Elliot, V. E., Miles, M. A., Jones, S., & Wang, W. C. (2002). Kindergarten readiness skills in children with sickle cell disease: Evidence of early neurocognitive damage? *Journal of Child Neurology, 17,* 111–116.

Steen, R. G., Hunte, M., Traipe, E., Hurh, P., Wu, S., Bilaniuk, L., et al. (2004). Brain T(1) in young children with sickle cell disease: Evidence of early abnormalities in brain development. *Magnetic Resonance Imaging, 22,* 299–306.

Steen, R. G., Miles, M. A., Helton, K. J., Strong, S., Wang, W. C., Xiong, X., et al. (2003). Cognitive impairment in children with hemoglobin SS sickle cell disease: Relationship to MR findings and hematocrit. *American Journal of Neuroradiology, 24,* 382–389.

Steen, R. G., Reddick, W. E., Mulhern, R. K., Langston, J. W., Ogg, R. J., Bieberich, A. A., et al. (1998). Quantitative MRI of the brain in children with sickle cell disease reveals abnormalities unseen by conventional MRI. *Journal of Magnetic Resonance Imaging, 8,* 535–543.

Steen, R. G., Xiong, X., Mulhern, R. K., Langston, J. W., & Wang, W. C. (1999). Subtle brain abnormalities in children with sickle cell disease: Relationship with blood hematocrit. *Annals of Neurology, 45,* 279–286.

Swift, A. V., Cohen, M. J., Hynd, G. W., Wisenbaker, J. M., McKie, K. M., Makari, G., et al. (1989). Neuropsychological impairment in children with sickle cell anemia. *Pediatrics, 84*(6), 1077–1085.

Switzer, J. A., Hess, D. C., Nichols, F. T., & Adams R. J. (2006). Pathophysiology and treatment of stroke in sickle-cell disease: Present and future. *Lancet Neurology, 5*(6), 501–512.

Tarazi, R. A., Grant, M. L., Ely, E., & Barakat, L. P. (2007). Neuropsychological functioning in preschool-age children with sickle cell disease: The role of illness-related and psychosocial factors. *Child Neuropsychology, 13,* 155–172.

Thompson, R. J., Armstrong, F. D., Link, C. L., Pegelow, C. H., Moser, F., & Wang, W. C. (2003). A prospective study of the relationship over time of behavior problems, intellectual functioning and family functioning in children with sickle cell disease: A report from the Cooperative Study of Sickle Cell Disease. *Journal of Pediatric Psychology, 28,* 59–65.

Thompson, R. J., Gustafson, K. E., Bonner, M. J., & Ware, R. E. (2002). Neurocognitive development of young children with sickle cell disease through three years of age. *Journal of Pediatric Psychology, 27*(3), 235–244.

Wang, W. C. (2007). Central nervous system complications of sickle cell disease in children: An overview. *Child Neuropsychology, 13,* 103–119.

Wang, W. C., Enos, L., Gallagher, D. M., Thompson, R., Guarini, L., Vichinsky, E., et al. (2001). Neuropsychological performance in school-aged children with sickle cell disease: A report from the Cooperative Study of Sickle Cell Disease. *Journal of Pediatrics, 139,* 391–397.

Wang, W. C., Langston, J. W., Steen, R. G., Wynn, L. W., Mulhern, R. K., Wilimas, J. A., et al. (1998). Abnormalities of the central nervous system in very young children with sickle cell anemia. *Journal of Pediatrics, 132,* 994–998.

Wasserman, A. L., Williams, J. A., Fairclough, D. L., Mulhern, R. K., & Wang, W. (1991). Subtle neuropsychological deficits in children with sickle cell disease. *American Journal of Pediatric Hematology/Oncology, 13,* 14–20.

White, D., Salorio, C., Schatz, J., & DeBaun, M. (2000). Preliminary study of working memory in children with stroke related to sickle cell disease. *Journal of Clinical and Experimental Neuropsychology, 22*(2), 257–264.

White, D. A., Saloria, C. F., Schatz, J., & DeBaun, M. R. (2000). Preliminary study of working memory in children with stroke related to sickle cell disease. *Journal of Clinical and Experimental Neuropsychology, 22,* 257–264.

Wiznitzer, M., Ruggeri, P. M., Masaryk, T. J., Ross, J. S., Modic, M. T., & Berman, B. (1990). Diagnosis of cerebrovascular disease in sickle cell anemia by magnetic resonance angiography. *Journal of Pediatrics, 117*(4), 551–555.

Woods, B. T. (1980). The restricted effects of right-hemisphere lesions after age one: Wechsler test data. *Neuropsychologia, 16,* 65–70.

Woods, B. T., & Teuber, H. L. (1973). Early onset of complimentary specialization of cerebral hemispheres in man. *Transactions of the American Neurological Association, 98,* 113–117.

Yang, Y. M., Cepeda, M., Price, C., Shah, A., & Mankad, V. (1994). Depression in children and adolescents with sickle cell disease. *Archives of Pediatrics and Adolescent Medicine, 148,* 457–460.

CHAPTER 19

Down Syndrome

HEATHER CODY HAZLETT
JULIE HAMMER
STEPHEN R. HOOPER
RANDY W. KAMPHAUS

Down syndrome was named after the physician John Langdon Down, who in 1866 published a description of patients he identified as "Mongolian." In addition to delineating the physical features of this syndrome, Down noted that these individuals were responsive to training and could benefit from intervention (Carr, 1995). International prevalence rates of Down syndrome are reported to be approximately 8.32 per 10,000 live births (Cocchi et al., 1988). This estimate is higher than earlier ones, due to efforts to screen pregnant women over the age of 35, who are felt to be at greater risk for giving birth to a child with Down syndrome. Nonetheless, because approximately 70% of babies born with Down syndrome are born to younger mothers, and because some women may refuse screening (Carr, 1995; Sadovnick & Baird, 1992), this figure is still high. Gender differences are evident, in that males commonly outnumber females (the sex ratio is 1.3:1); this may be due to a higher mortality rate in females during infancy (Carr, 1995).

GENETIC AND FAMILIAL ISSUES RELATED TO ETIOLOGY

Down syndrome is classified as one of the chromosomal disorders, meaning that the syndrome has been traced to malformations in the genes of individuals who display the syndrome. There are actually several different types of Down syndrome, with the most prevalent being trisomy 21 (94%), where there is actually a third chromosome 21 in addition to the usual two (Prescott, 1988). Trisomy occurs in approximately 4% of all pregnancies, making it the most common chromosomal abnormality in humans (Hassold, Sherman, & Hunt, 1995). Genetic anomalies have also been found on chromosome 21, in particular band q22. Specific regions of chromosome 21 have been mapped and are associated with the various features of Down syndrome. Currently, approximately 25–40 genes have been mapped to chromosome 21 through techniques such as gene linkage. This is one reason for the wide range of individual variation found in the population with Down syndrome (Korenberg, Pulst, & Gerwehr, 1992). Other types of Down syndrome consist of translocation 21, mosaicism, and partial trisomy 21 (Coleman, 1988; Pueschel, 1992b). Translocation 21 results when one part of chromosome 21 has been transferred to a different location. Mosaicism occurs when not all of the cells display the chromosomal trisomy, although a majority do display trisomy 21. Some research indicates that individuals with this condition have higher mean cognitive scores than those with trisomy 21.

Relative risk for giving birth to a child with Down syndrome is approximately 1%, plus the amount of risk associated with the mother's age during pregnancy. The risk for having a child with Down syndrome increases exponentially with maternal age. For example, a 20-year-old mother has a 1 in 1,923 chance of giving birth to an infant with Down syndrome, whereas the chance for a 49-year-old mother is 1 in 12 (Prescott, 1988). Prenatal procedures, such as amniocentesis and chorionic villi sampling, can be used to screen for Down syndrome. The etiology behind the maternal age effect has not yet been determined, although it appears to be related to an increase in trisomy at conception rather than a decrease in the ability to abort a trisomic fetus naturally (Hassold et al., 1995).

MEDICAL CONCERNS AND COMORBID DISORDERS

Although Down syndrome is primarily known as one of the chief causes of intellectual disabilities, it also includes distinctive physical characteristics, as Down noted in his 1866 report. These may include brachycephaly (broad head), a delay in the closure of the fontanels, hypoplasia of the midfacial bones, obliquely placed palpebral fissures, epicanthal folds, depressed nasal bridge, hyper- or hypotelorism, Brushfield spots (i.e., white spots on the periphery of the iris), an overlapping or folding of the helix of the ear, thickened lips, tongue protrusion and/or fissured tongue with increasing age, short and broad neck, umbilical hernias, broad and stubby hands and feet, a single palmar transverse crease, partial or complete syn-

dactyly, and a wide space between the first and second toes (Pueschel, 1992b). Certain features have been found to change over time. For example, the epicanthal folds and large neck may become less noticeable over time, while other features (e.g., a fissured tongue and dental problems) become more problematic with increasing age (Pueschel, 1992b). The intellectual disability evident with Down syndrome may range from mild to profound (according to the American Association on Intellectual and Developmental Disabilities classification), which adds to the heterogeneity of this population.

Ophthalmological Concerns

Ophthalmological problems can be major disabilities for individuals with Down syndrome. The most common causes of loss of vision are cataracts and acute keratoconus. Functionally, individuals may suffer from amblyopia, strabismus, blepharitis, and high refractive errors, which if untreated may be debilitating (Catalano, 1992; Niva, 1988; Tsiaras, Pueschel, Keller, Curran, & Giesswein, 1999). Fortunately, medical intervention is available for all of these conditions; therefore, parents, teachers, and health professionals should be aware of these potential difficulties and seek medical evaluation to determine the nature of the ophthalmological needs.

Oral Problems

Since the maxilla and mandible are smaller in persons with Down syndrome than in most individuals, the tongue may appear to be larger than normal. As a result of the smaller oral cavity and relatively larger tongue, oral hygiene may be difficult. In addition, individuals with Down syndrome may have a furrowed tongue or cleft palate, which may further complicate oral health. The tongue protrusion also contributes to the split, inflamed lips that are commonly seen in these individuals. Other common problems include malocclusions, anomalies in the dentition (e.g., congenitally missing teeth, delayed eruption of teeth, delayed shedding of primary teeth), and periodontal disease (e.g., gingivitis is seen in almost all persons with Down syndrome) (Vigild, 1992).

Cardiac Problems

The prevalence of congenital heart malformations in persons with Down syndrome has been reported to be as high as 50% (for trisomy 21), and cardiac anomalies remain the main cause of death, especially in the first few years of life (Marino, 1992). The most common types of anomalies found in these children are defects in the atrioventricular canal. These anomalies produce an increased risk of congestive heart failure. Certain types of cardiac defects result in decreased pulmonary blood flow, which may contribute to pulmonary artery hypertension and pulmonary vascular obstructive disease (Howenstein, 1992; Suzuki et al., 2000). Early diagnosis and corrective surgery may improve survival rates to 80–90% of children who may otherwise fail to reach their 15th year (Marino, 1992). A survival rate as high as 87.8% was reported for individuals with Down syndrome who had surgery for cardiovascular lesions. In contrast, a survival rate of 41.4% was reported for those who did not undergo surgery (Hijii, Fukushige, Igarashi, Takahashi, & Ueda, 1997).

Respiratory Concerns

Respiratory problems may result from the physical abnormalities observed in children with Down syndrome. For example, the small oral cavity and hypoplasia of the midfacial region create problems with airways. In addition, lungs in individuals with Down syndrome have been found to be smaller than average (Howenstein, 1992). Pneumonia continues to be one of the major causes of death, and there is an overall predisposition for contracting infectious diseases in the lower respiratory tract. Lower respiratory tract infections have also been linked to the increased mortality rates in this population. These conditions are related to the many structural and functional disorders associated with Down syndrome (Howenstein, 1992). Sinus infections and chronic rhinitis are common, and cases of bacterial pneumonia and viral infections are typically more severe in these individuals. Sleep apnea, which is characterized by snoring, restless sleep, interrupted breathing while asleep, mouth breathing, and daytime somnolence, has also been reported.

Gastrointestinal Anomalies

A number of gastrointestinal anomalies are associated with Down syndrome, but among the most common are esophageal atresia, tracheoesophageal fistula, duodenal atresia or stenosis, and Hirschsprung disease (Levy, 1992). The etiology of these conditions can be traced to malformation during embryonic development. A child with esophageal atresia may have difficulty breathing, due to the increased production of oropharyngeal secretions. Children may also exhibit a balky cough as a result of tracheoesophageal fistula. Both of these conditions are complicated by gastroesophageal reflux. Corrective surgery is available for these anomalies, and therefore early detection and intervention should prevail. Beasley, Allen, and Myers (1997) reported that despite treatment, individuals with Down syndrome who have esophageal atresia have a high mortality, perhaps due to the other physical anomalies associated with Down syndrome. There have been some claims that children with Down syndrome have difficulty with absorption of some foods (e.g., protein, fat, and vitamins). In that regard, Pueschel and colleagues (1999) found that approximately 3.8% of children with Down syndrome have celiac disease.

Dermatological Conditions

Although there is no dermatological condition that is characteristic of Down syndrome, several conditions are seen frequently (>50%) in this population. These maladies include dry skin, atopic dermatitis, fungal infections of the feet and nails, and mucosal anomalies (e.g., inflammation of the lip, scrotal tongue) (Benson & Scherbenske, 1992). Ercis, Balci, and Atakan (1996) found that 40.8% of children with Down syndrome had palmoplantar hyperkeratosis (hardened/dry skin on the palms of the hands and/or soles of the feet); 30.9% had seborrheic dermatitis (eczema, dandruff); 20% had a fissured tongue; 12.6% had cutis marmorata (discolored skin that may appear "marbled"); 11.2% had a geographic tongue (inflammation of the tongue); and 9.8% had xerosis (dry skin). With proper treatment, these conditions should not become disabling.

Other Physical Difficulties

In infancy and early childhood, ear infections are a significant problem for individuals with Down syndrome. This is an important medical concern, since frequent ear infections are known to contribute to developmental delays in language skills. The cause for the increased number of ear infections may be related to the abnormalities of the ear that are associated with Down syndrome. For this reason, hearing should be closely monitored and screened semiannually through age 8 (Downs & Balkany, 1988).

Disorders of the liver, such as hepatitis, have been linked to Down syndrome. Individuals with Down syndrome who are institutionalized are at particular risk for contracting hepatitis B. Proper hygiene and immunization may provide protection against hepatitis B. In addition, persons with Down syndrome seem to be susceptible to leukemia (Scola, 1992).

The genitourinary system may also be affected in persons with Down syndrome. Research has identified smaller-than-normal kidneys, obstructive lesions along the urinary tract, and difficulty with uric acid and creatinine clearance (Ariel & Shvil, 1992). Additional characteristics involve the genitalia. One commonly observed characteristic has been hypogenitalism, particularly with males. In addition, trisomy 21 has been found to be concomitant with other sex-related syndromes, such as Klinefelter, XYY, XXX, and Turner syndromes. At one time it was hypothesized that hypospadias and cryptorchidism were also linked to Down syndrome, but more recent findings have disproven such reports (Ariel & Shvil, 1992). In females, there may be the occurrence of hypermenorrhea or menorrhagia with the onset of puberty (Elkins, 1992). This problem may be due to a number of factors, such as hypothyroidism and/or obesity, both of which are associated with Down syndrome. Neuromuscular abnormalities are commonly reported in cases of Down syndrome, and often these contribute to the increased mortality rates within this population. Among the problems reported, subluxation and dislocation of the cervical spine, hip, and patella are the most life-threatening (Pueschel & Solga, 1992). Each of these conditions may impede physical activity by causing severe discomfort, which in turn contributes to decreased mobility and physical activity. Other orthopedic difficulties may arise from cervical spine instability in the atlanto-occipital and atlantoaxial regions (Frost et al., 1999). Persons with Down syndrome may suffer from severe scoliosis and typically have problems with collapsing flat feet and bunion deformity (Pueschel & Solga, 1992). Additional difficulties result from hypotonia, or low muscle tone, which is considered to be a major universal characteristic and is related to delays found in gross motor development.

Neurological and Psychiatric Conditions

Neurological Conditions

Down syndrome has been found to interfere with the fetal development of the central nervous system and to result in brain abnormalities. These abnormalities include a reduction in the total number of neurons throughout several cortical areas, abnormalities within the neurons themselves, and abnormalities in the ability of the neurons to communicate with each other (Florez, 1992). Although brain weight at birth is close to normal, brain weight for children with Down syndrome tends to fall in the below-average range over time. This condition may be related to a reduction in the neuronal density in cortical areas and decreased dendritic arborization (Florez, 1992). The most affected area of the brain in persons with Down syndrome is the cerebral cortex, where the reduction in the number of neurons, existence of dendritic spines, and poor synaptic connections contribute to difficulties in cognitive and learning processes (e.g., attention, information processing, integration, short- and long-term memory, and language skills) (Florez, 1992). Research using magnetic resonance imaging (MRI) to examine the brains of adults with Down syndrome and dementia indicated the presence of smaller total brain, left hippocampus, and left amygdala volumes, compared to nondemented individuals with Down syndrome (Pearlson et al., 1998). In addition, the adults with Down syndrome and dementia showed more generalized atrophy than their peers.

Other neurological problems that some children with Down syndrome face are seizure disorders. Increased rates of seizure disorders have been associated with Down syndrome, with prevalence rates reported as high as 33% in some studies (Pueschel, 1992b). Most seizures will begin before age 1 (40%) or after individuals reach their 30s (40%).

Psychiatric Conditions

Previous research by Myers (1992) showed the other psychiatric conditions that can be comorbid with Down syndrome. She found in children under the age of 20, that externalizing problems such as attention-deficit/hyperactivity disorder, oppositional defiant disorder, conduct disorder, and aggressive behaviors accounted for most of the disturbances. In persons over age 20, aggressive behaviors, major depressive disorder, and stereotypic behaviors were reported most frequently. Myers also stated that although children and adolescents with Down syndrome show lower risk for developing a psychiatric disorder than other individuals with intellectual disabilities, they are still at greater risk than the general population.

More recently, Dykens (2007) made similar observations about children with Down syndrome, again noting that they tend to be at lower risk for significant psychopathology than other groups of children with intellectual disabilities. In fact, Dykens and Kasari (1997) found that children with Down syndrome scored significantly lower on the Child Behavior Checklist than children with Prader–Willi syndrome and other nonspecific intellectual disabilities. Despite the suspected lower rates of psychopathology in individuals with Down syndrome, children and adolescents can still manifest behavioral and emotional problems. For example, Dykens, Shah, Sagun, Beck, and King (2002) found that although externalizing behavior was lower across community and clinic samples of children and adolescents with Down syndrome, internalizing behaviors were significantly higher in older adolescents ages 14–19 years, with particular increases in withdrawal. In fact, increases in withdrawal were found in 63% of community-based adolescents and 75% of clinic-referred adolescents. Coe and colleagues (1999) found that children with Down syndrome had significantly more behavior problems on parent and teacher ratings than matched controls without intellectual disabilities had; there were particular concerns in the areas of attention, conduct problems, and social withdrawal.

Finally, Einfeld, Tonge, Turner, Parmenter, and Smith (1999) examined the longitudinal course of behavior and emotional problems in young children with Down syndrome and found that these children had considerably fewer behavior problems than children with Prader–Willi syndrome and Williams syndrome. In addition, behavior problems did not change significantly over time for any of the syndromes. By contrast, McCarthy and Boyd (2001) found that the early childhood factors of presence of a psychiatric disorder and family environment did not predict adult psychopathology in young individuals with Down syndrome.

Systemic Problems

Persons with Down syndrome have a higher susceptibility to bacterial infections, malignancies, and autoimmune disturbances, as a result of a mild immune deficiency (Ugazio, Maccario, & Burgio, 1992). Further complications result from several hematological abnormalities that are unique to Down syndrome. These irregularities include transient myelodysplasia in infancy (the presentation of which resembles congenital leukemia), red cell macrocytosis, and increased susceptibility to leukemia (Lubin, Cahn, & Scott, 1992). At one time, Down syndrome was felt to be caused by generalized endocrine failure; however, the majority of persons with Down syndrome do not suffer from endocrine dysfunction (Pueschel & Bier, 1992). On the other hand, the prevalence rate for endocrine disturbances is greater for those with Down syndrome than for the general population. Among the most common findings are problems related to thyroid functioning, specifically hypothyroidism (Pueschel & Bier, 1992). This condition may predispose individuals with Down syndrome to become overweight, particularly when it is paired with the presence of hypotonia.

Mortality

The greatest likelihood of death resulting from medical complications, such as congenital anomalies, circulatory problems, and respiratory illness, occurs during the first year of life, with ages 1–9 being the largest age group at risk for early death (Sadovnick & Baird, 1992). With advances in medical treatment and early intervention for such difficulties, survival rates should improve in the future.

When Down originally characterized this syndrome in 1866, he commented on the shorter life expectancy for these individuals. This phenomenon held true until the 1940s, when average life expectancy rose from approximately 9 years to 12 years of age. It was estimated in the 1990s that about 44% of the children born between 1952 and 1981 would live to be at least 60 years old (Carr, 1995; Sadovnick & Baird, 1992). More recent estimates of life expectancy for males and females with Down syndrome were 61.1 years and 57.8 years, respectively (Glasson et al., 2003). Although the shorter life expectancy was at one time accounted for by the congenital heart defects that often accompany Down syndrome, this reason has not been substantiated in research comparing individuals with Down syndrome who did not have heart defects to a matched group with intellectual disabilities but not Down syndrome (Sadovnick & Baird, 1992). Strauss and Eyman (1996) noted in their large sample of individuals with Down syndrome that up to age 35, mortality rates were comparable to those for a sample of individuals with intellectual disabilities; however, after age 35, the mortality rates for the group with Down syndrome increased at a greater rate than for the group with intellectual disabilities.

DEVELOPMENTAL COURSE

Although the majority of children with Down syndrome display delayed motor function, cognitive development, and language acquisition, there are individual variations in rate and level of achievement. Children with Down syndrome experience a period of rapid growth and development during their first 3 years of life, much as other children do; however, their special needs may require some environmental supports in order for them to achieve their developmental milestones. Developmental stages generally mimic those found in normal children in the domains of sensorimotor functioning, conservation, and mastery of space, time, and moral judgment, although these skills are acquired at a slower rate (Hodapp & Zigler, 1990). This finding was supported by the work of Tingey, Mortensen, Matheson, and Doret (1991), who found that infants and young children with Down syndrome were more similar to normal children on the Personal, Social, and Adaptive domains of the Battelle Developmental Inventory, and less similar in the Communication and Cognitive domains. This discrepancy was found to widen as the children's age approached 36 months.

Temperament

Biological studies have found that children with Down syndrome may be less reactive to novelty, and thus may appear more passive or less generally reactive, than other children of similar age (Ganiban, Wagner, & Cicchetti, 1990). In many other regards, however, children with Down syndrome display the same temperamental variability as any other children. Zickler, Morrow, and Bull (1998) found that infants with Down syndrome were rated as more active, less intense, and more distractible, and tended to demonstrate more approach behaviors, when compared to typically developing infants. When maternal ratings of temperamental qualities for children with Down syndrome are compared to maternal ratings for nondisabled children, the descriptions appear to be relatively similar. However, mothers of a group with Down syndrome have reported lower adaptability and a greater need for stimulation for their children (Vaughn, Contreras, & Seiter, 1994). A study of older children and adolescents with Down syndrome, using maternal and teacher ratings of temperamental characteristics, found that mothers perceived their children as less active, more predictable, more positive in mood, less persistent, and more distractible (Gunn & Cuskelly, 1991). Mothers and teachers agreed on which children were viewed as easy or difficult overall, but the reports of individual characteristics constituting these categories varied for the two sets of raters. Ratekin (1996) found that children with Down syndrome were rated by their mothers as being higher in approachability, distractibility, and mood, but lower in persistence, than typically developing children were rated by their mothers.

Cognitive Development

Given that most children with Down syndrome suffer from some degree of intellectual disability (mild, moderate, severe, or profound), the degree of cognitive development that may be evident depends in part on how severe the cognitive deficits may be. The difficulty of using many standardized tests to evaluate a child with intellectual disabilities, and the problems with obtaining longitudinal data, make research in this area difficult to generalize to a population that is known for its heterogeneity. Although standardized intelligence tests have been found to be useful in classifying an individual as having intellectual disability or not, they are of more limited utility in discriminating between the various levels of intellectual disabilities (Kamphaus, 1993). For example, children with mosaicism have been found to score 10–30 points higher on IQ measures than those with trisomy 21, and have demonstrated normal visual-perceptual skills as well (Fishler & Koch, 1991); however, Wishart (1995) cautions that, generally speaking, there is no fixed "ceiling" of cognitive development for individuals with Down syndrome, and that learning for this population should continue well beyond adolescence.

Perhaps the most consistent finding regarding cognitive development in children with Down syndrome is that there is a general slowing, or perhaps decline, in their rate of development as they get older (Carr, 2005). Early accounts of Down syndrome portrayed a general decline in IQ over the lifespan. Carr (1995) summarized this research and found that there is actually little evidence that IQ, memory, or practical skills deteriorate significantly before the age of 50. In addition, fewer than 50% of individuals with Down syndrome show clear signs of dementia; however, many individuals with Down syndrome who live to be over

age 40 do show the characteristic features of Alzheimer disease in the central nervous system. These features consist of cortical atrophy, neurofibrillary tangles, and neuritic plaques (Lai, 1992; Mufson, Benzing, & Kordower, 1995). Visser, Aldenkamp, van Huffelen, and Kuilman (1997) found an increasing prevalence rate for dementia in a group with Down syndrome. After age 40, prevalence rates were about 11% between ages 40 and 49, but increased up to 77% between ages 60 and 69. Other studies have observed that adults with Down syndrome over the age of 50 are at substantial risk for the development of dementia associated with Alzheimer disease (e.g., Holland, Hon, Huppert, & Stevens, 2000; see Zigman & Lott, 2007, for a review).

Efforts to find a genetic link between Down syndrome and Alzheimer disease have had mixed results, with some indication that a gene for Alzheimer disease may be located on the long arm of chromosome 21. The dementia resulting from Alzheimer disease is difficult to establish in persons with intellectual disabilities, especially in severe cases; therefore, clinical studies attempting to establish the presence of dementia in Down syndrome populations are difficult to carry out. Moreover, hypothyroidism, poor nutrition, and depression may all masquerade as dementia, and all are common problems for persons with Down syndrome. This scenario makes differential diagnosis hard to accomplish. The clinical dementia associated with Alzheimer disease does, however, become evident in persons with Down syndrome who live to be 50 or older. The symptomatic presentation is essentially the same as that for groups without Down syndrome, but it may appear to be somewhat exaggerated, due to the physical and cognitive features already associated with Down syndrome (Lai, 1992).

Language Development

Language is closely linked to cognitive ability, in that the rate and degree of language attainment will depend heavily on the amount of cognitive deficit that exists. Some factors that lead to delays in language acquisition are related to the physical characteristics associated with Down syndrome. Problems with otitis media, cognitive dysfunction (e.g., memory, attention, arousal), and visual disturbances may impede a child's ability to gather auditory and visual cues concerning language. Compared to children without intellectual disabilities, children with Down syndrome acquire language skills more slowly than other motor or cognitive skills. In addition, language development fails to proceed at a consistent pace, but occurs in spurts, with a great deal of development occurring before the age of 7 (Fowler, 1988). This discrepancy can first be seen in infancy and grows larger as children become older. For example, although the rate of vocabulary learning in children with Down syndrome is typically consistent with their developmental age, it does not progress at a rate that is consistent with their other cognitive skills or consistent in relation to that of typically developing peers (Miller, 1995; for reviews, see Abbeduto, Warren, & Conners, 2007, and Roberts, Price, & Malkin, 2007). Recent studies have examined significant predictors of language outcomes in children with developmental disabilities and in children with Down syndrome in particular, and have found that parental responding significantly predicted language skills (Brady, Marquis, Fleming, & McLean, 2004; Yoder & Warren, 2004). More specifically, language production appears to be more impaired than language comprehension. Within expressive language, the grammatical/syntactical components of language rather than the lexical or nonverbal aspects seem to show the greatest impairments (Fowler, 1988; Miller, 1995). Children with Down syndrome have been described as having a specific language impairment characterized by fewer total words used in an utterance, fewer number of different words used, and less than average length of utterance (Chapman, Seung, Schwartz, & Bird, 1998). When adaptive behaviors were assessed with the Vineland Adaptive Behavior Scales in a group of children with Down syndrome from 1 to 11½ years of age, a relative weakness in communication (compared with daily living and socialization skills) was found (Dykens, Hodapp, & Evans, 1994). Within the communication domain, there was more deficiency in expressive language than in receptive language. This finding is supported by Miller's (1995) work. More recently, an examination of the linguistic and cognitive profile of individuals with

Down syndrome found that receptive and expressive language skills, along with theory of mind, were more severely impaired than in individuals with fragile X syndrome (Abbeduto et al., 2001).

Social Development

Because of the motor, perceptual, cognitive, and language delays that children with Down syndrome exhibit, their ability to gain social competence may also be diminished. For this reason, they may seek out developmentally matched rather than age-matched children for peer interactions. Play development has been reported to follow developmental trajectories as well (Beeghly, Perry, & Cicchetti, 1989). Earlier hypotheses that children with Down syndrome are more sociable than other children with intellectual disabilities, and that this feature is a defining quality of the whole group, have not been definitively supported by research, although some gender differences in sociability have been described. Ruskin, Kasari, Mundy, and Sigman (1994) found that young children with Down syndrome paid more attention to people during a social interaction paradigm than did mental-age-matched controls, demonstrating a greater focus of attention to the social cues provided. However, when presented with ambiguous stimuli paired with either positive or negative facial expressions from their parents, toddlers with Down syndrome were found to display significantly less appropriate responses (e.g., they responded with positive affect to negative expression) than did mental-age-matched controls (Knieps, Walden, & Baxter, 1994). Therefore, although children with Down syndrome may be as socially responsive as other children, they fail to learn socially referenced cues. These social-cognitive skills are essential to interpersonal skills and making friendships.

In a study on social-cognitive understanding in children with Down syndrome, Wishart (2007) found that in certain learning contexts (e.g., collaborative learning), the children with Down syndrome worked alongside other children, but engaged in more parallel working than collaborative working on a shared task. In addition, Wishart found relative weaknesses in emotional recognition in children with Down syndrome. Similarly,

Landry, Miller-Loncar, and Swank (1998) found that children with Down syndrome have a more difficult time than control children transferring goal-directed play skills used with their mothers in a joint play session to independent play situations. In other words, children with Down syndrome benefit from structured (directed) play, but have trouble using these skills on their own and may continue to need structured play time.

Growth and Motor Development

Individual factors (e.g., cardiac and skeletal problems, hypotonia, obesity, vision and hearing disturbances, and perceptual problems) may have an impact on the growth and motor development of any child with Down syndrome. Aspects of significance are height and weight. Prenatally, fetuses with Down syndrome have been found to be smaller than fetuses without disabilities. The largest deficit appears between birth and 36 months of age, where statistical differences have been found between children with Down syndrome (both males and females) and normal controls, with the children with Down syndrome being smaller than average. Potential factors affecting growth in infancy may include prematurity, cardiac disease, and genetics. During middle childhood, growth rates become closer to normal, although adolescents experience smaller pubertal growth spurts as well as delayed onset of menses for females (i.e., later than the typical onset of 10–14 years) (Elkins, 1992). They will, however, have normal development of secondary sex characteristics. By adulthood, individuals with Down syndrome are typically two standard deviations below normal in height (Cronk & Anneren, 1992). Individuals with Down syndrome are commonly found to be overweight because of excessive weight gain during infancy and childhood (Cronk & Anneren, 1992; Rubin, Rimmer, Chicoine, Braddock, & McGuire, 1998). The etiology of this weight gain has not yet been determined conclusively, though there are some indications that it may be a factor of hypothyroidism and/or hypotonia. Although their metabolic rates do not differ from normal, individuals with Down syndrome have less body mass and slower growth, and therefore require fewer calories (Pipes, 1992).

In general, motor development is delayed in children with Down syndrome, with the most frequently cited causal factors being the hypotonia and hyperflexia that can be seen in almost all of these children. There are individual variations in both the qualitative and quantitative aspects of motor skills. Dunst (1988) concluded that sensorimotor development in children with Down syndrome, despite their slower rate of development, was more like that of children without intellectual disabilities. In a cross-sectional study of 6- to 16-year olds with Down syndrome, using a range of manual tasks, Thombs and Sugden (1991) found evidence for an increased use of precision grips among older children. In addition, the older children were found to be faster on the speeded tasks. The authors concluded that on measures of speed, strategies, and types of grip, there are general developmental advances across age groups. Children with Down syndrome may display difficulty with gross and fine motor skills, balance, posture, strength, and flexibility (Brandt, 1996; Jobling, 1998), and subsequent interventions should be tailored to the children's individual needs, based on their medical and health conditions. An excellent review of the literature on motor development in children with Down syndrome was provided by Block (1991) approximately 20 years ago, and it continues to be pertinent to the present.

COGNITIVE, EMOTIONAL, AND BEHAVIORAL PRESENTATION

Cognitive Presentation

As noted earlier, a wide range of cognitive abilities can be observed in individuals with Down syndrome, creating a heterogeneous population. Interestingly, females have been found to have higher intellectual functioning than males in both childhood and adulthood (Carr, 1995). Many arguments have been made regarding this finding, but to date there are no established conclusions about the presence of gender differences. When compared to other groups of children with developmental disabilities, those with Down syndrome may not appear to be that different in the classroom. One study comparing the cognitive skills of adolescents with Down syndrome to those of children with cerebral palsy or nonspecific intellectual disabilities found no significant differences between any of the groups (Smith & Phillips, 1992). The group with Down syndrome did fail to show progress in language acquisition on a second assessment, but they also displayed some gains in cognition and copying skills, compared to the group with nonspecific intellectual disabilities. Other cognitive deficits noted in children with Down syndrome include limited memory functioning (particularly for spatial stimuli), reduced task persistence and distractibility, slowed reaction time and information-processing speed, and difficulty with reasoning and judgment (Gibson, 1991).

As noted above, almost all of the literature on Down syndrome discusses some type of language difficulty, particularly expressive language impairments, as constituting a hallmark of this disorder. Children with Down syndrome have been found to have delayed acquisition of language skills that is not commensurate with their mental age. This deficit may be due to the presence of central auditory processing abnormalities. For example, dichotic listening studies have found that individuals with Down syndrome have reversed hemispheric dominance (right- rather than left-hemisphere dominance) for processing speech (Dahle & Baldwin, 1992). Research using volumetric MRI measures has found that individuals with Down syndrome have a smaller left planum temporale (a region associated with language functioning) than controls (Frangou et al., 1997). The implications of a smaller planum in individuals with Down syndrome are still unclear, however, as the authors were unable to find a direct relationship between size and performance on their language testing.

Due to their neurological abnormalities, individuals with Down syndrome will display reduced short-term memory and will have greater difficulty recalling auditory than visual information (Florez, 1992). Difficulties in language development involve (1) an asynchrony in language production relative to language understanding and other cognitive skills; (2) an onset of productive deficits that coincides with vocabulary growth; (3) a slowness in the development of syntactic skills; and (4) heterogeneous language development for the population (Florez, 1992). In addition, difficulties with articulation may be exacerbated by hypotonia of facial muscles and related congenital abnormalities of the oral–peripheral region.

Emotional Presentation

As noted earlier, individuals with intellectual disabilities demonstrate greater susceptibility to stressors than the general population and can show a wide range of emotional expressions. The developmental delays and language impairments associated with intellectual disabilities may contribute to the finding that individuals with Down syndrome are at slightly greater risk for emotional problems than the general population (Myers, 1992). Children with Down syndrome will experience challenges in school, occupational, and social functioning, and these challenges may be manifested as mood disturbances (anxiety or depression), physical complaints, social withdrawal, or work inhibition (Myers, 1992). Although depression in children with Down syndrome has not been well documented in the literature, adults have been found to exhibit depression to a greater extent than children. The prevalence of major affective (mood) disorders in adults with intellectual disabilities has been estimated to be about 1–3.5% (Myers, 1992).

Behavioral Presentation

Cuskelly and Dadds (1992) performed a study of mother, father, and teacher ratings of behavior problems in children with Down syndrome compared to their siblings. On the Revised Behavior Problem Checklist, all raters reported that the group with Down syndrome exhibited significantly more total behavior problems and significantly more attention/immaturity problems than their siblings. There were also significant gender differences as viewed by the raters. Mothers reported the same level of problem behaviors for each gender, whereas fathers reported that the girls displayed more problems, and teachers experienced greater problems with boys. In an interesting follow-up study, Cuskelly and Gunn (1993) found that mothers of children with Down syndrome reported significantly more conduct problems in the female siblings than mothers who did not have a child with Down syndrome reported in their daughters. This finding may indicate that mothers of children with disabilities may have some misperceptions regarding "typical" behavior. It may also show that siblings of children with Down syndrome, especially girls, could experience greater adjustment problems and should be considered to be at risk for showing a variety of behavioral difficulties.

KEY ASSESSMENT ISSUES AND TOOLS

The diagnosis of Down syndrome is typically made at or before birth (35%), or within the first 2 years of life (46%), although there are some cases where a diagnosis has been made after the third year (Quine & Rutter, 1994). For this reason, most children enter preschool with a diagnosis. However, as Quine and Rutter (1994) found, parents are often not provided with detailed explanations of their children's impairments and the associated features of these. Health care professionals and school personnel should be aware of the need for education that parents and families may require to be informed participants in their children's medical care and related treatments.

Often parental reports constitute a chief source of assessment information regarding the developmental status of children with disabilities such as Down syndrome. When rating scales and interview data are being employed, estimates of a child's functioning must sometimes rely on the judgment of the parent who completes the forms. In a study comparing maternal and professional estimates of developmental status among children with disabilities, it was concluded that mothers provided higher estimates of ability across all developmental domains (Sexton, Thompson, Perez, & Rheams, 1990). Additional findings showed that maternal and professional ratings were highly correlated, with children's intellectual functioning being the most significant variable contributing to this correlation. In other words, mothers and professionals tended to agree more closely when children's intellectual functioning was closer to average.

Cognitive Assessment

In addition to the general intellectual deficits that are present in most children with Down syndrome, specific deficits have been described. For example, children with Down syndrome were found to exhibit a general deficit in their sequential processing, although selected deficits in simultaneous processing have also been noted (Hodapp et al., 1992). In general, variability has been found within this population, and failure to engage in tasks and response variability are factors that can add to the instability of findings (Wishart & Duffy, 1990).

At present, a number of well-standardized measures exist that can aide the examiner in gaining a reliable estimate of a child's intellectual functioning. A description of these tasks is beyond the scope of this chapter, but suffice it to say that most contemporary measures of cognitive functioning are multidimensional in nature. For example, the different dimensions provided by the Stanford–Binet Intelligence Scales, Fifth Edition (Roid, 2003) will provide not only the opportunity to gain an overall estimate of intellectual functioning (IQ), but an initial breakdown of specific cognitive functions as well (Fluid Reasoning, Knowledge, Quantitative Reasoning, Visual–Spatial Processing, Working Memory). Knowing the level *and* pattern of cognitive abilities should provide additional information with respect to describing the cognitive topography of Down syndrome, as well as the profile of relative strengths and weaknesses that may be present. This profile of abilities can also be complemented by more in-depth assessment using neuropsychological testing procedures in an effort to examine the specific cognitive dimensions in more detail (various executive functions, different kinds of memory, etc.).

Behavioral Assessment

There are no characteristic behaviors associated with Down syndrome. Rather, the full range of behaviors seen in nondisabled children may be exhibited by children with Down syndrome. Obstinacy, aggression, withdrawal, and self-injurious behaviors are among the most frequently seen behaviors, and they are also the ones that elicit the most frustration from parents and educators. Behavior management techniques such as positive and negative reinforcement have been shown to be effective in decreasing problem behaviors and increasing target behaviors. In a study using descriptive analysis to ascertain the function of problem behaviors in a small sample of children with intellectual disabilities, contingent reinforcement and teaching functionally equivalent behaviors were found to be effective in reducing problem behaviors for these children (Lalli, Browder, Mace, & Brown, 1993). In addition, because the students were required to communicate their requests, they concurrently improved their verbal skills.

Medical Assessment and Intervention

Approximately 20 years ago, the National Down Syndrome Society (NDSS) sponsored a conference on health care in Down syndrome, where suggestions were made for important medical interventions (Lott & McCoy, 1992). It was recommended that during the neonatal period and early infancy, there should be an attempt to establish chromosomal karyotype, communicate the diagnosis to parents, and refer parents to available support groups. In addition, several types of screenings were recommended, based on the known health concerns for children with Down syndrome. These included screening for cataracts, blockages in the gastrointestinal tract, congenital heart disease, thyroid dysfunction, and hearing problems. It was advised that these exams should continue annually into early adulthood. The NDSS also advocated enrolling these children in early intervention programs. These recommendations have set the stage for current clinical practice standards, with many of the original recommendations remaining in force.

During the preschool and school years, early efforts should focus on remediating common orthopedic problems (e.g., bunions, severe flat feet, dislocated hips) and dental problems, as well as on providing additional vaccinations (e.g., against influenza, pneumococcal infections, and hepatitis B) for at-risk children. Special behavioral programs may be beneficial to improve self-help skills, communication, and nutrition, as well as to ameliorate problems related to aggression, self-injurious behavior, and school adjustment. For example, some children with Down syndrome display food behavior problems, such as throwing or hoarding food (Pipes, 1992). Psychoeducational evaluation and remediation should also take place as early as possible, with routine developmental surveillance being provided throughout the school years.

Over the years, numerous treatments have been sought to help "cure" various dysfunctions caused by Down syndrome. Whereas some of these treatments have sought to improve intellectual functioning and others have attempted to alleviate physical conditions, they are considered unconventional, and practitioners may wish to familiarize themselves with these in order to discuss them competently with parents who show an interest in these therapies. Some of the more popular of these are as follows: (1) pituitary extract, given to improve intellectual and social development; (2) glutamic acid; (3) thyroid hormone, given to improve intellectual functioning; (4) 5-hydroxytryptophan, given to improve behavioral and motoric functioning; (5) dimethyl sulfoxide, given to improve behavior and learning; (6) sicca cells (fetal cell therapy), given to increase intellectual functioning and growth; (7) vitamins, minerals, enzymes, and hormones, administered to treat intellectual disabilities; and (8) facial plastic surgery, intended to improve characteristic features (for detailed reviews, see Pueschel, 1992a; Roizen, 2005). Parents may be willing to try these alternative therapies, despite evidence that demonstrates their lack of efficacy. Often parents are influenced by positive expectations of improvement and may attribute any change to the therapy. However, at all times, the health and best interest of a child should remain the primary focus.

OPTIONS FOR TREATMENT OF PSYCHOSOCIAL, EDUCATIONAL, AND EMOTIONAL PROBLEMS

Infants with Down syndrome commonly display delays in gross and fine motor, cognitive, personal, social, emotional, and language development (Dmitriev, 1988). These areas may be improved with training, and certain characteristics of children with Down syndrome facilitate such education. These factors include the following: (1) Infants with Down syndrome are more like normal infants than not and will respond to social gestures; (2) they will respond positively to physical assistance (e.g., shaping) while learning; (3) they are reinforced by their own successes; and (4) they have higher receptive than expressive language skills and good visual discrimination (Dmitriev, 1988). Interventions should also include a child's family, since there are some indications that maternal responsiveness to a preschooler with Down syndrome may be improved by the existence of available maternal supports (Lojkasek, Goldbert, Marcovitch, & MacGregor, 1990). The effectiveness of early intervention programs for children with disabilities has not gone without debate, since available research is often plagued by methodological flaws. Shonkoff, Hauser-Cram, Krauss, and Upshur (1992) reviewed the existing literature on the effects of early intervention services, and concluded that most programs for infants and toddlers with disabilities are only moderately effective in producing short-term benefits as measured by traditional cognitive or developmental measures. However, other studies suggest that longer, more intense interventions may be more effective in the age range from birth to 5 years. Not only has functioning been found to be closer to typical development with early infancy training programs, but there are indications that early entry into intervention programs is more cost-effective than later entry into such programs (Warfield, 1994). In other words, the earlier that treatment for developmental skills is available for infants, the better.

Dmitriev (1988) has advocated an interdisciplinary training model for effectively teaching children with Down syndrome—a model in which medical, educational, and parental participation is essential. The educational program should also include parent training in behavior management and developmental concerns. Developing a sequence of tasks and skills to be obtained will provide parents with a hierarchy of skills required for their child to master certain developmental goals. In one study, Wishart (1991) found that, compared to nondisabled infants, those with Down syndrome made inefficient use of the cognitive abilities that they did have and would often remain passive even when a task was within their ability level. The implications are that the delayed developmental rate seen in children with Down syndrome may be due to an interaction between inadequate

motivation levels and deficient learning. Fewell and Oelwein (1991) examined the effectiveness of the Model Preschool Program, which focused on children with Down syndrome and developmental delay. They found that of the six skill areas emphasized (gross motor skills, fine motor skills, cognition, receptive communication, expressive communication, and social/self-help skills), the children with Down syndrome made gains in all areas, with the exception of gross motor skills on the Classroom Assessment of Development Skills. However, on the Battelle Developmental Inventory, expressive language in addition to fine and gross motor skills failed to show developmental improvements. Nonetheless, the project presented evidence that early intervention could be successful in some areas of development.

Behavioral interventions designed to incorporate functional communication training have been shown to be effective (Arndorfer, Miltenberger, Woster, Rortvedt, & Gaffaney, 1994). Although the number of families involved in this study was limited, the researchers utilized behavioral interviews, direct observation, and experimental analysis to determine the functions of the children's problem behaviors. The researchers then used functional communication training as an intervention. This procedure involved teaching a child a response that resulted in the same desired consequence as a problem behavior. Others have endorsed the use of naturalistic teaching to gain acquisition of targeted skills (Fox & Hanline, 1993). A methodology of this nature would involve using the natural environment, natural consequences, and child initiation to teach new tasks. However, both approaches need to be researched empirically in order to determine whether these methods are truly successful. In another experiment designed to increase vocal responsiveness in preschoolers with Down syndrome, positive reinforcement (PR) was found to be successful (Drash, Raver, Murrin, & Tudor, 1989). Children were trained using PR alone, PR combined with dimming of lights, and PR combined with visual screening. All conditions were successful in increasing vocal responsiveness, with the two methods combining PR with other techniques producing the most improvement. It should be noted that a commonly used reinforcer (food) was not employed, in an effort to create a more socially valid paradigm. The results indicate that behavioral management techniques may be employed successfully to teach language skills. A small-scale study with three school-age children focused on increasing phonological awareness found that training could improve literacy skills (Kennedy & Flynn, 2003). Specific skills trained included alliteration detection, phoneme isolation, spelling of orthographically regular words, and rhyme detection.

Skills that preschool programs should concentrate on in order to increase independence include separation from parents, eating and drinking, handwashing, toileting, gross and fine motor skills, social skills, and language acquisition (see Love, 1988, and Oelwein, 1988, for model instructional plans). Cuskelly, Zhang, and Gilmore (1998) advocate training self-regulation skills, such as the ability to delay gratification and mastery motivation, early in development to help foster greater independence later in adulthood. Principles of applied behavior analysis are often successful when instructors are attempting to teach such tasks as feeding, toileting, cessation of habitual tongue protrusion, and gross and fine motor skills. Since the developmental age of children with Down syndrome often lags behind their chronological age, it is necessary to maintain an awareness of which activities a child is ready to perform successfully.

Placement in a regular classroom may also improve academic attainment in children with Down syndrome. One study of academic attainment in children with Down syndrome ages 6–14 years found that although cognitive ability level had the greatest impact on achievement, type of school attended was the next largest contributing factor (Sloper, Cunningham, Turner, & Knussen, 1990). Additional factors influencing academic attainment were gender (female), paternal locus-of-control ratings, and chronological age. In a naturalistic classroom setting, 3-year-olds with Down syndrome were compared to normal 2- and 3-year-olds, as well as to another group with mild to moderate intellectual disabilities, on some classroom behaviors (Bronson, Hauser-Cram, & Warfield, 1995). Both groups of children with developmental disabilities were found to perform lower on task mastery behaviors than either the typical 2-year-olds or 3-year-olds. The developmentally disabled groups completed only half as many tasks successfully as the typical children. In addition, both groups had higher rates of interaction with the teacher (i.e., more frequent demands for assistance). Compared to the other children with intellectual disabilities, the children with Down syndrome actually made fewer requests of the teacher and peers, but their requests were more successful. These findings indicate that children with Down syndrome may benefit from working within a buddy system, given that they experience lower task mastery but relatively advanced social interaction skills. Some research has indicated that developmental gains in children with Down syndrome are not associated with time spent in an integrated classroom, and in fact that slightly higher gains in expressive language are made in nonintegrated settings (Fewell & Oelwein, 1990).

The use of computers to teach language skills has been advocated as another teaching tool (Meyers, 1988). In this forum, the computer provides structure and scaffolding for the acquisition of spoken and written language skills such as vocabulary, spelling, comprehension, and sentence construction. Language intervention, as advocated by Miller (1995), should be family-based. Parents and siblings should encourage communication about daily activities and events, and should be responsive to a child's interests and initiation of communication.

Beginning in adolescence, the child's emotional health should be carefully monitored for symptoms of depression. Individuals with Down syndrome are at increased risk for developing major depression and have also been noted to develop learned helplessness (Harris, 1988). Activities to build self-esteem and self-concept, as well as to provide training in vocational matters, should be initiated during middle or high school.

Parents and families of children with Down syndrome may be in need of support services as well. These children, as a result of their cognitive and physical limitations, may require a great amount of parental care. Barnett and Boyce (1995) found that parents of children with Down syndrome devoted more time to child care and spent less time in social activities than parents without a disabled child. Both mothers and fathers made accommodations in the amount of time they spent doing daily household activities. Single parents, who were not sampled in this study, may therefore have even greater difficulty responding to the needs of children with Down syndrome. As mentioned earlier, the siblings of children with Down syndrome may be at risk for developing behavior problems and adjustment disorders. Another study that examined ratings of parental stress found that parents of a child with Down syndrome reported more stress than comparison families did (Cuskelly, Chant, & Hayes, 1998). For these reasons, it is important to provide these families with such resources as parent and sibling support groups.

ADOLESCENCE AND ADULTHOOD OUTCOMES

As a child with Down syndrome enters young adulthood, concerns regarding vocation and independent living emerge. Prior to the implementation of Public Law 94-142, the Education for All Handicapped Children Act of 1975, vocational training was not considered to be an integral part of service for adolescents with disabilities. Individuals should be prepared to function as independently as possible in society, and therefore should receive training in vocational and independent living skills. A greater range of opportunities currently exists for adolescents with Down syndrome as they approach completion of their educational careers. Sheltered workshops and other less restricted job sites are common places of eventual employment. On-the-job training may be provided through vocational schools, job coaches, community colleges, or sheltered workshops (Renzaglia & Hutchins, 1988). Additional counseling should focus on further development of social skills, on sexuality, and on separation from parents. Brown (1996) advocates training adaptive work and social behaviors early in development, to help prepare individuals for independent living later in life. Reproductive counseling for females is especially important, given the risk of producing a child with Down syndrome or congenital anomalies (Elkins, 1992). Most importantly, individuals with Down syndrome should be viewed as people first, with

the same desires as nondisabled individuals for developing relationships and becoming productive adults. Assistance should focus on the development of well-rounded persons who can live in the least restrictive environment possible—whether that means independently in the community, in supervised semi-independent settings, or within group homes.

CONCLUSION

Down syndrome is a genetic disorder with a distinct physical phenotype but a heterogeneous presentation of learning, behavioral, and medical conditions. It is the most common genetic cause of intellectual disabilities, and some degree of cognitive impairment is present in all individuals with Down syndrome. Despite a number of medical comorbidities, ranging from cardiac defects to dermatological conditions, improvements in management and intervention have extended the average lifespan of these individuals. Depending on adaptive behavior functioning and cognitive ability, individuals with Down syndrome can achieve a degree of independence within a supportive environment.

REFERENCES

Abbeduto, L., Pavetto, M., Kesin, E., Weissman, M. D., Karadottir, S., O'Brien, A., et al. (2001). The linguistic and cognitive profile of Down syndrome: Evidence from a comparison with fragile X syndrome. *Down Syndrome Research and Practice, 7,* 9–15.

Abbeduto, L., Warren, S. F., & Conners, F. A. (2007). Language development in Down syndrome: From the prelinguistic period to the acquisition of literacy. *Mental Retardation and Developmental Disabilities Research Reviews, 13,* 247–261.

Ariel, I., & Shvil, Y. (1992). Genitourinary system. In S. M. Pueschel & J. K. Pueschel (Eds.), *Biomedical concerns in persons with Down syndrome.* Baltimore: Brookes.

Arndorfer, R. E., Miltenberger, R. G., Woster, S. H., Rortvedt, A. K., & Gaffaney, T. (1994). Home-based descriptive and experimental analysis of problem behaviors in children. *Topics in Early Childhood Special Education, 14,* 64–87.

Barnett, W. S., & Boyce, G. C. (1995). Effects of children with Down syndrome on parents' activities. *American Journal on Mental Retardation, 100,* 115–127.

Beasley, S. W., Allen, M., & Myers, N. (1997). The effects of Down syndrome and other chromosomal abnormalities on survival and management in oesophageal atresia. *Pediatric Surgery International, 12*, 550–551.

Beeghly, M., Perry, B. W., & Cicchetti, D. (1989). Structural and affective dimensions of play development in young children with Down syndrome. *International Journal of Behavioral Development, 12*, 257–277.

Benson, P. M., & Scherbenske, J. M. (1992). In S. M. Pueschel & J. K. Pueschel (Eds.), *Biomedical concerns in persons with Down syndrome*. Baltimore: Brookes.

Block, M. E. (1991). Motor development in children with Down syndrome: A review of the literature. *Adapted Physical Activity Quarterly, 8*, 179–209.

Brady, N. C., Marquis, J., Fleming, K., McLean, L. (2004). Prelinguistic predictors of language growth in children with developmental disabilities. *Journal of Speech, Language, and Hearing Research, 47*, 663–677.

Brandt, B. R. (1996). Impaired tactual perception in children with Down's syndrome. *Scandinavian Journal of Psychology, 37*, 312–316.

Bronson, M. B., Hauser-Cram, P., & Warfield, M. E. (1995). Classroom behaviors of preschool children with and without developmental disabilities. *Journal of Applied Developmental Psychology, 16*, 371–390.

Carr, J. (1995). *Down's syndrome: Children growing up*. Cambridge, UK: Cambridge University Press.

Carr, J. (2005). Stability and change in cognitive ability over the life span: A comparison of populations with and without Down's syndrome. *Journal of Intellectual Disability Research, 49*, 915–928.

Catalano, R. A. (1992). Ophthalmologic concerns. In S. M. Pueschel & J. K. Pueschel (Eds.), *Biomedical concerns in persons with Down syndrome*. Baltimore: Brookes.

Chapman, R. S., Seung, H., Schwartz, S. E., & Bird, E. K. (1998). Language skills of children and adolescents with Down syndrome: II. Production deficits. *Journal of Speech, Language, and Hearing Research, 41*, 861–873.

Cocchi, G., Gualdi, S., Bower, C., Halliday, J., Jonsson, B., Myrelid, A., et al. (2010). International trends of Down syndrome 1993–2004: Births in relation to maternal age and terminations of pregnancies. *Birth Defects Research, Part A, 88*, 747–749.

Coe, D. A., Matson, J. L., Russell, D. W., Slifer, K. J., Capone, G. T., Baglio, C., et al. (1999). Behavior problems of with Down syndrome and life events. *Journal of Autism and Developmental Disorders, 29*, 149–156.

Coleman, M. (1988). Medical care of children and adults with Down syndrome. In V. Dmitriev & P. L. Oelwein (Eds.), *Advances in Down syndrome*. Seattle, WA: Special Child.

Cronk, C. E., & Anneren, G. (1992). Growth. In S. M. Pueschel & J. K. Pueschel (Eds.), *Biomedical concerns in persons with Down syndrome*. Baltimore: Brookes.

Cuskelly, M., Chant, D., & Hayes, A. (1998). Behaviour problems in the siblings of children with Down syndrome: Associations with family responsibilities and parental stress. *International Journal of Disability, Development and Education, 45*, 295–311.

Cuskelly, M., & Dadds, M. (1992). Behavioural problems in children with Down's syndrome and their siblings. *Journal of Child Psychology and Psychiatry, 33*, 749–761.

Cuskelly, M., & Gunn, P. (1993). Maternal reports of behavior of siblings of children with Down syndrome. *American Journal on Mental Retardation, 97*, 521–529.

Cuskelly, M., Zhang, A., & Gilmore, L. (1998). The importance of self-regulation in children with Down syndrome. *International Journal of Disability, Development and Education, 45*, 331–341.

Dahle, A. J., & Baldwin, R. L. (1992). Audiologic and otolaryngologic concerns. In S. M. Pueschel & J. K. Pueschel (Eds.), *Biomedical concerns in persons with Down syndrome*. Baltimore: Brookes.

Dmitriev, V. (1988). Programs for children with Down syndrome and other developmental delays: Development of an educational model. In V. Dmitriev & P. L. Oelwein (Eds.), *Advances in Down syndrome*. Seattle, WA: Special Child.

Downs, M. P., & Balkany, T. J. (1988). Otologic problems and hearing impairment in Down syndrome. In V. Dmitriev & P. L. Oelwein (Eds.), *Advances in Down syndrome*. Seattle, WA: Special Child.

Drash, P. W., Raver, S. A., Murrin, M. R., & Tudor, R. M. (1989). Three procedures for increasing vocal response to therapist prompt in infants and children with Down syndrome. *American Journal on Mental Retardation, 94*, 64–73.

Dunst, C. J. (1988). Sensorimotor development of infants with Down syndrome. In V. Dmitriev & P. L. Oelwein (Eds.), *Advances in Down syndrome*. Seattle, WA: Special Child.

Dykens, E. M. (2007). Psychiatric and behavioral disorders in persons with Down syndrome. *Mental Retardation and Developmental Disabilities Research Reviews, 13*, 272–278.

Dykens, E. M., Hodapp, R. M., & Evans, D. W. (1994). Profiles and development of adaptive behavior in children with Down syndrome. *American Journal on Mental Retardation, 98*, 580–587.

Dykens, E. M., & Kasari, C. (1997). Maladaptive

behavior in children with Prader–Willi syndrome, Down syndrome, and nonspecific mental retardation. *American Journal on Mental Retardation, 102,* 228–237.

Dykens, E. M., Shah, B., Sagun, J., Beck, T., & King, B. H. (2002). Maladaptive behaviour in children and adolescents with Down's syndrome. *Journal of Intellectual Disability Research, 46,* 484–492.

Einfeld, S., Tonge, B., Turner, G., Parmenter, T., & Smith, A. (1999). Longitudinal course of behavioural and emotional problems of young persons with Prader–Willi, fragile X, Williams and Down syndromes. *Journal of Intellectual and Developmental Disability, 24,* 349–354.

Elkins, T. E. (1992). Gynecologic care. In S. M. Pueschel & J. K. Pueschel (Eds.), *Biomedical concerns in persons with Down syndrome.* Baltimore: Brookes.

Ercis, M., Balci, S., & Atakan, N. (1996). Dermatological manifestations of 71 Down syndrome children admitted to a clinical genetics unit. *Clinical Genetics, 50,* 317–320.

Fewell, R. R., & Oelwein, P. L. (1990). The relationship between time in integrated environments and developmental gains in young children with special needs. *Topics in Early Childhood Special Education, 10,* 104–116.

Fewell, R. R., & Oelwein, P. L. (1991). Effective early intervention: Results from the Model Preschool Program for children with Down syndrome and other developmental delays. *Topics in Early Childhood Special Education, 11,* 56–68.

Fishler, K., & Koch, R. (1991). Mental development in Down syndrome mosaicism. *American Journal on Mental Retardation, 96,* 345–351.

Florez, J. (1992). Neurologic abnormalities. In S. M. Pueschel & J. K. Pueschel (Eds.), *Biomedical concerns in persons with Down syndrome.* Baltimore: Brookes.

Fowler, A. E. (1988). Language abilities in children with Down syndrome: Evidence for a specific syntactic delay. In V. Dmitriev & P. L. Oelwein (Eds.), *Advances in Down syndrome.* Seattle, WA: Special Child.

Fox, L., & Hanline, M. F. (1993). A preliminary evaluation of learning within developmentally appropriate early childhood settings. *Topics in Early Childhood Special Education, 13,* 308–327.

Frangou, S., Aylward, E., Warren, A., Sharma, T., Barta, P., & Pearlson, G. (1997). Small planum temporale volume in Down's syndrome: A volumetric MRI study. *American Journal of Psychiatry, 154,* 1424–1429.

Frost, M., Huffer, W. E., Sze, C. I., Badesch, D., Cajade-Law, A. G., & Kleinschmidt-DeMas. (1999). Cervical spine abnormalities in Down syndrome. *Clinical Neuropathology, 18,* 250–259.

Ganiban, J., Wagner, S., & Cicchetti, D. (1990).

Temperament and Down syndrome. In D. Cicchetti & M. Beeghly (Eds.), *Children with Down syndrome: A developmental perspective.* New York: Cambridge University Press.

Gibson, D. (1991). Searching for a life-span psychobiology of Down syndrome: Advancing educational and behavioral management strategies. *International Journal of Disability, Development and Education, 38,* 71–89.

Glasson, E. J., Sullivan, S. G., Hussain, R., Petterson, B. A., Montgomery, P. D., & Bittles, A. H. (2003). Comparative survival advantage of males with Down syndrome. *American Journal of Human Biology, 15,* 192–195.

Gunn, P., & Cuskelly, M. (1991). Down syndrome temperament: The stereotype at middle childhood and adolescence. *International Journal of Disability, Development and Education, 38,* 59–70.

Harris, J. C. (1988). Psychological adaptation and psychiatric disorders in adolescents and young adults with Down syndrome. In S. M. Pueschel (Ed.), *The young person with Down syndrome: Transition from adolescence to adulthood.* Baltimore: Brookes.

Hassold, T., Sherman, S., & Hunt, P. A. (1995). The origin of trisomy in humans. In C. J. Epstein, T. Hassold, I. T. Lott, L. Nadel, & D. Patterson (Eds.), *Etiology and pathogenesis of Down syndrome.* New York: Wiley-Less.

Hijii, T., Fukushige, J., Igarashi, H., Takahashi, N., & Ueda, K. (1997). Life expectancy and social adaptation in individuals with Down syndrome with and without surgery for congenital heart disease. *Clinical Pediatrics, 36,* 327–332.

Hodapp, R. M., Leckman, J. F., Dykens, E. M., Sparrow, S. S., Zelinsky, D. G., & Ort, S. I. (1992). K-ABC profiles in children with fragile X syndrome, Down syndrome, and nonspecific mental retardation. *American Journal on Mental Retardation, 97,* 39–46.

Hodapp, R. M., & Zigler, E. (1990). Applying the developmental perspective to individuals with Down syndrome. In D. Cicchetti & M. Beeghly (Eds.), *Children with Down syndrome: A developmental perspective.* New York: Cambridge University Press.

Holland, A. J., Hon, J., Huppert, F. A., & Stevens, F. (2000). Incidence and course of dementia in people with Down's syndrome: Findings from a population-based study. *Journal of Intellectual Disability Research, 44,* 138–146.

Howenstein, M. S. (1992). Pulmonary concerns. In I. T. Lott & E. E. McCoy (Eds.), *Down syndrome: Advances in medical care.* New York: Wiley-Liss.

Jobling, A. (1998). Motor development in school-aged children with Down syndrome: A longitudinal perspective. *International Journal of Disability, Development and Education, 45,* 283–293.

Kamphaus, R. W. (1993). *Clinical assessment of children's intelligence.* Needham Heights, MA: Allyn & Bacon.

Kennedy, E. J., & Flynn, M. C. (2003). Training in phonological awareness skills in children with Down syndrome. *Research in Developmental Disabilities, 24,* 44–57.

Kneips, L. J., Walden, T. A., & Baxter, A. (1994). Affective expressions of toddlers with and without Down syndrome in a social referencing context. *American Journal on Mental Retardation, 99,* 301–312.

Korenberg, J. R., Pulst, S. M., & Gerwehr, S. (1992). Advances in the understanding of chromosome 21 and Down syndrome. In I. T. Lott & E. E. McCoy (Eds.), *Down syndrome: Advances in medical care.* New York: Wiley-Liss.

Lai, F. (1992). Alzheimer disease. In S. M. Pueschel & J. K. Pueschel (Eds.), *Biomedical concerns in persons with Down syndrome.* Baltimore: Brookes.

Lalli, J. S., Browder, D. M., Mace, F. C., & Brown, D. K. (1993). Teacher use of descriptive analysis data to implement interventions to decrease students' problem behaviors. *Journal of Applied Behavior Analysis, 26,* 227–238.

Landry, S. H., Miller-Loncar, C. L., & Swank, P. R. (1998). Goal-directed behavior in children with Down syndrome: The role of joint play situations. *Early Education and Development, 9,* 375–392.

Levy, J. (1992). Gastrointestinal concerns. In S. M. Pueschel & J. K. Pueschel (Eds.), *Biomedical concerns in persons with Down syndrome.* Baltimore: Brookes.

Lojkasek, M., Goldberg, S., Marcovitch, S., & MacGregor, D. (1990). Influences on maternal responsiveness to developmentally delayed preschoolers. *Journal of Early Intervention, 14,* 260–273.

Lott, I. T., & McCoy, E. E. (Eds.). (1992). *Down syndrome: Advances in medical care.* New York: Wiley-Liss.

Love, P. L. (1988). The early preschool program: The bridge between infancy and childhood. In V. Dmitriev & P. L. Oelwein (Eds.), *Advances in Down syndrome.* Seattle, WA: Special Child.

Lubin, B. H., Cahn, S., & Scott, M. (1992). Hematologic manifestations. In S. M. Pueschel & J. K. Pueschel (Eds.), *Biomedical concerns in persons with Down syndrome.* Baltimore: Brookes.

Marino, B. (1992). Cardiac aspects. In S. M. Pueschel & J. K. Pueschel (Eds.), *Biomedical concerns in persons with Down syndrome.* Baltimore: Brookes.

McCarthy, J., & Boyd, J. (2001). Psychopathology and young people with Down's syndrome: Childhood predictors and adult outcome of disorder. *Journal of Intellectual Disability Research, 45,* 99–105.

Meyers, L. F. (1988). Using computers to teach children with Down syndrome spoken and written language skills. In L. Nadel (Ed.), *The psychobiology of Down Syndrome.* Cambridge, MA: MIT Press.

Miller, J. F. (1995). Individual differences in vocabulary acquisition in children with Down syndrome. In C. J. Epstein, T. Hassold, I. T. Lott, L. Nadel, & D. Patterson (Eds.), *Etiology and pathogenesis of Down syndrome.* New York: Wiley-Liss.

Mufson, E. J., Benzing, W. C., & Kordower, J. H. (1995). Dissociation of galaninergic and neurotrophic plasticity in Down syndrome and Alzheimer disease. In C. J. Epstein, T. Hassold, I. T. Lott, L. Nadel, & D. Patterson (Eds.), *Etiology and pathogenesis of Down syndrome.* New York: Wiley-Liss.

Myers, B. A. (1992). Psychiatric disorders. In S. M. Pueschel & J. K. Pueschel (Eds.), *Biomedical concerns in persons with Down syndrome.* Baltimore: Brookes.

Niva, R. A. (1988). Eye abnormalities and their treatment. In V. Dmitriev & P. L. Oelwein (Eds.), *Advances in Down syndrome.* Seattle, WA: Special Child.

Oelwein, P. L. (1988). Preschool and kindergarten programs: Strategies for meeting objectives. In V. Dmitriev & P. L. Oelwein (Eds.), *Advances in Down syndrome.* Seattle, WA: Special Child.

Pearlson, G. D., Breiter, S. N., Aylward, E. H., Warren, A. C., Grygorcewicz, M., Frangou, S., et al. (1998). MRI brain changes in subjects with Down syndrome with and without dementia. *Developmental Medicine and Child Neurology, 40,* 326–334.

Pipes, P. L. (1992). Nutritional aspects. In S. M. Pueschel & J. K. Pueschel (Eds.), *Biomedical concerns in persons with Down syndrome.* Baltimore: Brookes.

Prescott, G. H. (1988). Genetic counseling for families about Down syndrome. In V. Dmitriev & P. L. Oelwein (Eds.), *Advances in Down syndrome.* Seattle, WA: Special Child.

Pueschel, S. M. (1992a). General health care and therapeutic approaches. In S. M. Pueschel & J. K. Pueschel (Eds.), *Biomedical concerns in persons with Down syndrome.* Baltimore: Brookes.

Pueschel, S. M. (1992b). Phenotypic characteristics. In S. M. Pueschel & J. K. Pueschel (Eds.), *Biomedical concerns in persons with Down syndrome.* Baltimore: Brookes.

Pueschel, S. M., & Bier, J. B. (1992). Endrocrinologic aspects. In S. M. Pueschel & J. K. Pueschel (Eds.), *Biomedical concerns in persons with Down syndrome.* Baltimore: Brookes.

Pueschel, S. M., Romano, C., Failla, P., Barone, C., Pettinato, R., Castellano Chiodo, A., et al. (1999). A prevalence study of celiac disease in persons with Down syndrome residing in the

United States of America. *Acta Paediatrica, 88,* 953–966.

Pueschel, S. M., & Solga, P. M. (1992). Musculoskeletal disorders. In S. M. Pueschel & J. K. Pueschel (Eds.), *Biomedical concerns in persons with Down syndrome.* Baltimore: Brookes.

Quine, L., & Rutter, D. R. (1994). First diagnosis of severe mental and physical disability: A study of doctor-parent communication. *Journal of Child Psychology and Psychiatry, 35,* 1273–1287.

Ratekin, C. (1996). Temperament in children with Down syndrome. *Developmental Disabilities Bulletin, 24,* 18–32.

Renzaglia, A., & Hutchins, M. P. (1988). Establishing vocational training programs for school-age students with moderate and severe handicaps. In S. M. Pueschel (Ed.), *The young person with Down syndrome: Transition from adolescence to adulthood.* Baltimore: Brookes.

Roberts, J. E., Price, J., & Malkin, C. (2007). Language and communication development in Down syndrome. *Mental Retardation and Developmental Disabilities Research Reviews, 13,* 26–35.

Roid, G. H. (2003). *Stanford–Binet Intelligence Scales, Fifth Edition: Examiner's manual.* Itaska, IL: Riverside.

Roizen, N. J. (2005). Complementary and alternative therapies for Down syndrome. *Mental Retardation and Developmental Disabilities Research Reviee, 11*(2), 149–155.

Rubin, S. S., Rimmer, J. H., Chicoine, B., Braddock, D., & McGuire, D. E. (1998). Overweight prevalence in persons with Down syndrome. *Mental Retardation, 36,* 175–181.

Ruskin, E. M., Kasari, C., Mundy, P., & Sigman, M. (1994). Attention to people and toys during social and object mastery in children with Down syndrome. *American Journal on Mental Retardation, 99,* 103–111.

Sadovnick, A. D., & Baird, P. A. (1992). Life expectancy. In S. M. Pueschel & J. K. Pueschel (Eds.), *Biomedical concerns in persons with Down syndrome.* Baltimore: Brookes.

Scola, P. S. (1992). Disorders of the liver. In S. M. Pueschel & J. K. Pueschel (Eds.), *Biomedical concerns in persons with Down syndrome.* Baltimore: Brookes.

Sexton, D., Thompson, B., Perez, J., & Rheams, T. (1990). Maternal versus professional estimates of developmental status for young children with handicaps: An ecological approach. *Topics in Early Childhood Special Education, 10,* 80–95.

Shonkoff, J. P., Hauser-Cram, P., Krauss, M. W., & Upshur, C. C. (1992). Development of infants with disabilities and their families: Implications for theory and services delivery. *Monographs of the Society for Research in Child Development, 57*(6, Serial No. 230), 1–17.

Sloper, P., Cunningham, C., Turner, S., & Knussen, C. (1990). Factors related to the academic attainments of children with Down's syndrome. *British Journal of Educational Psychology, 60,* 284–298.

Smith, B., & Phillips, C. J. (1992). Attainments of severely mentally retarded adolescents by aetiology. *Journal of Child Psychology and Psychiatry, 33,* 1039–1058.

Strauss, D., & Eyman, R. K. (1996). Mortality of people with mental retardation in California with and without Down syndrome, 1986–1991. *American Journal on Mental Retardation, 100,* 643–653.

Suzuki, K., Yamaki, S., Mimori, S., Murakami, Y., Mori, K., Takahashi, Y., et al. (2000). Pulmonary vascular disease in Down's syndrome with complete atrioventricular septal defect. *American Journal of Cardiology, 86,* 434–437.

Thombs, B., & Sugden, D. (1991). Manual skills in Down syndrome children ages 6 to 16 years. *Adapted Physical Activity Quarterly, 8,* 242–254.

Tingey, C., Mortensen, L., Matheson, P., & Doret, W. (1991). Developmental attainment of infants and young children with Down syndrome. *International Journal of Disability, Development and Education, 38,* 15–26.

Tsiaras, W. G., Pueschel, S., Keller, C., Curran, R., & Giesswein, S. (1999). Amblyopia and visual acuity in children with Down's syndrome. *British Journal of Ophthalmology, 83,* 1112–1114.

Ugazio, A. G., Maccario, R., & Burgio, G. R. (1992). Immunologic features. In S. M. Pueschel & J. K. Pueschel (Eds.), *Biomedical concerns in persons with Down syndrome.* Baltimore: Brookes.

Vaughn, B. E., Contreras, J., & Seifer, R. (1994). Short-term longitudinal study of maternal ratings of temperament in samples of children with Down syndrome and children who are developing normally. *American Journal on Mental Retardation, 98,* 607–618.

Vigild, M. (1992). Oral health conditions. In S. M. Pueschel & J. K. Pueschel (Eds.), *Biomedical concerns in persons with Down syndrome.* Baltimore: Brookes.

Visser, F. E., Aldenkamp, A. P., van Huffelen, A. C., & Kuilman, M. (1997). Prospective study of the prevalence of Alzheimer-type dementia in institutionalized individuals with Down syndrome. *American Journal on Mental Retardation, 101,* 400–412.

Warfield, M. E. (1994). A cost-effectiveness analysis of early intervention services in Massachusetts: Implications for policy. *Educational Evaluation and Policy Analysis, 16,* 87–99.

Wishart, J. G. (1991). Taking the initiative in learning: A developmental investigation of infants with Down syndrome. *International Journal of Disability, Development and Education, 38,* 27–44.

Wishart, J. G. (1995). Cognitive abilities in children with Down syndrome: Developmental instability and motivational deficits. In C. J. Epstein, T. Hassold, I. T. Lott, L. Nadel, & D. Patterson (Eds.), *Etiology and pathogenesis of Down syndrome.* New York: Wiley-Liss.

Wishart, J. G. (2007). Socio-cognitive understanding: A strength or weakness in Down's syndrome? *Journal of Intellectual Disability Research, 51,* 996–1005.

Wishart, J. G., & Duffy, L. (1990). Instability of performance on cognitive tests in infants and young children with Down's syndrome. *British Journal of Educational Psychology, 60,* 10–22.

Yoder, P. J., & Warren, S. F. (2004). Early predictors of language in children with and without Down syndrome. *American Journal on Mental Retardation, 109,* 285–300.

Zickler, C. F., Morrow, J. D., & Bull, M. J. (1998). Infants with Down syndrome: A look at temperament. *Journal of Pediatric Health Care, 12,* 111–117.

Zigman, W. B., & Lott, I. T. (2007). Alzheimer's disease in Down syndrome: Neurobiology and risk. *Mental Retardation and Developmental Disabilities Research Reviews, 13,* 237–246.

CHAPTER 20

Klinefelter Syndrome

HEATHER CODY HAZLETT
MARIO GASPAR DE ALBA
STEPHEN R. HOOPER

Klinefelter syndrome (KS) is a disorder seen in males, resulting from an abnormality found at the chromosomal level. It was first described in 1942 by Klinefelter, Reifenstein, and Albright, who used the term to describe a small group of infertile men. More than a decade later, the discovery of an extra X chromosome was used to distinguish the syndrome further. Consequently, KS is considered a sex chromosome disorder. Normally, males are born with 46 chromosomes, with their gender being defined by a pairing of an X and a Y chromosome. Males born with KS, however, typically show an XXY pattern. There are some other variations, such as XXXY or XXXXY, and also cases considered to reflect mosaicism, which is characterized by having a combination of normal and abnormal cells. The prevalence of KS has been estimated at between 1 in 500 and 1 in 1,000 live-born males (Bojesen, Juul, & Gravholt, 2003; Lanfranco, Kamischke, Zitzmann, & Nieschlag, 2004). Estimates conducted in Denmark of all males born during a 13-year period have been reported to be as high as 1 in 426 (Nielsen & Wohlert, 1991).

Earlier studies of males with KS found an increased risk for psychiatric disorders, criminality, and intellectual disabilities (Forss-man, 1970; Schroder, Chapelle, Hokola, & Virkkunen, 1981). These studies, however, had serious methodological problems because they were generally conducted with populations that were already institutionalized or imprisoned (Cohen & Durham, 1985). Unfortunately, even some subsequent literature has relied on these early findings to describe individuals with KS as having high rates of incarceration and mental problems (Gilbert, 1993).

More recent research indicates that although there may be some significant cognitive, psychiatric, or behavioral problems in these individuals, outcomes are not as grim as the earlier conceptualizations indicated. Several longitudinal studies have contributed to our understanding of developmental outcomes in KS. For example, large prospective studies conducted during the late 1960s and early 1970s compiled outcome data for children born with sex chromosome abnormalities. Bender and Berch (1990) outlined the most important findings from this research. First, children with sex chromosome disorders appear to display increased risk for developmental, language, learning, and behavioral problems, compared to peers with a normal sex chromosome complement; however, their profiles appear relatively benign by comparison with earlier stereotypes, thus supporting the notion that earlier studies examined biased samples. Second, there is a great deal of variability in the phenotype of children with the same syndrome, and family/environmental influences may mediate the amount of dysfunction displayed because of the significant variability associated with KS. It is now widely accepted that the original description of males with KS is not entirely accurate and that they can actually present a wide spectrum of phenotypic variation (Lanfranco et al., 2004). Our description of KS in this chapter addresses the most recent and well-accepted findings regarding these children and their neuropsychological functioning. It must be noted that studies involving males with KS typically include only small cohorts, due to the limited number of affected individuals identified. Moreover, these findings must be considered carefully, given that an estimated 70–75% of these individuals are never diagnosed due to a lack of clinically significant signs, symptoms, and other manifestations (Bojesen et al., 2003; Lanfranco et al., 2004).

GENETIC AND FAMILIAL ISSUES RELATED TO ETIOLOGY

There are several different types of genetic disorders. These include autosomal dominant disorders (e.g., Huntington chorea), autosomal recessive disorders (e.g., phenylketonuria), X-linked disorders (e.g., Lesch–Nyhan syndrome), and those that involve chromosomal abnormalities. KS falls into this last category, since it is caused by sex chromosome abnormality. The phenomenon that results in a chromosomal abnormality is referred to a *nondisjunction*. This occurs when a pair of chromosomes fails to separate during either the first or second division of meiosis. When nondisjunction occurs, it results in *aneuploidy* (the absence or addition of a single chromosome—a *monosomy* or *trisomy*, respectively). Aneuploidy is the most common type of chromosome anomaly found in live births or spontaneous abortions, occurring in approximately 3% of all confirmed pregnancies (Evans, Drugan, Pryde, & Johnson, 1996). Some authors suggest that up to 10–25% of all fertilized human oocytes are either monosomic or trisomic (Pellestor, Andreo, Arnal, Humeau, & Demaille, 2002). Rather than the normal XY genotype that signifies the male gender, boys with KS will typically display a trisomy or XXY pattern of sex chromosomes. This trisomy can occur through various errors. If it is maternally derived, an XXY genotype can be due to an error during meiosis I, meiosis II, or the early mitotic division in the zygote (this last is referred to as a *postzygotic mitotic error*). The XXY pattern can result from paternal nondisjunction only during meiosis I (Thomas & Hassold, 2003). Roughly 50% of KS cases are caused by maternal meiotic errors, with three-fourths of these reported to show significant effects of maternal age (Gardner & Sutherland, 1996). Some have reported maternal age to be a contributing factor in approximately 60% of a sample of males with KS (Drugan, Isada, Johnson, & Evans, 1996b), while others have found rates of paternal nondisjunction to occur in slightly over half (57%) of the cases, with the exception of those directly linked to advanced maternal age (Evans et al., 1996). Several studies have shown an equal distribution of maternally and paternally derived KS. Advanced maternal age and, less clearly, paternal age have also been linked to an increased risk for KS (Lowe et al., 2001). Approximately 10% of individuals with KS exhibit mosaicism, meaning that not all cells examined display the XXY trisomy; instead, some show a normal XY pattern because the nondisjunction error occurred after fertilization (Pierce, 1990).

KS is one of the most frequently occurring sex chromosome abnormalities in males. In general, the sex chromosome abnormalities produce less significant impairments than those involving autosomal abnormalities (e.g., Down syndrome, Edwards syndrome). Hynd and Willis (1988) noted two hypotheses for this distinction. One is that the Y sex chromosome appears to carry only information necessary for gender determination. The second notes that any number of X chromosomes greater than the normal one appears to become relatively inactive in early fetal development.

A diagnosis of KS can be made by a thorough physical exam, by hormone testing, and most accurately through genetic testing. Genetic testing is done prenatally by amniocentesis or chorionic villus sampling, and postnatally through karyotyping (Pierce, 1990). There are no familial indicators that would suggest a higher risk for producing a child with KS, although females with trisomy XXX have been reported to be at greater risk for producing offspring with KS or XXX, and (in fewer cases) trisomy 21 and monosomy X0 (Drugan et al., 1996b). Advanced maternal age is a risk factor for any pregnancy, and in these cases a prenatal diagnosis of KS may be possible. Advanced paternal age has also been implicated as a risk factor for KS (Sloter, Nath, Eskenazi, & Wyrobek, 2004). Males with KS display a broad range of characteristic physical features and hormonal derangements, which are discussed below. Many of these may or may not be present at birth, and therefore the existence of an extra X chromosome may not be suspected or discovered until concerns about genital and pubertal development surface, or later during testing for infertility (Drugan, Isada, Johnson, & Evans, 1996a). In an overview of genetic disorders and their onset, Weatherall (1991) placed the average age for first appearance of KS-related impairments at 5 years. A more recent study suggested that fewer than 10% of boys with KS are diagnosed before puberty, and (as noted above) that possibly up to 70% of affected males with KS may never receive a diagnosis (Bojesen et al., 2003).

MEDICAL CONCERNS AND COMORBID DISORDERS

Generally speaking, the sex chromosome disorders have less of an impact on the phenotype than autosomal disorders do. With autosomal trisomies, as an example, there may be multiple affected systems and greater physical anomalies. The sex chromosome trisomies cause have less global impairment, but the development and function of the sex organs, hormonal production, and reproduction are all negatively affected by sex chromosome trisomies (Evans et al., 1996).

Genital Anomalies

In a review of the literature on the physical characteristics of KS, Theilgaard (1984) found several classic genital anomalies common among these individuals, and sub-sequent research has expanded on these observations. At birth, males have normal male genitalia without ambiguity, with occasional micropenis and hypospadias (Zeger et al., 2008). As they grow, decreased testicular size is the only consistent physical feature in KS (Visootsak & Graham, 2006). Cryptorchidism is also seen more frequently than in healthy controls (Bojesen, Juul, Birkebaek, & Gravholt, 2006). Hormonal disturbances become problematic during puberty, as secondary sex characteristics may be diminished by restricted levels of testosterone (see below). According to Schwartz and Root (1991), KS is the most common cause of hypogonadism in males. The testes initially enlarge normally to their peak size at midpuberty, but as the seminiferous tubules (which constitute 85% of the volume in the testes) hyalanize and fibrose, they decrease in size and become firm. Ultimately, the affected testes are smaller than average—typically less than 2.5 cm in diameter, and with a postpubertal volume of less than 10 ml (Smyth & Bremner, 1998; Tyler & Edman, 2004). Facial, axillary, and pubic hair tends to be sparse. Infertility is caused by progressive destruction of spermatogonia during puberty, which leads to azoospermia and is one of the primary disabling features of KS (Wikstrom et al., 2004). New assistive reproductive technologies, such as sperm recovery through testicular biopsy and *in vitro* fertilization using intracytoplasmic sperm injection, have given men with KS reproductive options that they did not previously have; these procedures have resulted in viable pregnancies (Denschlag, Tempfer, Kunze, Wolff, & Keck, 2004; Paduch, Fine, Bolyakov, & Kiper, 2008).

Hormonal Disturbances

Among the chief features of this syndrome are the endocrinological disturbances that impair normal genital and sexual development. Typically, a postpubertal patient will present with low to low-normal serum testosterone and inhibin B (marker of Sertoli cell function), higher concentrations of luteinizing hormone (LH) and follicle-stimulating hormone (FSH), and increased estradiol compared to genetically normal males (Lanfranco et al., 2004; Paduch et al., 2008). For the most part, authors have agreed that these hormone levels are normal during infancy and childhood, but recent studies have questioned this assertion. One study found that 75% of the cohort with KS had testosterone levels below the 25th percentile for age (Zeger et al., 2008). Other studies have presented conflicting information regarding the levels of testosterone seen during the hypothalamic–pituitary–gonadal axis surge that typically occurs in the first months of life (Aksglaede, Petersen, Main, Skakkebaek, & Juul, 2007; Ross et al., 2005). Regardless, testicular activity is minimal during typical childhood development; consequently, hypogonadism may remain clinically silent until the increased hormonal activity and expected changes at puberty are not seen. LH stimulates testosterone secretion, while FSH stimulates the development of sperm during puberty. Therefore, although males with KS will enter puberty at a normal age, inadequate testosterone secretion eventually prevents normal puberty from occurring (Styne, 1991). There have been some mixed accounts of thyroid conditions in these children, with some studies indicating an increased rate of congenital hypothyroidism, and others showing no significant findings (Schwartz & Root, 1991).

Neurological Findings

Some literature indicates that abnormal electroencephalograms (EEGs) and seizure activity are seen more frequently in males with KS than in the general population. Whether or not there is an increased rate of epilepsy in these males has not been determined conclusively. Essential tremor has been documented in a greater proportion of men with KS than in genetically normal controls (Harlow & Gonzalez-Alegre, 2009). Neuromuscular findings show that when compared to controls, boys with KS have lower scores on tasks involving fine and gross motor skills, coordination, agility, speed, dexterity, and strength (Robinson et al., 1986; Ross et al., 2008).

Other Physical Features

Boys with KS are typically taller than average because of elongated legs. The height increase is most dramatic between the ages of 5 and 8 years and is due to leg lengthening (Visootsak & Graham, 2006). Increased frequency of obesity has been described, and a tendency toward central obesity was found in 75% of affected males in one study (Ratcliffe, 1999). A relatively large study of 55 boys with KS found an increased prevalence of fifth-digit clinodactyly, hypertelorism, high arched palate, and elbow dysplasia (Zeger et al., 2008). Other associated findings seen more frequently in KS include diabetes mellitus, hyperlipidemia, hypercholesterolemia, gallbladder disease, chronic pulmonary infection, and peptic ulcer (Zuppinger, Engel, Forbes, Mantooth, & Claffey, 1967). Hypogonadism in KS may cause an unfavorable change in body composition and result in the metabolic syndrome, which includes abdominal obesity, atherogenic dyslipidemia, elevated blood pressure, insulin resistance or glucose intolerance, prothrombotic state, and proinflammatory state (Ishikawa, Yamaguchi, Kondo, Takenaka, & Fujisawa, 2008). Evans and colleagues (1996) found diabetes to occur in 8% of their total population of individuals with KS, as well as increased rates of elbow dysplasia, elongated limbs, chronic bronchitis, and poor fine motor coordination. There is also an increased risk of decreased bone mineral content due to the androgen deficiency, which results in osteopenia and osteoporosis (Schwartz & Root, 1991). Some variants of KS (e.g., XXXY and XXXXY) have been associated with short stature or radioulnar synostosis (Schwartz & Root, 1991). In general, individuals with 46,XY/47,XXY mosaicism have fewer phenotypic findings; as the number of X chromosomes increases (XXXY, XXXXY), the frequency of nearly all phenotypic anomalies increases (Lanfranco et al., 2004). The one exception is height, which is inversely proportional to the number of X chromosomes (Visootsak, Aylstock, & Graham, 2001).

Other nonspecific features include increased rates of fatigue, venous stasis ulcers, and essential tremor (Schwartz & Root, 1991). Of the few accounts of cardiac defects associated with KS, these appear to occur more frequently in the rarer cases of polysomy (e.g., XXXXY) than in the more common XXY presentation (Elias & Yanagi, 1981). In addition, the number and severity of these cardiac defects may be directly correlated with the degree of polysomy. A study that followed more than 600 men with KS and documented the cause of death for 163 of them demonstrated increased mortality rates from diabetes, cerebrovascular, cardiovascular, pulmonary, and gastrointestinal diseases, as well as increased risks of lung and breast cancer (Swerdlow et al., 2001). Increased morbidity from ischemic heart disease, deep vein thrombosis, pulmonary embolism, and intestinal thrombosis has also been seen (Bojesen et al., 2006). Furthermore, the rate of meditational germ cell tumors is increased (Volkl et al., 2006). Other studies have not shown a significant comorbidity of renal or lymphatic conditions in this population (Evans et al., 1996).

DEVELOPMENTAL COURSE

About two decades ago, Schwartz and Root (1991) outlined common clinical presentations of KS at the various developmental stages, and their description remains useful today. Specifically, during infancy, KS may be discovered during routine evaluations for the presence of cryptorchidism, microphallus, or hypospadias. School-age children may present with learning or behavioral/social problems. During adolescents, clinical presentations may result from gynecomastia, delayed onset of puberty, abnormally tall stature, small testes, or eunuchoid habitus. Adults are most often discovered during investigations of infertility, but may be identified during evaluations for malignancies and/or tumors.

Physical Development and Puberty

The majority of infants with KS are indistinguishable from unaffected infants at birth. However, Diamond and Watson (2004) cited information from an Edinburgh study that found babies with KS to be smaller in weight, length, and head circumference than controls; their head circumference remained between the 10th and the 25th percentiles. Fifth-finger and/or fifth-toe clinodactyly has also been seen in greater frequency (Simpson, 2003). Samango-Sprouse (2001) found the presence of decreased muscle tone and delayed ambulation, particularly in those children who had not received therapy. In childhood, physical development generally follows normal patterns, and motor developmental milestones are not significantly different. As noted earlier, an increased height velocity (owing to greater leg growth seen between the ages of 5 and 8 years) has been reported, as well as a tendency toward central obesity (Ratcliffe, 1999). It is not until puberty, however, that more specific disturbances are noted. Bender and Berch (1990) noted that the males in their sample displayed reduced sensory–motor integration and motor strength. Others have found a variety of motor difficulties, including decreased running speed, overall agility, and dexterity in visual–motor tasks (Ross et al., 2008). Gynecomastia has been noted in a greater percentage of boys with KS than of controls (Ratcliffe, 1999; Smyth & Bremner, 1998).

For the purposes of comparison, typical pubertal development is briefly reviewed. Normal secondary sexual development in males involves genital development and pubic hair growth, and features of puberty related to the external genitalia may begin to develop at any time from age 11 to 15 years (Wheeler, 1991). This process involves the growth of the testes, maturation of the scrotum, and growth of the penis. In males with KS, the size of the penis is within normal limits, but often on the smaller side, while the testes begin to be distinguished by more obviously diminished size and maturation. Androgens control pubic hair growth, and (as mentioned above) males with KS have decreased androgen production, which results in diminished or absent pubic hair growth. Normally, pubic, axillary, and facial hair growth follows on the heels of genital development; in KS, this growth may be delayed, diminished, or absent. During puberty, the voice normally deepens and the bulbourethral glands enlarge. Both processes may be abnormal in KS. In addition, although some breast enlargement is typical in normal adolescence, in KS there may be significant gynecomastia (also as mentioned above). Other major characteristics of normal pubertal development in males involve alterations in lean body mass and fat distribution, and rapid skeletal growth. In KS, fat deposition may be increased centrally, and the distribution may mimic that of girls (e.g., hip and thigh) (Wheeler, 1991). Boys tend to take on a eunuchoid body habitus (long legs and arms, narrow shoulders, wide hips, etc.).

Therefore, physical features at puberty may involve absent or diminished growth of facial, chest, and pubic hair. Gynecomastia, small testes, central obesity, feminine fat distribution, and poor muscle tone may also be present in these males, although varying degrees of these conditions have been reported (Pierce, 1990). Schwartz and Root (1991) estimate that 30–60% of all children with KS will exhibit gynecomastia by late puberty, and they place the prevalence of later-developing carcinoma of the breast at 9 in 1,000. They are careful to note that although this rate is above that for genetically normal men and one-fifth the rate for women, the role of the extra X chromosome in this higher risk for carcinoma in KS is unknown. Severe gynecomastia is not improved with androgen therapy, and mastectomy is often recommended when there are significant physical or psychological concerns. Ratcliffe (1999) found that gynecomastia was often transient and rarely required surgical correction.

Neurological Development

Two hypotheses regarding neurological development have been put forth by Bender and Berch (1990) to explain the characteristics seen in sex chromosome disorders. One hypothesis is that the presence of a sex chromosome anomaly may alter normal patterns of brain growth, resulting in abnormal rates of brain tissue growth and maturation, which in turn will have an impact on functioning. This causal pattern, implicated in cases of extra X chromosomes, is that the extra chromosome interferes with left-hemisphere specialization for language, resulting in decreased language functioning. The second hypothesis involves the impact that hormones may have on brain growth and functioning. For example, the abnormal testosterone levels seen in individuals with KS may be related to their impairments in verbal ability. Bender and Berch have been careful to point out, however, that neither hypothesis has been proven conclusively with physiological, empirical evidence. Some implications for differences in brain growth patterns have been made by studying dermal ridges. These may be used as indicators of prenatal growth because they become differentiated during midfetal development and remain constant from that point. Netley

and Rovet (1982) found evidence for diminished dermal ridge counts in a group of children with KS, indicating that their prenatal growth is slower.

Hemispheric specialization in KS has been studied by observing differences in their performance on verbal and nonverbal tasks. Netley and Rovet (1984) found that a group of boys with KS performed more poorly than controls on a number of tasks involving lateral presentation of material. For example, the boys with KS did more poorly on dichotic stop consonants, whereas their performance was better than that of controls on dichotic melodies and half-field dots. The authors interpreted these findings to mean that boys with KS have difficulty in dealing efficiently with information normally preferentially processed by the left hemisphere, and that their right-hemispheric functions appear to play a larger role in both nonverbal and verbal processing. Overall, when compared to age-matched controls, children with KS have been found to display diminished left-hemisphere specialization for language and enhanced right-hemisphere specialization for nonverbal processing (Netley, 1990). This finding is supported by the fact that language deficits also are seen in females with XXX, particularly in expressive language and auditory processing (Walzer et al., 1986). A study examining dichotic listening performance found that for a group with KS compared to a control group, left-hemispheric processing was impaired when they were presented with dichotic syllables (Theilgaard, 1984). Narrowing even further the potential structural basis for the neuropsychological deficits seen in KS, a magnetic resonance imaging (MRI) case–control study of 42 individuals with KS demonstrated diminished total cerebral volume and all lobar volumes, as well as a larger lateral ventricle volume, compared to those of controls. The cortex was significantly thinner in the group with KS in left inferior frontal, temporal, and superior motor regions (Giedd et al., 2007). A smaller study of 10 individuals with KS found reduced volume of the left temporal lobe gray matter (Patwardhan, Eliez, Bender, Linden, & Reiss, 2000), and another study cited reduced volume of the insula, amygdala, hippocampus, cingulate, and occipital gyri, as well as diminished right parietal lobe white matter (Shen et al., 2004).

Cognitive Development

There are distinctions between the cognitive deficits seen in trisomies of the sex chromosome and those associated with the autosomal trisomies. Individuals with sex chromosome trisomies may have normal or above-average intelligence, and if intellectual disabilities are present, they are typically found to be in the mild range. Autosomal trisomies, on the other hand, usually result in profound intellectual disabilities (Evans et al., 1996). Generally, studies have shown that children with KS may display a wide range of intellectual ability, ranging from mild intellectual disabilities to above-average intelligence. Reviewing a 37-year prospective study, Bender and Berch (1991) noted that the cohort of 11 persons with KS had normal Verbal IQ (VIQ) and Performance IQ (PIQ) scores, although they were skewed lower than those of their euploid siblings. Walzer, Bashir, and Silbert (1990) found IQs to be 10–15 points lower than those of typical peers in a group of 13 boys with KS. Of these, 11 had demonstrated learning problems in reading and spelling throughout their academic histories. In an exhaustive literature review on the cognitive profile of boys with KS, Rovet, Netley, Keenan, Bailey, and Stewart (1996) concluded that a chronic cognitive deficit in verbal abilities and language processing was consistent across 27 independent research studies. In addition, a pattern of general underachievement in school and risk for dyslexia was evident in these children. Rovet and colleagues conducted their own longitudinal study of cognitive functioning in KS; they followed 36 boys with KS and 33 sibling controls for 20 years. Their findings indicated that compared to the controls, the boys with KS demonstrated significantly depressed verbal ability contrasted with normal nonverbal ability.

Most studies agree that children with KS have significant deficits in their verbal abilities. VIQ scores on traditional measures (e.g., the Wechsler scales) are generally below average, while PIQ scores are within the average range (Ratcliffe, Masera, & McKie, 1994). Rovet and colleagues (1996) found VIQ scores to be about 20 points lower than those of unaffected siblings. Newer studies estimate that both VIQ and PIQ scores are normal and usually range from the low 90s to 100 (Simpson, 2003), but these studies may not have included sibling controls for comparison. Netley (1987) sought to predict intellectual attainment in children with KS from observing the psychometric data of their siblings. He found that compared to their siblings, the boys with KS had lower intelligence test scores, particularly in verbal abilities, although their IQ scores were highly correlated with that of their unaffected siblings. This would indicate that aptitude in young boys with KS might be predicted from that of their siblings. Some have hypothesized that the presence of an extra X chromosome is what deflates the verbal skills, since females with an extra X chromosome also display impaired verbal abilities (Cohen & Durham, 1985; Netley & Rovet, 1982). Others propose that the extra X chromosome represents a risk factor for a specific developmental reading disorder (Bender, Puck, Salbenblatt, & Robinson, 1986).

In cases of polysomies (e.g., XXXY, XXXXY), the level of intellectual impairment appears to increase with the number of additional X chromosomes, with approximately a 15-point IQ decrease per extra X chromosome (Simpson, 2003). Intellectual disabilities are frequent in those individuals who have four or more X chromosomes (Gardner & Sutherland, 1996). Behavioral difficulties also appear more frequently in this population. One case of a child with XXXXY has been reported where the child did not display severe intellectual disability or abnormal social development (Sheridan & Radlinski, 1988); however, the authors noted that early intervention for learning and a supportive home environment may have contributed to this atypical presentation.

Language Development

Young boys with KS have also been noted to display delayed speech and language development, with the first words spoken at between 18 and 24 months versus the more typical 12 months (Simpson, 2003). Specific deficits have been discovered in the areas of articulation, phonemic processing, word finding, language comprehension, verbal memory, oral expression, and linguistic processing speed (Geschwind, Boone, Miller, & Swerdloff, 2000). Language delays have been demonstrated to last up to 8 or 9 years of age, and some research indicates that they may continue through adulthood. In the longitudinal study mentioned above, Rovet and colleagues (1996) determined that males with KS had greater difficulty on tasks involving auditory memory, language comprehension, and language expression. This finding supports an earlier report by Leonard and Sparrow (1986), who found language delays in a small sample of males with KS. These individuals displayed delayed language development, limited vocabulary and syntax, difficulty with verbal concepts, and lack of fluency. In the prospective study by Walzer and colleagues (1986), speech and language delays were evident by the third year of life. Specifically, parents reported problems with articulation, word finding, sentence formation, and expressive language. Assessment of these children indicated that whereas receptive language was age-appropriate, deficits existed in auditory memory and expressive language (e.g., syntax, dysnomia, narrative production).

Other studies have suggested that men with KS have problems with the prosody of language, as well as the semantic problems described above. In a Dutch study comparing men with KS to 20 controls, the cohort with KS demonstrated relative difficulties discriminating emotions in verbal content, and even more so in tone of voice (van Rijn et al., 2007). These types of difficulties are more likely to affect the ability to develop the appropriate social use of language.

BEHAVIORAL, ACADEMIC, AND EMOTIONAL PRESENTATION

Behavioral Presentation

Behavioral development is felt to be the result of certain predispositions and environmental influences. With children who have genetic disorders, the physical consequences of the genetic abnormalities often result in certain behaviors. However, as with all behaviors, the transactional interaction between the children's characteristics and their environment must be considered in the etiology of their behavioral presentation (Hynd & Willis, 1988). Research studies conducted in the 1960s and early 1970s with adult populations tended to find increased rates of

aggressiveness, alcohol and other substance abuse, arson, criminal behavior, depression, personality disorders, and schizophrenia in persons with KS (Schwartz & Root, 1991). As mentioned earlier, however, these studies possessed methodological flaws. Chiefly, they were limited to individuals who were already in psychiatric hospitals or penal institutions. More recent studies have suggested that KS does not appear to be associated with criminal behavior or sociopathy (Wodrich, 2008), and in fact that psychiatric problems are rare among men with KS (Geschwind et al., 2000). Interestingly, the behavioral characteristics associated with KS (e.g., low activity, high pliancy) have led some researchers to find that teachers may view these children as warm, likeable, anxious to please, and helpful. The general tendency of many individuals with KS to withdraw in novel situations and to be less assertive may tend to cause teachers to view these children as lazy, unmotivated, or unwilling to try, however (Walzer et al., 1986).

Academic Performance

Academic difficulties have been found in the areas of reading, spelling, and arithmetic; these are probably related to specific language deficits in the area of auditory–verbal processing (Schwartz & Root, 1991). Poor school performance is typical in children with KS, particularly in reading and spelling. In one study, 92% of individuals with KS reported difficulties in learning to read, and 70% had an absolute reading deficit (Geschwind et al., 2000). Difficulties with speech production, language processing, and sentence structuring are thought to interfere with both reading and spelling (Mandoki, Sumner, Hoffman, & Riconda, 1991). Research looking at the development of reading and spelling in KS proposes that the course follows normal developmental patterns, but becomes arrested at some point (Seymour & Evans, 1988). Prospective and longitudinal research (Robinson et al., 1986; Walzer et al., 1986) indicates that children with KS are more likely to be referred for special education evaluations by their classroom teachers, and also more likely to be enrolled in a learning disability classroom. In their longitudinal study, Rovet and colleagues (1996) found boys with KS to perform significantly worse on measures of word decoding, reading comprehension, spelling, written language skills, arithmetic, math problem solving, and the acquisition of conceptual knowledge in areas such as science and humanities. In addition, the boys with KS were found to perform lower on standardized achievement tests, and they tended to fall further behind grade and age level expectations as they grew older. Interestingly, Rovet and colleagues noted that most of the boys with KS were equally impaired on measures of reading and arithmetic; however, they characterized the learning disability seen in KS as primarily language-based. The specific deficits demonstrated throughout all their findings appeared to reside in the area of auditory–verbal processing. This hypothesis is supported by earlier research (Bender et al., 1986), which demonstrated significant impairments in reading recognition, reading comprehension, and auditory short-term memory in a group of boys with KS. Bender and colleagues' (1986) sample was characterized by average intelligence, language dysfunction associated with slow processing and poor short-term memory, and a history of reading difficulty in school.

Emotional Presentation

Various prospective studies done within this population describe children with KS as less active, less assertive, and more susceptible to stress than controls (Bender & Berch, 1990). Temperamentally, these boys are also depicted as introverted, lacking ambition, pliant, less sociable, and socially inappropriate (Netley, 1990; Wodrich, 2008). In a longitudinal study, specific temperamental characteristics were observed in a cohort of XXY males from birth to age 7 (Walzer et al., 1986). Interview and observational data were obtained on variables such as activity level, intensity of responding, pliancy (e.g., easy to manage, assertiveness), approach–withdrawal, adaptability, and capacity to relate. Compared to a control group, the children with KS were again consistently rated as lower in activity and intensity, more pliant, and more withdrawn in new situations.

On the Personality Inventory for Children (Lachar & Gruber, 1994), boys with KS were found to differ significantly from controls on ratings of achievement, intelligence, and development, in addition to ratings of lower-than-average activity (Stewart, Bailey, Netley, Rovet, & Park, 1986). Another study of the psychological nature of adults with KS found them to be less teasing and sarcastic and more submissive than either controls or a group of XYY men (Schiavi, Theilgaard, Owen, & White, 1984).

van Rijn, Swaab, Aleman, and Kahn (2006) have suggested that, compared to genetically normal controls, men with KS have greater difficulty with the accurate perception of social-emotional cues (e.g., angry facial expressions) and experience greater emotional arousal in response to emotion-inducing events; these factors may cause them to be more influenced by their emotions when making decisions under these circumstances. Adding to their difficulty, men with KS seem to be less able to identify and verbalize the emotions they experience. These deficits impair social-cognitive processing and play an important role in the social difficulties that have been previously described in this syndrome.

Social Problems

As mentioned above, men with KS may display many characteristics that make social interactions problematic. These include social withdrawal, social anxiety, and shyness, as well as poor interpretation of the emotional content of facial expressions and verbal communication (Ratcliffe, 1999; Robinson, Bender, & Linden, 1990; van Rijn et al., 2006). This assortment of traits has lead some researches to question whether an increased level of autistic traits exists in men with KS. Using the Autism Spectrum Quotient, a self-administered questionnaire that assesses features of the core autistic phenotype in adults of typical intelligence, one study found that men with KS displayed more autistic traits in all domains than controls did. Increased autistic traits were associated with more distress during social interactions, and consequently less frequent participation in social interactions (van Rijn, Swaab, Aleman, & Kahn, 2008). There have been a few case reports in the literature of a dual diagnosis of autism and KS (Jha, Sheth, & Ghaziuddin, 2007). Deficits in response inhibition have also been documented (Temple & Sanfilippo, 2003) and can have deleterious effects on social interactions.

KEY ASSESSMENT ISSUES

Several issues are relevant to KS within the context of diagnosis and assessment. First, if a diagnosis of KS is made upon birth or shortly thereafter through genetic testing, both physiological development and learning capabilities can be assessed early and monitored over the course of the child's schooling. Developmental surveillance is critical following an early diagnosis and should facilitate early intervention services if problems surface. This developmental surveillance should continue as the individual grows older and can be assessed with more specific types of tools. This assessment can include comprehensive psychoeducational testing, which can help determine which, if any, impairments are present. Of special importance is careful assessment of language, motor skills, and social-emotional functioning (Wodrich, 2008). A detailed neuropsychological evaluation may also prove useful in documenting a profile of abilities and assisting in ongoing treatment planning.

However, a child may not carry a diagnosis, since many of the features most typical of KS (e.g., delayed puberty, diminished testes, absent secondary sex characteristics) do not appear until the beginning of adolescence. Therefore, child care professionals should be familiar with the characteristic learning, behavioral, and physical presentation of KS in order to recognize affected individuals, refer them for genetic evaluation and appropriate psychoeducational testing, and then implement interventions as early as possible. Again, such testing should include an evaluation of verbal abilities with an emphasis on expressive versus receptive language functioning, verbal memory, and auditory–verbal processing, as children with KS are at risk for reading and spelling disabilities.

OPTIONS FOR TREATMENT

Physiological Issues

In infants born with hypospadias, cryptorchidism, or a significantly small phallus, appropriate and timely treatment and/or surgical correction should be sought. Again, however, a majority of individuals with KS are not diagnosed until adolescence, when a paucity of testosterone causes a pubertal delay and a delay in the development of some secondary sexual characteristics.

Testosterone replacement therapy can have many beneficial effects, including regression of gynecomastia, improved development of masculine secondary sexual characteristics, increase in muscle bulk and bone marrow density, increased energy and endurance, improved mood and concentration, and decreased psychosocial problems (Bojesen & Gravholt, 2007; Nielsen, Pelsen, & Sorensen, 1988; Simm & Zacharin, 2006). Testosterone has been shown to have positive effects on fat mass, muscle mass, and muscle strength, as well as sexual activity, and it improves positive aspects of mood in young hypogonadal men (Wang et al., 2000). It has been suggested that treatment begin in early adolescence and continue lifelong, in order to prevent osteoporosis, obesity, the metabolic syndrome, and diabetes (Bojesen & Gravholt, 2007). It is important to recall that most patients with KS have only low-normal levels of testosterone, but that virtually all have increased gonadotropin levels. For this reason, testosterone replacement has been recommended if gonadotropin levels are elevated, even if testosterone levels are in the low end of the normal range. The aim of testosterone supplementation is normalization of LH and testosterone levels to the middle of the normal range, rather than just the low-normal range (Bojesen & Gravholt, 2007). Interestingly, a small imaging study of 10 individuals with KS also found relative preservation of the gray matter in the left temporal region associated with exposure to exogenous androgen, and a subsequent association with increased verbal fluency scores (Patwardhan et al., 2000).

Psychosocial Problems

Reviewing several studies of psychosocial adjustment in boys with KS, Robinson, Bender, Linden, and Salbenblatt (1990) provided common personality descriptors from these studies, which included "shy," "immature," "restrained," "reserved," and "poor peer relationships." The presence of a supportive and stable family environment was noted to have positive effects on psychosocial adjustment for these children. Other studies have described this population as cautious in new situations, low in motor activity, and possessing an easy disposition (Walzer et al., 1990). Walzer and colleagues (1990) commented that these characteristics predisposed children with KS to present as "low-key" children who were well liked by their teachers and who had few behavioral management problems. One problem with this study, and a characteristic that plagues much research with the sex chromosome disorders, is that the study examined both XXY and XYY boys.

Bender, Linden, and Robinson (1990) described a high-risk profile for children with sex chromosome disorders, based on the results of a prospective study. These high-risk children tended to be those who had problems communicating with peers; academic problems marked by low achievement; few hobbies or little participation in extracurricular activities; behavioral immaturity; and social isolation. This profile was viewed as a risk for poor psychosocial functioning as well as adult psychopathology. The authors also recognized the importance of environmental factors in determining outcome.

Emotional Problems

The abnormal sexual characteristics as well as the academic difficulties associated with KS often result in low self-esteem and poor self-concept in later adolescence or young adulthood. A follow-up study indicated that adult males with KS are often lonely, immature, and passive, and that they may have few friends (Nielsen, Johnsen, & Sorensen, 1980). Testosterone treatment's therapeutic effects on sexual development have also been found to improve problems stemming from low self-esteem (Nielsen et al., 1988; Schwartz & Root, 1991). Mazur and Clopper (1991) reviewed clinic cases they had seen with gynecomastia and determined that one of the greatest related concerns was the impact on psychosocial functioning. They reported that their patients had a history of being teased by peers regarding their breast development, which in turn resulted in social isolation and withdrawal in approximately 70% of these children. Cases of anorexia nervosa have been described in conjunction with KS, with poor body image and problems with puberty implicated in the etiology

(El-Badri & Lewis, 1991; Hindler & Norris, 1986). There are also accounts of schizophrenia in KS, with the hypothesis that the presence of an extra X chromosome and/or the abnormal hormonal levels during prenatal development may be the cause of this association (Pomeroy, 1980; Roy, 1981). Other types of psychopathology, such as bipolar disorders, have been linked to KS, but there is less of a consensus regarding this relationship (Everman & Stoudemire, 1994). When bipolar disorders are present, however, most accounts trace the etiology of these disorders to the presence of the extra X chromosome.

In an older study examining the sexual development of individuals with KS, these males were found to date and become sexually involved at a later age than their peers (Raboch, Mellan, & Starka, 1979). In view of the KS-related tendencies toward withdrawal and negative peer interactions, this relative delay is understandable. A survey of men seen at an infertility clinic who were determined to have KS reported below-average school performance, little energy, poor relations with parents or siblings, and more mental illness than seen in a control group (Kessler & Moos, 1973); however, it should be noted that many individuals with KS do marry and have successful relationships as adults.

As noted earlier, no current research supports the older contention that these individuals have higher rates of criminality or mental health problems. Although earlier studies asserted this possibility (Murken, 1973; Zuppinger et al., 1967), these studies had significant methodological flaws (e.g., problems with sample size and selection bias), which more recent work has attempted to correct. In fact, more recent studies have reported results showing no increased rates of mental health problems, and indeed a rarity of psychiatric problems, among men with KS (Geschwind et al., 2000). Other studies, however, continue to demonstrate a significantly increased risk of discharge from hospitals with a psychiatric diagnosis (Bojesen et al., 2006). Still, the consensus is that there appears to be a significant increase in psychosocial problems due to impulsivity and social inappropriateness in this subpopulation, as well as introversion, unassertiveness, and lack of ambition (Geschwind &

Dykens, 2004). There is no evidence indicating increased sociopathy or criminal intent in this population.

Educational Problems

Given the difficulty identifying infants with KS who may not display any abnormal features (e.g., congenital abnormalities), teachers may come across these undiagnosed children later once they enter the regular classroom setting. For example, Mandoki and Sumner (1991) described the case of a 14-year-old male who was diagnosed with KS only after suffering from years of academic failure, interpersonal problems, and emotional disturbance. Some physical features that may indicate KS include a small head circumference, greater-than-average height, small genitals, and proportionately long legs (Mandoki et al., 1991). When these characteristics are coupled with learning difficulties specific to reading and spelling, a referral for diagnostic testing (i.e., by karyotype) may be in order. The most common presenting problems of undiagnosed boys with KS are school underachievement, poor peer relationships, impulsivity, aggressiveness, withdrawal, apathy, and immaturity. Some treatment with medication and hormones is available to address the abnormal sexual development and aggressive behaviors in these males (see above). Although the learning disability will not be "cured" by this treatment, both medical and academic interventions are important for preventing these features from developing.

Some specific implications for the classroom have been offered by Rovet and colleagues (1996). Generally, they feel that intervention efforts should center on the language-based learning disorder. Speech–language therapy is recommended, with a special emphasis on vocabulary building, improving sentence understanding, comprehension skills, and word finding. Additional training to enhance memory functioning can be provided by presenting advance organizers for reading comprehension tasks, structuring lessons into smaller chunks to learn, and providing drilling on math facts. Obviously, a detailed assessment of reading and spelling skills will provide specific, targeted areas for educational intervention.

ADOLESCENCE AND ADULTHOOD OUTCOMES

Onset of adolescence is typically not delayed, but it is during this period that the major implications of this disorder become manifest. As discussed above, among the chief signs are the smaller testes. An androgen deficiency may also be determined by testing blood levels, with typical treatments involving testosterone replacement. Although some literature recommends that this treatment begin at age 12 for all children with KS, this policy remains debated (Gardner & Sutherland, 1996). The beneficial results of this treatment have been described earlier. A small study examining both physiological and psychological changes as a result of testosterone treatments found that the males with KS not only began to develop a more masculine physique and secondary sex characteristics, but also had improved perceptions of body image, increased assertiveness and goal-directed behavior, and heightened sexual drive (Johnson, Myhre, Ruvalcaba, Thuline, & Kelley, 1970). Approximately 50% of adolescents with KS will display gynecomastia, which can be treated surgically.

Although infertility has been found to be the general rule in individuals with KS, and a cause of social-emotional strain, some exceptions have been reported in the literature. Gardner and Sutherland (1996) hypothesized that these reports were probably attributable to cases of mosaicism. A more important point made by these authors is that there is a lack of information regarding the risk of having children with sex chromosome anomalies for individuals with KS who may produce children.

Genetic counseling for the family and the individual with KS can play an important role in ameliorating fears and improving outcomes. If KS is detected *in utero* through amniocentesis or chorionic villus sampling, counseling should emphasize the expected phenotype and its wide variability, as well as a 10% increase in the risk of pregnancy loss. Recurrence risk also should be discussed. Although little empirical evidence exists in this relatively small subpopulation to show any recurrence risk at all, some have suggested that the recurrence risk is probably close to that of trisomy 21 and trisomy 18—syndromes resulting from similar age-related meiotic nondisjunction errors (Simpson, 2003). The issue of sterility should be discussed with the parents and the male with KS. Robinson and colleagues (1986) found that parents of children with KS expressed worry about communicating information about the chromosomal abnormality and resulting infertility to their children. Furthermore, parents feel a sense of loss and grief themselves regarding their children's probable infertility. An individual with KS should be educated early about the issue of sterility. Recent advances in sperm recovery through testicular biopsy and viable pregnancy through intracytoplasmic sperm injection should be described, and referrals to the appropriate centers should be made in a timely manner (optimally in early adolescence or sooner). Alternatives such as adoption can also be discussed as options for raising children. Nielsen and colleagues (1980) found that within a group of individuals with KS, those who sought adoption or insemination by donor as alternatives were happier and had more stable marriages. Since it is not uncommon for individuals with KS to be discovered when infertility is the referral problem, marriage counseling may also be critical in these cases identified later.

CONCLUSION

KS is a sex-linked chromosomal disorder that has distinct learning, behavioral, and physiological features. Language-based learning disabilities are perhaps the most challenging academic problems, and language-processing deficits can persist into adulthood. The physical anomalies and hormonal disturbances present in this disorder can create both social and emotional challenges, particularly with the onset of puberty. Advances in testosterone replacement therapies have provided treatment for many of the hormone-related problems, and there is evidence that early treatment may also serve as a protective mechanism against some of the cognitive and neurological impairments. Early genetic identification, perhaps even prenatally, can help lead to earlier intervention for both the learning and physiological features. As further advances are made in the years to come, it is likely that there will be additional gains in the treatment outcomes for individuals with KS.

REFERENCES

Aksglaede, L., Petersen, J. H., Main, K. M., Skakkebaek, N. E., & Juul, A. (2007). High normal testosterone levels in infants with non-mosaic Klinefelter's syndrome. *European Journal of Endocrinology/European Federation of Endocrine Societies, 157*(3), 345–350.

Bender, B. G., & Berch, D. B. (1990). Overview: Psychological phenotypes and sex chromosome abnormalities. In D. B. Berch & B. G. Bender (Eds.), *Sex chromosome abnormalities and human behavior.* Boulder, CO: Westview Press.

Bender, B. G., & Berch, D. B. (1991). Overview: Psychological phenotypes and sex chromosome abnormalities. In D. B. Berch & B. G. Bender (Eds.), *Sex chromosome abnormalities and human behavior.* Boulder, CO: Westview Press.

Bender, B. G., Linden, M., & Robinson, A. (1990). Sex chromosome abnormalities: In search of developmental patterns. In D. B. Berch & B. G. Bender (Eds.), *Sex chromosome abnormalities and human behavior.* Boulder, CO: Westview Press.

Bender, B. G., Puck, M. H., Salbenblatt, J. A., & Robinson, A. (1986). Dyslexia in 47,XXY boys identified at birth. *Behavior Genetics, 16,* 343–354.

Bojesen, A., & Gravholt, C. H. (2007). Klinefelter syndrome in clinical practice. *Nature Clinical Practice. Urology, 4*(4), 192–204.

Bojesen, A., Juul, S., Birkebaek, N. H., & Gravholt, C. H. (2006). Morbidity in Klinefelter syndrome: A Danish register study based on hospital discharge diagnoses. *Journal of Clinical Endocrinology and Metabolism, 91*(4), 1254–1260.

Bojesen, A., Juul, S., & Gravholt, C. H. (2003). Prenatal and postnatal prevalence of Klinefelter syndrome: A national registry study. *Journal of Clinical Endocrinology and Metabolism, 88*(2), 622–626.

Cohen, F. L., & Durham, J. D. (1985). Update your knowledge of Klinefelter syndrome. *Journal of Psychosocial Nursing and Mental Health Services, 23,* 19–25.

Denschlag, D., Tempfer, C., Kunze, M., Wolff, G., & Keck, C. (2004). Assisted reproductive techniques in patients with Klinefelter syndrome: A critical review. *Fertility and Sterility, 82*(4), 775–779.

Diamond, M., & Watson, L. A. (2004). Androgen insensitivity syndrome and Klinefelter's syndrome: Sex and gender considerations. *Child and Adolescent Psychiatric Clinics of North America, 13*(3), 623–640.

Drugan, A., Isada, N. B., Johnson, M. P., & Evans,

M. I. (1996a). Genetics: An overview. In N. B. Isada, A. Drugan, M. P. Johnson, & M. I. Evans (Eds.), *Maternal genetic disease*. Stamford, CT: Appleton & Lange.

Drugan, A., Isada, N. B., Johnson, M. P., & Evans, M. I. (1996b). Parental chromosomal anomalies. In N. B. Isada, A. Drugan, M. P. Johnson, & M. I. Evans (Eds.), *Maternal genetic disease*. Stamford, CT: Appleton & Lange.

El-Badri, S. M., & Lewis, M. A. (1991). Anorexia nervosa associated with Klinefelter's syndrome. *Comprehensive Psychiatry, 32*(4), 317–319.

Elias, S., & Yanangi, R. M. (1981). Cardiovascular defects. In J. D. Schulman & J. L. Simpson (Eds.), *Genetic diseases in pregnancy: Maternal effects and fetal outcome*. New York: Academic Press.

Evans, M.I., Drugan, A., Pryde, P.G., & Johnson, M.P. (1996). Genetics and the obstetrician. In N. B. Isada, A. Drugan, M. P. Johnson, & M. I. Evans (Eds.), *Maternal genetic disease*. Stamford, CT: Appleton & Lange.

Everman, D. B., & Stoudemire, A. (1994). Bipolar disorder associated with Klinefelter's syndrome and other chromosomal abnormalities. *Psychosomatics, 35*, 35–40.

Forssman, H. (1970). The mental implications of sex chromosome aberrations. *British Journal of Psychiatry, 117*, 353–363.

Gardner, R. J. M., & Sutherland, G. R. (1996). *Chromosome abnormalities and genetic counseling* (2nd ed.). New York: Oxford University Press.

Geschwind, D. H., Boone, K. B., Miller, B. L., & Swerdloff, R. S. (2000). Neurobehavioral phenotype of Klinefelter syndrome. *Mental Retardation and Developmental Disabilities Research Reviews, 6*(2), 107–116.

Geschwind, D. H., & Dykens, E. (2004). Neurobehavioral and psychosocial issues in Klinefelter syndrome. *Learning Disabilities Research and Practice, 19*(3), 166–173.

Giedd, J. N., Clasen, L. S., Wallace, G. L., Lenroot, R. K., Lerch, J. P., Wells, E. M., et al. (2007). XXY (Klinefelter syndrome): A pediatric quantitative brain magnetic resonance imaging case-control study. *Pediatrics, 119*(1), e232–e240.

Gilbert, P. (1993). *The A–Z reference book of syndromes and inherited disorders*. New York: Chapman & Hall.

Harlow, T. L., & Gonzalez-Alegre, P. (2009). High prevalence of reported tremor in Klinefelter syndrome. *Parkinsonism and Related Disorders, 15*(5), 393–395.

Hindler, C.G., & Norris, D.L. (1986). A case of anorexia nervosa with Klinefelter's syndrome. *British Journal of Psychiatry, 149*, 659–660.

Hynd, G.W., & Willis, W. G. (1988). *Pediatric neuropsychology*. Needham Heights, MA: Allyn & Bacon.

Ishikawa, T., Yamaguchi, K., Kondo, Y., Takenaka, A., & Fujisawa, M. (2008). Metabolic syndrome in men with Klinefelter's syndrome. *Urology, 71*(6), 1109–1113.

Jha, P., Sheth, D., & Ghaziuddin, M. (2007). Autism spectrum disorder and Klinefelter syndrome. *European Child and Adolescent Psychiatry, 16*(5), 305–308.

Johnson, H. R., Myhre, S. A., Ruvalcaba, R. H. A., Thuline, H. C., & Kelley, V. C. (1970). Effects of testosterone on body image and behavior in Klinefelter's syndrome: A pilot study. *Developmental Medicine and Child Neurology, 12*, 454–460.

Kessler, S., & Moos, R. (1973). Behavioral aspects of chromosomal disorders. *Annual Review of Medicine, 24*, 89–102.

Klinefelter, H. F., Reifenstein, E. C., & Albright, F. (1942). Syndrome characterized by gynecomastia, aspermatogenesis without A-Leydigism, and increased excretion of follicle-stimulating hormone. *Journal of Clinical Endocrinology, 2*, 615–627.

Lachar, D., & Gruber, C. P. (1994). *The Personality Inventory for Youth*. Los Angeles, CA: Western Psychological Services.

Lanfranco, F., Kamischke, A., Zitzmann, M., & Nieschlag, E. (2004). Klinefelter's syndrome. *Lancet, 364*, 273–283.

Leonard, M. F., & Sparrow, S. (1986). Prospective study of development of children with sex chromosome anomalies: New Haven Study IV. Adolescence. *Birth Defects: Original Article Series, 22*, 221–249.

Lowe, X., Eskenazi, B., Nelson, D. O., Kidd, S., Alme, A., & Wyrobek, A. J. (2001). Frequency of XY sperm increases with age in fathers of boys with Klinefelter syndrome. *American Journal of Human Genetics, 69*(5), 1046–1054.

Mandoki, M. W., & Sumner, G. S. (1991). Klinefelter syndrome: The need for early identification and treatment. *Clinical Pediatrics, 30*, 161–164.

Mandoki, M. W., Sumner, G. S., Hoffman, R. P., & Riconda, D. L. (1991). A review of Klinefelter's syndrome in children and adolescents. *Journal of the American Academy of Child and Adolescent Psychiatry, 30*, 160–172.

Mazur, T., & Clopper, R. R. (1991). Pubertal disorders: Psychology and clinical management. *Endocrinology and Metabolism Clinics of North America, 20*(1), 211–230.

Murken, J.D. (1973). The XYY syndrome and Klinefelter's syndrome. In P. E. Becker, W. Lenz, F. Vogel, & G. G. Wendt (Eds.), *Topics in human genetics* (Vol. 2). Stuttgart, Germany: Grammlich.

Netley, C. (1987). Predicting intellectual functioning in 47,XXY boys from characteristics of siblings. *Clinical Genetics, 32*, 24–27.

Netley, C. (1990). Behavior and extra X aneuploid states. In D. B. Berch & B. G. Bender (Eds.), *Sex chromosome abnormalities and human behavior.* Boulder, CO: Westview Press.

Netley, C., & Rovet, J. (1982). Verbal deficits in children with 47,XXY and 47,XXX karyotypes: A descriptive and experimental study. *Brain and Language, 17,* 58–72.

Netley, C., & Rovet, J. (1984). Hemispheric lateralization in 47,XXY Klinefelter's syndrome boys. *Brain and Cognition, 3,* 10–18.

Nielsen, J., Johnsen, S. G., & Sorensen, K. (1980). Follow-up 10 years later of 34 Klinefelter males with karyotype 47,XXY and 16 hypogonadal males with karyotype 46,XY. *Psychological Medicine, 10,* 345–352.

Nielsen, J., Pelsen, B., & Sorensen, K. (1988). Follow-up of 30 Klinefelter males treated with testosterone. *Clinical Genetics, 33*(4), 262–269.

Nielsen, J., & Wohlert, M. (1991). Chromosome abnormalities found among 34910 newborn children: Results from a 13–year incidence study in Arhus, Denmark. *Human Genetics, 87,* 81–83.

Paduch, D. A., Fine, R. G., Bolyakov, A., & Kiper, J. (2008). New concepts in Klinefelter syndrome. *Current Opinion in Urology, 18*(6), 621–627.

Patwardhan, A. J., Eliez, S., Bender, B., Linden, M. G., & Reiss, A. L. (2000). Brain morphology in Klinefelter syndrome: Extra X chromosome and testosterone supplementation. *Neurology, 54*(12), 2218–2223.

Pellestor, F., Andreo, B., Arnal, F., Humeau, C., & Demaille, J. (2002). Mechanisms of nondisjunction in human female meiosis: The co-existence of two modes of malsegregation evidenced by the karyotyping of 1397 in-vitro unfertilized oocytes. *Human Reproduction, 17*(8), 2134–2145.

Pierce, B. A. (1990). *The family genetic sourcebook.* New York: Wiley.

Pomeroy, J. C. (1980). Klinefelter's syndrome and schizophrenia. *British Journal of Psychiatry, 136,* 597–599.

Raboch, J., Mellan, J., & Starka, L. (1979). Klinefelter's syndrome: Sexual development and activity. *Archives of Sexual Behavior, 8*(4), 333–339.

Ratcliffe, S. (1999). Long-term outcome in children of sex chromosome abnormalities. *Archives of Disease in Childhood, 80*(2), 192–195.

Ratcliffe, S. G., Masera, N., Pan, H., & McKie, M. (1994). Head circumference and IQ of children with sex chromosome abnormalities. *Developmental Medicine and Child Neurology, 36,* 533–544.

Robinson, A., Bender, B. G., Borelli, J. B., Puck, M. H., Salbenblatt, J. A., & Winter, J. S. D. (1986). Sex chromosomal aneuploidy: Prospective and longitudinal studies. In S. G. Ratcliffe & N. Paul (Eds.), *Prospective studies on children with sex chromosome aneuploidy.* New York: Alan R. Liss.

Robinson, A., Bender, B. G., & Linden, M. G. (1990). Summary of clinical findings in children and young adults with sex chromosome anomalies. *Birth Defects Original Article Series, 26*(4), 225–228.

Robinson, A., Bender, B. G., Linden, M. G,, & Salbenblatt, J. (1990). Sex chromosome aneuploidy: The Denver prospective study. *Birth Defects: Original Article Series, 26*(4), 59–115.

Ross, J. L., Roeltgen, D. P., Stefanatos, G., Benecke, R., Zeger, M. P., Kushner, H., et al. (2008). Cognitive and motor development during childhood in boys with Klinefelter syndrome. *American Journal of Medical Genetics, Part A, 146A*(6), 708–719.

Ross, J. L., Samango-Sprouse, C., Lahlou, N., Kowal, K., Elder, F. F., & Zinn, A. (2005). Early androgen deficiency in infants and young boys with 47,XXY Klinefelter syndrome. *Hormone Research, 64*(1), 39–45.

Rovet, J., Netley, C., Keenan, M., Bailey, J., & Stewart, D. (1996). The psychoeducational profile of boys with Klinefelter syndrome. *Journal of Learning Disabilities, 29*(2), 180–196.

Roy, A. (1981). Schizophrenia and Klinefelter syndrome. *Canadian Journal of Psychiatry, 26,* 262–264.

Samango-Sprouse, C. (2001). Mental development in polysomy X Klinefelter syndrome (47,XXY; 48,XXXY): Effects of incomplete X inactivation. *Seminars in Reproductive Medicine, 19*(2), 193–202.

Schiavi, R. C., Theilgaard, A., Owen, D. R., & White, D. (1984). Sex chromosome anomalies, hormones, and aggressivity. *Archives of General Psychiatry, 41,* 93–99.

Schroder, J., Chapelle, A., Hakola, P., & Virkkunen, M. (1981). The frequency of XYY and XXY men among criminal offenders. *Acta Psychiatrica Scandinavica, 63,* 272–276.

Schwartz, I. D., & Root, A. W. (1991). The Klinefelter syndrome of testicular dysgenesis. *Endocrinology and Metabolism Clinics of North America, 20*(1), 153–163.

Seymour, P. H. K., & Evans, H. M. (1988). Developmental arrest at the logographic stage: Impaired literacy functions in Klinefelter's XXXY syndrome. *Journal of Research in Reading, 11*(2), 133–151.

Shen, D., Liu, D., Liu, H., Clasen, L., Giedd, J., & Davatzikos, C. (2004). Automated morphometric study of brain variation in XXY males. *NeuroImage, 23*(2), 648–653.

Sheridan, M. K., & Radlinski, S. (1988). Brief report: A case study of an adolescent male with XXXXY Klinefelter's syndrome. *Journal of Autism and Developmental Disorders, 18*(3), 449–456.

Simm, P. J., & Zacharin, M. R. (2006). The psychosocial impact of Klinefelter syndrome—A 10 year review. *Journal of Pediatric Endocrinology and Metabolism, 19*(4), 499–505.

Simpson, J. J. (2003). Klinefelter syndrome: Expanding the phenotype and identifying new research directions. *Genetics in Medicine, 5*(6), 460–468.

Sloter, E., Nath, J., Eskenazi, B., & Wyrobek, A. J. (2004). Effects of male age on the frequencies of germinal and heritable chromosomal abnormalities in humans and rodents. *Fertility and Sterility, 81*(4), 925–943.

Smyth, C. M., & Bremner, W. J. (1998). Klinefelter syndrome. *Archives of Internal Medicine, 158*(12), 1309–1314.

Stewart, D., Bailey, J., Netley, C., Rovet, J., & Park, E. (1986). Growth and development from early to midadolescence of children with X and Y chromosome aneuploidy: The Toronto study. *Birth Defects: Original Article Series, 22*(3), 119–182.

Styne, D. M. (1991). Puberty and its disorders in boys. *Endocrinology and Metabolism Clinics of North America, 20*(1), 43–69.

Swerdlow, A. J., Hermon, C., Jacobs, P. A., Alberman, E., Beral, V., Daker, M., et al. (2001). Mortality and cancer incidence in persons with numerical sex chromosome abnormalities: A cohort study. *Annals of Human Genetics, 65*(Pt. 2), 177–188.

Temple, C. M., & Sanfilippo, P. M. (2003). Executive skills in Klinefelter's syndrome. *Neuropsychologia, 41*(11), 1547–1559.

Theilgaard, A. (1984). A psychological study of the personalities of XYY and XXY men. *Acta Psychiatrica Scandinavica, 69*(Suppl. 315), 1–132.

Thomas, N. S., & Hassold, T. J. (2003). Aberrant recombination and the origin of Klinefelter syndrome. *Human Reproduction Update, 9*(4), 309–317.

Tyler, C., & Edman, J. C. (2004). Down syndrome, Turner syndrome, and Klinefelter syndrome: Primary care throughout the life span. *Primary Care, 31*(3), 627–648, x–xi.

van Rijn, S., Aleman, A., Swaab, H., Krijn, T., Vingerhoets, G., & Kahn, R. S. (2007). What it is said versus how it is said: Comprehension of affective prosody in men with Klinefelter (47,XXY) syndrome. *Journal of the International Neuropsychological Society, 13*(6), 1065–1070.

van Rijn, S., Swaab, H., Aleman, A., & Kahn, R. S. (2008). Social behavior and autism traits in a sex chromosomal disorder: Klinefelter (47XXY) syndrome. *Journal of Autism and Developmental Disorders, 38*(9), 1634–1641.

van Rijn, S., Swaab, H., Aleman, A., & Kahn, R. S. (2006). X chromosomal effects on social cognitive processing and emotion regulation: A study with Klinefelter men (47,XXY). *Schizophrenia Research, 84*(2–3), 194–203.

Visootsak, J., Aylstock, M., & Graham, J. M., Jr. (2001). Klinefelter syndrome and its variants: An update and review for the primary pediatrician. *Clinical Pediatrics, 40*(12), 639–651.

Visootsak, J., & Graham, J. M., Jr. (2006). Klinefelter syndrome and other sex chromosomal aneuploidies. *Orphanet Journal of Rare Diseases, 1*, 42.

Volkl, T. M., Langer, T., Aigner, T., Greess, H., Beck, J. D., Rauch, A. M., et al. (2006). Klinefelter syndrome and mediastinal germ cell tumors. *American Journal of Medical Genetics, Part A, 140*(5), 471–481.

Walzer, S., Bashir, A. S., Graham, J. M., Silbert, A. R., Lange, N. T., DeNapoli, M. F., et al. (1986). Behavioral development of boys with X chromosome aneuploidy: Impact of reactive style on the educational intervention for learning deficits. In S. G. Ratcliffe & N. Paul (Eds.), *Prospective studies on children with sex chromosome aneuploidy.* New York: Liss.

Walzer, S., Bashir, A. S., & Silbert, A. R. (1990). Cognitive and behavioral factors in the learning disabilities of 47,XXY and 47,XYY boys. *Birth Defects: Original Article Series, 26*, 45–58.

Wang, C., Swerdloff, R. S., Iranmanesh, A., Dobs, A., Snyder, P. J., Cunningham, G., et al. (2000). Transdermal testosterone gel improves sexual function, mood, muscle strength, and body composition parameters in hypogonadal men. *Journal of Clinical Endocrinology and Metabolism, 85*(8), 2839–2853.

Weatherall, D. J. (1991). *The new genetics and clinical practice* (3rd ed.). New York: Oxford University Press.

Wheeler, M. D. (1991). Physical changes of puberty. *Endocrinology and Metabolism Clinics of North America, 20*(1), 1–14.

Wikstrom, A. M., Raivio, T., Hadziselimovic, F., Wikstrom, S., Tuuri, T., & Dunkel, L. (2004). Klinefelter syndrome in adolescence: Onset of puberty is associated with accelerated germ cell depletion. *Journal of Clinical Endocrinology and Metabolism, 89*(5), 2263–2270.

Wodrich, D. D. (2008). Psychoeducational implications of sex chromosome anomalies. *School Psychology Quarterly, 23*(2), 301–311.

Zeger, M. P., Zinn, A. R., Lahlou, N., Ramos, P., Kowal, K., Samango-Sprouse, C., et al. (2008). Effect of ascertainment and genetic features on the phenotype of Klinefelter syndrome. *Journal of Pediatrics, 152*(5), 716–722.

Zuppinger, K., Engel, E., Forbes, A. P., Mantooth, L., & Claffey, J. (1967). Klinefelter's syndrome: A clinical and cytogenetic study in twenty-four cases. *Acta Endocrinologica, 54*(Suppl. 113), 5–48.

CHAPTER 21

Phenylketonuria

SUSAN E. WAISBREN

HISTORICAL AND THEORETICAL BACKGROUND

Religion, politics, geography, and genetics all pertain to the study of phenylketonuria (PKU). An isolated community in San'a, the capital of Yemen more than 300 years ago, was probably home to the bearer of an unusual gene for PKU. The Jews of Yemen were forbidden to marry persons of other faiths, and others were punished by death if they converted to Judaism. Consequently, the gene spread only within this community, and it has been possible to trace cases of PKU among Israelis of Yemenite Jewish origin to the one family in San'a (Wright, 1990). Different mutations for PKU have been traced to the Vikings and to gene bearers in Japan, Italy, Denmark, Scotland, Ireland, Kuwait, South America, and South Africa. Each of these mutations leads to an obstruction in the metabolism of phenylalanine, an essential amino acid abundant in protein. As an autosomal recessive disorder, PKU is inherited from each parent and affects males and females at an equal rate. The mutant gene produces a defect in the liver enzyme phenylalanine hydroxylase (PAH), resulting in a block in the conversion of phenylalanine to tyrosine. The only cure presently available for this disorder is liver transplantation (Vajro et al., 1993). Given the risks inherent in liver transplantation, this "cure" is generally not considered. Moreover, treatments exist that prevent mental retardation, the most severe consequence of PKU.

In 1934, Asbjorn Følling, a Norwegian physician, discovered PKU. A mother of two children with intellectual disabilities came to see him after consulting many other doctors. She insisted that both her children had a similar degree of mental retardation and patterns of behavior; in addition, she pointed out that both excreted urine with a unique odor. Følling, who had also trained in chemistry, studied the children's urine using a wide variety of agents until he discovered that it contained a large amount of phenylpyruvic acid. He knew that phenylpyruvic acid is a metabolite of phenylalanine, and he suspected that the defect in this disorder involves phenylalanine metabolism (Følling, 1934). Others demonstrated that the disorder is inherited and that excess phenylalanine is present in blood.

It was not until 1954, however, that a treatment was discovered. Again a persistent mother, this time in England, provided the impetus for the discovery (see Koch, 1997). She brought to a physician named Hørst

Bickel her 17-month-old daughter, who had the typical features of PKU: intellectual disability, eczema, awkward gait, spastic reflexes, and no language abilities. The child took no interest in her surroundings, moaned incessantly, and banged her head. The young doctor reasoned that perhaps if the child's phenylalanine intake were limited, the buildup of the toxic amino acid could be prevented. Along with Louis Woolf, in London, he created an amino acid mixture containing all the necessary parts of protein except for phenylalanine (Bickel, Gerrard, & Hickmans, 1954). He advised the mother to feed her daughter the special formula and to avoid all other protein foods or drinks. Two weeks later, the mother returned, claiming a miracle. The little girl had learned to crawl and pull herself to a stand, and was bright and cheerful instead of dull and irritable. Bickel prescribed continuation of the treatment, but this time added phenylalanine to the formula. The mother returned 2 days later to report that her daughter had reverted to the previous state and that the formula no longer worked (Gerrard, 1994). Through this experiment, Bickel proved that phenylalanine caused the neurological problems and that dietary treatment was beneficial. He also realized that the sooner the special diet could be started, the greater the benefit.

The scene then shifted to the United States, where Robert Guthrie met Robert MacCready at a meeting of the National Association for Retarded Children. Each was a father of a child with intellectual disabilities. MacCready was also the director of the Diagnostic Division of the Massachusetts Public Health Laboratories in Boston, and Guthrie was a physician and microbiologist from Buffalo, New York. Guthrie told MacCready about a test he had invented, the now famous Guthrie bacterial assay for the filter paper blood test (Guthrie & Susi, 1963). From a drop of blood obtained from the heel of a newborn infant, PKU could be identified within the first few days of life. Treatment started at this early age prevented intellectual disabilities. MacCready was so impressed by this new technology that he spent a week in Buffalo learning the test. He brought it back to Boston, installed it in the Bacteriology Laboratory, and started the first newborn screening program for PKU (MacCready, 1963).

Despite the straightforward results, the simplicity of the method, and the clear rationale for newborn screening, its acceptance was far from easy. With persistence equal to that of the mothers from Norway and England, Guthrie and MacCready lobbied in Washington and traveled throughout the United States arguing for mandatory, government-supported newborn screening (Koch, 1997). By 1964 they had succeeded in Massachusetts, and 11 years later 43 states had enacted a newborn screening law (Paul, 1999). Today laws mandating newborn screening for PKU exist throughout North America and most of Europe.

The reasons why PKU causes neurological problems remain unproven. Pathology reports, neuroimaging, research into biochemical pathways, and studies using animal models suggest that the accumulation of phenylalanine metabolites in blood is not directly related to neuropsychological deficits in PKU, but rather indirectly linked to aberrations in myelin, competition across the blood–brain barrier, and reductions in neurotransmitters (Surtees & Blau, 2000). These hypotheses are described below.

- *Myelin synthesis and turnover.* Phenylalanine or its metabolites in large quantities may be toxic to the brain by inhibiting myelin development (Scriver & Kaufman, 2001). Magnetic resonance imaging (MRI) studies suggest that when phenylalanine levels are high, myelination in the brain is reduced (Scarabino et al., 2009). In untreated or poorly treated children with PKU, myelination is delayed; in adults who discontinue the diet, dysmyelination occurs. Since, however, the degree of myelin in the brain has not been clearly associated with IQ or clinical symptoms in PKU, the precise mechanism of phenylalanine toxicity has eluded investigators (Jones et al., 1995).

- *Competition for transport.* Phenylalanine competes with several other essential amino acids (large neutral amino acids, or LNAAs) for transport across the blood–brain barrier. Since the transport across the blood–brain barrier tends to have a higher affinity for phenylalanine than for the other LNAAs in the presence of a high level of blood phenylalanine, the usual amounts of other amino acids, such as tyrosine and tryptophan, fail to reach the brain (Miller,

Braun, Pardridge, & Oldendorf, 1985). Tyrosine and tryptophan are precursors of the neurotransmitters dopamine and serotonin, respectively, which are consequently reduced in the brain (Güttler & Lou, 1986; Krause et al., 1985). Moreover, reduction of important amino acids is likely to inhibit protein synthesis in the brain, which is critical for cognitive functioning (Hoeksma et al., 2009).

• *Dopamine reduction.* Since phenylalanine cannot be metabolized to tyrosine in PKU, tyrosine is reduced, and the metabolites of tyrosine are also reduced. One of these metabolites is the neurotransmitter dopamine, and, as expected, dopamine levels are reduced in the cerebrospinal fluid of people with PKU. Moreover, certain parts of the brain, specifically the prefrontal cortex, are highly sensitive to even modest reductions in dopamine; this explains why specific functions related to these brain areas are selectively impaired in patients with PKU (Diamond, Ciaramitaro, Donner, Djali, & Robinson, 1994). Treatment with large doses of tyrosine, however, do not prevent the neurological effects of PKU. Years ago, a child was not treated with the phenylalanine-restricted diet, but instead was treated only with high doses of tyrosine. Unfortunately, the treatment was unsuccessful, and the child developed severe intellectual disability (Batshaw, Valle, & Bessman, 1981). In a more recent study, adults with PKU who had discontinued or relaxed treatment were administered high doses of tyrosine or a placebo in a double-blind crossover study. Despite increases in plasma tyrosine (and presumed increases in brain dopamine) during tyrosine supplementation, no beneficial effects were noted (Pietz, Landwehr, Schmidt, de Sonneville, & Trefz, 1995). Thus high phenylalanine levels are still considered the most likely pathological agent in PKU.

Questions about neuropathology in PKU led investigators to search for animal models, where brain chemistry could be studied directly. Until the 1990s, no monkeys, mice, rabbits, or any other animals with PKU could be found. It was possible to raise the blood phenylalanine levels of normal animals by loading the diet with phenylalanine, often in conjunction with an inhibitor of the PAH enzyme. However, the conversion of phenylalanine to tyrosine could not be blocked

sufficiently to prevent some increase in the tyrosine level; hence these experimental animals were never very similar to humans with PKU, who had chronically low levels of tyrosine. Using classical mutagenesis and selective breeding, researchers began to "create" the PKU mouse. When a known mutagen was fed to hundreds of pregnant mice, and when a phenylalanine-loaded diet was then fed to the offspring, mice suspected of being carriers of the mutant PAH gene could be identified. After cross-breeding carriers for three generations, the researchers eventually created a strain of mice with PKU. These mice, when fed a normal-protein diet, had elevated phenylalanine levels and appeared to have intellectual disabilities; for instance, they could not swim, while their littermates without PKU did so easily. Moreover, these mice had lighter-colored coats and were smaller in size—features corresponding to the lighter hair and smaller stature of children with untreated PKU. When fed a phenylalanine- restricted but otherwise nutritionally balanced diet, the mice began to look more like their siblings without PKU. Some probably even learned to swim (McDonald, Bode, Dove, & Shedlovsky, 1990; Shedlovsky, McDonald, Symula, & Dove, 1993).

With these mice, researchers have begun to study more closely the parts of the brain affected by PKU. Myelin abnormalities were found to be a result of increased myelin turnover and decreased myelin production (Surtees & Blau, 2000). Moyle, Fox, Arthur, Bynevelt, and Burnett (2007) found that in mice with PKU there is significant hypomyelination, as well as decreased activity of an enzyme that contributes to cholesterol biosynthesis regulation. Regions of the brain that are known to myelinate before birth do not show this decreased activity, whereas regions that develop after birth do.

Cabib, Pascucci, Ventura, Romano, and Puglisi-Allegra (2003) found that mice with untreated PKU had an impaired ability to encode spatial and nonspatial information, whereas healthy mice showed no impairments, suggesting a profile of learning disabilities similar to that found in children with PKU. Pascucci, Andolina, Ventura, Puglisi-Allegra, and Cabib (2008) later explained these deficits as potentially related to reduced availability of brain amines during postnatal development. Mihalick, Langlois, Krienke, and Dube (2000) reported on a study in which mice searched for a treat hidden in one of two different scented areas of sand. The task required learning where the treat was most likely to be hidden, based on previous trials. Although healthy mice were able to complete this task without difficulties, mice with untreated PKU were slower to find the hidden treat, suggesting slower mental processing abilities.

Although devastating effects usually occur when PKU is untreated, and close-to-normal development is attained when PKU is treated within the first weeks of life, there are exceptions. A few individuals with untreated PKU and high phenylalanine levels have average intelligence, and some individuals with well-treated PKU suffer neurological effects and have lower IQs than their siblings. Two individuals in the same family occasionally have dramatically different outcomes. None of the theories regarding the pathology in PKU can yet explain these exceptional cases.

GENETICS

The small warning label on diet soda cans containing the artificial sweetener aspartame reads, "Phenylketonurics: Contains phenylalanine." This warning has greatly increased the public awareness of PKU. In reality, PKU is one of the most common genetic disorders known. In the United States, 1 out of 50 people are carriers. Results of newborn screening of over 5 million neonates from throughout the world indicate varying rates. PKU is almost unknown among individuals of African descent, but fairly common among those of European descent, with prevalence rates ranging from 1 in 5,400 in Ireland to 1 in 11,000 in the United States and 1 in 16,000 in Switzerland (Woo, Lidsky, Guttler, Chandra, & Robson, 1983). As an autosomal recessive disorder, PKU is inherited from both parents. When both the mother and father are carriers, the chance of each child's inheriting PKU is 1 in 4.

Soon after PKU was discovered, physicians and parents noted that not all children with PKU were the same in their phenylalanine levels when off diet, or in their tolerance for phenylalanine before their blood levels rose. People in Italy, for example, appeared to have a milder form of PKU than people in Ireland: They could tolerate more protein, they had lower blood phenylalanine levels, and they seemed to be less affected by their PKU. In the 1980s, the answer to this puzzling picture appeared. Woo and colleagues (1983) cloned the gene for PAH, the enzyme responsible for the conversion of phenylalanine to tyrosine. When this gene is defective, the enzyme does not function or does not function completely; as a consequence, a rise in phenylalanine occurs. The investigators eventually realized that many mutations exist in the PAH gene. Mapped to chromosome 12, the PAH gene is 90 kb in length (12q22–24.2; 13 exons). Most children inherit two different mutations, resulting in substantial genetic heterogeneity in those with PKU (Scriver, Kaufman, Eisensmith, & Woo, 1995). By 1996, there were over 250 known mutations linked to PKU (Guldberg et al., 1996); by 2009, 560 different mutations had been identified (*www. PAHdb.mcgill.ca*).

Does genotype make a difference? The answer is yes and no. Studies (e.g., Trefz et al., 1993) suggest that patients with classic PKU, who have blood phenylalanine levels greater than 20 mg/dl on a normal diet and no activity of the PAH enzyme, have genotypes differing from those patients with mild PKU (with blood phenylalanine levels of 10–20 mg/dl and 5–15% residual activity of the enzyme) and of patients with non-PKU hyperphenylalaninemia (with blood phenylalanine levels of 2–10 mg/dl and an estimated 25% residual activity of PAH).

The phenotype, however, depends primarily on the particular combination of genes inherited from the mother and father. For example, a patient with the genotype of R408W/IVS-12 will have a more severe biochemical defect (and probably a lower IQ) than a patient with the genotype R408W/Y414C, even though the two patients share the R408W gene. The reason is that although the R408W mutation confers no PAH enzyme activity, the Y414C allows for enough of the enzyme activity to produce mild PKU, whereas the IVS-12 mutation also confers no PAH activity and thus results in severe PKU. In addition to the genetic factors related to the PAH genotype, however, other physiological and genetic factors affect the phenotypic outcome in PKU (Ozalp et al., 1994).

An intriguing question is that of the persistence of PKU in the population. Some people have argued that the disease should have "died out," since before the era of newborn screening, amost all individuals with PKU had severe intellectual disabilities, and few reproduced. One explanation is that new mutations occur frequently enough to replace mutations that have disappeared through lack of reproduction (Levy, 1989). Others believe that there must be a selective advantage to carrier status for PKU (Kidd, 1987), possibly including a lower spontaneous abortion rate (Woolf, 1976). Most likely, carrier status is sufficiently high to remain constant, despite the rates at which affected individuals reproduce (Kirkman, 1982). Prenatal diagnosis is available for PKU (Scriver et al., 1995), but is not commonly requested.

DEVELOPMENTAL COURSE UNDER VARIOUS CONDITIONS

No Treatment or Late Treatment

Children with classic PKU, if untreated, have severe intellectual disabilities, eczema, seizures, ataxia, motor deficits, and behavioral problems. Autism is often prominent. Although they appear normal until about age 6 months, infants with untreated PKU gradually exhibit developmental problems and can display self-mutilation, aggression, impulsivity, and psychosis (Penrose, 1972).

Parents and caretakers today now introduce the special phenylalanine-restricted diet to adults with untreated PKU when medications and behavioral programs fail to control psychotic symptoms, aggression, or self-abuse. Follow-up studies document little or no improvement in cognitive performance. However, case reports suggest moderate and sometimes even dramatic improvement in behavior if metabolic control is achieved and maintained on a long-term basis (Adams, 2009; Baumeister & Baumeister, 1998; Harper & Reid, 1987; Yannicelli & Ryan, 1995).

Even today, an infant with PKU is occasionally missed in newborn screening because of laboratory or hospital error. Not receiving the benefit of early dietary therapy, the child soon exhibits early signs of developmental delay. Most of these "missed" children are eventually diagnosed in early childhood. Treatment at this stage often results in improvement, with some children who neither walked nor talked at age 3 or 4 years reaching these developmental milestones shortly after restriction of their phenylalanine intake. Eventual developmental outcome in these children is variable, with some attaining an IQ within the average range, but most others performing within the range of mild to moderate intellectual disability. Late treatment such as this, however, is almost always associated with significant learning disabilities, even when IQ is within the average range.

Dietary Treatment

Dietary treatment for PKU consists of a phenylalanine-restricted diet, including a special formula and foods low in phenylalanine. Until recently, the only formula options have been amino-acid-based formulas that contain all of the necessary nutrients (amino acids) in protein, apart from phenylalanine. Unfortunately, amino acids in this form have a distinctive, strong taste and odor. Almost all infants accept the formula without difficulties; however, some children find it distasteful as they grow older, and many adults returning to the diet deem it unpalatable.

The diet permits sugars and fats; measured amounts of fruits and vegetables; and special low-protein pastas, grains, and breads. Meats, fish, eggs, dairy products, nuts, soy products, regular grains, and corn are not allowed. When children or adults "cheat" or consume more than the allocated amount of protein, they do not immediately feel ill, although a few individuals report feeling tired or distracted. Most experience no immediate side effects. It is only the cumulative effect of increased phenylalanine intake that is noticeable. Dietary control is monitored through frequent sampling of blood phenylalanine levels.

Until the 1980s, most clinics in North America and Europe recommended diet discontinuation during middle childhood (Schuett & Brown, 1984). At about age 5 or 6 years, most children with PKU were suddenly allowed to eat as much protein as they desired. Although it was known that their blood phenylalanine levels would rise, it was thought that their cognitive abilities would be unaffected. The fact that high phenylalanine levels are known to affect myelin in the brain, and that myelination is essentially complete after infancy, provided the rationale for this approach to treatment of PKU. Moreover, children who did not adhere to the diet despite medical recommendations did not develop intellectual disabilities. Thus the policy of diet discontinuation was adopted.

Despite the early enthusiasm for considering PKU a disease of early childhood, evidence gradually mounted demonstrating that diet discontinuation resulted in diminished IQ in a sizable proportion of these children (Waisbren, Schnell, & Levy, 1980). A North American PKU Collaborative Study was established to determine the effects of diet discontinuation in early-treated children with PKU (Koch, Azen, Friedman, & Williamson, 1982). The results of the follow-up study indicated that the age at which blood phenylalanine levels consistently exceeded 15 mg/dl was the best predictor of IQ and school achievement at ages 8 and 10 years (Holtzman, Kronmal, van Doorninck, Azen, & Koch, 1986). A retrospective study of 46 patients in Pennsylvania followed beyond age 12 years reported similar results (Legido et al., 1993). On the other hand, a policy of diet discontinuation at age 10 years was instituted in Scotland, and no declines in cognitive and motor functioning were noted after diet discontinuation in adolescents and young adults at a median age of 20 years. However, the individuals with PKU performed less well on all tests than age-matched subjects without PKU (Griffiths, Paterson, & Harvie, 1995).

A National Institutes of Health (NIH) Consensus Conference with a multidisciplinary panel convened in 2000 in Washington, DC, to prepare guidelines for the treatment of PKU. Lifelong diet continuation was recommended, with the understanding that the diet may be relaxed in older patients, depending on individual needs. Patients being treated for maternal PKU were advised to maintain blood phenylalanine levels at 2–6 mg/dl beginning 3 months before pregnancy and continuing throughout pregnancy (NIH Consensus Development Panel, 2001). These guidelines are currently being reconsidered, as more has become known since 2000 about the specific neuropsychological deficits that occur even in early and continuously treated individuals with PKU (von Spronsen & Burgard, 2008).

New and Emerging Treatments

Oral administration of sapropterin dihydrochloride (BH4), commercially known as Kuvan, recently received approval from the U.S. Food and Drug Administration for the treatment of PKU. BH4 is a cofactor of PAH, the enzyme responsible for converting phenylalanine to tyrosine. BH4 boosts the activity of this enzyme in individuals with PKU who have residual enzyme activity. Approximately 80% of patients with mild PKU and about 10% of patients with classic PKU who take BH4 respond with lowered phenylalanine levels and increased tolerance of phenylalanine (protein), without negative physical or neurological effects (Blau et al., 2009; Levy et al., 2007). Increased dietary flexibility may lead to increased metabolic control in noncompliant patients with PKU and in women with PKU who are pregnant (Ficge & Blau, 2007). Some clinicians encourage a trial of BH4 therapy in all patients with PKU, since it appears to have results independent of patients' genotype, phenotype, or age (Bóveda et al., 2007), although some genotypes may be associated with BH4 responsiveness (Blau et al., 2009).

LNAA therapy is another supplemental therapy, known commercially as Lanoflex, PreKUnil, or Neophe. In large quantities, LNAAs can compete with phenylalanine at the blood–brain barrier, so that less phenylalanine and more LNAAs cross into the brain (Matalon et al., 2003, 2007; Schindeler et al., 2007). Unlike BH4, LNAA therapy does not reduce the blood phenylalanine level, although it may lower brain phenylalanine concentrations (Matalon et al., 2007).

Recently a new phenylalanine-free source of protein has been identified. This protein, called glycomacropeptide (GMP), is produced during cheese making; when isolated from cheese whey, it contains virtually no phenylalanine (Ney et al., 2009). GMP formulas and foods are an alternative to the current amino acid formulas (LaClaire et al., 2009). GMP has been noted to improve protein retention and phenylalanine utilization, as well as to lower phenylalanine levels in the brain (van Calcar et al., 2009). GMP foods increase satiety and have a more palatable taste and odor than the amino acid formulas do, and may thus increase adherence to dietary recommendations (Mcleod, Clayton, van Calcar, & Ney, in press; Ney et al., 2009; van Calcar et al., 2009; van Spronsen & Enns, 2010).

Pegylated recombinant phenylalanine ammonia lyase is an investigational enzyme substitution therapy for the treatment of PKU that would theoretically reduce blood phenylalanine levels in all individuals with PKU. Studies in mice suggest that phenylalanine levels could be controlled without diet (Sarkissian et al., 2008). Known commercially as Peg-Pal, this potential therapy involving weekly subcutaneous injections is currently undergoing clinical trials in humans.

Gene therapy for PKU has not been ignored. To date, researchers have successfully introduced into the liver of a PKU mouse a recombinant adenoviral vector containing a normal gene for PAH. Within a week, the mouse was "cured" of PKU, but the effect did not persist. Moreover, mice once treated did not respond to repeated injections of the adenovirus vector (Eisensmith & Woo, 1994; Fang et al., 1994; Jung et al., 2008). In another study, PAH-based fusion proteins and fragments of human hepatocyte growth factor were put together to induce PAH in the liver. Not only did this result in lowering phenylalanine levels in mice, but the new proteins remained active, unlike the recombinant adenoviral vector (Eavri & Lorberboum-Galski, 2007).

Neuropsychological Effects despite Treatment

Early diagnosis and treatment for PKU unquestionably prevent the severe neurological complications from PKU; however, subtle psychological consequences have been exposed. Early studies from a clinical perspective focused on IQ, since it was documented that children with PKU usually attained IQ scores 6–9 points lower than those of their siblings and parents (Fishler, Azen, Henderson, Friedman, & Koch, 1987), and that IQ diminished when diet was discontinued (Seashore, Friedman, Novelly, & Bapat, 1985). A recent meta-analysis of studies that focused on overall intelligence in chil-

dren and adults with PKU confirmed the relationship between blood phenylalanine levels and IQ. The combined results of 40 studies showed that in children with PKU, mean lifetime blood phenylalanine levels were significantly correlated with Full Scale IQ ($r = -.34$). A similar correlation ($r = -.35$) was noted between IQ and blood phenylalanine levels during the "critical period" (0–12 years of age), and with the concurrent blood phenylalanine level ($r = -.31$) (Waisbren et al., 2007).

In addition to lowered IQ, visual–motor deficits (Koff, Boyle, & Pueschel, 1977), global processing problems (Waisbren, Brown, de Sonneville, & Levy, 1994), and executive functioning deficits (Pennington, van Doorninck, McCabe, & McCabe, 1985; van Zutphen et al., 2007) have been reported. Even early-treated children tend to have awkward pencil grips and poor handwriting. Fine motor speed is diminished, copying letters or figures is a laborious process, and work takes longer to complete. When asked to copy geometric designs, many children with PKU have notable difficulties, particularly when they are required to integrate figures. Visual demonstrations, diagrams, and models are less effective than verbal explanations. The children have difficulties remembering the location of objects in space. The "number line" may be incomprehensible for years after it has been taught in arithmetic class.

The Prefrontal Cortex Hypothesis and Dopamine

The pattern of deficits noted in treated PKU led to a suspicion that the prefrontal cortex is involved (Welsh, Pennington, Ozonoff, Rouse, & McCabe, 1990). Projections of dopaminergic neurons in the neocortex are found primarily in the frontal lobes (Porrino & Goldman-Rakic, 1982), and the prefrontal cortex has one of the highest levels of dopamine turnover in the brain (Diamond et al., 1994; Diamond, Prevor, Callender, & Druin, 1997; Tam, Elsworth, Bradberry, & Roth, 1990). Diamond and her colleagues (1997) demonstrated that subjects with blood phenylalanine levels greater than 360 μmol/L (6 mg/dl) performed less well on tasks of executive functions (working memory and inhibitory abilities dependent on the dorsalateral prefrontal cortex) than on non-executive-function tasks. Other investigations supported these findings (Weglage, Pietsch, Fünders, Koch, & Ullrich, 1996; Welsh et al., 1990). In early and continuously treated children (ages 7–14 years) compared to age-matched peers, the ability to inhibit a "prepotent" (or expected) response was significantly poorer (Huijbregts, de Sonneville, Licht, Sergeant, & von Spronsen, 2002). Children with early-treated PKU compared to control samples have also shown lessened attention, impaired problem-solving abilities, hyperactivity, impulsivity, poor planning, and disorganization (DeRoche et al., 2008; Gassio et al., 2008; Moyle, Fox, Arthur, et al., 2007). Stemerdink (1996) found that in 36 older patients (ages 8–19 years) treated early and continuously, neuropsychological performance on three out of four prefrontal tasks was impaired. The same pattern has been found in another study of adults with early-treated PKU (Ris, Williams, Hunt, Berry, & Leslie, 1994).

Researchers have also found evidence for impairment in visual contrast sensitivity when blood phenylalanine levels are elevated. This is relevant, since it is hypothesized that the retina is also highly sensitive to moderate reductions in brain dopamine (Diamond, 1994; Stemerdink, 1996).

Not all studies, however, support the dopamine–prefrontal dysfunction hypothesis. Mazzocco and colleagues (1994), using the Tower of Hanoi and visual search tests, found that children ages 6–13 years who were treated early and continuously showed no deficits on the neuropsychological tests, despite a range of blood phenylalanine levels.

Variations of the dopamine hypothesis have also been proposed. Krause and colleagues (1985) reported a correlation between increased reaction time and decreased urinary dopamine in patients with PKU. Since brain dopamine is concentrated in the corpus striatum, and since choice reaction time tests require a motor response as well as integration of stimuli, they speculated that the nigrostriatal and corticostriatal pathways are affected. Faust, Libon, and Pueschel (1986–1987) obtained similar results; they suspected that the deficits are associated with complex areas of the brain, such as the anterior frontal regions, and in

motor areas that represent less advanced functions.

Although recent studies have generally supported Diamond's work, they also suggest a more complex neuropsychological profile in PKU. Channon, German, Cassina, and Lee (2004) noted impairments in attention, working memory, and fluency, but performance did not decline with increased cognitive load. In a study focusing on inhibitory control in well-treated children with PKU, Christ, Steiner, Grange, Abrams, and White (2006) found only subtle differences between subjects and matched controls. These authors suggested that discrepant results could be attributed to the age at which testing was performed, since there is evidence that some executive abilities are more apparent in older than in younger children with PKU (White, Nortz, Mandernach, Huntington, & Steiner, 2002).

The White Matter Abnormalities Hypothesis

Inconsistent results from tests of executive functioning have prompted research on white matter abnormalities and slow processing speed as probable causes of cognitive deficits in PKU (Channon, Mockler, & Lee, 2005). Some studies have used MRI to investigate the relevance of myelin abnormalities in PKU. Reports conclude that the severity of the MRI changes is significantly and independently associated with the phenylalanine concentration at the time of the investigation. When metabolic control improves, the MRI picture also improves. The area of the brain in which white matter abnormalities are most commonly noted is the parieto-occipital region. Despite the provocative nature of these results, MRI findings have not always been found to correlate with IQ, neuropsychological functioning, or neurological symptoms (Jones et al., 1995; Thompson et al., 1993).

In a meta-analytic review of past research (Moyle, Fox, Bynevelt, et al., 2007) and in recent studies (Huijbregts et al., 2003; Moyle, Fox, Bynevelt, Arthur, & Burnett, 2007), the largest effect sizes derived from tests of processing speed. White matter abnormalities detected on MRI were found in association with high blood phenylalanine levels and slow processing speed (Anderson et al., 2007).

Elevated blood phenylalanine levels clearly compromise neuropsychological performance in individuals with PKU. Early-treated children who maintain treatment beyond early childhood and have controlled blood phenylalanine levels function better on cognitive tests (Schmidt, Rupp, Burgard, & Pietz, 1992; Antshel & Waisbren, 2003a, 2003b; Moyle, Fox, Bynevelt, et al., 2007). IQ loss occurs in early-treated adolescents with elevated phenylalanine levels (Beasley, Costello, & Smith, 1994). Recommendations from the various PKU clinics vary with regard to what constitutes metabolic control in children over 6 years of age. The target for most clinics is now 2–6 mg/dl. However, due to the restrictiveness of the diet, few teenagers are able to maintain levels within this range (Walter et al., 2002). In a follow-up study of children in the United Kingdom, only 12% of the children were following a strict diet by age 14 years, and only 4% were following a strict diet by age 18 years (Beasley et al., 1994). One research group suggests that levels as high as 15 mg/dl may be benign in teenagers and young adults (Griffiths et al., 1995). Other investigators contend that any elevation above 6 mg/dl may have adverse effects (Diamond, 1994).

Concurrent blood phenylalanine levels in individuals with PKU have been correlated with reaction time (Clarke, Gates, Hogan, Barrett, & McDonald, 1987; Schmidt et al., 1994) and were once thought to reflect the level of brain phenylalanine (Jordan, Brunner, Hunt, & Berry, 1985). In one study, short-term dietary intervention and reductions in blood phenylalanine led to improved performance on tasks assessing speed of information processing in adults (Huijbregts, de Sonneville, Licht, von Spronsen, & Sergeant, 2002). However, not all investigators reported clear-cut associations between blood phenylalanine levels and neuropsychological outcomes. In a study of children at approximately age 11 years, blood phenylalanine correlated with performance on tests of attention, fine motor coordination, and IQ, but blood phenylalanine was no longer related to performance on any test 3 years later (Weglage et al., 1999). Similarly, in a study in which phenylalanine intake was manipulated to increase phenylalanine levels, no change was found in performance for individual children under lower or higher

phenylalanine levels (Griffiths, Ward, Harvie, & Cockburn, 1998). In a study of adults both on and off diet, most neuropsychological test results correlated with phenylalanine levels during childhood and not with concurrent levels (Brumm et al., 2004).

One novel approach to explaining variability in neurocognitive functioning among individuals with PKU posits an association between stability of blood phenylalanine levels and functioning. In a retrospective study of 45 early and well-treated children with PKU, stability of blood phenylalanine level was a better predictor of IQ ($r = -.37$, $p = .06$) than lifetime mean blood phenylalanine level ($r = -.18$, $p = .34$) (Anastasoaie, Kurzias, Forbes, & Waisbren, 2008).

Developmental Domains Usually Unaffected in PKU

Infants with early-treated PKU generally attain developmental milestones at the appropriate ages. Most sit up at about 6 months of age, walk at a year, and begin talking at 18–24 months. Although some do not want to give up the bottle, most graduate to a cup and demonstrate appropriate table manners. They learn to tie their shoes in kindergarten, and can ride a two-wheeler, count by twos, and recite the alphabet at the same times as most of their peers. Most do not have difficulties learning to read. They interact well with peers, try to please their teachers, and spend hours on the computer as teenagers. And many children treated early and continuously show no impairments on a wide variety of tests of information processing (Stemerdink et al., 1995). Thus, in many respects, children with early-treated PKU are indistinguishable from other children their age.

BEHAVIORAL, ACADEMIC, AND EMOTIONAL PRESENTATION

Attention-Deficit/ Hyperactivity Disorder

Often linked to the underlying neuropsychological deficits in PKU is attention-deficit/hyperactity disorder (ADHD). Researchers and clinicians have alluded to an increased prevalence of attentional problems in PKU (Burgard, Rey, Rupp, Avadie, & Rey, 1997; Lou,

1994). More recent studies have supported the idea that elevated phenylalanine levels are toxic to neurological systems, resulting in symptoms of ADHD, with exposure earlier in life leading to increased risk for ADHD (Antshel & Waisbren, 2003a). An estimated 26% of children with early-treated PKU received medication for ADHD, compared to 7% of children with diabetes (Arnold, Vladutin, Orlowski, Blakely, & DeLuca, 2004). This is significantly higher than the rate of 4.3% of children who received medication for ADHD in the general population (Visser & Lesesne, 2003). Methylphenidate (Ritalin) and other medications do not appear to result in significant improvements in attention and school achievements, although some parents report that their children exhibit greater self-control when on medication. However, careful studies of the effects of medications for ADHD in children with PKU need to be conducted.

School Achievement

Difficulties in arithmetic typify the learning profile among young children with PKU (Weglage, Fünders, Wilken, Schubert, & Ullrich, 1993). Achievement spans the full range, with some children placed in special programs, others struggling in regular classes, still others proceeding at the same rate as peers, and a few gaining honors in law school. Nonetheless, when children with PKU confront problems in school, they invariably falter in math class. The North American PKU Collaborative Study documents a steady decline in arithmetic scores in both diet-continued and diet-discontinued children from ages 6 to 10 years (Fishler et al., 1987). By age 12 years, achievement scores in arithmetic fall again in 90% of children, regardless of dietary control (Azen et al., 1991). A study by Gassio and colleagues (2008) found that children with PKU were twice as likely as their peers to experience school problems. Thirty-nine percent required special tutoring, and 12% repeated grades. In patients whose phenylalanine levels were elevated, these issues were amplified.

With arithmetic, the underlying cause for difficulties seems to be twofold. First is the issue of spatial perception. Simply put, the children fail to perceive the number line in their "mind's eye." The concepts *more than*

and *less than*, equal distances between numbers, and fixed sequences are not secure ideas. One-to-one correspondence between numbers and objects comes slowly. Addition and subtraction can be drilled, but an intuitive sense of sums and differences may be forever lacking. Multiplication facts can be learned with considerable effort, but without frequent use, they are easily lost. Fractions present almost insurmountable obstacles, as do geometric shapes and formulas. A good sense of spatial arrangement is also needed to line up numbers for performing calculations with paper and pencil. Children with PKU commonly turn in disorganized papers, with wrong answers because numbers are lined up improperly. A second impediment to success in arithmetic is a weakness in executive functioning. Because of their difficulties maintaining information in memory, children with PKU struggle with calculations requiring more than one step. Word problems are especially challenging because they require a child to decide on the appropriate operation and to remember numbers for computing the answer.

As the children grow older, difficulties in reading comprehension become apparent. Decoding skills come readily to most children with PKU, and the first through third grades pass uneventfully. Fourth grade brings new demands for reading comprehension and application of rote skills; suddenly many children with PKU fall behind their classmates and are referred for psychological evaluations. In actuality, the underlying weaknesses have always been there, but simple compensatory strategies have sufficed to keep the children at grade level. By fourth grade, problems in executive functioning and sustaining attention interfere with the acquisition of new knowledge and the ability to master new skills. Science and social studies, as well as arithmetic and reading, become difficult subjects.

Spelling continues to be a strength for most of these children, although for some the sequencing issue hinders visualization of the correct order of letters. In fourth grade, homework increases, as does the amount of written work required. Again, the problem in visual–motor coordination that could once be overcome by hard work now overwhelms the children's coping mechanisms. Occupational therapy is sometimes recommended for children with poor visual–motor skills. If teachers do not recognize such a child's underlying learning difficulties, they may deem the child lazy, dull, inattentive, or obstinate. Even if teachers do suspect a learning disability, they may assume that the child has a typical form of dyslexia or ADHD. However, this may not be the case. Careful evaluation of the child is important to identify the specific pattern of deficits and the particular factors related to PKU that may have an impact on the child's behavior in the classroom. The child's level of PKU, treatment history, and current degree of metabolic control need to be considered, along with the psychosocial stresses the child may be experiencing.

Emotional Disturbances

The effects of PKU on personality and temperament were noted by early researchers (Fisch, Sines, & Chang, 1981). Measures of "persistence," "intensity," and "rhythmicity" were observed to be lower in children with PKU (Schor, 1983). Early-treated school children were rated as more clumsy, talkative, and hypersensitive than their peers (Siegel, Balow, Risch, & Anderson, 1968). On the other hand, patience, sociability, and obedience to the law were also attributed to the genetic defect. In untreated and late-treated PKU, bizarre behaviors were noted, including obsessive–compulsive rituals, self-abuse, and extreme tactile sensitivity. Although such attributions are rare today, they presaged interest in the effects of metabolic disequilibrium on personality and emotion. Today parents note that their children sometimes undergo personality changes when their phenylalanine levels rise (Schuett, 1997).

The long-term consequences of early-treated PKU are relatively unknown. Woolf (1979) speculated that if diet was discontinued in middle childhood an insidious process would begin, culminating in loss of IQ, antisocial behavior, and severe emotional disturbance (including frank psychosis). Although such consequences are rare, effects of a less serious nature are common. One study of young women with PKU revealed that they were less mature than their peers: They obtained a driver's license at a later age and tended to remain longer in their parents' homes (Waisbren, Hamilton, St. James, Shiloh, & Levy, 1995). Other studies of adolescents with PKU have indicated that they are less independent, less achievement-oriented, lower in self-esteem, and more frustrated than peers (Weglage et al., 1992). Off-diet individuals with PKU function poorly in social situations (Schuett 1997), but those who remain on diet experience a positive quality of life (Bosch et al., 2007; Koch et al., 2002).

Agoraphobia has been identified as a complication of elevated phenylalanine levels. Among five adults who experienced panic attacks and were unable to venture more than a short distance from their homes, the two who returned to the phenylalanine-restricted diet experienced dramatic improvement in symptoms (Waisbren & Levy, 1991).

Adolescents and young women with PKU who either were late-treated (i.e., treatment was initiated after 90 days of age) or had terminated the diet for a period of at least 5 years were compared to women who were early-treated and had remained continuously on the diet. The women who had extended exposure to elevated phenylalanine levels evidenced significantly greater psychopathology as measured by the Minnesota Multiphasic Personality Inventory. The pattern of scores was remarkably consistent, with a tendency toward elevations on scales related to thought disorder and mood. Although they were not actively psychotic, the women who had experienced extended exposure to high blood phenylalanine levels were poor assessors of the emotions or expectations of others. They were also prone to feelings of alienation, depression, and social isolation, and had difficulties thinking and communicating (Waisbren & Zaff, 1994). For patients who remain on the diet, the future appears brighter (Weglage et al., 1992).

Researchers from the German Collaborative Study (Pietz et al., 1997) reported that the rate of psychiatric disorders in the adults with PKU was 35.7%, compared to 16.1% in controls. Patients with PKU showed exclusively "internalizing" disturbances (especially depression and anxiety), whereas control subjects demonstrated both internalizing and externalizing (antisocial) symptoms. Females with PKU were more likely than males to experience depression. No correlation has been found between the severity or pattern of psychopathology and biochemical control (Weglage et al., 2000). Moreover, no correlations between psychiatric symptoms and MRI abnormalities have been observed. However, a restrictive, controlling style of parenting is a risk factor for the development of psychiatric symptoms, prompting the German researchers to conclude that psychiatric disturbances in adults with PKU may be related to psychological factors rather than to biochemical or neurological sources. Researchers also report high rates of depression and anxiety in adults with PKU in association with elevated blood phenylalanine levels (Brumm et al, 2004; Smith & Knowles, 2000).

MEDICAL COMORBIDITY

In the past, children with untreated PKU were often diagnosed with autism, and indeed presented with the hallmark features of this disorder (Koch, Acosta, Fishler, Schaeffler, & Wohlers, 1967). Even today, the few children in the United States missed by newborn screening and therefore not treated are often diagnosed with autism, as well as developmental delays.

If "overtreated," with extreme limitation of protein intake resulting in phenylalanine depletion, a child with PKU can experience significant growth retardation, lethargy, and even death. Fortunately, the need to monitor metabolic status carefully to avoid overrestriction was recognized early in the history of treatment for PKU (Hanley, Linsao, Davidson, & Moes, 1970).

Some individuals who discontinue treatment experience dramatic consequences, including seizures, problems with balance, hallucinations, and paralysis of the legs. These reports, though quite alarming, do not represent the usual course of PKU in diet-discontinued individuals. Nonetheless, when they do occur, there is little doubt that phenylalanine toxicity is a contributing factor, since returning to treatment alleviates (though it may not cure) the problems (Schuett, 1997).

Single-case reports of distinct medical conditions in association with PKU have also been published. These include anorexia nervosa (Clarke & Yapa, 1991), congenital hypothyroidism (Schmidt, Solberg, Dia-ment, & Pimentel, 1981), diabetes (Webster & Wallace, 1995), Down syndrome (Blehova, Pazoutova, & Subrt, 1970; Fisch & Horrobin, 1968), Duchenne muscular dystrophy (Roth, Cohn, Berman, & Segal, 1976), Hartnup disease (Jonxis, 1957), hereditary fructose intolerance (Celiker, Dural, & Erdem, 1993), histidinemia (Walker et al., 1981), and lymphoblastic leukemia (Wang et al., 2007). Genetic linkages have been sought, but not found, between PKU and these disorders.

MATERNAL PKU

In a single generation, the benefits of newborn screening for PKU in terms of preventing intellectual disability could be erased by the effects of maternal PKU (Kirkman, 1982). *Maternal PKU* refers to the risks to the fetus when the mother has PKU. The damage to the fetus occurs because of the intrauterine environment, since the fetus relies on the mother to metabolize phenylalanine. There are no particular risks inherent in paternal PKU, apart from the possibility of the child's having PKU if the mother is a carrier (Fisch, Matalon, Weisberg, & Michals, 1991). On the other hand, when the mother has PKU and does not receive treatment, her fetus is exposed to toxic levels of phenylalanine. Among the birth defects that result from phenylalanine exposure in untreated maternal PKU are intellectual disability (95%), microcephaly (90%), and congenital heart disease (17%) (Lenke & Levy, 1980). The precise mechanism of fetal damage in maternal PKU is still unknown, although it is clear that the fetus is harmed by the abnormal intrauterine environment produced by the genetically abnormal mother (Ghavami & Levy, 1986; Levy & Ghavami, 1996).

The risks in maternal PKU are significantly reduced if the mother initiates strict dietary treatment prior to pregnancy and maintains metabolic control throughout pregnancy (Hanley, Clarke, & Schoonheyt, 1987; Koch et al., 1990, 1994; Lynch, Pitt, Maddison, Wraith, & Danks, 1988). Women with non-PKU mild hyperphenylalaninemia, whose natural blood phenylalanine levels are much less elevated than those in women with PKU, incur little or no risk for adverse pregnancy outcomes (Levy & Waisbren, 1983; Levy et al., 1994). This finding underscores the importance of metabolic control in maternal PKU.

Given the known benefits of dietary therapy, delivery of treatment for maternal PKU should be a straightforward process. However, this is not the case. Since many young women with PKU deviate from medical recommendations in adolescence, they must significantly modify their diet for pregnancy. Many have difficulties resuming the highly restricted diet and tolerating the special formula. Many have not been followed by a metabolic clinic since childhood, and some may not even remember that they have PKU. Despite tracking and educational efforts, metabolic control is often not achieved adequately or in time to prevent damage to the fetus.

The International Collaborative Study of Maternal Phenylketonuria was a longitudinal, prospective study of the effects of dietary treatment during pregnancy in women with PKU in the United States, Canada, and Germany (Koch et al., 1993, 1994). The pregnant women received ultrasound examinations, nutrition consultation, and metabolic monitoring as part of the study protocol. Offspring received developmental evaluations in the neonatal period and at 12 and 24 months; thereafter, they were evaluated every 2 or 3 years through age 10 years. Results indicated that the number of gestational weeks until a mother reduced her blood phenylalanine level predicted a child's neonatal course, developmental quotient (DQ), and IQ. Birth head circumference was significantly related to maternal phenylalanine levels during weeks 8–12 of gestation (Rouse et al., 1997). Examiner ratings of infants on the Dubowitz Neurological Assessment of the Preterm and Full-Term Newborn Infant suggested that 29% evidenced signs of abnormalities in muscle tone, head control, reflexes, and responsiveness. Those who attained abnormal ratings had poor responses on measures of axial tone: posterior head control, anterior head control, head lag, and ventral suspension. Scores on the Dubowitz Neurological Assessment were significantly influenced by the gestational age at which a mother with PKU attained metabolic control (Waisbren et al., 1998). The DQ at age 6–12 months in maternal PKU offspring whose mothers attained metabolic control by 20 weeks' gestation was within the average range, whereas the DQ of offspring whose mothers were not in metabolic control until after 20 weeks' gestation was below 85. Assessments at age 4 years confirmed the association between offspring outcome and timing of maternal metabolic control. A total of 253 children of women with PKU (n = 149) were assessed with the McCarthy Scales of Children's Abilities. The General Cognitive Index (similar to an IQ) decreased as weeks to metabolic control increased (r = −.58; p < .001). The mean IQ was 93 for offspring whose mothers attained metabolic control by 10 weeks, 88 for those whose mothers attained metabolic control between 10 and 20 weeks, and 73 for those whose mothers were not in control until after 20 weeks (Hanley et al., 1996; Waisbren et al., 2000). Among all children born to mothers with PKU, 30% had social and behavioral problems (Waisbren et al., 2000).

In a study that included some offspring through 10 years of age, 44% were noted to exhibit significant behavioral problems (Ng, Rae, Wright, Gurry, & Wray, 2003). The most recent large-scale study of maternal PKU (Maillot, Lilburn, Baudin, Morley, & Lee, 2008) included 105 children born to 67 mothers with PKU, the majority of whom were in relatively good metabolic control during pregnancy. The sample was divided into two groups: offspring of mothers who received a low-phenylalanine diet prior to pregnancy, and offspring of mothers who initiated the diet after they became pregnant (usually within the first trimester). Although birth head circumference did not differ between the two groups of offspring, DQ at 1 year of age was 107 for offspring of mothers treated prior to pregnancy and 99 for offspring whose mothers were treated after pregnancy began. At 8 years of age, the difference in IQ between the two groups was more than 15 points (111 vs. 91). Variability in the blood phenylalanine level during pregnancy also correlated negatively with IQ scores, even when the blood phenylalanine level was within the recommended range, with correlations as high as −.71 at age 14 years.

The neurodevelopmental picture of maternal PKU offspring is not yet complete. However, there are indications that it is similar to that found in fetal alcohol syndrome. Not only are there similarities in facial dysmorphology (Levy & Ghavami, 1996), but the neuropsychological profile may be similar, with increased rates of language deficits, hyperactivity, and deficient motor skills (Janzen, Nanson, & Block, 1995).

Thus, despite treatment, offspring from maternal PKU pregnancies often function developmentally and cognitively below normal levels (Koch et al., 1990). One reason for this is that more than 60% of women with PKU who become pregnant do so unintentionally and are not in metabolic control (Waisbren et al., 1995). Although this rate of unplanned pregnancies is similar to that in the general population in the United States (Harrison & Rosenfield, 1996), it has serious consequences for women with PKU (Hanley et al., 1987; Koch et al., 1994; Levy & Ghavami, 1996).

The factors found to be most highly correlated with adherence to medical recommendations in maternal PKU are social support and positive attitudes about the efficacy and acceptability of treatment. Programs to enhance social support and positive attitudes have had promising results (Levy & Waisbren, 1994; Waisbren, Shiloh, St. James, & Levy, 1991; Waisbren et al., 1995, 1997). In addition, compliance can sometimes be improved through changes in the type of formula prescribed, the use of gelatin capsules containing the formula (Kecskemethy, Lobbregt, & Levy, 1993), or supplementation with BH4 (Cunningham, Pridjian, Smith, & Anderson, 2009; Koch, Moseley, & Güttler, 2005). Use of a gastrostomy tube led to good metabolic control in a pregnant woman suffering from severe nausea and poor tolerance of formula (Schwoerer, Bingen, van Calcar, Heighway, & Rice, 2009).

The deficits in offspring from treated maternal PKU pregnancies may also be caused in part by suboptimal home environments. Of concern are the limited intellectual abilities, reduced social resources, and emotional difficulties of women with PKU. In a study of adolescents and young adult women with PKU, the mean IQ was 85, and a substantial proportion of the women were of low socioeconomic status (Waisbren et al., 1995). These discouraging demographics persist today in the subgroup of individuals who have discontinued treatment (Brumm et al., 2004).

ASSESSMENT

Children with PKU require careful monitoring, especially during infancy and school years. As described earlier, even those children who maintain excellent metabolic control are at risk for learning disabilities. Annual testing in the preschool years should be followed with biennial testing during elementary school, preferably by a psychologist familiar with metabolic disorders. Thereafter, testing is recommended when a child experiences difficulties or when metabolic control changes. The frequency with which problems in executive functioning and attention occur suggests that neuropsychological testing should also be performed. Assessments are critical for prevention of future learning disabilities, since it is now clear that early intervention can lead to improved neuronal structures, even in babies with disrupted brain development—and, by extrapolation, in infants and children at risk for frontal lobe or white matter abnormalities (Shonkoff, 2003). Assessments are also important for determining treatment efficacy and the need for modifications in diet or supplementation with medications to reduce phenylalanine exposure or variability. In addition, neuropsychological evaluations identify the types of remedial educational services that may be needed.

It is critical for the psychologist to communicate with the parents and schools about the specific learning profiles of students with PKU. Their difficulties in arithmetic may not be the same as the deficits noted in children without PKU. A recurring theme in the treatment of PKU is the importance of metabolic control. In almost all situations, the test results must be interpreted in association with the current blood phenylalanine level and the degree of metabolic control in previous years. Early history must also be taken into account.

Table 21.1 presents instruments that have been used to identify deficits common in PKU. After the preschool years, a full Wechsler Intelligence Scale for Children should be administered to establish a baseline. Thereafter, the Wechsler Abbreviated Scales of Intelligence may be used, since IQ tends to remain stable for those who maintain metabolic control (Waisbren et al., 2007). Emphasis shoud be placed on tests of executive

TABLE 21.1. Instruments for Assessment of Various Domains Affected by PKU

Domain	Age group	Instrument
Infant development	6 months to 36 months	Bayley Scales of Infant and Child Development, Third Edition; Adaptive Behavior Assessment System—Second Edition
Preschool intelligence	> 30 months to 6 years, 11 months	Wechsler Preschool and Primary Scale of Intelligence—Third Edition
Child intelligence	7 years to 16 years, 11 months	Wechsler Intelligence Scale for Children—Fourth Edition; Wechsler Abbreviated Scales of Intelligence
Adult intelligence	> 17 years	Wechsler Adult Intelligence Scale—Third Edition; Wechsler Abbreviated Scales of Intelligence
Achievement	5 years to adult	Wechsler Individual Achievement Test—Second Edition
Language	> 5 years	Boston Naming Test
Executive functioning	4 years to adult	Behavior Rating Index of Executive Function; California Verbal Learning Test
Visual–motor skills	3 years to adult	Beery–Buktenica Developmental Test of Visual–Motor Integration; Rey–Osterreith Complex Figure
Attention	3 years to 17 years	Conners 3rd Edition
Adaptive behavior	2 years to adult	Adaptive Behavior Assessment System, Second Edition
Emotional well-being	4 years to adult	Behavior Assessment System for Children, Second Edition; Beck Depression Inventory, Second Edition; Beck Anxiety Inventory

functioning, processing speed, behavior (including attention) and emotional well-being, since these areas present challenges for most children and adults with PKU.

Current efforts are underway to develop a uniform assessment method for PKU and other metabolic/genetic disorders (Waisbren & White, 2010). A Genetics and Metabolism Psychology Network has recently been organized to accomplish this task and will post the recommended test battery on its website (*www.GMPsych.org*).

In addition to neuropsychological testing, assessment techniques aimed at uncovering physiological correlates of functioning have been employed. Electroencephalographic examinations traditionally identified slow-wave abnormalities, but only in late-treated or off-diet children. Evoked potentials appeared promising in the 1980s (Pueschel, Fogelson-Doyle, Kammerer, & Matsumiya, 1983), but other studies using evoked potentials revealed no correlations between these and current clinical, biochemical, and neurophysiological parameters (Leuzzi, Cardona, Antonozzi, & Loizzo, 1994). MRI and other brain imaging techniques (Cleary et al., 1994; Johannik et al., 1994; Jones et al., 1995; Peng et al., 2004), have been used primarily for research purposes. White matter abnormalities (reflecting reduced myelin) have consistently appeared, but not in association with reduced IQ (Peng et al., 2004). The MRI examinations indicate that myelin reduction in PKU results from a reversible condition of reduced myelin synthesis rather than from excessive myelin loss. The term *dysmyelination* is more appropriate than *demyelination* for describing what occurs in PKU (Pearsen, Gean-Martin, Levy, & Davis, 1990).

In a recent study using T2-weighted and fluid-attenuated inversion recovery scans, white matter in the parietal region was consistently affected. Myelin reduction in the occipital region ranked second in frequency, followed by frontal and temporal regions. The authors concluded that MRI abnormalities in PKU reflect intracellular accumulation of a hydrophilic metabolite, but do not indicate abnormalities in white matter architecture and structure (Leuzzi et al., 2007). Another study using more advanced imaging techniques have contributed additional information about white matter changes in 32 subjects with classic PKU. Using MRI, plus proton magnetic resonance spectroscopy and diffusion MRI with a 3.0-tesla scanner, investigators detected periventricular and subcortical white matter changes in all subjects. In 29 patients, proton magnetic resonance spectroscopy documented pronounced abnormal signal elevation at 7.36 ppm, corresponding to phenylalanine, despite its low concentration. Diffusion MRI revealed hyperintensity in the areas exhibiting MRI changes. The investigators concluded that the 3.0-tesla diffusion MRI was the most suitable imaging technique in PKU (Scarabino et al., 2009).

TREATMENT IMPLEMENTATION

Treatment Adherence: Emotional and Developmental Issues

The biggest challenge in PKU is adherence to treatment. Maintaining metabolic control necessitates massive adjustments in daily life once a child is beyond infancy. Every social gathering, school lunch period, travel plan, summer activity, and nightly meal must be planned. Adolescents with PKU describe their social lives and emotional development as much more restricted than those of their peers (Weglage et al., 1992). Despite the best efforts of parents, most children and adolescents reject the formula or deviate from the diet at some periods. At different ages, the emotional issues vary, but the result is similar: a rise in blood phenylalanine levels and an increase in the risk for attentional, cognitive, and emotional problems.

The impact of PKU on neuropsychological functioning may lead to behaviors or personality styles in children that, in turn, elicit certain types of responses from parents or teachers. These responses may exacerbate the problem. For example, the hyperactive or impulsive behavior common in children with PKU may lead to poor self-control with the diet. This produces an anxious or overly controlling response from the parents, which may lead to an increase in poor dietary compliance and oppositional behavior in the children (Hendrikx, van der Schot, Slijper, Huisman, & Kalverboer, 1994).

When resistance to the diet occurs, various strategies may be employed. Usually parents can help their children regain equanimity, but sometimes psychological counseling is needed. The rebellious children who refuse formula, cheat on the diet, fuss, and complain are well known to every clinic. These children frighten their parents and siblings by their nonchalant attitude about the consequences of elevated phenylalanine levels. Parents try rewards, punishments, and pleas. They ask doctors, nutritionists, and other professionals to talk to their children. They may drink the formula themselves to show that it is not distasteful. They may involve the children's friends to encourage dietary compliance. Nothing seems to alter the situation.

One interpretation of the time of rebellion is that it represents a struggle for identity— a sense of oneself apart from one's parents. This struggle can occur at many different ages. Some 2-year-olds go through this stage. Some 10-year-olds or teenagers suddenly appear incorrigible with regard to the diet. The best strategy at this time is to validate the struggle for independence. The topic should be discussed in age-appropriate terms, and the need for greater autonomy should be acknowledged. Greater independence should then be granted in areas that are unrelated to food. For young children, this may mean later bedtimes or more choices about activities, friends, or clothing. In older children, encouragement to attend camp or to pursue a new hobby or skill may satisfy the need for independence without placing the children at risk. In every case, when the struggle for independence is at its height, there is a need to engage the child. This can be in the form of more special time with parents and extra support from professionals. A direct focus on the diet will be of little benefit, since the underlying issue is elsewhere.

For children who have generally been reasonable about the treatment but suddenly reject the diet, a cognitive approach may be best. A trip to the laboratory to see how blood specimens are analyzed, participation in PKU conferences, exposure to articles in newsletters or scientific journals, or discussions about the genetics and consequences of PKU may be helpful. Some children benefit from writing reports on their disorder or from learning to cook low-protein foods, prepare the recipes, and maintain food records. A change in formula, a trial of using capsules, or a new schedule for drinking the formula can renew the commitment to the diet.

In adults, difficulties in executive functioning (planning abilities, organization, memory, and impulse control) increase the challenges of adherence to diet. A vicious cycle ensues, with poor metabolic control leading to increased executive functioning deficits, which in turn make it even more difficult to plan meals, organize schedules to include drinking the formula, remember protein allowance, and resist disallowed foods.

Suggestions for Developing Treatment Plans

An achievement protocol for knowledge and skills can serve as a guide for parents, patients and professionals. Below is an outline of one such protocol. This protocol can be referred to whenever a child or adolescent attends a clinic, in order to assess the level of knowledge and self-management that the young person has achieved.

Infants and toddlers (2–3 years)

- Eats with rest of the family at dinner
- Names foods (in general)
- Asks before eating uncertain foods
- Shows awareness of difference between his or her diet and that of family and friends
- Has knowledge of "yes" and "no" foods
- Has knowledge of procedural methods for blood sampling
- Drinks formula out of a cup
- Helps prepare formula—child can pour and stir/shake/blend
- Begins to count food items
- Reports foods consumed that day
- Has basic knowledge of reasons for PKU diet

Preschool (4–6 years)

- Handles social situations concerning food
- Prepares formula (with assistance)
- Can explain PKU and PKU diet in simple terms
- Is knowledgeable about the daily schedule for formula intake
- Takes blood sample with help
- Has knowledge of basic reasons for his or her clinic visits

- Understands basic number concepts necessary for measuring foods
- Is knowledgeable about the daily phenylalanine allowance
- Identifies and serves proper portions of allowed food

School age (7–11 years)

- Prepares formula (with parents' supervision)
- Is beginning to list foods on food record
- Understands untreated versus poorly treated versus treated PKU
- Acknowledges having PKU to peers
- Has knowledge of PKU and PKU diet
- Follows a low-phenylalanine recipe
- Performs blood sampling with parental support
- Monitors own blood levels and understands recommended range
- Understands basic genetics of PKU
- Can determine phenylalanine content of foods from manual or label

Adolescence (12–18 years)

- Prepares formula independently
- Prepares low-protein recipe
- Performs blood sampling independently
- Explains the genetics of PKU
- Explains the rationale of dietary therapy
- Understands whom to consult about PKU or the PKU diet
- Demonstrates ability to cope with social pressures
- Maintains diet record independently
- (For a girl) Demonstrates knowledge of maternal PKU

Some clinics now offer a "PKU school," in which several children of similar age attend a clinic together and participate in a group learning activity, such as preparing a low-protein recipe or taking a finger stick blood specimen (Heffernan & Trahms, 1981). This provides social support, as well as practical experience with some aspects of self-monitoring.

Making the Transition to Adult Health Care

Making a smooth transition from pediatric to adult health care is important for any adolescent or adult with a chronic health condition (Lotstein, McPherson, Strickland, & Newacheck, 2005; McManus, Fox, O'Connor, Chapman, & MacKinnon, 2008; Reiss et al., 2005). Moreover, there are special issues for adults with PKU, including vitamin deficiencies, osteoporosis, and the maternal PKU syndrome (Hoeks, den Heijer, & Janssen, 2009). In order to make sure patients have a successful transition to adult health care, six critical steps have been identified for patients and health care providers to follow: (1) Patients should have an identified health care professional to oversee their individual transition; (2) patients and providers should identify the knowledge and skills required for developmentally appropriate care; (3) an up-to-date and portable medical record (personal health summary) should be kept by patients; (4) health care providers should assist patients in writing a health care transition plan by the time a patient is 14 years of age; (5) all patients should receive the necessary care to protect and optimize their health; and (6) continuous and affordable health insurance should be guaranteed, so that all costs of the transition planning and care are covered (American Academy of Pediatrics, American Academy of Family Physicians, & American College of Physicians–American Society of Internal Medicine, 2002). These steps are reasonable, but many patients and their families are not prepared to make the transition to adult health care (Reiss, Gibson, & Walker, 2005). In addition, many physicians do not discuss the steps of this transition. The majority of pediatric practices do not employ designated transition staff; offer transition services, referrals for adult health care physicians, or transition plans; or create portable medical records (McManus et al., 2008). Reasons behind this failure to implement a transition procedure include a lack of communication between physicians and patients regarding the transition, adult health care providers who are unequipped for dealing with pediatric-onset conditions, and lack of funds for transition teams in pediatric clinics. Many patients and families also express anxiety about leaving their familiar pediatric care providers (McManus et al., 2008; Reiss et al., 2005). To address these problems, some programs provide an identified transition "navigator," educational materials, and a written transition plan (McPherson, Than-

iel, & Minniti, 2009; Rubin, 2008; Tuchman, Slap, & Britto, 2008). Psychologists can contribute to this process by supporting patients in considering their feelings about taking on greater responsibilities and overcoming barriers to continued treatment.

SUMMARY AND CONCLUSIONS

PKU exemplifies the challenges inherent in the study of neurodevelopment in genetic disorders. In one of nature's best-designed experiments (Roth, 1986), a defect in a single gene leads to disruptions in brain development that affect behavior, cognition, personality, social relationships, and even the health of the next generation. PKU is a disorder that has bred controversy since its discovery. Følling (1934), the doctor who first discovered the disorder, worked hard to convince colleagues that the musty smell noted in the urine of some children with intellectual disabilities represented a metabolic disorder. Bickel and colleagues (1954), who discovered a treatment for PKU, fought skeptics who discounted their contention that high phenylalanine levels were harmful and that a low-phenylalanine diet could prevent brain damage in children with PKU. Guthrie, who discovered the simple bacterial assay to measure phenylalanine in filter paper blood specimens (Guthrie & Susi, 1963), and MacCready (1963), who worked for the Massachusetts Public Health Laboratories, at first faced ridicule for insisting on mandatory newborn screening. The replacement of the Guthrie test with tandem mass spectrometry for newborn screening sparked controversy as well (Tarini, 2007). Later arguments arose over the safety of diet discontinuation, the value of dietary therapy for untreated adults with intellectual disabilities, and the benefits of a return to diet for apparently well-functioning adults on a regular diet. Current debate surrounds the introduction of nondietary treatments for PKU, such as BH4 (sapropterin) (Schuett, 2008). Much still needs to be discussed about the theory that attributes deficits in frontal lobe functioning to moderate reductions of brain dopamine in children with PKU who are treated early and continuously. Investigations continue to clarify the meaning of abnormal MRI findings, the relevance of genotype, and the feasibility of gene therapy and enzyme replacement therapy.

Research on neuropsychological outcomes in early-treated PKU over the past 25 years has identified a typical profile of learning deficits and behavioral problems, despite considerable inconsistency in results. Failure to replicate some findings reflects diversity in study designs and limitations due to lack of control populations, disparities in instruments used, small sample sizes, and reliance on cross-sectional rather than longitudinal studies (DeRoche & Welsh, 2008). Nevertheless, despite uncertainty in some areas, much is now known about PKU. The following list summarizes the key information useful to psychologists:

• PKU is an inherited disorder of phenylalanine metabolism, which inhibits the conversion of phenylalanine to tyrosine. In PKU, the gene controlling PAH (the enzyme responsible for this conversion) is defective.

• Treatment with a diet low in phenylalanine (and a synthetic protein supplement) prevents the most severe consequences of PKU if started within the first few weeks of life. Newborn screening provides the best means for identifying babies with PKU, so that the diet can be initiated before significant brain damage occurs.

• Despite treatment, learning disabilities and deficits in neuropsychological functioning are common in children with PKU.

• Some adolescents and adults with PKU experience agoraphobia, anxiety, depression, social withdrawal, and other emotional disturbances as a consequence of diet discontinuation.

• Treatment for PKU must not be too strict or too lax. Since different individuals appear to have different tolerances for phenylalanine and varying responses to elevated levels, predictions about future complications are impossible. Some individuals experience dramatic consequences after diet discontinuation, while others appear to be relatively unaffected.

• Occasionally other disorders coexist with PKU, but no genetic linkages have been discovered.

• Damage to the fetus from untreated maternal PKU is caused by the intrauterine environment and is associated with micro-cephaly, congenital heart disease, low birthweight, and intellectual disability in the offspring. Treatment largely prevents these adverse outcomes. However, the majority of maternal PKU pregnancies continue to be inadequately treated because of psychosocial factors.

• Assessment of children with PKU permits the early identification of learning difficulties and indicates directions for alternative interventions or supplemental treatments. Particular attention needs to be give to executive functioning, information-processing speed, visual–motor skills, arithmetic, and reading comprehension.

• The degree of metabolic control is usually correlated with neuropsychological outcome. Stability of blood phenylalanine levels may also be critical.

• Neuropsychological testing, along with neuroimaging, can provide information about the brain effects associated with PKU. Neuropsychological testing suggests specific deficits in the prefrontal cortex, an area of the brain selectively sensitive to diminished levels of brain dopamine. MRI studies suggest myelin abnormalities that do not appear to be related to IQ but may affect processing speed.

• Dietary compliance remains the critical factor in PKU treatment. Different strategies for maintaining metabolic control need to be employed, depending on the child's age and psychological issues.

• Treatment plans for PKU must address biochemical, nutritional, and psychosocial issues. Social support and positive attitude toward treatment appear to be the most important factors associated with adherence to medical recommendations in PKU and maternal PKU.

• This field is rapidly changing as innovative therapies, more sophisticated neuropsychological testing, and advanced neuroimaging become available.

Three key conclusions emerge:

1. The first 3–5 years of life represent the most critical period to maintain blood phenylalanine levels within the recommended range with as little variability as possible.
2. Current treatments do not prevent deficits in mental processing speed and ex-

ecutive functioning, which affect nearly all aspects of life and inhibit adherence to diet for PKU.

3. Lifelong treatment for PKU leads to more positive outcomes in intellectual functioning, emotional well-being, and quality of life.

The field remains open for research. With technological advances in genotyping, biochemical analysis, neuroimaging, treatment alternatives, and neuropsychological testing, answers should be forthcoming to some of the basic questions regarding the underlying pathology in PKU and the nature of optimal therapies for this disorder.

ACKNOWLEDGMENT

Rebecca Owens and Lydia Carr are acknowledged for their help in revising and editing this chapter.

REFERENCES

Adams D. J. (2009) Treatment of an individual with phenylketonuria and neurological impairment with sapropterin. *Molecular Genetics and Metabolism, 98*, 25.

American Academy of Pediatrics, American Academy of Family Physicians, & American College of Physicians–American Society of Internal Medicine. (2002). A consensus statement on health care transitions for young adults with special health care needs. *Pediatrics, 110*, 1304–1305.

Anderson, P. J., Wood, S. J., Francis, D. E., Coleman, L., Anderson, V., & Boneh, A. (2007). Are neuropsychological impairments in children with early-treated phenylketonuria (PKU) related to white matter abnormalities or elevated phenylalanine levels? *Developmental Neuropsychology, 32*, 645–668.

Anastasoaie, V., Kurzias, L., Forbes, P., & Waisbren, S. (2008). Stability of blood phenylalanine levels and IQ in children with phenylketonuria. *Molecular Genetics and Metabolism, 95*, 17–20.

Antshel, K. M., & Waisbren, S. E. (2003a). Developmental timing of exposure to elevated levels of phenylalanine is associated with ADHD symptom expression. *Journal of Abnormal Child Psychology, 31*, 565–574.

Antshel, K. M., & Waisbren, S. E. (2003b). Timing is everything: Executive functions in children exposed to elevated levels of phenylalanine. *Neuropsychology, 17*, 458–468.

Arnold, G. L., Vladutiu, C. J., Orlowski, C. C., Blakely, E. M., & DeLuca, J. (2004). Prevalence of stimulant use for attentional dysfunction in children with phenylketonuria. *Journal of Inherited Metabolic Disease, 27*, 137–143.

Azen, C. G., Koch, R., Friedman, E. G., Berlow, S., Caldwell, J., Krause, W., et al. (1991). Intellectual development in 12-year-old children treated for phenylketonuria. *American Journal of Diseases of Children, 145*, 35–39.

Batshaw, M. L., Valle, D., & Bessman, S. P. (1981). Unsuccessful treatment of phenylketonuria with tyrosine. *Journal of Pediatrics, 99*, 159–162.

Baumeister, A. A., & Baumeister, A. A. (1998). Dietary treatment of destructive behavior associated with hyperphenylalanineuria. *Clinical Neuropharmacology, 21*, 18–27.

Beasley, M. G., Costello, P. M., & Smith, I. (1994). Outcome of treatment in young adults with phenylketonuria detected by routine neonatal screening between 1964 and 1971. *Quarterly Journal of Medicine, 87*, 155–160.

Bickel, H., Gerrard, J., & Hickmans, E. M. (1954). The influence of phenylalanine intake on the chemistry and behavior of a phenylketonuric child. *Acta Paediatrica, 43*, 64–73.

Blau, N., Bélanger-Quintana, A., Demirkol, M., Feillet, F., Giovannini, M., MacDonald, A., et al. (2009). Optimizing the use of sapropterin (BH(4)) in the management of phenylketonuria. *Molecular Genetics and Metabolism, 96*, 158–163.

Blehova, B., Pazoutova, N., & Subrt, I. (1970). Phenylketonuria associated with Down's syndrome. *Journal of Mental Deficiency Research, 14*, 274–275.

Bosch, A. M., Tybout, W., von Spronsen, F. J., de Valk, H. W., Wijburg, F. A., & Grootenhuis, M. A. (2007). The course of life and quality of life of early and continuously treated Dutch patients with phenylketonuria. *Journal of Inherited Metabolic Disease, 30*, 29–34.

Bóveda, M. D., Couce, M. L., Castiñeiras, D. E., Cocho, J. A., Pérez, B., Ugarte, M., et al. (2007). The tetrahydrobiopterin loading test in 36 patients with hyperphenylalaninaemia: Evaluation of response and subsequent treatment. *Journal of Inherited Metabolic Disease, 30*, 812.

Brumm, V. L., Azen, C., Moats, R. A., Stern, A. M., Broomand, C., Nelson, M. D., et al. (2004). Neuropsychological outcome of subjects participating in the PKU adult collaborative study: A preliminary review. *Journal of Inherited Metabolic Disease, 27*, 549–566.

Burgard, P., Rey, F., Rupp, A., Avadie, V., & Rey, J. (1997). Neuropsychologic functions of early treated patients with phenylketonuria, on and off diet: Results of a cross-national and cross-sectional study. *Pediatric Research, 41*, 368–374.

Cabib, S., Pascucci, T., Ventura, R., Romano, V., & Puglisi-Allegra, S. (2003). The behavioral profile of severe mental retardation in a genetic mouse model of phenylketonuria. *Behavioral Genetics, 33*, 301–310.

Celiker, V., Dural, O., & Erdem, K. (1993). Anesthetic management of a patient with hereditary fructose intolerance and phenylketonuria. *Turkish Journal of Pediatrics, 35*, 127–130.

Channon, S., German, E., Cassina, C., & Lee, P. (2004). Executive functioning, memory, and learning in phenylketonuria. *Neuropsychology, 18*, 613–620.

Channon, S., Mockler, C., & Lee, P. (2005). Executive functioning and speed of processing in phenylketonuria. *Neuropsychology, 25*, 679–686.

Christ, S. E., Steiner, R. D., Grange, D. K., Abrams, R. A., & White, D. A. (2006). Inhibitory control in children with phenylketonuria. *Developmental Neuropsychology, 30*, 845–864.

Clarke, D. J., & Yapa, P. (1991). Phenylketonuria and anorexia nervosa. *Journal of Mental Deficiency Research, 35*, 165–170.

Clarke, J. T. R., Gates, R. D., Hogan, S. E., Barrett, M., & MacDonald, G. W. (1987). Neuropsychological studies on adolescents with PKU returned to phenylalanine-restricted diets. *American Journal of Mental Retardation, 92*, 255–262.

Cleary, M. A., Walter, J. H., Wraith, J. E., Jenkins, J. P. R., Alani, S. M., & Whittle, T. K. (1994). Magnetic resonance imaging of the brain in phenylketonuria. *Lancet, 344*, 87–90.

Cunningham, A., Pridjian, G., Smith, J., & Anderson, H. C. (2009). PKU treatment with tetrahydrobiopterin (Sapropterin) during pregnancy. *Molecular Genetics and Metabolism, 98*, 24.

DeRoche, K., & Welsh, M. (2008). Twenty-five years of research on neurocognitive outcomes in early-treated phenylketonuria: Intelligence and executive function. *Developmental Neuropsychology, 33*, 474–504.

Diamond, A. (1994). Phenylalanine levels of 6–10 mg/dl may not be as benign as once thought. *Acta Paediatrica, 83*(Suppl. 407), 89–91.

Diamond, A., Ciaramitaro, V., Donner, E., Djali, S., & Robinson, R. M. (1994). An animal model of early-treated PKU. *Journal of Neuroscience, 14*, 3072–3082.

Diamond, A., Prevor, M. B., Callender, G., & Druin, D. P. (1997). Prefrontal cortex cognitive deficits in children treated early and continuously for PKU. *Monographs of the Society for Research in Child Development, 62*(4, Serial No. 252), 1–208.

Eavri, R., & Lorberboum-Galski, H. (2007). A novel approach for enzyme replacement therapy: The use of phenylalanine hydroxylase-based fusion proteins for the treatment of phenylketonuria. *Journal of Biological Chemistry, 282*, 23402–23409.

Eisensmith, R. C., & Woo, S. L. C. (1994). Gene therapy for phenylketonuria. *Acta Paediatrica, 83*(Suppl. 407), 124–129.

Fang, B., Eisensmith, R. C., Li, X. H. C., Shedlovsky, A., Dove, W., & Woo, S. L. C. (1994). Gene therapy for phenylketonuria: Phenotypic correction in a genetically deficient mouse model by adenovirus-mediated hepatic gene transfer. *Gene Therapy, 1*, 247–254.

Faust, D., Libon, D., & Pueschel, S. (1986–1987). Neuropsychological functioning in treated phenylketonuria. *International Journal of Psychiatry in Medicine, 16*, 169–177.

Fiege, B., & Blau, N. (2007). Assessment of tetrahydrobiopterin (BH4) responsiveness in phenylketonuria. *Journal of Pediatrics, 150*, 627–630.

Fisch, R. O., & Horrobin, J. M. (1968). Down's syndrome with phenylketonuria. *Clinical Pediatrics, 7*, 226–227.

Fisch, R. O., Matalon, R., Weisberg, S., & Michals, K. (1991). Children of fathers with phenylketonuria: An international survey. *Journal of Pediatrics, 118*, 739–741.

Fisch, R. O., Sines, L. K., & Chang, P. (1981). Personality characteristics of nonretarded phenylketonurics and their family members. *Journal of Clinical Psychiatry, 42*, 106–113.

Fishler, K., Azen, C. G., Henderson, R., Friedman, E., & Koch, R. (1987). Psychoeducational findings among children treated for phenylketonuria. *American Journal of Mental Deficiency, 92*, 65–73.

Følling, A. (1934). Utskillelse av fenylpyrodruesyre i urinen som stoffskifteanomali i forbindelse med imbecillitet. *Nordisk Median Tikskiift, 8*, 1054–1059.

Gassió, R., Artuch, R., Vilaseca, M. A., Fusté, E., Colome, R., & Campistol, J. (2008). Cognitive functions and the antioxidant system in phenylketonuric patients. *Neuropsychology, 22*, 426–431.

Ghavami, M., & Levy, H. L. (1986). Prevention of fetal damage through dietary control of maternal hyperphenylalaninemia. *Clinical Obstetrics and Gynecology, 29*, 580–585.

Griffiths, P., Paterson, L., & Harvie, A. (1995). Neuropsychological effects of subsequent exposure to phenylalanine in adolescents and young adults with early-treated phenylketonuria. *Journal of Intellectual Disability Research, 39*, 365–372.

Griffiths, P., Ward, N., Varvie, A., & Cockburn, F. (1998). Neuropsychological outcome of experimental manipulation of phenylalanine intake in treated phenylketonuria. *Journal of Inherited Metabolic Disease, 21*, 29–38.

Guldberg, P., Levy, H. L., Hanley, W. B., Koch, R., Matalon, R., Rouse, B. M., et al. (1996). Phenylalanine hydroxylase gene mutations in the United States: Report from the Maternal PKU Collaborative Study. *American Journal of Human Genetics, 59*, 84–94.

Guthrie, R., & Susi, A. (1963). A simple phenylalanine method for detecting phenylketonuria in large populations of newborn infants. *Pediatrics, 32,* 338–343.

Güttler, F., & Lou, H. (1986). Dietary problems of phenylketonuria: Effect on CNS transmitters and their possible role in behaviour and neuropsychological function. *Journal of Inherited Metabolic Disease, 9*(Suppl. 2), 169–177.

Hanley, W. B., Clarke, J. T. R., & Schoonheyt, W. E. (1987). Maternal phenylketonuria (PKU): A review. *Clinical Biochemistry, 20,* 149–156.

Hanley, W. B., Koch, R., Levy, H. L., Matalon, R., Rouse, B., Azen, C. G., et al. (1996). The North American Maternal Phenylketonuria Collaborative Study, developmental assessment of the offspring: Preliminary report. *European Journal of Pediatrics, 255*(Suppl. 1), S169–S172.

Hanley, W. B., Linsao, L., Davidson, W., & Moes, C. A. (1970). Malnutrition with early treatment of phenylketonuria. *Pediatric Research, 4,* 318–327.

Harper, M., & Reid, A. H. (1987). Use of a restricted protein diet in the treatment of behaviour disorder in a severely mentally retarded adult female phenylketonuric patient. *Journal of Mental Deficiency Research, 31,* 209–212.

Harrison, P. F., & Rosenfield, A. (Eds.). (1996). *Contraceptive research and development: Looking to the future.* Washington, DC: National Academy Press.

Heffernan, J. F., & Trahms, C. M. (1981). A model preschool for patients with phenylketonuria. *Journal of the American Dietetic Association, 79,* 306–308.

Hendrikx, M. M., van der Schot, L. W., Slijper, F. M., Huisman, J., & Kalverboer, A. F. (1994). Phenylketonuria and some aspects of emotional development. *European Journal of Pediatrics, 153,* 832–835.

Hoeks, M. P., den Heijer, M., & Janssen, M. C. (2009). Adult issues in phenylketonuria. *Netherlands Journal of Medicine, 67,* 2–7.

Hoeksma, M., Reijngoud, D. J., Pruim, J., de Valk, H. W., Paans, A. M., & von Spronsen, F. J. (2009). Phenylketonuria: High plasma phenylalanine decreases cerebral protein synthesis. *Molecular Genetics and Metabolism, 96,* 177–182.

Holtzman, N. A., Kronmal, R. A., van Doorninck, W., Azen, C. G., & Koch, R. (1986). Effect of age at loss of dietary control on intellectual performance and behavior of children with phenylketonuria. *New England Journal of Medicine, 314,* 593–598.

Huijbregts, S., de Sonneville, L. M., Licht, R., Sergeant, J., & von Spronsen, F. (2002). Inhibition and prepotent responding and attentional flexibility in treated phenylketonuria. *Developmental Neuropsychology, 22,* 481–499.

Huijbregts, S., de Sonneville, L. M., Licht, R., von Spronsen, F. J., & Sergeant, J. A. (2002). Short term dietary intervention children and adolescents with treated phenylketonuria: Effects on neuropyschological outcome of a well-controlled population. *Journal of Inherited Metabolic Disease, 25,* 419–430.

Huijbregts, S. C., de Sonneville, L. M., van Spronsen, F. J., Berends, I. E., Licht, R., Verkerk, P. H., et al. (2003). Motor function under lower and higher controlled processing demands in early and continuously treated phenylketonuria. *Neuropsychology, 17,* 369–379.

Janzen, L. A., Nanson, J. L., & Block, G. W. (1995). Neuropsychological evaluation of preschoolers with fetal alcohol syndrome. *Neurotoxicology and Teratology, 17,* 273–279.

Johannik, K., Van Hecke, P., Francois, B., Marchal, G., Smet, M. H., Jaeken, J., et al. (1994). Localized brain proton NRM spectroscopy in young adult phenylketonuria patients. *Magnetic Resonance in Medicine, 31,* 53–57.

Jones, S. J., Turano, G., Kriss, A., Shawkat, F., Kendall, B., & Thompson, A. J. (1995). Visual evoked potentials in phenylketonuria: Association with brain MRI, dietary state, and IQ. *Journal of Neurology, Neurosurgery and Psychiatry, 59,* 260–265.

Jonxis, J. H. P. (1957). Oligophrenia phenylpyruvica en de hartnupziekte. *Nederlands Tijdschrift voor Geneeskunde, 101,* 569–574.

Jordan, M. K., Brunner, R. L., Hunt, M. M., & Berry, H. K. (1985). Preliminary support for the oral administration of valine, isoleucine and leucine for phenylketonuria. *Developmental Medicine and Child Neurology, 27,* 33–39.

Jung, S. C., Park, J. W., Oh, H. J., Choi, J. O., Seo, K. I., Park, E. S., et al. (2008). Protective effect of recombinant adeno-associated virus 2/8–mediated gene therapy from the maternal hyperphenylalaninemia in offsprings of a mouse model of phenylketonuria. *Journal of Korean Medical Science, 23,* 877–883.

Kecskemethy, H. H., Lobbregt, D., & Levy, H. L. (1993). The use of gelatin capsules for ingestion of formula in dietary treatment of maternal phenylketonuria. *Journal of Inherited Metabolic Disease, 16,* 111–118.

Kidd, K. K. (1987). Population genetics of a disease. *Nature, 327,* 282–283.

Kirkman, H. N. (1982). Projections of a rebound in frequency of mental retardation from phenylketonuria. *Applied Research in Mental Retardation, 3,* 319–328.

Koch, J. H. (1997). *Robert Guthrie: The PKU story, a crusade against mental retardation.* Pasadena, CA: Hope.

Koch, R., Acosta, P., Fishler, K., Schaeffler, G., & Wohlers, A. (1967). Clinical observations on phenylketonuria. *American Journal of Diseases of Children, 113,* 6–15.

Koch, R., Azen, C. G., Friedman, E. G., & Williamson, M. L. (1982). Preliminary report on the effects of diet discontinuation in PKU. *Journal of Pediatrics, 100*, 870–875.

Koch, R., Burton, B., Hoganson, G., Peterson, R., Rhead, W., Rouse, B., et al. (2002). Phenylketonuria in adulthood: A collaborative study. *Journal of Inherited Metabolic Disease, 25*, 333–346.

Koch, R., Hanley, W., Levy, W., Matalon, R., Rouse, B., de la Cruz, F., et al. (1990). A preliminary report of the Collaborative Study of Maternal Phenylketonuria in the United States and Canada. *Journal of Inherited Metabolic Disease, 13*, 641–650.

Koch, R., Levy, H., Matalon, R., Rouse, B., Hanley, W., & Azen, C. G. (1993). The North American Collaborative Study of Maternal Phenylketonuria: Status report, 1993. *American Journal of Diseases of Children, 147*, 1224–1230.

Koch, R., Levy, H. L., Matalon, R., Rouse, B., Hanley, W., Trefz, F., et al. (1994). The International Collaborative Study of Maternal Phenylketonuria: Status report, 1994. *Acta Pediatrica, 83*(Suppl. 402), 111–119.

Koch, R., Moseley, K., & Güttler, F. (2005). Tetrahydrobiopterin and maternal PKU. *Molecular Genetics and Metabolism, 86*(Suppl. 1), S139–S141.

Koff, E., Boyle, P., & Pueschel, S. (1977). Perceptual–motor functioning in children with phenylketonuria. *American Journal of Diseases of Children, 131*, 1084–1087.

Krause, W., Halminski, M., McDonald, L., Dembure, P., Salvo, R., Freides, D., et al. (1985). Biochemical and neuropsychological effects of elevated plasma phenylalanine in patients with treated phenylketonuria: A model for the study of phenylalanine and brain function in man. *Journal of Clinical Investigation, 75*, 40–48.

LaClaire, C. E., Ney, D. M., MacLeod, E. L., & Etzel, M. R. (2009). Purification and use of glycomacropeptide for nutritional management of phenylketonuria. *Journal of Food Science, 74*, E199–E206.

Legido, A., Tonyes, L., Carter, D., Schoemaker, A., Di George, A., & Grover, W. D. (1993). Treatment variables and intellectual outcome in children with classic phenylketonuria. *Clinical Pediatrics, 32*, 417–425.

Lenke, R. R., & Levy, H. L. (1980). Maternal phenylketonuria and hyperphenylalaninemia: An international survey of the outcome of untreated and treated pregnancies. *New England Journal of Medicine, 303*, 1202–1208.

Leuzzi, V., Cardona, F., Antonozzi, I., & Loizzo, A. (1994). Visual, auditory and somatosensorial evoked potentials in early and late treated adolescents with phenylketonuria. *Journal of Clinical Neurophysiology, 11*, 602–606.

Leuzzi, V., Tosetti, M., Montanaro, D., Carducci, C., Artiola, C., Carducci, C., et al. (2007). The pathogenesis of the white matter abnormalities in phenylketonuria: A multimodal 3.0 tesla MRI

and magnetic resonance spectroscopy (1H MRS) study. *Journal of Inherited Metabolic Disease, 30*, 209–216.

Levy, H. L. (1989). Molecular genetics of phenylketonuria and its implications. *American Journal of Human Genetics, 45*, 667–670.

Levy, H. L., & Ghavami, M. (1996). Maternal phenylketonuria: A metabolic teratogen. *Teratology, 53*, 176–184.

Levy, H. L., Goss, B. S., Sullivan, D. K., Michals-Matalon, K., Dobbs, J. M., Guldberg, P., et al. (1994). Maternal mild hyperphenylalaninemia: Results of treated and untreated pregnancies in two sisters. *Journal of Pediatrics, 125*, 467–469.

Levy, H. L., Milanowski, A., Chakrapani, A., Cleary, M., Lee, P., Trefz, F. K., et al. (2007). Efficacy of sapropterin dihydrochloride (tetrahydrobiopterin, 6R-BH4) for reduction of phenylalanine concentration in patients with phenylketonuria: a phase III randomised placebo-controlled study. *Lancet, 370*, 504–510.

Levy, H. L., & Waisbren, S. E. (1983). Effects of untreated maternal phenylketonuria and hyperphenylalaninemia in the fetus. *New England Journal of Medicine, 309*, 1269–1274.

Levy, H. L., & Waisbren, S. E. (1994). PKU in adolescents: Rationale and psychosocial factors in diet continuation. *Acta Paediatrica, 83*(Suppl. 407), 92–97.

Lotstein, D. S., McPherson, M., Strickland, B., & Newacheck, P. W. (2005). Transition planning for youth with special health care needs: Results from the National Survey of Children with Special Health Care Needs. *Pediatrics, 115*, 1162–1568.

Lou, H. C. (1994). Dopamine precursors and brain function in phenylalanine hydroxylase deficiency. *Acta Paediatrica, 83*(Suppl. 407), 86–88.

Lynch, B. C., Pitt, D. B., Maddison, T. G., Wraith, J. E., & Danks, D. M. (1988). Maternal phenylketonuria: Successful outcome in four pregnancies treated prior to conception. *European Journal of Pediatrics, 148*, 72–75.

MacCready, R. A. (1963). Phenylketonuria screening programs. *New England Journal of Medicine, 269*, 52.

Maillot, F., Lilburn, M., Baudin, J., Morley, D. W., & Lee, P. J. (2008). Factors influencing outcomes in the offspring of mothers with phenylketonuria during pregnancy: The importance of variation in maternal blood phenylalanine. *American Journal of Clinical Nutrition, 88*(3), 700–705.

Matalon, R., Michals-Matalon, K., Bhatia, G., Burlina, A. B., Burlina, A. P., Braga, C., et al. (2007). Double blind placebo control trial of large neutral amino acids in treatment of PKU: Effect on blood phenylalanine. *Journal of Inherited Metabolic Disease, 30*, 153–158.

Matalon, R., Surendran, S., Matalon, K. M., Tyring, S., Quast, M., Jinga, W., et al. (2003). Future role of large neutral amino acids in transport of phenylalanine into the brain. *Pediatrics, 112,* 1570–1574.

Mazzocco, M. M., Nord, A. M., Van Doorninck, W., Greene, C. L., Kovar, C. G., & Pennington, B. F. (1994). Cognitive development among children with early-treated phenylketonuria. *Developmental Neuropsychology, 10,* 133–151.

McDonald, J. D., Bode, V. C, Dove, W. F., & Shedlovsky, A. (1990). Pah^{hPh}-5: A mouse mutant deficient in phenylalanine hydroxylase. *Proceedings of the National Academy of Sciences USA, 87,* 1965–1967.

Mcleod, E. L., Clayton, M. K., Van Calear, S. C., & Ney, D. M. (in press). Breakfast with glycomacropeptide compared with amino acids suppresses plasma ghrelin in individuals with phenylketonuria. *Molecular and Genetic Metabolism.*

McManus, M., Fox, H., O'Connor, K., Chapman, T., & MacKinnon, J. (2008). *Pediatric perspectives and practices on transitioning adolescents with special needs to adult health care* (Vol. 6) [Brochure]. Washington, DC: National Alliance to Advance Adolescent Health.

McPherson, M., Thaniel, L., & Minniti, C. P. (2009). Transition of patients with sickle cell disease from pediatric to adult care: Assessing patient readiness. *Pediatric Blood Cancer, 52,* 838–541.

Mihalick, S. M., Langlois, J. C., Krienke, J. D., & Dube, W. V. (2000). An olfactory discrimination procedure for mice. *Journal of Experimental Animal Behavior, 73,* 305–318.

Miller, L., Braun, L. D., Pardridge, W. M., & Oldendorf, W. H. (1985). Kinetic constants for blood–brain barrier amino acid transport in conscious rats. *Journal of Neurochemistry, 45,* 1427–1432.

Moyle, J. J., Fox, A. M., Arthur, M., Bynevelt, M., Burnett, J. R. (2007). Meta-analysis of neuropsychological symptoms of adolescents and adults with PKU. *Neuropsychology Review, 17,* 91–101.

Moyle, J. J., Fox, A. M., Bynevelt, M., Arthur, M., & Burnett, J. R. (2007). A neuropsychological profile of off-diet adults with phenylketonuria. *Journal of Clinical and Experimental Neuropsychology, 29,* 436–441.

National Institutes of Health (NIH) Consensus Development Panel. (2001). National Institutes of Health Consensus Development Conference Statement: Phenylketonuria: Screening and management, October 16–18, 2000. *Pediatrics, 108,* 972–982.

Ney, D. M., Gleason, S. T., van Calcar, S. C., MacLeod, E. L., Nelson, K. L., Etzel, M. R., et al. (2009). Nutritional management of PKU with glycomacropeptide from cheese whey. *Journal of Inherited Metabolic Disease, 32,* 32–39.

Ng, T. W., Rae, A., Wright, H., Gurry, D., & Wray, J. (2003). Maternal phenylketonuria in Western Australia: Pregnancy outcomes and developmental outcomes in offspring. *Journal of Pediatric Child Health, 39,* 358–363.

Ozalp, I., Coskum, T., Ozguc, M., Tokath, A., Yalaz, K., Vanh, L., et al. (1994). The PAH gene: Genetic and neurological evaluation of untreated and late-treated patients with phenylketonuria. *Journal of Inherited Metabolic Disease, 17,* 371.

Paul, D. B. (1999). PKU screening: Competing agendas, converging stories. In M. Fortun & E. Mendelsohn (Eds.), *The practices of human genetics* (pp. 185–195). Dordvecht, The Netherlands: Kluwer Academic.

Pascucci, T., Andolina, D., Ventura, R., Puglisi-Allegra, S., & Cabib, S. (2008). Reduced availability of brain amines during critical phases of postnatal development in a genetic mouse model of cognitive delay. *Brain Research, 1217,* 232–238.

Pearsen, K. D., Gean-Marton, A. D., Levy, H. L., & Davis, K. R. (1990). Phenylketonuria: MR imaging of the brain with clinical correlation. *Radiology, 177,* 437–440.

Peng, S. S., Tseng, W. Y., Chien, Y. H., Hwu, W. L., & Liu, H. M. (2004). Diffusion tensor images in children with early-treated, chronic, malignant phenylketonuria: Correlation with intelligence assessment. *American Journal of Neuroradiology, 25,* 1569–1574.

Pennington, B. F., van Doorninck, J. W., McCabe, L. L., & McCabe, E. R. B. (1985). Neuropsychological deficits in early treated phenylketonuric children. *American Journal of Mental Deficiency, 89,* 467–474.

Penrose, L. S. (1972). *The biology of mental defect* (4th ed.). London: Sidgwick & Jackson.

Pietz, J., Fatkenheuer, B., Burgard, P., Armbruster, M., Esser, G., & Schmidt, H. (1997). Psychiatric disorders in adult patients with early-treated phenylketonuria. *Pediatrics, 99,* 345–350.

Pietz, J., Landwehr, A., Schmidt, H., de Sonneville, L., & Trefz, F. K. (1995). Effect of high-dose supplementation on brain function in adults with phenylketonuria. *Journal of Pediatrics, 127,* 936–943.

Porrino, L. J., & Goldman-Rakic, P. S. (1982). Brain stem innervation of prefrontal and anterior cingulate cortex in the rhesus monkey revealed by retrograde transport of HRP. *Journal of Comparative Neurology, 205,* 63–76.

Pueschel, S. M., Fogelson-Doyle, L., Kammerer, B., & Matsumiya, Y. (1983). Neurophysiological, psychological and nutritional investigations during discontinuation of the phenylalanine-restricted diet in children with classic phenylketonuria. *Journal of Mental Deficiency Research, 27,* 61–67.

Reiss, J. G., Gibson, R. W., & Walker, L. R. (2005). Health care transition: Youth, family, and provider perspectives. *Pediatrics, 115,* 112–120.

Ris, M. D., Williams, S. E., Hunt, M. M., Berry, H. K., & Leslie, N. (1994). Early-treated phenylketonuria: Adult neuropsychologic outcome. *Journal of Pediatrics, 124,* 388–392.

Roth, K. S. (1986). Newborn metabolic screening: A search for "nature's experiments." *Southern Medical Journal, 79,* 47–54.

Roth, K. S., Cohn, R. M., Berman, P., & Segal, S. (1976). Phenylketonuria and Duchenne muscular dystrophy: A case report. *Journal of Pediatrics, 88,* 689–705.

Rouse, B., Azen, C., Koch, R., Matalon, R., Hanley, W., de la Cruz, F., et al. (1997). Maternal Phenylketonuria Collaborative Study (MPKUCS) offspring: Facial anomalies, malformations, and early neurological sequelae. *American Journal of Medical Genetics, 69,* 89–95.

Rubin, K. R. (2008). Turner syndrome: Transition from pediatrics to adulthood. *Endocrine Practice, 14,* 775–781

Sarkissian, C. N., Gámez, A., Wang, L., Charbonneau, M., Fitzpatrick, P., Lemontt, J. F., et al. (2008). Preclinical evaluation of multiple species of PEGylated recombinant phenylalanine ammonia lyase for the treatment of phenylketonuria. *Proceedings of the National Academy of Sciences USA, 105,* 20894–20899.

Scarabino, T., Popolizio, T., Tosetti, M., Montanaro, D., Giannatempo, G. M., Terlizzi, R., et al. (2009). Phenylketonuria: white-matter changes assessed by 3. 0–T magnetic resonance (MR) imaging, MR spectroscopy and MR diffusion. *La Radiologica Medica, 114,* 461–744.

Schindeler, S., Ghosh-Jerath, S., Thompson, S., Rocca, A., Joy, P., Kemp, A., et al. (2007). The effects of large neutral amino acid supplements in PKU: An MRS and neuropsychological study. *Molecular Genetics and Metabolism, 91,* 48–54.

Schmidt, B. J., Solberg, A. J., Diament, A. J., & Pimentel, H. (1981). Phenylketonuria in patients with congenital hypothyroidism. *Pediatric Research, 15,* 176.

Schmidt, E., Rupp, A., Burgard, P., & Pietz, J. (1992). Information processing in early treated phenylketonuria. *Journal of Clinical and Experimental Neuropsychology, 14,* 388.

Schmidt, E., Rupp, A., Burgard, P., Pietz, J., Weglage, J., & de Sonneville, L. M. J. (1994). Sustained attention in adult phenylketonuria: The influence of the concurrent phenylalanine-blood-level. *Journal of Clinical and Experimental Neuropsychology, 16,* 681–688.

Schor, D. P. (1983). PKU and temperament: Rating children three through seven years old in PKU families. *Clinical Pediatrics, 22,* 807–811.

Schuett, V. E. (1997). Off-diet young adults with PKU: Lives in danger. *National PKU News, 8,* 1–5.

Schuett, V. E. (2008). Message from the editor of *National PKU News* regarding Kuvan's FDA Approval. *National PKU News, 20,* 1.

Schuett, V. E., & Brown, E. S. (1984). Diet policies of PKU clinics in the United States. *American Journal of Public Health, 74,* 501–503.

Schwoerer, J. A. S., Bingen, L. M., van Calcar, S., Heighway, S., & Rice, G. M. (2009). Use of gastrostomy tube to prevent maternal PKU syndrome (Abstract No. 160). *Molecular Genetics and Metabolism, 98,* 18.

Scriver, C. R., & Kaufman, S. (2001). Hyperphenylalaninemias: Phenylalanine hydroxylase deficiency. In C. R. Scriver, A. L. Baudet, W. S. Sly, & D. Valle (Eds.), *The metabolic and molecular bases of inherited disease* (8th ed., pp. 1667–1724). New York: McGraw-Hill.

Scriver, C. R., Kaufman, S., Eisensmith, R. C., & Woo, S. L. C. (1995). The hyperphenylalaninemias. In C. R. Scriver, A. L. Beaudet, W. S. Sly, & E. Valle (Eds.), *The metabolic and molecular bases of inherited disease* (7th ed., pp. 1025–1075). New York: McGraw-Hill.

Seashore, M. R., Friedman, E., Novelly, R. A., & Bapat, V. (1985). Loss of intellectual function in children with phenylketonuria after relaxation of dietary phenylalanine restriction. *Pediatrics, 75,* 226–232.

Shedlovsky, A., McDonald, J. D., Symula, D., & Dove, W. F. (1993). Mouse models of human phenylketonuria. *Genetics, 134,* 1205–1210.

Shonkoff. J. P. (2003). From neurons to neighborhoods: Old and new challenges for developmental and behavioral pediatrics. *Journal of Developmental and Behavioral Pediatrics, 24,* 70–76.

Siegel, F., Balow, B., Risch, R. O., & Anderson, V. E. (1968). School behavior profile ratings of phenylketonuric children. *American Journal of Mental Deficiency, 72,* 937–943.

Smith, I., & Knowles J. (2000). Behaviour in early treated phenylketonuria: A systematic review. *European Journal of Pediatrics, 159*(Suppl. 2), S89–S93.

Stemerdink, B. A., van der Meere, J. J., van der Molen, M. W., Kalverboer, A. F., Hendrikx, M. M. T., Huisman, J., et al. (1995). Information processing in patients with early and continuously-treated phenylketonuria. *European Journal of Pediatrics, 154,* 739–746.

Stemerdink, N. (1996). *Early and continuously treated phenylketonuria: An experimental neuropsychological approach.* Amsterdam: Academisch Proefschrift.

Surtees, R., & Blau, N. (2000). The neurochemistry of phenylketonuria. *European Journal of Pediatrics, 159*(Suppl. 2), S109–S113.

Tam, S. Y., Elsworth, J. D., Bradberry, C. W., & Roth, R. H. (1990). Mesocortical dopamine neurons: High basal firing frequency predicts tyrosine dependence of dopamine synthesis. *Journal of Neural Transmission, 81,* 97–110.

Tarini B. A. (2007). The current revolution in newborn screening: New technology, old controversies. *Archives of Pediatrics and Adolescent Medicine, 161,* 767–772.

Thompson, A. J., Tillotson, S., Smith, I., Kendall, B., Moore, S. G., & Brenton, D. P. (1993). Brain MRI changes in phenylketonuria: Associations with dietary status. *Brain, 116,* 811–821.

Tuchman, L. K., Slap, G. B., & Britto, M. T. (2008). Transition to adult care: Experiences and expectations of adolescents with a chronic illness. *Child: Care, Health, and Development, 5,* 557–563.

Vajro, P., Strisciuglio, P., Houssin, D., Huault, G., Laurent, J., Alvarez, F., et al. (1993). Correction of phenylketonuria after liver transplantation in a child with cirrhosis. *New England Journal of Medicine, 329,* 363–366.

van Calcar, S. C., MacLeod, E. L., Gleason, S. T., Etzel, M. R., Clayton, M. K., Wolff, J. A., et al. (2009). Improved nutritional management of phenylketonuria by using a diet containing glycomacropeptide compared with amino acids. *Amerian Journal of Clinical Nutrition, 89*(4), 1068–1077.

van Zutphen, K. H., Packman, W., Sporri, L., Needham, M. C., Morgan, C., Weisiger, K., et al. (2007). Executive functioning in children and adolescents with phenylketonuria. *Clinical Genetics. 72,* 13–18.

Visser, S. N., & Lesesne, C. A. (2003). Mental health in the United States: Prevalence of diagnosis and medication treatment for attention-deficit/hyperactivity disorder—United States. *Morbidity and Mortality Weekly Report, 54,* 842–847.

von Spronsen, F. J., & Burgard, P. (2008). The truth of treating patients with phenylketonuria after childhood: the need for a new guideline. *Journal of Inherited Metabolic Disease, 31,* 673–679.

von Spronsen, F. J., & Enns, G. M. (2010). Future treatment strategies in phenylketonuria. *Molecular Genetics and Metabolism, 99*(Suppl. 1), S90–S95.

Waisbren, S. E., Brown, M. J., de Sonneville, L. M. J., & Levy, H. L. (1994). Review of neuropsychological functioning in treated phenylketonuria: An information processing approach. *Acta Paediatrica, 84*(Suppl. 408), 98–103.

Waisbren, S. E., Chang, P. N., Levy, H. L., Shifrin, H., Allred, E., Azen, C., et al. (1998). Neonatal neurological assessment of offspring in maternal PKU. *Journal of Inherited Metabolic Disease, 21,* 39–48.

Waisbren, S. E., Hamilton, B. D., St. James, P. J., Shiloh, S., & Levy, H. L. (1995). Psychosocial factors in maternal phenylketonuria: Women's adherence to medical recommendations. *American Journal of Public Health, 85,* 1636–1641.

Waisbren, S. E., Hanley, W., Levy, H. L., Shifrin, H., Allred, E., Azen, C., et al. (2000). Outcome at age 4 years in offspring of women with maternal phenylketonuria: The Maternal PKU Collaborative Study. *Journal of the American Medical Association, 283,* 756–762.

Waisbren, S. E., & Levy, H. L. (1991). Agoraphobia in phenylketonuria. *Journal of Inherited Metabolic Disease, 14,* 755–764.

Waisbren, S. E., Noel, K., Fahrbach, K., Cella, C., Frame, D. Dorenbaum, A., et al. (2007). Phenylalanine blood levels and clinical outcomes in phenylketonuria: A systematic literature review and meta-analysis. *Molecular Genetics and Metabolism, 92,* 63–70.

Waisbren, S. E., Rokni, H., Bailey, I., Rohr, F., Brown, T., & Warner-Rogers, J. (1997). Social factors and the meaning of food in adherence to medical diets: Results of a maternal phenylketonuria summer camp. *Journal of Inherited Metabolic Disease, 20,* 21–27.

Waisbren, S. E., Schnell, R. R., & Levy, H. L. (1980). Diet termination in children with phenylketonuria: A review of psychological assessments used to determine outcome. *Journal of Inherited Metabolic Disease, 3,* 149–153.

Waisbren, S. E., Shiloh, S., St. James, P. J., & Levy, H. L. (1991). Psychosocial factors in maternal phenylketonuria: Prevention of unplanned pregnancies. *American Journal of Public Health, 81,* 299–304.

Waisbren, S. E., & White, D. A. (2010). Screening for cognitive and social-emotional problems in individuals with PKU: Tools for use in the metabolic clinic. *Molecular Genetics and Metabolism, 99*(Suppl. 1), S96–S99.

Waisbren, S. E., & Zaff, J. (1994). Personality disorder in young women with treated phenylketonuria. *Journal of Inherited Metabolic Disease, 17,* 584–592.

Walker, V., Clayton, B. E., Ersser, R. S., Francis, D. E. M., Lilly, P., Seakins, J. W. T., et al. (1981). Hyperphenylalaninaemia of various types among three-quarters of a million neonates tested in a screening program. *Archives of Disease in Childhood, 56,* 759–764.

Walter, J. H., White, F. J., Hall, S. K., MacDonald, A., Rylance, G., Boneh, A., et al. (2002). How practical are recommendations for dietary control in phenylketonuria? *Lancet, 360,* 55–57.

Wang, C., Camfield, C. S., Fernandez, C. V., Hurley, T., & Campbell, K. (2007). Successful neurological outcome of a child with classical phenylketonuria and acute lymphoblastic leukemia: A 7-year follow-up. *American Journal of Medical Genetics, Part A, 143A,* 3324–3327.

Webster, D. R., & Wallace, J. (1995). PKU and diabetes: Help requested. *Journal of Inherited Metabolic Disease, 18,* 649.

Weglage, J., Fünders, B., Wilken, B., Schubert, D., Schmidt, E., Burgard, P., et al. (1992). Psychological and social findings in adolescents with phenylketonuria. *European Journal of Pediatrics, 151*, 522–525.

Weglage, J., Fünders, B., Wilken, B., Schubert, D., & Ullrich, K. (1993). School performance and intellectual outcome in adolescents with phenylketonuria. *Acta Paediatrica, 81*, 582–586.

Weglage J., Grenzebach M., Pietsch M., Feldmann, R. N., Linnenbank, R., Denecke, J., et al. (2000). Behavioural and emotional problems in early-treated adolescents with phenylketonuria in comparison with diabetic patients and healthy controls. *Journal of Inherited Metabolic Disease, 23*, 487–496.

Weglage, J., Pietsch, M., Denecke, J. Sprinz, A., Feldmann, R., Grenzebach, M., et al. (1999). Regression of neuropsychological deficits in early treated phenylketonuria during adolescence. *Journal of Inherited Metabolic Disease, 22*, 693–705.

Weglage, J., Pietsch, M., Fünders, B., Koch, H. G., & Ullrich, K. (1996). Deficits in selective and sustained attention processes in early treated children with phenylketonuria: Result of impaired frontal lobe functions? *European Journal of Pediatrics, 155*, 200–204.

Welsh, M. C., Pennington, B. F., Ozonoff, S., Rouse, B., & McCabe, E. R. B. (1990). Neuropsychology of early-treated phenylketonuria: Specific executive function deficits. *Child Development, 61*, 1697–1713.

White, D., Nortz, M., Mandernach, T., Huntington, K., & Steiner, R. D. (2002). Age-related working memory impairments in children with prefrontal dysfunction associated with phenylketonuria. *Journal of the International Neuropsychological Society, 8*, 1–11.

Woo, S. L. C., Lidsky, A. S., Guttier, F., Chandra, T., & Robson, K. J. H. (1983). Cloned human phenylalanine hydroxylase gene allows prenatal diagnosis and carrier detection of classical phenylketonuria. *Nature, 306*, 151–155.

Woolf, L. I. (1976). A study of the cause of the high incidence of phenylketonuria in Ireland and west Scotland. *Irish Medical Journal, 69*, 398–401.

Woolf, L. I. (1979). Late onset phenylalanine intoxication. *Journal of Inherited Metabolic Disease, 2*, 19–20.

Wright, K. (1990, September). Cradle of mutation. *Discover*, pp. 22–23.

Yannicelli, S., & Ryan, A. (1995). Improvements in behaviour and physical manifestations in previously untreated adults with phenylketonuria using a phenylalanine-restricted diet: A national survey. *Journal of Inherited Metabolic Disease, 18*, 131–134.

CHAPTER 22

Rett Syndrome

A Truly Pervasive Developmental Disorder

ROBERT T. BROWN
KATHLEEN K. McMILLAN

Rett syndrome (abbreviated RTT in the present chapter, but also often as RS) is a genetically based neurodevelopmental disorder that presents in infancy or early childhood as a striking deterioration after apparently normal initial development. The *Diagnostic and Statistical Manual of Mental Disorders*, fourth edition, text revision (DSM-IV-TR; American Psychiatric Association, 2000) terms it Rett's disorder and classifies it as a pervasive developmental disorder (PDD). Classic RTT is the most severe and the most truly pervasive PDD, affecting virtually all domains of functioning. Although it has been the subject of hundreds of original articles and reviews, RTT is little known to many professionals (Percy, 2008a). This situation is unfortunate, as RTT is in some ways unique among PDDs, and those working with clinical populations should have a basic knowledge of its characteristics.

Classic RTT involves dramatic slowdowns in normal development, deceleration of growth, lack of interest in the environment, deterioration of motor functioning, hand stereotypies, loss of expressive language, abnormal sleep and breathing, seizure disorders, abnormal social interactions, self-injurious behaviors, orthopedic abnormalities (particularly scoliosis), and eventual severe/profound mental retarda-tion. Although RTT is a rare disorder, with a prevalence of approximately 1 in 15,000 females, it may be the second most common form (after Down syndrome) of severe mental retardation (Hagberg, 1995b), and the most common cause of profound mental retardation (Percy, 2002), in females. The many thousand known cases occur apparently equally in all parts of the world and all ethnic groups. Over 4,400 cases have been diagnosed in the United States (Percy, 2009); many older cases may be undiagnosed (Smeets et al., 2003). Major increases in our understanding of RTT's genetic basis, genotype–phenotype relations, cases in males, and potential treatments have occurred since the chapters on it in the first edition of this handbook (Brown & Hoadley, 1999) and the more recent *Handbook of Neurodevelopmental and Genetic Disorders in Adults* (Brown, McMillan, & Herschthal, 2005) were published.

RTT is unique in several ways:

1. Apparently normal initial development is *only* apparent; it is frequently marked by growth retardation from birth and passivity in early infancy.
2. Rapid mental and physical deterioration is often followed by stabilization or reduction of some symptoms.

3. Classic RTT develops through a series of four stages.
4. Initially thought to affect only females, RTT and RTT-like disorders occur in males.
5. At least 95% of female cases have a mutation in the MECP2 gene; however, such mutations are involved in other conditions.
6. RTT occurs in both classic and specific variant forms.
7. Although classic RTT symptoms are severe, variability is higher than was first realized.
8. Physical appearance in childhood and life expectancy are generally nearly normal.

HISTORY AND BACKGROUND

In the early 1960s, in his pediatric clinic at the University of Vienna, Andreas Rett by chance saw two unrelated thin girls who were wringing their hands in an unusual manner and rocking in autistic-like movements. In 1966, he published descriptions of several girls with similar symptoms and developmental histories in an obscure German journal. Although Rett (1977) subsequently published a chapter in English, his findings were largely overlooked. Hagberg (1995b) has summarized Rett's work.

Also in the early 1960s, Bengt Hagberg in Sweden was independently studying similar cases. Rett and Hagberg met by chance at a conference in Canada and discussed their common observations (Percy, 2009). That discussion led to the first widely circulated description of RTT in English (Hagberg, Aicardi, Dias, & Ramos, 1983). In a sense, two chance events—Rett's initial observations, and Rett and Hagberg's meeting—led to RTT's becoming widely known. The story supports Louis Pasteur's classic statement that in fields of observation, chance favors the prepared mind.

DIAGNOSIS OF CLASSIC RTT AND RTT VARIANTS

Classic RTT

Necessary, supportive, and exclusionary criteria for classic RTT are given in Table 22.1 (International Rett Syndrome Foundation

[IRSF], 2008). These criteria were developed by an expert panel sponsored by the International Rett Syndrome Association, the IRSF's predecessor (Hagberg, Hanefeld, Percy, & Skjeldal, 2002). Particularly important is criterion 6: "The almost continuous repetitive wringing, twisting or clapping hand automatisms during wakefulness constitute the hallmark of the condition," according to Hagberg (1995b, p. 973). Overall growth retardation is also generally seen: 95% of girls with RTT are below the 5th

TABLE 22.1. Classic RTT: Necessary, Supportive, and Exclusionary Diagnostic Criteria

Necessary criteria (must occur)

1. Apparently normal prenatal/perinatal history
2. Psychomotor development delayed from birth or apparently normal to about age 6 months
3. Normal head circumference at birth
4. Postnatal deceleration of head growth in most cases
5. Loss of purposeful hand skills between 6 and 30 months of age
6. Persistent stereotypic hand wringing/squeezing, clapping/tapping, mouthing, and/or washing/rubbing
7. Progressive social withdrawal, verbal/nonverbal communication loss and/or dysfunction, and cognitive impairment
8. Impaired locomotion or loss of locomotion

Supportive criteria (may occur)

1. Disturbed breathing (hyperventilation, breath-holding, forced expulsion of air/saliva, air gulping) while awake
2. Bruxism
3. Impaired sleep patterns from early infancy
4. Abnormal muscle tone resulting in muscle wasting and dystonia
5. Peripheral vasomotor disturbances (cold, blue hands and feet)
6. Progressive scoliosis/kyphosis
7. Overall growth retardation
8. Hypotrophic (small) feet; small, thin hands

Exclusionary criteria (must not occur)

1. Enlarged organs or other signs of storage disease
2. Retinopathy, optic atrophy, or cataract
3. Pre-, peri-, and/or postnatal brain damage
4. Identified metabolic or other progressive neurological disorder
5. Neurological disorder owing to severe infection or head trauma

Note. Adapted from IRSF (2008). Copyright 2008 by the International Rett Syndrome Foundation.

percentile in height and weight by 2 years of age (Percy & Lane, 2005).

Diagnosis of RTT is based on clinical signs, not genetic analysis (e.g., Hagberg et al., 2002; Percy, 2008a). The relationship between RTT and MECP2 gene mutations is not perfect, as described in more detail in a later section. Some individuals diagnosed with RTT do not have a known mutation, and some with a mutation do not show RTT.

Atypical RTT

The realization that females diagnosed with RTT were more heterogeneous than was originally thought led to the category of atypical RTT or RTT variants (Hagberg, 1995a, 1995b). Main and supportive criteria for atypical RTT are given in Table 22.2. Atypical RTT should be diagnosed only in girls of 10 years or older, although criterion behaviors may appear throughout childhood. Girls with atypical RTT generally show less severe symptoms than those with classic RTT. Gross and fine motor control and mental retardation may be less severe;

TABLE 22.2. Atypical RTT: Main and Supportive Diagnostic Criteria

Main criteria (must meet at least three)

1. Absence or reduction of hand skills
2. Reduction or loss of babble speech
3. Monotonous pattern of hand stereotypies
4. Reduction or loss of communication skills
5. Deceleraton of head growth from first years of life
6. RTT disease profile: a regression stage followed by a recovery of interaction contrasting with slow neuromotor regression

Supportive criteria (must meet at least five)

1. Breathing irregularities
2. Bloating/air swallowing
3. Teeth grinding (harsh-sounding type)
4. Abnormal locomotion
5. Scoliosis/kyphosis
6. Lower-limb muscle atrophy
7. Cold, purplish feet, usually growth-impaired
8. Sleep disturbances, including night screaming outbursts
9. Laughing/screaming spells
10. Diminished response to pain
11. Intense eye contact/eye pointing

Note. Adapted from IRSF (2008). Copyright 2008 by the International Rett Syndrome Foundation.

---

some girls retain language, although it tends to be atypical and telegraphic. Several specific variants have been identified, including early-onset seizure, congenital with abnormal early development, delayed, and Zappella variant/preserved speech (e.g., Percy, 2008a). Since girls with the last-mentioned variant show actual, although slow, motor and language development in childhood and can draw and speak in sentences, the term *Zappella variant* may be preferable to *preserved speech* (e.g., Renieri et al., 2009).

Diagnostic Concerns

Of importance for parents and therapists is accurate diagnosis as early as possible. Some professionals may be reluctant to diagnose RTT early because of its eventual severity, but many parents are frustrated by the lack of a diagnosis that fits their children's behaviors or has implications for treatment and care. A parent checklist and video technique may be useful in making a detailed diagnosis (Fyfe et al., 2007), and a symptom checklist may help determine whether a girl should be referred for testing for a *MECP2* mutation (Huppke, Köhler, Laccone, & Hanefeld, 2003). Classification and diagnosis are still controversial issues (e.g., Matson, Fodstad, & Boisjoli, 2008).

DEVELOPMENTAL TREND OF CLASSIC RTT

Classic RTT develops through a four-stage sequence of behavioral and physical changes first described by Hagberg and Witt Engerström (1986). Kerr and Witt Engerström (2001) provide a useful table of the stages. Age of onset, transition time from one stage to the next, manifestation of features, and duration of all stages are variable. This section draws on Budden (1997), Hagberg (1995b), Hagberg and Witt Engerström (1986), Kerr (1995), Moser and Naidu (1996), and Naidu (1997) to describe major characteristics of early development prior to onset of symptoms and at each stage, along with disorders from which RTT should be differentiated.

Pre-Stage 1: Early Development

Development appears largely normal until at least 5–6 months of age. Early motor skills, including reaching for objects, usually appear. Infants commonly develop self-feeding and can be weaned onto solid foods. Many babble and walk, although their gait is often unusual. However, subtle signs of RTT appear early. Newborns who later manifest RTT generally have below-normal occipital frontal circumference, length, and weight, suggesting prenatal effects of *MECP2* mutations (Huppke, Held, Laccone, & Hanefeld, 2003). Many developmental milestones are delayed. Feeding difficulties, floppiness, jerkiness, delays in babbling and motor development, poor mobility, repetitive limb movement, failure to recognize familiar adults, limited play, repeated facial and mouth twitching, and repeated opening/closing of hands when trying to grasp an object may appear in early infancy (e.g., Kerr, 1995).

Many girls use single words, and a few use short phrases (Tams-Little & Holdgrafer, 1996). Of interest for potential early awareness of the disorder, these authors also found that parents of only 1 of 17 girls with RTT reported use of three nonverbal communication gestures (giving, pointing, and showing) that typically develop at about 9–10 months of age.

Stage 1: Early-Onset Stagnation

The first stage begins at 6–18 months of age and lasts for months. Overall, an infant appears to hit a developmental wall, although some advances (particularly in gross motor control) may occur. Much cognitive development ceases. Deceleration of head growth leads to below-normal head circumference by the end of the second year (Kerr, 1995). Although no obvious pattern of abnormalities is apparent, hypotonia, loss of interest in play and the environment, loss of acquired hand functions, and random hand movements are typical. Differential diagnoses include benign congenital hypotonia, cerebral palsy, Prader–Willi syndrome, and metabolic disorders.

Stage 2: Rapid Destructive

At about 18 months of age (range = 1–4 years), affected children's general functioning deteriorates so rapidly that onset "may be so acute that parents can sometimes give a specific date after which their child was no longer 'normal'" (Budden, 1997, p. 2).

Cognitive functioning, purposeful hand use, and expressive language deteriorate further. Hand stereotypies typically appear and may be continuous during waking hours. Walking may deteriorate or not develop. Girls who do walk generally show gait abnormalities, particularly a spread-legged stance. Hyperventilation, bruxism, and breath holding are common, as are behaviors characteristic of autism. Seizures and vacant spells resembling seizures may occur, and virtually all girls with RTT have abnormal electroencephalograms (EEGs) by the end of stage 2. Sleep patterns may become erratic and accompanied by bouts of screaming and inappropriate laughter (Kerr & Witt Engerström, 2001). Differential diagnoses include autism, encephalitis, metabolic disorders (including inborn errors of metabolism), and neurodegenerative disorders.

Stage 3: Plateau

Stage 3 generally lasts until about 10 years of age. Hand stereotypies continue, and mobility may further deteriorate. Measured mental retardation is generally in the severe/profound range, but assessment is difficult because of communication and motor impairments. Tremulousness, ataxia, bruxism, hyperventilation or breath holding, seizures, overall rigidity (hypertonia), and scoliosis may appear or increase. However, autistic symptoms may diminish, and social interactions, hand use, communication, alertness, and self-initiated behavior may increase. Nonverbal communication through eye pointing is claimed to improve, but this claim is controversial. Using a "blind" procedure, Meyer, Kennedy, Shulka, and Cushing (1999) found that caretakers of an adolescent with RTT did not accurately interpret her eye pointing, but made inferences based on their familiarity with her. Unfortunately, many studies that claim to have demonstrated choice behavior through eye pointing have not controlled for potential confounding effects. In one study (Baptista, Mercadante, Macedo, & Schwartzman, 2006) claiming that girls with classic RTT answered correctly on cognitive tasks via eye pointing and looking time, the girls sat on their mothers' laps, allowing for subtle cueing. Researchers measuring eye pointing or gazing need to control for confounding sources of cueing and experimenter effects.

Differential diagnoses include cerebral palsy and other motor disorders, Angelman and Lennox–Gastaut syndromes, and spinocerebellar degeneration.

Stage 4: Late Motor Deterioration

Final phenotypes of classic RTT vary widely (e.g., Hagberg, 1995b), but virtually all older patients will be dependent on others for meeting basic needs. Physical size, including brain size, is dramatically below normal (e.g., Cass et al., 2003). Motor function decreases further, with increased rigidity, muscle wasting, and scoliosis. Mobility also decreases further; many girls will need to use wheelchairs, although others will walk with altered gait throughout life. Repetitive hand stereotypies, drooling, feeding/sleeping problems, skeletal deformities, seizures, joint problems, gastrointestinal problems (including constipation), and breathing abnormalities are almost universal (e.g., Percy, 2008a). Puberty is often delayed, but otherwise normal. Girls may be unable to convey pain from menstrual discomfort or vaginal infection. Remaining expressive language generally disappears, and receptive language decreases. Eye pointing as communication is claimed to continue, and girls often seek social interaction. Chewing and swallowing problems may necessitate artificial feeding (e.g., Lava, Slotte, Jochym-Nygren, van Doorn, & Witt Engerstrom, 2006; Leonard, Fyfe, Leonard, & Msall, 2001). The girls have likes and dislikes, and can indicate likes through such behaviors as facial expressions and laughter (Cass et al., 2003; Kerr & Witt Engerström, 2001). Survival rate is essentially normal to 10 years of age, but then begins to drop. Survival at ages 20, 35, and 50 years is 80%, 70%, and 50%, respectively (Percy, 2008a).

GENETICS

For many years, RTT was assumed to be a single-gene X-linked dominant disorder, for many reasons: (1) Concordance is close to 100% in monozygotic twins and 0% in dizygotic twins; (2) only about 0.5% of RTT cases are familial; and (3) early findings indicated that RTT fully appeared only in females, with a few cases of males with Rett-like symptoms.

The breakthrough occurred in 1999, when Amir and colleagues reported mutations in several cases of RTT of *MECP2,* a large gene at the tip of the long arm of the X chromosome. *MECP2* (pronounced meck-pea-two [National Institute of Neurological Diseases and Stroke, 2003]) encodes a protein, MeCP2, a transcriptional repressor that controls expression of other genes. Most mutations reduce or eliminate function of MeCP2. Impaired MeCP2 in turn may disrupt normal developmental pathways by leading other genes to turn and/or stay on at inappropriate times, resulting in uncontrolled gene expression (Johnston, 2004). Given MeCP2's broad role in regulating gene action, one should not be surprised that *MECP2* mutations may have severe effects. As Armstrong (2005, p. 751) stated: "The abnormalities in the anatomy, chemistry, and clinical manifestations of Rett syndrome all suggest that *MECP2* is essential for neuronal maturation."

More than 200 mutations have been identified on the four *MECP2* exons. About 95% of females with RTT have a *MECP2* mutation. However, some with RTT have no known mutation, and some with mutations do not show RTT. About 39% of all cases are associated with four missense *MECP2* mutations (T158M, R306C, R133C, and R106W); 35% with four nonsense mutations (R168X, R255X, R294X, and R270X); 8.8% with C-terminal deletions; and 6.4% with large deletions (e.g., Percy, 2008a; Percy & Lane, 2009).

Severity of RTT symptomatology varies with type of *MECP2* mutation (e.g., Naidu et al., 2003). Relatively mild symptoms are associated with R133C, R294X, R306C, and C-terminal deletion mutations. Girls with the T158M mutation may show only RTT behavioral symptoms in infancy and childhood, but slowly deteriorate into classic RTT in adolescence. The R306X mutation appears largely to impair only language. On the other hand, R168X mutations are associated with more severe outcomes, particularly in walking, hand use, and language (Neul et al., 2008; Smeets, Chenaul, Curfs, Schrander-Stumpel, & Frijns, 2009). Considerable variability in severity occurs in girls with the same mutation, suggesting that additional factors, such as skewed X chromosome inactivation or action of other mutated genes, influence severity (e.g., Naidu et al.,

2003). About 2 weeks after conception, one of the two X chromosomes in female zygotes is inactivated. In some cases, the inactivation may be skewed or partial, leading to over- or underrepresentation of some genes.

Several nonclassic RTT phenotypes are associated with *MECP2* mutations in both males and females. Female phenotypes include the preserved speech/Zappella variant, the delayed-onset variant, mild learning disability, Angelman syndrome, and unaffected carriers. Male phenotypes include fatal encephalopathy (most cases), Rett/Klinefelter syndrome (47,XXY genotype), Angelman syndrome, X-linked mental retardation/progressive spasticity, and somatic mosaicism/neurodevelopmental delay (Hagberg et al., 2002; Online Mendelian Inheritance in Man [OMIM], 2004). However, detailed analysis of the DNA sequence of the *MECP2* gene in 28 males with Rett-like characteristics, 13 of whom met criteria for a RTT variant, failed to find any *MECP2* mutations (Santos et al., 2009). If other mutated genes are found to be responsible for cases such as those of Santos and colleagues (2009), efforts should be made to determine whether they exacerbate symptoms in those who also have a *MECP2* mutation. For example, the congenital RTT variant has recently been attributed to a mutation on the FOXG1 gene (Ariani et al., 2008).

MOUSE MODELS

Basic Aspects

Research using mouse models of RTT, developed through several means of reducing levels of *MECP2*, has advanced our understanding of the effects of *MECP2* mutations on development of Rett-like symptoms that complement many findings on human cases (for summaries of earlier models, see Armstrong, 2005; Percy, 2008b). Increasing numbers and types of models are being reported, to the extent that only summaries can be provided here. Because the different models have been formed by using different techniques of reducing MECP2, each has its specific characteristics. In general, they develop apparently normally until about 3–8 weeks of age, but then develop various RTT symptoms. Following Armstrong (2005), we describe mutants in terms of the laboratories in which they were developed. Zoghbi mutant mice

developed tremors, motor impairments, low general activity, apparent anxiety, seizures, curvature of the spine, and stereotypic forelimb movements (Shahbazian et al., 2002). Jaenisch mutant mice developed apparently normally initially and were fertile, but at about age 5 weeks began to show progressive RTT-like symptoms such as nervousness, tremors, cold limbs, and breathing problems. Brain size and neuronal cell size were both reduced. Death occurred at about 10 weeks of age. Females heterozygous for *MECP2* developed normally for about 4 months, but then showed reduced activity, gait abnormalities, and weight gain (Chen, Akbarian, Tudor, & Jaenisch, 2001). Bird *MECP2*-null male and female mice developed an unnatural gait and reduced movement at ages 3–8 weeks, followed by hindlimb clasping, irregular breathing, and teeth/jaw abnormalities. Increasingly severe symptoms led to death at about 54 days. Bird female mice heterozygotic for *MECP2* behaved normally until about age 12 weeks, when they began to show hindlimb clasping and reduced movement. By age 9 months, about half showed additional symptoms, but then largely stabilized (Guy, Hendrich, Holmes, Martin, & Bird, 2001). Tam mice have virtually no *MECP2* and show severe early motor deficits, stereotyped hindlimb clasping, impaired motor learning, fear conditioning, and memory. Analyses revealed impaired amygdaloid and hippocampal formation, as well as impaired activity of several specific genes involved in nervous system development and functioning (Pelka et al., 2006). Another Rett mouse model (Stearns et al., 2007) showed similar patterns: Males without *MECP2* showed low activity, abnormal gait, paw stereotypies, relatively high fear, and deficits in learning. Brain volumes overall and in the amygdala, hippocampus, and striatum were smaller than those of controls. Females with one normal and one mutant *MECP2* gene showed similar, but less severe, abnormalities

In mice, MeCP2 regulates brain-derived neurotrophic factor (BDNF). BDNF encodes a protein essential for adult neuronal plasticity, which in turn is essential for learning and memory. *MECP2* mutations deregulate this protein in mice, and this deregulation, through action on BDNF, may be at least partly responsible for RTT (e.g., Chen et al., 2003; Gabellini, Green, & Tupler, 2004).

Implications for Potential Therapy

Various manipulations reduce the effects of *MECP2* mutations in mouse models. Giacometti, Luikenhuis, Beard, and Jaenisch (2007) provided Jaenisch mice with a "rescue transgene" that postnatally activated MeCP2 in the mice's brains. Rescued mice showed delayed development of RTT-like symptoms and lived longer than untreated ones. Furthermore, the brains of rescued Jaenisch mice were similar to those of typical nonmutant mice. Thus postnatal remediation of MeCP2 deficiency may reduce severity of subsequent brain damage and RTT.

At least two studies support Giacometti and colleagues' (2007) suggestion. In the first study, rearing heterozygous female Tam *MECP2*-deleted mutant mice in enriched environments improved their performance on several behavioral tests and showed increased cerebellar levels of BDNF, relative to those of such mice reared in standard cages. Male mice with no *MECP2* gene raised in enriched environments showed no improvements in behavioral tests or brain measures over such mice raised in standard cages. The authors (Kondo et al., 2008) infer from these findings that a normal *MECP2* gene is needed for the enriched environment to have a positive effect.

In the second study, injections of a substance reactivating the *MECP2* gene in Bird mutant male and female mice that were several weeks old and manifesting Rett-like symptoms considerably reduced the symptoms, prolonged life, and reversed hippocampal long-term potentiation deficits present in untreated mutant mice (Guy, Gan, Selfridge, Cobb, & Bird. 2007). These findings indicate considerable malleability in the structure of the nervous system even in adult mutant mice. Obviously these findings have implications for, if not direct applicability to, human RTT (see, e.g., Percy, 2008a, 2008b).

RTT IN MALES

Basic Aspects

RTT for many years was thought to occur only in females, but then Coleman (1990) and Philippart (1990) independently reported two possible cases in males. Subsequent research has confirmed both classic and atypical RTT in males, but at extremely low rates.

As might be expected, classic RTT has been reported in boys with the 47,XXY karyotype of Klinefelter syndrome or 47,XXY/46,XY mosaicism. One boy with Klinefelter syndrome initially developed normal sitting, grasping, playing, and feeding, and had begun to say a few words appropriately. By a year of age, he was losing hand, language, and social skills, and was developing stereotyped hand movements, bruxism, and constipation. By age 3, he had severe mental retardation, had lost purposeful hand movements, and exhibited general hypotonia—all characteristic of RTT, but not Klinefelter. Genetic tests indicated that the second X chromosome came from the father through nondisjunction (Schwartzman et al., 1999). In a highly unusual case (Maiwald et al., 2002), a boy who was identified as male by prenatal sonogram and postnatal phenotype, but who had a female 46,XX genotype, showed RTT-like symptoms (delayed motor development, lack of language, hypotonia, microcephaly, and loss of purposeful hand movements) by age 24 months.

RTT-like symptoms, including growth and mental retardation, hypotonia, absent or lost language, microcephaly, seizures, scoliosis, abnormal EEG patterns, and respiratory irregularities, have been reported in boys from families with recurrent RTT in their daughters (Schanen et al., 1998) and boys with somatic *MECP2* mutations (Clayton-Smith, Watson, Ramsden, & Black, 2000; Topcu et al., 2002). One of Schanen and colleagues' (1998) cases died at age 18 months, apparently from respiratory failure; the other showed motor and other delays and a head circumference below the 5th percentile at 9 months of age. Clayton-Smith and colleagues' (2000) case developed hand stereotypies, whereas Topcu and colleagues' (2002) did not. 46,XY males with nonmosaic *MECP2* mutations may manifest a variety of disorders: classic and atypical RTT, congenital encephalopathy and early death, mild to severe mental retardation, neurological disorders (e.g., ataxia, seizures, and hypotonia), and PPM-X syndrome (mental retardation, pyramidal signs, psychosis, and macro-orchidism) (Moog et al., 2003).

Why Is RTT Rare in Males?

Two explanations have been offered for the very low prevalence of RTT in males. The more generally supported is that males' shorter Y chromosome lacks a normal gene to moderate the effects of an *MECP2* mutation on the X chromosome. 46,XY males would be nonviable, dying either prenatally or early postnatally. The other explanation (Thomas, 1996) was based on evidence that RTT is a dominant X chromosome disorder largely caused by spontaneous mutations that are more frequent in sperm than in eggs. Since chromosomally normal women (46,XX) get one X chromosome from their fathers, and chromosomally normal males (46,XY) always get their X chromosome from their mothers, more affected females than males would be expected, owing to normal patterns of inheritance.

Evidence supports both explanations. Akesson, Hagberg, and Wahlström (1997) reported significantly fewer male siblings among girls with RTT than would be expected. Since males' X chromosome is received from the mother, maternal transmission was indicated in these cases. Furthermore, early postnatal death of males with *MECP2* mutations suggests more prenatal deaths. Finally, a knockout *MECP2* mouse model produced no surviving male offspring (see Trappe et al., 2001, for details and references). Trappe and colleagues' (2001) research also provides support for Thomas's (1996) explanation. Of 27 females with RTT owing to spontaneous *MECP2* mutations, 26 had the mutation on the X chromosome from the father. Given that most male and female cases of familial RTT and RTT-like conditions arise from maternal *MECP2* mutations, most of the 99.5% of cases of RTT that are nonfamilial probably originate from a spontaneous *MECP2* mutation on the paternal X chromosome. The rarity of familial cases also supports Thomas. Since they are not mutually exclusive, both explanations could be involved in the low prevalence of RTT in males.

NEUROPATHOLOGY

RTT is associated with dramatic global and localized neurological, neurochemical, and neurophysiological effects. Areas involved in motor control are greatly affected. As would be expected from the fact that seizures and sleep disorders are common in RTT, EEG patterns tend to be abnormal (e.g., Jellinger, 2003). Perhaps the most striking effect is small brain size, which appears to be about that of a normal 12-month infant virtually throughout life.

On initial inspection, many parts of the brains of those with RTT appear normal (Armstrong & Kinney, 2001), and the brains show no abnormal neuronal migration or obvious cell loss or atrophy (Neul & Zoghbi, 2004). However, numerous abnormalities have been documented. The cerebral hemispheres progressively atrophy, with overall reduction of gray and white matter, particularly in the frontal and temporal lobes (e.g., Kaufmann, 2001). The corpus callosum may be 30% below normal size. The brains of those with RTT also have small dendritic trees in pyramidal neurons of layers III and V in the frontal, motor, and temporal lobes; small neurons with increased neuronal packing density in the cerebral cortex, thalamus, basal ganglia, amygdala, and hippocampus; and reduced numbers of synapses in many areas (e.g., Armstrong, 2005; Jellinger, 2003; Neul & Zoghbi, 2004). Blood flow is reduced throughout the cortex (e.g., Armstrong & Kinney, 2001), particularly in prefrontal and temporoparietal areas (e.g., Jellinger, 2003). The midbrain, cerebellum, and basal ganglia, particularly the caudate nucleus and thalami, are smaller (e.g., Dunn et al., 2002; Jellinger, 2003). Cerebellar abnormalities suggest prenatally arrested development (Jellinger, 2003). Positron emission tomography scans show reduced uptake of fluorodopa and increased dopamine D2 receptor binding in the caudate and putamen of girls with RTT relative to those of normal controls (Dunn et al., 2002). Dunn and colleagues (2002) suggest that RTT involves a presynaptic deficit of nigrostriatal activity.

Substance P, a neuromodulator, is substantially reduced in girls with RTT. Its reduction in spinal cord areas involved in transmission of pain stimuli could be involved in these girls' often reported reduced pain perception. It is also involved in control of many other functions affecting those with RTT, including respiration, transmission of visual and olfactory information, heart rate and rhythm, growth, and sleep (e.g., Armstrong & Kinney, 2001).

Levels of many neurotransmitters are also reduced in those with RTT (e.g., Armstrong, 2005; Neul & Zoghbi, 2004). Dysfunction of the cholinergic forebrain system, which causes reduced choline acetyltransferase activity, is often found (e.g., Jellinger, 2003). The brains of those with RTT generally have low levels of dopamine, norepinephrine, serotonin, and their metabolites. Consistently found is reduced pigmentation in the substantia nigra (Jellinger, 2003). Some of these abnormalities may owe to the reduced concentrations of nerve growth factor found in the cerebrospinal fluid of girls with RTT (Riikonen, 2001). As reported by Percy (2008a), abnormal development of brainstem serotonin transporter binding has been observed in brainstem tissue of human cases of RTT, which may lead to characteristic dysregulation of gastrointestinal and respiratory systems. Percy suggests that clinical trials of serotonin and/or norepinephrine inhibitors are warranted in an attempt to remediate this dysregulation.

The variety of respiratory and cardiovascular conditions led Julu (2001) to suggest that RTT is a "congenital dysautonomia" and that "early brainstem dysfunction underlies the respiratory disturbance and may contribute to sudden deaths" (p. 132). Levels of cardiac sensitivity to baroflex and cardiac vagal tone in girls with RTT are almost 50% lower than normal, indicating a lack of integration in the brainstem, particularly in the nucleus tractus solitarius (Julu, 2001).

Of interest, brainstem neural systems that develop between 36 weeks' gestational age and 2–3 months postnatally appear to be abnormal, whereas those developing earlier appear normal. Thus RTT onset may occur in late fetal or early postnatal development and may involve early lesions of monoamine neurons (Nomura & Segawa, 2001). According to Nomura and Segawa (2001), low functioning of the noradrenergic and serotonergic neurons that develop during that period may be responsible for RTT-associated sleep disorders, and deficiencies in dopaminergic neurons may follow. They propose that early lesions of monoamine neurons in brainstem and midbrain may lead to arrested or inadequate synaptogenesis at all brain levels (including the cortex) that

occurs in a caudal-to-rostral direction. This directionality in turn may underlie the developmental course of RTT symptoms. This "monoamine hypothesis" seems in keeping with Naidu and colleagues' (2003) proposal that *MECP2* mutations lead to failure of appropriate timing of MeCP2 in developing cerebellar neurons and increased glutamate and N-methyl-D-aspartate (NMDA) receptors. High levels of glutamate and NMDA receptors in turn lead to hyperexcitability of neurons in the brain, contributing to many RTT symptoms.

TREATMENT AND MANAGEMENT

Although no completely and generally effective treatment regimen for RTT is available, intense intervention may delay the appearance of some symptoms and alleviate others (e.g., Glaze, 1995). Given RTT's multidimensional and generally severe effects, a multidisciplinary treatment team of professionals should be available either directly or through connection with a regional RTT center to develop a fully accurate diagnosis, including identification of specific MECP2 mutations, and course of treatment. This team is likely to include a pediatrician, neurologist, neuropsychologist, geneticist, orthopedic surgeon, gastroenterologist, endocrinologist, physical therapist, speech–language therapist, and family therapist.

Several factors need to be considered in planning interventions:

1. Those with RTT typically have very long latencies, as long as a minute, to respond to directions. Therapists and parents must allow time for response.

2. Accurate diagnosis is important to ensure effective, and avoid ineffective, treatment. For example, three girls with RTT, initially diagnosed with autism, were inadvertent participants in Lovaas's intensive behavior modification program (Smith, Klevstrand, & Lovaas, 1995). The program, although demonstrably effective with autistic children, had few positive effects on these girls, and gains tended to be offset by losses. More targeted behavioral treatment may be effective, however, as described below.

3. Individual differences in degree and type of impairments, and in responsiveness

to (as well as tolerance of) various interventions, necessitate individualized treatment programs (e.g., Van Acker, 1991).

4. Most reports of successful interventions have had few participants, making generality of findings uncertain.

5. Most behavioral interventions involve extensive training. Much effort, persistence, and tolerance for frustration are required, since the changes reported in some studies have been slow and even difficult to see. Indeed, Piazza, Anderson, and Fisher (1993) suggest that parents be warned about the effort involved and the need to keep careful response records in order to see progress.

6. Generally, those with RTT appear to respond strongly to music (e.g., Kerr, Belichenkob, Woodcock, & Woodcock, 2001). It facilitates learning and development of skills to such an extent that "music therapy should now be regarded as an essential part of communication assessment and therapy" (Kerr, 2002, p. 283). Preferred music may be a reinforcer (e.g., Merker & Wallin, 2001).

7. Some with RTT show hearing loss, particularly with increasing age (e.g., Pillion, Rawool, Bibat, & Naidu, 2003). They may benefit from hearing aids, but caretakers need to attend carefully to their use. Parents, therapists, and teachers may need to adjust oral communication and music therapy to the auditory functioning of those with RTT.

8. Claims that girls with RTT can communicate through eye pointing must be interpreted with caution, as discussed above.

In the studies described here, all participants had been formally diagnosed with RTT. Specialized behaviorally based programs have successfully modified various behaviors in persons of different ages with RTT, often in institutional settings. Using verbal and physical prompts and reinforcement (praise), Piazza and colleagues (1993) attempted to teach five girls who initially had very limited self-feeding skills to scoop food onto a spoon, bring the spoon to their mouths, and put the spoon in their mouths. The girls' self-feeding improved to varying degrees both during the 8-week program and in later follow-up. One girl was almost completely feeding herself 18 months after the end of the program. Through use of shaping, graduated guidance, and hand regulation, Bat-Haee (1994) increased self-feeding,

ambulation, and use of an adaptive switch in an adult woman who had been completely dependent on staff members.

Of interest is a program (Roane, Piazza, Sgro, Volkert, & Anderson, 2001) that successfully reduced stereotyped hand movements in an adolescent and an adult who engaged in chronic stereotyped hand movements—behaviors thought to be inherent to RTT. Initial observations indicated that the stereotyped behaviors occurred almost continuously across situations and regardless of external contingencies, suggesting that they were under "automatic reinforcement" (Roane et al., 2001, p. 142) that produced or alleviated stimulation. The most successful treatment involved response interruption: Whenever one of the girls engaged in a stereotyped hand movement, a therapist said, "Hands down, [girl's name]," while moving her hands away from her face and holding them for 20 seconds. During treatment sessions, both girls' stereotyped hand movements declined to near zero levels. However, treatment involved some 65–100 10-minute sessions given 8–10 times daily, 5 days a week, and the effects showed little generalization to other settings.

Mechanical and computer-based devices have been used to modify girls' behavior. Using a computer fitted with a touch-sensitive screen and voice synthesizer, Van Acker and Grant (1995) presented combined visual–auditory representations of favored (and, in a subsequent phase, nonfavored) foods to three girls. In the first phase of training, a picture of a favored food item appeared on the computer screen as the voice synthesizer asked, "Would you like some _____?" To varying extents, the girls learned, with initial guidance, to touch the screen to receive a small amount of a favored food. Acquisition took weeks at two sessions a day. In the later phase, two of the girls clearly discriminated between favored and nonfavored foods, learning relatively quickly to respond at a high rate for favored foods and at a low rate for nonpreferred foods. In subsequent generalization testing, the same two girls responded appropriately in lunchroom and home settings.

Working with a 3-year-old, Sullivan, Laverick, and Lewis (1995) tried to increase contingent responding for music and musical toys. They fitted the girl's orthopedic chair with two pad switches, one behind her head and one between her hands. Pressing on either pad led to presentation of a toy for as long as the switch was depressed. The child rapidly acquired the head-pressing response, keeping the switch closed for minutes at a time. Hand responses also occurred at a lower frequency. Subsequent introduction of novel toys increased responding. After 6 months of training, the girl showed positive anticipatory emotions at the outset of sessions and smiling, laughter, and vocalizations during sessions; after 9 months, she began to show similar responses in anticipation of a session. Other (and more easily implemented) procedures may reduce stereotyped hand clasping and other movements. These include physical restraints that prevent hand-to-mouth movements, simply holding a girl's hand, or allowing the girl to hold a favored toy. Giving one girl a set of baby keys, which she manipulated for long periods of time, reduced her hand wringing (Hanks, 1990).

Adaptive technology may help to overcome some RTT-associated motor and language impairments. For example, Skotko, Koppenhaver, and Erickson (2004) successfully increased communication between girls and their mothers while the mothers read storybooks to the girls. The researchers restrained each girl's nondominant hand in order to increase functional use of the dominant hand, and gave the girls augmentative and alternative communication (AAC) devices with material related to their storybooks. Mothers began asking their daughters more questions, which the daughters could answer with the AAC devices. Communication between each mother and daughter subsequently became synchronized into actual dialogue. Mothers also increased their responses to their daughters' AAC communications.

The Halliwick method of hydrotherapy has shown promising results in reducing stereotyped behaviors and increasing motor skills (Bumin, Uyanik, Yilmaz, Kayihan, & Topçu, 2003). In the Halliwick method, a therapist guides an individual client through a structured four-phase sequence: (1) mental and physical adjustment to water; (2) rotation control, designed to increase control over balance; (3) controlled movement in water, teaching the client to float and lie flat in both still and turbulent water; and

(4) movement in water, teaching the client elementary swimming (e.g., Starfish Club, 2004). An 11-year-old girl with RTT was given weekly treatment sessions of unspecified length. Her stereotypical hand movements declined after the first session and continued to decline across sessions. After 8 weeks, she showed improved hand use in feeding, holding objects, and transferring objects from hand to hand; improved balance; increased interaction with the environment; and reduced hyperactivity and anxiety. This technique obviously warrants evaluation with more subjects over a longer period of time.

As apraxia and other distortions of motor movements are virtually universal in RTT, physical therapy is critical (e.g., Hanks, 1990). It helps girls to maintain or reacquire ambulation, an obviously important skill (Van Acker, 1991), and to develop or maintain transitional behaviors needed to stand up from sitting or lying positions. Such therapy may involve use of a therapy ball and activities to stimulate balance, weight shifting and bearing, and gait. Gait is further impaired by rigidity in the heels of the feet, leading to toe walking. Ankle–foot orthoses and physical therapy help to maintain more normal walking (Budden, 1997). Whirlpool baths may be helpful. Most girls begin to develop scoliosis before age 8, and many also show kyphosis (hunchback) (Huang, Lubicky, & Hammerberg, 1994). Physical therapy and careful positioning in seated positions may slow the development of scoliosis, but corrective surgery is often required.

RTT is often characterized by abnormal sleep patterns. Two quite different approaches have successfully helped to increase normal sleep. Using a behavioral approach with three cases, Piazza, Fisher, and Moser (1991) woke the girls from daytime sleep that occurred outside of their usual naptimes, removed them from bed for 1 hour if they showed delayed sleep (response cost), and gradually advanced bedtimes (fading). Treatment increased regular sleep patterns and nighttime sleep, and decreased daytime sleep and nighttime waking. Using a 4-week melatonin treatment for nine girls with RTT, McArthur and Budden (1998) reported that during baseline, subjects had long sleep onset and short, interrupted total sleep time. Overall, melatonin decreased sleep onset and increased total sleep time and efficiency in girls whose baseline sleep was most impaired, but their response to melatonin was highly variable.

Mobility and feeding generally require the most day-to-day intervention by caregivers. According to Percy (2008a), gastrointestinal problems may be the most difficult medical issue. In extreme cases, tube feeding may be necessary. Owing to feeding difficulties, many with RTT will be underweight. Those who can feed themselves, on the other hand, may become overweight. A detailed food intake record may help identify foods that are consistently accepted or refused. Chewing and swallowing problems, as well as gastroesophageal reflux and digestive problems, can contribute to growth retardation. Speech therapy may be helpful not so much for retaining language as for facilitating chewing and swallowing. Supplementary tube feedings may be necessary to help increase growth (Glaze & Schultz, 1997), and some older girls may need to be fitted with gastric tubes, as in the case history near the end of this chapter. Further complicating feeding issues is frequent constipation, which may be difficult to correct through diet or additional fluids (e.g., Kerr & Witt Engerström, 2001). Laxatives or enemas may be necessary.

Seizures occur in most cases, particularly in stage 3 (Glaze & Schultz, 1997). Unfortunately, parents may overestimate daytime seizure activity, some of which may be behaviorally based, but may miss actual seizures, many of which occur during sleep (e.g., Budden, 1997; Glaze & Schultz, 1997). Most seizures can be controlled with antiseizure medication, most frequently carbamazepine and/or valproic acid. Occasionally, in otherwise intractable cases, a ketogenic diet may be used (Budden, 1997; Liebhaber, Riemann, & Baumeister, 2003), although it presents management problems.

Agitation, screaming, and tantrums are frequently reported. The rapid neurological and physical changes associated with the onset of the disease may understandably provoke emotional outbursts. Girls with RTT frequently respond negatively to stimulus or routine change, so transitions from one setting or pattern to another should be gradual and accompanied by a parent if possible. Agitation or screaming may also reflect physical pain or irritation for which the girls have

no other signal. Gastrointestinal problems are a potential cause of such agitation (e.g., Percy, 2008a). After the girls go through puberty, caretakers need to be sensitive to their menstrual cycles; agitation in older individuals may reflect premenstrual discomfort or a gynecological disorder that may be easily treatable (Budden, 1997). Behavior modification may be helpful; one of us (Kathleen K. McMillan) successfully used behavior modification to reduce her daughter's tantrums, as described later. Other suggested treatments include medication (particularly at night), music, quiet settings, massage, and hydrotherapy (particularly warm baths) (see, e.g., Van Acker, 1991).

Clinical trials of various treatments are underway.

Effects on Parents and Siblings

Descriptions relying predominantly on medical terminology barely convey the extent to which families are challenged. After a fairly normal period of development, parents ... witness their infant suddenly lose hand skills, not progress, lose words she had already learned, and start to withdraw. The search for a diagnosis and for therapeutic help can be time consuming and emotionally challenging. Because Rett syndrome is usually the result of a spontaneous mutation, the diagnosis of a genetic disorder is totally unexpected. In the middle phase of adjustment, families have to deal with extremely distressing behaviors associated with the disorder.... For parents, this means that they have to rearrange their life to make space for a child with many cognitive, physical, and communicative impairments. Having a child with Rett syndrome requires multiple medical and educational visits that limit parents' abilities to hold jobs or advance in their careers. (Retzlaff, 2007, p. 249)

Retzlaff's (2007) description trenchantly captures the difficulties facing those who deal with an individual with RTT. He might only have added that siblings are affected as well. Daily caretaking tasks may both call for the assistance of siblings (and other relatives) and lead to parents' having limited interactions with those siblings. As in the case history described below, aggressive behaviors may not only produce immediate pain, but leave permanent physical scars. Many of the effects of RTT can be ameliorated only with use of well-focused behavioral therapy, which requires extensive parental involvement, and multiple medications, delivery of which may be difficult owing to the affected girls' swallowing problems. Sleep problems are common—and, as Percy (2009) so tellingly stated, if a child does not sleep, neither do the parents. The stressors suffered by families of an individual with RTT all too often lead to fatigue and burnout.

In an interview study, Retzlaff (2007) described six categories of stress reported by parents of children with RTT: emotional, symptom-related (e.g., seizures, screaming bouts), uncertainty about RTT's effects, rejection by others, incompetent or unavailable professionals, and comparisons with healthy children and families. Not surprisingly, parents differed in their success in dealing with the stresses. Those who had other family members with serious medical problems, had strong social supports, spoke positively about the child with RTT and the family as a whole, and took charge of working with the child coped well. In particular, they described their daughter with RTT as having enriched the family. On the other hand, those who viewed the child from the outset as a burden, were rejected by others (including extended family and friends), had negative experiences with professionals, and focused almost exclusively on the negative impact of dealing with their child took far longer and were less successful overall in adjusting to their situation.

Owing to the lifelong impact of RTT on parents and other family members, counseling for them will be particularly important (Lieb-Lundell, 1988). Of importance, given the degree of care that adults with RTT require and their relative longevity, parents are likely to face issues of lifelong care and financial arrangements for their adult child after they can no longer care for her.

The IRSF makes available numerous resources for professionals and families dealing with those affected by RTT, and its website (*www.rettsyndrome.org*) should be routinely consulted. It publishes the *Rett Syndrome Handbook* (Hunter, 2007), a detailed presentation of virtually all aspects of RTT; provides a Regional Representative Program, made up of individuals who serve as human resources to families; and lists diagnostic clinics. OMIM (2004), which is routinely updated, should be consulted for current research findings.

MAGGIE: FROM INFANCY TO ADULTHOOD

Coauthor of this chapter and mother of Maggie, a 36-year-old woman with RTT, I (Kathleen K. McMillan) have lived through much of what is described in this chapter. Maggie was our first child, born when my husband was in military service in 1974, years before RTT became known. My pregnancy was uncomplicated, and she weighed 7 pounds, 9 ounces after a normal birth. She reached milestones at the following months of age: She sat at 4, wound up toys by 7, said her first word at 10, had a vocabulary of about 16 words and showed interest in books at 16, and somersaulted independently at 21. But her behavior had started to deteriorate at 12 months, when she began having violent temper tantrums. At 16 months, her language skills started to regress. She learned no new words and used old ones less and less. At 20 months, Maggie said only "mama," "papa," and "baby." She also aggressively threw toys and ate everything from cigarette butts to dirt and plants. Maggie pushed, hit, and scratched her younger sister, born when Maggie was 20 months old, severely enough to scar her face. She not only lost the ability to wind up toys, but by 24 months could not even pick them up. Her pediatrician told me that Maggie was showing "normal regression" owing to the birth of her sister, but months later said he felt she showed some autistic characteristics.

Growth retardation became prominent and persistent. Maggie entered an apparently autistic phase, smearing feces on herself and her surroundings. At 28 months, if I did not attend to her, she often defecated in her hands and threw the feces at me. If I left her bed at night, she screamed and vomited. Her eating behaviors became bizarre: She chewed ice, bit and chewed glass, and put everything in her mouth, including a dead animal she found in the yard. One of her grandmothers urged me to spank her. But when spanked, Maggie laughed, suggesting insensitivity to pain. At one point, when I was afraid of becoming abusive, a physician recommended a course in behavior modification. My use of behavioral principles led Maggie to stop vomiting and reduce other attention-getting behaviors, helping me deal with her for the first time since her infancy. At age 7 years, she was placed in a class for autistic children. A year later, although on medication, she began to have about 20 tonic–clonic seizures daily. Tests indicated multiple allergies, but changes in diet had little effect. At about age 9 years, she began again behaving aggressively toward herself and others. Once she slapped her face so hard that she deformed her jaw and began to cry hysterically. When I tried to soothe her, Maggie bit me so hard that I had to pry her off.

Physicians proposed various diagnoses, including schizophrenia, autism, mental retardation, childhood aphasia, and hyperactivity. Because Maggie was small and not gaining weight even though she ate a lot, malnutrition was also suggested, and I felt accused of being a neglectful mother. At about the time my husband and I were considering residential treatment, Maggie had a severe seizure, fell down a flight of stairs, and was admitted to a hospital. Having read about RTT, I shortly thereafter described it to some of her physicians. Fortunately, her neurologist had recently attended an RTT conference and diagnosed her correctly. She was among the first 250 girls diagnosed worldwide with RTT. Depakote, which had been found effective for girls with RTT, reduced her seizures and aggressive behavior. We dropped plans for residential treatment, although she still showed severe mood swings. Speech therapy was not effective, but Maggie's continued walking may owe a great deal to the physical therapy she received.

Maggie met virtually all diagnostic criteria for RTT and went through the four developmental stages described earlier. Her cognitive development became largely arrested, and her hands became infected from stereotyped hand mouthing. Bruxism, air swallowing, and breath holding were common. She still walked, but had gait apraxia and jerky body movements. She had surgery for scoliosis at age 15 years. Growth retardation continued. Compared to her earlier "Jekyll–Hyde" behavior, her temperament became calmer, and by her late teens, she was easygoing most of the time, had fewer seizures, and had regained some lost skills;

however, she was still totally dependent on others for basic needs.

Near the end of Maggie's last year in public school, my husband and I began to worry about her long-term future in light of her need for care and our own ages. At home, we could provide Maggie with love and support, but residential care provided many services that we could not: frequent bed checks at night; full-time nursing; physical, speech, occupational, and aquatic therapy; and a degree of both independence and inclusion. At age 19, while still in public school, Maggie moved into her own room in a residential home. The timing was important because she was used to being away from the family. If she had become accustomed to living full-time at home, adjustment to the residential home would have been more difficult. The residential home provides many activities. Her favorite was going out to eat, and she gained 17 pounds in her first year. Unfortunately, she later developed a serious swallowing problem; her weight began to plummet, and a gastric tube was implanted in 1998.

Maggie now participates in the adult day program at the residential home, which creates jobs to meet residents' individual needs and abilities. Maggie helps make pet biscuits and beds that are sold to local pet stores. For example, she stuffs pet beds, which are held in place with an adaptive frame. The program also has pet therapy, computer learning, horticulture, and aquatics.

At this writing, Maggie can see and hear, but not talk. Unlike many adults with RTT, she can walk, but with gait problems. Her hands are often clasped at her mouth, leading to balance problems. She drools, leaving her hands wet and subject to fungal infections; she gulps air and has H-pyloris, both of which lead to gastric distress; she has gastroesophageal reflux, eating difficulties, and swallowing problems; and she still has occasional tonic–clonic seizures, only partially controlled by medication. Because she also continues to fall during seizures, she now wears a staff-designed vest to reduce injury. She appears to communicate through eye gaze and finger pointing, but with long response latency. Generally loving and appreciative, she occasionally lashes out, apparently to communicate pain from gastric distress. Recent genetic analysis has revealed that she has a *MECP2* C-terminal deletion.

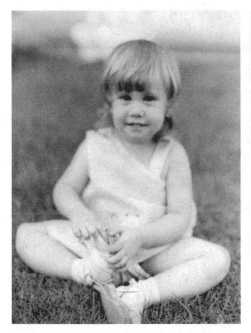

FIGURE 22.1

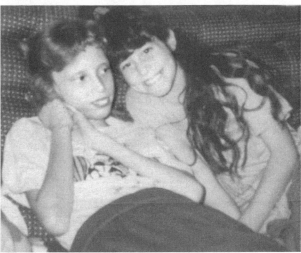

FIGURE 22.2

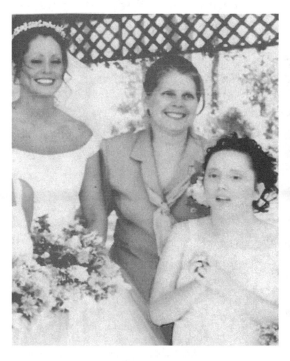

FIGURE 22.3

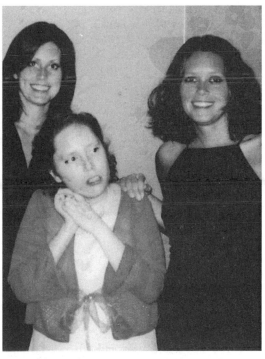

FIGURE 22.4

FIGURES 22.1–22.4. Photographs of Maggie at ages 22 months, 15 years, 26 years, and 30 years, respectively. Note (1) stereotyped hand clasping even at 22 months; (2) change in relative height (in Figure 22.2, Maggie is taller than her 10-year-old sister, but in Figure 22.3, 11 years later at the same sister's wedding, she is far shorter); (3) diminished growth and the still common hand clasping near her mouth—both apparent in Figure 22.4 (in 2005), where she is between her two younger sisters.

Is RTT a PDD, an Autism Spectrum Disorder, Both, or Neither?

An unfortunate current tendency is to use the term autism spectrum disorders (ASDs) interchangeably with, or even use it to replace, the DSM-IV-TR (American Psychiatric Association, 2000) category of PDDs. A brief summary of current terminology problems follows.

Two U.S. National Institutes of Health agencies have taken contradictory positions. The National Institute of Mental Health (NIMH) "Autism Spectrum Disorders (Pervasive Developmental Disorders)" webpage (NIMH, 2009, p. 1) states that "ASDs [are] also known as PDDs.... These disorders ... range from a severe form, called autistic disorder ... to a much milder form, Asperger syndrome. They also include two rare disorders, Rett syndrome and childhood disintegrative disorder." Thus NIMH uses ASDs and PDDs interchangeably and implies that autistic disorder is the most severe form—a highly questionable implication, given classic RTT's severity.

On the other hand, the National Institute of Child Health and Human Development (NICHD) has it both ways. Its "Autism Spectrum Disorders (ASDs)" webpage (NICHD, 2008, p. 1) states: "Health care providers think of autism as a 'spectrum' disorder, a group of disorders with similar features.... Currently, the ASD category includes: Autistic disorder ..., Asperger syndrome, and PDD-NOS (or atypical autism). In some cases, health care providers use a broader term, *pervasive developmental disorder* [emphasis in original], to describe autism. This category includes the ASDs above, plus Childhood Disintegrative Disorder and Rett syndrome." But NICHD's "Rett Syndrome" webpage (NICHD, 2006, p. 1) treats RTT as an ASD. Thus NICHD describes RTT as a PDD, but not an ASD on one webpage; on another, it terms it an ASD.

ASD and PDD as presently used are fuzzy concepts with no clear boundaries. In the extreme, one could claim that the term ASD has no commonly agreed-upon meaning, is essentially incoherent, and thus should be either clarified or discarded. In any event, RTT should not be described as an ASD because it has a far broader range of effects, is generally more severe than ASDs, and usually has an identified genetic basis. In short, it does not fall on the same spectrum (i.e., continuum or range) as do ASDs.

Concluding Remarks

In recent years, much progress has been made in understanding RTT's genetic basis, phenotypic variability, and neurological correlates. Unfortunately, similar progress has not occurred in treatment. Indeed, those involved with treatment may feel as Ignaz Semmelweis (1861/1981) did when he was searching for the cause of childbed fever: that their attempts are "like a drowning man, who grasps at a straw." Although several promising treatments are now available, all have been used in only small numbers of cases, and most require extensive training. Greatly needed are larger-sample, well-controlled evaluations with long-term follow-up of these programs, particularly those that can be relatively easily implemented.

What we can state with most confidence is that, given the rate of new findings, some material in this chapter will turn out not to be accurate. Indeed, it is quite likely that this will be the case at publication. We wish we knew which material this will be. We hope, of course, that the first to be discarded will be what we have said about the lack of generally effective treatment.

References

Akesson, H. O., Hagberg, B., & Wahlström, J. (1997). Rett syndrome: Presumptive carriers of the gene effect. Sex ratio among their siblings. *European Child and Adolescent Psychiatry, 6*(Suppl. 1), 101–102.

American Psychiatric Association. (2000). *Diagnostic and statistical manual of mental disorders* (4th ed., text rev.). Washington, DC: Author.

Amir, R. E., Van den Veyver, I. B., Wan, M., Tran, C. Q., Francke, U., & Zoghbi, H. Y. (1999). Rett syndrome is caused by mutations in X-linked MECP2, encoding methyl CpG-binding protein 2. *Nature Genetics, 23*, 185–188.

Ariani, F., Hayek, G, Rondinella, D., Artuso R., Mencarelli, M. A., Spanhol-Rosseto, A., et al. (2008). *FOXG1* is responsible for the congenital variant of Rett syndrome. *American Journal of Human Genetics, 83*, 89–93.

Armstrong, D. D. (2005). Neuropathology of Rett syndrome. *Journal of Child Neurology, 20,* 747–753.

Armstrong, D. D., & Kinney, H. C. (2001). The neuropathology of the Rett disorder. In A. Kerr & I. Witt Engerström (Eds.), *Rett disorder and the developing brain* (pp. 57–84). Oxford, UK: Oxford University Press.

Baptista, P. M., Mercadante, M. T., Macedo, E. C., & Schwartzman, J. S. (2006). Cognitive performance in Rett syndrome girls: A pilot study using eyetracking technology. *Journal of Intellectual Disability Research, 50,* 662–666.

Bat-Haee, M. A. (1994). Behavioral training of a young woman with Rett syndrome. *Perceptual and Motor Skills, 78,* 314.

Brown, R. T., & Hoadley, S. L. (1999). Rett syndrome. In S. Goldstein & C. R. Reynolds (Eds.), *Handbook of neurodevelopmental and genetic disorders in children* (pp. 459–477). New York: Guilford Press.

Brown, R. T., McMillan, K. K., & Herschthal, A. (2005). Rett syndrome. In S. Goldstein & C. R. Reynolds (Eds.), *Handbook of neurodevelopmental and genetic disorders in adults* (pp. 383–409). New York: Guilford Press.

Budden, S. S. (1997). Understanding, recognizing, and treating Rett syndrome. *Medscape Women's Health, 2*(3), 1–11.

Bumin, G., Uyanik, M., Yilmaz, I., Kayihan, H., & Topçu, M. (2003). Hydrotherapy for Rett syndrome. *Journal of Rehabilitation Medicine, 35,* 44–45.

Cass, H., Reilly, S., Owen, L., Wisbeach, A., Weekes, L., Wigram, T., et al. (2003). Findings from a multidisciplinary clinical case series of females with Rett syndrome. *Developmental Medicine and Child Neurology, 45,* 325–337.

Chen, W. G., Chang, Q., Lin, Y., Meissner, A., West, A. E., Griffith, E. C., et al. (2003). Derepression of BDNF transcription involves calcium-dependent phosphorylation of MeCP2. *Science, 302,* 885–889.

Chen, R. Z., Akbarian, S., Tudor, M., & Jaenisch, R. (2001). Deficiency of methyl-CpG binding protein-2 in CNS neurons results in a Rett-like phenotype in mice. *Nature Genetics, 27,* 327–331.

Clayton-Smith, J., Watson, P., Ramsden, S., & Black, G. C. M. (2000). Somatic mutation in MECP2 as a non-fatal neurodevelopmental disorder in males. *Lancet, 356,* 830–832.

Coleman, M. (1990). Is classical Rett syndrome ever present in males? *Brain and Development, 12,* 31–32.

Dunn, H. G., Stoessl, A. J., Ho, H. H., MacLeod, P. M., Poskitt, K. J., Doudet, D. J., et al. (2002). Rett syndrome: Investigation of nine patients, including PET scan. *Canadian Journal of Neurological Sciences, 29,* 345–357.

Fyfe, S., Downs, J., McIlroy, O., Burford, B., Lister, J., Reilly, S., et al. (2007). Development of a video-based evaluation tool in Rett syndrome. *Journal of Autism and Developmental Disorders, 37,* 1636–1646.

Gabellini, D., Green, M. R., & Tupler, R. (2004). When enough is enough: Genetic diseases associated with transcriptional derepression. *Current Opinion in Genetics and Development, 14,* 301–307.

Giacometti, E., Luikenhuis, S., Beard, C., & Jaenisch, R. (2007). Partial rescue of MeCP2 deficiency by postnatal activation of MeCP2. *Proceedings of the National Academy of Sciences, USA, 104*(6), 1931–1936.

Glaze, D. G. (1995). Commentary: The challenge of Rett syndrome. *Neuropediatrics, 26,* 78–80.

Glaze, D. G., & Schultz, R. J. (1997). Rett syndrome: Meeting the challenge of this gender-specific neurodevelopmental disorder. *Medscape Women's Health, 2*(1), 1–9.

Guy, J., Gan, J., Selfridge, J., Cobb, S., & Bird, A. (2007). Reversal of neurological defects in a mouse model of Rett syndrome. *Science, 315,* 1143–1147.

Guy, J., Hendrich, B. Holmes, M., Martin, J. E., & Bird, A. (2001). A mouse Mecp2-null mutation causes neurological symptoms that mimic Rett syndrome. *Nature Genetics, 27,* 322–326.

Hagberg, B. (1995a). Clinical delineation of Rett syndrome variants. *Neuropediatrics, 26,* 62.

Hagberg, B. (1995b). Rett syndrome: Clinical peculiarities and biological mysteries. *Acta Paediatrica, 84,* 971–976.

Hagberg, B., Aicardi, J., Dias, K., & Ramos, O. (1983). A progressive syndrome of autism, dementia, ataxia, and loss of purposeful hand use in girls: Rett's syndrome. Report of 35 cases. *Annals of Neurology, 14,* 471–479.

Hagberg, B., Hanefeld, F., Percy, A., & Skjeldal, O. (2002). An update on clinically applicable diagnostic criteria in Rett syndrome. *European Journal of Paediatric Neurology, 6,* 293–297.

Hagberg, B., & Witt Engerström, I. (1986). Rett syndrome: A suggested staging system for describing impairment profile with increasing age toward adolescence. *American Journal of Medical Genetics, 24*(Suppl. 1), 47–59.

Hanks, S. (1990). Motor disabilities in the Rett syndrome and physical therapy strategies. *Brain and Development, 12,* 157–161.

Huang, T.-J., Lubicky, J. P., & Hammerberg, K. W. (1994). Scoliosis in Rett syndrome. *Orthopaedic Review, 23,* 931–937.

Hunter, K. (2007). *Rett syndrome handbook* (2nd ed.). Cincinnati, OH: International Rett Syndrome Foundation.

Huppke, P., Held, M., Laccone, F., & Hanefeld, F. (2003). The spectrum of phenotypes in females with Rett syndrome. *Brain and Development, 25,* 346–351.

Huppke, P., Köhler, K., Laccone, F., & Hanefeld, F. (2003). Indication for genetic testing: A checklist for Rett syndrome. *Journal of Pediatrics, 142,* 332–335.

International Rett Syndrome Foundation (IRSF). (2008). Testing and diagnosis. Retrieved May 19, 2010, from *www.rett syndrome.org/about-rett-syndrome/testing-and-diagnosis.html*

Jellinger, K. A. (2003). Rett syndrome—an update. *Journal of Neural Transmission, 110,* 681–701.

Johnston, M. V. (2004). Clinical disorders of brain plasticity. *Brain and Development, 26,* 73–80.

Julu, P. O. O. (2001). The central autonomic disturbance in Rett syndrome. In A. Kerr & I. Witt Engerström (Eds.), *Rett disorder and the developing brain* (pp. 131–181). Oxford, UK: Oxford University Press.

Kaufmann, W. F. (2001). Cortical development in Rett syndrome: Molecular, neurochemical, and anatomical aspects. In A. Kerr & I. Witt Engerström (Eds.), *Rett disorder and the developing brain* (pp. 85–106). Oxford, UK: Oxford University Press.

Kerr, A. M. (1995). Early clinical signs in the Rett syndrome. *Neuropediatrics, 26,* 67–71.

Kerr, A. M. (2002). Annotation: Rett syndrome: Recent progress and implications for research and clinical practice. *Journal of Child Psychology and Psychiatry, 43,* 277–287.

Kerr, A. M., Belichenkob, P., Woodcock, T., & Woodcock, M. (2001). Mind and brain in Rett disorder. *Brain and Development, 23*(Suppl. 1), S44–S49.

Kerr, A. M., & Witt Engerström, I. (2001). The clinical background to the Rett disorder. In A. Kerr & I. Witt Engerström (Eds.), *Rett disorder and the developing brain* (pp. 1–26). Oxford,UK: Oxford University Press.

Kondo, M., Gray, L. J., Pelka, G. J., Christodoulou, J., Tam, P. P. L., & Hannan, A. J. (2008). Environmental enrichment ameliorates a motor coordination deficit in a mouse model of Rett syndrome— Mecp2 gene dosage effects and BDNF expression. *European Journal of Neuroscience, 27,* 3342–3350.

Lava, J., Slotte, A., Jochym-Nygren, M., van Doorn, J., & Witt Engerstrom, I. (2006). Communication and eating proficiency in 125 females with Rett syndrome: The Swedish Rett Center Survey. *Disability and Rehabilitation, 28,* 1267–1279.

Leonard, H., Fyfe, S., Leonard, S., & Msall, M. (2001). Functional status, medical impairments, and rehabilitation resources in 84 females with Rett syndrome: A snapshot across the world from the parental perspective. *Disability and Rehabilitation, 23,* 107–117.

Liebhaber, G. M., Riemann, E., & Baumeister, F. A. (2003). Ketogenic diet in Rett syndrome. *Journal of Child Neurology, 18,* 74–75.

Lieb-Lundell, C. (1988). The therapist's role in the management of girls with Rett syndrome. *Journal of Child Neurology, 3*(Suppl.), S31–S34.

Maiwald, R., Bonte, A., Jung, H., Bitter, P., Storm, Z., Laccone, F., et al. (2002). De novo MECP2 mutation in a 46,XX male patient with Rett syndrome [Letter]. *Neurogenetics, 4,* 107–108.

Matson, J. L., Fodstad, J. C., & Boisjoli, J. A. (2008). Nosology and diagnosis of Rett syndrome. *Research in Autism Spectrum Disorders, 2,* 601–611.

McArthur, A. J., & Budden, S. S. (1998). Sleep dysfunction in Rett syndrome: A trial of exogenous melatonin treatment. *Developmental Medicine and Child Neurology, 40,* 186–192.

Merker, B., & Wallin, N. L. (2001). Musical responsiveness in the Rett syndrome. In A. Kerr & I. Witt Engerström (Eds.), *Rett disorder and the developing brain* (pp. 327–338). Oxford, UK: Oxford University Press.

Meyer, K. A., Kennedy, C. H., Shulka, S., & Cushing, L. S. (1999). Receptive communication in late-stage Rett syndrome: A cautionary note. *Journal of Autism and Developmental Disorders, 29,* 93–94.

Moog, U., Smeets, E. E. J., van Roozendaal, K. E. P., Schoenmakers, S., Herbergs, J., Schoonbrood-Lenssen, A. M. J., et al. (2003). Neurodevelopmental disorders in males related to the gene causing Rett syndrome in females (*MECP2*). *European Journal of Paediatric Neurology, 7,* 5–12.

Moser, H. W., & Naidu, S. (1996). The discovery and study of Rett syndrome. In A. J. Capute & P. J. Accardo (Eds.), *Developmental disabilities in infancy and childhood* (2nd ed., pp. 379–386). Baltimore: Brookes.

Naidu, S. (1997). Rett syndrome: A disorder affecting early brain growth. *Annals of Neurology, 42,* 3–10.

Naidu, S., Bibat, G., Kratz, L., Kelley, R. I., Pevsner, J., Hoffman, E., et al. (2003). Clinical variability in Rett syndrome. *Journal of Child Neurology, 18,* 662–668.

National Institute of Child Health and Human Development (NICHD). (2008). Autism spectrum disorders (ASDs). Retrieved July 20, 2009, from *www.nichd.nih. gov/health/topics/asd.cfm*

National Institute of Child Health and Human Development (NICHD). (2006). Rett syndrome. Retrieved July 20, 2009, from *www.nichd.nih.gov/ health/topics/rett_syndrome.cfm*

National Institute of Mental Health (NIMH). (2009). Autism spectrum disorders (pervasive developmental disorders). Retrieved July 20, 2009, from *www.nimh.nih.gov/health/topics/autism-spectrum-disorders-pervasive-developmental-disorders/index.shtml*

National Institute of Neurological Disorders and Stroke. (2003). Rett syndrome fact sheet. Retrieved July 20, 2009, from *www.ninds.nih.gov/health_and_medical/pubs/rett.htm*

Neul, J. L., Fang, P., Barrish, J., Lane, J., Caeg, E. B., Smith, E. O., et al. (2008). Specific mutations in methyl-CpG-binding protein 2 confer different severity in Rett syndrome. *Neurology, 70,* 1313–1321.

Neul, J. L., & Zoghbi, H. Y. (2004). Rett syndrome: A prototypical neurodevelopmental disorder. *The Neuroscientist, 10,* 118–128.

Nomura, Y., & Segawa, M. (2001). The monoamine hypothesis in Rett syndrome. In A. Kerr & I. Witt Engerström (Eds.), *Rett disorder and the developing brain* (pp. 205–225). Oxford, UK: Oxford University Press.

Online Mendelian Inheritance in Man (OMIM). (2004). Rett syndrome; RTT. MIM #312750. Retrieved May 19, 2010, from *www.ncbi.nlm.nih.gov/omim/312750*

Pelka, G. J., Watson, C. M., Radziewic, T., Hayward, M., Lahooti, H., Christodoulou, J., et al. (2006). Mecp2 deficiency is associated with learning and cognitive deficits and altered gene activity in the hippocampal region of mice. *Brain, 129,* 887–898.

Percy, A. K. (2002). Rett syndrome: Current status and new vistas. *Neurologic Clinics, 20,* 1125–1141.

Percy, A. K. (2008a). Rett syndrome: From recognition to diagnosis to intervention. *Expert Review of Endocrinology and Metabolism, 3,* 327–336.

Percy, A. K. (2008b). Rett syndrome: Recent research progress. *Journal of Child Neurology, 23,* 543–549.

Percy, A. K. (2009). *Rett syndrome 101: Current illuminations.* Paper presented at the annual conference of the International Rett Syndrome Foundation, Leesburg, VA.

Percy, A. K., & Lane, J. B. (2005). Rett syndrome: Model of neurodevelopmental disorders. *Journal of Child Neurology, 20,* 718–721.

Percy, A. K., & Lane, J. B. (2009). *Rett syndrome after twenty-five years: Where it started and where it is today.* Paper presented at the annual conference of the International Rett Syndrome Foundation, Leesburg, VA.

Philippart, M. (1990). The Rett syndrome in males. *Brain and Development, 12,* 33–36.

Piazza, C. C., Anderson, C., & Fisher, W. (1993). Teaching self-feeding skills to patients with Rett syndrome. *Developmental Medicine and Child Neurology, 35,* 991–996.

Piazza, C. C., Fisher, W. W., & Moser, H. W. (1991). Behavioural treatment of sleep dysfunction in patients with the Rett syndrome. *Brain and Development, 13,* 232–237.

Pillion, J. P., Rawool, V. W., Bibat, G., & Naidu, S. (2003). Prevalence of hearing loss in Rett syndrome. *Developmental Medicine and Child Neurology, 45,* 338–343.

Renieri, A., Mari, F., Mencarelli, M. A., Scala, E., Ariani, F., Longo, I., et al. (2009). Diagnostic criteria for the Zappella variant of Rett syndrome. *Brain and Development, 31,* 208–216.

Rett, A. (1966). Uber ein eigenartiges Hirnatrophisches Syndrom bei Hyperammonamie im Kindes alter [On an unusual brain atropic syndrome with hyperammonia in childhood]. *Wiener Medizinische Wochenschrift, 116,* 425–428. (As cited in Moser & Naidu, 1996, and Rett Syndrome Diagnostic Criteria Work Group, 1988.)

Rett, A. (1977). Cerebral atrophy associated with hyperammonaemia. In P. J. Vinken & G. W Bruyn (Eds.), *Handbook of Clinical Neurology: Vol. 29. Metabolic and deficiency diseases of the nervous system* (Part III, pp. 305–329). Amsterdam: North-Holland.

Retzlaff, R. (2007). Families of children with Rett syndrome: Stories of coherence and resilience. *Families, Systems, and Health, 25,* 246–262.

Riikonen, R. (2001). Neurotrophic factors in the pathogenesis of Rett syndrome. In A. Kerr & I. Witt Engerström (Eds.), *Rett disorder and the developing brain* (pp. 125–129). Oxford, UK: Oxford University Press.

Roane, H. S., Piazza, C. C., Sgro, G. M., Volkert, V. M., & Anderson, C. M. (2001). Analysis of aberrant behaviour associated with Rett syndrome. *Disability and Rehabilitation, 23,* 139–148.

Santos, M., Temudo, T., Kay, T., Carrilho, I., Medeira, A., Cabral, H., et al. (2009). Neurodevelopmental phenotype in male patients: Mutations in the MECP2 gene are not a major cause of Rett syndrome-like or related neurodevelopmental phenotype in male patients. *Journal of Child Neurology, 24,* 49–55.

Schanen, N. C., Kurczynski, T. W., Brunnelle, D., Woodcock, M. M., Dure, L. S., IV, & Percy, A. K. (1998). Neonatal encephalopathy in two boys in families with recurrent Rett syndrome. *Journal of Child Neurology, 13,* 229–231.

Schwartzman, J. S., Zatz, M., Vasquez, L. R., Gomes, R. R., Koiffmann, C. P., Fridman, C., et al. (1999). Rett syndrome in a boy with a 47,XXY karyotype [Letter]. *American Journal of Human Genetics, 64,* 1781–1785.

Semmelweis, I. P. (1981). *The etiology, the concept and the prophylaxis of childbed fever* (F. P. Murphy, Trans.). Birmingham, AL: Classics of Medicine Library. (Original work published 1861)

Shahbazian, M. D., Young, J. I., Yuva-Paylor, L. A., Spencer, C. M., Antalffy, B. A., Noebels, J. L., et al. (2002). Mice with truncated MeCP2 recapitulate many Rett syndrome features and display hyperacetylation of histone H3. *Neuron, 35,* 243–254.

Skotko, B. G., Koppenhaver, D. E., & Erickson, K. A. (2004). Parent reading behaviors and communication outcomes with girls with Rett syndrome. *Exceptional Children, 70,* 145–166.

Smeets, E. E., Chenaul, M., Curfs, L. M., Schrander-Stumpel, C. T., & Frijns, J. P. (2009). Rett syndrome and long-term disorder profile. *American Journal of Medical Genetics, Part A, 149A,* 199–205.

Smeets, E. E., Schollen, E., Moog, U., Matthijs, G., Herbergs, J., Smeets, H., et al. (2003). Rett syndrome in adolescent and adult females: Clinical and molecular genetic findings. *American Journal of Medical Genetics, 122A,* 227–233.

Smith, T., Klevstrand, M., & Lovaas, O. I. (1995). Behavioral treatment of Rett's disorder: Ineffectiveness in three cases. *American Journal of Mental Retardation, 100,* 317–322.

Starfish Club. (2004). The Halliwick method. Retrieved from *kildare.ie/starfish/the-halliwick-method.htm*

Stearns, N. A., Schaevitz, L. R., Bowling, H., Nag, N., Berger, U. V., & Berger-Sweeney, J. (2007). Behavioral and anatomical abnormalities in *Mecp2* mutant mice: A model for Rett syndrome. *Neuroscience, 146,* 907–921.

Sullivan, M. W., Laverick, D. H., & Lewis, M. (1995). Brief report: Fostering environmental control in a young child with Rett syndrome:

A case study. *Journal of Autism and Developmental Disabilities, 25,* 215–221.

Tams-Little, S., & Holdgrafer, G. (1996). Early communication development in children with Rett syndrome. *Brain and Development, 18,* 376–378.

Thomas, G. H. (1996). High male:female ratio of germline mutations: An alternative explanation for postulated gestational lethality in males in X-linked dominant disorders. *American Journal of Human Genetics, 58,* 647–653.

Topcu, M., Akyerli, C., Sayi, A., Toruner, G. A., Kocoglu, S. R., Cimbis, M., et al. (2002). Somatic mosaicism for a MECP2 mutation associated with classic Rett syndrome in a boy. *European Journal of Human Genetics, 10,* 77–81.

Trappe, R., Laccone, F., Cobilanschi, J., Meins, M., Huppke, P., Hanefeld, F., et al. (2001). MECP2 mutations in sporadic cases of Rett syndrome are almost exclusively of paternal origin. *American Journal of Human Genetics, 68,* 1093–1101.

Van Acker, R. (1991). Rett syndrome: A review of current knowledge. *Journal of Autism and Developmental Disabilities, 21,* 381–406.

Van Acker, R., & Grant, S. H. (1995). An effective computer-based requesting system for persons with Rett syndrome. *Journal of Childhood Communication Disorders, 16,* 31–38.

CHAPTER 23

Lesch–Nyhan Syndrome
A Sex-Linked Inborn Error of Metabolism

DAVID L. WODRICH
LORI A. LONG

Lesch–Nyhan syndrome (LNS) is a rare inborn error of metabolism (estimated to be present in 1 of 380,000 live births). In LNS, mutations in the gene coding for the enzyme hypoxanthine–guanine phosphoribosyltransferase (HPRT) on the X chromosome lead to deficient enzyme activity. This results in abnormal purine metabolism, and therefore in elevated levels of uric acid, the end product of purine metabolism. Several physiological problems may ensue, including chronic kidney disease and central nervous system (CNS) impairments (Nyhan & Wong, 1996). It now appears that neurotransmitter deficiencies in dopamine underlie the CNS impairments, and thus the developmental, behavioral, and motoric impairments, that characterize LNS. Anatomically, dopaminergic pathways are known to encompass basal ganglia (symmetrical masses composed of gray matter) and connected structures (e.g., frontal lobes). Behaviorally, dopamine is understood to be associated with movement, reward, planning, and response inhibition. Neuropsychiatrically, dopamine and dopaminergic pathways are central to the expression of various movement disorders (e.g., Parkinson disease) and psychiatric disorders in which compulsions and impulse dysregulation are hallmarks (e.g., Tourette

syndrome). These same characteristics appear in LNS.

HISTORY AND BACKGROUND

LNS has an interesting history. Its understanding has potential relevance for diverse professional groups seeking to clarify the causes of particular neurodevelopmental disorders (of which LNS is one), as well as the broader topics of genetic, biochemical, and neurological underpinnings of behavior and development. In 1962, William Nyhan had completed pediatric training at Yale and earned a PhD at the University of Illinois before receiving an appointment at Johns Hopkins. Michael Lesch was a medical student on his service at Johns Hopkins when the two men encountered a 4-year-old patient who presented with recurrent hematuria (blood in the urine) and, on closer inspection, crystals in his urine (Nyhan, 2005). When the crystals were identified as uric acid, and elevated uric acid was also found in the blood, a problem with metabolism of purine was deduced. Coupling these unexpected findings with the patient's developmental and behavioral presentation prompted further contemplation. This boy suffered from significantly delayed motor development and, apparently, cerebral palsy. More striking were a badly mutilated lip and fingertips. The detection of a brother with the same phenotype, a typically developing sister, and two phenotypically normal parents suggested to Nyhan and Lesch the presence of a genetic disorder, later documented to be an X-linked recessive disorder. An examination of the patient revealed abnormal reflexes, spasticity, and involuntary movements, suggesting a syndrome that was neurological in nature.

Michael Lesch devoted himself full-time to the study of the disorder. He and Nyhan detected extreme elevations of serum uric acid in both brothers; their results were published in 1964 (Nyhan, 2005). When patients from around the world were subsequently reported, all of whom were boys, the X-linked basis of the disorder was substantiated. Within a few years, the nature of the enzymatic error was understood and shared with the scientific community (Nyhan, Sweetman, Carpenier, Carter, & Hoefnagel, 1968; Seegmiller, Rosenbloom, & Kelley, 1967). In part, the role of HPRT was discovered when a widely used antirejection drug, azathioprine, failed to produce its typical effect among boys with LNS. Important clues included the facts that azathioprine was known to undergo conversation to 6-mercaptopurine via involvement of HPRT, and that azathiopine was known to reduce uric acid levels. However, in patients with LNS, azathiopine exerted none of the expected effect on uric acid levels. This helped to implicate HPRT as the underlying metabolic error in LNS (see Figure 23.1).

It was soon discovered, however, that a subgroup of patients existed in whom HPRT metabolism was disordered, but who expressed none of the classic LNS symptoms. This latter group still had gout (as did all boys with full LNS) and the previously mentioned crystals in their urine. It was found that this group had 1–50% of the normal HPRT activity, but no CNS involvement. Males with zero HPRT activity remain the rule, but other variations have been found (Nyhan, 2005). By the early 1980s, the gene involved in production of HPRT was understood to be located on the long arm of the X chromosome (Jolly et al., 1983). Later research suggested dopaminc abnormalities

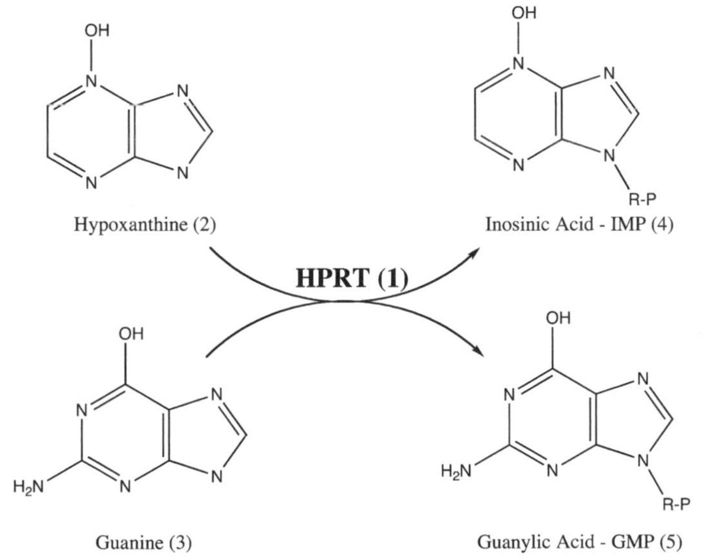

FIGURE 23.1. Disordered metabolic pathway associated with LNS. The inborn error of metabolism concerns the absence of HPRT (1). Because in patients with LNS the HPRT enzyme is unavailable to accomplish its typical task of enabling hypoxanthine (2) and guanine (3) to be converted to inosinic acid (4) and guanylic acid (5), hypoxanthine and guanine accumulate to excessive levels, which results in excessive accumulation of uric acid when they are converted to uric acid by xanthine oxidase (an enzyme not depicted in this figure). The accumulation of excess hypoxanthine may directly produce adverse neurological consequences. Data from Torres and Puig (2007).

and basal ganglia dysfunction, and broadly stimulated questions about the relationship of biochemistry and behavior.

LNS is unique in terms of its metabolic–behavioral links. As seen below, quite noteworthy self-abuse behavior characterizes nearly all boys with LNS. LNS represents the first metabolic disease in which there existed a clear set of behaviors. In part, this prompted Nyhan in 1971 to coin the term *behavioral phenotype* (see Nyhan, 2005). Crucially, Nyhan pointed out that a behavioral phenotype, "a characteristic pattern of behavior consistently associated with a biologic disorder" (Nyhan, 2005, p. 1), sometimes permits professionals to establish a syndromal diagnosis, just as physical signs (i.e., dysmorphic signs) do.

In the end, Nyhan went on to found the Department of Pediatrics at the University of California–San Diego. He remains there, actively studying LNS and many other inherited diseases of metabolism. Lesch's later career path led to internal medicine and cardiology; he never returned to the disorder that bears his name (Nyhan, 2005).

Diverse research efforts have continued to reveal the makeup of LNS. By the 1990s, the location and extent of dopamine anomalies were documented. For example, Wong and colleagues (1996) used positron emission tomography (PET) and MRI to study a small group of men (ages 19–35 years) with LNS. PET results, established by using a ligand that binds to dopamine, showed between 50% and 63% reduced dopamine-binding potential in the caudate and between 64% and 75% reduction in the putamen (both basal ganglia structures) compared to controls. MRI results failed to detect differences in putamen volume, but detected a 30% reduction in caudate volume compared to controls. This information fits with small-scale autopsy findings, in which documented anomalies in the dopamine system were associated with caudate and putamen. It also appears to match animal studies in which the HPRT system was altered (producing a reduction in striatal dopamine transporters) or in neonatal rats that underwent intentional dopamine depletion procedures (producing LNS-like self-abusive behavior; see Wong et al., 1996, for details). Cumulative information like this suggests that the dopamine system is central to producing LNS signs and symptoms.

DEVELOPMENTAL COURSE

Children with LNS develop such severe impairments that extremely early detection of abnormalities is the rule; however, the disorder presents so rarely that precise LNS diagnosis may be at risk. For example, in presenting an interesting case from Slovenia, Levart (2007) commented that only a single case would be expected in her country every 20 years. Consequently, children may be incorrectly diagnosed. For instance, the presentation of significant motor delays may result in a cerebral palsy diagnosis (Nyhan, 2005). It may not be until children present with self-injurious behaviors that physicians consider other diagnoses. The "gold standard" for diagnosis is laboratory testing that determines less than 1.5% HPRT activity in erythrocytes (Nyhan, 2005). Research suggests that analysis of erythrocytes, or red blood cells, permits detection of minute levels of HPRT that may be missed if other cells alone are studied. To date, no known studies are available to offer descriptive statistics about diagnosis.

The hallmark features of LNS are quite striking, and they encompass both biological and behavioral–developmental dimensions. During the first 6–8 months, however, developmental milestones may appear to be grossly normal (Nyhan, 1973). Typically, the first indication of abnormality may occur when orange crystals appear in diapers, indicating the presence of urate crystals in the urine. Later, children will present with motor and cognitive developmental delays, as well as begin engaging in self-injurious behaviors. The developmental course of each of these phenomena is reviewed.

Essentially every patient with full LNS expresses the following set of neurological signs and impairments: increased muscle tone, associated with a scissor position of the lower extremities; extremely delayed motor development; spasticity with deep tendon reflexes and Babinski signs; and involuntary movements (Nyhan, 1997). Thus a particular motor phenotype appears evident in individuals with LNS and is distinguishable from the phenotypes of other motor disorders. Jinnah and colleagues (2006) studied a group of 44 patients with LNS (ages 2–38) who expressed the full syndrome (i.e., mental retardation, self-injurious behaviors, motor disability, and overproduction of uric acid). Examinations included a complete medical history, standardized written protocols focusing on motor features, and assessments of muscle tone. A scale was also used to index the severity of motor deficits (1 = motor abnormality absent; 2 = motor abnormality mild; 3 = motor abnormality severe enough to preclude meaningful function). The developmental progression of motor impairments began at 3–6 months with hypotonia and failure to sit upright. Typically by 6–12 months, involuntary movements appeared (although some parents reported this to be delayed up to 4 years). No significant progression of motor impairments was noted beyond ages 5–6 years. The primary feature of the motor disorder in all patients was dystonia (i.e., a disabling movement disorder characterized by sustained contraction of muscles, leading to twisting, distorted postures). Mild to moderate forms of choreoathetosis (50%) and ballismus (30%) were also found.

As motor deficits intensify, most babies either lose the ability to sit or fail to master sitting at all. No patients with full LNS walk or sit independently (Nyhan, 1997). Gout may also appear when uric acid is deposited on the articular cartilage of joints, tendons, and surrounding tissues. Wheelchair use (usually a narrow chair, with supports at the chest) is then nearly universal, and it follows that executing activities of daily living depends on assistance from others.

LNS is also associated with speech and eating problems. For example, Jinnah and colleagues (2006) found that speech was delayed in all 44 of their patients with LNS (first words by age 2–4 years). All speech was dysarthric, resulting in slowed expression and constrained intelligibility. Chewing and swallowing were difficult for most patients; 20% of the sample required a gastrostomy tube. Eating problems may also compromise caloric intake for many, and aspiration, accompanied by pneumonia, is a looming risk.

Cognitive impairments are often present in individuals with LNS; however, relatively little is known about the development of these impairments over time. A study by Matthews, Solan, Barabas, and Robey (1999) compared the initial results on the Stanford–Binet Intelligence Scale: Fourth Edition (SB-IV; Thorndike, Hagen, & Sattler, 1986) among six individuals (ages 14–23 years) with follow-up scores earned at 2 and 4 years later. Overall, scores on the SB-IV declined. Initial scores averaged 61.3 (range = 40–81); scores at the 2-year follow-up averaged 59.2 (range = 39–77); and scores at the 4-year follow-up averaged 54.7 (range = 36–75). Though the decline in scores from initial testing to the 2-year follow-up was not statistically significant, the scores at the 4-year follow-up were statistically significantly different from those at both the initial ($p < .02$) and the 2-year follow-up ($p < .02$) assessments. Mental age of the sample did not meaningfully increase over 4 years (i.e., it rose from 7.0 to just 7.9). The greatest gains were seen in children under the age of 13, with a plateau apparently reached between ages 13 and 17 years concerning abstract visual reasoning and aspects of short-term memory. The plateau may occur because older boys suffer decreases in attentiveness and flexibility of thinking with age. However, many of the teenage boys in this study enjoyed continued growth in some areas (e.g., vocabulary and memory for objects). Quite variable mental abilities are reported by parents, and some boys appear to maintain surprisingly well-preserved skills and assorted interests (Anderson, Ernst, & Davis, 1992).

LNS's most troubling aspect is extreme self-injurious behavior. Nyhan (1973) has long argued that this behavioral feature itself helps suggest LNS, and is often implied quite quickly by observation of missing tissue. Nyhan points out that although self-abusive behavior is common among individuals with developmental delay, patients with LNS are unique in their tendency to cause loss of their own tissue. Virtually all patients have bitten their lips destructively upon eruption of their primary teeth. These are well documented photographically in numerous case reports appearing in the literature. Paradoxically, these children remain sensitive to pain (e.g., screaming with pain upon biting themselves). Thus one might speculate that a disturbance in the subjective experience of pain or in the body's response to pain (e.g., release of pain-induced endorphins) exists in those with LNS. This line of thinking is visited again in discussion of some LNS treatments (i.e., botulinum toxin; see below).

In an extensive study of 64 individuals with LNS (ages 1–40 years), parents/caregivers reported on types of self-injurious behaviors (Robey, Reck, Giacomini, Barabas, & Eddey, 2003). Ninety-one percent of parents/caregivers reported self-mutilating behaviors, with the age at emergence of these behaviors ranging from 5 months to 10 years. Over half of the sample (53%) reported that the first behaviors observed included lip and finger biting. The behaviors reported included biting fingers (78%), biting lips and mouth (77%), extending arms in doorways (66%), banging head (56%), tipping wheelchair (33%), poking eyes (31%), inserting fingers in wheelchair spokes (30%), rubbing head on wheelchair headrest (27%), and rubbing arms on restraints (17%). Hierarchical cluster analyses were performed to examine the degree of co-occurrence among self-injurious behaviors. The strongest association was found between insertion of fingers in wheelchair spokes and the rubbing of arms on restraints. Finger biting and lip biting were also closely associated. Likewise, older patients with LNS displayed more varied self-injurious behaviors in the past than did younger patients, indicating that these behaviors continue over time, but may change in appearance.

For some individuals with LNS, aggression may also be outwardly directed, especially toward caregivers. For instance, children may vomit and spit to express interpersonal aggression (McCarthy, 2004). Both self-mutilation and aggression, however, are compulsive in that afterward children typically report feeling powerless to have stopped themselves, and many communicate remorse (Morales, 1999). A unique finding concerns a phenomenon called *emotional self-injury*, which caregivers have referred to when describing outwardly directed behaviors (i.e., a child's saying no when he actually wants something, caregiver-directed verbal abuse) that appears to eventuate in negative emotional consequences for the patient himself (Robey et al., 2003). This potential aspect of self-directed aggression may be an important component of the behavioral phenotype; however, there is currently no research detailing such consequences.

The behavioral phenotype of LNS may extend beyond self-injurious and aggressive behaviors. Schretlen and colleagues (2005) used the Child Behavior Checklist (CBCL; Achenbach, 1991) and the American Association on Mental Retardation's Adaptive Behavior Scale—Residential and Community, Second Edition (ABS-RC2; Nihira, Leland, & Lambert, 1993) to evaluate emotional and behavior status. They studied individuals with full LNS, individuals with a variant of LNS including no self-injurious behaviors, and healthy controls. Boys with full LNS were found to have higher levels of anxiety, depression, social problems, disrupted thinking, inattention, and distraction, as well as stereotyped, hyperactive, attention-seeking, and aggressive behaviors, compared to healthy controls (Schretlen et al., 2005). In contrast, those individuals with the variant of LNS free of self-injurious behavior were generally more similar to healthy controls on most behavioral dimensions, but they showed levels of inattention similar to those of individuals with LNS. These findings suggest the possibility of a behavioral phenotype that is broader and includes more than just self-injury.

Why changes may occur over time is not well known. Certainly accumulation of frustration is one possibility. CNS changes, such as cerebral atrophy, may occur in individuals with LNS. Neuroimaging studies of 25 patients found that three experienced atrophy—reduction in cerebral (17%) and basal ganglia (34%) volumes (Jinnah et al., 2006). These findings are consistent with those of Matthews and colleagues (1999), who identified declines in cognitive functioning as these individuals moved into adulthood.

As a group, individuals experience reduced life expectancy. Causes of death include pneumonia and various infectious diseases. With the use of medication (allopurinol), kidney function can be preserved. Patients often survive into the second or third decade (Torres & Puig, 2007).

GENETICS AND FAMILY PATTERNS

Because LNS is an X-linked recessive disorder, the disorder is almost exclusively evident among boys and young men (five anomalous female cases have apparently been reported, however; see Torres & Puig, 2007). The gene responsible for HPRT production is located on the long arm of the X chromosome (at Xq26) and consists of nine exons. Mutations are known to be quite heterogeneous in both location and type, and include deletions, insertions, duplications, and point mutations

(Torres & Puig, 2007). A second X chromosome (XX) in females with LNS typically results in a favorable outcome of adequate production of the enzyme HPRT. Consequently, normal brain development occurs in most girls with the LNS genotype, although rare cases of females expressing the phenotype have been reported (McCarthy, 2004). In 1989, Gibbs, Nguyen, McBride, Koepf, and Caskey found among 15 cases the occurrence of DNA base substitutions, small DNA deletions, a single DNA base insertion, and an error in RNA splicing. It is possible to use DNA as a means of diagnosis and carrier identification; that is, mutant alleles within individual families are directly detectable. Nonetheless, because nearly all families have their own mutation, there are practical limitations imposed on clinical diagnosis. Molecular methods of prenatal diagnosis and heterozygote detection are viewed as laborious. Thus physicians use them only when working with families in which there is an affected individual whose mutation has been determined (Nyhan, 2005).

RISK FACTORS FOR PHENOTYPIC EXPRESSION

The range of phenotypic expression in LNS now appears to be larger than might have originally been anticipated. In part, this derives from a more diverse underlying genotype. As noted above, it was recognized fairly early in the course of studying LNS that a few individuals experience HPRT deficiency representing more than zero activity, whereas the vast majority of patients with LNS have no HPRT activity. This means that, broadly, three variations in HPRT deficiency can be recognized: LNS variants, so-called neurological variants, and partial variants (Nyhan, 2005). Those with any of the LNS variants have virtually no HPRT activity detectable; they express the classic LNS syndrome described in this chapter. Those few individuals with the neurological variants may have essentially no HPRT in erythrocyte assay, but some activity in whole-cell assay. These males have a phenotype characterized by neurological signs, but not classic behavioral features of LNS or frank mental retardation. Those with partial variants have 0–50% HPRT activity in erythrocyte assay, but HPRT activity in whole-cell as-

says. Patients with partial variants lack both the classic LNS behavioral features and the hallmark spasticity and choreoathetosis of those with the neurological variants.

Hladnik, Nyhan, and Bertolli (2008) recently published an article with important implications for the genotype–phenotype correlations in LNS. Typically, families with a mutation in the HPRT gene express this in the same, or a similar, phenotype. This article describes a single family with an HPRT gene variant that permits some enzyme activity, and associated milder clinical expressions, rather than the full LNS syndrome. This family, however, was characterized by three discernible phenotypes. One family member expressed the classic LNS syndrome, whereas this patient's brother and an uncle had a much milder disease and associated symptom expression. These individuals' clinical presentation was difficult to distinguish from that of disease-free individuals. Finally, two cousins of the patient with classic LNS had an intermediate level of expressed disease. As a result, the authors concluded, it is no longer possible to assume that a given mutation in the HPRT gene will predictably lead to "a reproducible pattern of clinical expression."

ASSESSMENT

Of special concern for psychologists is the fact that valid cognitive assessments of children with LNS are difficult to accomplish. Assessment techniques that can circumvent each child's impairments—such as observation techniques, untimed items that can be answered by pointing/eye gaze, or other appropriate nonverbal response measure (e.g., the Peabody Picture Vocabulary Test, Fourth Edition; Dunn & Dunn, 2007)—may represent the best hope for valid appraisal. On the other hand, Anderson and colleagues (1992) used a parent survey as an alternative to intelligence tests to identify cognitive functioning and characteristics specific to patients with LNS (Anderson & Ernst, 1994). The questionnaire consisted of 176 items organized into 18 sections, including family genetics, patient health, motor ability, school achievement, verbal ability, and self-injury. Such a survey may be useful in obtaining baseline measures of cognitive functioning that would otherwise be impossible to collect via examiner-administered cognitive assessments.

Nonetheless, standard IQ tests have been used and may provide some insight. For example, as part of a National Institute of Mental Health study that concerned neurotransmitter anomalies in LNS, Ernst and colleagues (2000) collected SB-IV (Thorndike et al., 1986) IQ test scores on 11 males with LNS (ages 10–20 years). The mean IQ score was 67.9 (standard deviation = 17.7). The degree to which these individuals were representative of the population with LNS as a whole, or how much their observed IQ scores were influenced by motor or behavioral problems, is unknown. Nonetheless, this information provides some evidence to support parents' speculation that many of these individuals are often spared cognitive impairment as severe as their motor dysfunction and behavioral disturbances. Also using the SB-IV, Matthews, Solan, and Barabas (1995) found that composite scores ranged from those indicating the moderate range of mental retardation to the low-average range (see "Developmental Course," above, for more details of this study). Again, cognitive ability may be variable in this patient population, and mental retardation does not appear to be universal.

Though self-injurious behaviors are the most characteristic of the disorder, a broader spectrum of emotional and behavioral problems may exist. Parents and other caregivers can provide information on both adaptive behaviors and psychosocial adjustment. For instance, as noted earlier, Schretlen and colleagues (2005) used the CBCL (Achenbach, 1991) and the ABS-RC2 (Nihira et al., 1993) to evaluate the emotional and behavioral impact of the disorder. Various internalizing and externalizing behaviors, as well as social difficulties, were present. The findings suggested the usefulness of psychosocial and adaptive behavior measures in the assessment of LNS.

TREATMENT

It is understandable that those concerned with the care of patients with LNS are intensely interested in treatment. A host of related questions about school, developmental therapies, and the like also routinely arise, even when direct ways to ameliorate symptoms or promote development are unavailable. One aspect of care that professionals often overlook is the importance of informing and supporting parents. The salience of parents' needs, which concern primarily bottom-line issues of dealing with difficult behavior, is eloquently summarized by William Nyhan (2005) himself:

> The realization that there is a biological basis of behavior could be very helpful to parents in understanding their children and learning ways to deal with such children. Parents want to know what their children will be like as the years go on and this is particularly true for behavior that must be lived with day to day. It is behavior that can destroy a family or lead to admission to an institution, not intelligence or a cytogenetic or enzymatic status. Appropriate counseling as to what to expect and introduction to parent support groups and to others with the same phenotype lead to realistic ways to cope with an unusual child. (p. 2)

Beyond these compelling informational/support needs, most treatment can be considered biological, behavioral, or preventative in nature. These three classes of treatments are covered below, and summarized in Table 23.1, in that order. Recommendations for educational interventions are also presented.

Biological Treatments

Seeking to remedy LNS's core HPRT enzyme deficiency would be a logical starting point for any treatment. Unfortunately, this deficit cannot be remedied. In fact, failure of a medication (azathioprine) that was known to lower uric acid levels in kidney transplant patients to produce an effect in the urine or blood of patients with LNS was one early cue to the presence of the HPRT enzyme deficiency (Nyhan, 2005). Still, controlling an immediate consequence of HPRT deficiency, overproduction of uric acid, is possible. Allopurinol is a xanthine oxidase inhibitor, which is administered as an oral medication. Because xanthine oxidase converts the excess of hypoxanthine and guanine found in patients with LNS into uric acid, its inhibition can diminish uric acid levels in serum and urine. This has the effect of reducing the development of gout-related symptoms and helping to preserve kidney function. Consequently, allopurinol is advocated for use at

TABLE 23.1. Summary of Interventions for Patients with LNS

Reference	Intervention type	Patients studied	Symptom reductions and other improvements
Biological			
Kirkpatrick-Sanchez et al. (1998)	Serotonergic diet[a], paroxetine (SSRI), and sertraline (SSRI)	6-year-old male	Decrease in lip and tongue biting, finger biting, kicking, scratching, and rubbing face; reduced use of mouth guard and limb restraints
McManaman and Tam (1999)	Gabapentine (antiepileptic)	3-year-old male	Decreases in cheek and lip biting
Harris (2008)	Deep brain stimulation	Four patients (ages not reported)	Decreases in dystonia and self-injurious behavior
Cif et al. (2007)	Deep brain stimulation	16-year-old male	Decreases in dystonia and self-injurious behavior; teeth extraction no longer under consideration; reduced limb restraint
Dabrowski et al. (2005)	Botulinum toxin A (BTX-A)	10-year-old male	Decreases in self-injury to hands, lip, and tongue; reportedly improved speech; return to school
Gutierrez, Pellene, and Micheli (2008)	Botulinum toxin A	30-year-old male	Decreases in lip and finger biting
Serrano et al. (2008)	Levodopa/carbidopa	3-year-old male	Improved head control; able to pick up objects
Behavioral			
Duker (1975)	Extinction and DRO	9-year-old male	Decreases in finger biting and crying following self-induced bite[b]
Bull and LaVecchio (1978)	Systematic desensitization, extinction, and play therapy	10-year-old male	Decreases in coprolalia, biting, head banging, injury to others, neck snapping, spitting, and vomiting
Anderson et al. (1978)	Punishment[a], time-out, DRO, and positive reinforcement of self-injurious behavior[a]	Males ages 3, 5, 11, 12, and 13 years	Decreases in finger biting, head banging, and use of restraints
Gilbert et al. (1979)	Extinction and DRO	4½-year-old male	Decreases in leg, arm, head, face, and nose banging, as well as nose and face scratching; splints removed
Buzas et al. (1981)	DRI	14-year-old male	Decreases in lip damage, finger-to-mouth responses, crying, and vocalizations of wanting to be restrained
Wurtele et al. (1984)	Extinction, self-instruction, and relaxation	13-year-old male	Decreases in finger biting[b]
McGreevy and Arthur (1987)	DRI and punishment	2-year-old male	Decreases in biting arms, forearms, and back of hands[b]
Grace et al. (1988)	Self-instruction, positive reinforcement, and time-out	14-year-old male	Decreases in lip biting; freedom from restraints

Note. Interventions listed are confined to those that were the subjects of peer-reviewed journal articles (other interventions coincidentally mentioned in the articles are not listed separately in the table). Despite our efforts to search medical and psychological journals, some articles may have been missed.
[a]Denotes an intervention that failed to improve target symptoms (whereas other listed interventions produced improvement).
[b]This study included other variables that failed to improve, besides those noted.

the first detection of HPRT deficiency (Torres & Puig, 2007). Unfortunately, this treatment does not have an effect on CNS-related symptoms.

When one reads the background of patients with LNS in case studies, use of psychotropic medication is commonly noted. Summaries of LNS typically confirm that physician experts also often use medications to address neurological and behavioral signs/symptoms. For example, Torres and Puig (2007) confirm that medication affecting gamma-aminobutyric acid (GABA) receptors, such as benzodiazepines and baclofen, are used to address spasticity and dystonia as well as anxiety. Moreover, parents report that their children have frequently been tried on various medications to diminish the almost universal array of behavioral and neurological symptoms (Anderson & Ernst, 1994). Despite their apparently frequent case-by-case use, little has been published regarding the efficacy of these medications in LNS.

In 1998, a U.S. group (Kirkpatrick-Sanchez, Williams, Gualtieri, & Raichman, 1998) reported a case in which psychotropic medication was augmented by behavioral treatment (see also "Behavioral Treatments," below). The patient was a 6-year-old African American male with LNS who presented with unmanageable behavior in a group setting. He had been placed in this setting at age 3 years because of his behavior, although he also had mild mental retardation. His lengthy behavioral problem list included lip and tongue biting, finger biting, kicking, scratching, and rubbing his face against solid objects to the point of bleeding. Like many boys with LNS, he required restraints. During the night, these consisted of tight bedsheet wrapping, the use of arm splints, and a face mask (to prevent him from rubbing his face on the bed); during the day, wrist restraints (on his wheelchair), arm splints, a neck roll head support, and a mouth guard were used. After behavioral treatments had reduced baseline aggressive behavior by 71%, medication and other biological options were considered because the boy's aggressive behavior remained at clinically unacceptable levels. An attempt at a serotonergic diet (e.g., accentuation of fruit, curtailment of caffeine and salt) produced no discernible effect on behavior, however. Subsequently, paroxetine (a selective serotonin reuptake inhibitor [SSRI]) was introduced at 5 mg and increased stepwise to 30 mg at the end of 4 weeks. It appears that subsequently paroxetine was discontinued, and sertraline was introduced and increased eventually to 200 mg. The authors indicate that paroxetine was associated with a 32% reduction in self-injurious behaviors occurring when the patient was unrestrained (measured by rate per minute recorded by an observer). The more effective medication, however, appeared to be sertraline, adjusted to 200 mg. No percentage of reduction was reported in the article, however, and the authors reported that no reliability checks were available for this portion of the data set. Remaining on 200 mg of sertaline (and with a change of residential setting), the patient appeared to show significant overall improvement, such as reduced mouth guard and limb restraint use.

Gabapentine, an antiepileptic drug affecting the GABA system, was reportedly efficacious in reducing lip and cheek biting in a 3-year-old boy with LNS (McManaman & Tam, 1999). Following a gastrostomy (i.e., surgical insertion of a feeding tube), self-injurious behavior increased in severity and frequency. The patient was initially prescribed diazepam, which proved ineffective. Gabapentine was then added at 400 mg daily, leading to decreased biting within the first week; consequently, diazepam was discontinued. At 3 weeks, the gabapentine dose was increased to 800 mg daily, and the boy's parents reported that the self-injurious behaviors ceased. When a bowel obstruction occurred several weeks later, gabapentine treatment was discontinued, resulting in an immediate reappearance of self-injurious behaviors. Once the obstruction was treated, gabapentine was reintroduced, resulting in immediate reduction of self-injurious behaviors.

Another medication approach involves dopamine, the key neurotransmitter that is anomalous. An interesting single case is reported by a Spanish group (Serrano et al., 2008). This involved a child with LNS who had the expected low dopamine metabolite values in his cerebrospinal fluid. He had been first identified because of conspicuous motor problems evident for four months. With early introduction of levodopa/carbidopa (L-dopa) therapy, clinical improvement was noted. For example, by 18 months the patient reportedly demonstrated improved head control, and he was able to pick up objects, although dyskinetic movements remained. The authors propose that L-dopa treatment begun very early in the lives of children with LNS may have the potential to improve neurological symptoms and contribute to better outcome. More controlled investigations of medication appear to be in order (see also Cif et al., 2007, below, for a list of medications that apparently proved ineffective in a case ultimately treated by other means).

The extreme disabilities accompanying LNS have no doubt contributed to the wide-ranging search for viable treatments. This search has been extended to the realm of neurosurgical procedures, which at first may seem surprising or disquieting to readers who associate such procedures with the unfortunate psychosurgical history of frontal lobotomy. On reconsideration, however, the use of such techniques may make more sense if one recalls that the profoundly debilitating symptoms characterizing LNS may be attributable to known brain dysfunctions, and that reversible treatments involving neuropacemakers to accomplish deep brain stimulation are already approved by the U.S. Food and Drug Administration for essential tremor and Parkinson disease (U.S. Department of Health and Human Services, 1997). James Harris at Johns Hopkins (2008) reported a series of four patients who underwent implantation of electrodes to stimulate both motor and limbic circuits in the globus pallidus. The procedure is accomplished in a consciously sedated or fully anesthetized state and is guided by the use of MRI. The implanted electrodes enable deep brain stimulation in a process aimed to represent "neuromodulatory treatment." Compared to baseline, at follow-up patients expressed reduced dystonia and complete elimination of self-injurious behavior. One patient reportedly remained free of self-injurious behaviors 7 years after the intervention. A clinical trial of the procedure is reportedly scheduled to begin.

A similar approach was reported by a French group (Cif et al., 2007). A 16-year-old male with severe LNS was diagnosed at age 6 months and expressed generalized dystonia, athetosis of all four limbs, and dysarthria. It was the psychosocial/behavioral presentation, however, that proved most troubling. This involved frequent hand, tongue, and lip biting; lip amputation; eye poking; spitting; and coprolalia. He required constant limb restraint. Efforts to treat him with medications (baclofen, diazepam, clomipramine, cyamemazine) proved ineffective. Deep brain stimulation was accomplished via double bilateral simultaneous stimulation to limbic and motor internal pallidum. Dystonia (measured by the Burke–Fahn–Marsden Dystonia Rating Scale; Burke et al., 1985) and self-injurious and aggressive behavior (measured by the Behavior Problems Inventory; Rojahn, Matson, Lott, Esbensen, & Smalls, 2001) improved during the first week of stimulation. The patient's caregivers were also eventually able to abandon consideration of extracting his teeth (to prevent mutilation). Moreover, the patient no longer required attachment to his bed or wheelchair and was ultimately able to drive his own wheelchair.

An alternative biological treatment, botulinum toxin A (BTX-A), was recently reported by two research groups. BTX-A is well known to temporarily inhibit release of acetylcholine from presynaptic neurons; this ultimately results in muscle weakness or paralysis, as occurs in the cosmetic use of Botox. In the first study, Dabrowski, Smathers, Ralstrom, Nigro, and Leleszi (2005) used BTX-A injection in both masseter muscles (i.e., muscles in the cheek that close the jaws during chewing) at two sites. The subject was a 10-year-old male with developmental delay from infancy and apparent cerebral palsy, but an LNS diagnosis was not confirmed until age 8 years. Self-mutilation began before 8 years and comprised ulceration of hands, lips, and tongue. Within a few days of initiating treatment, self-mutation diminished to the point that the wounds healed and the boy was able to return to school. Speech also reportedly improved (no objective measurements were undertaken, however). Injections were required each 12 weeks to maintain effects. Equivalent results were obtained with a 30-year-old with LNS who was also treated with BTX-A (Gutierrez, Pellene, & Micheli, 2008). The mechanism by which injections of BTX-A work is not clear. Peripheral action alone (production of muscle weakness at the injection site) is not a plausible explanation. Among the speculative possibilities are that BTX-A exerts a CNS sensory effect via altered feedback that is somehow instrumental in diminished self-abusive behavior; inhibition of substance P or glutamate is another possibility (Dabrowski et al., 2005).

Behavioral Treatments

Considering the severity of the self-injurious behaviors exhibited in LNS, it is not surprising that the most common form of intervention is mechanical restraints. In behavioral terms, this practice might be viewed as an example of response prevention. A study executed over a decade ago ascertained that nearly one-half of affected boys were restrained 100% of the time (Anderson & Ernst, 1994). Such restraints are often welcomed by children who feel unable to inhibit their self-injury (i.e., there is a compulsive quality to their acts). Commonly used restraints include arm and elbow splints, wrist and leg restraints on the wheelchair, finger guards, mouth guards, face masks, helmets, and bed straps. Coverings have also been used to prevent injury, including dishwashing gloves, biking gloves, and towels and Ace bandages wrapped around thumbs. The use of restraints, however, is not a preferred intervention because they may diminish quality of life; furthermore, clinicians are legally and ethically obligated to provide patients with the least restrictive method of controlling behavior (Olson & Houlihan, 2000).

Another form of response prevention is extraction of teeth, which is often useful in cases when children engage in lip, finger, and cheek biting. Anderson and Ernst (1994) confirmed that 24 of 40 children with LNS had undergone teeth extraction. Parents and patients in the study overwhelmingly supported teeth extraction to manage biting and had no regrets following the procedure. Following extraction, a child's ability to chew food should be largely unaffected. Likewise, because articulation in most patients with LNS is poor to begin with, it may not worsen speech, although no known study provides objective evidence for this speculation.

Wide use of restrictive practices aside, it is advantageous to employ alternative behavioral treatments that do not jeopardize quality of life. In an early study, Anderson, Dancis, and Alpert (1978) examined the effect of several behavioral treatments in five male patients with LNS ages 3, 5, 11, 12, and 13 years. The patients wore arm restraints due to frequent finger biting, lip biting, head banging, or neck snapping. To address these self-injurious behaviors, four behavioral treatments were evaluated: aversive consequences (i.e., an electric finger shock contingent on self-injurious behavior); differential reinforcement of other behavior (DRO—i.e., smiling, talking, and playing while a child was not engaging in self-injurious behavior); positive reinforcement of attempts at self-injurious behavior (i.e., preventing the self-injurious behavior, and then making reassuring statements and stroking the child—a common response of parents); and time-out contingent on self-injury (i.e., withdrawal of adult attention following self-injurious behavior). In all treatment conditions (with the exception of time-out), a response prevention procedure was used, wherein an adult intercepted the child's attempts at self-injury. Though not all subjects in the study received all four treatments, results indicated that the DRO and time-out procedures resulted in decreases in self-injurious behavior. The most substantive effects resulted from a combination of time-out and DRO: Self-injury was eliminated in all four subjects that were evaluated. Aversive consequences (i.e., finger shock) were unsuccessful in suppressing self-injurious behaviors and in some cases accelerated behaviors (as measured by two raters using frequency counts). As would be expected, reinforcement contingent on attempts at self-injurious behavior resulted in a rapid increase in self-injury. To sustain improvements in self-injurious behaviors, therapists trained parents to use time-out and positive reinforcement and provided home visits to ensure proper implementation. Follow-up at 22–24 months indicated that all children were free of restraints at school and that three of the five children were placed in restraints at night.

Anderson and colleagues' (1978) finding that aversive consequences (i.e., finger shocks) may facilitate self-injurious behavior highlights the importance of developing behavioral treatments that are responsive to the unique needs of patients with LNS. In response to these findings, Zilli and Hasselmo (2008) developed a model of behavioral treatments specific to patients with LNS.

Consistent with the hypothesized dopamine signal dysfunction in individuals with LNS, they demonstrated that painful consequences act as reinforcement. Though this model provides an explanation for the results of behavioral treatments in patients with LNS, how it can be used to improve interventions remains unclear. Nonetheless, this study underscores that painful consequences may not have the desired effect of decreasing behaviors in these individuals, thus emphasizing the necessity of techniques such as differential reinforcement.

The effectiveness of differential reinforcement compared to aversive procedures for children with LNS was a consistent finding in a recent review of seven behavioral treatment studies (Olson & Houlihan, 2000). The most common interventions, and indeed those shown to be most effective, were DRO, differential reinforcement of incompatible behaviors (DRI), and extinction. Reinforcement was offered through verbal praise, attention, hugs, or dispensing cola into the mouth when a child was engaged in either non-self-injurious or incompatible behaviors (i.e., drawing, playing games, eating candy, learning sign language, and touching toys). Extinction involved ignoring the children (i.e., withdrawing attention) when they engaged in self-injurious behaviors. Though extinction appears to be effective, serious damage can occur during extinction bursts; therefore, that technique may be best used in combination with response prevention (i.e., mouth guards, wraps) and DRI or DRO (Wurtele, King, & Drabman, 1984). Aversive techniques (e.g., finger shocks) were also studied, but these procedures paradoxically intensified self-injury (see discussion above). Parents corroborated these results, confirming that positive reinforcement was useful in controlling self-injury, whereas punitive techniques such as time-out or loss of reinforcement were not (Anderson & Ernst, 1994).

Many patients and parents have reported that anxiety is an antecedent to self-injury. Moreover, many patients have reported feeling anxiety when restraints are removed (Gilbert, Spellacy, & Watts, 1979); when presented with new situations, tasks, or people; or when ill (Anderson & Ernst, 1994). The role of anxiety in triggering self-injurious behaviors suggests a need for interventions targeted at reducing emotional distress. Two studies have evaluated the effectiveness of such interventions. Wurtele and colleagues (1984) identified the antecedents of a 13-year-old boy's self-injurious behavior as muscle tension and an internal voice telling him to bite. Intervention included extinction, wearing of a mouth guard and gloves, relaxation training, self-instruction to refrain from self-injurious behavior, and social support. In addition, the parents received training in how to use the procedures and ways to prompt their son. At a 6-month follow-up, attempts at self-injury had markedly decreased, and the boy only occasionally wore the mouth guard (although he still wore gloves). Likewise, Bull and LaVecchio (1978) used a combination of extinction, systematic desensitization (e.g., relaxation exercises, exposure to a hierarchy of anxiety-provoking situations, and removal of restraints), and play therapy for a 10-year-old boy with LNS. After 10 sessions, the child no longer engaged in self-injury. Results at an 18-month follow-up indicated the boy no longer used restraints, did not engage in coprolalia, and was learning to walk on crutches. Interventions aimed at preventing anxiety in order to prevent self-injurious behavior thus appear promising for patients with LNS, but more systematic, controlled research seems warranted.

One issue threatening the use of behavioral techniques in patients with LNS is the prospect of symptom substitution (i.e., as one self-injurious behavior decreases, it may be replaced with another; Olson & Houlihan, 2000). For example, Duker (1975) found that a combination of DRO and extinction resulted in decreased self-biting, but concomitant increases in head banging. Similarly, McGreevy and Arthur (1987) reported that a combination of DRI and punishment decreased biting of forearms, arms, and the backs of hands; however, finger biting increased, and the boy in their study began a new self-injurious behavior of biting the palms of his hands. Unfortunately, procedures to address the problem of symptom substitution do not exist. Crucially, studies that systematically used generalization procedures across both change agents and settings did not report such problems, either during active study phases or at follow-up (Anderson et al., 1978; Buzas, Ayllon, & Collins, 1981). Thus it may be advantageous to include generalization procedures in behavioral treatments to help preclude the occurrence of symptom substitution.

In general, the studies on behavioral modification techniques indicate short-term decreases in self-injurious behaviors in individuals with LNS; however, concerns about maintenance and generalization remain. Generalization procedures were used in four of the seven studies reviewed by Olson and Houlihan (2000), which included training staff and parents, and employing interventions across multiple settings. These studies showed improvements at 6-week to 24-month follow-ups (Anderson et al., 1978; Grace, Cowart, & Matson, 1988; McGreevy & Arthur, 1987; Wurtele et al., 1984). In addition to staff and parent training, procedures to enhance generalization and maintenance might include pairing natural reinforcers with artificial ones or training individuals in self-instruction and evaluation. In this regard, Grace and colleagues (1988) used a self-assessment procedure with a 14-year-old male with LNS who engaged in compulsive self-biting. The youngster was taught to point to a happy face when he engaged in a non-self-injurious behavior and a sad face for a self-injurious behavior. Correct self-assessments were reinforced with hugs, whereas incorrect ones were punished with a 30-second time-out from positive reinforcement. Three days following the intervention, rates of biting behaviors went from an initial range of 1 to 60 bites (hospital) and a range of 1 to 37 bites (bedroom) per 30-minute session down to zero bites in each setting. At a 19-week follow-up assessment, no recurrence of self-biting was noted. Such procedures appear to offer patients with LNS the skills to monitor and control their own self-injurious behaviors, thereby leading to increased generalization and maintenance of treatment effects.

In summary, behavioral treatments appear efficacious for an array of self-injurious behaviors; however, this conclusion arises from research conducted primarily in highly controlled settings with considerable expert/researcher support. Thus additional studies examining the effectiveness of standard behavioral techniques in diverse settings on the one hand, and the use of additional techniques (e.g., overcorrection) on the other hand, are needed. Furthermore, broader treatment outcomes, such as the impact of documented behavior changes on overall qualify of life,

do not appear to have been addressed yet (see Kazdin, 2001, for discussion). The impact of any procedure or combination of procedures (e.g., pharmacotherapy and behavior techniques) that reduces the need for more invasive practices, such as mechanical restraints, seems to be especially compelling.

Preventative Treatments

Genetic counseling may have a role in prevention of LNS. Because LNS is inherited in an X-linked fashion, fathers of boys with LNS will not have LNS, and they are not carriers of a mutant HPRT allele. The risk to unborn siblings of a patient with LNS depends on the mother's carrier status. If she is documented to carry a mutant HPRT allele, then she has a 50% chance of transmitting the HPRT mutation in each pregnancy. Sons who inherit the mutation will be affected, whereas daughters who inherit the mutation are themselves carriers but will not express the LNS phenotype (just as is true of their mothers). If the nature of a family's mutation (as in an affected male family member) is known, then a woman's carrier status can be determined by biochemical and enzymatic testing procedures (Torres & Puig, 2007). Interestingly, however, approximately 30% of patients' mothers do not carry a mutant HPRT allele. It is presumed that such patients carry a de novo mutation arising from germinal cell mutation (Torres & Puig, 2007). For pregnancies at risk of LNS, prenatal testing is possible by amniotic cells at approximately 15–18 weeks of gestation or by chorionic villus cells acquired at an earlier point during pregnancy. Either enzyme (HPRT) analysis or molecular (DNA) analysis can be conducted.

Educational Interventions

Unfortunately, to date, no known studies have been published reviewing common educational services and classroom interventions for patients with LNS. Considering the severity of cognitive and behavioral symptoms often associated with the syndrome, most children with LNS are likely to qualify for special education services. Early intervention services might focus on eating and drinking, followed later by communication skills and play. Many children with LNS suffer from poor articulation; thus it is often recommended that they attend regular sessions with a speech–language therapist, especially a therapist knowledgeable about related disorders (e.g., cerebral palsy; McCarthy, 2004). Documentation of the effectiveness of these services, however, has not yet appeared in the literature.

CONCLUSION

LNS is an X-linked inborn error of metabolism that is rare but causes profound impairments in the boys and men affected by it. Although substantial progress has occurred in understanding the causes and expression of the disorder, its treatments remain limited, and the efficacy of these treatments is largely undocumented in well-controlled studies. Nonetheless, if systematically applied and monitored in individual cases, behavioral interventions may reduce symptoms. Promising biological treatments may also be on the horizon. Furthermore, LNS continues to hold promise for researchers hoping to understand the relationship among biochemistry, brain function, behavior, and development.

ACKNOWLEDGMENTS

Thanks to Mark Joseph, MD, Phoenix Children's Hospital, and Matthew D. Wodrich, PhD, Université de Genève, for reviewing and commenting on portions of this chapter.

REFERENCES

Achenbach, T. M. (1991) *Manual for the Child Behavior Checklist/4–18 and 1991 Profile*. Burlington: University of Vermont, Department of Psychiatry.

Anderson, L. T., Dancis, J., & Alpert, M. (1978). Behavioral contingencies and self-mutilation in Lesch–Nyhan disease. *Journal of Consulting and Clinical Psychology, 46*, 529–536.

Anderson, L. T., & Ernst, M. (1994). Self-injury in Lesch–Nyhan disease. *Journal of Autism and Developmental Disorders, 24*, 67–81.

Anderson, L. T., Ernst, M., & Davis, S. V. (1992). Cognitive abilities of patients with Lesch–Nyhan disease. *Journal of Autism and Developmental Disorders, 22*, 189–203.

Bull, M., & LaVecchio, F. (1978). Behavior therapy for a child with Lesch–Nyhan syndrome. *Developmental Medicine and Child Neurology, 20*, 368–375.

Burke, R. E., Fahn, S., Marsden, C. D., Bressman, S. B., Moskowitz, C., & Friedman, J. (1985). Validity and reliability of a rating scale for the primary torsion dystonias. *Neurology, 35*, 73–77.

Buzas, H. P., Ayllon, T., & Collins, F. (1981). A behavioral approach to eliminate self-mutilative behavior in a Lesch–Nyhan patient. *Journal of Mind and Behavior, 2*, 47–56.

Cif, L., Biolsi, B., Gavarini, S., Saux, A., Robles, S. G., Tancu, C., et al. (2007). Antero-ventral internal pallidum stimulation improves behavioral disorders in Lesch–Nyhan disease. *Movement Disorders, 22*, 2126–2129.

Dabrowski, E., Smathers, S. A., Nigro, M. A., & Leleszi, J. P. (2005). Botulinum toxin as a novel treatment for self-mutilation in Lesch–Nyhan syndrome. *Developmental Medicine and Child Neurology, 47*, 636–639.

Duker, P. (1975). Behavior control of self-biting in a Lesch–Nyhan patient. *Journal of Mental Deficiencies Research, 19*, 11–19.

Dunn, L. M., & Dunn, L. M. (2007). *Peabody Picture Vocabulary Test, Fourth Edition*. San Antonio, TX: Pearson Assessments.

Ernst, M., Zametkin, A. J., Pascualvaca, D., Matochik, J. A., Eisenhofer, G., & Murphy, D. L., et al. (2000). Adrenergic and noradrenergic plasma levels in Lesch–Nyhan disease. *Neuropsychopharmacology, 22*, 320–326.

Gibbs, R. A., Nguyen, P., McBride, L. J., Koepf, S. M., & Caskey, C. T. (1989). Identification of mutations leading to Lesch–Nyhan syndrome by automated direct DNA sequencing *in vitro* amplified cDNA. *Proceedings of the National Academy of Sciences USA, 86*, 1919–1923.

Gilbert, S., Spellacy, E., & Watts, R. W. E. (1979). Problems in the behavioral treatment of self-injury in Lesch–Nyhan syndrome. *Developmental Medicine and Child Neurology, 21*, 795–799.

Grace, N., Cowart, C., & Matson, J. (1988). Reinforcement and self-control for treating a chronic case of self injury in Lesch–Nyhan syndrome. *Journal of the Multihandicapped Person, 1*, 53–59.

Gutierrez, C., Pellene, A., & Micheli, F. (2008). Botulinum toxin: Treatment of self-mutilation in patients with Lesch–Nyhan syndrome. *Clinical Neuropharmacology, 31*, 180–183.

Hladnik, U., Nyhan, W. L., & Bertolli, M. (2008). Variable expression of HPRT deficiency in 5 members of a family with the same mutation. *Archives of Neurology, 65*, 1240–1243.

Harris, J. C. (2008). Neuromodulatory treatment (DBS) for dystonia and self-injurious behavior in Lesch–Nyhan disease. *Journal of Intellectual Disability Research, 52*(8–9), 656.

Jinnah, H. A., Visser, J. E., Harris, J. C., Verdu, A., Larovere, L., & Ceballos-Picot, I. (2006). Delineation of the motor disorder of Lesch–Nyhan disease. *Brain, 129*, 1201–1217.

Jolly, D. J., Okayama, H., Berg, P., Esty, A. C., Filpula, D., Bohlen, G. G., et al. (1983). Isolation and characterization of a full length, expressible cDNA human hypoxanthine-guanine phosphoribosyl transferase. *Processings of the National Academy of Sciences USA, 80*, 477–481.

Kazdin, A. E. (2001). *Behavior modification in applied settings* (6th ed.). Belmont, CA: Wadsworth/Thomson.

Kirkpatrick-Sanchez, S., Williams, D. E., Gualtieri, C. T., & Raichman, J. A. (1998). Case report: The effects of selective serotonergic reuptake inhibitors combined with behavioral treatment on self-injury associated with Lesch–Nyhan syndrome. *Journal of Developmental and Physical Disabilities, 10*, 283–290.

Levart, T. K. (2007). Rare variant of Lesch–Nyhan syndrome without self-mutilation or nephrolithiasis. *Pediatric Nephrology, 22*, 1975–1978.

Matthews, W. S., Solan, A., & Barabas, G. (1995). Cognitive functioning in Lesch–Nyhan syndrome. *Developmental Medicine and Child Neurology, 37*, 715–722.

Matthews, W. S., Solan, A., Barabas, G., & Robey, K. (1999). Cognitive functioning in Lesch–Nyhan syndrome: A 4–year follow-up study. *Developmental Medicine and Child Neurology, 41*, 260–262.

McCarthy, G. (2004). Medical diagnosis, management, and treatment of Lesch–Nyhan disease. *Nucleosides, Nucleotides, and Nucleic Acids, 23*, 1147–1152.

McGreevy, P., & Arthur, M. (1987). Effective behavioral treatment of self-biting by a child with Lesch–Nyhan syndrome. *Developmental Medicine and Child Neurology, 29*, 536–540.

McManaman, J., & Tam, D. J. (1999). Gabapentin for self-injurious behavior in Lesch–Nyhan syndrome. *Journal of Pediatric Neurology, 20*, 381–382.

Morales, P. C. (1999). Lesch–Nyhan syndrome. In S. Goldstein & C. R. Reynolds (Eds.), *Handbook of neurodevelopmental and genetic disorders in children* (pp. 478–498). New York: Guilford Press.

Nihira, K., Leland, H., & Lambert, N. (1993). *AAMR Adaptive Behavior Scale—Residential and Community examiner's manual*. Austin, TX: PRO-ED.

Nyhan, W. L. (1973). The Lesch–Nyhan syndrome. *Annual Review of Medicine, 24*, 41–60.

Nyhan, W. L. (1997). The recognition of Lesch–Nyhan syndrome as an inborn error of purine metabolism. *Journal of Inherited and Metabolic Diseases, 29*, 171–178.

Nyhan, W. L. (2005). Lesch–Nyhan disease. *Journal of the History of the Neurosciences, 14*, 1–10.

Nyhan, W. L., Sweetman, L., Carpenier, D. G., Carter, C. H., & Hoefnagel, D. (1968). Effects of azathioprine in a disorder of uric acid metabolism and cerebral function. *Journal of Pediatrics, 72*, 111–118.

Nyhan, W. L., & Wong, D. F. (1996). New approaches to understanding Lesch–Nyhan disease. *New England Journal of Medicine, 334*, 1602–1604.

Olson, L., & Houlihan, D. (2000). A review of behavioral treatments used for Lesch–Nyhan syndrome. *Behavior Modification, 24*, 202–222.

Robey, K. L., Reck, J. F., Giacomini, K. D., Barabas, C., & Eddey, G. E. (2003). Modes and patterns of self-mutilation in persons with Lesch–Nyhan disease. *Developmental Medicine and Child Neurology, 45*, 167–171.

Rojahn, J., Matson, J. L., Lott, D., Esbensen, A. J., & Smalls, Y. (2001). The behavior problems inventory: an instrument for the assessment of self-injury, stereotyped behavior, and aggression/destruction in individuals with developmental disabilities. *Journal of Autism and Developmental Disorders, 31*, 577–578.

Schretlen, D. J., Ward, J., Meyer, S. M., Yun, J., Puig, J. G., Nyhan, W. L., et al. (2005). Behavioral aspects of Lesch–Nyhan disease and its variants. *Developmental Medicine and Child Neurology, 47*, 673–677.

Seegmiller, J. E., Rosenbloom, F. M., & Kelley, W. N (1967). Enzyme defect associated with a sex-linked human neurological disorder and excessive purine synthesis. *Science, 155*, 1682–1684.

Serrano, M., Perez-Duenas, B., Ormzabal, A., Artuch, R., Campistol, J., Torres, R. J., et al. (2008). Levodopa therapy in a Lesch–Nyhan disease patient: Pathological, biochemical, neuroimaging, and therapeutic remarks. *Movement Disorders, 23*, 1297–1300.

Thorndike, R. L., Hagen, E. P., & Sattler, J. M. (1986). *Stanford–Binet Intelligence Scale* (4th ed.). Chicago: Riverside.

Torres, R. J., & Puig, J. G. (2007). Hypoxanthine–guanine phosophoribosyltransferase (HPRT) deficiency: Lesch–Nyhan syndrome. *Orphanet Journal of Rare Diseases, 2*, 1–10.

U.S. Department of Health and Human Services. (1997, August). FDA approves implanted brain stimulator to control tremors. Retrieved May 5, 2009, from *www.fda.gov/bbs/topics/NEWS/NEW00580.html*

Wong, D. F., Harris, J. C., Naidu, S., Yokoi, F., Marenco, S., Dannals, R. F., et al. (1996). Dopamine transporters are markedly reduced in Lesch–Nyhan disease *in vivo*. *Proceedings of the National Academy of Sciences USA, 93*, 5539–5543.

Wurtele, S. K., King, A. C., & Drabman, R. S. (1984). Treatment package to reduce self-injurious behavior in a Lesch–Nyhan patient. *Journal of Mental Deficiency Research, 28*, 227–234.

Zilli, E. A., & Hasselmo, M. E. (2008). A model of behavior treatments for self-mutilation behavior in Lesch–Nyhan syndrome. *NeuroReport, 19*, 459–462.

CHAPTER 24

Seizure Disorders

THOMAS L. BENNETT
DEANA B. DAVALOS
MAILE HO-TURNER
BARBARA C. BANZ

Seizures are transient symptoms of abnormal neuronal activity in the brain triggered by a variety of etiologies. Although the causes of seizures are poorly understood, it is clear that the prevalence of seizures in infants, children, and adolescents is quite high. It has been estimated that approximately 5% of the world's population may experience a seizure at some point in life, with nearly one-third of these individuals developing epilepsy (World Health Organization, 2001). The global population with epilepsy has been estimated at 50 million. *Epilepsy* has been defined as a brain disorder characterized by recurrent disturbances in the electrical functions of the brain that result in seizures (Kobau et al., 2008). The prevalence of epilepsy in people from Europe and North America across the lifespan has been reported at 5–8 per 1,000 (Forsgren, 2004). Studies assessing a wide range of age groups suggest that general prevalence rates presented in the literature should also be interpreted with the understanding that the risk for developing epilepsy is not equal across the lifespan. Instead, infants and children under the age of 5 may be at the greatest risk for both initial seizures and epilepsy (Annegers, Dubinsky, Coan, Newmark, & Roht, 1999). Childhood epilepsy syndromes have long been clinically observed to have some genetic or hereditary component. It has not been until the past two decades that increasing pathological and neurodevelopmental data supporting these observations have been linked to clinical observations (Marini et al., 2004).

Furthermore, a child's immature brain is not simply a miniature of an adult brain; it is both anatomically and physiologically different. Thus one needs to look to, and specifically study, the immature brain in order to understand childhood epilepsy disorders. The appearance of epilepsy through different stages of cortical development in the fetus and through the early childhood years has differential implications and manifestations, as well as outcome prognoses and treatment implications.

What we do know about childhood epilepsy is that many factors appear to contribute to seizure thresholds. Seizure thresholds have a major impact on the child's propensity to develop a recurrent seizure disorder (epilepsy), which will in turn have resulting cognitive deficits associated with the epileptic syndrome. Three major factors affecting the occurrence of seizures are (1) genetic predispositions/familial history, (2) age at onset, and (3) environmental stressors. The effect of these factors is cumulative. That is, a child of a particular age who has a familial history of epilepsy and who is exposed to environmental stressors (e.g., fever) has a greater chance of developing a seizure disorder than a child of the same age without the familial history and/or the environmental stressors.

MAJOR PRECIPITATING FACTORS

Genetics

As early as 1960, Lennox and Lennox noted a strong concordance rate for childhood absence epilepsy in identical twins, as well as higher rates of electroencephalographic (EEG) spike-and-wave patterns in families with a family history of epilepsy. Since then, both partial and generalized seizure types have been linked to genetic causes. Animal studies in which genetic mutations result in familial strain occurrences of epilepsy have also contributed to the increased awareness of the contribution of genetics to epilepsy syndromes. However, the exact effects of these mutations and inheritances on the neuroanatomical development and physiology of the brain and seizure thresholds are still unclear.

The occurrence and development of some forms of epilepsy have been definitively linked to genetic inheritance, while others have a weaker connection. Febrile seizures, childhood absence epilepsy, juvenile myoclonic epilepsy, Rasmussen syndrome, generalized tonic–clonic epilepsy, and complex partial seizures, among others, have all been shown to have definite genetic contributions in their development. That is, familial history increases the occurrence of the seizures types, although it is not the sole determinant of its manifestation.

Age at Onset

Newborns have a very high cortical threshold, and elicitation of a seizure response is very difficult. However, as children progress into infancy and toddlerhood (up to about age 2), they have a much higher susceptibility to febrile and other seizures; in other words, their seizure threshold has lowered. This is the time period when most childhood epilepsy syndromes begin, although each ep-

ilepsy syndrome has its own peak incidence age ranges. Through childhood and adolescence (age 2 and beyond), the seizure threshold increases proportionally until it reaches adult levels.

Environmental Stressors

Environmental stressors include fever spiking, fatigue, excitement, ionic concentrations/metabolism, and other factors. Fevers as agents precipitating seizures are especially notable in febrile seizures, as their name implies. A fever's rate of rise and amplitude are directly related to a seizure's onset and intensity.

This chapter continues with a brief description of the stages of neurodevelopment and associated neuropathologies that have been recently linked together to provide a better understanding of childhood epilepsy. We then describe the various classification schemes of childhood seizures and epilepsy syndromes. Finally, the manifestation of childhood seizure syndromes and their behavioral, cognitive, and neuropsychological issues are considered.

NEURODEVELOPMENTAL AND NEUROPATHOLOGICAL ASPECTS

There are four relatively distinct stages of neural development, which can each serve as a point of disruption and which have specific implications for the appearance of seizure disorders. The first three stages of neural development (regional determination and segmentmation, cytogenesis, and cell migration) are completed by the end of the second trimester of pregnancy. The last stage of development (growth and differentiation) begins late in the second trimester and continues through the early years of postnatal development, when many epilepsy syndromes manifest themselves. Generally, the earlier the pathology occurs, the graver the outcome.

Deviance in the earliest stages of neural development is so grave, in fact, that the fertilized egg may not even be implanted in the uteral lining for development, or miscarriage may occur. Fetuses that do survive the first stage of regional determination and segmentation with deviant neural development often do not survive to term. If such a fetus does survive to term, the infant usually has severe malformations of the cerebrum. Any further neural development is also deviant and probably will produce seizure disorders. Deviance in the cytogenic and migratory stages of development is more survivable than earlier deviance, but it produces neuroanatomical anomalies that are grossly and microscopically apparent. Displaced neural tissue (heterotopia) defects such as agyria and microgyria occur in these stages. Also possible with deviant development in these stages, but not grossly visible, is the clustering of neurons in the wrong areas of the brain (microdysgenesis).

Generally, these heterotopic and microdysgenetic disorders are due to defects in the development of the neuronal guidance tracts (also known as [a.k.a.] radial glides) or the migrating neurons themselves. Microdysgenetic patterns have been histologically linked to childhood epileptic disorders and to various cognitive problems in childhood (e.g., dyslexia, mental retardation). Cell transformation and interactions to produce a mature brain are the major activities in the last stage (growth and differentiation) of development. Again, this stage begins only after three stages of development are complete and continues through infancy until about age 2. This is the "fine-tuning" stage. Of notable interest here is that many childhood epilepsy syndromes appear in infancy and up to age 2, although recent research indicates that this stage of cortical development may be largely complete by the first year of life.

Cepeda and colleagues (2006) have utilized clinical-pathological techniques suggesting that the mechanisms involved in epileptogenesis may begin as early as during the prenatal developmental period through the first year of life. Others have utilized both animal and human models supporting the argument that the factors precipitating epileptogenesis may emerge as early as the prenatal period through the first weeks of life (Velisek & Moshe, 2003).

A number of studies during the past three decades have sought to understand the developmental neural mechanisms involved in epilepsy. In the 1980s Meencke and colleagues conducted a series of studies of neuropathologies associated with childhood epilepsy syndromes, and their findings were strikingly parallel to findings regarding the developmental stages of the fetal brain (Meencke, 1985, 1989). Meencke's group studied the brains of infants and children with a variety of childhood epilepsies, including infantile spasms (a.k.a. West syndrome), Lennox–Gastaut syndrome, and primary generalized seizure disorders (including childhood and juvenile myoclonic epilepsies). From the patterns of pathologies he observed, Meencke drew the following inferences: (1) Pathoanatomical abnormality of the brain is reflective of an increased likelihood of epilepsy, and vice versa; (2) the younger a child is at the age of onset, the greater the gravity of the pathoanatomical disruption; and (3) the younger the child is at the age of onset, the more aggressive the syndrome is, and the greater the gravity of the seizure disorder and behavioral disability. Although facets of Meencke's findings have been revised throughout the years, the argument persists that certain abnormalities in the developing brain increase the likelihood of experiencing seizures, and, conversely, experiencing seizures at different developmental stages can alter the trajectory of the developing brain (Sanchez & Jensen, 2001).

The conclusion that is beginning to emerge is that epileptic syndromes are largely genetically based, and that their etiologies and pathologies may eventually be explained in terms of inherited or acquired neurodevelopmental anomalies. These genetically acquired, anomalous developmental sequences of the brain may have long-term repercussions in the form of (frequently) lifelong epileptic syndromes.

CLASSIFICATION SCHEMES

In general, a *seizure* may be conceptualized as a sudden discharge of electrical activity in the brain that results in alterations of sensation, behavior, or consciousness. *Epilepsy*, as noted earlier, is a condition of recurrent seizures. An *epileptic syndrome* is characterized by a recurrence of consistent symptoms and behavioral manifestations.

There are three major ways in which childhood seizures and epilepsy can be studied and classified. In this section, we discuss seizure classification by (1) the cause of the seizure, (2) the seizure syndrome presentation, and (3) the epilepsy syndrome (this type of classification is generally more age- and behavior-based). These methods of classifying seizures are not mutually exclusive, and terms from more than one scheme are frequently used concurrently to discuss a single epileptic syndrome.

Classification by Cause of Seizure

Symptomatic Seizures

Symptomatic seizures and epileptic syndromes have a known cause, such as trauma, metabolic imbalance, developmental abnormality, or fever. Symptomatic seizures are also called *reactive* or *provoked* seizures when they occur in response to some irritation (e.g., fever or trauma) to the brain. The cause of a symptomatic seizure, therefore, can be either developmental in nature or acquired.

Cryptogenic Seizures

Cryptogenic seizures have a cause that is undetermined, but that appears to be related in occurrence to some other neurological or cognitive condition. The seizures are presumed to be symptomatic, but their exact cause is as yet hidden.

Idiopathic Seizures

Idiopathic seizures are those for which the cause is completely unknown and there is no evidence of an underlying abnormality. The child with epilepsy is essentially normal except for the occurrence of seizures. Idiopathic seizures are presumed to be inherited and are defined by age-related onsets.

Classification by Seizure Syndrome Presentation

Prenatal Seizures

Prenatal seizures are extremely rare (Usta, Adra, & Nassar, 2007). In the past, prenatal seizures that were readily recognized and reported (by the mother) were those induced by pyridoxine dependence, resulting in a generalized tonic–clonic seizure of the fetus. Even massive cortical damage to the fetal brain will rarely produce recognizable seizures in the fetus. And although recent advances in ultrasonographic diagnosis have been made, there is still speculation that fetal seizures are likely to be grossly underrepresented (Maouris, 1987) and generally indiscernible to the mother or otherwise mistaken for normal fetal movement unless they are generalized tonic–clonic seizures.

Neonatal Seizures

A neonatal seizure can occur from birth up to about 1 month of age. Most neonatal seizures occur over a short span of time (e.g. several days), and fewer than half of infants experiencing neonatal seizures develop seizures later in life (Scher, Trucco, Beggarly, Steppe, & Macpherson, 1998). These benign seizures have been categorized as a separate epileptic syndrome and are referred to as either *benign nonfamilial neonatal seizures* or *benign idiopathic neonatal seizures* when there is not a family history, or *benign familial neonatal convulsions* or *benign familial neonatal seizures* (Claes et al., 2004). Although there is speculation that benign neonatal idiopathic seizures may differ from benign familial neonatal seizures, the diagnostic criteria used to differentiate the groups are mainly based on the presence of a family history of seizures or epilepsy in the familial group (Plouin & Anderson, 2002).

Benign familial neonatal seizures usually begin 2 or 3 days after birth and spontaneously resolve by 6 months of age. Minimal or no intellectual or cognitive sequelae are known to result. Nonfamilial neonatal seizures are extremely rare after 2 months of age, and the neonatal seizure is typically symptomatic of some central nervous system (CNS) disturbance (e.g., neurodevelopmental anomalies, withdrawal from maternal drug addiction, pyridoxine dependence, metabolic disturbance, intracranial infection). Diagnosis of neonatal seizures is difficult, due to both the variation in seizure expression and the need for astute and careful behavioral observation.

Drawing on his observations and clinical studies, Volpe (1989) proposed a separate neonate seizure classification, based on a newborn's limited behavioral repertoire and resulting seizure manifestation. The neonate not only has a more limited behavioral repertoire than the older child, but also has a vastly different level of cortical maturity. This neuronal immaturity has implications for the newborn brain's ability to propagate, spread, and inhibit abnormal firing that could result in a seizure. Neurodevelopmental aspects of seizures in the neonate are also evidenced by the differential manifestation of seizures in full-term versus premature infants. In general, the younger the neonate is (neurodevelopmentally speaking), the more primitive is the seizure manifestation.

There are four major classes of neonatal seizures (*subtle, tonic, clonic,* and *myoclonic*). Subtle seizures appear to be the most commonly observed type of neonatal seizure. Subtle seizures can be subclassified, according to their manifestations, into those with motor, oral buccal, eye, or apneic involvement. Subtle motor seizures manifest themselves as repetitive swimming, rowing, and pedaling behaviors of the upper or lower extremities. Subtle oral buccal seizures are manifested as lip-smacking, chewing, and sucking behaviors. Subtle eye seizures manifest themselves as deviant horizontal eye movements and sustained blinking or opening of eyes. Subtle seizures that are manifested as apnea are very rare, and most neonatal apnea is not indicative of seizures unless there are other symptoms present suggesting seizure activity (Simeonsson & Hillenbrand, 2007). Tonic, clonic, and myoclonic neonatal seizures may be subclassified into focal and generalized seizures, and myoclonic seizures may also be multifocal. There is some limited evidence of lesional relationship to seizure manifestations. Focal clonic seizures in the neonate may occur with local cortical lesions or may be due to metabolic abnormality (Simeonsson & Hillenbrand, 2007). Widespread cortical lesions may result in generalized tonic or multifocal clonic seizures. Myoclonic seizures are also observed in the neonate, and generalized tonic–clonic seizures are very rarely observed. The classification of neonatal seizures proposed by Volpe (1989) and diagnostic notes are presented in Table 24.1.

International Classification of Seizures

The international classification scheme is the most widely accepted and utilized format for clinical classification of epileptic seizure disorders. Its rough division of seizure types was first conceived by Gowers in 1885 (see the reprinted original—Gowers, 1885/1964), but was further developed and refined by the International League Against Epilepsy's

TABLE 24.1. Neonatal Seizure Classification

Seizure type	Behavioral manifestation and general diagnostic notes
Subtle	Stereotyped and involuntary movements; normal EEG
Motor	Swimming, rowing, pedaling in upper or lower extremities
Oral	Lip smacking, chewing, sucking
Eyes	Horizontal deviation, blinking, sustained open eyes
Apneic	Rare on their own but may occur with subtle oral seizures
Clonic	Abnormal EEG associated with underlying pathology
Focal	Rhythmic unilateral involvement of the limbs, face, or trunk
Generalized	Bilateral or shifting involvement
Tonic	More common in premature infants; normal EEG
Focal	Sustained posturing of one limb
Generalized	Sustained posturing of all limbs
Myoclonic	
Focal	Sudden flexion or extension of large muscle groups; normal EEG
Multifocal	More than one muscle group involved; normal EEG
Generalized	All muscle groups; may be accompanied by abnormal EEG

Note. From Volpe (1989). Copyright 1989 by *Pediatrics.* Adapted by permission of *Pediatrics.*

(ILAE's) Commission on Classification and Terminology in 1989. Although the ILAE is currently working on an updated or entirely new classification, the guidelines set forth in 1989 are those currently used in research and practice. In this conceptualization, seizures are broadly classified as being either partial or generalized, and then further subclassified according to their behavioral manifestations. Although many variations of this classification system exist, one such variation is presented here as Table 24.2.

Partial seizures (previously referred to as *focal* or *local* seizures) are initially limited to one hemisphere. The onset of a seizure and most of its initial manifestation are limited. Partial seizures can be further subclassified into *simple* and *complex* partial seizures, depending on whether consciousness is altered. When consciousness remains intact, the seizure is termed a simple partial seizure. The manifestations of these types of seizures can then be further subclassified into those affecting motor skills or those involving sensory symptoms. Complex partial seizures affect consciousness.

Seizures whose onset involves both hemispheres are termed *primary generalized* seizures. These seizures can be convulsive or nonconvulsive and can also be subclassified into *absence* (petit mal or staring spells), *myoclonic*, and *tonic–clonic* (grand mal) seizures. Partial seizures of any type may become generalized seizures and are thus

TABLE 24.2. International Classification of Seizures

I. Partial/focal epilepsies
  A. Symptomatic (note that as imaging technology improves, more and more epilepsies are being reclassified as being symptomatic)
    1. Rasmussen syndrome
    2. Syndromes characterized by seizures with specific modes of precipitation
    3. Partial epilepsies with a lobe of origin (e.g., temporal lobe epilepsy)
  B. Idiopathic (including, but not limited to the following)
    1. Benign childhood epilepsy with centrotemporal spike
    2. Childhood epilepsy with occipital paroxysms
    3. Primary reading epilepsy
  C. Cryptogenic

II. Generalized epilepsies
  A. Symptomatic (note that as imaging technology improves, more and more epilepsies are being reclassified as being symptomatic)
    1. Nonspecific etiologies
    2. Specific etiologies
  B. Idiopathic
    1. Benign neonatal convulsions (familial and nonfamilial)
    2. Benign myoclonic epilepsy in infancy
    3. Childhood absence epilepsy
    4. Juvenile absence epilepsy
    5. Juvenile myoclonic epilepsy
  C. Cryptogenic
    1. Infantile spasms (West syndrome)
    2. Lennox–Gastaut syndrome
    3. Epilepsy with myoclonic–astatic seizures
    4. Epilepsy with myoclonic absences

III. Epileptic syndromes with undetermined focal or generalized seizures
  A. Neonatal seizures (see Table 22.1)
  B. Severe myoclonic epilepsy in infancy

IV. Special syndromes
  A. Febrile seizures
  B. Status epilepticus
  C. Seizures in reaction to specific environmental stressors

Note. Adapted from Commission on Classification and Terminology (1989). Not all syndromes addressed by the Commission are included here.

termed *secondary generalized* seizures or *secondary generalizations*.

Classification by Specific Childhood Epilepsy Syndromes

The third method of classification is probably the most useful when one is considering childhood epilepsy because virtually all of these syndromes are age-related. Table 24.3 provides a quick reference of childhood epilepsy syndromes, along with the peak onset ages and hallmark features of each syndrome.

Infantile Spasms/West Syndrome

Infantile spasms usually appear between the ages of 4 and 8 months. They rarely occur before 2 months of age or after 1 year. Etiology may be genetic (e.g., an inherited condition called tuberous sclerosis), or it may be attributable to a host of other etiologies, including birth injury or metabolic imbalances. Approximately 60% of infantile spasms are generally considered to be symptomatic of brain disorder or brain injury; the remaining cases are considered idiopathic or cryptogenic.

Infantile spasms are characterized by a very specific seizure manifestation. The infant experiences a sudden flexion of the entire body, with knees flexed, arms extended, and head tucked. This position is held for a couple of seconds and is repeated every few seconds. The spasms occur in definite sets of 5, 10, or 15. That is, the alternations between flexion and relaxation (separated by a few seconds) occur in sets of 5, 10, or 15. They most often occur in the transitional period between sleep and wakefulness. These seizures are most often treated with medications such as adrenocorticotropic hormone or traditional antiepileptic drugs (AEDs), and if uncontrolled, the child's epilepsy may evolve into the Lennox–Gastaut syndrome (at about age 3 or 4). Uncontrolled infantile spasms progressing into Lennox–Gastaut syndrome can result in some degree of impaired intellectual functioning, behavioral disturbances, and developmental delays or a regression in developmental milestones.

TABLE 24.3. Childhood Epilepsy Syndromes, Their Peak Onset Range, and Hallmark Features

Epilepsy syndrome	Peak age at onset	Hallmark features
Infantile spasms/West syndrome	4 to 8 months	Definite sets (5, 10, or 15) of flexion–extension
Infantile myoclonic epilepsy	1 to 2 years	Flexion–extension in single or cluster events, not sets
Febrile seizures	6 to 24 months	Precipitated by a high fever with a fast rise
Myoclonic–astatic epilepsy/ Doose syndrome	2 to 5 years	Manifestation is complex and can include all seizure types
Lennox–Gastaut syndrome	3 to 4 years	Specific triad: tonic–clonic seizures, abnormal EEG, mental retardation
Progressive unilateral encephalopathy/ Rasmussen syndrome	3 to 10 years	Focal seizures that move to produce a series of distinct focal seizures; moderate intellectual decline
Benign rolandic epilepsy	4 to 10 years	Seizure occurrence during sleep or onset; remits in adolescence
Epilepsy with myoclonic absences	6 to 7 years	Absence seizures with bilateral clonic jerks
Childhood absence epilepsy	7 years	Frequent staring spells daily
Juvenile absence epilepsy	12 to 13 years	Less frequent staring spells, fewer than one per day
Juvenile myoclonic epilepsy	14 to 15 years	Bilateral, irregular jerking on awakening from sleep; frequently elicited by sleep deprivation and fatigue

Infantile Myoclonic Epilepsy

Infantile myoclonic epilepsy occurs in children during their first or second year of life who are otherwise normal in development but who have a familial history of epilepsy. Its etiology is usually symptomatic of some CNS abnormality, but may remain cryptogenic for some time.

The seizure manifestation, as its name suggests, involves brief episodes of muscular contractions that can occur as one brief episode or in clusters. The classic form of it consists of a sudden flexion or extension of the trunk and/or limbs. It is differentiated from infantile spasms by the lack of dependable serial clustering in contraction. The EEG is often normal initially, but may later be characterized by bursts of spike–wave and polyspike–wave complexes. Intellectual development may be mildly delayed, and some minor personality change may occur (Commission on Classification and Terminology, 1989), but the general outlook is good.

Febrile Seizures

It is estimated that the prevalence of febrile seizures is between 3% and 8% in children under the age of 8 years old (Sadlier & Scheffer, 2007). The onset of febrile seizures most commonly occurs between the ages of 6 months and 6 years; the median age of onset is 18 months. More than half of the cases of febrile seizures occur between 12 and 30 months (American Academy of Pediatrics, Committee on Quality Improvement, 1999; Offringa et al., 1994). They are reliably elicited by a rapidly evolving and very high fever, but their occurrence is also dependent on age and cortical maturity, as well as familial history/genetic predisposition (Degan, Degan, & Hans, 1991). Thus febrile seizures are often considered the paradigm for age-dependent epilepsies because of their consistent and direct interdependence on three factors; age, genetics, and environmental factors.

Febrile seizures can be subclassified into simple and complex categories, although the use of the terms *simple* and *complex* can be misleading. A simple febrile seizure is a purely reactive, single, uncomplicated febrile seizure episode. Complex febrile seizures start with a focal seizure, and the seizure episode lasts longer than 15 minutes and occurs repeatedly within a 24-hour period. In approximately 90% of children, the duration of the febrile seizure is less than 10 minutes; only approximately 10% of children experience seizures lasting longer than 15 minutes (Berg & Shinnar, 1996).

Febrile seizures typically have an excellent outcome and are associated with normal intellect and the absence of long-lasting, detrimental effects. Therefore, treatment of febrile seizures with AEDs is often discouraged unless children exhibit recurrent prolonged seizures, due to the adverse effects AEDs may have on behavior, cognitive processes, and intellectual development, as well as other health factors (e.g., they can cause liver damage). However, acute treatment may be indicated for prolonged seizures lasting longer than 5 minutes, including rectal diazepam and buccal or intranasal midazolam (Bhattacharyya, Kalra, & Gulati, 2006; McIntyre et al., 2005).

Up to 30% of all children who experience a febrile seizure may experience a second febrile seizure (depending on a variety of predisposing factors). Between 2% and 20% of children who experience febrile seizures will develop a nonfebrile seizure disorder (epilepsy).

Myoclonic–Astatic Epilepsy (Doose Syndrome)

Myoclonic–astatic epilepsy (a.k.a. Doose syndrome) has a complex seizure manifestation, which can include myoclonic, astatic, myoclonic–astatic, tonic absence, clonic absence, and tonic–clonic seizures. It occurs in children between the ages of 7 months and 6 years, but prevalence rates peak in children between the ages of 2 and 5 years who have developed normally up to that point. Those with myoclonic–astatic epilepsy usually have a family history of idiopathic generalized epilepsy. The progression of the syndrome is variable, but status frequently occurs, and the progression into a tonic epilepsy syndrome is not associated with a favorable prognosis.

Lennox–Gastaut Syndrome

Lennox–Gastaut syndrome usually appears in children at about age 3 or 4 (but spans the ages from 1 to 8) who have previously experienced uncontrolled infantile spasms. However, the syndrome can also appear in otherwise healthy children and adolescents without any apparent precursor. The onset of the syndrome may be accompanied by a cessation of intellectual development. Development after onset for some children may be severely arrested; for other affected children, it may be less severely affected. The syndrome is accompanied by a very abnormal and easily recognizable EEG of spike-and-wave discharge superimposed on abnormal background activity. Thus it is characterized by a specific triad: seizures, abnormal EEG, and some degree of mental retardation.

The seizure manifestation is similar to infantile spasms (sudden flexion of the body), but does not appear in definitive series. The child, who is now walking, experiences the sudden body flexion (a.k.a. myoclonic, atonic, or akinetic seizures) and often falls to the ground. The syndrome is severe and appears to be a combination of seizure types, including focal and/or multifocal generalized tonic, tonic–clonic, myoclonic, atonic, and absence seizures. These seizures are unpredictable, are difficult to control, and occur with increased frequency as the syndrome progresses. Thus many children with this syndrome are very sheltered and wear protective headgear.

It is notable, however, that although most of the literature supports this severe sequence of events associated with Lennox–Gastaut syndrome, there have been reports of less severe developmental sequelae. Longitudinal studies following children with the syndrome indicate that they may be capable of attaining low-average intellect and full-time work. It thus seems that these children can fare reasonably well with a combination of educational, psychosocial, and pharmaceutical intervention (S. Goldstein, personal communication, September 22, 1997; Yagi, 1996).

Progressive Unilateral Encephalopathy/ Rasmussen Syndrome

Progressive unilateral encephalopathy (a.k.a. Rasmussen syndrome) is a devastating syndrome that appears in healthy and apparently typically developing children between the ages of 3 and 10. It strikes without warning, and the initial episode is usually a severe generalized seizure that has no precipitating incident. A child then experiences focal seizures that increase in frequency. These focal seizures will gradually become more intense (but will not become multifocal), until more than half of these children experience a continuous focal seizure (epilepsy partialis continua).

The syndrome then progresses to surrounding areas of the initial foci and will spread in concentric circles until the entire hemisphere is involved. Note, however, that the seizure does not generalize. Rather, the focal seizure will move from the initial loci to a conjoining area, and the function associated with that cortical area will become the manifestation of the seizure. The manifestation will eventually change again to whatever behavior or function is associated with the area adjoining the second foci.

The progressive deterioration occurring with Rasmussen syndrome usually results in a variable degree of intellectual and language impairment that ranges from mild to severe. Its progression appears unstoppable, but some children have responded well to radical hemispherectomy. Such children often experience some improvement in intellectual functioning. Research has also pointed to the cause of Rasmussen encephalopathy as being an autoimmune disorder in which antibodies bind to and overstimulate gluatamate receptors in the brain. Promising but not yet definitive research has indicated that effective short-term treatment may be found in techniques such as plasma exchange, in which the antibodies are filtered from the blood (Palcoux et al., 2007). Thus far, however, this treatment has had limited success, and patients have relapsed after a few months. Although there does not appear to be one course of action that is effective for all individuals with Rasmussen syndrome, the European consensus group has provided a well thought-out algorithm for the clinical management of these patients. The treatment model proposes immunotherapy, hemispherectomy, medication, or minimal therapy, based on the needs of each individual patient (Bien et al., 2005).

Benign Rolandic Epilepsy

The onset of benign rolandic epilepsy typically occurs between the ages of 4 and 10. There is frequently a genetic component involved in cases of benign rolandic epilepsy, and it is thought to be an autosomal dominant inherited disorder. Seizures most frequently occur at night, during sleep or sleep onset, and can be partial or generalized seizures that are accompanied by centrotemporal spikes in the EEG. The seizure disorder usually remits on its own in adolescence.

Epilepsy with Myoclonic Absences

The combination of absence seizures interspersed with bilateral clonic jerks defines epilepsy with myoclonic absences. Seizures may occur frequently throughout a typical day, but are thought to decrease in frequency as sleep stages progress. AED therapy is difficult, and cognitive impairment and progression to other forms of epilepsy (such as Lennox–Gastaut syndrome) may occur. The EEG is strikingly characteristic in that the abnormal activity, similar to that of childhood absence epilepsy, is characterized by reliably occurring bilateral synchronous spike-and-wave discharges.

Childhood Absence Epilepsy

Childhood absence epilepsy (a.k.a. pyknoepilepsy or petit mal epilepsy) typically occurs in children between the ages of 4 and 8, with peak manifestation between the ages of 6 and 7. It is thought to be a complex polygenic disorder, and prevalence rates for childhood absence epilepsy are higher for those with a family history of epilepsy. Concordance studies in monozygotic twins have been reported at 70–85% (Berkovic, 1998). The prevalence is thought to be higher in females than in males, although equal prevalence in girls and boys has been reported in numerous studies. Several absences (staring spells) a day are experienced, and EEG study may reveal spike-and-wave activity superimposed on a normal background. Generalized tonic–clonic seizures may surface during adolescence in approximately 40% of children with absence seizures.

Juvenile Absence Epilepsy

The seizure manifestation of juvenile absence epilepsy looks very much like that of childhood absence epilepsy, but the frequency of seizure occurrence is much lower. Seizures typically are fewer than one per day. Onset occurs between the ages of 10 and 17, with a peak onset at about age 12. Absence seizures may be accompanied by generalized tonic–clonic seizures or myoclonus seizures. Generalized tonic–clonic seizures also frequently precede the onset of a juvenile absence epilepsy syndrome. EEG study may reveal spike-and-wave discharges that are greater than 3 Hz in frequency.

Juvenile Myoclonic Epilepsy

Juvenile myoclonic epilepsy is characterized by bilateral, irregular jerking in the upper extremities upon awakening. It appears at about puberty in normal adolescents and frequently persists into adulthood. It typically manifests itself between the ages of 12 and 18, with a peak onset between the ages of 14 and 15. Juvenile myoclonic epilepsy is frequently (approximately 90–95% of cases) accompanied by generalized tonic–clonic seizures, and less frequently (approximately 30% of cases) also by absence seizures (Baykan et al., 2008; Panayiotopoulos, Obeid, & Waheed, 1989; Renganathan & Delaney, 2003). It has a fairly strong familial occurrence rate; it is thought to be transmitted as a Mendelian dominant or recessive trait or possibly as complex oligogenic traits (Delgado-Escueta, 2007). Over half of individuals with juvenile myoclonic epilepsy have first- and second-degree relatives with some form of epilepsy (Delgado-Escueta et al., 1989). Heavy consumption of alcohol, photosensitizing lights, fatigue, and sleep deprivation have all been identified as possible precipitating factors, but sleep deprivation has been identified as the most common trigger, accounting for approximately 75–90% of juvenile myoclonic seizures (Dhanuka, Jain, Daljit, & Maheshwari, 2001; Panayiotopoulos, Obeid, & Tahan, 1994). The prognosis for intellectual development is good. The presence of intellectual or neurological decline should lead one to suspect progressive myoclonic epilepsy rather than juvenile myoclonic epilepsy.

NEUROPSYCHOLOGICAL SEQUELAE ASSOCIATED WITH EPILEPSY

Intellectual and cognitive impairments in people with epilepsy, especially memory deficits, were observed and noted in the literature over 100 years ago. Unfortunately, there is increasing evidence that cognitive deficits result not only from seizures themselves, but from the use of many (if not most) AEDs. Therefore, AEDs may compound the cognitive difficulties and behavioral problems seen in persons with epilepsy (American Academy of Pediatrics, Committee on Drugs, 1985; Bootsma et al., 2006; Drane & Meador, 2002; Loring & Meador, 2001; Ortinski & Meador, 2004). The following discussion is based in large part on Bennett (1992) and Bennett and Ho (1997). The specific cognitive effects of AEDs are not addressed here, and the interested reader is referred to Bennett and Ho for specific information.

The apparent association between cognitive impairment and epilepsy has been observed for several centuries. Dewhurst (1980) uncovered a reference in Thomas Willis's 17th-century lectures at Oxford University to the losses in memory, intellect, and reality testing that persons experience during and after seizures. Physicians continued to note the frequent co-occurrence of cognitive impairment with epilepsy throughout the 19th century and into the middle of the 20th century. As research continued to examine the relationship of epilepsy and cognitive impairment, it became apparent that intellectual decline was not as pervasive as was formerly believed. Various sampling errors and design methodology oversights (e.g., studying institutionalized patients, lack of control for medication types and levels, lack of control for type of seizures studied) were proffered as explanations. Another major issue was the rather primitive means of assessing cognitive functioning available in that era. Early studies largely depended on IQ testing as their major objective measure. Although IQ testing can provide a relatively sound measure of a person's biological level of adaptive functioning, it is highly dependent on achievement. In addition, IQ testing is not sensitive to the cognitive effects of brain injury, and the relationship of recurrent seizure disorders to brain injury is obvious.

Neuropsychological Assessment in Childhood Epilepsy

Rather than using IQ as a measure of cognitive functions, recent research has adopted a cognitive process approach to evaluating cognitive abilities in epileptic populations. The cognitive processes investigated have included sensory functions, attention and sustained concentration, learning and memory, language skills, perceptual abilities, conceptualization and reasoning, and motor abilities. The majority of studies have not investigated all of these processes, and within a given process such as attention, one is struck by the fact that few investigators use the same task. Second, a test may not evaluate what it purports to evaluate; for instance, a "test of memory" may require high levels of attention for success. Poor performance may also be a consequence of impaired language or conceptualization processes.

This last difficulty can potentially be circumvented by utilizing a comprehensive battery approach in assessment, such as the Halstead–Reitan Neuropsychological Test Battery (Reitan & Wolfson, 1985). Reitan (1974) believed that this approach would be sensitive to the aggregate of cognitive impairments that might characterize a particular type of epilepsy under investigation. Carl Dodrill further refined the battery approach in the assessment of individuals with epilepsy (see Dodrill, 1978, 1981) by expanding the Halstead–Reitan Battery to optimally assess cognitive deficits associated with epilepsy. His Neuropsychological Battery for Epilepsy uses 16 measures of performance (as well as other psychosocial and empirically pertinent measures, such as familial history of seizure disorders), and he established norms that reliably distinguish the performance of patients with epilepsy from that of closely matched control subjects. Dodrill's battery, and the general application of neuropsychological test battery approaches to evaluate the cognitive effects associated with epilepsy, represent advances. Unfortunately, the most common approach still remains narrow, and the majority of inquiries on this topic have continued to focus on a single type, or only a few types, of cognitive ability.

When competently provided, a neuropsychological assessment can be a valuable aid in establishing a severity of cognitive impairments and monitoring the effects of treatments for a seizure disorder. Although the vast majority of children with epilepsy retain normal levels of intellectual functioning, they are disproportionately skewed toward the lower end of average IQ levels. This is presumably due to the underlying pathophysiology of the epileptic syndrome.

The importance of understanding a child's intellectual capabilities is key to being able to decipher underlying causes of poor academic performance. Material beyond a child's difficulty level, or boredom with material beneath his or her level, can each lead to poor academic performance. Frustration with these academic difficulties and with misplaced parental and teacher expectations can lead the child to behave in improper manners during school and thus to be classified as having behavioral problems. Pressures to perform at unrealistic levels by parents and teachers may be alleviated early in the child's academic career by recognizing the contributions and appropriateness of intelligence testing to academic placement and performance. Learning problems due to interrupted auditory or visual information processing secondary to the seizure activity are common. Lack of concentration and distractibility are also more common in children with epilepsy than in children without such conditions. Particular care must be taken to evaluate the possible influences of AEDs on learning, behavioral, and attentional deficiencies, as they all can cause problems (Loring, Marino, & Meador, 2007; Vermeulen & Aldenkamp, 1995). Such sequelae are common causes of academic difficulties in children with epilepsy, and careful evaluation of the causes of academic problems must be made.

A Neuropsychological Model of Brain Functioning

To appreciate fully the effects of epilepsy on cognitive processes, it is helpful to consider these processes within a theoretical or conceptual model of the behavioral correlates of brain functioning. In our own conceptualizations, we have found it helpful to expand on and modify the model presented by Reitan and Wolfson (1985), which denotes six categories of brain–behavior relationships. Bennett (1988) has expanded the number of categories to seven, in order to separate attention from memory and to emphasize the dependence of memory on attention and concentration. He has also expanded on their level of logical analysis and renamed it

executive functions. Note that this is a process model, not an anatomical model. With the exceptions of (1) language skills and (2) visual–spatial skills, visual construction, and perceptual–motor skills—which are primarily represented in the left and right hemispheres, respectively—these processes are bilaterally represented. This model is diagrammed in Figure 24.1.

According to this model, the first level of neuropsychological processing is input to the brain via one of the sensory systems. It should be remembered that input can also arise endogenously from within the brain. The input must be attended to or concentrated on for information processing to occur and for the significance of the input to be ascertained (second level). Determining the significance of the stimulus or remembering it for later reference requires involvement of the memory system (third level).

The interdependence of attention and memory illustrates the fact that this neural system is dynamic, with activity flowing in both directions. In general, if information is to be remembered, it must be attended to (although, on the other hand, attention is no guarantee for memory). Similarly, attention is dependent on memory in terms of attentional processes' being involved in such activities as habituation and filtering of gated-out, irrelevant information.

Input material that is verbal in nature requires the processing activities of a fourth neuropsychological category, language skills. Nonverbal material similarly requires processing mechanisms of a fifth category: visual–spatial skills, visual construction, and perceptual–motor skills.

Executive functions represent the highest level of information processing. These activities are involved in logical analysis, conceptualization, planning, self-monitoring, and flexibility of thinking. Poor performance on tests of executive functions can result from a primary deficit in these functions themselves, or it can result from a primary deficit in one of the lower levels of processing on which executive functions depend. Executive functions quickly become quite impaired in a person who is distractible, forgetful, and/or language-impaired, or who cannot perform higher-level perceptual processes.

Motor functions are the basis for responding and represent the final common path of

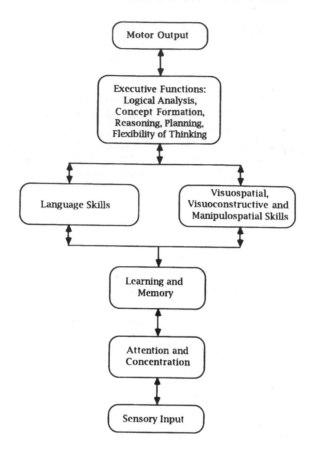

FIGURE 24.1. Conceptual model of the behavioral correlates of brain functioning (after Reitan & Wolfson, 1985). From Bennett (1988). Copyright 1988 by *Journal of Cognitive Rehabilitation*. Reprinted by permission.

the neuropsychological processes. They reflect the output capabilities of the system. This is the rationale for placing motor output at the top of the diagram. With this neuropsychological model as a backdrop, the effects of epilepsy on specific cognitive processes can be discussed.

Effects of Epilepsy on Specific Cognitive Processes

Sensory Input

Both impairment and exaggeration of sensory input can be said to result from seizures. Absence or petit mal attacks are generalized nonconvulsive seizures that occur particularly in children. They are characterized by brief episodes of loss of consciousness lasting approximately 5–15 seconds. During these episodes, a child seems to be unaware of his or her surroundings, and stares with a vacant expression. Sensory input occurring during these periods is neither attended to nor registered.

Complex partial seizures, on the other hand, may be manifested as sensory misperceptions and/or hallucinations. Misperceptions are often visual and complex. They typically involve distortions in depth perceptions or size. Size misperceptions can result in objects' being perceived as much smaller (micropsia) or larger (macropsia) than they are. Visual misperceptions reflect a posterior temporal lobe seizure focus. For example, they were observed to occur in a patient of ours prior to discovery of a right temporal lobe astrocytoma, and they diminished following its removal.

Misperception of voices results from a focal discharge of the anterior temporal lobe neocortex, especially from the left hemisphere. Voices may be perceived as too high or too low in pitch, or as being too loud or soft. The patient may complain that the voices around him or her sound as if they are "coming out of a tunnel."

Hallucinations or auras that are experienced by patients with complex partial seizures are typically simple. In general, olfactory–gustatory sensations, which are often quite displeasing, result from a focal discharge in the uncus of the hippocampus. Our patients who experience these auras most typically report salty or bitter taste sensations, and/or olfactory sensations best described as "burning flesh" or "putrid." One patient—whose seizures were particularly refractory to AED therapy, and who experienced secondary generalized seizures that were correlated with menstruation—was anosmic except when she experienced olfactory auras just prior to and during menstruation each month.

Abdominal and epigastric sensations typically arise from an amygdala focus. Simple auditory phenomena, such as buzzing, ringing, and hissing sounds, are produced by focal activity on the surface of the temporal lobe, especially the primary auditory reception area. Complex visual hallucinations, although uncommon, arise from pathological excitation of visual cortical areas, especially the posterior parietal or temporal association cortex (Manford & Andermann, 1998).

Cephalgic auras reflect discharge originating in the central regions of the temporal lobes. They consist of severe, sharp, stabbing, knife-like head pains that are often associated with the head's feeling too big, too small, or off the body. Cephalgic auras will occasionally be misdiagnosed as migraine headaches and subsequently incorrectly medicated.

An important feature of auras is that they are passive experiences. The patient feels like an observer of these ictal (seizure-related) events, dissociated from the actual experience. This is different from the experience of an individual with schizophrenia, who firmly believes that his or her hallucinations are "real" experiences. The ictal events are unrelated to the environment, except for rare seizures that are triggered by specific stimuli (e.g., musicogenic seizures, sexual seizures). We once had a patient whose seizures were reliably triggered whenever he played the arcade game Foosball! More typically for the patient with complex partial seizures, the ictal events begin spontaneously with an arrest of all activity, and the aura and/or psychomotor responses follow. Finally, while attention is usually paid to the most salient attribute of the epileptic patient's aura, the dream-like quality of the epileptic aura will often encompass many experiences. For example, a patient of ours regularly experienced a series of events including epigastric sensations, time distortion, detachment from her surroundings, and olfactory sensations as components of her seizure episodes.

Attention and Concentration

Impairment of attention and concentration, in the absence of overt clinical seizures, has been documented by several writers. Teacher and caretaker ratings for children with epilepsy frequently note marked inattentiveness and the detrimental effects of epilepsy-associated inattention on academic success (Huberty, Austin, Harczlak, Dunn, & Ambrosius, 2000; Titus, Kanive, Sanders, & Blackburn, 2008).

Keene and colleagues (2005) studied 158 children with epilepsy of varying etiologies and found that attentional deficits were one of the key problems noted in these children. Specifically, approximately 30% of the children with epilepsy in this study were described by their parents as having attention problems that were more than two standard deviations above the mean for the normative sample. Fastenau and colleagues (2004) also found poorer performance on attentional measures in children with chronic seizures than in normative samples.

Specific attentional difficulties in epilepsy appear to be related to seizure type. Patients with generalized seizures show greater impairment on measures of sustained attention than patients with focal seizures do. It has been argued that this occurs because generalized seizures are more likely than focal seizures to affect the central subcortical structures that are responsible for maintaining attention.

In contrast, limited studies have suggested that patients with focal seizures show more impairment on tests of selective attention than patients with generalized seizures do

(Loiseau, Signoret, & Strube, 1984). One argument for this finding is that subcortical structures are important in determining what to pay attention to (selective attention) (Stores, 1984). However, more recent research has argued that despite the significant literature suggesting that individuals with epilepsy are at significant risk for attentional deficits, results from studies assessing specific risk factors in terms of seizure type have not been consistent (Dunn & Kronenberger, 2006). Specifically, an example from Dunn and Kronenberger's review addresses seizure focus—a facet of seizures that might be expected to predict different types of attentional deficits depending on the foci, but does not consistently suggest a fixed pattern of deficits across studies. For example, past findings suggest that frontal lobe foci may pose a greater risk for attentional deficits (Hernandez et al., 2003; Sherman, Armitage, Connolly, Wambera, & Strauss, 2000); other researchers argue that in fact temporal lobe foci may pose more risk (Stores, 1978); and the authors of two larger studies argue that there is no association between foci and attentional problems (Dunn, Austin, Harezlak, & Ambrosius, 2003; Hesdorffer et al., 2004). Therefore, while there is consensus regarding the role of attentional deficits in epilepsy, there is still further research needed to elucidate the role of chronicity, foci, medication, and comorbidity in the development of attentional deficits in this population.

Learning and Memory

Deficits in the ability to learn and remember material on a daily basis have been noted by teachers and parents of children with epilepsy for many years. Wilson, Ivani-Chalain, Besag, and Bryant (1993) have used a children's version of the Rivermead Behavioral Memory Test to demonstrate everyday memory difficulties encountered by children with severe epilepsies. More recent research suggested that everyday memory problems may be a problem in children with epilepsy, but noted that attention problems may be the core cognitive deficit underlying these problems (Kadis, Stollstorff, Elliott, Lach, & Smith, 2003).

Evidence has accumulated associating memory deficits with temporal lobe epilepsy (TLE). In an early study that compared cognitive abilities in patients with generalized seizures to patients with focal complex partial seizures of temporal lobe origin, Quadfasel and Pruyser (1955) found that memory impairment was significant only in the group with focal seizures. Since that original study, a multitude of studies have been published supporting the key role of the hippocampus and temporal lobe in relationship to memory problems in epilepsy (Adda, Castro, Alem-Mar, de Manreza, & Kashiara, 2008; Messas, Mansur, & Castro, 2008; Powell et al., 2007).

There has also been a great deal of research on both adults and children suggesting that focal seizures of left temporal lobe origin yield greater verbal than nonverbal deficits, and that the opposite pattern is obtained with right temporal lobe dysfunction (Jambaque, Dellatolas, Dulac, Ponsot, & Signoret, 1993; Majdan, Sziklas, & Jones-Gotman, 1996; Powell et al., 2007). The lateralizing effect on memory has also been supported in studies utilizing EEG and functional magnetic resonance imaging (Binder et al., 2008; Vannucci, 2007). However, in children specifically, several studies suggest that the lateralization effects seen in adults are not as robust in early development (Bell & Davies, 1998; Giovagnoli, Erbetta, Villani, & Avanzini, 2005; Gonzalez, Anderson, Mitchell, & Harvey, 2007).

One potential argument for the discordant findings in the literature regarding lateralization focuses on the disparity in tests that have been used to assess verbal and nonverbal skills. Gonzalez and colleagues (2007) point out that tests assessing nonverbal skills (specifically, nonverbal memory measures) are likely to recruit several different neural mechanisms, depending on the requirements of each task. For example, within the epilepsy literature, nonverbal memory tests requiring memory for the location of objects relative to the environment (i.e., allocentric memory) and facial recognition have shown impairment more consistently than nonverbal memory measures requiring recall of geometric designs have (Abrahams, Pickering, Polkey, & Morris, 1997; Barr et al., 1997; Chiaravalloti & Glosser, 2004; Feigenbaum & Morris, 2004). These disparities are probably due to specific cognitive requirements involved in each type of task and the areas of the brain recruited for each task. Gonzalez and colleagues point out that children with mesial versus lateral temporal lobe epilepsy may exhibit very different types of memory impairment, similar to the pattern seen in adults (Helmstaedter, Grunwald, Lehnertz, Gleißner, & Elger, 1997).

An additional difficulty in detecting and addressing the memory difficulties experienced by persons with epilepsy is evidenced by their lack of insight into their own memory difficulties. This "metamemory" deficit in association with temporal lobe seizure foci has been noted over the years and suggests that individuals with TLE have poorer insight and self-monitoring skills with regard to memory (Deutsch, Saykin, & Sperling, 1996; Prevey, Delaney, & Mattson, 1988).

Taken together, these studies suggest a significant impairment of memory functions in patients with seizures of temporal lobe origin. However, the vast research on memory processes alone illustrates the difficulties encountered in attempting to evaluate specific cognitive processes in patients with epilepsy.

Language Skills

Both experimental inquiry and clinical observation have long indicated that epilepsy may adversely affect language skills and reading acquisition. Williams and colleagues (1996) found that children with uncontrolled seizures (absence or complex partial) had more difficulty with complex verbal materials than children whose seizures were well controlled. Butterbaugh and colleagues (2004) noted learning disabilities in reading comprehension and written language in approximately half of presurgical patients with left temporal lobe epilepsy (52.6% and 42.1%, respectively). An interesting case reported by Vargha-Khadem and colleagues (1997) involved an 8½-year-old child with uncontrolled seizures who underwent radical hemispherectomy of the left hemisphere. Prior to his surgery, the child was mute and had the language comprehension skills of a 3- to 4-year-old. Not only did his seizures remit following the surgery, but he spontaneously regained language development a month after withdrawal of AEDs! These results, among others, have prompted new questions regarding whether the mechanisms of seizure control (usually AEDs) actually have detrimental effects on language skills as severe as those of the epilepsy itself.

Regardless of the mechanisms by which language skills are affected, it is well established that specific language skills can be affected in epilepsy. Robinson (1991) has noted that over 20% of children with language impairment have some history of seizures. This number is significantly greater than the 5–7% seizure prevalence that has been noted in the general childhood population. The possible explanations for the high prevalence in this population have included the following: Seizures may disturb language functioning in the brain; there may be a genetic link between language disability and epilepsy; or brain abnormalities associated with seizures may also contribute to dysfunction in language related skills (Robinson, 1991).

In regard to specific types of language impairment, Parkinson (2002) studied language and communication skills in over 100 children with epilepsy between the ages of 5 and 17 years and found that more than 37% of the children had undiagnosed language impairments. These impairments included (among others) overgeneralized use of grammatical rules and structures; ignoring morphological features and inflectional word endings in the absence of hearing loss; difficulties in comprehension of words with more than one meaning or syntactic role; pragmatic impairment; and anomia. Anomia and dysnomia have been reported in individuals with epilepsy for years, and it has been suggested that dysnomia in this population may be confused with poor memory by both an individual with epilepsy and others (Mayeux, Brandt, Rosen, & Benson, 1980). Mayeux and colleagues (1980) further suggest that the verbosity and circumstantiality observed in some patients with complex partial seizures (e.g., Bennett, 1987) may be the expression of a compensatory mechanism for dysnomia.

Circumstantiality is seen in both the spoken and written communication of these patients. Their spoken communications are often overinclusive and include excessive background detailing, in addition to using excessive words and taking too much time to convey a thought (Bear, Freeman, & Greenberg, 1984; Field, Saling, & Berkovic, 2000). These tendencies can prevent conversations from reaching a normal end, and this style can lead to such patients' being shunned. Hypergraphia (i.e., a tendency toward excessive and compulsive writing) is also often seen in patients with complex partial seizures and was first comprehensively documented in these patients by Waxman and Geschwind (1980). It is often characterized by verbosity and circumstantiality, but it facilitated the writing of the legendary author and victim of complex partial seizures, Feodor Dostoievsky (Geschwind, 1984).

Perceptual–Motor Skills

There has not been a great deal of research investigating the effects of epilepsy on perceptual–motor skills, but the following has been reported. Early research noted total time, memory, and localization scores from the Tactual Performance Test as sensitive measures of the effects of epilepsy on cognitive processes (Dodrill, 1978, 1981). The total time score is a measure of perceptual–motor (manipulospatial) ability. A deficit in spatial memory can be evaluated via the localization score if a significant discrepancy exists between the localization score and the memory score from this task.

More recently, multiple studies have noted visual-perceptual deficits in epilepsy, including facial recognition and spatial judgment. Some studies localize these deficits to the right hippocampal region in TLE, and suggest notably greater deficits in those whose seizures began earlier in life than in those with later onsets (Getz et al., 2002; Hermann et al., 2002; Martin et al., 1999).

Executive Functions

Because of their dependence on lower-level neuropsychological functions, executive functions of the brain involved in such processes as conceptualization, logical analysis, reasoning, planning, sequential thinking, flexibility of thinking, and self-monitoring are especially sensitive to dysfunction, including the types of dysfunction associated with epilepsy. As indicated earlier in this chapter, executive functions will typically be impaired in a person who exhibits distractibility, a poor memory, language impairment, and/or difficulty with perceptual–motor skills. In a general sense, executive functions are the basis for a person's ability to meet the demands of his or her environment effectively. Although these impairments may be easily overlooked, they are commonly seen in individuals with epilepsy, as indicated by

performance on such tests as the Trail Making Tests, the Wisconsin Card Sorting Test (WCST), and the Category Test.

An interesting study by Martin and colleagues (2002) investigated the relationship of various clinical variables and neuroanatomic correlates in TLE to performance on the WCST. Specifically, 89 patients with lateralized TLE (47 left, 42 right) underwent baseline testing on the WCST. Seventy-two patients completed both presurgical and postsurgical assessment following an anterior temporal lobectomy (ATL). The results indicated that those patients with a history of secondary generalized seizures performed worse on the preoperative WCST than did patients without such a history. A more surprising finding was that those patients who were seizure-free after ATL did not perform better on the WCST than those who did not become seizure-free. The authors postulate that the results suggest that temporal lobe structural abnormalities associated with epilepsy do not significantly affect executive function as measured by the WCST. These findings suggest that the critical neurocorrelates of WCST performance in patients with TLE probably lie outside the temporal lobe and most likely are related to metabolic disruption to frontostriatal neural network systems.

Martin and colleagues (2000) also examined the role of bilateral hippocampal sclerosis, extrahippocampal mesial temporal atrophy, and temporal neocortical lesions on WCST performance and found that performance was not significantly affected by any of the types of lesions or atrophy. This finding is in contrast to that of Corcoran and Upton (1993), who utilized a modified WCST with patients who had hippocampal sclerosis associated with TLE. The authors speculated that working memory might play a critical role in WCST performance after they found that patients with hippocampal sclerosis (particularly the patients with right foci) performed more poorly than those with frontal lobe seizure foci (Upton & Corcoran, 1995).

The debate continues regarding the impact of TLE on tasks that are thought to assess frontal or executive functions, as well as in the conceptualization of executive functions. In fact, the *central* executive functions conceptualized and referred to by many authors often overlap with working memory and attention. Thus, amidst the ongoing debates concerning conceptualization and testing of executive functions, there still is no consensus regarding the effects of epilepsy on executive functions independent of other cognitive functions.

Motor Output

Decreased reaction time and psychomotor speed are common difficulties for individuals with epilepsy. Mitchell, Zhou, Chavez, and Guzman (1992) studied simple reaction time, forced-choice reaction time, and choice reaction time with distraction in 112 children with epilepsy. The children with epilepsy were significantly slower, were more variable, and made more omission errors than the controls. This pattern of performance was maintained even when the analysis was limited to only those patients with epilepsy who had IQs greater than 90. And although it was observed that reaction times were related to IQ, they were not generally related to seizure severity, duration of seizure disorder, or duration of medication use. In addition, untreated patients did not differ from those with AED levels in the therapeutic range on the day of testing, but they did differ significantly from controls.

Although reaction time does not typically garner much attention as a core cognitive deficit associated with dysfunction in daily life, McGuckin (1980) has proposed that lack of speed is one of the four main barriers to competitive employment faced by adults with epilepsy, and this same lack of speed may also be conceptualized as a barrier to academic success in children and adolescents (Bennett-Levy & Stores, 1984).

ETIOLOGICAL FACTORS IN THE COGNITIVE DEFICITS ASSOCIATED WITH EPILEPSY

The same factors that influence the development of epilepsy (age, genetics, and environmental stressors) are also related to the cognitive sequelae associated with epilepsy. In addition, the etiology and type of seizures associated with a child's epileptic syndrome have some differential effects on cognition. These differential cognitive sequelae are discussed here.

In general, more significant effects are thought to result if they seizure disorder starts at an early age, if a patient has poor seizure control, if the individual has had the disorder for a relatively long period of time, and if the person exhibits multiple seizure types. Complex partial seizures, particularly those of temporal lobe origin, are typically believed to produce more obvious cognitive and behavioral changes than most other seizure types.

Etiology of the Seizure Disorder

Of the intellectual correlates associated with epilepsy and the variables that alter them, one of the most predictable relationships is that between seizure etiology and IQ. The IQ scores of individuals whose seizures are idiopathic have long been established to be significantly higher than scores attained by patients whose seizures have known etiologies; this is true of both institutionalized and noninstitutionalized children and adults.

The types of cognitive deficits associated with epilepsy vary significantly, depending on the origin of the seizures. A general decline in cognitive functioning has been described as highly comorbid with epilepsy, but particularly so for those individuals who have partial epilepsy with a temporal or frontal lobe origin (Oyegbile et al., 2004). The literature focusing on the relationship between the temporal lobes and cognitive dysfunction is clearly the largest, given that TLE has been the most frequently studied type of epilepsy. Even within this literature, however, there is great disparity by the localization of the focus. Gonzalez and colleagues (2007) studied 43 children with lesional TLE and noted significant differences on a number of cognitive tasks, depending on the localization of the lesion (i.e., left, right, or intratemporal). Among the specific deficits noted, facial recognition was significantly worse in individuals with right TLE than in those with left TLE. Notable differences were noted within the intratemporal group (i.e., mesial or lateral) in terms of arbitrary associative learning and complex figure recall.

In adults, the task of determining cognitive deficits resulting from specific areas of localization becomes even more complicated, due to the influence of other types of pathology and insult that may be introduced with age. Research in our laboratory on the cognitive effects of epilepsy in adults with clear evidence of focal left versus right temporal lobe seizures, but without prior head injury or neurological disease, indicated no lateralized deficits (Haynes & Bennett, 1991). The only trend that appeared was that the subjects with epilepsy as a group exhibited generalized deficits in the areas of psychomotor speed, selective attention, and reasoning ability. This study emphasizes the importance of ruling out underlying cerebral pathology due to head injury or other neurological disease in studying cognitive processes in persons with epilepsy per se.

Seizure Type and Frequency

In addition to seizure etiology, the type and frequency of seizures constitute important variables influencing the nature and extent of intellectual and cognitive dysfunction. A number of studies have shown generalized tonic–clonic seizures to be associated with greater intellectual and cognitive impairment than other types of seizures. Studies over the years have also repeatedly demonstrated, in both children and adults, that frequent generalized seizures are associated with the highest levels of cognitive impairment (vs. less frequent seizures and other types of seizures). The detrimental effect of frequency of seizures on intellectual and cognitive functioning has been shown to be consistent across all seizure types.

Bulteau and colleagues (2000) evaluated 251 children (98 girls and 153 boys) who ranged in age from 3 to 17 years and who all had documented diagnoses of an epileptic syndrome. Information was obtained regarding IQ, school placement, age of onset of seizures, duration of epilepsy, seizure frequency, and number of AEDs. Results suggested that, similar to past findings, age of onset and seizure frequency were both associated with poor outcome. The children with idiopathic generalized or localization-related epilepsy not only had higher IQ scores, but they also had a higher probability of mainstream schooling, than those with symptomatic or cryptogenic generalized epilepsies or those whose etiologies were classified as "undetermined." When the researchers looked at performance on measures within the Wechsler Intelligence Scale for Children—Revised (WISC-R), they found that subtests profile in localization-related epilepsies were different, depending on the location of the epileptic focus. In regard to AEDs, findings suggested that those children receiving two or more AEDs were less likely to receive mainstream schooling even when seizure frequency and severity of the epilepsy were taken into account. Lastly, in terms of the effects of duration on cognitive functioning, the authors found that IQ decreased with duration of epilepsy only in the individuals with symptomatic or cryptogenic generalized epilepsies and epilepsies of undetermined origin; IQ remained stable with duration in the two other types of epileptic syndromes.

Early studies also found seizure type to affect selected cognitive functions differentially. Regardless of seizure type, the performance of children with epilepsy was below that of the control group. Of greater interest, however, were past findings suggesting that children with left temporal lobe foci showed learning and memory deficits on measures requiring delayed recall of verbal material, whereas children with right temporal lobe foci had greater difficulty with recall tasks involving visual–spatial abilities. Significant differences between performances on measures of recent memory were not evident between groups. Furthermore, children whose seizures were centrecephalic in nature performed at a significantly lower level on tasks of sustained attention than those in the temporal lobe groups, without exhibiting either short-term or long-term memory impairment.

Patterns of intellectual performance on the Wechsler Adult Intelligence Scale—Revised (WAIS-R) or WISC-R that varied with seizure type have been observed in multiple studies (Bulteau et al., 2000; Giordani et al., 1985, 1993). Bulteau and colleagues (2000) found that in children, depending on the etiology of the seizure, different patterns of performances emerged. Specifically, those individuals within the frontal epilepsy group showed relative deficits on WISC-R Arithmetic and Coding compared to other subtests. Those with occipital epilepsy exhibited relative weaknesses on image completion, image arrangement, and the Coding subtest. Those with multifocal epilepsy exhibited varied performance across all subtests, and those with TLE and rolandic epilepsy exhibited rather consistent performance across subtests. Giordani and colleagues (1993) studied adults and found that patients with focal (temporal) seizures showed compromised performance on WAIS-R Vocabulary when compared to patients with generalized seizures, whereas the generalized group performed less well on Block Design.

Because seizure classification and their inclusion criteria have not been consistent, particularly in the earlier studies, and because populations tested have not been uniform across investigations (institutionalized vs. noninstitutionalized), direct comparisons between studies are not always possible. The study of seizure type and frequency and its effect on intellectual and cognitive functioning is further complicated by the severity of seizures and the levels of AEDs necessary to achieve adequate seizure control. It is also possible that in some cases, the association between observed cognitive deficits and frequency of seizures is due to the extent of cerebral damage that is responsible for both. When considered as a whole, however, current studies suggest that the extent of intellectual and cognitive dysfunction in epilepsy varies with the type of seizure and increases with greater seizure frequency.

Age at Onset and Duration of Disorder

The relationship between early onset of a seizure disorder and poor prognosis for mental functioning has been noted for over a century, and current research continues to support this observation. Studies of intellectual and neuropsychological functions in children with epilepsy, regardless of seizure type, indicate that onset of seizures early in life with a consequently long duration of seizure disorders place children at higher risk for cognitive dysfunction.

Oyegbile and colleagues (2004) assessed cognitive dysfunction in individuals with chronic TLE compared to healthy control subjects and determined that chronicity of epilepsy was related to greater impairment in mental status, specifically in terms of intelligence, memory, language, visual-perceptual skills, and motor skills. This finding was even more striking for those with chronic epilepsy and less educational attainment.

To assess the role of early-onset versus late-onset TLE on brain structure and cognitive processing, Hermann and colleagues (2002) compared healthy controls to patients with early-onset and late-onset TLE. The findings suggested that the patients with early-onset TLE (mean onset age, 7.8 years) exhibited substantial reduction in brain tissue volumes and significantly impaired performance on a number of cognitive measures when compared to the patients with late-onset TLE (mean onset age, 23.3 years). On the neuropsychological battery administered to the groups, the early-onset patients performed significantly worse on 7 of the 12 tests (Full Scale IQ; Performance IQ; naming; spatial orientation; verbal and visual memory; problem solving). Similar trends were noted on a number of other measures.

Dodrill (1993) is careful to point out the need for careful consideration of other possible factors that contribute to the poorer cognitive outcome associated with early onset, such as the fact that a lower age at onset usually means a much higher number of total seizure occurrences. In fact, Dodrill (1986) has previously found evidence that the total number of tonic–clonic seizures a person experiences may be as important as, if not more important than, the age at onset.

SUMMARY

Childhood epilepsy syndromes are wide and varied. Their seizure and behavioral manifestations span the possibilities of syndromes classified by the ILAE (listed in Table 24.2). Moreover, childhood epilepsies have been shown to exist both neonatally and even prenatally. Seizures at these age ranges have their own manifestation and classification. What we know to be common about most childhood epilepsy disorders is that their onset, whether a single seizure occurrence or a long-lasting epileptic disorder, usually has some genetic component (i.e., there is a close relative with a history of some type of seizure disorder). We know more about the genetic inheritance modes of some epileptic disorders than we do about others. We also know more about the cognitive and neuropsychological consequences of some syndromes than we do about others. However, it does appear that the age at which the disorder began, the duration of the disorder, and the frequency and duration of the seizures are all factors in a child's long-term outcome. As basic and applied scientists continue to collaborate and compare notes, we come closer to reaching answers about the neurodevelopmental and physiological underpinnings of epilepsy and their impact on cognitive development.

REFERENCES

Abrahams, S., Pickering, A., Polkey, C. E., & Morris, R. G. (1997). Spatial memory deficits in patients with unilateral damage to the right hippocampal formation. *Neuropsychologia, 35,* 11–24.

Adda, C. C., Castro, L. H., Alem-Mar, S., de Manreza, M. L., & Kashiara, R. (2008). Prospective memory and mesial temporal epilepsy associated with hippocampal sclerosis. *Neuropsychologia, 46,* 1954–1964.

American Academy of Pediatrics, Committee on Drugs. (1985). Behavioral and cognitive effects of anticonvulsant therapy. *Pediatrics, 76,* 644–647.

American Academy of Pediatrics, Committee on Quality Improvement, Subcommittee on Febrile Seizures. (1999). Practice parameter: Long-term treatment of the child with simple febrile seizures. *Pediatrics, 103,* 1307–1309.

Annegers, J. F., Dubinsky, S., Coan, S. P., Newmark, M. E., & Roht, L. (1999). The incidence of epilepsy and unprovoked seizures in multiethnic, urban health maintenance organizations. *Epilepsia, 40*(4), 502–506.

Barr, W. B., Chelune, G. J., Hermann, B. P., Loring, D. W., Perrine, K., Strauss, E., et al. (1997). The use of figural reproduction tests as measures of nonverbal memory in epilepsy surgery candidates. *Journal of the International Neuropsychology Society, 3,* 435–443.

Baykan, B., Altindag, E. A., Bebek, N., Ozturk, A. Y., Aslantas, B., Gurses, C., et al. (2008). Myoclonic seizures subside in the fourth decade in juvenile myoclonic epilepsy. *Neurology, 70,* 2123–2129.

Bear, D. M., Freeman, R., & Greenberg, M. (1984). Behavioral alterations in patients with temporal lobe epilepsy. In D. Blumer (Ed.), *Psychiatric aspects of epilepsy* (pp. 197–227). Washington, DC: American Psychiatric Press.

Bell, B. D., & Davies, K. G. (1998). Anterior temporal lobectomy, hippocampal sclerosis, and memory: Recent neuropsychological findings. *Neuropsychology Reviews, 8,* 25–41.

Bennett, T. L. (1987). Neuropsychological aspects of complex partial seizures: Diagnostic and treatment issues. *International Journal of Clinical Neuropsychology, 9,* 37–45.

Bennett, T. L. (1988). Use of the Halstead–Reitan Neuropsychological Test Battery in the assessment of head injury. *Journal of Cognitive Rehabilitation, 3,* 18–24.

Bennett, T. L. (1992). Cognitive effects of epilepsy and anticonvulsant medications. In T. L. Bennett (Ed.), *The neuropsychology of epilepsy.* New York: Plenum Press.

Bennett, T. L., & Ho, M. R. (1997). The neuropsychology of pediatric epilepsy and antiepileptic drugs. In C. R. Reynolds & E. Fletcher-Janzen (Eds.), *Handbook of clinical child neuropsychol-ogy* (2nd ed., pp. 517–538). New York: Plenum Press.

Bennett-Levy, J., & Stores, G. (1984). The nature of cognitive dysfunction in schoolchildren with epilepsy. *Acta Neurologica Scandinavica, 69*(Suppl. 99), 79–82.

Berg, A. T., & Shinnar, S. (1996). Unprovoked seizures in children with febrile seizures: Short-term outcome. *Neurology, 47,* 562–568.

Berkovic, S. F. (1998). Genetics of epilepsy syndromes. In J. Engel, Jr., & T. A. Pedley (Eds.), *Epilepsy: A comprehensive textbook* (pp. 217–224). Philadelphia: Lippincott–Raven.

Bhattacharyya, M., Kalra, V., & Gulati, S. (2006). Intranasal midazolam versus rectal diazepam in acute childhood seizures. *Pediatric Neurology, 34,* 355–359.

Bien, C. G., Granata, T., Antozzi, C., Cross, J. H., Dulac, O., Kurthen, M., et al. (2005). Pathogenesis, diagnosis and treatment of Rasmussen encephalitis: A European consensus statement. *Brain, 128,* 454–471.

Binder, J. R., Sabsevitz, D. S., Swanson, S. J., Hammeke, T. A., Raghavan, M., & Mueller, W. M. (2008). Use of preoperative functional MRI to predict verbal memory decline after temporal lobe epilepsy surgery, *Epilepsia, 49,* 1377–1394.

Bootsma, H., Aldenkamp, A. P., Diepman, L., Hulsman, J., Lambrechts, D., Leenen, L., et al. (2006). The effect of antiepileptic drugs on cognition: Patient perceived cognitive problems of topiramate versus levetiracetam in clinical practice. *Epilepsia, 47,* 24–27.

Bulteau, C., Jambaque, I., Viguier, D., Kieffer, V., Dellatolas, G., & Dulac, O. (2000). Epileptic syndromes, cognitive assessment and school placement: A study of 251 children. *Developmental Medicine and Child Neurology, 42,* 319–327.

Butterbaugh, G., Olejniczak, P., Roques, B., Costa, R., Rose, M., Fisch, B., et al. (2004). Lateralization of temporal lobe epilepsy and learning disabilities, as defined by disability-related civil rights law. *Epilepsia, 45,* 963–970.

Cepeda, C., André, V. M., Levine, M. S., Salamon, N., Miyata, H., Vinters, H. V., et al. (2006). Epileptogenesis in pediatric cortical dysplasia: The dysmature cerebral developmental hypothesis. *Epilepsy and Behavior, 9,* 213–225.

Chiaravalloti, N. D., & Glosser, G. (2004). Memory for faces dissociates from memory for location following anterior temporal lobectomy. *Brain and Cognition, 54,* 35–42.

Claes, L., Ceulemans, B., Audenaert, D., Deprez, L., Jansen, A., Hasaerts, D., et al. (2004). De novo KCNQ2 mutations in patients with benign neonatal seizures. *Neurology, 63,* 2155–2158.

Commission on Classification and Terminology, International League Against Epilepsy. (1989). Proposal for revised classification of epilepsies and epileptic syndromes. *Epilepsia, 30,* 389–399.

Corcoran, R., & Upton, D. (1993). A role for the hippocampus in card sorting? *Cortex, 29*, 293–304.

Degan, R., Degan, H. E., & Hans, K. A. (1991). A contribution to the genetics of febrile seizures: Waking and sleeping EEG in siblings. *Epilepsia, 32*, 515–522.

Delgado-Escueta, A. V. (2007). Advances in genetics of juvenile myoclonic epilepsies. *Epilepsy Currents, 7*, 61–67.

Delgado-Escueta, A. V., Greenberg, D. A., Treiman, L., Liu, A., Sparkes, R. S., Barbetti, A., et al. (1989). Mapping the gene for juvenile myoclonic epilepsy. *Epilepsia, 30*, S8–S18.

Deutsch, G. K., Saykin, A., & Sperling, M. R. (1996). Metamemory in temporal lobe epilepsy. *Assessment, 3*, 255–263.

Dewhurst, K. (Ed.). (1980). *Thomas Willis' Oxford lectures*. Oxford, UK: Sanford.

Dhanuka, A. K., Jain, B. K., Daljit, S., & Maheshwari, D. (2001). Juvenile myoclonic epilepsy: A clinical and sleep EEG study. *Seizure, 10*, 374–378.

Dodrill, C. B. (1978). A neuropsychological battery for epilepsy. *Epilepsia, 19*, 611–623.

Dodrill, C. B. (1981). Neuropsychology of epilepsy. In S. B. Filskov & T. J. Boll (Eds.), *Handbook of clinical neuropsychology* (pp. 366–395). New York: Wiley.

Dodrill, C. B. (1986). Correlates of generalized tonic-clonic seizures with intellectual, neuropsychological, emotional, and social function in patients with epilepsy. *Epilepsia, 27*, 399–411.

Dodrill, C. B. (1993). Neuropsychology. In J. Laidlaw, A. Richens, & D. Chadwick (Eds.), *A textbook of epilepsy* (4th ed., pp. 459–473). New York: Churchill Livingstone.

Drane, D. L., & Meador, K. J. (2002). Cognitive and behavioral effects of antiepileptic drugs. *Epilepsy and Behavior, 3*, 49–53.

Dunn, D., & Kronenberger (2006). Childhood epilepsy, attention problems, and ADHD: Review and practical considerations. *Seminars in Pediatric Neurology, 12*, 222–228.

Dunn, D. W., Austin, J. K., Harezlak, J., & Ambrosius, W. T. (2003). ADHD and epilepsy in childhood. *Developmental Medicine and Child Neurology, 45*, 50–54.

Fastenau, P. S., Shen, J., Dunn, D. W., Perkins, S. M., Hermann, B. P., & Austin, J. K. (2004). Neuropsychological predictors of academic underachievement in pediatric epilepsy: Moderating roles of demographic, seizure, and psychosocial variables. *Epilepsia, 45*, 1261–1272.

Feigenbaum, J. D., & Morris, R. G. (2004). Allocentric versus egocentric spatial memory after unilateral temporal lobectomy in humans. *Neuropsychology, 18*, 462–472.

Field, S. J., Saling, M. M., & Berkovic, S. F. (2000). Interictal discourse production in temporal lobe epilepsy. *Brain and Language, 74*, 213–222.

Forsgren, L. (2004). Epidemiology and prognosis of epilepsy and its treatment. In S. Shorvon, D. Fish, E. Perucca, & W. E. Dodson (Eds.), *The treatment of epilepsy* (2nd ed., pp. 21–42). Malden, MA: Blackwell Science.

Geschwind, N. (1984). Dostoievsky's epilepsy. In D. Blumer (Ed.), *Psychiatric aspects of epilepsy* (pp. 325–334). Washington, DC: American Psychiatric Press.

Getz, K., Hermann, B. Seidenberg, M., Bell, B., Dow, C., Jones, J., et al. (2002). Negative symptoms in temporal lobe epilepsy. *American Journal of Psychiatry, 159*, 644–651.

Giordani, B., Berent, S., Sackellares, J. C., Rourke, D., Seidenberg, M., O'Leary, D. S., et al. (1985). Intelligence test performance of patients with partial and generalized seizures. *Epilepsia, 26*, 37–42.

Giordani, B., Rourke, D., Berent, S., Sackllares, J. C., Seidenberg, M., Butterbaugh, G., et al. (1993). Comparison of WAIS subtest performance of patients with complex partial (temporal lobe) and generalized seizures. *Psychological Assessment, 5*, 159–163.

Giovagnoli, A. R., Erbetta, A., Villani, F., & Avanzini, G. (2005). Semantic memory in partial epilepsy: Verbal and non-verbal deficits and neuroanatomical relationships. *Neuropsychologia, 43*, 1482–1492.

Gonzalez, L. M., Anderson, V. A., Mitchell, L. A., & Harvey, A. S. (2007). The localization and lateralization of memory deficits in children with temporal lobe epilepsy. *Epilepsia, 48*, 124–132.

Gowers, W. R. (1964). *Epilepsy and other chronic convulsive disorders* (American Academy of Neurology Reprint Series). New York: Dover. (Original work published 1885)

Haynes, S., & Bennett, T. L. (1991). Cognitive impairment in adults with complex partial seizures. *International Journal of Clinical Neuropsychology, 12*, 74–81.

Helmstaedter, C., Grunwald, T., Lehnertz, K., Gleißner, U., & Elger, C. E. (1997). Differential involvement of left temporolateral and temporomesial structures in verbal declarative learning and memory: evidence from temporal lobe epilepsy. *Brain and Cognition, 35*, 110–131.

Hermann, B., Seidenberg, M., Bell, B., Rutecki, P., Sheth, R., Ruggles, K., et al. (2002). The neurodevelopment impact of childhood-onset temporal lobe epilepsy on brain structure and function. *Epilepsia, 43*, 1062–1071.

Hernandez, M. T., Sauerwein, H. C., Jambaque, I., de Guise, E., Lussier, F., Lortie, A., et al. (2003). Attention, memory, and behavioral adjustment in children with frontal lobe epilepsy. *Epilepsy and Behavior, 4*, 522–536.

Hesdorffer, D. C., Ludvigsson, P., Olafsson, E., Gudmundsson, G., Kjartansson, O., & Hauser, W. A. (2004). ADHD as a risk factor for incident unprovoked seizures and epilepsy in children. *Archives of General Psychiatry, 61*, 731–736.

Huberty, T. J., Austin, J. K., Harezlak, J., Dunn, D.W., & Ambrosius, W. T. (2000). Informant agreement in behavior ratings for children with epilepsy. *Epilepsy and Behavior, 1*, 427–435.

Jambaque, I., Dellatolas, G., Dulac, O., Ponsot, G., & Signoret, J. (1993). Verbal and visual memory impairment in children with epilepsy. *Neuropsychologia, 31*, 1321–1337.

Kadis, D. S., Stollstorff, M., Elliott, I., Lach, L., & Smith, M. L. (2003). Cognitive and psychological predictors of everyday memory in children with intractable epilepsy. *Epilepsy and Behavior, 5*, 37–43.

Keene, D. L., Manion, I., Whiting, S., Belanger, E., Brennan, R., Jacob, P., et al. (2005). A survey of behavior problems in children with epilepsy. *Epilepsy Behavior, 6*, 581–586.

Kobau, R., Zahran, H., Thurman, D. J., Zack, M. M., Henry, T. R., Schachter, S. C., et al. (2008). Epilepsy surveillance among adults—19 states, behavioral risk factor surveillance system. *Morbidity and Mortality Weekly Report, 57*, 1–20.

Lennox, W. G., & Lennox, M. A. (1960). *Epilepsy and related disorders.* Boston: Little, Brown.

Loiseau, P., Signoret, J. L., & Strube, E. (1984). Attention problems in adult epileptic patients. *Acta Neurologica Scandinavica, 69*(Suppl. 99), 31–34.

Loring, D. W., Marino, S., & Meador, K. J. (2007). Neuropsychological and behavioral effects of antiepilepsy drugs. *Neuropsychology Review, 17*, 413–425.

Loring, D. W., & Meador, K. J. (2001). Cognitive and behavioral effects of epilepsy treatment. *Epilepsia, 42*, 24–32.

Majdan, A., Sziklas, V., & Jones-Gotman, M. (1996). Performance of healthy subjects and patients with resection from the anterior temporal lobe on matched tests of verbal and visuoperceptual learning. *Journal of Clinical and Experimental Neuropsychology, 18*, 416–430.

Manford, M., & Andermann, F. (1998). Complex visual hallucinations: Clinical and neurobiological insights. *Brain, 121*, 1819–1840.

Maouris, P. G. (1987). Spontaneous fetal seizures in utero. *American Journal of Obstetrics and Gynecology, 157*, 1009–1010.

Marini, C., Scheffer, I. E., Crossland, K. M., Grinton, B. E., Phillips, F. L., McMahon, J. M., et al. (2004). Genetic architecture of idiopathic generalized epilepsy: Clinical genetic analysis of 55 multiplex families. *Epilepsia, 45*(5), 467–478.

Martin, R. C., Sawrie, S., Hugg, J., Gilliam, F., Faught, E., & Kuzniecky, R. (1999). Cognitive correlates of 1H MRSI-detected hippocampal abnormalities in temporal lobe epilepsy. *Neurology, 53*, 2052.

Martin, R. C., Sawrie, S. M., Gilliam, F. G., Palmer, C. A., Faught, E., Morawetz, R. B., et al. (2002). Wisconsin Card Sorting performance in patients with temporal lobe epilepsy: Clinical and neuroanatomical correlates. *Epilepsia, 41*, 1626–1632.

Mayeux, R., Brandt, J., Rosen, J., & Benson, F. (1980). Interictal and language impairment in temporal lobe epilepsy. *Neurology, 30*, 120–125.

McGuckin, H. M. (1980). Changing the world view of those with epilepsy. In R. Canger, F. Angeleri, & J. K. Perry (Eds.), *Advances in epileptology: XIth Epilepsy International Symposium, 1980* (pp. 205–208). New York: Raven Press.

McIntyre, J., Robertson, S., Norris, E., Appleton, R., Whitehouse, W. P., Phillips, B., et al. (2005). Safety and efficacy of buccal midazolam versus rectal diazepam for emergency treatment for seizures in children: A randomized controlled trial, *Lancet, 366*, 205–210.

Meencke, H. J. (1985). Neuron density in the molecular layer of the frontal cortex in primary generalized epilepsy. *Epilepsia, 26*, 450–454.

Meencke, H. J. (1989). Pathology of childhood epilepsies. *Cleveland Clinic Journal of Medicine, 56*(Suppl. 1), S111–S120.

Messas, C. S., Mansur, L. L., & Castro, L. H. (2008). Semantic memory impairment in temporal lobe epilepsy associated with hippocampal sclerosis. *Epilepsy and Behavior, 12*, 311–316.

Mitchell, W. G., Zhou, Y., Chavez, J. M., & Guzman, B. L. (1992). Reaction time, attention, and impulsivity in epilepsy. *Pediatric Neurology, 8*, 19–24.

Offringa, M., Bossuyt, P. M., Lubsen, J., Ellenberg, J. H., Nelson, K. B., Knudsen, F. U., et al. (1994). Risk factors for seizure recurrence in children with febrile seizures: A pooled analysis of individual patient data from five studies. *Journal of Pediatrics, 124*, 574–584.

Ortinski, P., & Meador, K. J. (2004). Cognitive side effects of antiepileptic drugs. *Epilepsy and Behavior, 5*(Suppl. 1), S60–S65.

Oyegbile, T. O., Jones, J., Bell, B., Rutecki, P., Sheteh, R., et al. (2004). The nature and course of neuropsychological morbidity in chronic temporal lobe epilepsy. *Neurology, 62*, 1736–1742.

Palcoux, J., Carla, H., Tardieu, M., Carpentier, C., Sebire, G., Garcier, J., et al. (2007). Plasma exchange in Rasmussen's encephalitis. *Therapeutic Apheresis and Dialysis, 1*, 79–82.

Panayiotopoulos, C. P., Obeid, T., & Tahan, A. R. (1994). Juvenile myoclonic epilepsy: A 5-year prospective study. *Epilepsia, 35*, 285–296.

Panayiotopoulos, C. P., Obeid, T., & Waheed, G. (1989). Absences in juvenile myoclonic epilepsy: A clinical and video-electroencephalographic study. *Annals of Neurology, 25*, 391–397.

Parkinson, G. M. (2002). High incidence of language disorder in children with focal epilepsies. *Developmental Medicine and Child Neurology, 44*, 533–537.

Plouin, P., & Anderson, E. (2002). *Epileptic symptoms in infancy, childhood and adolescence* (3rd ed., pp. 3–13). New York: Libbey.

Powell, H. W., Richardson, M. P., Symms, M. R., Boulby, P. A., Thompson, P. J., Duncan, J. S., et al. (2007). Reorganization of verbal and nonverbal memory in temporal lobe epilepsy due to unilateral hippocampal sclerosis. *Epilepsia, 48,* 1512–1525.

Prevey, M. L., Delaney, R. C., & Mattson, R. H. (1988). Metamemory in temporal lobe epilepsy: Self monitoring of memory functions. *Brain and Cognition, 7,* 298–311.

Quadfasel, A. F., & Pruyser, P. W. (1955). Cognitive deficits in patients with psychomotor epilepsy. *Epilepsia, 4,* 80–90.

Reitan, R. M. (1974). Psychological testing of epileptic patients. In O. Magnus & L. de Haas (Eds.), *Handbook of clinical neurology: Vol. 15. The epilepsies* (pp. 559–575). Amsterdam: Elsevier.

Reitan, R. M., & Wolfson, D. (1985). *The Halstead–Reitan Neuropsychological Test Battery: Theory and clinical interpretation* (2nd ed.). Tucson, AZ: Neuropsychology Press.

Renganathan, R., & Delanty, N. (2003). Juvenile myoclonic epilepsy: Under-appreciated and under-diagnosed. *Postgraduate Medical Journal, 79,* 78–80.

Robinson, R. J. (1991). Causes and associations of severe and persistent specific speech and language disorders in children. *Developmental Medicine and Child Neurology, 33,* 943–962.

Sadlier, L. G., & Scheffer, I. E. (2007). Febrile seizures. *British Medical Journal, 334,* 307–311.

Sanchez, R. M., & Jensen, F. E. (2001). Maturational aspects of epilepsy mechanisms and consequences for the immature brain. *Epilepsia, 42*(5), 577–585.

Scher, M. S., Trucco, G. S., Beggarly, M. E., Steppe, D. A., & Macpherson, T. A. (1998). Neonates with electrically confirmed seizures and possible placental associations. *Pediatric Neurology, 19*(1), 37–41.

Sherman, E. M. S., Armitage, L. L., Connolly, M. B., Wambera, K. M., & Strauss, E. (2000). Behaviors symptomatic of ADHD in pediatric epilepsy: Relationship to frontal lobe epileptiform abnormalities and other neurological predictors. *Epilepsia, 41,* 191.

Simeonsson, K. L., & Hillenbrand, K. M. (2007). Neonatal seizures. In R. M. Perkin, J. D. Swift, D. A. Newton, & N. G. Anas (Eds.), *Pediatric hospital medicine: Textbook of inpatient management* (2nd ed., pp. 578–582). Philadelphia: Lippincott Williams & Wilkins.

Stores, G. (1978). School children with epilepsy at risk for learning and behavior problems. *Developmental Medicine and Child Neurology, 20,* 502–508.

Stores, G. (1984). Intensive EEG monitoring in paediatrics. *Developmental Medicine and Child Neurology, 26,* 231–234.

Titus, J. B., Kanive, R., Sanders, S. J., & Blackburn, L. B. (2008). Behavioral profiles of children with epilepsy: Parent and teacher reports of emotional, behavioral, and educational concerns on the BASC-2. *Psychology in the Schools, 45*(9), 893–904.

Upton, D., & Corcoran, R. (1995). The role of the right temporal lobe in card sorting: A case study. *Cortex, 31,* 405–409.

Usta, I. M., Adra, A. M., & Nassar, A. H. (2007). Ultrasonographic diagnosis of fetal seizures: A case report and review of the literature. *BJOG: An International Journal of Obstetrics and Gynaecology, 114,* 1031–1033.

Vannucci, M. (2007). Visual memory deficits in temporal lobe epilepsy: Toward a multifactorial approach. *Clinical EEG and Neuroscience, 38,* 18–24.

Vargha-Khadem, F., Carr, L. J., Isaacs, E., Brett, E., Adams, C., & Mishkin, M. (1997). Onset of speech after left hemispherectomy in a nine-year-old boy. *Brain, 120,* 159–182.

Velisek, L., & Moshe, S. L. (2003). Temporal lobe epileptogenesis and epilepsy in the developing brain: Bridging the gap between the laboratory and the clinic. Progression, but in what direction? *Epilepsia, 44,* 51–39.

Vermeulen, J., & Aldenkamp, A. P. (1995). Cognitive side-effects of chronic antiepileptic drug treatment: A review of 25 years of research. *Epilepsy Research, 22,* 65–95.

Volpe, J. J. (1989). Neonatal seizures: Current concepts and revised classification. *Pediatrics, 84,* 422–428.

Waxman, S. A., & Geschwind, N. (1980). Hypergraphia in temporal lobe epilepsy. *Neurology, 30,* 314–317.

Williams, J., Sharp, G., Lange, B., Bates, S., Griebel, M., Spence, G. T., et al. (1996). The effects of seizure type, level of seizure control, and antiepileptic drugs on memory and attention skills in children with epilepsy. *Developmental Neuropsychology, 12,* 241–253.

Wilson, B. A., Ivani-Chalain, R., Besag, F. M. C., & Bryant, T. (1993). Adapting the Rivermead Behavioural Memory Test for use with children aged 5 to 10 years. *Journal of Clinical and Experimental Neuropsychology, 15,* 474–486.

World Health Organization. (2001, February). Epilepsy: Aetiology, epidemiology and prognosis (Fact sheet No. 165). Geneva: Author.

Yagi, K. (1996). Evolution of Lennox–Gastaut syndrome: A long-term longitudinal study. *Epilepsia, 37,* 48–51.

CHAPTER 25

Prader–Willi Syndrome

ELISABETH M. DYKENS
SUZANNE B. CASSIDY
MELISSA L. DeVRIES

Prader–Willi syndrome is a complex, multisystem disorder whose intriguing genetic and behavioral features have attracted renewed interest from researchers and clinicians alike. The major manifestations of Prader–Willi syndrome include hypotonia; early failure to thrive, followed by later excessive appetite and obesity; hypogonadism; short stature; characteristic appearance; developmental disability; and significant behavioral dysfunction. Approximately 1 in 10,000–15,000 individuals is diagnosed with Prader–Willi syndrome (Burd, Vesely, Martsolf, & Kerbeshian, 1990; Wigren & Hansen, 2003a), and it occurs in both sexes and all races.

Prader–Willi syndrome was first described in 1956 (Prader, Labhart, & Willi, 1956). Twenty-five years later, the syndrome captured the interest of human geneticists because it was the first syndrome that was found to be caused by a small missing piece of chromosomal material called a *microdeletion*; this discovery was made by researchers using the newly developed technique of high-resolution chromosome analysis (Ledbetter et al., 1981). Prader–Willi syndrome is now known to be one of the most common microdeletion syndromes, one of the most frequent disorders seen in genetics clinics, and the most common recognized genetic form of obesity.

Prader–Willi syndrome is also the first recognized human disorder in which it was appreciated that the relevant genes are expressed differently, depending on whether they are inherited from the mother or the father (Nicholls, Knoll, Butler, Karam, & Lalande, 1989). This phenomenon of differential gene expression is known as *genomic imprinting*. In addition, Prader–Willi syndrome is distinctive in being caused by several different genetic alterations of the relevant chromosomal region, which is the long arm of chromosome 15. Prader–Willi syndrome thus occupies an important place in the contemporary history of human genetic disorders.

Clinical diagnostic criteria for Prader–Willi syndrome have been developed (Holm et al., 1993; Whittington et al., 2002), and accurate, specific genetic testing has become available (American Society of Human Genetics [ASHG] & American College of Medical Genetics [ACMG], 1996; Crinò et al., 2003). However, the diagnosis is still delayed in many cases because of a failure to recognize the syndrome's characteristic physical and behavioral manifestations. In addition to a distinctive physical phenotype,

Prader–Willi syndrome has a characteristic behavioral phenotype, which includes a blend of unusual cognitive findings, psychiatric vulnerabilities, and maladaptive behaviors (e.g., temper tantrums and argumentativeness). These features are as important to quality of life and morbidity as are some of the syndrome's medical problems, and they are often the focus of intervention and treatment (Bellon-Harn, 2005; Cassidy, 1984; Durst, Rubin-Jabotinsky, Raskin, Katz, & Zislin, 2000; Dykens & Cassidy, 1995; Dykens, Hodapp, Walsh, & Nash, 1992a; Holm et al., 1993).

Since its identification over 50 years ago, then, Prader–Willi syndrome has emerged as a complicated disorder that highlights the need for a multidisciplinary approach to research and management. This chapter reviews many aspects of Prader–Willi syndrome, including its medical, genetic, cognitive, behavioral, developmental, and psychiatric features. As appropriate management often has a positive impact on the health and quality of life of people affected with Prader–Willi syndrome, the chapter also summarizes commonly used medical and behavioral interventions, especially those aimed at controlling the syndrome's characteristic obesity and behavioral/psychiatric dysfunction.

CLINICAL FINDINGS AND NATURAL HISTORY

Although many of the physical manifestations of Prader–Willi syndrome are related to functional hypothalamic deficiency, the disorder's clinical appearance in infancy differs considerably from that in childhood and adulthood.

Hypotonia

Hypotonia of prenatal onset is nearly uniformly present and is the likely cause of decreased fetal movement, frequent abnormal fetal position, and difficulty at the time of delivery, often necessitating cesarean section (Cassidy, 1984; Cassidy & Driscoll, 2009; Holm et al., 1993). The neonatal central hypotonia is almost invariably associated with poor suck, with consequent failure to thrive and the necessity for gavage or other special feeding techniques. Infantile lethargy, with decreased arousal and weak cry, are also prominent findings, often leading to the necessity to awaken the child to feed. Reflexes may be decreased or absent. Neuromuscular electrophysiological and biopsy studies are normal or nonspecific, and the hypotonia gradually improves. Delayed motor milestones are evident; the average age of sitting is 12 months and of walking is 24 months. Adults remain mildly hypotonic, with decreased muscle bulk and tone.

Hypogonadism

Hypogonadism is prenatal in onset (Eiholzer & Lee, 2006; Lee, 1995), and is evident at birth as small genitalia. Males generally have undescended testes; a small, hypopigmented, and poorly rugated scrotum; and sometimes a small penis. In females, the labia minora and clitoris are small. These findings persist throughout life, though spontaneous descent of testes has been observed up to adolescence. There is also evidence of hypogonadism in abnormal pubertal development. Although pubic and axillary hair may develop early or normally, the remainder of pubertal development is delayed and usually incomplete. Adult males only occasionally have voice change, male body habitus, or substantial facial or body hair. In females, breast development generally begins at a normal age, but menstrual periods are either absent or infrequent (and, if occurring, they are late in onset). In both males and females, sexual activity is relatively rare, and infertility is the rule.

The hypogonadism is hypothalamic in origin, and both pituitary and gonadal hormones are generally deficient (Cassidy, 1984; Lee, 1995). Since the pituitary gland and gonads are normal but understimulated, treatment with pituitary or gonadal hormones can increase the development of secondary sex characteristics.

Obesity

Obesity is the major cause of morbidity and mortality in Prader–Willi syndrome, and longevity may be nearly normal if obesity is avoided (Cassidy, Devi, & Mukaida, 1994; Einfeld et al., 2006; Greenswag, 1987). Significant weight excess, if allowed to occur, follows the early period of failure to thrive; the onset of excessive eating, or *hyperphagia*, typically begins between 1 and 6 years of age. Food-seeking behaviors are common, including hoarding or foraging for food; eating unappealing substances such as garbage, pet food, and frozen food and may vary by genetic subtype, based on differences in how visual food stimuli are perceived—see Key & Dykens, 2008); and stealing food or money to buy food. Low muscle tone and a disinclination to exercise add to the effects of the drive to eat excessively. A high threshold for vomiting may complicate bingeing on spoiled food from the garbage or items such as boxes of sugar or frozen uncooked meat. Toxicity has occurred from ineffective ipecac used to induce vomiting.

As shown in Figure 25.1, the obesity in Prader–Willi syndrome is central in distribution, with relative sparing of the distal extremities; even individuals who are not overweight tend to deposit fat on the abdomen, buttocks, and thighs. Cardiopulmonary compromise can result from excessive obesity, as can type 2 diabetes mellitus, hypertension, thrombophlebitis, and chronic leg edema. Sleep apnea occurs at increased frequency.

The hyperphagia in Prader–Willi syndrome is due to a hypothalamic abnormality that results in lack of satiety (DelParigi et al., 2002; Holland et al., 1993; Zipf & Bernston, 1987). In addition, there is a decreased caloric requirement (Holm & Pipes, 1976; Kundert, 2008), probably related to hypotonia and decreased activity.

Facial Features

Characteristic facial features either are present from birth or evolve over time (Aughton & Cassidy, 1990; Butler, Hanchett, & Thompson, 2006). As shown in Figure 25.2, facial features include narrow bifrontal diameter, almond-shaped palpebral fissures, narrow nasal bridge, and downturned mouth with a thin upper lip. Small, narrow hands with a straight ulnar border and sometimes tapering fingers are usually present by age 10, as are short, often broad feet, with an average adult female shoe size of 3 and male shoe size of 5 (Hudgins, McKillop, & Cassidy,

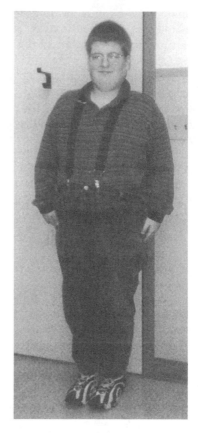

FIGURE 25.1. A 27-year-old man with Prader–Willi syndrome. Note the narrow bifrontal diameter and typical body habitus, with central obesity and small hands. Photograph used by permission of the patient and his family.

1991). African Americans with Prader–Willi syndrome are less likely to have small hands and feet, and they may also lack the typical facial phenotype (Cassidy, Geer, Holm, & Hudgins, 1996; Hudgins, Geer, & Cassidy, 1998).

A characteristic body habitus, including sloping shoulders, heavy midsection, and genu valgus with straight lower-leg borders, is usually present from toddlerhood (see Figure 25.1). Fairer coloring than other family members, manifested as lighter skin, hair, and eye color, occurs in about a third of affected individuals (Butler, 1989; Butler, Hanchett, & Thompson, 2006). Strabismus is often present. Scoliosis, kyphosis, or both are common; the former can occur at any age, and the latter develops in early adulthood.

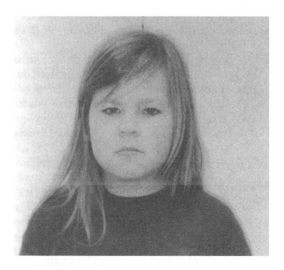

FIGURE 25.2. Face of a typical 10-year-old girl with Prader–Willi syndrome. Note the relatively narrow bifrontal diameter, almond-shaped eyes, and downturned corners of the mouth. Photograph used by permission of the patient's family.

Short Stature

Birthweight and birth length are usually within normal limits, but the early period of failure to thrive may mean that both weight and length fall below the 3rd percentile. Short stature, if not apparent in childhood, is almost always present by the second half of the second decade, associated with lack of a pubertal growth spurt. Average height is 155 cm for males and 148 cm for females. African Americans tend to be taller (Cassidy et al., 1996; Hudgins et al., 1998). Growth hormone deficiency has been demonstrated in most tested patients with Prader–Willi syndrome, and treatment with growth hormone increases height and lean body mass, often resulting in decreased body mass index (Angulo et al., 1996; Dudley, McManus, Vogels, Whittington, & Muscatelli, 2008; Lee, 1995).

Other Medical Issues

Numerous more minofr physical findings characterize this condition, including thick, viscous saliva that may predispose to dental caries and contribute to articulation abnormalities; high pain threshold; skin picking; and high threshold for vomiting. Sleep disturbances, especially excessive daytime sleepiness and oxygen desaturation in rapid-eye-movement sleep, are common even in the absence of obesity (Cotton & Richdale, 2006; Hertz, Cataletto, Feinsilver, & Angulo, 1995). Osteoporosis is also frequent.

Despite the multisystem nature of Prader–Willi syndrome, people with this condition generally enjoy good health if morbid obesity is avoided. Indeed, parents often report that their child with Prader–Willi syndrome is healthier than the child's unaffected siblings.

ORIGIN AND GENETIC BASIS

Since the first description of Prader–Willi syndrome, it has been apparent that many of its features arise from insufficient functioning of the hypothalamus. Thus many of the functions of this part of the brain are disturbed in Prader–Willi syndrome, including control of homeostatic functions such as hunger, thirst, sleep–wake cycles, and temperature regulation. The hypothalamus also releases hormones that travel to the pituitary gland, controlling the release of other hormones such as growth hormone, the sex hormones (gonadotropins), and thyroid-stimulating hormones (which regulate basal metabolic rate). Studies of the destruction of the hypothalamus in animals, particularly cats, show that many of the functional abnormalities seen in Prader–Willi syndrome occur in these animals. Prader–Willi syndrome symptoms are seen as well in cases of previously normal persons with acquired damage to the hypothalamus due to an injury, stroke, or tumor. Even the personality characteristics seen in Prader–Willi syndrome, including the temper tantrums, may result.

Because the hypothalamus was a logical place to look for a structural defect in Prader–Willi syndrome, the few reported autopsy studies have focused on that part of the brain. Unfortunately, no visible gross or microscopic structural defect or other abnormality has been documented that could explain the clinical features of the syndrome. The hypothalamic deficiency is thus likely to be functional, with preliminary findings suggesting altered function of oxytocin-secreting neurons (putative satiety cells) in the hypothalamic paraventricular nucleus (Swaab, 2004; Swaab, Purba, & Hofman, 1995).

Although the exact hypothalamic deficit has yet to be identified, considerable progress has been made in identifying the genetic basis of Prader–Willi syndrome. At the end of the 1970s, a new technique, high-resolution chromosome banding, was developed for analyzing chromosomes in more detail than was previously possible. This technique operates by capturing the chromosome in an earlier stage of the cell cycle, when it is more elongated, thus allowing much greater visibility of fine chromosome structure. Prior to this time, researchers had noted that a number of people with Prader–Willi syndrome had a rearrangement of the chromosomes that involved chromosome 15. Using high-resolution chromosome analysis, Ledbetter and colleagues (1981) reported the presence of a small deletion within the long arm of chromosome 15—called del 15(q11–13) in standard chromosome nomenclature—in about half the people with Prader–Willi syndrome whom they studied. This deletion was found to represent a new change in an affected individual (de novo deletion), since neither parent was found to have it. Subsequently, many workers studied series of patients to further delineate the exact location and frequency of the deletion, which is now known to occur in approximately 70% of those with Prader–Willi syndrome (ASHG & ACMG, 1996; Butler, 1996). With a few exceptions, the remainder of patients with Prader–Willi syndrome have normal-appearing chromosomes under the microscope.

The development of molecular genetic technology in the late 1980s allowed determination of the basis for Prader–Willi syndrome in patients with normal chromosomes. First, molecular techniques allowed investigators to confirm the observation previously made under the microscope that the deletion, when it was found, occurred solely in the paternally inherited chromosome 15, even though the blood chromosomes of the father were normal (Butler, 1990; Nicholls et al., 1989). Second, as expected, it was found that some people who did not have a deletion visible with chromosomal techniques did have a deletion that could be de-

termined with the more accurate molecular techniques (Delach et al., 1994). However, this was the case in only a small proportion of individuals without a visible deletion. More interestingly, a seminal study by Nicholls and colleagues (1989) found via molecular techniques that most of the remaining patients without a deletion had two maternally derived chromosome 15s and no paternally derived chromosome 15—a situation called *uniparental disomy* (UPD). Thus, instead of inheriting one paternal and one maternal chromosome 15 (which is the usual situation), people with Prader–Willi syndrome who do not have a deletion have the syndrome because they have received no paternal chromosome 15, but instead have two maternal chromosome 15s. The chromosomes themselves are normal in number and structure, but the inheritance pattern is wrong.

In effect, whether there is a paternal deletion or maternal UPD, Prader–Willi syndrome results from the lack of paternal contribution to the specific region of chromosome 15's long arm associated with this disorder. Sometimes a person with Prader–Willi syndrome due to maternal UPD has two copies of the same member of the maternal chromosome 15 pair (isodisomy), sometimes both members of the maternal chromosome 15 pair (heterodisomy), and sometimes a complicated combination of the two. However, the composition of the maternal chromosomes really does not affect the final result, since all the chromosome 15s are normal.

The genetic findings in Prader–Willi syndrome can be explained by a phenomenon called *genomic imprinting*. This is a process whereby genes or groups of neighboring genes are modified differently, and thereby expressed differently, depending on the sex of the parent from whom they were inherited. The genes themselves are not altered, since imprinting is a reversible process. Rather, some genes are inactivated or switched off, so that they no longer produce RNA and then protein in the process of decoding that constitutes gene expression. Although imprinting has been recognized for several years in some genes of other animals and plants, Prader–Willi syndrome was the first human disorder in which it was recognized. Several other human conditions have subsequently been found to be related to imprinting. The maternally derived copies of chromosome 15 in the region critical for Prader–Willi syndrome are inactivated in the normal situation, and only the paternally derived region is expressed in cells. When the paternal copy of this region is missing—by deletion or by complete absence, as in maternal UPD—there is no active copy of the genetic information, and an abnormality in development therefore results in Prader–Willi syndrome (Kundert, 2008; Nicholls, 1993).

Thus, again, Prader–Willi syndrome is caused by the absence of the normally active paternally inherited genes at chromosome 15(q11-13). In about 70% of cases, it is due to a deletion; in most individuals the deletion is of the same size, with the same breakpoints on the chromosome. Most of the remaining patients have maternal UPD for chromosome 15 (Nicholls et al., 1989; Mascari et al., 1992; Poyatos et al., 2009; Robinson et al., 1991). Approximately 5% of patients with Prader–Willi syndrome have a translocation or other structural abnormality involving chromosome 15 that has caused either a deletion or maternal UPD for the critical region. UPD usually affects the whole chromosome 15, but only in the small region of imprinted genes related to Prader–Willi syndrome does it matter which parent the chromosome comes from.

Approximately 1–5% of patients with Prader–Willi syndrome—including virtually all studied families in which there has been a recurrence of the syndrome—have neither deletion nor UPD, but rather have a very small deletion in the center controlling the imprinting process within 15q11–13 (Buiting et al., 1994; Poyatos et al., 2009; Saitoh et al., 1997). Methylation is one mechanism by which genomic imprinting can occur, and methylation has been demonstrated for several genes identified within the Prader–Willi critical region. Interestingly, a clinically very different disorder, Angelman syndrome, is the result of an oppositely imprinted gene in the same region of chromosome 15 (Williams et al., 1995). In contrast to Prader–Willi syndrome, people with Angelman syndrome typically have severe to profound mental retardation, limited expressive language, seizure disorder, an ataxic gait, and bouts of inappropriate laughter.

Several genes have been mapped within the Prader–Willi/Angelman region, and others that are not maternally inactivated have been mapped between the common deletion breakpoints. The first mapped gene, considered an important candidate gene, is small nuclear ribonucleoprotein N (SNRPN). This gene is expressed from the paternally inherited chromosome only (Glenn et al., 1996; Ozcelik et al., 1992), and is expressed abundantly in the brain. The other identified genes are currently of unknown function. The nonimprinted P gene, which also resides in this region, codes for tyrosinase-positive albinism, and its deletion probably causes the hypopigmentation seen in one-third of patients with Prader–Willi syndrome (Spritz et al., 1997).

Recently, some clinical differences have been reported between patients with Prader–Willi syndrome due to deletion and those with the syndrome due to UPD (Cassidy et al., 1997; Gillessen-Kaesbach et al., 1995; Kundert, 2008; Mitchell et al., 1996). Perhaps the most clinically significant of these are that patients with UPD may lack the typical facial phenotype (Cassidy et al., 1997), and that they may have delayed diagnosis (Gunay-Aygun & Cassidy, 1997).

DIAGNOSIS, DIFFERENTIAL DIAGNOSIS, AND DIAGNOSTIC TESTING

Prior to the availability of complete sensitive and specific laboratory testing, diagnostic criteria for Prader–Willi syndrome were developed through a consensus process (Butler, Hanchett, & Thompson, 2006; Hagerman, 1999; Holm et al., 1993). These criteria, listed in Table 25.1, are still extremely valuable in suggesting the diagnosis and indicating the need for diagnostic testing. It should be emphasized that no one individual will have all the manifestations of the disorder, and that there is considerable variability in the severity of each of the findings.

The differential diagnosis for Prader–Willi syndrome in infancy includes many causes of neonatal hypotonia, particularly neuromuscular disorders. Later in childhood and adulthood, a number of conditions involving mental retardation with associated obesity may be included in the differential diagnosis, including Bardet–Biedl syndrome, Albright

TABLE 25.1. Summary of the Clinical Diagnostic Criteria for Prader–Willi Syndrome

Major criteria (1 point each)	Minor criteria (½ point each)	Supportive criteria (no points)
Infantile central hypotonia	Decreased fetal movement and infantile lethargy	High pain threshold
Infantile feeding problems/failure to thrive	Typical behavior problems	Decreased vomiting
Rapid weight gain between 1 and 6 years	Sleep disturbance/sleep apnea	Temperature control problems
Characteristic facial features	Short stature for the family by age 15 years	Scoliosis and/or kyphosis
Hypogonadism: genital hypoplasia, pubertal deficiency	Hypopigmentation	Early adrenarche
Developmental delay/mental retardation	Small hands and feet for height, age	Osteoporosis
	Narrow hands with straight ulnar border	Unusual skill with jigsaw puzzles
	Esotropia, myopia	Normal neuromuscular studies
	Thick, viscous saliva	
	Speech articulation difficulties	
	Skin picking	

Note. The diagnosis should be strongly suspected in children under 3 years of age with 5 points, 3 from major criteria; or in those above 3 years of age with 8 points, 4 from major criteria. The original diagnostic criteria, developed before the availability of sensitive and specific genetic testing, included a major criteria of chromosome 15 deletion or other chromosome 15 anomaly. Items from Holm et al. (1993).

hereditary osteodystrophy, and Cohen syndrome (see Gunay-Aygun, Cassidy, & Nicholls, 1997, for a review). Other disorders causing mental retardation in which obesity is an occasional finding, such as fragile X, Smith–Magenis, and Angelman syndromes, may also be confused with Prader–Willi syndrome. Acquired hypothalamic injury from accidents, tumors, or surgical complications can closely mimic Prader–Willi syndrome.

Two important organizations in genetic research, the ASHG and the ACMG, published a statement in 1996 regarding the status of genetic testing for Prader–Willi and Angelman syndromes. Currently, the most efficient molecular diagnostic test for Prader–Willi syndrome examines the parent-specific methylation pattern within the Prader–Willi/Angelman region, using Southern hybridization and methylation-sensitive probes (SNRPN and PW71) (ASHG & ACMG, 1996). If the methylation pattern is characteristic of maternal-only inheritance, Prader–Willi syndrome is confirmed; if not, Prader–Willi due to deletion, UPD, or an imprinting mutation is ruled out. Knowing whether the Prader–Willi syndrome is due to deletion, UPD, or an imprinting mutation is important for genetic counseling purposes, as well as for identifying those few cases

with a translocation or inherited microdeletion. High-resolution cytogenetic analysis can often detect the 15q11–13 deletion; however, this technique has unacceptably high false-negative and false-positive rates, and it is no longer considered sufficient for diagnostic purposes. The definitive diagnostic test for the common size deletion causing Prader–Willi syndrome is fluorescent *in situ* hybridization (FISH), using probes within the Prader–Willi/Angelman critical region (SNRPN or D15S11). UPD can be detected with polymerase chain reaction; informative microsatellite markers from the Prader–Willi/Angelman region are used to study both parents and the child. Additional markers from other chromosomes can confirm correct paternity.

Prenatal detection of Prader–Willi syndrome is now possible. FISH is indicated when a cytogenetic 15q deletion is suspected after chorionic villus sampling (CVS) or amniocentesis. If trisomy 15 is detected on CVS and the fetus survives, parent-of-origin studies (methylation analysis or microsatellite marker) are indicated and validated (Christian et al., 1996; Kubota et al., 1996). FISH and parent-of-origin studies are also indicated if an inherited or de novo translocation involving chromosome 15 is detected prenatally. Parents should be studied in cases with an identified imprinting mutation, since a healthy parent can carry this abnormality and may be at increased risk for recurrence (Saitoh et al., 1997). Prenatal detection is possible through identification of the mutation or maternal-only methylation pattern in a fetus (Kubota et al., 1996).

Prader–Willi syndrome due either to the large deletion in the absence of a structural chromosome abnormality or to UPD has not been reported to recur, though a theoretical recurrence risk of approximately 1% or less is appropriate for genetic counseling purposes. UPD is caused by nondisjunction, as evidenced by advanced maternal age in this group (Dudley & Muscatelli, 2007; Mascari et al., 1992; Robinson et al., 1991), and by documentation of cases of trisomy 15 on CVS and maternal UPD at birth. Since nondisjunction can recur, a recurrence risk of 1% is appropriate for genetic counseling. In families with an imprinting mutation, a recurrence risk of up to 50% pertains, as this probably involves a dominant mutation in the paternal grandmother's germ line.

In many ways, then, Prader–Willi syndrome is a model genetic disorder—the source of remarkable new genetic discoveries. Now cast as the most common recognized genetic form of obesity, Prader–Willi has also made genetic history by being the first recognized human disease associated with UPD, with genomic imprinting, and with a clinically distinct yet genetically related "sister" syndrome (Angelman syndrome). Furthermore, the search for specific genes in the Prader–Willi/Angelman critical region is now well underway.

In contrast to these genetic advances, we know much less about Prader–Willi's complex cognitive and behavioral phenotype. Findings to date, however, suggest that Prader–Willi syndrome is also a promising condition for studying behavioral phenotypes of mental retardation syndromes in general (Dykens, 1995; Hodapp & Fidler, 1999; Holland et al., 2003; Martin et al., 1998). As described in the remainder of the chapter, many people with Prader–Willi syndrome show a blend of unusual cognitive styles, maladaptive behaviors, and psychiatric vulnerabilities that may prove unique, and that open up specific avenues of treatment and intervention.

COGNITIVE, ADAPTIVE, AND BEHAVIORAL PHENOTYPE

Cognitive and Adaptive Functioning

Cognitive and Adaptive Levels

The average IQ reported in most studies of people with Prader–Willi syndrome is about 70 (e.g., Butler, Hanchett, & Thompson, 2006; Dykens, Hodapp, Walsh, & Nash, 1992b). The mean IQ in Prader–Willi syndrome is thus high relative to those in other genetic disorders (Rosner, Hodapp, Fidler, Sagun, & Dykens, 2004), including prevalent conditions such as fragile X syndrome (Dykens, Hodapp, & Leckman, 1994) or Down syndrome (Hodapp, 1996), and less prevalent disorders, such as 5p– syndrome (Dykens & Clarke, 1997) or Smith–Magenis syndrome (Dykens, Finucane, & Gayley, 1997).

Although on average people with Prader–Willi syndrome show mild levels of mental retardation, their IQ scores range from average levels to profound mental retardation. Extrapolating IQ data from 575 subjects in 57 published studies, Curfs (1992) found that 34% showed mild mental retardation, 27% had moderate delays, and only 6% showed severe to profound levels of impairment. Approximately one-third of subjects were relatively high-functioning, or with IQs above 70; 27% showed borderline levels of intelligence (IQs of 70–84); and 5% showed average IQ scores. Whitman and Thompson (2006) have noted a similar distribution.

Whittington, Holland, and Webb (2009) have demonstrated that the IQs of patients with Prader–Willi syndrome, considered as one diagnostic group, have a low correlation with the IQs of their siblings. However, when genetic subtypes are considered, the IQ scores of patients with UPD are just as correlated with those of their siblings as the IQs of siblings without the syndrome would be, whereas the IQ scores of patients with the deletion subtype show almost no correlation with those of their siblings.

Even high-functioning individuals, however, rarely perform adaptively at a level commensurate with their IQs. *Adaptive functioning* is typically viewed as the performance of behaviors required for personal or social sufficiency (Sparrow, Balla, & Cicchetti, 1984). Clinical observations in Prader–Willi syndrome often suggest impaired adaptive functioning, yet only one study has formally assessed adaptive behavior in this population. Dykens and colleagues (1992b) administered a standardized assessment instrument, the Vineland Adaptive Behavior Scales (Sparrow et al., 1984), to caregivers of 21 adolescents and young adults with Prader–Willi syndrome. These subjects showed adaptive behavior composite standard scores that ranged from 20 to 50, all in the moderate to severe range of delay. The mean Vineland composite standard score was 37, which fell more than two standard deviations (31 points) below subjects' mean IQ of 68. As discussed later, low adaptive performance is probably associated with interference from significant behavioral dysfunction and a persistent drive to eat.

Cognitive Level and Weight

Early work in Prader–Willi syndrome suggested a significant inverse correlation between IQ and weight (Crnic, Sulzbacher, Snow, & Holm, 1980); that is, lower IQ scores were believed to be associated with increased weight. It was even suggested that prevention of obesity might also prevent mental retardation. Yet common lore in the Prader–Willi syndrome community actually suggests the opposite relationship; that is, brighter individuals may be more clever or ingenious about obtaining food, and thus may be at increased risk of obesity. More recent data do not support either hypothesis: Dykens and colleagues (1992b) and Whittington and colleagues (2004b) found no significant relations between IQ and body mass index (a measure of obesity). Persons with relatively high versus low IQ scores thus seem similarly vulnerable to the syndrome's problems with obesity.

Cognitive Profiles

Early clinical observations suggested that many children with Prader–Willi syndrome showed significant relative strengths in reading and weaknesses in arithmetic (e.g., Holm, 1981; Sulzbacher, Crnic, & Snow, 1981). These informal observations led to the idea that cognition in this syndrome was best characterized by uneven academic performance, as found in youngsters with learning disabilities.

Achievement studies, however, do not provide overwhelming support for a specific learning disability profile in Prader–Willi syndrome. Administering the Kaufman Assessment Battery for Children (K-ABC; Kaufman & Kaufman, 1983) to 21 adolescents and adults with Prader–Willi syndrome, Dykens and colleagues (1992b) found a nonsignificant discrepancy in age-equivalent scores in arithmetic versus reading (7.68 years vs. 8.55 years, respectively). Furthermore, Taylor (1988) examined an unspecified number of individuals with Prader–Willi syndrome, and reported a mean standard achievement test score of 70 in math and 73 in reading. More recent data from studies by Whittington and colleagues (2004a), which demonstrated a pattern of greater academic underachievement in arithmetic as compared to reading or spelling in a population-based sample of individuals with Prader–Willi syndrome, and by Bartella and colleagues (2005), which documented impairments in mathematical abilities in a sample of individuals with Prader–Willi syndrome, support findings from earlier studies. However, such findings only hint at uneven academic performance. Clearly, more studies are needed on the extent to which individuals with Prader–Willi syndrome show discrepancies across areas of academic achievement, as well as between achievement and IQ.

Only a few studies have moved beyond academic achievement to identify other aspects of cognitive processing in people with Prader–Willi syndrome. Examining global cognitive patterns on Wechsler tests, Borghgraef, Fryns, and Van den Berghe (1990) reported "great differences" (p. 148) in Verbal versus Performance IQ scores in 8 of their 12 subjects with Prader–Willi syndrome. Three of these individuals showed at least a 15-point discrepancy in favor of the Verbal IQ. Significant Verbal versus Performance IQ differences were also found in a study of 26 children with Prader–Willi syndrome (ages 7–15 years); 10 subjects showed elevations in the Performance IQ, and 3 in the Verbal IQ (Curfs, Wiegers, Sommers, Borghgraef, & Fryns, 1991). In contrast, Whittington and colleagues (2004b) noted that individuals with Prader–Willi syndrome due to deletion performed better on verbal measures. Findings are thus inconsistent.

More detailed studies of specific cognitive processes shed some light on these inconsistent findings. Table 25.2 summarizes these studies. Taylor (1988) compared Wechsler subtest scores in an unspecified number of subjects with Prader–Willi syndrome to those in a sample of individuals with obesity and mental retardation but without Prader–Willi syndrome. The two groups showed comparable subtest scores, with just one exception: Relative to the controls, the subjects with Prader–Willi syndrome showed significantly higher scores on Block Design, a task tapping visual–motor integration. Similarly, Curfs and colleagues (1991) found that one-half of their sample showed significant Wechsler subtest scatter, and that 9 of these 13 children had relative strengths in Block Design. These findings suggest strengths in some individuals in perceptual–spatial organization and visual–motor integration.

Consistent with these strengths, many people with Prader–Willi syndrome show an unusual facility with jigsaw puzzles (Dykens, 2002). In addition, engaging these skills in the form of leisure activities has been correlated with decreased maladaptive behaviors in such individuals (Sellinger, Hodapp, & Dykens, 2006). This skill is so striking that it is noted as a supportive finding in the consensus diagnostic criteria for Prader–Willi syndrome (Holm et al., 1993). Clinically, we observe as well that many adolescents and young adults have a strong propensity for "word search" puzzles, often carrying their word-finding books with them to school or work. Individuals with Prader–Willi syndrome have been noted to perform on par with their typical peers on word search tasks (Dykens, 2002). We also found that subject performance on a visual memory task was correlated with parental reports of subject interest and facility with jigsaw and word search puzzles. Recent studies have examined parents' attributions of jigsaw puzzle performance and how performance is related to parent assistance on such visual–spatial tasks (Ly & Hodapp, 2005a, 2005b), as well

TABLE 25.2. Summary of Cognitive and Adaptive Studies in People with Prader–Willi Syndrome

Study	Number and age of subjects	Key findings
Cognitive processing		
Curfs et al. (1991)	26 with PWS, 7–15 years	WISC-R Performance IQ > Verbal IQ in 10 subjects. Verbal IQ > Performance IQ in 3 subjects. Block Design high in 9 subjects.
Dykens et al. (1992a)	21 with PWS, 13–26 years 31 with PWS, 5–30 years	K-ABC Simultaneous Processing > Sequential Processing. Strengths: Visual-perceptual. Weaknesses: Visual–motor short-term memory. Stable IQ in childhood and adulthood.
Gabel et al. (1986)	15 with PWS, M = 12 years 15 nondisabled controls	Controls exceeded PWS on all measures. For PWS on Detroit Test of Learning Aptitude, visual recall of objects, letters > auditory recall of words.
Taylor (1988)	Unspecified with PWS Controls with obesity/mental retardation	On WISC-R, PWS > controls on Block Design only.
Warren and Hunt (1981)	11 with PWS, age unknown 12 with nonspecific etiologies, matched on age and IQ	On pictorial memory tasks, PWS < nonspecific group in visual short-term memory; PWS had no improvements in Performance with increasing age or IQ; PWS on par with nonspecific group in long-term memory for well-known information.
Adaptive behavior		
Dykens et al. (1992b)	21 with PWS, 13–26 years	On Vineland, strengths in Daily Living Skills (especially domestic skills), weaknesses in Socialization (especially coping skills); modest increases in adaptive skills with advancing age.

Note. PWS, Prader–Willi syndrome; WISC-R, Wechsler Intelligence Scale for Children—Revised; K-ABC, Kaufman Assessment Battery for Children.

as strategies and correlates of jigsaw puzzle performance in individuals with Prader–Willi syndrome (Verdine, Troseth, Hodapp, & Dykens, 2008). However, additional studies are needed that better relate facility with puzzles to cognitive profiles, and that determine exactly how widespread puzzle-solving skills are in this population.

Visual processing strengths are also suggested by Gabel and colleagues (1986), who administered a battery of attentional, visual–spatial, and psychomotor tasks to 15 children with Prader–Willi syndrome and 15 age- and sex-matched nondisabled children. Not surprisingly, the children with Prader–Willi scored consistently lower than the controls; however, they also showed discrepancies in scores on subtests of the Detroit Tests of Learning Aptitude (Baker & Leland, 1967). Specifically, these subjects had relatively low scores on tasks assessing auditory attention and recall for words, and high scores on tasks measuring visual attention and recall for objects and letters. Gabel and colleagues conclude that youngsters with Prader–Willi syndrome may have strengths in visual processing relative to auditory processing.

Further work has clarified and expanded certain aspects of the apparent strengths in visual processing. In the administration of the K-ABC to 21 subjects, Dykens and colleagues (1992b) found that Simultaneous Processing was better developed than Sequential Processing. High scores were noted in tasks assessing perceptual closure, long-term memory, spatial organization, attention to visual detail, and visual–motor integration. Among the Sequential Processing tasks, which rely on short-term memory, subjects showed particular difficulties with visual–motor and auditory–visual short-term memory. A profile is thus suggested for some individuals with Prader–Willi syndrome: relative strengths in perceptual organization, and difficulties in visual and other short-term memory tasks.

Indeed, visual processing strengths may not always be readily apparent, especially in short-term memory tasks. In a series of studies assessing pictorial short-term memory, Warren and Hunt (1981) compared 11 children with Prader–Willi syndrome to age- and IQ-matched children with mental retardation of nonspecific etiologies. Rela-

tive to their counterparts, the children with Prader–Willi syndrome showed more difficulties with immediate visual memory, no improvements in recall of stimuli with either increasing mental or chronological age, and a greater loss of information over time. In contrast to these short-term memory deficits, the children with Prader–Willi performed on par with the control group in a long-term memory task assessing how quickly subjects recalled well-known information. Interestingly, parents often report that their offspring with Prader–Willi syndrome can recall well-known or more obscure facts with a remarkable level of detail (e.g., where people parked as they arrived for a family party years ago). As suggested by Warren and Hunt's (1981) findings, however, this type of recall is not likely to prove unique to Prader–Willi syndrome.

In summary, then, some people with Prader–Willi syndrome show relative strengths in spatial–perceptual organization and visual processing. Relative weaknesses may be apparent in short-term memory, including visual, motoric, and auditory short-term processing. Although findings suggest a distinctive cognitive profile, not all persons with Prader–Willi syndrome show this profile. Studies are needed that identify the range of cognitive profiles seen in this syndrome, including how variables such as age or IQ may relate to different cognitive patterns. Cognitive profiles identified to date in Prader–Willi syndrome may be shared among people with other genetic syndromes or with nonspecific etiologies. Additional comparative studies are thus necessary to settle the issue of whether Prader–Willi syndrome is associated with a unique profile of cognitive or academic strengths or weaknesses.

Adaptive Profiles

Deficits in specific domains of adaptive behavior are salient in the definition and diagnosis of mental retardation (see Hodapp & Dykens, 1994, for a review). Despite their nosological prominence, however, little is known about the adaptive strengths and weaknesses of people with specific syndromes, including those with Prader–Willi syndrome (Dykens, 1995). In one study of adolescents and adults with Prader–Willi syndrome, relative strengths were found on the Daily Living Skills domain of the Vineland Adaptive Behavior Scales, especially in domestic skills such as cooking and cleaning (Dykens et al., 1992a). As noted in Table 25.2, these same subjects showed significant relative weaknesses in the Socialization domain, notably in the coping skills subdomain.

Although distinctive, these profiles are not unique to Prader–Willi syndrome. Males with fragile X syndrome, for example, showed relative strengths in Daily Living Skills on the Vineland (Dykens, Hodapp, & Leckman, 1994), and females with fragile X syndrome had relative weaknesses in Socialization (Freund, Reiss, & Abrams, 1993). However, the reasons for these similar profiles are likely to be different across syndromes. In individuals with Prader–Willi syndrome, strengths in cooking or cleaning seem consistent with interests in food, whereas these same skills in males with fragile X syndrome may be related to the repetitive, rote nature of these daily living tasks (Dykens, Hodapp, & Leckman, 1994). The weaknesses in coping skills seen in Prader–Willi syndrome are likely to be associated with the impulsivity, temper tantrums, and compulsive tendencies that characterize this syndrome (Dykens & Cassidy, 1995; Oliver, Woodcock, & Humphreys, 2009; Woodcock, Oliver, & Humphreys, 2009). Among females with fragile X syndrome, however, problems with Socialization are seen primarily in the interpersonal subdomain, and are probably related to that syndrome's proneness to shyness, gaze aversion, and social anxiety (Freund et al., 1993). Although Vineland profiles may thus be similar across these or other syndromes, the factors associated with these profiles are likely to be different.

Linguistic Profiles

Language development in children with Prader–Willi syndrome is typically delayed, though expressive vocabulary and language may eventually emerge as areas of strength for many youngsters with the syndrome. Studies that have examined speech–language issues in people with Prader–Willi syndrome have noted significant variability across individuals with regard to speech–language development and patterns of strengths and weaknesses (e.g., Van Borsel, Defloor, & Curfs, 2007). Branson (1981) found no common features in the language profiles of 21 children with Prader–Willi syndrome. Similarly, various linguistic profiles were observed in 18 children by Kleppe, Katayama, Shipley, and Foushee (1990). Differences were seen across subjects' severity of speech and language problems, and in the range of their intelligibility, fluency, and voice problems. Kleppe and colleagues did, however, find some common speech–language characteristics, primarily hypernasality, errors with certain speech sounds and complex syntax, and reduced vocabulary skills relative to age expectations. The speech and articulation difficulties are likely to be associated with hypotonia, and perhaps with thick, viscous saliva (Kleppe et al., 1990). More recent findings further support the presence of articulation errors, oral–motor difficulties, and hypernasality in young children with Prader–Willi syndrome (Lewis, Freebairn, Heeger, & Cassidy, 2002). Speech problems, primarily with articulation and intelligibility, were also noted by 33 out of 43 parents of children with Prader–Willi syndrome ages 4–19 years (Dykens & Kasari, 1997). Akefeldt, Akefeldt, and Gillberg (1997), in addition to Defloor, Van Borsel, and Curfs (2000), have documented significant impairments in word recall and syntax. In addition, individuals with Prader–Willi syndrome often talk too much and verbally perseverate on a narrow range of topics (Dykens, Leckman, & Cassidy, 1996). It remains unknown, however, how perseveration relates to such linguistic features as pragmatics, discourse, and the social uses of language.

Cognitive and Adaptive Development

Data are limited on how cognition in people with Prader–Willi syndrome changes over the course of development. An early study of eight children with the syndrome reported that IQ declined in early childhood (Dunn, 1968). It was unclear, however, whether these declines were assessed by formal IQ tests or by a failure to achieve certain developmental milestones.

Using standardized IQ scores, Dykens and colleagues (1992b) conducted both cross-sectional and longitudinal analyses of IQ change in children and adults. IQ scores were cross-sectionally examined in 21 adolescents and adults, and longitudinal analyses included 31 subjects ages 5–30 years who had been given the same IQ test twice. IQ scores showed nonsignificant fluctuations in both cross-sectional and longitudinal analyses, with no evidence of IQ declines in childhood or early adulthood. Overall IQ scores thus appear relatively stable in school-age children with Prader–Willi syndrome, reflecting slow and steady gains in mental age that then stabilize in the adult years.

Regarding their levels of adaptive skills, adolescents and young adults with Prader–Willi syndrome seem to show steady gains in certain aspects of their adaptive behavior, primarily their daily living and socialization skills (Dykens et al., 1992a; Holland et al., 2003). Longitudinal studies are necessary to clarify these preliminary findings, as well as to identify how gains in adaptive skills relate to age, IQ, residential placement, and educational or vocational programming.

Findings to date thus point to a different course of cognitive and adaptive development in people with Prader–Willi syndrome, compared to people with some other genetic syndromes. Some children with Down syndrome, for example, show alternating periods of growth and stability in their cognitive, adaptive, and linguistic development (Dykens, Hodapp, & Evans, 1994; Hodapp & Zigler, 1990). Many males with fragile X syndrome show slow, steady gains in cognitive and adaptive functioning that seem to stabilize in late childhood or early adolescence, resulting in a plateau in mental age scores and decline in IQ and adaptive behavior standard scores (Dykens, Hodapp, & Leckman, 1994). Different trajectories across Prader–Willi and other syndromes call into question the idea that people with mental retardation are uniform in their course of slowed development, regardless of their etiology (Hodapp, 2004; Hodapp & Fidler, 1999; Silverstein, 1982).

In addition to comparative studies, longitudinal work is sorely needed that relates cognitive and adaptive development to the onset of hyperphagia in young children with Prader–Willi syndrome. The severity of non-food-related maladaptive behaviors has been shown to be related to the severity of eating behavior (Dimitropoulos, Blackford, Walden, & Thompson, 2006). More stud-

ies need to be conducted that examine how the onset or severity of hyperphagia affects a young child's developing cognitive or behavioral schemas. Given the central role of hyperphagia in Prader–Willi syndrome, we suspect that this effect is far-reaching. It may be, for example, that the young child with Prader–Willi syndrome develops cognitive or behavioral schemas to accommodate to hyperphagia, such as more attention to some stimuli than to others, or tantrums or anxiety when food is denied. These strategies may then stay with the child over time; may spill over into areas unrelated to food; and may ultimately contribute to the perseverative, compulsive-like behaviors, tantrums, and other problems that characterize Prader–Willi syndrome.

Maladaptive Behavior and Psychopathology

Range of Maladaptive Behavior

Most behavioral work in Prader–Willi syndrome focuses on maladaptive features and psychopathology. These problems are often severe, and they immediately capture our attention as both clinicians and researchers. Although the behavioral dysfunction is compelling, studies of it have been accomplished at the expense of research on the personality and psychosocial strengths of people with Prader–Willi syndrome. Although studies of strengths in people with Prader–Willi syndrome are now underway, at this time we know very little about how social competencies or personality strengths relate to behavioral dysfunction and psychopathology.

Anecdotally, young children with Prader–Willi syndrome are described as pleasant, friendly, social, and somewhat placid (Cassidy, 1984). These features do not necessarily disappear, but older children and adults are routinely described as showing a host of negative or maladaptive behaviors, with young adults showing the greatest risk (Dykens, 2004; Steinhausen, Eiholzer, Hauffa, & Malin, 2004). Often these behaviors are more difficult to manage than food seeking, and they pose multiple challenges to families, teachers, and clinicians (Dykens & Hodapp, 1997).

Characteristic behavior problems are noted as minor criteria in the consensus diagnostic criteria for Prader–Willi syndrome (Holm et al., 1993), with often-noted problems including temper tantrums, stubbornness, oppositionality, rigidity, lying, and stealing. Many persons with this syndrome are also described as quite clever and manipulative, especially in regard to obtaining food.

The frequency and severity of maladaptive behaviors were examined in more detail in two different samples of subjects with Prader–Willi syndrome. We administered the Child Behavior Checklist (CBCL; Achenbach, 1991) to parents and caregivers of 91 subjects with Prader–Willi syndrome (subjects were ages 4–47 years). Maladaptive behaviors that occurred in 50% or more of the sample are summarized in Table 25.3. Certain behaviors were seen in 75% to almost 100% of subjects, including skin picking, argumentativeness, stubbornness, obsessions, tantrums, underactivity, excessive sleep, compulsions, and anxiety.

We administered a different measure, the Reiss Screen for Maladaptive Behavior, to parents and caregivers of 61 adolescents and adults with Prader–Willi syndrome (subjects were ages 13–49 years) (Dykens & Cassidy, 1995). Certain behaviors were remarkably consistent across samples and measures, including temper tantrums (84%), overeating (81%), impulsivity (74%), and aggression (64%).

The majority of subjects in both samples had scores that reached clinically significant levels. Among the 91 children and adults, 82% had CBCL T-scores consistent with those of Achenbach's (1991) clinically referred sample. Among the 61 adolescents and adults, 85% had one or more clinically elevated subtest scores on the Reiss Screen, with most (72%) showing two or more clinical elevations (Dykens & Cassidy, 1995). Maladaptive behaviors thus often reach a point where further clinical evaluation and interventions are necessary (Dykens & Hodapp, 1997).

Specificity of Maladaptive Features

Although certain behaviors are both salient and clinically significant in Prader–Willi syndrome, studies have yet to compare these features to those of other persons with mental retardation. In particular, we do not know which maladaptive features are specific to Prader–Willi syndrome, which are shown by many persons with mental retardation, and which are shared by persons with only a few other etiologies of mental retardation.

At first glance, hyperphagia appears a unique aspect of Prader–Willi syndrome. Although some people with mental retardation show increased interests in food or propensities to being overweight (Prasher, 1995), these generally do not occur to the same degree as in Prader–Willi syndrome. Other behaviors, such as temper tantrums, argumentativeness, or stubbornness, are seen in many persons with mental retardation in general.

Although persons with Prader–Willi syndrome are not unique in all aspects of mal-

TABLE 25.3. Frequently Occurring CBCL Behaviors in 91 Individuals with Prader–Willi Syndrome (Ages 4–47 Years)

Behavior	%	Behavior	%
Skin picking	97	Mood changes	76
Argues a lot	95	Excessive sleep	75
Stubborn	95	Steals (food)	71
Obsessions	94	Compulsions	71
Overeating	93	Worried, anxious	70
Tantrums	88	Talks too much	68
Underactive	87	Prefers being alone	67
Overtired	81	Can't concentrate	66
Clumsy	80	Gets teased a lot	65
Disobedient	78	Speech problems	65
Demands attention	78	Peers don't like	60
Lies (food-related)	78	Hoards	55
Overweight	77	Withdrawn	53
Impulsive	76	Unhappy, sad	51

adaptive behavior, certain behaviors may be more common in this population than in others with mental retardation. Dykens and Kasari (1997) compared 43 subjects with Prader–Willi syndrome (ages 4–19 years) to age- and sex-matched subjects with Down syndrome and nonspecific mental retardation. On the CBCL (Achenbach, 1991), subjects with Prader–Willi syndrome showed significantly higher levels of internalizing, externalizing, and overall problem behaviors. These individuals were also more apt to overeat and be overweight; to be teased by peers; and to show skin picking, argumentativeness, verbal perseveration, obsessions, compulsions, fatigue, sleep problems, underactivity, and stealing at home (primarily food or money to buy food).

A discriminant-function analysis of these CBCL data suggested a relatively distinct Prader–Willi syndrome behavioral phenotype, with 91% of the persons with Prader–Willi syndrome correctly classified, and just 3 of the 86 comparison group subjects mistakenly assigned to the Prader–Willi group. As shown in Table 25.4, seven behaviors best discriminated the three groups, with the Prader–Willi group being singularly high in skin picking, fatigue, obsessions, and talking too much. Thus a blend of certain maladaptive behaviors appears quite distinctive to Prader–Willi syndrome, and may be highly predictive of this disorder. Overeating, food obsessions, and sleep disturbances are salient in Prader–Willi syndrome; yet other obsessions and repetitive, compulsion-like behaviors also seem to be central distinguishing features of this syndrome.

Correlates of Maladaptive Behavior

Most studies do not find significant gender differences in the maladaptive behavior of people with Prader–Willi syndrome. Three other variables, however, do relate to maladaptive behavior, sometimes in unexpected ways: IQ scores, weight, and family stress.

IQ SCORES

A central issue is whether people with relatively high IQ scores are somehow protected from some of the syndrome's more troublesome maladaptive behaviors. A high IQ often emerges as a protective factor in children who are at risk for delay or adjustment problems, or who are experiencing psychosocial adversities (Garmezy, Masten, & Tellegen, 1984; although see also Luthar, 1991, and Werner, 2005). We (Dykens & Cassidy, 1995) tested this possibility by comparing 43 subjects with relatively high IQs (mean IQ of 79) to 43 subjects with lower IQs (mean IQ of 59). No significant differences were found in either the type or severity of maladaptive behavior across groups.

These data, which are consistent with clinical observations of patients with Prader–Willi syndrome, have important implications for service delivery. In particular, state or other agencies that use low IQ scores (usually below 70) as a service eligibility re-

TABLE 25.4. Seven Behaviors That Discriminated Children with Prader–Willi Syndrome from Those with Down Syndrome and Nonspecific Mental Retardation with 91% Accuracy

Behavior	Prader–Willi syndrome	Down syndrome	Nonspecific mental retardation
Skin picking	High	Low	Low
Overtired	High	Low	Low
Obsessions	High	Low	Low
Impulsivity	High	Low	High
Speech problem	High	Low	Low/high[a]
Hyperactive	Low	Low	High

Note. Items from Dykens and Kasari (1997).
[a]"Lower than subjects with Prader–Willi syndrome, higher than subjects with Down syndrome.

quirement may exclude higher-functioning persons whose treatment needs are similar to those of lower-functioning persons. In Prader–Willi syndrome, then, IQ may be a less meaningful entry point into state or other systems of care than are the behavioral needs of the persons being served.

WEIGHT

Unlike IQ, maladaptive behavior may be related to weight, but in a way that is opposite to general expectations. Dykens and Cassidy (1995) found that thinner adults (i.e., those with lower body mass indices) had significantly higher maladaptive behavior scores than heavier persons (i.e., those with higher body mass indices), notably in internalizing symptoms. Specifically, thinner subjects showed more distressful affect and problems in thinking—confused and distorted thinking, anxiety, sadness, fearfulness, and crying. These findings need to be further explored, including how they relate to the stress of losing weight, as well as to changes in brain chemistry and physical activity level.

FAMILY STRESS

Finally, maladaptive behaviors are significantly related to heightened levels of familial stress (Dykens et al., 1996; Hodapp, Dykens, & Masino, 1997). Behavior problems in offspring with Prader–Willi syndrome (especially externalizing problems, such as tantrums and aggression) are the best predictors of familial stress, even in comparison with such features as the offspring's age, sex, IQ level, or degree of obesity. Furthermore, stress in families of children with Prader–Willi syndrome is high relative to stress in families of children with other types of mental retardation (Hodapp et al., 1997). Although parents are often most concerned about their children's tantrums and compulsiveness, these problems probably interact with hyperphagia and the lifelong need for dietary management to create high levels of stress.

Development of Maladaptive Behavior

It is not yet clear how maladaptive features in persons with Prader–Willi syndrome

shift and change over the course of development. The beginning of hyperphagia in early childhood is often associated with the onset or worsening of such behaviors as temper tantrums and aggression (Dimitropoulos, Fuerer, Butler, & Thompson, 2001; Dykens, Maxwell, Pantino, Kossler, & Roof, 2007). These behaviors then seem fairly stable across the developmental years. Dykens and Cassidy (1995) found similar rates of tantrums and other "externalizing" behaviors in young children (ages 4–7 years) and in older children (ages 8–12 years). Yet advancing age in these same children was correlated with heightened internal distress and features of depression, including withdrawal, isolation, negative self-image, and pessimism.

Some clinical reports note that behavioral problems increase in the adolescent and adult years, due to growing physical and psychosocial pressures (Greenswag, 1987; Whitman & Accardo, 1987). In contrast, others observe clinically that behavioral and emotional problems lessen with advancing age, and that older adults with Prader Willi syndrome may be more amenable to intervention (Waters, 1990).

Yet changes in maladaptive behavior may not follow a simple linear function. Instead, these behaviors may wax and wane throughout adulthood (Dykens & Cassidy, 1995; Dykens et al., 1992a). Whereas some behaviors may increase with age, others may improve or remain fairly stable. Examining 21 adolescents and adults cross-sectionally with the CBCL, Dykens and colleagues (1992a) found that underactivity and fatigue increased with age, whereas certain "externalizing" difficulties (e.g., running away and destroying property) decreased from adolescence to adulthood. Still other behaviors seemed to be fairly stable, such as temper tantrums, stubbornness, skin picking, and hoarding (Dykens et al., 1992a).

The waxing and waning of behavior problems may sometimes be associated with specific psychosocial stressors. Many young adults, for example, experience increased behavioral difficulties when they leave home and move into a group home setting, or when they make the transition from one job to another. In other persons, however, psychosocial precipitants for behavioral shifts are not apparent.

Psychiatric Features

The vast majority of studies in *dual diagnosis,* or co-occurring mental retardation and psychiatric illness, have used heterogeneous groups of subjects with mental retardation of mixed or unknown etiologies (Dykens, 1996). As a result, more is known about psychiatric illness in the general, heterogeneous population of people with mental retardation than in persons whose mental retardation has specific genetic etiologies.

Partly because of this mixed-group approach, little is yet known about the prevalence rates of psychiatric disorders in the population of persons with Prader–Willi syndrome. Although population-based prevalence studies have yet to be done, clinically we find that certain psychiatric disorders occur infrequently. For example, although many people with Prader–Willi syndrome steal food, and are impulsive and distractible, rates seem low for full-blown conduct disorder or attention-deficit/hyperactivity disorder. Tic disorders, dementia, and schizophrenia also appear relatively infrequently in this population. However, Clarke (1993) and Clarke, Webb, and Brachmann-Clarke (1995) reported on psychotic episodes in four young adults with Prader–Willi syndrome; all cases showed a paternal deletion of chromosome 15. These patients had a sudden onset of hallucinations and other psychotic symptoms, with no obvious precipitating events. All showed good outcome following milieu and pharmacological treatment. These cases suggest a need for large-scale studies that can identify whether Prader–Willi syndrome involves a particular vulnerability to schizophrenia-spectrum disorders, above and beyond the risk associated with mental retardation.

Reddy and Pfeiffer (2007) compared a sample of patients with Prader–Willi syndrome to a sample with mental retardation only and another having mental retardation and comorbid psychiatric disorder. Their findings suggested that youth with Prader–Willi syndrome displayed significantly higher rates of psychopathology, both of an internalizing and externalizing nature, when compared to peers with mental retardation only. In fact, the behaviors noted in the sample with Prader–Willi were comparable to those seen in the sample with comorbid mental retardation and psychiatric disorder across behavioral domains; an exception was that the Prader–Willi sample displayed less severe mood symptoms than the dual-diagnosis group.

Furthermore, Prader–Willi syndrome does not appear to include a heightened risk of autism or pervasive developmental disorder not otherwise specified (PDD-NOS), beyond the risk due to mental retardation. Of the handful of patients with Prader–Willi syndrome and co-occurring autism or PDD NOS that we have seen in the clinical setting, however, all had maternal UPD of chromosome 15. These clinical observations are consistent with those of Rogan and colleagues (1994) and Veltman and colleagues (2004), who suggested increased risks of autism or other, rare disorders in Prader–Willi syndrome cases involving maternal UPD of chromosome 15.

However, several other psychiatric disorders may occur with increased frequency in persons with Prader–Willi syndrome. These include mood disorders, as well as obsessive–compulsive disorder (OCD) and other anxiety disorders. Depressive features such as sadness and low self-esteem, as well as anxiety, fears, and worries, have all been noted in several studies of maladaptive behavior in Prader–Willi syndrome (e.g., Dykens et al., 1992a; Dykens & Cassidy, 1995; Dykens & Kasari, 1997; Stein, Keating, Zar, & Hollander, 1994; Whitman & Accardo, 1987). Among 91 children and adults assessed with the CBCL, for example, we found that 76% showed mood lability; 70% were worried or anxious; and 51% showed sadness, depression, and withdrawal.

Only recently have studies examined samples with Prader–Willi syndrome using formal *Diagnostic and Statistical Manual of Mental Disorders,* fourth edition, text revision (DSM-IV-TR; American Psychiatric Association [APA], 2000) or *International Classification of Diseases,* 10th revision (ICD-10; World Health Organization, 1992) diagnostic criteria for depressive disorders, or for anxiety disorders other than OCD. Soni and colleagues (2007) confirmed earlier work suggesting that psychiatric illness in individuals with Prader–Willi is predominantly mood- or anxiety-related in nature. In addition, those participants with UPD were shown to have greater severity, risk of recurrence, and number of episodes, and a worse response to medication, than the participants with deletion had. It thus remains unknown to what extent the sadness or worry shown by some persons with Prader–Willi syndrome might lead to full-blown cases of these disorders. It is also unclear what factors might predispose some persons with the syndrome to be more or less susceptible to mood or anxiety disorders.

Increased risks of OCD have been found in persons with Prader–Willi syndrome. Compulsive-like symptoms have long been hallmark features of Prader–Willi syndrome—primarily skin picking, food preoccupations, and repetitive food-seeking behaviors (e.g., Didden, Korzilius, & Curfs, 2007; Dykens et al., 1992a; Hellings & Warnock, 1994; Holm et al., 1993; Stein et al., 1994). Yet many persons show repetitive thoughts and compulsive behaviors not related to skin picking or food (Clarke et al., 2002; Greaves, Prince, Evans, & Charman, 2006; Wigren & Hansen, 2005) that may not subside with age (Wigren & Hansen, 2003b).

Dykens and colleagues (1996) identified a wide range of non-food-related obsessions and compulsions in a study of 91 children and adults with Prader–Willi syndrome. As measured by the Yale–Brown Obsessive–Compulsive Scale (Goodman et al., 1989), prominent compulsions in this sample included hoarding items such as paper, pens,

trash, and toiletries (58%); rewriting and redoing things (37%); and concerns with symmetry, exactness, ordering, and arranging (35–40%). Over half of the subjects (53%) also had to tell, ask, or say things, often perseverating on a narrow range of topics. Relatively fewer subjects had cleaning, contamination, or checking symptoms (15–24%). Thus, for instance, many subjects in this study often ordered and arranged toys or objects according to specific rules based on size, shape, or color, or simply until they were "just right." Others rewrote letters or words until they were just right, or could not tolerate slight imperfections in the environment.

Furthermore, as specified in the DSM-IV criteria for OCD (APA, 1994), a remarkably high proportion of subjects had moderate to severe levels of obsessive and compulsive symptomatology. Indeed, 64% showed at least a moderate level of symptom-related distress, and 80% had symptom-related adaptive impairment. Other ties between Prader–Willi syndrome and OCD were found by comparing 43 adults with Prader–Willi syndrome to age- and sex-matched nonretarded adults with OCD (Dykens et al., 1996). As shown in Table 25.5, the two groups showed similar levels of symptom severity, similar numbers of compulsions, and more areas of symptom similarity than difference.

TABLE 25.5. Comparison of Compulsions in 43 Adults with Prader–Willi Syndrome versus Age- and Gender-Matched Adults with OCD

	PWS		OCD		
Y-BOCS features	M	SD	M	SD	F
Number of compulsions	3.75	2.11	4.02	2.81	NS
Severity of compulsions	10.77	3.90	9.09	4.44	NS
Specific symptoms	%		%		χ^2
Cleaning	33%		37%		NS
Checking	16%		55%		21.16**
Repeating rituals	40%		54%		NS
Counting	19%		28%		NS
Ordering/arranging	29%		28%		NS
Hoarding	79%		7%		46.75**
Need to tell, ask	51%		23%		7.16*

Note. Y-BOCS, Yale–Brown Obsessive–Compulsive Scale; NS, nonsignificant. Items from Dykens, Leckman, and Cassidy (1996).
*$p < .01$; **$p < .001$.

Increased risks of OCD are thus strongly indicated in persons with Prader–Willi syndrome (State, Dykens, Rosner, Martin, & King, 1999); these individuals exhibit a wide range of severe symptoms, and are similar to adults without mental retardation but with OCD. In contrast, studies with heterogeneous groups of persons with mental retardation find that only 1–3% meet criteria for OCD (e.g., Davis, Saeed, & Antonacci, 2008; Meyers, 1987; Vitiello, Spreat, & Behar, 1989). It may be that one or more genes associated with this increased vulnerability to OCD will be found in the Prader–Willi critical region on chromosome 15, or that the pathogenesis of Prader–Willi syndrome in some way predisposes individuals to obsessive and compulsive behaviors.

Further work needs to identify the extent to which Prader–Willi syndrome also involves heightened risks of mood, non-OCD anxiety, impulse control, or psychotic disorders, above and beyond the risks associated with mental retardation per se. It also remains unknown how any of these psychiatric features relate to molecular genetic status. Behavioral or cognitive differences have generally not been found between subjects with chromosome 15 paternal deletion and those with maternal UPD (Cassidy et al., 1997). Although Cassidy (1995) reported that those with deletion may be more prone to repetitive skin picking and perhaps other compulsive symptoms, other findings fail to support this conclusion (Milner et al., 2005). Persons with maternal UPD may be more prone to autism or PDD symptoms (Milner et al., 2005; Rogan et al., 1994), however, more research is still needed to clarify these preliminary observations.

INTERVENTIONS: MEDICAL AND BEHAVIORAL

Managing Prader–Willi syndrome's characteristic obesity and significant behavioral/psychiatric dysfunction constitutes a major treatment challenge, requiring cooperative input from geneticists, primary care physicians, endocrinologists, nutritionists, psychologists, psychiatrists, educators, families, group home staff members, and other care providers. It is often helpful for a health or mental health professional to follow an individual with Prader–Willi syndrome on a long-term basis, to help maintain continuity of care and to coordinate services. Table 25.6 summarizes many of the intervention recommendations discussed below. More detailed information on the management of Prader–Willi syndrome may be found in an edited volume written for care providers of all types, now in its third edition (Butler, Lee, & Whitman, 2006).

TABLE 25.6. Salient Treatment Recommendations in Prader–Willi Syndrome

- Maintain well-balanced, reduced-calorie diet (1,000–1,200 kilocalories/day), assuring adequate calcium intake.
- Encourage regular, sustained exercise (30 minutes daily).
- Restrict access to food (e.g., locked cabinets, refrigerator).
- Provide close supervision, especially in the school cafeteria, at work, and in the community.
- Maintain external food supports even when people lose weight or have high IQs.
- Be aware of possible conflict between food restrictions and choice/personal rights.
- Assess feasibility of growth hormone treatment.
- Consider over-the-counter products to increase saliva production.
- Appreciate impact of tantrums and other maladaptive behaviors on family stress.
- Provide clear behavioral expectations and limits, beginning at an early age; apply consistent limits across home and school or work.
- Maintain consistency in daily routines.
- Assess for increased risks of OCD/other anxiety disorders, impulse control problems, and depressive disorders.
- Determine whether compulsive tendencies lead to getting "stuck," and provide extra support with transitions.
- Check for sadness even in persons with adequate weight control.
- Ensure appropriate special education, and be sure that IEPs address needs for speech and physical therapies, as well as needs for increased physical activity.
- Provide ample planning for school-to-work transition; consider need for food supports in transition plans; assess feasibility of dedicated group homes versus other living settings.

Medical Management

Obesity

With good reason, weight and dietary management have long been targets of intervention in Prader–Willi syndrome. Experience in almost 30 years of managing Prader–Willi syndrome in an interdisciplinary clinic has demonstrated that obesity prevention or weight reduction and maintenance can be achieved with the following:

- A well-balanced, low-calorie diet of about 1,000–1,200 kilocalories/day (assuring adequate calcium intake).
- Periodic weigh-ins (e.g., once a week).
- Regular exercise to increase muscle mass and thus efficiently burn calories (30 minutes per day is an appropriate goal).
- Environmental modification as needed, such as locking kitchen cabinets and the refrigerator.
- Close supervision to minimize access to food (e.g., supervision of spending money; supervision of meals in the school cafeteria, on the job, or in the community).

Although these techniques are considered state-of-the-art in treating hyperphagia in Prader–Willi syndrome, they are increasingly viewed by advocates in the developmental disability field as being too restrictive, and as limiting the personal rights and choices of adults with this syndrome (see Dykens, Goff, et al., 1997, for a discussion). Clinicians thus need to be aware of possible conflicts between some interventions (e.g., locking the refrigerator or limiting spending money) with their clients' right to food and to their paychecks. Furthermore, external food supports and interventions should be continued even when people lose weight or show needs for less supervision in the non-food-related parts of their lives.

To date, no medication has shown long-term effectiveness in controlling appetites in people with Prader–Willi syndrome, despite the widespread interest in such a medication in the Prader–Willi syndrome community. Therefore, behavioral approaches continue to be of considerable value in helping parents and other care providers set limits concerning food, and supporting them in the lifelong effort to prevent the health consequences of obesity (Dykens & Cassidy, 1995).

Other Medical Concerns

Management of other physical problems associated with Prader–Willi syndrome is largely problem-oriented. Although the use of growth hormone in Prader–Willi syndrome is still somewhat controversial, ongoing controlled studies suggest great benefit from growth hormone replacement therapy. Not only does such treatment result in increased height; perhaps more importantly, it causes an improvement in body composition and increased muscle mass, thus decreasing the body mass index (Angulo et al., 1996).

Sex hormone replacement therapy will increase the development of secondary sex characteristics and theoretically may improve osteoporosis, but testosterone treatment is sometimes associated with an increase in aggressive behavior. No controlled trials of treatment with sex hormones have yet been published.

Products to increase saliva production have proved of benefit in treating the dry mouth associated with Prader–Willi syndrome, and are also likely to improve dental hygiene and perhaps articulation as well. Speech therapy can be beneficial to people with Prader–Willi syndrome of all ages to address speech production abnormalities, and physical and occupational therapies have also proven helpful in treating hypotonia and poor coordination.

Educational, Behavioral, and Psychiatric Management

Educational and Vocational Management

Most children with Prader–Willi syndrome need special education services that address their unique cognitive and behavioral needs (Fidler, Hodapp, & Dykens, 2002; Levine & Wharton, 1993). Although individualized education programs (IEPs) should be based on a careful assessment of each student's cognitive strengths and weaknesses, most IEPs include speech–language and physical therapies; supervision around food; and extra physical education classes or other ways of increasing physical activity during the school day (e.g., walking). Many students do well with "hands-on" lessons and techniques that capitalize on their visual–spatial strengths, and that minimize their weaknesses in auditory–verbal short-term memory and sequential processing.

Students with Prader–Willi syndrome are placed in both inclusive and specialized or segregated educational settings; often a combination of these settings works well. Parents of students with Prader–Willi syndrome tend to view their children's ideal educational placement as specialized rather than inclusive (Hodapp, Freeman, & Kasari, 1998). Compared to parents of children with Down syndrome, parents of students with Prader–Willi syndrome request more specialized services (e.g., speech or physical therapies), even if this means leaving their local neighborhood school; they are also more concerned with the transition from school to work in the adolescent years (Hodapp et al., 1998).

Adults with Prader–Willi syndrome need careful vocational planning. Successful job placements typically require job coaches and extra support to address food seeking and other behavioral difficulties. Many adults also do well in group homes, especially ones designed specifically for persons with Prader–Willi syndrome. Compared to family homes or less supervised community settings, group homes dedicated to adults with Prader–Willi syndrome appear to be the most effective in reducing and maintaining weight over time, as well as in managing behavioral difficulties (Cassidy et al., 1994; Greenswag, 1987).

Behavioral and Psychiatric Management

Clinicians need to be aware that even though food-related behavior is a significant issue in Prader–Willi syndrome, other maladaptive behaviors are likely to be the major reasons why many families seek professional help. We have noted earlier that even as compared to food issues, obesity, age, or IQ level, the best predictors of family stress are maladaptive behaviors such as temper tantrums, compulsion, and needs for sameness in routine (Dykens et al., 1996; Hodapp et al., 1997).

Improved behavior both at home and at school is often the result of strict reinforcement of behavioral limits, clear delineation of behavioral expectations, and establishment of regular routines. Establishing clear limits regarding food and behavior is especially important with the emergence of hyperphagia in the toddler or preschool years. Clinically, we find that setting behavioral limits at a young age paves the way for more successful responses to limit setting over the developmental and adolescent years.

But families often have difficulty adhering to and enforcing behavioral and food limits over the long term. Some families benefit from occasional or more sustained support from behavioral, family, and other therapists, as well as from the support of other families of persons with Prader–Willi syndrome. Ongoing parent support groups are now offered through the state chapters of the Prader–Willi Syndrome Association (*www.pwsausa.org*) and through the Prader–Willi Foundation (*www.fpwr.org*); toll-free numbers for these organizations are 800-926-4797 and 800-253-7993, respectively. Support groups can also be accessed through state and national meetings, as well as the Internet. These formal and informal parent-to-parent support mechanisms are often of enormous help to families.

In addition to behavioral interventions and family support, many persons with Prader–Willi syndrome need extra help getting "unstuck" from their obsessions and compulsions. Indeed, tantrums and stubbornness in persons with this syndrome often seem related to their being "stuck" and unable to move from one activity or thought to the next. Consistent limit setting across home and school settings often helps reduce tantrums, as do predictable daily routines. Other tantrums may be circumvented by distraction and by giving individuals ample warning about transitions, including special auditory or visual transitional cues. If tantrums are inevitable, it is typically helpful for parents or teachers to avoid talking about the issue until well after the individual has settled down.

Although the prevalence of mood disorders in the population with Prader–Willi syndrome remains unknown, depressive features need to be carefully assessed in clients with this syndrome (Deescheemaeker et al., 2002). As they develop, children may be particularly vulnerable to increased negative self-evaluation, isolation, and withdrawal (Dykens & Cassidy, 1995); these features may reflect the children's growing awareness of their differences from peers. Depressive features and disorganized thinking may also be heightened among adolescents and adults who have achieved adequate weight control (Dykens & Cassidy, 1995). Many children and adults benefit from school, clinic, or recreational programs that target improved self-esteem, social skills, and peer relations (Dykens & Cassidy, 1995; Kundert, 2008; Levine & Wharton, 1993).

In addition, pharmacology is often used to address depressive or obsessive–compulsive features, as well as severe aggression and temper tantrums. Several case studies report that selective serotonin reuptake inhibitors (SSRIs) have helped some individuals gain better control of tantrums and compulsive symptoms such as skin picking (Benjamin & Buot-Smith, 1993; Dech & Budow, 1991; Eiholzer, 2001; Hellings & Warnock, 1994; Warnock & Kestenbaum, 1992). Although SSRIs are currently quite popular in the Prader–Willi syndrome community, controlled studies have yet to be published. More recently, open-label small-scale studies have documented the effectiveness of topiramate, an anticonvulsant, in the reduction of self-injurious behavior among individuals with Prader–Willi syndrome (Shapira, Lessig, Lewis, Goodman, & Driscoll, 2004; Shapira, Lessig, Murphy, Driscoll, & Goodman, 2002). Risperidone has also been used in the reduction of disruptive behavioral symptoms (Durst et al., 2000).

NEXT STEPS

Although Prader–Willi syndrome was identified just over 50 years ago, research on it is accumulating at a growing rate, particularly on the genetic aspects of this disorder. Work is now well underway that aims to identify specific genes in the Prader–Willi/Angelman critical region, as well as mechanisms associated with genomic imprinting. In comparison, research on Prader–Willi syndrome's behavioral phenotype lags behind. This gap is probably attributable to the predominant practice in behavioral studies of using heterogeneous groups of subjects with mental retardation (Dykens, 1995, 1996; Hodapp & Dykens, 1994). We thus know more about behavior and development in people with mental retardation in general than we do about people with distinctive etiologies such as Prader–Willi or other syndromes.

With its genetic and behavioral complexities, Prader–Willi syndrome is an ideal condition to pave the way for more syndrome-specific behavioral research. Although studies on maladaptive behavior and psychiatric problems are now emerging, research is also needed on the strengths and competencies of people with this disorder. Furthermore, approaches are needed that tie together genetics and behavior in Prader–Willi syndrome. Studies might, for example, systematically compare behavior, development, and hypothalamic function across persons with deletions as opposed to UPD. Finally, treatment outcome research is sorely needed, including studies of how early diagnosis and intervention affect subsequent health, mental health, and quality of life. Such research offers much promise for improving the long-term success of people with Prader–Willi syndrome and their families.

ACKNOWLEDGMENTS

We are grateful to the families of patients affected with Prader–Willi syndrome for their continuing support and participation in Prader–Willi syndrome clinics and clinical research. Particular appreciation goes to those who are willing to have photographs published. We are grateful as well to the many professionals who help run the Prader–Willi syndrome clinics at the University of Connecticut, the University of California at Los Angeles, and Case Western Reserve University. We also thank Robert M. Hodapp for his helpful comments on this chapter. This work was supported in part by Grant No. 03008 from the National Institute of Child Health and Human Development.

REFERENCES

Achenbach, T. M. (1991). *Manual for the Child Behavior Checklist/4–18 and 1991 Profile.* Burlington: University of Vermont, Department of Psychiatry.

Akefeldt, A., Akefeldt, B., & Gillberg, C. (1997). Voice, speech, and language characteristics of children with Prader–Willi syndrome. *Journal of Intellectual Disability Research, 41,* 302–311.

American Psychiatric Association (APA). (1994). *Diagnostic and statistical manual of mental disorders* (4th ed.). Washington, DC: Author.

American Psychiatric Association (APA). (2000). *Diagnostic and statistical manual of mental disorders* (4th ed., text rev.). Washington, DC: Author.

American Society of Human Genetics (ASHG) &

American College of Medical Genetics (ACMG). (1996). Diagnostic testing for Prader–Willi and Angelman syndromes: Report of the ASHG/ACMG Test and Technology Transfer Committee. *American Journal of Human Genetics, 58,* 1085–1088.

Angulo, M., Castro-Magana, M., Mazur, B., Canas, J. A., Vitollo, P. M., & Sarrantonio, M. (1996). Growth hormone secretion and effects of growth hormone therapy on growth velocity and weight gain in children with Prader–Willi syndrome. *Journal of Pediatric Endocrinology and Metabolism, 9,* 393–400.

Aughton, D. A., & Cassidy, S. B. (1990). Physical features of Prader–Willi syndrome in neonates. *American Journal of Diseases of Children, 144,* 1251–1254.

Baker, H. J., & Leland, B. (1967). *Detroit Tests of Learning Aptitude.* Indianapolis, IN: Bobbs-Merrill.

Bartella, L., Girelli, L., Grungi, G., Marchi, S., Molinari, E., & Semenza, C. (2005). Mathematical skills in Prader–Willi syndrome. *Journal of Intellectual Disability Research, 49,* 159–169.

Bellon-Harn, M. L. (2005). Clinical management of a child with Prader–Willi syndrome from maternal uniparental disomy (UPD) genetic inheritance. *Journal of Communication Disorders, 38,* 459–472.

Benjamin, E., & Buot-Smith, T. (1993). Naltrexone and fluoxetine in Prader–Willi syndrome. *Journal of the American Academy of Child and Adolescent Psychiatry, 32,* 870–873.

Borghgraef, M., Fryns, J. P., & Van den Berghe, V. D. (1990). Psychological profile and behavioral characteristics in 12 patients with Prader–Willi syndrome. *Genetic Counseling, 38,* 141–150.

Branson, C. (1981). Speech and language characteristics of children with Prader–Willi syndrome. In V. A. Holm, S. Sulzbacher, & P. Pipes (Eds.), *The Prader–Willi syndrome* (pp. 179–183). Baltimore: University Park Press.

Buiting, K., Saitoh, S., Gross, S., Dittrich, B., Schwartz, S., Nicholas, R. D., & Horsthemke, B. (1994). Inherited microdeletions in the Angelman and Prader–Willi syndromes define an imprinting centre on human chromosome 15. *Nature Genetics, 9,* 395–400.

Burd, L., Vesely, B., Martsolf, J., & Kerbeshian, J. (1990). Prevalence study of Prader–Willi syndrome in North Dakota. *American Journal of Medical Genetics, 37,* 97–99.

Butler, M. G. (1989). Hypopigmentation: A common feature of the Prader–Labhart–Willi syndrome. *American Journal of Human Genetics, 45,* 140–146.

Butler, M. G. (1990). Prader–Willi syndrome: Current understanding of cause and diagnosis. *American Journal of Medical Genetics, 35,* 319–332.

Butler, M. G. (1996). Molecular diagnosis of Prader–Willi syndrome: Comparison of cytogenetic and molecular genetic data including parent of origin dependent methylation DNA patterns. *American Journal of Medical Genetics, 61,* 188–190.

Butler, M. G., Hanchett, J. M., & Thompson, T. (2006). Clinical findings and natural history of Prader–Willi syndrome. In M. G. Butler, P. D. K. Lee, & B. Y. Whitman (Eds.), *Management of Prader–Willi syndrome* (3rd ed., pp. 201–241). New York: Springer-Verlag.

Butler, M. G., Lee, P. D. K., & Whitman, B. Y. (Eds.). (2006). *Management of Prader–Willi syndrome* (3rd ed.). New York: Springer-Verlag.

Cassidy, S. B. (1984). Prader–Willi syndrome. *Current Problems in Pediatrics, 14,* 1–55.

Cassidy, S. B. (1995, June). *Complexities of clinical diagnosis of Prader–Willi syndrome.* Paper presented at the 2nd Prader–Willi Syndrome International Conference, Oslo, Norway.

Cassidy, S. B., Devi, A., & Mukaida, C. (1994). Aging in Prader–Willi syndrome: 22 patients over age 30 years. *Proceedings of the Greenwood Genetics Center, 13,* 102–103.

Cassidy, S. B., & Driscoll, D. J. (2009). Prader–Willi syndrome. *European Journal of Human Genetics, 17,* 3–13.

Cassidy, S. B., Forsythe, M., Heeger, S., Nicholls, R. D., Schork, N., Benn, P., et al. (1997). Comparison of phenotype between patients with Prader–Willi syndrome due to deletion 15q and uniparental disomy 15. *American Journal of Medical Genetics, 68,* 433–440.

Cassidy, S. B., Geer, J. S., Holm, V. A., & Hudgins, L. (1996). African-Americans with Prader–Willi syndrome are phenotypically different. *American Journal of Human Genetics, 59,* A21.

Christian, S. L., Smith, A. C. M., Macha, M., Black, S. H., Elder, F. F. B., Johnson, J. M. P., et al. (1996). Prenatal diagnosis of uniparental disomy 15 following trisomy 15 mosaicism. *Prenatal Diagnosis, 16,* 323–332.

Clarke, D. J. (1993). Prader–Willi syndrome and psychoses. *British Journal of Psychiatry, 163,* 680–684.

Clarke, D. J., Boer, H., Whittington, J., Holland, A., Butler, J., & Webb, T. (2002). Prader–Willi syndrome, compulsive and ritualistic behaviors: The first population-based survey. *British Journal of Psychiatry, 180,* 358–362.

Clarke, D. J., Webb, T., & Bachmann-Clarke, J. P. (1995). Prader–Willi syndrome and psychotic symptoms: Report of a further case. *Irish Journal of Psychological Medicine, 12,* 27–29.

Cotton, S., & Richdale, A. (2006). Brief report: Parental descriptions of sleep problems in children with autism, Down syndrome, and Prader–Willi syndrome. *Research in Developmental Disabilities, 27,* 151–161.

Crinò, A., Schiaffini, R., Ciampalimni, P., Spera, S., Beccaria, L., Benzi, L., et al. (2003). Hypogonadism and pubertal development in Prader–Willi syndrome. *European Journal of Pediatrics, 162,* 327–333.

Crnic, K. A., Sulzbacher, S., Snow, J., & Holm, V. A. (1980). Preventing mental retardation associated with gross obesity in the Prader–Willi syndrome. *Pediatrics, 66,* 787–789.

Curfs, L. G. (1992). Psychological profile and behavioral characteristics in Prader–Willi syndrome. In S. B. Cassidy (Ed.), *Prader–Willi syndrome and other 15q deletion disorders* (pp. 211–222). Berlin: Springer-Verlag.

Curfs, L. G., Wiegers, A. M., Sommers, J. R., Borghgraef, M., & Fryns, J. P. (1991). Strengths and weaknesses in the cognitive profile of youngsters with Prader–Willi syndrome. *Clinical Genetics, 40,* 430–434.

Davis, E., Saeed, S. A., & Antonacci, D. J. (2008). Anxiety disorders in persons with developmental disabilities: Empirically informed diagnosis and treatment: Reviews literature on anxiety disorders in DD population with practical take-home messages for the clinician. *Psychiatric Quarterly, 79,* 249–263.

Dech, B., & Budow, L. (1991). The use of fluoxetine in an adolescent with Prader–Willi syndrome. *Journal of the American Academy of Child and Adolescent Psychiatry, 30,* 298–302.

Deescheemaeker, M. J., Vogels, A., Govers, V., Borghgraef, M., Willekens, D., Swillen, A., et al. (2002). Prader–Willi syndrome: New insights in the behavioural and psychiatric spectrum. *Journal of Intellectual Disability Research, 46,* 41–50.

Defloor, T., Van Borsel, J., & Curfs, L. M. G. (2000). Speech fluency in Prader–Willi syndrome. *Journal of Fluency Disorders, 25,* 85–98.

Delach, J. A., Rosengren, S. S., Kaplan, L., Greenstein, R. M., Cassidy, S. B., & Benn, P. A. (1994). Comparison of high resolution chromosome banding and fluorescence *in situ* hybridization (FISH) for the laboratory evaluation of Prader–Willi syndrome and Angelman syndrome. *American Journal of Medical Genetics, 52,* 85–91.

DelParigi, A., Tschöp, M., Heiman, M. L., Salbe, A. D., Vozarova, B., Sell, S. M., et al. (2002). High circulating ghrelin: A potential cause for hyperphagia and obesity in Prader–Willi syndrome. *Journal of Clinical Endocrinology and Metabolism, 87,* 5461–5464.

Didden, R., Korzilius, H., & Curfs, L. M. G. (2007). Skin-picking in individuals with Prader–Willi syndrome: Prevalence, functional assessment, and its comorbidity with compulsive and self-injurious behaviors. *Journal of Applied Research in Intellectual Disabilities, 20,* 409–419.

Dimitropoulos, A., Blackford, J., Walden, T., & Thompson, T. (2006). Compulsive behavior in Prader–Willi syndrome: Examining severity in early childhood. *Research in Developmental Disabilities, 27,* 190–202.

Dimitropoulos, A., Fuerer, I. D., Butler, M. G., & Thompson, T. (2001). Emergence of compulsive behavior and tantrums in children with Prader–Willi syndrome. *American Journal on Mental Retardation, 106,* 39–51.

Dudley, O., McManus, B., Vogels, A., Whittington, J., & Musciatelli, F. (2008). Cross-cultural comparisons of obesity and growth in Prader–Willi syndrome. *Journal of Intellectual Disability Research, 52,* 426–436.

Dudley, O., & Muscatelli, F. (2007). Clinical evidence of intrauterine disturbance in Prader–Willi syndrome, a genetically imprinted neurodevelopmental disorder. *Early Human Development, 83,* 471–478.

Dunn, H. G. (1968). The Prader–Labhart–Willi syndrome: Review of the literature and report of nine cases. *Acta Paediatrica Scandinavica, 186,* 1–38.

Durst, R., Rubin-Jabotinsky, K., Raskin, S., Katz, G., & Zislin, J. (2000). Risperidone in treating behavioural disturbances of Prader–Willi syndrome. *Acta Psychiatrica Scandinavica, 102,* 461–465.

Dykens, E. M. (1995). Measuring behavioral phenotypes: Provocations from the "new genetics." *American Journal of Mental Retardation, 99,* 522–532.

Dykens, E. M. (1996). DNA meets DSM: Genetic syndromes' growing importance in dual diagnosis. *Mental Retardation, 34,* 125–127.

Dykens, E. M. (2002). Are jigsaw puzzle skills "spared" in persons with Prader–Willi syndrome? *Journal of Child Psychology and Psychiatry, 43,* 343–352.

Dykens, E. M. (2004). Maladaptive and compulsive behavior in Prader–Willi syndrome: New insights from older adults. *American Journal on Mental Retardation, 109,* 142–153.

Dykens, E. M., & Cassidy, S. B. (1995). Correlates of maladaptive behavior in children and adults with Prader–Willi syndrome. *American Journal of Medical Genetics, 60,* 546–549.

Dykens, E. M., & Clarke, D. J. (1997). Correlates of maladaptive behavior in individuals with 5p- (cri-du-chat) syndrome. *Developmental Medicine and Child Neurology, 39,* 752–756.

Dykens, E. M., Finucane, B. M., & Gayley, C. (1997). Cognitive and behavioral profiles in persons with Smith–Magenis syndrome. *Journal of Autism and Developmental Disorders, 27,* 203–211.

Dykens, E. M., Goff, B. J., Hodapp, R. M., Davis, L., Devanzo, P., Moss, F., et al. (1997). Eating themselves to death: Have "personal rights" gone too far in treating people with Prader–Willi syndrome? *Mental Retardation, 35,* 312–314.

Dykens, E. M., & Hodapp, R. M. (1997). Treatment issues in genetic mental retardation syndromes. *Professional Psychology: Research and Practice, 28,* 263–270.

Dykens, E. M., Hodapp, R. M., & Evans, P. W. (1994). Profiles and development of adaptive behavior in children with Down syndrome. *American Journal of Mental Retardation, 98,* 580–587.

Dykens, E. M., Hodapp, R. M., & Leckman, J. F. (1994). *Behavior and development in fragile X syndrome.* Newbury Park, CA: Sage.

Dykens, E. M., Hodapp, R. M., Walsh, K., & Nash, L. J. (1992a). Adaptive and maladaptive behavior in Prader–Willi syndrome. *Journal of the American Academy of Child and Adolescent Psychiatry, 31,* 1131–1136.

Dykens, E. M., Hodapp, R. M., Walsh, K., & Nash, L. J. (1992b). Profiles, correlates and trajectories of intelligence in individuals with Prader–Willi syndrome. *Journal of the American Academy of Child and Adolescent Psychiatry, 31,* 1125–1130.

Dykens, E. M., & Kasari, C. (1997). Maladaptive behavior in children with Prader–Willi syndrome, Down syndrome and non-specific mental retardation. *American Journal of Mental Retardation, 102,* 228–237.

Dykens, E. M., Leckman, J. F., & Cassidy, S. B. (1996). Obsessions and compulsions in Prader–Willi syndrome. *Journal of Child Psychology and Psychiatry, 37,* 995–1002.

Dykens, E. M., Maxwell, M. A., Pantino, E., Kossler, R., & Roof, F. (2007). Assessment of hyperphagia in Prader–Willi syndrome. *Obesity, 15,* 1816–1826.

Eiholzer, U. (2001). *A comprehensive team approach to the management of Prader–Willi syndrome.* Retrieved January 12, 2009, from *www.ipwso.org*

Eiholzer, U., & Lee, P. D. K. (2006). Medical considerations in Prader–Willi syndrome. In M. G. Butler, P. D. K. Lee, & B. Y. Whitman (Eds.), *Management of Prader–Willi syndrome* (3rd ed., pp. 97–152). New York: Springer-Verlag.

Einfeld, S. L., Kavanagh, S. J., Smith, A., Evans, E. J., Tonge, B. J., et al. (2006). Mortality in Prader–Willi syndrome. *American Journal on Mental Retardation, 111,* 193–198.

Fidler, D. J., Hodapp, R. M., & Dykens, E. M. (2002). Behavioral phenotypes and special education: Parent report of education isues for children with Down syndrome, Prader–Willi syndrome, and Williams syndrome. *Journal of Special Education, 36,* 80–88.

Freund, L. S., Reiss, A. L., & Abrams, M. T. (1993). Psychiatric disorders associated with fragile X in the young female. *Pediatrics, 91,* 321–329.

Gabel, S., Tarter, R. E., Gavaler, J., Golden, W., Hegedus, A. M., & Mair, B. (1986). Neuropsychological capacity of Prader–Willi children: General and specific aspects of impairment. *Applied Research in Mental Retardation, 7,* 459–466.

Garmezy, N., Masten, A. S., & Tellegen, A. (1984). The study of stress and competence in children: A building block for developmental psychopathology. *Child Development, 55,* 97–111.

Gillessen-Kaesbach, G., Robinson, W., Lohmann, D., Kaya-Westerloh, S., Passarge, E., & Horsthemke, B. (1995). Genotype–phenotype correlation in a series of 167 deletion and non-deletion patients with Prader–Willi syndrome. *Human Genetics, 96,* 638–643.

Glenn, C. C, Saitoh, S., Jong, M. T., Filbrandt, M. M., Surti, U., Driscoll, D. J., et al. (1996). Gene structure, DNA methylation and imprinted expression of the human *SNRPN* gene. *American Journal of Human Genetics, 58,* 335–346.

Goodman, W. K., Price, L. H., Rasmussen, S. A., Mazure, C, Fleischmann, R. L., Hill, C. L., et al. (1989). The Yale–Brown Obsessive–Compulsive Scale: Development, use and reliability. *Archives of General Psychiatry, 46,* 1006–1011.

Greaves, N., Prince, E., Evans, D. W., & Charman, T. (2006). Repetitive and ritualistic behavior in children with Prader–Willi syndrome and children with autism. *Journal of Intellectual Disability Research, 50,* 92–100.

Greenswag, L. R. (1987). Adults with Prader–Willi syndrome: A survey of 232 cases. *Developmental Medicine and Child Neurology, 29,* 145–152.

Gunay-Aygun, M., & Cassidy, S. B. (1997). Delayed diagnosis in Prader–Willi syndrome due to uniparental disomy. *American Journal of Medical Genetics, 71,* 106–110.

Gunay-Aygun, M., Cassidy, S. B., & Nicholls, R. D. (1997). Prader–Willi and other syndromes associated with obesity and mental retardation. *Behavior Genetics, 27,* 307–324.

Hagerman, R. J. (1999). *Neurodevelopmental disorders: Diagnosis and treatment.* New York: Oxford University Press.

Hellings, J. A., & Warnock, J. K. (1994). Self-injurious behavior and serotonin in Prader–Willi syndrome. *Psychopharmacology Bulletin, 30,* 245–250.

Hertz, G., Cataletto, M., Feinsilver, S. H., & Angulo, M. (1995). Developmental trends of sleep-disordered breathing in Prader–Willi syndrome: The role of obesity. *American Journal of Medical Genetics, 56,* 188–190.

Hodapp, R. M. (1996). Cross-domain relations in Down syndrome. In J. A. Rondal, J. Perera, L. Nadel, & A. Comblain (Eds.), *Down syndrome: Psychological, biopsychological and socioeducational perspectives* (pp. 65–79). London: Whurr.

Hodapp, R. M. (2004). Studying interactions, reactions, and perceptions: Can genetic disorders serve as behavioral proxies? *Journal of Autism and Developmental Disorders, 34,* 29–34.

Hodapp, R. M., & Dykens, E. M. (1994). Mental retardation's two cultures of behavioral research.

American Journal of Mental Retardation, 98, 675–687.

Hodapp, R. M., Dykens, E. M., & Masino, L. (1997). Stress and support in families of persons with Prader–Willi syndrome. *Journal of Autism and Developmental Disorders, 27,* 11–23.

Hodapp, R. M., & Fidler, D. J. (1999). Special education and genetics: Connections for the 21st century. *Journal of Special Education, 33,* 130–137.

Hodapp, R. M., Freeman, S. F., & Kasari, C. (1998). Parental educational preferences for students with mental retardation: Effects of etiology and current placement. *Education and Training in Mental Retardation and Developmental Disabilities, 33*(4), 342–349.

Hodapp, R. M., & Zigler, E. (1990). Applying the developmental perspective to individuals with Down syndrome. In D. Cicchetti & M. Beeghly (Eds.), *Children with Down syndrome: A developmental perspective* (pp. 1–28). New York: Cambridge University Press.

Holland, A. J., Treasure, J., Coskeran, P., Dallow, J., Milton, N., & Hillhouse, E. (1993). Measurement of excessive appetite and metabolic changes in Prader–Willi syndrome. *International Journal of Obesity, 17,* 526–532.

Holland, A. J., Whittington, J. E., Butler, J., Webb, T., Boer, H., & Clarke, D. (2003). Behavioral phenotypes associated with specific genetic disorders. Evidence from population-based study of people with Prader–Willi syndrome. *Psychological Medicine, 33,* 141–153.

Holm, V. A. (1981). The diagnosis of Prader–Willi syndrome. In V. A. Holm, S. Sulzbacher, & P. L. Pipes (Eds.), *The Prader–Willi syndrome* (pp. 27–44). Baltimore: University Park Press.

Holm, V. A., Cassidy, S. B., Butler, M. G., Hanchett, J. M., Greenswag, L. R., Whitman, B. Y., et al. (1993). Prader–Willi syndrome: Consensus diagnostic criteria. *Pediatrics, 91,* 398–402.

Holm, V. A., & Pipes, P. L. (1976). Food and children with Prader–Willi syndrome. *American Journal of Diseases of Children, 130,* 1063–1067.

Hudgins, L., Geer, J. S., & Cassidy, S. B. (1998). Phenotypic differences in African Americans with Prader–Willi syndrome. *Genetic Medicine, 1,* 49–51.

Hudgins, L. H., McKillop, J. A., & Cassidy, S. B. (1991). Hand and foot lengths in Prader–Willi syndrome. *American Journal of Medical Genetics, 41,* 5–9.

Kaufman, A. S., & Kaufman, N. L. (1983). *Kaufman Assessment Battery for Children.* Circle Pines, MN: American Guidance Service.

Key, A. P. F., & Dykens, E. M. (2008). 'Hungry eyes': Visual processing of food images in adults with Prader–Willi syndrome. *Journal of Intellectual Disability Research, 52,* 536–546.

Kleppe, S. A., Katayama, K. M., Shipley, K. G., & Foushee, D. R. (1990). The speech and language characteristics of children with Prader–Willi syndrome. *Journal of Speech and Hearing Disorders, 55,* 300–309.

Kubota, T., Sutcliffe, J. S., Aradhya, S., Gillessen-Kaesbach, G., Christian, S. L., Horsthemke, B., et al. (1996). Validation studies of *SNRPN* methylation as a diagnostic test for Prader–Willi syndrome. *American Journal of Medical Genetics, 66,* 77–80.

Kundert, D. K. (2008). Prader–Willi syndrome. *School Psychology Quarterly, 23,* 246–257.

Ledbetter, D. H., Riccardi, V. M., Airhart, S. D., Strobel, R. J., Keenen, S. B., & Crawford, J. D. (1981). Deletion of chromosome 15 as a cause of Prader–Willi syndrome. *New England Journal of Medicine, 304,* 325–329.

Lee, P. D. (1995). Endocrine and metabolic aspects of Prader–Willi syndrome. In L. Greenswag & R. Alexander (Eds.), *Management of Prader–Willi syndrome* (pp. 32–57). New York: Springer-Verlag.

Levine, K., & Wharton, R. K. (1993). *Children with Prader–Willi syndrome: Information for school staff.* Rosyln Heights, NY: Visible Ink.

Lewis, B. A., Freebairn, L. Heeger, S., & Cassidy, S. B. (2002). Speech and language skills of individuals with Prader–Willi syndrome. *American Journal of Speech-Language Pathology, 11,* 285–294.

Luthar, S. S. (1991). Vulnerability and resilience: A study of at risk adolescents. *Child Development, 62,* 600–616.

Ly, T. M., & Hodapp, R. M. (2005a). Children with Prader–Willi syndrome versus Williams syndrome: Indirect effects on parents during a jigsaw puzzle task. *Journal of Intellectual Disability Research, 49,* 929–939.

Ly, T. M., & Hodapp, R. M. (2005b). Parents' attributions of their child's jigsaw-puzzle performance: Comparing two genetic syndromes. *Mental Retardation, 43,* 135–144.

Martin, A., State, M., Koenig, K., Schultz, R., Dykens, E. M., Cassidy, S. B., et al. (1998). Prader–Willi syndrome. *American Journal of Psychiatry, 155,* 1265–1273.

Mascari, M. J., Gottlieb, W., Rogan, P. K., Butler, M. G., Waller, D. A., Armour, J. A. L., et al. (1992). The frequency of uniparental disomy in Prader–Willi syndrome. *New England Journal of Medicine, 326,* 599–607.

Meyers, B. A. (1987). Psychiatric problems in adolescents with developmental disabilities. *Journal of the American Academy of Child and Adolescent Psychiatry, 26,* 74–79.

Milner, K. M., Craig, E. E., Thompson, R. J., Veltman, M. W. M., Thomas, N. S., Roberts, S., et al. (2005). Prader–Willi syndrome: Intellectual abilities and behavioral features by genetic subtype. *Journal of Child Psychology and Psychiatry, 46,* 1089–1096.

Mitchell, J., Schinzel, A., Langlois, S., Gillessen-Kaesbach, G., Michaelis, R. C, Abeliovich, D., et al. (1996). Comparison of phenotype in uniparental disomy and deletion Prader–Willi syndrome: Sex specific differences. *American Journal of Medical Genetics, 65,* 133–136.

Nicholls, R. D. (1993). Genomic imprinting and uniparental disomy in Angelman and Prader–Willi syndrome: A review. *American Journal of Medical Genetics, 46,* 16–25.

Nicholls, R. D., Knoll, J. H., Butler, M. G., Karam, S., & Lalande, M. (1989). Genetic imprinting suggested by maternal heterodisomy in nondeletion Prader–Willi syndrome. *Nature, 342,* 281–285.

Oliver, C., Woodcock, K. A., & Humphreys, G. W. (2009). The relationship between components of the behavioural phenotype in Prader–Willi syndrome. *Journal of Applied Research in Intellectual Disabilities, 22(4),* 403–407.

Ozcelik, T., Leff, S., Robinson, W., Donlon, T., Lalande, M., Sanjines, E., et al. (1992). Small nuclear ribonucleoprotein polypeptide N (*SNRPN*), an expressed gene in the Prader–Willi syndrome critical region. *Nature Genetics, 2,* 265–269.

Prader, A., Labhart, A., & Willi, A. (1956). Ein syndrom von aidositas, kleinwuchs, kryptorchismus und oligophrenic nach myotonieartigem zustand im neugeborenenalter. *Schweizerische Medizinische Wochenschrift, 86,* 1260–1261.

Prasher, V. P. (1995). Overweight and obesity amongst Down syndrome adults. *Journal of Intellectual Disability Research, 39,* 437–441.

Poyatos, D., Camprubí, C., Gabau, E., Nosas, R., Villatoro, S., Coll, M. D., et al. (2009). Prader–Willi syndrome patients: Study of 77 patients. *Medicina Clinica, 133,* 649–656.

Reddy, L. A., & Pfeiffer, S. I. (2007). Behavioral and emotional symptoms of children and adolescents with Prader–Willi syndrome. *Journal of Autism and Developmental Disorders, 37,* 830–839.

Robinson, W. P., Bottani, A., Yagang, X., Balakrishman, J., Binkert, F., Machler, M., et al. (1991). Molecular, cytogenetic and clinical investigations of Prader–Willi syndrome patients. *American Journal of Human Genetics, 49,* 1219–1234.

Rogan, P. K., Mascari, J., Ladda, R. L., Woodage, T., Trent, R. J., Smith, A., et al. (1994, July). *Coinheritance of other chromosome 15 abnormalities with Prader–Willi syndrome: Genetic risk estimation and mapping.* Paper presented at the 16th Annual PWS(USA) National Scientific Day, Atlanta, GA.

Rosner, B. A., Hodapp, R. M., Fidler, D. J., Sagun, J. N., & Dykens, E. M. (2004). Social competence in persons with Prader–Willi, Williams, and Down's syndromes. *Journal of Applied Research in Intellectual Disabilities, 17,* 209–217.

Saitoh, S., Buiting, K., Cassidy, S. B., Conroy, J. M., Driscoll, D. J., Gabriel, J. M., et al. (1997). Clinical spectrum and molecular diagnosis of Angelman and Prader–Willi syndrome imprinting mutation patients. *American Journal of Medical Genetics, 68,* 195–206.

Sellinger, M. H., Hodapp, R. M., & Dykens, E. M. (2006). Leisure activities in individuals with Prader–Willi, Williams, and Down syndromes. *Journal of Developmental and Physical Disabilities, 18,* 59–71.

Shapira, N. A., Lessig, M. C., Lewis, M. H., Goodman, W. K., & Driscoll, D. J. (2004). Effects of topiramate in adults with Prader–Willi syndrome. *American Journal on Mental Retardation, 109,* 301–309.

Shapira, N. A., Lessig, M. C., Murphy, T. K., Driscoll, D. J., & Goodman, W. K. (2002). Topiramate attenuates self-injurious behavior in Prader–Willi syndrome. *International Journal of Neuropsychopharmacology, 5,* 141–145.

Silverstein, A. B. (1982). A note on the constancy of IQ. *American Journal of Mental Deficiency, 87,* 227–229.

Soni, S., Whittington, J., Holland, A. J., Webb, T., Maina, E., Boer, H., et al. (2007). The course and outcome of psychiatric illness in people with Prader–Willi syndrome: Implications for management and treatment. *Journal of Intellectual Disability Research, 51,* 32–42.

Sparrow, S. S., Balla, D., & Cicchetti, D. V. (1984). *Vineland Adaptive Behavior Scales.* Circle Pines, MN: American Guidance Service.

Spritz, R. A., Bailin, T., Nicholls, R. D., Lee, S. T., Park, S. K., Mascari, M. J., et al. (1997). Hypopigmentation in the Prader–Willi syndrome correlates with *P* gene deletion but not with haplotype of the hemizygous *P* allele. *American Journal of Medical Genetics, 71,* 57–62.

State, M. W., Dykens, E. M., Rosner, B., Martin, A., & King, B. H. (1999). Obsessive–compulsive symptoms in Prader–Willi and 'Prader–Willi-like' patients. *Journal of the American Academy of Child and Adolescent Psychiatry, 38,* 329–334.

Stein, D. J., Keating, K., Zar, H. J., & Hollander, E. (1994). A survey of the phenomenology and pharmacotherapy of compulsive and impulsive–aggressive symptoms in Prader–Willi syndrome. *Journal of Neuropsychiatry and Clinical Neuroscience, 6,* 23–29.

Steinhausen, H.-C., Eiholzer, U., Hauffa, B. P., & Malin, Z. (2004). Behavioral and emotional disturbances in people with Prader–Willi syndrome. *Journal of Intellectual Disability Research, 48,* 47–52.

Sulzbacher, S., Crnic, K., & Snow, J. (1981). Behavioral and cognitive disabilities in Prader–Willi syndrome. In V. Holm, S. Sulzbacher, & P. Pipes (Eds.), *The Prader–Willi syndrome* (pp. 147–169). Baltimore: University Park Press.

Swaab, D. F. (2004). Neuropeptides in hypothalamic neuronal disorders. *International Review of Cytology, 240,* 305–375.

Swaab, D. F., Purba, J. S., & Hofman, M. A. (1995). Alterations in the hypothalamic paraventricular nucleus and its oxytocin neurons (putative satiety cells) in Prader–Willi syndrome: A study of 5 cases. *Journal of Clinical Endocrinology and Metabolism, 80,* 573–579.

Taylor, R. L. (1988). Cognitive and behavioral features. In M. L. Caldwell & R. L. Taylor (Eds.), *Prader–Willi syndrome: Selected research and management issues* (pp. 29–42). New York: Springer-Verlag.

Van Borsel, J., Defloor, T., & Curfs, L. M. G. (2007). Expressive language in persons with Prader–Willi syndrome. *Genetic Counseling, 18,* 17–28.

Veltman, M. W. M., Thompson, R. J., Roberts, S. E., Thomas, N., S., Whittington, J., & Bolton, P. F. (2004). Prader–Willi syndrome: A study comparing deletion with uniparental disomy cases with reference to autism spectrum disorders. *European Child and Adolescents Psychiatry, 13,* 42–50.

Verdine, B. N., Troseth, G. L., Hodapp, R. M., & Dykens, E. M. (2008). Strategies and correlates of jigsaw puzzle and visuospatial performance by persons with Prader–Willi syndrome. *American Journal on Mental Retardation, 113,* 343–355.

Vitiello, B., Spreat, S., & Behar, D. (1989). Obsessive–compulsive disorder in mentally retarded patients. *Journal of Nervous and Mental Disease, 177,* 232–236.

Warnock, J. K., & Kestenbaum, T. (1992). Pharmacologic treatment of severe skin picking behaviors in Prader–Willi syndrome. *Archives of Dermatology, 128,* 1623–1625.

Warren, J., & Hunt, E. (1981). Cognitive processing in children with Prader–Willi syndrome. In V. Holm, S. Sulzbacher, & P. Pipes (Eds.), *The Prader–Willi syndrome* (pp. 161–177). Baltimore: University Park Press.

Waters, J. (1990). Prader–Willi syndrome. In J. Hogg, J. Sebba, & L. Lambe (Eds.), *Profound mental retardation and multiple impairment: Vol. 3. Medical and physical care and management* (pp. 54–67). London: Chapman & Hall.

Werner, E. E. (2005). What can we learn about resilience from large-scale longitudinal studies. In S. Goldstein & R. B. Brooks (Eds.), *Handbook of resilience in children* (pp. 91–105). New York: Springer.

Whitman, B. Y., & Accardo, P. (1987). Emotional problems in Prader–Willi adolescents. *American Journal of Medical Genetics, 28,* 897–905.

Whitman, B. Y., & Thompson, T. (2006). Neurodevelopmental and neuropsychological aspects of Prader–Willi syndrome. In M. G. Butler, P. D.

K. Lee, & B. Y. Whitman (Eds.), *Management of Prader–Willi syndrome* (3rd ed., pp. 245–271). New York: Springer-Verlag.

Whittington, J., Holland, A., & Webb, T. (2009). Relationship between the IQ of people with Prader–Willi syndrome and that of their siblings: Evidence for imprinted gene effects. *Journal of Intellectual Disability Research, 53,* 411–418.

Whittington, J. E., Holland, A. J., Webb, T., Butler, J., Clarke, D., & Boer, H. (2002). Relationship between clinical and genetic diagnosis of Prader–Willi syndrome. *Journal of Medical Genetics, 39,* 926–932.

Whittington, J. E., Holland, A. J., Webb, T., Butler, J., Clarke, D., & Boer, H. (2004a). Academic underachievement by people with Prader–Willi syndrome. *Journal of Intellectual Disability Research, 48,* 188–200.

Whittington, J. E., Holland, A. J., Webb, T., Butler, J., Clarke, D., & Boer, H. (2004b). Cognitive abilities and genotype in a population-based sample of people with Prader–Willi syndrome. *Journal of Intellectual Disability Research, 48,* 172–187.

Wigren, M., & Hansen, S. (2003a). Prader–Willi syndrome: Clinical picture, psychosocial support, and current management. *Child: Care, Health, and Development, 29,* 449–456.

Wigren, M., & Hansen, S. (2003b). Rituals and compulsivity in Prader–Willi syndrome: Profile and stability. *Journal of Intellectual Disability Research, 47,* 428–438.

Wigren, M., & Hansen, S. (2005). ADHD symptoms and insistence on sameness in Prader-Will syndrome. *Journal of Intellectual Disability Research, 49,* 449–456.

Williams, C. A., Angelman, H., Clayton-Smith, J., Driscoll, D. J., Hendrickson, J. E., Knoll, J. H., et al. (1995). Angelman syndrome: Consensus for diagnostic criteria. *American Journal of Medical Genetics, 56,* 237–238.

Woodcock, K., Oliver, C., & Humphreys, G. (2009). Associations between repetitive questioning, resistance to change, temper outbursts, and anxiety in Prader–Willi and fragile X syndromes. *Journal of Intellectual Disability Research, 53,* 265–278.

World Health Organization. (1992). *International classification of diseases* (10th rev.). Geneva: Author.

Zipf, W. B., & Bernston, G. G. (1987). Characteristics of abnormal food-intake patterns in children with Prader–Willi syndrome and study of effects of naloxone. *American Journal of Clinical Nutrition, 46,* 277–281.

CHAPTER 26

Disorders of Mitochondrial Metabolism

RUSSELL P. SANETO

Mitochondria are eukaryotic cytoplasmic organelles that are essential for almost all of a cell's energy production, via oxidative phosphorylation (OXPHOS). Disorders that alter OXPHOS function can compromise energy-demanding cellular functions. When critically low adenosine triphosphate (ATP) levels are reached, cellular function is altered, and organ failure can ultimately occur. The most vulnerable organs, such as brain and muscle, are those that rely on high levels of energy. So many mitochondrial disorders involve brain and muscle dysfunction that mitochondrial diseases were once exclusively labeled *mitochondrial encephalomyopathies*. As the field of mitochondrial medicine has evolved with enhanced and expanded diagnostic testing, and as research on mitochondrial function unfolds, it is becoming clear that this small organelle plays a very important role in multisystemic disease and not just diseases related to direct OXPHOS function. Diseases due to impaired importation of mitochondrial proteins, defects of mitochondrial dynamics (e.g., fusion and fission), and alteration of maintenance and expression of mitochondrial DNA (mtDNA) have all become more evident in infants and children. Ultimately, however, all true primary mitochondrial disorders are associated with abnormalities of OXPHOS.

The unique genetics and physiology of mitochondrial function create a variety of clinical manifestations, which range from single-organ defects to multisystemic involvement. Disease onset ranges from the neonatal period to old age. The variety of phenotypic expression is impressive, yet many diverse genetic and biochemical defects have similar presentations. These diseases are truly "a puzzle wrapped in an enigma." This chapter focuses on mitochondrial diseases that are significantly expressed during infancy and childhood. I highlight putative genotype–phenotype correlations when they exist, as well as the pathophysiology for each group of diseases when appropriate.

BACKGROUND

I begin by describing some clinical aspects of mitochondrial physiology and genetics, to shed some light on the reasons for the variety and breadth of mitochondrial disease.

Mitochondrial Biology

The mitochondria are double-membrane organelles found in every cell type, with the exception of the mature red blood cell. There are from two to thousands of mitochondria within each cell, depending on the bioenergetic needs of the cell. The inner membrane provides a highly efficient barrier to ionic diffusion, which is an important factor in generating the proton electromagnetic gradient responsible for the final step of ATP generation (Saraste, 1999). Within the inner mitochondrial membrane lies the matrix. The matrix contains multiple enzymes involved in the tricarboxylic acid cycle and beta-oxidation (carbohydrate and fat metabolism, respectively). There are also components for lipid and cholesterol synthesis, as well as multiple copies of mtDNA that provide specific mitochondrion proteins.

The electron transport chain is composed of five enzymatic multisubunit polypeptide complexes located within the inner mitochondrial membrane. Approximately 88 proteins make up this chain. With the exception of complex II, all of the complexes have subunits that are encoded by nuclear and mitochondrial genomes. Only 13 of these polypeptides are encoded by mtDNA (Figure 26.1); the rest are nuclear-encoded. Complex II is entirely encoded by the nuclear genome. Subunits are assembled with prosthetic groups and metal-containing centers by a set of assembly factors, which are unique to each subunit. Together with specific "electron shuttles" of coenzyme Q10 (ubiquinone) and cytochrome c, electrons are shuttled among complexes I–IV in the oxidative process to reduce molecular oxygen (Wallace, 1999). Utilizing the produced proton gradient, complex V (ATP synthase) forms ATP from adenosine diphosphate (ADP) and inorganic phosphate—the phosphorylation step in the process of OXPHOS.

Mitochondrial DNA

The mtDNA genome is extraordinarily concise and is distinct from nuclear DNA. Unlike nuclear DNA, mtDNA is almost entirely (93%) made up of exons and consists of several thousand copies per cell (polyploidy) with distinct codons. It lacks histones, and genes are transcribed from both strands as large polycistrons. All of the exons are continuous with each other (Anderson et al., 1981). Furthermore, mtDNA is almost exclusively maternally inherited (Taylor & Turnbull, 2005). In humans, the mitochondrial genome is a 16,569-base-pair, multicopy, double-stranded molecule (Figure 26.1). It encodes 13 polypeptides of the OXPHOS system, 7 subunits of complex I, 1 subunit of complex III, 3 subunits of complex IV, and 2 subunits of complex V. The other (approximately 75) subunits are encoded by the nuclear genome. In addition, the mtDNA encodes 2 ribosomal RNA (rRNA) and 22 transfer RNA (tRNA) genes, which are necessary for the intramitochondrial synthesis of the 13 mitochondrial proteins. Both rRNA and tRNA are specific to mitochondria and are distinct from cellular RNA.

The mitochondrion remains entirely dependent on the nuclear genome for most of its functional machinery. It requires nuclear-encoded products for provision of enzymes for replication, DNA repair, transcription, and translation. In fact, integrative analysis estimates the mitochondrial proteome to be approximately 1,500 gene products (Calvo et al., 2006). This dependency on two genomes creates some very interesting functional consequences of mtDNA and nuclear mutations, in the form of heterogeneous diseases seemingly unexplained by their genetic abnormalities.

mtDNA Replication

mtDNA undergoes continuous replication, which is independent from the cell cycle and occurs in dividing and nondividing cells (Taanman, Muddle, & Muntau, 2003). The replisome consists of unique proteins: the heterodimeric mtDNA specific polymerase gamma (POLG), containing a polymerase subunit, linker region, and proofreading subunit (Graziewicz, Longley, & Copeland, 2006); accessory protein polymerase gamma B (POLG 2; Carrodeguas, Theis, Bogenhagen, & Kisker, 2001); 5'-3' helicase Twinkle (Spelbrink et al., 2001); and other single-stranded replication factors (Copeland, 2008). The exact process and complete structure are still unclear (Holt, 2009).

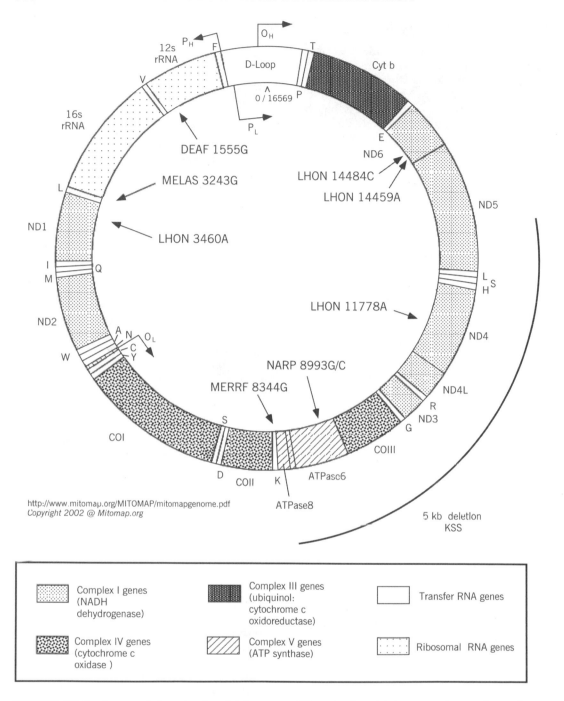

FIGURE 26.1. A map of the mitochondrial genome. The mitochondrial genome is circular and comprises 16,569 base pairs. It codes for 7 subunits of complex I (ND1–ND6 and ND4L), 1 subunit of complex III (cytochrome b), 3 subunits of complex IV (COI–COIII), and 2 subunits of complex V (ATPase 6 and 8). It also codes for 2 ribosomal RNA (rRNA) genes and 22 transfer RNA (tRNA) genes, which are required for intramitochondrial protein synthesis. Nine of the most common mitochondrial mutations are given at their approximate positions within the genome. The displacement loop (D-loop), or noncoding region, contains sequences needed for the initiation of both mtDNA replication and transcription. The proposed origin of the heavy-strand replication is shown as O_H, and that of the light-strand replication is noted as O_L. From *mitomap.org*. Copyright 2002 by mitomap.org. Reprinted by permission.

Homoplasmy, Heteroplasmy, and Threshold

There are up to several thousand copies of mtDNA molecules (*polyploidy*) per cell. When all the copies of the mtDNA genome are identical, this is termed *homoplasmy*. When there are two or more mtDNA genotypes mixed within a cell, the term *heteroplasmy* is used. A mutation within mtDNA can be considered either a homoplasmic mutation (all the mtDNA contain the mutation) or a heteroplasmic mutation (a mixed population of normal and mutated mtDNA is present). An important concept is *threshold*. Threshold represents the percentage (or load) of mutation mtDNA that determines or contributes to disease expression—both clinical and biochemical defects of a particular tissue. Numerous studies have shown that almost all mutations are functionally recessive, and that a biochemical phenotype is associated with high levels of mutations above a critical threshold, usually in the range of 70–95% (Rossignol et al., 2003; Sciacco, Bonilla, Schon, DiMauro, & Moraes, 1994). There has been a single report of a dominant mutation-inducing disease with low levels of heteroplasmy (Sacconi et al., 2008).

mtDNA Inheritance and Bottleneck Effect

The current model of mtDNA inheritance is that all mtDNA is inherited through the maternal line and is therefore clonal (Giles, Blanc, Cann, & Wallace, 1980). However, there has been a single report of paternal transmission of a 2-base-pair deletion in subunit ND2 of complex I in muscle of a patient with mitochondrial myopathy (Schwart & Vissing, 2002). Haplotype analysis proved that this deletion was from the father's mtDNA, although the deletion was not found in the father, nor was it found in any tissue in the patient other than the muscle. Subsequent studies have not shown evidence of paternal mtDNA transmission in myopathies, demonstrating the rare occurrence of paternal inheritance (Filosto et al., 2003; Schwartz & Vissing, 2004). There is some evidence that paternal mtDNA is selected for degradation by the ovum (Sutovsky, Van Leyen, McCauley, Day, & Sutovsky, 2004).

The evidence is overwhelming that paternal inheritance is exceedingly rare.

During cell division, the proportion of mutant mtDNA may shift, resulting in daughter cells with varying heteroplasmy ratios. Presumably this process is random, and during oogenesis the predicted 100,000–150,000 mtDNA molecules within a single oocyte are segregated through a "bottleneck," where only a small proportion of mtDNA is transmitted to the primary oocyte. Thus one daughter oocyte may inherit significantly more or less mutated mtDNA, with the resulting offspring having a significant variation in the mutational load of mtDNA compared to the mother. Not only can whole organisms develop with various levels of heteroplasmy, but during organogenesis, mitotic segregation can lead to significantly altered levels of mutated mtDNA in some tissues compared to others (Lightowlers, Chinnery, & Howell, 1997). In postmitotic tissues (e.g., muscle and brain), the proportion of heteroplasmy can increase over time; in rapidly dividing cells (e.g., blood), some mutations may be lost (Rahman, Brown, Chong, Wilson, & Brown, 2001). This process of mtDNA segregation may not be random. There is animal evidence suggesting that segregation of mtDNA is not a random event (Battersby, Loredo-Osti, & Shoubridge, 2003). Whether this exists and can alter pathological mutations in humans is not clear, but the process of bottleneck in oocytes and mitotic segregation in tissues has important implications for varying phenotypic expression within various tissues as well as among patients.

A recent study demonstrated that putative pathological mtDNA mutations may be present at higher than expected levels in the healthy population. Elliott, Samuels, Eden, Relton, and Chinnery (2008) found that in over 3,000 sequential samples of umbilical cord blood, 1 in 200 live births harbored one of the 10 most common pathological mtDNA mutations. The most common pathological mutation, m.3243A>G, had a mutational load of roughly 30%, which is well below the putative disease threshold of 70–80% (DiMauro & Schon, 2008). Of these live births, only 0.00107% harbored a mutation not detected in the mother's blood. This suggests that pathological mtDNA mutations are common in the healthy population. Since population studies suggest that the prevalence of patients with mitochondrial encephalopathy, lactic acidosis, and stroke-like episodes (MELAS) who have the m.3243A>G mutation is approximately 3.65 per 100,000 (Di Donato, 2009), the factors modifying disease expression remain unknown. Certainly the numbers of carriers would predict a larger population.

Nuclear DNA Mutations

The genetic etiology responsible for the presentation of mitochondrial disease changes with age: mtDNA mutations are more likely to be found with increased age, compared to nuclear DNA mutations (Schaefer, Taylor, Turnbull, & Chinnery, 2004; Tulinius, Holme, Kristiansson, Larsson, & Oldfors, 1991). Molecular investigation thus far has failed to identify the responsible gene defect in 50% of adults and 80–90% of pediatric disorders (Zeviani & Di Donato, 2004). Partial responsibility for this discrepancy may be the high proportion of pediatric patients having nuclear DNA mutations, which are estimated to cause 75–90% of primary mitochondrial disease (DiMauro & Hirano, 2008). An interesting study evaluated the clinical differences in young patients with nuclear versus mtDNA mutations in OXPHOS (Rubio-Gozalbo et al., 2000). Siblings with nuclear mutations showed similar clinical manifestations, a more severe clinical course, and an earlier onset of disease, compared to siblings with mtDNA mutations. Although only small numbers were investigated, this study suggests that diseases due to nuclear mutations occur earlier and are more severe, whereas mtDNA mutations cause a more diverse set of clinical findings and expressed later in life.

Nuclear–Mitochondrial Intergenomic Communication

Proper mtDNA replication, maintenance, and translation rely on the coordinated interaction between nuclear- and mtDNA-synthesized products. When nuclear mutations alter these processes, qualitative (multiple deletions) or quantitative (depletion) alterations of mtDNA or defective translations of mtDNA products occur. These defects are almost all caused by alterations in the nucleotide pools required to synthesize mtDNA or in the enzymes associated with mtDNA replication that function at the replication fork (Spinazzola & Zeviani, 2005).

Multiple mtDNA deletions are due to failure of homeostasis of mitochondrial nucleotide pools. However, the exact mechanism underlying the formation of mtDNA deletions is unclear. There is a close association with accumulation of deletions and segmental ragged red fibers in complex IV negative fibers. Deletions are usually absent in rapidly dividing cells, but are detected in heart, brain, muscle, and kidney cells (Spinazzola & Zeviani, 2009). Clinically, mtDNA deletion syndromes are almost always associated with ocular problems (progressive external ophthalmoplegia and ptosis) and limb myopathy (proximal weakness), and invariably with peripheral neuropathy, brain dysfunction (ataxia, dementia, and psychosis), sensorineural hearing loss, and cataracts. Biochemically, most of the deletion syndromes, as well as mtDNA depletion syndromes, are involved in the salvage pathways of mitochondrial deoxynucleotides, which constitute the major source of DNA precursors in liver, brain, and muscle.

Depletion of mtDNA results in severe reduction of the mtDNA copy number. This group of mitochondrial diseases is transmitted as autosomal recessive disorders. They are phenotypically heterogeneous and invariably affect infants and children. The depletion of mtDNA copy number may affect either a specific tissue (usually muscle or liver and brain) or a combination of tissues (including muscle, liver, brain, and kidney). Three main clinical presentations are described: myopathic, encephalomyopathic, and hepatocerebral. Myopathic phenotype is associated with mutations in the thymidine kinase 2 (TK2) and p53-induced ribonucleotide reductase B subunit (RRM2B) genes. Encephalomyopathies are associated with the succinate synthase A and B genes. The hepatocerebral phenotype is associated with mutations in the Twinkle, POLG, DGUOK, and MPV17 genes. Not all gene mutations are in proteins involved with nucleotide pool homeostasis; for example, some children with hepatocerebral syndrome have mutations in MPV17, a gene that encodes an inner mitochondrial matrix protein of unclear function. Furthermore, there remain unknown genes responsible for mtDNA depletion syndromes, as patients having severely reduced mtDNA copy number have no mutations in known depletion genes (Spinazzola et al., 2008).

Epidemiology

The minimum prevalence of OXPHOS disease is estimated to be 1 in 5,000 live births (Smeitink, Zeviani, Turnbull, & Jackobs, 2006). This is probably a low estimate, due to the wide spectrum of clinical presentations, which may elude diagnosis in some patients. Diagnostic modalities also may lower detection rates. For example, muscle biopsy is often used for diagnosis, especially in children; parents will sometimes decline this surgical procedure for their children, thereby limiting diagnosis. Gene testing is still in its infancy in mitochondrial disease, as only recently has whole mtDNA genome sequencing become available. Furthermore, gene analysis in the pediatric population is difficult to perform, in part because unidentified nuclear mutations account for the majority of cases. Gene testing is also expensive, and insurance companies often do not cover costs, which can restrict the use of genetic analysis. These epidemiological problems are further complicated by early infant deaths and ethical considerations of presymptomatic genetic testing. All these factors impede accurate epidemiological determination of prevalence.

The estimate of mtDNA contribution to the prevalence of mitochondrial disease in England has revealed the minimum prevalence of pathological mutations for adults to be 9.2 in 100,000 (Schaefer et al., 2008). As described above, although a relatively high percentage of healthy females carry one of the 10 most common mtDNA pathological mutations, the frequency of mtDNA disease in England is not proportional to the prevalence of mtDNA mutations (Elliott et al., 2008). This is another piece of this puzzle of mitochondrial disease.

The two most common mtDNA diseases are Leber hereditary optic neuropathy (LHON), estimated to have a minimum point prevalence in northern England of 3.13 per 100,000, and MELAS, estimated to have a miminum prevalence of 3.65 per 100,000 (Schaefer et al., 2008). The most common childhood presentation of a mitochondrial disease is Leigh syndrome, but this syndrome has multiple etiologies of mtDNA and nuclear mutations (Castro-Gago et al., 2006).

HISTORY

The field of mitochondrial medicine has a long history, but its evolution into an independent specialty is only in its infancy. The study of mitochondrial physiology is filled with Nobel Prize laureates who described the structure, location, and bioenergetics of mitochondria. These studies formed the foundation of our present knowledge about the mechanisms of ATP production via OXPHOS coupled to proton motive force. However, the understanding of how errors in these mechanisms translate into disease is only beginning to be unraveled. The two seminal discoveries that have been the building blocks of mitochondrial medicine were that mitochondria possess their own DNA (Nass & Nass, 1963) and that ragged red fibers are present in some mitochondrial diseases (Engel & Cunningham, 1963).

Although this can be debated, the initial clinical descriptions of mitochondrial diseases were published by Theodore Leber (1871) for mtDNA-based disorders and Bernard Alpers (1931) for nuclear-DNA-based diseases. Leber described four families with a unique and characteristic pattern of visual loss that contradicted the traditional concept of Mendelian inheritance. It would be over 100 years until the genetic era of mitochondrial disease was ushered in by Wallace and colleagues (1988), who showed that the mutation m.11778G>A in mtDNA was the cause of what was called LHON. Alpers (1931) described three children who displayed rapidly progressive neurodegeneration with liver involvement. It was not until Naviaux and Nguyen (2004) determined that Alpers–Huttenlocher syndrome, also called Alpers syndrome, was caused by mutations in the POLG gene.

The initial protocols of mitochondrial disease diagnosis have remained essentially unchanged over the years; they have traditionally consisted of a muscle biopsy, enzyme assays of the five electron transport chain complexes, and histochemical analysis of the muscle specimen for ragged red fibers. The genetic era has enabled diagnosis of a wide variety of pathological mtDNA mutations, numbering over 200 at this writing (consult *mitomap.org* for the current number). Only 55 or so nuclear genes have been described to cause disease (Haas et al., 2008), but between 1,300 and 1,500 genes involved in mitochondrion structure and function remain unknown. So the genetic tools to diagnose mitochondrial disease are still evolving. I think we are in a very exciting period of improved diagnosis and understanding of mitochondrial disease.

DEVELOPMENTAL COURSE

The expression of mitochondrial disease can occur at any time during life, with involvement of any organ system. As with most other diseases that are expressed at various times of life, the earlier the presentation, the more severe the mitochondrial disease. Onset of mitochondrial disease seems to occur mainly at two distinct time periods: the neonatal period and later infancy/childhood. As noted numerous times in this chapter, however, there are no firm rules regarding either the presentation of symptoms or the time periods of onset. The constellation of signs and symptoms is what alerts a clinician that a possible mitochondrial disease exists in an individual patient.

Neonatal Presentation

Mitochondrial diseases that present in the neonatal period are severe. Such diseases can present very soon after birth, and most involve multiple systems (Table 26.1). Mortality is high. Males and females are equally affected. Most neonatal presentations are thought to have nuclear DNA mutations; only a small percentage have been found to have mtDNA mutations. Because many infants are not tested and many unknown nuclear genes may be responsible for such diseases, the true prevalence of these diseases is unknown.

TABLE 26.1. Clinical Manifestations of Mitochondrial Disease in the Neonatal Period

Neurological

Unexplained encephalopathy
Nystagmus/abnormal eye movement
Seizures
Hypotonia
Coma
Basal ganglia disease
    MRI abnormalities (Leigh syndrome)
    Abnormal movements
Microcephaly
Hearing loss
Ataxia

Respiratory

Breathing abnormalities

Cardiovascular

Cardiomyopathy (especially hypertrophic)
Unexplained cardiac failure
Superventricular tachycardia

Gastroenterological

Intestinal dysmotility
Cyclic vomiting
Hepatomegaly
Liver failure
Hypoglycemia
Poor feeding and failure to thrive

Hematological

Anemia (especially sideroblastic)
Pancytopenia
Other
Arhrogryposis
Unexplained clinical collapse

Note. The more systems involved, the greater the clinical suspicion of mitochondrial disease.

Demographics

The male–female ratio across studies of patients presenting during the neonatal period is approximately 1:1 (Table 26.2). Studies that include older children show a greater male–female ratio, 1.5:1 (Table 26.3).

Pregnancy

Prematurity (gestational age < 37 weeks) was noted in 8 of 32 neonatal patients reported by an Australian group (Gibson, Halliday, Kirby, Yaplito-Lee, & Thorburn, 2008). The population rate for prematurity

TABLE 26.2. Neonatal Onset of Mitochondrial Disease

	Skadal et al. (2003)	Gibson et al. (2008)	Garcia-Cazorla et al. (2005)	Wortmann et al. (2009)
Patients	29	32	57	6
Male–female ratio	1.8:1[a]	1:1	1:1	1:1
ETC	21	24[b]	56	3[c]
mtDNA	0	2	1	0
nDNA	8	6	0	3
Neurological symptoms[d]	29	17	48	6
Death (<3 years)	20	28	33	1

Note. Studies listed are representative studies investigating neonatal onset of disease. Two studies (Skadal et al., 2003; Wortmann et al., 2009) represent data derived from larger pediatric cohorts. SUCLA2, gene encoding the ATP-dependent succinyl-CoA synthase; RYR1, gene encoding the type 1 ryanodine receptor; ETC, electron transport chain; mtDNA, mitochondrial DNA; nDNA: nuclear DNA.
[a]Data are derived from neonatal- and childhood-onset populations.
[b]Data represents patients with ETC abnormalities, minus one patient with a complex I defect and a mutation in a nuclear-DNA-encoded subunit of complex I, NDUFS6.
[c]Data represent ETC abnormalities, minus 1 patient with a complex I defect and 1 patient with a mutation in a nuclear-encoded protein, SUCLA2; and 1 patient with a complex V defect and mutation in a nuclear-encoded protein, RYR1. The nuclear mutations in the Skladal et al. (2003) paper represent 8 patients with pyruvate dehydrogenase deficiency. Nuclear mutations cited in Gibson et al. (2008) represent patients with mutations in NDUFS6, polymerase gamma 1, and tafazzin genes.
[d]Movement disorder (dystonia, choreoathetoid, myoclonus), encephalopathy, epilepsy, hearing loss, peripheral neuropathy, developmental delay, ophthalmological disease, ataxia, and migraine.

TABLE 26.3. Childhood Onset of Mitochondrial Disease

	Skladal et al. (2003)	Scaglia et al. (2004)	Darin et al. (2001)	Kirby et al. (1999)	Debray et al. (2007)
Patients	44	113[a]	32	51	73[a]
Male–female ratio	1.8:1[b]	1.4:1	1:1	1.4:1	1.4:1[b]
ETC	28[c]	80	23[d]	45[e]	44[f]
mtDNA	11	13	6	6	15
nDNA	5	2	2	0	13
Neurological symptoms[g]	37	99	29	40	66
Death (< 3 years)	32	4	5	16	27

Note. Studies listed are retrospective studies of pediatric patients referred to specialty centers for diagnosis and treatment. Two studies represent studies derived from pediatric cohorts, including significant percentages from neonatal onset (see Table 26.2). The other studies have a small percentage, but not completely identified, of patients who presented during the neonatal period. See Table 26.2 for abbreviations.
[a]Designation of mitochondrial disease is based on modified Walker criteria (Bernier et al., 2002) and not exclusively on ETC defect or pathological mtDNA or nDNA mutation.
[b]Data represent both neonatal- and childhood-onset patients.
[c]Data represents patients with ETC abnormalities, minus 11 patients with mtDNA mutations (p.3243A>G, p.8344A>G, p.8993T>C) and large mtDNA deletions.
[d]Data represent one pair of twins (one of the twins was not formally tested) and three siblings of index cases, who demonstrated phenotypes similar to those of the tested siblings.
[e]Data represent all patients with complex I defects at a single referral center. ETC data represent ETC abnormalities minus 6 patients with mtDNA mutations (m.3243A>G, m.14459G>A, m.3303C>T, m.3242G>A).
[f]Data represent three sets of siblings where one of the siblings had an enzymatically proven ETC defect. mtDNA defects: m.3243A>G, m.8993T>G, m.8993A>C, m.14484T>C, m.9984G>A, m.260G>X, 7466_747delC, and large mtDNA deletions.
[g]Movement disorder (dystonia, choreoathetoid, myoclonus), encephalopathy, epilepsy, hearing loss, peripheral neuropathy, developmental delay, ophthalmological disease, ataxia, and migraine.

for the general population in Victoria, Australia, was approximately 8% (Riley, Davey, & King, 2005). Even compared to the prematurity rate in the United States during a similar time period of 11.1% of single births (Martin et al., 2010), the rate of prematurity in this patient group was more than double that in the general population. In the Gibson and colleagues (2008) study, there was no significant association between prematurity and any particular clinical, enzymatic, or molecular defect. Although there was a higher rate of prematurity and intrauterine growth retardation observed in complex I deficiency, this was not statistically significant. Low birthweight (<10% mean weight) was seen in 7 of the 32 patients (Gibson et al., 2008). The low-birthweight data described by von Kleist-Retzow and colleagues (2003) were similar to those for the Australian cohort. Larger cohort studies are needed to verify and extend the Australian data.

Mortality

The data from the literature (Table 26.2) suggest that mortality has a break at the 3-year mark; that is, if an infant survives beyond 3 years of age, the prognosis for longer survival is good. However, neonatal onset is accompanied by a high early mortality rate (66% mortality by age 3 years). In one study, onset after the neonatal period, but before 6 months of age, was also predictive of early mortality (Debray et al., 2007). Death within 3 months of birth is common—13 of 32 infants in one study (Gibson et al., 2008) and 16 of 57 in another (Garcia-Cazorla et al., 2005). Mortality was not related to organ system involved, prematurity, or birthweight in the Australian group (Gibson et al., 2008). However, another study showed that higher mortality was related to initial hyperlactacidemia and combined enzyme deficiencies (Garcia-Cazorla et al., 2005). Further research is needed before conclusions about specific biochemical markers for early mortality can be drawn.

There are limited data on prognosis for survivors after the 3-year mark, but patient survival up to 18 years of age (6 out of 57 patients) has been reported (Garcia-Cazorla et al., 2005). The high mortality rate in the neonatal presentation group suggests that mitochondrial disease may account for a high proportion of neonatal deaths. Early death may preclude diagnostic attempts, and therefore the true prevalence of neonatal-onset mitochondrial disease is likely to remain underestimated.

Clinical Manifestations

Initial presentations usually evolves into multisystemic involvement in the neonatal period (Table 26.1). Nonspecific features of feeding difficulties, failure to thrive, seizures, hypotonia, persistent vomiting, and respiratory symptoms are common initial manifestations (Garcia-Cazorla et al., 2005; Gibson et al., 2008; Skladal et al., 2003; Sue, Hirano, DiMauro, & De Vivo, 1999; Wortmann et al., 2009). As time passes, most cases either segregate into three categories, with major involvement in specific organ systems (encephalomyopathic, hepatodigestive, and isolated myopathic) (Gibson et al., 2008) or are diagnosed with a common mitochondrial syndromic disease. My experience, however, is that most patients have at least minor involvement in other systems, so although disease expression may predominantly involve specific organ systems, most cases include involvement of other organs.

Some patients present very early, even on the first day of life. A "collapse" on day 1 of life was reported in 8 of 32 neonates, most of whom required full resuscitation (Gibson et al., 2008). Skladal and colleagues (2003) described a "fulminant course" in 10 out of 29 neonates (symptomatic in the first month of life), with death occurring by 6 months of age. Unfortunately, this latter report did not indicate the age of symptom onset. Other reports do not identify this category of neonatal presentation. It may reflect the catastrophic presentation just after birth, so that a diagnostic workup did not or could not occur.

Most patients develop neurological symptoms, including hypotonia, seizures, and global developmental delay/encephalopathy. In the studies reviewed here, 17 of 32 patients (Gibson et al., 2008), 21 of 57 (Garcia-Cazorla et al., 2005), 28 of 29 (Skladal et al., 2003), and 5 out of 6 (Wortmann et al., 2009) presented with neurological symptoms. As time procedes, up to 97% develop developmental delay/encephalopathy (Garcia-Cazorla et al., 2005). However, again, multisystemic involvement is the rule (Table 26.1). In several studies, those presenting in the neonatal period and having the best outcomes tended to have multisystemic manifestations without significant accentuated encephalomyopathy, or primarily hepatodigestive (Garcia-Cazorla et al., 2005; Gibson et al., 2008) or primarily myopathic involvement (Garcia-Cazorla et al., 2005). Unfortunately, even in this population, only rare patients had normal IQ (Garcia-Cazorla et al., 2005). The vast majority of patients did not express classic mitochondrial syndrome phenotypes, with the exception of Leigh and Alpers syndromes.

Most patients have deficits in enzyme activity of one or multiple electron transport chain complexes (Darin et al., 2001; Garcia-Cazorla et al, 2005; Rubio-Gozalbo et al., 2000; Skladal et al., 2003; Wortmann et al., 2009). The electron transport chain complex I is the most commonly involved (Garcia-Cazorla et al., 2005; Gibson ct al., 2008; Skladal et al., 2003). In total, isolated electron transport chain complex defects outnumbered combined complex deficiencies in these studies: 67 of 93 patients had single-complex deficiencies. Unfortunately, the genetics of all the components of the five electron transport chain complexes remain unknown.

Genetic Etiologies

Presumably most of the electron transport chain complex defects represent nuclear mutations. In the majority of studies citing specific mtDNA mutations, the extent of analysis was not given, suggesting that full mtDNA sequencing was not performed. Full sequencing has only become commercially available in the last several years. So mtDNA-derived electron transport chain complex gene mutations cannot be completely ruled out; however, the probability is low, given that these mutations are relatively rare (Zeviani & Di Donato, 2004).

LEIGH SYNDROME

The only mtDNA syndrome described in the neonatal-onset group is Leigh syndrome. All neonates described to date with mtDNA-derived Leigh syndrome have had the mtDNA mutation m.8996A>G. At least 26 mtDNA mutations have been described to produce Leigh syndrome (Finsterer, 2008), but whether all of these mutations can give rise to Leigh syndrome during the neonatal period remains unknown.

Denis Leigh (1951) described a syndrome of focal, bilaterally symmetrical, spongiform, necrotic lesions associated with demyelination, vascular proliferation, and gliosis in the brainstem, diencephalons, basal ganglia, and cerebellum, with or without cerebral white matter changes. Magnetic resonance imaging (MRI) mimics pathological findings and shows hallmark progressive signal abnormalities within the lentiform and caudate nuclei, with changes in the thalamus, periaquiductal gray, tementum, red nuclei, and dentate nuclei (Figure 26.2; Saneto, Friedman, & Shaw, 2008). Typically, onset is within the first 2 years of life (Ostergaard et al., 2007), but adult onset has been described (Van Maldergem et al., 2002). However, most patients present in the first month of life (Piao, Tang, Yang, & Liu, 2006). Phenotypically, there is a range of findings from severe neurological involvement (e.g.,

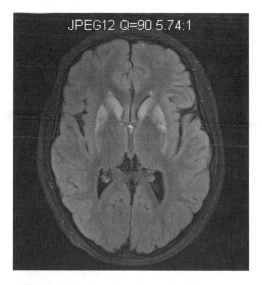

FIGURE 26.2. Magnetic resonance imaging (MRI) of a boy with Leigh syndrome. This is an axial image acquired using a 3-tesla MRI scanner (Siemens Trio). The patient was 6 years of age and had an mtDNA mutation in the ATPase 6 subunit of complex V. The axial image demonstrates hyperintense signal on fluid-attenuated inversion recovery (FLAIR) sequence bilaterally within the putamen and caudate.

psychomotor delay, muscle weakness, hypotonia, truncal ataxia, intention tremor, seizures, ophthalmoparesis, optic atrophy, or dystonia) to near-normal neurological findings (Bugiani, Tiranti, Farina, Uziel, & Zeviani, 2005; Finsterer, 2008). Some patients demonstrate multisystem disease with minimal neurological involvement (Martin et al., 1990). Non-neurological manifestations include short stature, cardiomyopathy, severe constipation/diarrhea, respiratory failure, and dysmorphic features (Finsterer, 2008). Due to such phenotypic heterogeneity, criteria for specific diagnosis of Leigh syndrome has been proposed (Rahman et al., 1996).

There is also marked genetic heterogeneity in Leigh syndrome. In addition to the more than 26 mtDNA mutations, at least 22 nuclear gene mutations can be involved in the etiology of Leigh syndrome (Finsterer, 2008). Nuclear mutations in electron transport chain subunits (complex I and complex II) and in assembly factors (complex I and complex IV) have been described. In addition, mutations in the heme synthesis enzyme (complex IV function), coenzyme Q10 production, pyruvate dehydrogenase complex, elongation factors G1 and Tu, transcriptional coactivator LRP130, succinate coenzyme-A ligase A2 (SUCLA2), and biotinidase have been found to produce Leigh syndrome. The fairly consistent pathological findings in the context of such a wide variety of genetic and phenotypic presentations suggest that a developmentally sensitive period of mitochondrial insult gives rise to many cases of Leigh syndrome. However, adult-onset cases are also seen, so alternative mechanisms for pathological development of lesions must exist.

One of the nuclear DNA etiologies of Leigh syndrome is a class of mitochondrial diseases known as disorders of mtDNA maintenance or nuclear–mitochondrial intergenomic communication (Table 26.4). These disorders are so called because the primary disorder resides in a nuclear gene, but the target is mtDNA. Gene mutation results in multiple mtDNA deletions or depletion of mtDNA copy number. SUCLA2 is a mitochondrial matrix enzyme that catalyzes the formation of succinate and ATP from succinyl-CoA and ADP in the tricarboxylic acid cycle. SUCLA2 is the ß-subunit of succinyl-CoA synthase. A founder effect mutation within the Faroe Island population was found in patients with phenotypic Leigh syndrome, with an incidence of 1 in 1,700 (Ostergaard et al., 2007). However, other mutations within the SUCLA2 gene are found in other ethnic groups, suggesting a wider occurrence (Wortmann et al., 2009). It is not clear how a defect in the tricarboxylic acid cycle can cause depletion in mtDNA.

PYRUVATE DEHYDROGENASE COMPLEX DEFICITS

Several case series have noted defects in the pyruvate dehydrogenase complex (PDHC) as a source of neonatal mitochondrial disease (Skladal et al., 2003). These patients presented mainly during the neonatal period ($n = 8$ of 13). Only several hundred cases of these defects have been reported. Most mutations are sporadic, and recurrence rate is very low. The most common form, a mutation in E1α, behaves as an X-linked dominant disorder; other causes are due to autosomal recessive genes within the protein supercomplex. This complex catalyzes the oxidation of pyruvate to CO_2 and acetyl CoA and generates nicotinamide adenine dinucleotide. The most severe presentation occurs during the neonatal period, with metabolic acidosis and lactic acidemia. There is often hyperammonemia, and death occurs prior to 6 months of age (Stromme, Borud, & Moe, 1976). There is a more indolent presentation with a chronic modest lactate acidemia that initially comes to medical attention due to delayed psychomotor development (Hansen, Christensen, & Brandt, 1982). The majority of these patients have clinical, MRI, and neuropathological findings similar to those in Leigh syndrome (Leigh, 1951). Most will die between 10 months and 3 years of age. Patients with milder presentations tend to be females with a slowly progressive Leigh syndrome or males with ataxia (Blass, Lansdale, Uhlendorf, & Hom, 1971).

DELETION AND DEPLETION mtDNA DISORDERS

In addition to Leigh syndrome due to SUCLA2 mutations (see above), there are at least four other enzyme defects that induce neonatal mitochondrial disease and mtDNA depletion. Mutations in succinate-CoA synthase B (SUCLG1), deoxyguanosine kinase

TABLE 26.4. Disorders of Mitochondrial Maintenance (Nuclear–Mitochondrial Intergenomic Communication)

Gene	Age at onset	CNS features	Systemic features	Depletion organ(s)
POLG1	Infancy–adulthood	Ataxia, seizures, dementia, blindness, PEO, neuropathy	Liver failure[a], gastrointestinal dysmotility, vomiting, myopathy	Liver, muscle
DGUOK	Neonatal	Dystonia, nystagmus, hypotonia	Liver failure	Liver
MPV17	Neonatal–adulthood	Ataxia, neuropathy, dystonia, hypotonia	Liver failure, mental retardation, scoliosis, corneal scarring	Liver
Twinkle	Infancy	Athetosis, seizures, myopathy, mental retardation, PEO, psychosis, neuropathy, ataxia, hypotonia	Liver failure	Liver
TK2	Infancy–childhood	Seizures, PEO	Myopathy	Muscle
RRM2B	Neonatal	Microcephaly, mental retardation, hearing loss, hypotonia	Myopathy, tubulopathy, nephrocalcinosis	Muscle, kidney
SUCLG1	Neonatal	Hypotonia, severe early encephalopathy	Lactic acidosis hepatomegaly	Liver, muscle
SUCLA2	Neonatal–infancy	Dystonia, hearing loss, encephalopathy, PEO, neuropathy, mental retardation, hypotonia	Short stature	Muscle

Note. POLG1, polymerase gamma 1; PEO, progressive external opthalmoplegia; DGUOK, deoxyguanosine kinase; MPV17, encodes a small mitochondrial membrane protein of unclear function; TWINKLE, mitochondrial DNA helicase; TK2, thymidine kinase; RRM2B, p53-dependent ribonucleotide reductase; SUCLG1, GTP-dependent succinyl-CoA synthase; SUCLA2, ATP-dependent succinyl-CoA synthase.
[a]Liver failure is induced by valproic acid exposure, but will occur without exposure. All mitochondrial DNA depletion syndromes are inherited as autosomal recessive traits. There are also autosomal dominant forms of POLG1 mutations that have adult onset.

(DGUOK), MPV17, and RRM2B have all been found to cause neonatal-onset disease (Table 26.4). The depletion disorders are presented here because they are of recent discovery, and their description may help clinical investigators diagnose early-onset mitochondrial disorders.

There is a single report of a rare disorder involving early onset of severe lactic acidosis on the first day of life and death within several days of life. This disorder presents with dysfunction in multiple electron transport chains and mtDNA depletion. The mutation was found in SUCLG1 in multiple members of a consanguineous family (Ostergaard et

al., 2007). Patients demonstrated intrauterine growth retardation, premature birth, dysmorphic features, and a combination of muscle and liver electron transport chain abnormalities; this is similar to other early neonatal presentations. Whether other neonates with this disorder will be found remains unknown.

Two depletion hepatocerebral syndromes are caused by mutations in DGUOK and MPV17. Both syndromes present with combinations of persistent vomiting, failure to thrive, hypotonia, hypoglycemia, and progressive neurological symptoms, especially nystagmus (Copeland, 2008; Dimmock et al., 2007; Freisinger et al., 2006; Parini et al., 2009; Spinazzola et al., 2008). In DGUOK deficiency, liver cirrhosis leads to early-onset liver failure and is the most prominent feature. The type of mutation seems to determine age of onset; frameshift or nonsense mutations have neonatal onset, whereas missense mutations present later in infancy (Freisinger et al., 2006). A rare neonatal-onset hepatocerebral syndrome arises from mutations in MPV17, with hepatomegaly and progressive liver failure in the first weeks of life. There is also a milder form with less liver involvement, but progressive neurological involvement, and survival into adulthood; this is known as Navajo neurohepatopathy (Karadimas et al., 2006).

The fourth depletion syndrome in the neonatal age group results from mutations in RRM2B. The most severe form is a homozygous loss-of-function mutation inducing severe mtDNA depletion in muscle. Clinical presentation varies, but often includes hypotonia, diarrhea, renal tubulopathy, seizures, respiratory distress, and lactic acidosis (Bornstein et al., 2008; Bourdon et al., 2007). In the majority, death can occur before 4 months of age. However, there is a range of disease from early infancy to adulthood, with varying symptoms (Tyynismaa et al., 2009).

INFANTILE REVERSIBLE CYTOCHROME C OXIDASE DEFICIENCY MYOPATHY

One very interesting and important neonatal mitochondrial disease needs to be mentioned. It is rare, but the identification of this entity can literally be life-saving. As described throughout this section, children with early-onset disease often die early. A particular form of complex IV deficiency presents soon after birth with severe muscle weakness and hypotonia in the first few days to weeks of life, often requiring mechanical ventilation. What is surprising about this disorder is that it spontaneously remits, with recovery to normal (in most cases) by 2–3 years of age (DiMauro et al., 1981; Horvath et al., 2009). At presentation, this disorder is potentially life-threatening and often necessitates life-sustaining measures. The defect that induces complex IV deficiency, ragged red fibers within muscle, and often other electron transport chain defects has been proven to be a homoplasmic tRNA-Glu mutation, m.14674T>C. If clinicians are not aware of this mutation, withdrawal of medical care may occur. Infants presenting with severe muscle weakness and hypotonia should be actively worked up for this possible mutation, as prognosis and further heroic medical efforts are warranted if the m.14674T>C mutation is found.

Infancy and Childhood

After the neonatal period, the median age of mitochondrial disease onset was 7 months in one study (Debray et al., 2007) and 44 months in another (Scaglia et al., 2004), with a range of presentation from 2 weeks to 18 years (Darin et al., 2001; Debray et al., 2007; Kirby et al., 1999; Scaglia et al., 2004; Skladal et al., 2003). Nuclear mutations represent the majority of disease etiology, with a small proportion of mtDNA-derived mitochondrial syndromes (but larger and more diverse than the proportion in the neonatal presentation) (Table 26.3). Those patients having nuclear mutations tend to present with symptoms during early childhood, whereas those possessing mtDNA mutations tend to present later in life (Rubio-Gozalbo et al., 2000; Skladal et al., 2003).

Demographics

There is a male–female ratio of approximately 1.5:1 across most studies in patients presenting during infancy and childhood (Table 26.3). The reason for the slight male predominance is not clear.

Pregnancy and Delivery

In one study, birthweight was below the 3rd percentile in 13 of 66 patients (Debray et al., 2007). This would be significantly higher than the proportion of such births in the general population, if compared to the United States and Australian data (see above). This facet of mitochondrial disease in this age group needs further study, but when taken together with neonatal-onset data, it suggests that *in utero* growth compromise may be significant in some forms of mitochondrial disease.

Mortality

Mortality is lower in the infancy/childhood-onset population than in the neonatal-onset population but still high, with median age at death 13 months in one study (Debray et al., 2007) and 5.3 years in another (Scaglia et al., 2004). Approximately 50% live beyond 3 years of age, without any association with biochemical defect associated with mortality (Table 26.3). Debray and colleagues (2007) found that patients having their first symptoms before 6 months of age were 10 times more likely to die early, and that even when patients with LHON were excluded, the presence of a pathological mtDNA mutation was associated with a lower mortality rate.

Clinical Manifestations

There is a wide spectrum of clinical manifestations (Table 26.5) in this group of patients, from multisystemic disorders to isolated myopathy or liver disease. The most frequent presentation involves the central nervous system (CNS) and muscle; CNS involvement is mostly diagnosed as developmental delay, encephalopathy, and hypotonia, and muscle involvement is described as myopathy or exercise intolerance (Darin et al., 2001; Debray et al., 2007; Kirby et al., 1999; Scaglia et al., 2004; Skladal et al., 2003). Neurological involvement was as high as 90% in two studies (Debray et al., 2007; Scaglia et al., 2004). Cerebral involvement, noted as developmental delay, was less common in patients with pure myopathy (50%) and not found in the group with LHON (Debray et al., 2007), which may cause the prevalence of mitochondrial disease to be underestimated in these groups. Common problems cited were liver and gastrointestinal tract difficulties; sensorineural hearing loss; ophthalmological abnormalities; renal problems; and heart problems, including cardiomyopathy and cardiac arrhythmias. There do not seem to be significant associations between type of electron transport chain defect and clinical presentation or organ involvement. Microcephaly, though only described in one study, was found in 32% of patients and was progressive in 20% (Debray et al., 2007).

The clinical phenotypes within the group of electron transport chain defects are broad,

TABLE 26.5. Clinical Manifestations of Mitochondrial Disease in Children

Neurological

Encephalopathy
  Encephalopathy with low/moderate dosing of valproate
  Nonspecific psychomotor delay
Basal ganglia disease
  MRI abnormalities (Leigh syndrome)
  Abnormal movements (especially dystonia)
Seizures
  Epilepsia partialis continua
  Status epilepticus (especially if unexplained)
  Myoclonic seizures
Myoclonus
Myopathy
Peripheral neuropathy
Ataxia
Migraine headache
Cerebellar
  Hypotonia
  Loss of deep tendon reflexes
  Atrophy (especially vermial)
Neurodegeneration (especially after a viral illness)
Stroke-like events (nonvascular territory)
Proton resonance spectroscopy finding of lactate peaks
Hearing loss

Cardiovascular

Cardiomyopathy (hypertrophic, dilated, noncompaction)
Unexplained heart block
Wolff–Parkinson–White arrhythmia

Ophthalmological

Retinal degeneration with signs of night blindness, color vision defects, or pigmentary retinopathy
Ophthalmoplegia/paresis
Ptosis
Eye movement abnormalities
Sudden or insidious optic neuropathy/atrophy

Gastroenterological

Unexplained valproate-induced liver failure
Gastrointestinal dysmotility
Pseudo-obstructive episodes

Renal

Fanconi syndrome
Glomerular proteinuria

Endocrine

Diabetes
Exocrine pancreas dysfunction

Note. As abnormalities are found in multiple systems, the more systems involved, the greater the clinical suspicion of mitochondrial disease.

with no clearly demarcated subgroups. Most involve muscle and brain, but various other organ systems are also involved. The exceptions are mostly mtDNA syndromes, deletion/depletion syndromes, and the more classical mitochondrial syndromes. There are a few rare exceptions in children presenting in this age group, with some patients presenting solely with cardiomyopathy (Kirby et al., 1999). As noted above, pure myopathy with or without cerebral involvement is possible (Debray et al., 2007).

The presence of cardiomyopathy deserves special mention because of its high frequency (18–40%) and increased mortality (Debray et al., 2007; Scaglia et al., 2004). In the largest pediatric study, 40% of patients demonstrated cardiac disease (Scaglia et al., 2004). The majority of these patients exhibited hypertrophic cardiomyopathy (58%), with dilated cardiomyopathy and left ventricular noncompaction seen in the rest. This patient group had only an 18% survival rate at 16 years of age, whereas patients without cardiomyopathy had a 95% survival rate at the same age. Eleven percent of patients with a complex I defect presented with cardiomyopathy, 4% with hypertrophic cardiomyopathy, and 2% with dilated cardiomyopathy (Kirby et al., 1999). In this latter study, all presented within the first year of life and died early, with the exception of one patient alive at 11 years of age. Treatment options such as cardiac transplant may be possible in this group (see "Treatment," below).

In this patient population (Table 26.3), the majority of patients had electron transport chain defects (without mtDNA or nuclear mutations), with percentages ranging from 56% to 86%. In two studies, complex IV defects were the most common (27% and 46%), and complex I defects were the most common in the other three studies (39%, 32%, and 86%). It should be noted that the Kirby and colleagues (1999) study represented a cohort of patients with complex I defects, and the percentage was calculated based on those patients with complex I defects without pathological mtDNA mutation. When this latter study is excluded, the next most common electron transport chain defects were combinations of dysfunctional complexes.

Genetic Etiologies (mtDNA)

mtDNA mutation diseases account for 14–20%, with a mean of 17.2%, of the infancy/childhood-onset population. One must remember that these diseases are almost all classic mitochondrial disease syndromes (Table 26.6). One of these syndromes found in this population is LHON, described above.

The most common mitochondrial syndrome in infancy and childhood is MELAS. Approximately 80% of cases have a mutation at position m.3243A>G within the tRNA for leucine (tRNA[leu]; Goto, Nonaka, & Horai, 1990). The other genetic etiologies of MELAS involve other mtDNA and nuclear DNA mutations (Janssen, Nijtmans, van den Heuvel, & Smeitink, 2006; Malfatti et al., 2007). The age of onset varies, but the syndrome usually occurs before the age of 40 years. MELAS presents as a progressive neurodegenerative disorder associated with headache, treatment resistant partial seizures, short stature, exercise intolerance and muscle weakness, sensorineural hearing loss, diabetes, and slowly progressing dementia (Hirano & Pavlakis, 1994; Hirano et al., 1992). Migraine headache with nausea and vomiting is common and often precedes stroke-like events. Respiratory depression may be the presenting symptom, particularly in the context of a viral infection (Saneto & Bouldin, 2006). Partial seizures or epilepsia partialis continua may also precede or accompany stroke-like events (Ribacoba, Salas-Puig, Gonzalez, & Astudillo, 2006). On MRI, the stroke-like lesions are often transient, with lesions predominantly affecting gray matter and not confined to vascular territories (Figure 26.3; Barkovich, Good, Koch, & Berg, 1993; Hirano & Pavlakis, 1994; Saneto et al., 2008).

The second most frequent mtDNA syndrome is Kearns–Sayre syndrome, with rare cases evolving into this syndrome from Pearson syndrome. Of historical interest, the mtDNA deletion causing Kearns–Sayre syndrome was one of the first mutations to be described and associated with human disease (Holt, Harding, & Morgan-Hughes, 1988; Kearns & Sayre, 1958). Although not usually presenting during childhood, progressive external ophthalmoplegia (PEO) falls into this deletion syndrome. Pearson,

TABLE 26.6. Classic Mitochondrial Disease Syndromes

Syndrome	Age of onset	Neurological phenotype	Systemic phenotype
PEO	Adolescence	PEO, myopathy, ptosis	Cardiomyopathy
KSS	Childhood	PEO, retinitis pigmentosa, ataxia, neuropathy	Cardiomyopathy, conduction block, short stature, diabetes
Pearson	Infancy	None	Siderblastic anemia, exocrine pancreatic insufficiency
MELAS	Childhood	Stroke-like episodes, seizures, ataxia, myoclonus, cortical blindness, migraine, ragged red fibers	Cardiomyopathy, short stature, gastrointestinal dysmotility
MERRF	Childhood	Myoclonus, seizures, ataxia, ragged red fibers, dementia, sensorineural hearing loss	Diabetes
NARP	Adult	Ataxia, neuropathy, myopathy, retinitis pigmentosa	Neuropathy
Leigh	Infancy	Seizures, neuropathy, developmental delay, dystonia, hypotonia	Cardiomyopathy, respiratory failure
LHON	Adolescent	Blindness (central), circumpapillary telangiectatic microangiopathy	None

Note. PEO, progressive external ophthalmoplegia; KSS, Kearns–Sayre syndrome; MELAS, mitochondrial, encephalopathy, lactic acidosis, and stroke-like episodes; MELAS, mitochondrial encephalomyopathy, lactic acidosis, and strokelike episodes; MERRF, myoclonus, epilepsy with ragged red fibers; NARP, neuropathy, ataxia, retinitis pigmentosa; LHON, Leber hereditary optic neuropathy.

Kearns–Sayre, and PEO syndromes can represent a continuum from infancy through childhood/early adolescence. All three syndromes are due to mtDNA deletion/duplication. The size of mtDNA rearrangement can vary from a few base pairs to seven kilobases, with the large deletions spanning the genes between cytochrome b and cytochrome oxidase subunit II (Holt et al., 1988; McShane et al., 1991; Moraes et al., 1989; Rotig et al., 1989). Disease severity is due to the degree of heteroplasmy and not to the size of the deletion. Heteroplasmy varies between tissues, and the degree of it shifts over time (Larsson, Holme, Kristiansson, Oldfors, & Tulinius, 1990). This is due to the postfertilization origin of the deletion/duplication. The higher the percentage of heteroplasmy, the more severe and earlier the onset of the clinical syndrome, from Pearson syndrome to PEO. Pearson syndrome presents during infancy (Pearson et al., 1979; Rotig et al., 1990); if the infant survives, then the disorder often develops into Kearns–Sayre syndrome. Isolated Kearns–Sayre syndrome usually presents in childhood (< 20 years of age), whereas PEO is most often an adult disorder but rarely is seen during childhood (Scaglia et al., 2004). Again, symptoms reflect the degree of heteroplasmy. Pearson syndrome is characterized by refractory siderblastic anemia, vaculization of bone marrow precursor cells, and often death during infancy. Kearns–Sayre syndrome presents with ophthalmoplegia, ptosis, retinitis pigmentosa, and multisystemic involvement including complete heart block. PEO usually only involves muscle problems of ophthalmoplegia, ptosis, and possibly proximal muscle weakness. The single deletions/duplications arise as primary mtDNA mutational events within the oocyte and therefore, are usually not maternally transmitted. The risk of subsequent transmission from an affected woman has been estimated to be 4% (Chinnery et al., 2000).

Myoclonus, epilepsy with ragged red fibers (MERRF) is maternally inherited from a mutation of mtDNA at position m.8344A>G in the tRNA^{Lys} (Wallace et al., 1988). Other

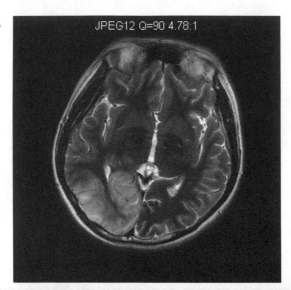

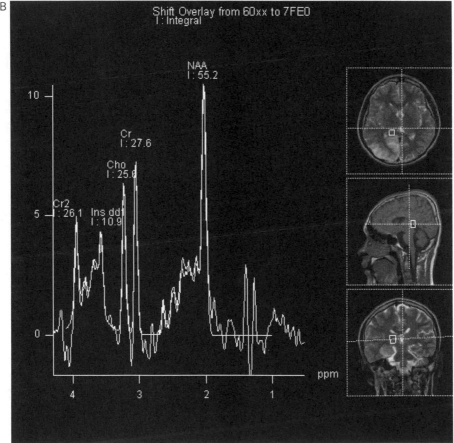

FIGURE 26.3. MRI and [^{1}H] proton magnetic resonance spectroscopy (MRS) of a patient with mitochondrial encephalopathy, lactic acidosis, and stroke-like episodes (MELAS). Panel A is an MRS axial image acquired with a 3-tesla MRI scanner (Siemens Trio, TE 80, TR 1700, FOV, 16 cm) showing dramatically elevated lactate. The voxel is placed in the deep gray matter just superior to the midtemporal structures. Panel B is an axial view of an 11-year-old boy who presented with headache that progressed to focal seizures. This T2-weighted image acquired with a 3-tesla MRI scanner (Siemens Trio) demonstrates hyperintense T2 signal within the cortical gray matter of the occipital region that does not correspond to a known vascular territory. There is also some subcortical white matter involvement.

mutations with the tRNA[Lys] have been associated with MERRF (Silvestri, Moraes, Shanske, Oh, & DiMauro, 1992). This mitochondrial syndrome is the most clearly correlated with clinical, biochemical, and molecular findings. There are positive correlations with age of onset, severity of disease, mtDNA heteroplasmy, and reduced activity of electron transport chain complex activity (Hammans et al., 1993). This syndrome is clinically characterized by myoclonus, myoclonic seizures, muscle weakness, dementia, and wasting (Shoffner et al., 1990). Unlike most mitochondrial diseases expressed in childhood, this syndrome usually demonstrates ragged red fibers on muscle biopsy (Shoffner et al., 1990). Although not completely understood, symmetrical lipomatosis, especially in the trunk, is frequently found (Zeviani & Di Donato, 2004).

The onset of Leigh syndrome can be seen in this age range as well. Whereas the mutation of m.8993T>G within mtDNA and PDHC mutations in nuclear DNA cause the vast majority of neonatal-onset cases of Leigh syndrome, other mutations in mtDNA and nuclear DNA begin to be expressed as Leigh syndrome during infancy and childhood (see the earlier discussion). More than 26 mtDNA mutations and 22 nuclear DNA mutations have been described; mutations in the SURF1 gene are the most common nuclear mutations (Finsterer, 2008). The mutation at 8993 demonstrates the concept of heteroplasmy: Two mitochondrial syndromes can arise from the same mtDNA mutation—in this case, Leigh syndrome and neurogenic weakness, ataxia, and retinitis pigmentosa (NARP). NARP is associated with a heteroplasmic T>G transversion at position 8993 (Holt et al., 1990). In patients with over 90% heteroplasmy, Leigh syndrome is expressed, whereas those with a lower percentage of heteroplasmy express NARP. NARP is uncommonly seen in the infant and child population (Debray et al., 2007; Scaglia et al., 2004).

Genetic Etiologies (Nuclear DNA)

A large group of disorders result from faulty intergenomic communication producing depletion of mtDNA. Five mtDNA depletion disorders due to mutations within MPV17, RRM2B, DGUOK, SUCLA2, and SCULG1 can be seen in infancy and childhood (Table 26.4). One distinctive disorder presenting in the first year of life with severe myopathy is caused by mutations in TK2 (Spinazzola & Zeviani, 2009). This syndrome presents with feeding difficulty, failure to thrive, hypotonia, and muscle weakness, and infrequently with ophthalmoplegia. For unclear reasons, a spectrum of muscle involvement can produce spinal muscular atrophy-like motor neuron disease (Mancuso et al., 2002), rigid spine myopathy (Oskoui et al., 2006), isolated myopathy (Oskoui et al., 2006), or a severe myopathy with marked weakness that may be accompanied by encephalopathy and seizures (Galbiati et al., 2006). Unfortunately, death usually occurs in infancy or childhood, but some patients live into the teenage years (Moraes et al., 1991; Oskoui et al., 2006). A helpful lab finding is elevated serum creatine kinase with multiple electron transport chain complex defects (Spinazzola & Zeviani, 2009). Organ specificity is related to the need of nondividing cells for deoxynucleosiol triphosphates (dNTP) pool synthesis via the salvage pathway and the activity of the mitochondrial enzyme TK2 in muscle (Copeland, 2008). There are unknown genes involved in the myopathic form of mtDNA depletion, as fewer than 30% of the cases are associated with TK2 mutations (Spinazzola & Zeviani, 2009).

Mitochondrial neurogastrointestinal encephalopathy (MNGIE) is an autosomal recessive multisystem syndrome that is characterized by both mtDNA deletions and partial mtDNA depletion (Hirano et al., 2001). Patients demonstrate PEO, peripheral neuropathy, leukodystrophy, and severe gastrointestinal dysmotility (Hirano et al., 1994). The severe gastrointestinal dysmotility produces frequent diarrhea and intestinal pseudo-obstruction, leading to severe cachexia and early death. This dysmotility is due to mtDNA depletion in the external layer of muscularis propria. The onset of MNGIE is usually in the second to fifth decade, but it has been reported to occur in childhood (Debray et al., 2007; Scaglia et al., 2004). The genetic defect lies in the pyrimidine salvage pathway required for the conversion of thymidine and phosphate to thymine and deoxyribose-1-phosphate (Nishino, Spinazzola, & Hirano, 1999). Autosomal recessive or compound heterozygous mutations in the thymidine phosphoryalase gene, ECGF1, cause accumulation of thymidine and uracil in blood. The increased concentration in circulating deoxythymidine results in increased mtDNA mutagenesis (Song, Wheeler, & Matthews, 2003). MNGIE is one of the few mitochondrial diseases with an effective treatment (see "Treatment," below).

Mutations in the POLG gene result in a spectrum of neurological syndromes, encompassing hepatocerebral, encephalomyopathic, and isolated-PEO phenotypes. When such mutations are expressed during infancy to early childhood, the severe disorder of Alpers–Huttenlocher or Alpers syndrome occurs. This syndrome is defined by the triad of progressive neurological degeneration; explosive onset of seizures, often presenting as status epilepticus or epilepticus partialis continua; and liver failure (Naviaux et al., 1999). Liver failure is almost universally induced by exposure to valproic acid. Death usually occurs during childhood, but it can occur as late as in the second decade, depending on mutation and other unclear factors (Stewart et al., 2009). In all cases, the POLG mutations in Alpers syndrome are recessive. Multiple combinations of mutations within POLG have been reported to induce Alpers syndrome (*dir-apps.niehs. nih.gov/polg*). Interestingly, the same mutations that induce an Alpers phenotype can also be responsible for autosomal recessive PEO or the syndrome of ataxia–neuropathy described next (Copeland, 2008; Weiss & Saneto, 2010; Wong et al., 2008). The reason for this remains unknown.

In the phenotypic continuum of POLG disorders, a syndrome of ataxia–neuropathy with its onset in the early teenage years has been described. This disorder has many names: mitochondrial–ataxic syndrome; spinocerebellar ataxia–epilepsy syndrome; and sensory neuropathy, ataxia, dysarthria, ophthalmoplegia syndrome. Clinical symptoms occur in various combinations of peripheral neuropathy, ataxia, cognitive impairment, dysarthria, involuntary movements, psychiatric abnormalities, myoclonus, and epileptic seizures. Various mutations in POLG can give rise to this group of disorders but most contain the mutation c.467A>T in one allele (reviewed in Copeland, 2008). This spectrum of symptoms typlify the difficulties in correlation of phenotype and genotype in

mitochondrial diseases. POLG mutations can cause Alpers syndrome in the infant (Naviaux & Nguyen, 2004) and either autosomal recessive or dominant PEO in the adult population (Hirano et al., 2001; Van Goethem, Dermaut, Lofgren, Martin, & Van Broeckhoven, 2001). Mutations in the POLG gene alter its activity, but the mechanisms involved in producing various phenotypes and onset of symptoms is unknown.

Special comments on POLG are needed. This protein is the only DNA polymerase found in mitochondria. The POLG gene has two domains: the N-terminal exonuclease and C-terminal polymerase domains, held together by a linker region. Mutations in the two most common "hot spots," c.467A>T and c.848G>T, are found in approximately 1% of the northern European population (Hakonen et al., 2007). It is estimated that POLG mutations occur in 0.05% of other ethnic groups. In the most recent consortium meeting concerning POLG diseases, it was estimated that these diseases account for 25% of all mitochondrial diseases, reflecting the high POLG mutation rate (Chinnery & Zeviani, 2008).

BARTH SYNDROME

Barth syndrome is an X-linked recessive disorder caused by mutations in the tafazzin gene, located at Xq28 (Bione et al., 1996). Tafazzin is responsible for remodeling of cardiolipins in the mitochondrial inner membrane. Cardiolipins play a modulatory role in the activities of several electron transport chain complexes, suggesting alterations of electron transport chain activities as the etiology of disease (Valianpour et al., 2002). The cardinal features of this syndrome are cardiac and skeletal myopathy with neutropenia, and short stature (Barth et al., 1983). The cardiomyopathy is classically a dilated cardiomyopathy with endocardial fibroelastosis. Isolated left ventricular noncompaction can also be found. Barth syndrome usually occurs during infancy, but can present at any time during the first decade of life. The cardiomyopathy may improve with age, if it does not prove fatal during early childhood. However, its severity can fluctuate and worsen again in adolescence.

Not reported in the cohort studies above are mutations in the C10orf2 gene or the mtDNA helicase Twinkle (Lonnqvist, Pae-tau, Valanne, & Pihko, 2009). I add this because of the early onset of disorders due to these mutations and their similarity to POLG disease. Initial symptoms of ataxia, muscle hypotonia, athetoid movements, and loss of deep tendon reflexes occur at about 1 year of age in patients with homozygote mutations and 6 months of age in patients with compound heterozygote mutations. Around the teenage years, sensory axonal neuropathy and female hypergonadotro-phic hypogonadism occur. There is a range of learning difficulties from moderate to severe. Type of mutation is associated with morbidity; in the compound heterozy-gote type, death occurs before 5 years of age. Thus far, only the 23 children in the Lonnquist and colleagues cohort have been described, and these mutations may thus be due to a founder effect.

GENETIC AND FAMILY PATTERNS

Inheritance of mitochondrial diseases fol-lows the rules of Mendelian inheritance of autosomal recessive, autosomal dominant, or X-linked recessive disorders. In addition, mitochondrial disease can be inherited by the unique pattern of maternal inheritance. The range of inheritance patterns, together with the variability in disease expression, makes disease patterns unpredictable and hard to recognize. For example, a single disorder such as Leigh syndrome can result from mul-tiple genetic abnormalities. As noted earlier, over 26 pathological mutations in mtDNA and over 22 nuclear gene mutations can give rise to Leigh syndrome. In contrast, multiple phenotypes may arise from mutations in a single gene. For example, mutations in the single gene POLG can give rise to at least eight syndromes that are expressed from in-fancy to old age (>75 years). This variability in both phenotype and genotype creates a spectrum of disorders that are often difficult to diagnose and limits specific recognition of disease patterns.

However, there are some patterns that seem to hold true, at least in the data we have to date. As in so many metabolic dis-orders, the earlier the onset of the disease, the more involved the disease. In the case of mitochondrial disease, the more severe the disorder, the earlier the mortality of the infant or child. Earlier onset usually means that a nuclear mutation is responsible for a disorder. Within a particular family, nuclear mutations usually give rise to similar symp-toms, time of onset, and outcome, whereas pathological mutations in mtDNA usually give rise to onset of disease later in life and to milder symptoms. Furthermore, a range of symptoms can be found within families with a pathological mtDNA mutation, from no symptoms to complete manifestation of the disorder. However, there are some ex-ceptions even to these patterns, as described above.

BIOLOGICAL AND NEUROPSYCHOLOGICAL MARKERS

Although most large cohort studies (see above) have indicated that the majority of patients have neurological involvement, the true prevalence of cognitive defects in mito-chondrial disorders remains unknown. CNS involvement varied from 70% to 90% in cohort studies. Patients expressing primar-ily cardiomyopathy may have less promi-nent cognitive delays; in one study, only 20% had delays (Scaglia et al., 2004). Defi-cits in the overall group included decreased Performance IQ and short-term memory deficits. One study demonstrated higher rates of cerebral dysfunction and intellec-tual deterioration (Kartsounis, Truong, Morgan-Hughes, & Harding, 1992). In another group of children, Performance IQ was found to be lower than Verbal IQ, with nonverbal cognitive impairment and com-promised visual–spatial abilities (Turconi et al., 1999). Further studies on this aspect of mitochondrial disease, in a larger group of patients with defined mitochondrial dis-orders, is needed.

There are no highly specific and sensitive biological markers in mitochondrial disease. Historically, elevated lactate and the pres-ence of ragged red fibers have been used as markers for mitochondrial disease; however, both of these can occur in other disorders, and thus their specificity and sensitivity for mitochondrial disease are limited. Neverthe-less, in the correct clinical context, elevated lactate and/or pyruvate can be an important biological indicator of mitochondrial disease, so such elevations must be considered in the context of other signs and symptoms. An excellent explanation of lactate and pyruvate in mitochondrial disease can be found in the article by Haas and colleagues (2007). By contrast, ragged red fibers have not been shown to be sensitive for mitochondrial disease in the neonatal to young adult populations (Vogel, 2001). So, although many patients with mitochondrial disease may have specific biological abnormalities, there are no highly specific markers of such disease. The constellation of findings—clinical, biochemical, and neuroimaging—is what leads the clinician to an appropriate diagnosis (Haas et al., 2007, 2008).

ASSESSMENT

Over the years, there have been multiple approaches to the diagnosis of mitochondrial disease (Bernier et al., 2002; Nissenkorn et al., 1999; Nonaka, 2002; Taylor, Schaefer, Barron, McFarland, & Turnbull, 2004; Wolf & Smeitink, 2002). These systematic approaches use a combination of clinical, biochemical, and morphological criteria. None of these systems are perfect; the certainty of diagnosis is stratified into "definite," "probable," "possible," and "unlikely." A nice summary of the limitations to these approaches has been published (Naviaux, 2004). In this summary, Naviaux makes the astute statement that "none of these systems has yet been applied to a mixed population of patients with mitochondrial disease and similar, but non-mitochondrial disease" (p. 354). Although this is true, most in the field have selected their "favorite" diagnostic paradigm and adhere to this system as their diagnostic tool. Two helpful review articles on the diagnosis of mitochondrial disorders have been published by a collaborative effort of the Mitochondrial Medicine Society (Haas et al., 2007, 2008). Because several databases now exist, the rigorous testing of systems across patient populations should allow investigators to become more precise in diagnosing mitochondrial diseases and in differentiating these from nonmitochondrial diseases. Ideally, the eventual results will be more precise definitions of mitochondrial diseases and refined criteria for their diagnosis.

TREATMENT

Treatment of mitochondrial disorders has been limited for a variety of reasons, one of which is that the lack of diagnostic consensus has made it difficult to create a standardized pool of patients for clinical trials. However, there are other reasons why treatment remains in its infancy. These diseases have been only been widely described since the late 1980s; research dollars have been limited; most current treatments are considered medical foods, and therefore the incentive for clinical trials is small; and the mitochondrial disease spectrum is broad.

Currently, most mitochondrial medicine physicians use a combination of vitamins and cofactors to optimize nutrition and general health, and to prevent worsening (catabolism) of symptoms during times of illness and physiological stress. The current goals for medical intervention are to increase energy production (ATP) and reduce abnormal free-radical production. A review of this subject has recently been published by the Mitochondrial Medicine Society (Parikh et al., 2009).

Organ Transplantation

The multiorgan involvement of most mitochondrial diseases would preclude the transplant of single organs. However, there are three circumstances in which specific organ transplantation may be considered. Two involve mtDNA depletion syndromes, one causing gastrointestinal dysfunction and the other liver dysfunction. The third situation involves isolated cardiomyopathy.

MNGIE may be the single mitochondrial disease for which organ transplant may be the "cure." This disorder, as described above, is a disorder of nucleotide utilization that results in severe gastrointestinal malabsorption, encephalopathy, leukodystrophy, and myopathy. Stem cell transplant has proven to be efficacious in the long-term reversal of symptoms (Hirano et al., 2006). At this writing, the initial stem cell transplant patient is demonstrating clinical improvements about 60 months after transplant (M. Hirano, personal communication, April 2009). A total of nine patients with MNGIE have undergone stem cell transplant, with some mixed results (Schupbach et al., 2009). Two of the patients have shown significant clinical improvement. Three patients were showing some improvement less than 2 years after transplant. The other four patients suffered transplant complications and expired. Multiple factors need to be considered in severely compromised patients with MNGIE. Optimizing treatment, such as timing transplantation to occur when patients are relatively healthy, may improve outcome.

Patients with the hepatocerebral depletion syndrome caused by DGUOK mutations may represent candidates for liver transplantation. In a meta-analysis, a Kaplan–Meier analysis showed that the lack of neurological involvement is associated with long-term survival (Dimmock et al., 2007). *Neurological involvement* was defined in this review as profound hypotonia, significant psychomotor retardation, and nystagmus. In this meta-analysis, liver transplant in patients with neurological symptoms was not associated with improved survival. However, of the three patients with no neurological symptoms, one patient had died but two others were still alive. The numbers are too small to permit any judgments on transplantation, and caution should be used at this time. Dimmock and colleagues (2007) strongly suggest that neurological involvement should preclude transplant, and this has been echoed in the literature by others.

The third possible clinical scenario in which transplantation may be considered is isolated cardiomyopathy. As noted above, these patients seem to have limited neurological involvement, and patients with isolated myopathy (noncardiac) have long-term survival compared to those with other types of mitochondrial disease. My colleagues and I have transplanted four patients with isolated cardiomyopathy who had developed cardiac failure (Saneto, 2010). All of these patients had electron transport chain defects. Each of these patients is currently alive and thriving 4–9 years after transplant.

Concluding Remarks

Mitochondrial disorders are relatively common and can present at any time throughout the lifespan. The expression of dual genomes and the unique physiology of mitochondria produce a wide spectrum of diseases, usually with multiple organ involvement. As in many other metabolic disorders, the more severe the disease, the earlier the presentation and the more devastating the disorder. Neonatal onset usually confers high morbidity with early mortality; patients typically die within 3 years of diagnosis. The mortality and morbidity caused by infancy/childhood-onset disorders are also high, but lower than those of the neonatal-onset disorders. Due to the high energy demand, the CNS and muscular system are usually involved, with high morbidity. The most common neurological dysfunction is cognitive delay, and most patients have some compromise in cognitive functioning. Only limited neuropsychological testing has been performed in this population. The extent of cognitive involvement within mitochondrial disease in general, and specific syndromes in particular, remains to be better studied.

Unfortunately, there is no single test that is sensitive or specific for any mitochondrial disease; therefore, diagnosis remains dependent on a combination of biochemical, structural, and neuroimaging testing, together with clinical exam and history. As genetic testing becomes more readily available, diagnosis should become more precise. However, given the possible combinations of genetic and physiological interactions, these diseases are likely to remain spectrum disorders. The multiplicity of symptoms within varying disease presentations makes clinicial acumen essential in diagnosis.

The most pressing needs in mitochondrial medicine are to stratify various diseases into a classification scheme based on phenotype and genetics, to uncover the natural history of these diseases, and to develop treatment strategies for specific disease types. I think that this is the right time for these possibilities to begin becoming realities. The next few years will be an exciting adventure for the development of mitochondrial medicine.

Acknowledgments

I wish to thank the families of my patients who have allowed me to care for their loved ones. In addition, I thank the Mitochondrial Research Guild at Seattle Children's Hospital for donating its time and funds to help me care better for my patients.

REFERENCES

Alpers, B. J. (1931). Diffuse progressive degeneration of the gray matter of the cerebrum. *Archives of Neurology and Psychiatry, 25,* 469–505.

Anderson, S., Bankier, A. T., Barrell, B. G., de Bruijn, M. H., Coulson, A. R., Drouin, J., et al. (1981). Sequence and organization of human mitochondrial genome. *Nature, 290,* 457–465.

Barkovich, A. J., Good, W. V., Koch, T. K., & Berg, B. O. (1993). Mitochondrial disorders: Analysis of their clinical and imaging characteristics. *American Journal of Neuroradiology, 14,* 1119–1137.

Barth, P. G., Scholte, H. R., Berden, J. A., Van der Klei-Van Moorsel, J. M., Luyt-Houwen, I. E. M., Van't Veer-Korthol, E. T., et al. (1983). An X-linked mitochondrial disease affecting cardiac muscle, skeletal muscle and neutrophil leucocytes. *Journal of Neurological Sciences, 62,* 327–355.

Battersby, B. J., Loredo-Osti, J. C., & Shoubridge, E. A. (2003). Nuclear genetic control of mitochondrial DNA segregation. *Nature Genetics, 33,* 183–186.

Bernier, F. P., Boneh, A., Dennett, X., Chow, C. W., Cleary, M. A., & Thornburn, D. R. (2002). Diagnostic criteria for respiratory chain disorders in adults and children. *Neurology, 59,* 1406–1411.

Bione, S., D'Adams, P., Maestrini, E., Gedeon, A. K., Bolhuis, P. A., & Toniolo, D. A. (1996). A novel X-linked genc, G4. 5 is responsible for Barth syndrome. *Nature Genetics, 12,* 385–389.

Blass, J. P., Lonsdale, D., Uhlendorf, B. W., & Hom, E. (1971). Intermediate ataxia with pyruvate decarboxylase deficiency. *Lancet, 1,* 1302.

Bornstein, B., Area, E., Flanigan, K. M., Ganesh, J., Jayakar, P., Swohoda, K. J., et al. (2008). Mitochondrial DNA depletion syndrome due to mutations in the RRM2B gene. *Neuromuscular Disorders, 18,* 453–459.

Bourdon, A., Minai, L., Serre, V., Jais, J. P., Sarzi, E., Aubert, S., et al. (2007). Mutation of RRM2B, encoding p53-controlled ribonucleotide reductase (p53R2), causes severe mitochondrial DNA depletion. *Nature Genetics, 39,* 776–780.

Bugiani, M., Tiranti, V., Farina, L., Uziel, G., & Zeviani, M. (2005). Novel mutations in COX15 in a long surviving Leigh syndrome patient with cytochrome c oxidase deficiency. *Journal of Medical Genetics, 42,* e28.

Calvo, S., Jain, M., Xie, X., Sheth, S. A, Chang, B., Goldberger, O. A., et al. (2006). Systematic identification of human mitochondrial disease genes through integrative genomics. *Nature Genetics, 38,* 576–582.

Carrodeguas, J. A., Theis, K., Bogenhagen, D. F., & Kisker, C. (2001). Crystal structure and deletion analysis show that the accessory subunit of mammalian DNA polymerase gamma POL gamma B functions as a homodimer. *Molecular Cell, 7,* 43–54.

Castro-Gogo, Blanco-Barca, M. O., Campos-Gonzalez, Y., Arenas-Barbero, J., Pintos-Martinex, E., & Eiris-Punal, J. (2006). Epidemiology of pediatric mitochondrial respiratory chain disorders in normthwest Spain. *Pediatric Neurology, 34,* 204–211.

Chinnery, P. F., Johnson, M. A., Wardell, T. M., Singh-Kler, R., Hayes, C., Brown, D. T., et al. (2000). The epidemiology of pathogenic mitochondrial DNA mutation. *Annals of Neurology, 48,* 188–193.

Chinnery, P. F., & Zeviani, M. (2008). 155th ENMC workshop: Polymerase gamma and disorders of mitochondrial DNA synthesis, 21–23 September 2007, Naarden, The Netherlands. *Neuromuscular Disorders, 18,* 259–267.

Copeland, W. C. (2008). Inherited mitochondrial disease of DNA replication. *Annual Review of Medicine, 59,* 131–146.

Darin, N., Oldfors, A., Moslemi, A.-R., Holme, E., & Tulinius, M. (2001). The incidence of mitochondrial encephalomyopathies in childhood: Clinical features and morphological, biochemical, and DNA abnormalities. *Annals of Neurology, 49,* 377–383.

Debray, F.-G., Lambert, M., Chevalier, I., Robitaille, Y., Decarle, J.-C., Shoubridge, E. A., et al. (2007). Long-term outcome and clinical spectrum of 73 pediatric patients with mitochondrial diseases. *Pediatrics, 119,* 722–733.

Di Donato, S. (2009). Multisystem manifestations of mitochonrial disorders. *Journal of Neurology, 256,* 693–710.

DiMauro, S., & Hirano, M. (2008). Pedaling from genotype to phenotype. *Archives of Neurology, 63,* 1125–1129.

DiMauro, S., Nicholson, J. F., Hays, A. P., Eastwood, A. B., Koenigsberger, R., & DeVivo, D. C. (1981). Benign infantile mitochondrial myopathy due to reversible cytochrome c oxidase deficiency. *Transactions of the American Neurological Association, 106,* 205–207.

DiMauro, S., & Schon, E. A. (2008). Mitochondrial disorders in the nervous system. *Annual Review of Neuroscience, 31,* 91–123.

Dimmock, D. P., Zhang, Q., Dionisi-Vici, C., Carrozzo, R., Shieh, J., Tang, L-Y., et al. (2007). Clinical and molecular features of mitochondrial DNA depletion due to mutations in deoxyguanosine kinase. *Human Mutation: Mutation in Brief 990,* 1–15.

Elliott, H. R., Samuels, D. C., Eden, J. A., Relton, C. L., & Chinnery, P. F. (2008). Pathogenic mitochondrial DNA mutations are common in the general population. *American Journal of Human Genetics, 83,* 254–260.

Engel, W. K., & Cunningham, G. G. (1963). Rapid examination of muscle tissue: An improved trichrome method for fresh-frozen biopsy sections. *Neurology, 13,* 919–923.

Filosto, M., Mancuso, M., Vives-Bauza, C., Vila, M. R., Shanske, S., Hirano, M., et al. (2003). Lack of paternal inheritance of muscle mitochondrial DNA in sporadic mitochondrial myopathies. *Annals of Neurology, 54*, 524–526.

Finsterer, J. (2008). Leigh and Leigh-like syndrome in children and adults. *Pediatric Neurology, 39*, 223–235.

Freisinger, P., Futterer, N., Lankes, E., Gempel, K., Berger, T. M., Spalinger, J., et al. (2006). Hepatocerebral mitochondrial DNA depletion syndrome caused by deoxyguanosine kinase (DGUOK) mutations. *Archives of Neurology, 63*, 1129–1134.

Galbiati, S., Bordoni, A., Papadimitriou, D., Toscano, A., Rodolico, C., Katsarou, E., et al. (2006). Hepatocerebral mitochondrial DNA depletion syndrome caused by deoxyguanosine kinase (DGUOK) mutations. *Pediatric Neurology, 34*, 177–185.

Garcia-Cazorla, A., De Lonlay, P., Nassogne, M. C., Rustin, P., Touati, G., & Saudubray, J. M. (2005). Long-term follow-up of neonatal mitochondrial cytopathies: A study of 57 patients. *Pediatrics, 116*, 1170–1177.

Gibson, K., Halliday, J. L., Kirby, D. M., Yaplito-Lee, J., & Thorburn, D. R. (2008). Mitochondrial oxidative phosphorylation disorders presenting in neonates: Clinical manifestations and enzymatic and molecular diagnoses. *Pediatrics, 122*, 1003–1008.

Giles, R. E., Blanc, H., Cann, H. M., & Wallace, D. C. (1980) Maternal inheritance of human mitochondrial DNA. *Proceedings of the National Academy of Sciences USA, 77*, 6715–6719.

Goto, Y., Nonaka, I., & Horai, S. (1990). A mutation in tRNA(Leu(UUR)) gene associated with the MELAS subgroup of mitochondrial encephalopathies. *Nature, 348*, 651–653.

Graziewicz, M. A., Longley, M. J., & Copeland, W. C. (2006). DNA polymerase gamma in mitochondrial DNA replication and repair. *Chemical Reviews, 106*, 383–405.

Haas, R. H., Parikh, S., Falk, M. J., Saneto, R. P., Wolf, N. I., Darin, N., et al. (2007). Mitochondrial disease: A practical approach for primary care physicians. *Pediatrics, 120*, 1326–1333.

Haas, R. H., Parikh, S., Falk, M. J., Saneto, R. P., Wolf, N. I., Darin, N., et al. (2008). The in-depth evaluation of suspected mitochondrial disease. *Molecular Genetics and Metabolism, 94*, 16–37.

Hakonen, A. H., Davidzon, G., Salemi, R., Bindoff, L. A., Van Goethem, G., DiMauro, S., et al. (2007). Abundance of the POLG disease mutations in Europe, Australia, New Zealand, and the United States explained by single ancient European founders. *European Journal of Human Genetics, 15*, 779–783.

Hammans, S. R., Sweeney, M. G., Brockington, M., Lennox, G. G., Lawton, M. F., Kennedy, C. R., et al. (1993). The mitochondrial DNA transfer RNA (Lys)A>G(8344) mutation and the syndrome of myoclonic epilepsy with ragged red fibers (MERRF): Relationship of clinical phenotype to proportion of mutant mitochondrial DNA. *Brain, 116*, 617–632.

Hansen, T. L., Christensen, E., & Brandt, N. H. (1982). Studies on pyruvate carboxylase, pyruvate decarboxylase and lipoamide dehydrogenase in subacute necrotizing encephalomyelopathy. *Acta Paediatrica Scandinavica, 71*, 263–267.

Hirano, M., Marti, R., Casali, C., Tadesse, S., Uldrick, T., Fine, B., et al. (2006). Allogenic stem cell transplantation corrects biochemical derangements in MNGIE. *Neurology, 67*, 1458–1460.

Hirano, M., Marti, R., Ferreiro-Barros, C., Vila, M. R., Tadesse, S., Nishigaki, Y., et al. (2001). Defects of intergenomic communication: Autosomal disorders that cause multiple deletions and depletion of mitochondrial DNA. *Seminars in Cell and Developmental Biology, 11*, 417–427.

Hirano, M., & Pavlakis, S. G. (1994). Mitochondrial myopathy, encephalopathy, lactic acidosis, and strokelike episodes (MELAS): Current concepts. *Journal of Child Neurology, 9*, 4–13.

Hirano, M., Ricci, E., Koenigsberger, M. R., Defendini, R., Pavlakis, S. G., DeVivo, D. C., et al. (1992). MELAS: An original case and clinical criteria for diagnosis. *Neuromuscular Disorders, 2*, 125–135.

Holt, I. J. (2009). Mitochondrial DNA replication and repair: All a flap. *Trends in Biochemical Sciences, 34*, 358–365.

Holt, I. J., Harding, A. E., Petty, R. K., & Morgan-Hughes, J. A. (1990). A new mitochondrial disease associated with mitochondrial DNA heteroplasmy. *American Journal of Human Genetics, 46*, 428–433.

Holt, I. J., Harding, A. E., & Morgan-Hughes, J. A. (1988). Deletions of muscle mitochondrial DNA in patients with mitochondrial myopathies. *Nature, 331*, 717–719.

Horvath, R., Kemp, J. P., Tuppen, H. A. L., Hudson, G., Oldfors, A., Marie, S. K. N., et al. (2009). Molecular basis of infantile reversible cytochrome c oxidase deficiency myopathy. *Brain, 132*(Pt. 11), 3165–3174.

Janssen, R. J. R. J., Nijtmans, I. G., van den Heuvel, L. P., & Smeitink, J. A. M. (2006). Mitochondrial complex I: Structure, function and pathology. *Journal of Inherited Metabolic Disease, 29*, 499–515.

Karadimas, C. L., Vu, T. H., Holve, S. A., Chronopulou, P., Quinzii, C., Johnsen, S. D., et al. (2006). Navajo neurohepatopathy is caused by a mutation in the MPV17 gene. *American Journal of Human Genetics, 79*, 544–548.

Kartsounis, L. D., Troung, D. D., Morgan-Hughes, J. A., & Harding, A. E. (1992). The neuropsychological features of mitochondrial myopathies and encephalomyopathies. *Archives of Neurology, 49*, 158–160.

Kearns, T. P., & Sayre, G. P. (1958). Retinitis pigmentosa, external ophthalmoplegia and complete heart block. *Archives of Ophthalmology, 60*, 280–289.

Kirby, D. M., Crawford, M., Cleary, M. A., Dahl, H.-H. M., Dennett, X., & Thorburn, D. R. (1999). Respiratory chain complex I deficiency. *Neurology, 52*, 1255–1264.

Larsson, M.-G., Holme, E., Kristiansson, B., Oldfors, A., & Tulinius, M. (1990). Progressive increase of the mutated mitochondrial DNA fraction in Kearns–Sayre syndrome. *Pediatric Research, 28*, 131–136.

Leber, T. (1871). Ueber hereditacre und congenital angelegte schnervenleiden. *Graefe's Archive for Opthalmology, 17*, 249–291.

Leigh, D. (1951). Subacute necrotizing encephalomyelopathy in an infant. *Journal of Neurology, Neurosurgery and Psychiatry, 14*, 216–221.

Lightowlers, R. N., Chinnery, P. F., & Howell, N. (1997). Mammalian mitochondrial genetics: Heredity, heteroplasmy and disease. *Trends in Genetics, 13*, 450–455.

Lonnqvist, T., Paetau, A., Valanne, L., & Pihko, H. (2009). Recessive Twinkle mutations cause severe epileptic encephalopathy. *Brain, 132*, 1553–1562.

Malfatti, E., Bugiani, M., Ivernizzi, F., Fichinger-Moura de Souza, C., Sanseverino, M. T., Glugliana, R., et al. (2007). Novel mutations of ND genes in complex I deficiency associated with mitochondrial encephalopathy. *Brain, 130*, 1894–1904.

Mancuso, M., Salviati, L., Sacconi, S., Otaegul, D., Camano, P., Marina, A., et al. (2002). Mitochondrial DNA depletion mutations in thymidine kinase gene with myopathy and SMA. *Neurology, 59*, 1197–1202.

Martin, E., Burger, R., Wiestler, O. D., Caduff, R., Boltshauser, E., & Boesch, C. (1990). Brainstem lesion revealed by MRI in a case of Leigh's disease with respiratory failure. *Pediatric Radiology, 20*, 349–350.

Martin, J. A., Hamilton, B. E., Sutton, R, D,, Ventura, S. J., Menacker, D., Kimeyer, S., et al. (2009). Births: Final data for 2006. *National Vital Statistics Reports, 57*, 1–86.

McShane, M. A., Hammans, S. R., Sweeney, M., Holt, I. J., Beattie, T. J., Brett, E. M., et al. (1991). Pearson syndrome and mitochondrial encephalomyopathy in a patient with deletion of mtDNA. *American Journal of Human Genetics, 48*, 39–42.

Moraes, C. T., DiMauro, S., Zeviani, M., Lombes, A., Shanske, S., Miranda, A. F., et al. (1989). Mitochondrial DNA deletions in progressive external ophthalmoplegia and Kearns–Sayre syndrome. *New England Journal of Medicine, 320*, 1293–1299.

Moraes, C. T., Shanske, S., Tritschler, H. J., Aprille, J. R., Andreetta, F., Bonilla, E., et al. (1991). mtDNA depletion with variable tissue expression: A novel genetic abnormality in mitochondrial diseases. *American Journal of Human Genetics, 48*, 492–501.

Nass, M. M., & Nass, S. (1963). Intrmitochondrial fibers with DNA characteristics: I. Fixation and electron staining reactions. *Journal of Cell Biology, 19*, 593–611.

Naviaux, R. K. (2004). Developing a systematic approach to the diagnosis and classification of mitochondrial disease. *Mitochondrion, 4*, 351–361.

Naviaux, R. K., & Nguyen, K. V. (2004). POLG mutations associated with Alpers' syndrome and mitochondrial DNA depletion. *Annals of Neurology, 55*, 706–712.

Naviaux, R. K., Nyhan, W. L., Barshop, B. A., Poulton, J., Markusic, D., Karpinski, N. C., et al. (1999). Mitochondrial DNA polymerase gamma deficiency and mtDNA depletion in a child with Alpers' syndrome. *Annals of Neurology, 45*, 54–58.

Nishino, I., Spinazzola, A., & Hirano, M. (1999). Thymidine phosphorylase gene mutations in MNGIE, a human mitochondrial disorder. *Science, 283*, 689–692.

Nissenkorn, A., Zeharia, A., Lev, D., Watemberg, N., Fattal-Valevski, A., Barash, V., et al. (2000). Neurologic presentations of mitochondrial disorders. *Journal of Child Neurology, 15*, 44–48.

Nonaka, I. (2002). Approach for a final diagnosis of mitochondrial disease. *Nippon Rinsho, 60*(Suppl. 4), 224–228.

Oskoui, M., Davidson, G., Pascual, J., Erazo, R., Gurgel-Giannetti, J., Krishna, S., et al. (2006). Clinical spectrum of mitochondrial DNA depletion due to mutations in the thymidine kinase 2 gene. *Archives of Neurology, 63*, 1122–1126.

Ostergaard, E., Hansen, F. J., Sorensen, N., Duno, M., Vissing, J., Larsen, P. L., et al. (2007). Mitochondrial encephalomyopathy with elevated methylmalonic acid is caused by SUCLA2 mutations. *Brain, 130*, 853–861.

Parikh, S., Saneto, R., Falk, M. J., Anselm, I., Cohen, B. H., & Haas, R. (2009). A modern approach to the treatment of mitochondrial disease. *Current Treatment Options in Neurology, 11*, 414–430.

Parini, R., Furlan, F., Notarangelo, L., Spinazzola, A., Uziel, G., Strisciuglio, P., et al. (2009). Glucose metabolism and diet-based prevention of liver dysfunction in MPV17 mutant patients. *Journal of Hepatology, 50*, 215–221.

Pearson, H. A., Lobel, J. S., Kocoshis, S. A., Naiman, J. L., Windmiller, J., Lammi, A. T., et al. (1979). A new syndrome of refractory sideroblastic anemia with vacuolization of marrow precursors and exocrine pancreatic dysfunction. *Journal of Pediatrics, 95*, 976–984.

Piao, Y. S., Tang, G. C., Yang, H., & Lu, D. H. (2006). Clinico-neuropathological study of a Chinese case of familial adult Leigh syndrome. *Neuropathology, 26,* 218–221.

Rahman, S., Brown, R. M., Chong, W. K., Wilson, C. J., & Brown, G. K. (2001). A SURF1 gene mutation presenting as isolated leukodystrophy. *Annals of Neurology, 49,* 797–800.

Rahman, S., Blok, R. B., Dahl, H. H. M., Danks, D. M., Kirby, D. M., Chow, C. W., et al. (1996). Leigh syndrome: Clinical features and biochemical and DNA abnormalities. *Annals of Neurology, 39,* 343–351.

Ribacoba, R., Salas-Puig, J., Gonzalez, C., & Astudillo, A. (2006). Characteristics of status epilepticus in MELAS: Analysis of four cases. *Neurology, 21,* 1–11.

Riley, M. H., Davey, M. A., & King, J. (2005). *Births in Victoria 2003–2004.* Melbourne, Australia: Victorian Perinatal Data Collection Unit, Victorian Government Department of Human Services.

Rossignol, R., Faustin, B., Rocher, C., Malgat, M., Mazat, J. P., & Letellier, T. (2003). Mitochondrial threshold effects. *Biochemical Journal, 370,* 751–762.

Rotig, A., Colonna, V., Bonnefont, J. P., Blanch, S., Fischer, A., Saudubray, J. M., et al. (1989). Mitochondrial DNA deletion in Pearson's marrow/pancreas syndrome. *Lancet, 1,* 902–903.

Rotig, A., Cormier, V., Blanche, S., Bonnefont, J. P., Ledeist, F., Romero, N., et al. (1990). Pearson's marrow-pancreas syndrome: A multisystem mitochondrial disorder in infancy. *Journal of Clinical Investigation, 86,* 1601–1608.

Rubio-Gozalbo, M. E., Kijkman, K. P., van den Heuvel, L. P., Sengers, R. C. A., Wendel, U., & Smeitink, J. A. M. (2000). Clinical differences in patients with mitochondriocytopathies due to nuclear versus mitochondrial DNA mutations. *Human Mutation, 15,* 522–532.

Sacconi, S., Salviati, L., Nishigaki, Y., Walker, W. F., Hernandez-Rosa, E., Trevission, E., et al. (2008). A functionally dominant mitochondrial DNA mutation. *Human Molecular Genetics, 17,* 1814–1820.

Saneto, R. P., & Bouldin, A. (2006). A boy with muscle weakness, hypercarbia, and the mitochondrial DNA A3243G mutation. *Journal of Child Neurology, 21,* 77–79.

Saneto, R. P., Friedman, S. D., & Shaw, D. W. W. (2008). Neuroimaging of mitochondrial disease. *Mitochondrion, 8,* 396–413.

Saneto, R. P., & Law, Y. (2010). [Cardiac transplant in patients with mitochondrial disease]. Unpublished raw data.

Saraste, M. (1999). Oxidative phosphorylation at the fin de siecle. *Science, 283,* 579–587.

Scaglia, F., Towbin, J. A., Craigen, W, J., Belmont, J. W., Smith, E. O., Neish, S. R., et al. (2004). Clinical spectrum, morbidity, and mortality in 113 pediatric patients with mitochondrial disease. *Pediatrics, 114,* 925–931.

Schaefer, A. M., McFarland, R., Blakely, E. L. He, L., Whittaker, R. G., Taylor, R. W., et al. (2008). Prevalence of mitochondrial DNA disease in adults. *Annals of Neurology, 63,* 35–39.

Schaefer, A. M., Taylor, R. W., Turnbull, D. M., & Chinnery, P. F. (2004). The epidemiology of mitochondrial disorders—past, present and future. *Biochimica et Biophysica Acta, 1659,* 115–120.

Schupbach, M., Benoist, J.-F., Casali, C., Elhasid, R., Fay, K., Hahn, D., et al. (2009). Allogenic hematopoietic stem cell transplantation (HSCT) for mitochondrial neurogastrointestinal encephalomyopathy (MNGIE). *Neurology, 73,* 332.

Schwartz, M., & Vissing, J. (2002). Paternal inheritance of mitochondrial DNA. *New England Journal of Medicine, 347,* 576–580.

Schwartz, M., & Vissing, J. (2004). No evidence for paternal inheritance of mtDNA in patients with soradic mtDNA mutations. *Journal of the Neurological Sciences, 218,* 99–101.

Sciacco, M., Bonilla, E., Schon, E. A. ., DiMauro, S., & Moraes, C. T. (1994). Distribution of wild-type and common deletion forms of mtDNA in normal and respiration-deficient muscle fibers from patients with mitochondrial myopathy. *Human Molecular Genetics, 3,* 13–19.

Shoffner, J. M., Lott, M. T., Lezza, A. M., Seibel, P., Ballinger, S. W., & Wallace, D. C. (1990). Myoclonic epilepsy and ragged-red fibers disease (MERRF) is associated with a mitochondrial DNA tRNA[lys] mutation. *Cell, 61,* 931–937.

Silvestri, G., Moraes, C. T., Shanske, S., Oh, S. J., & DiMauro, S. (1991). A new mtDNA mutation in the tRNA lys gene associated with myoclonic epilepsy and ragged-red fibers (MERRF). *American Journal of Human Genetics, 51,* 1213–1217.

Skladal, D., Sudmeier, C., Konstantopoulou, V., Stockler-Ipsiroglu, S., Plecko-Startinig, B., Bernert, G., et al. (2003). The clinical spectrum of mitochondrial disease in 75 pediatric patients. *Clinical Pediatrics, 42,* 703–710.

Smeitink, J. A., Zeviani, M., Turnbull, D. M., & Jackobs, H. T. (2006). Mitochondrial medicine: A metabolic perspective on the pathology of oxidative phosphorylation disorders. *Cell Metabolism, 3,* 9–13.

Song, S., Wheeler, L. J., & Mathews, C. K. (2003). Deoxyribonucleotide pool imbalance stimulates deletions in HeLa cell mitochondrial DNA. *Journal of Biological Chemistry, 278,* 43893–43896.

Spelbrink, J. N., Li, F. Y., Tiranti, V., Nikali, K., Yuan, Q. P., Tariq, M., et al. (2001). Human mitochondrial DNA deletions associatd with mutations in the gene encoding Twinkle, a phage T7 gene 4-like protein localized in mitochondria. *Nature Genetics, 28,* 223–231.

Spinazzola, A., Santer, R., Akman, O. H., Tsiakas, K., Schaefer, H., Ding, X., et al. (2008). Hepatocerebral from of mitochondrial DNA depletion syndrome. *Archives of Neurology, 65*, 1108–1113.

Spinazzola, A., & Zeviani, M. (2005). Disorders of nuclear–mitochondrial intergenomic signaling. *Gene, 354*, 162–168.

Spinazzola, A., & Zeviani, M. (2009). Disorders from perturbations of nuclear–mitochondrial intergenomic cross-talk. *Journal of Internal Medicine, 265*, 174–192.

Stewart, J. D., Tennant, S., Powell, H., Pyle, A., Blakely, K. L., He, L., et al. (2009). Novel POLG1 mutations associated with neuromuscular and liver phenotypes in adults and children. *Journal of Medical Genetics, 46*, 209–214.

Stromme, J. H., Borud, O., & Moe, P. J. (1976). Fatal lactic acidosis in a newborn attributable to a congenital defect of pyruvate dehydrogenase. *Pediatric Research, 10*, 60–66.

Sue, C. M., Hirano, M., DiMauro, S., & De Vivo, D. C. (1999). Neonatal presentations of mitochondrial metabolic disorders. *Seminars in Perinatalology, 23*, 113–124.

Sutovsky, P., Van Leyen, K., McCauley, T., Day, B. N., & Sutovsky, M. (2004). Degradation of paternal mitochondria after fertilization: Implications for heteroplasmy, assisted reproductive technologies and mtDNA inhcritance. *Reproductive BioMedicine Online, 8*, 24–33.

Taanman, J. W., Muddle, J. R., & Muntau, A. C. (2003). Mitochondrial DNA depletion can be prevented by cGMP and dAMP supplementation in a resting culture of deoxyguanosine kinase-deficient fibroblasts. *Human Molecular Genetics, 12*, 1839–1845.

Taylor, R. W., Schaefer, A. M., Barron, M. J., McFarland, R., & Turnbull, D. M. (2004). The diagnosis of mitochondrial muscle disease. *Neuromuscular Disorders, 14*, 237–245.

Taylor, R. W., & Turnbull, D. M. (2005). Mitochondrial DNA mutations in human disease. *Nature Reviews Genetics, 6*, 389–402.

Tulinius, M. H., Holme, E., Kristiansson, B., Larsson, N. G., & Oldfors, A. (1991). Mitochondrial encephalomyopathies in childhood: 1. Biochemical and morphologic investigations. *Journal of Pediatrics, 119*, 242–250.

Turconi, A. C., Benti, R., Castelli, E., Pochintesta, S., Felsari, G., Comi, G., et al. (1999). Focal cognitive impairment in mitochondrial encephalomyopathies: A neuropsychological and neuroimaging study. *Journal of the Neurological Sciences, 170*, 57–63.

Tyynismaa, H., Ylikallio, E. M., Patel, M., Molnar, M. J., Haller, R. G., & Suomalainen, A. (2009). A heterozygous truncation mutation in RRM2B causes autosomal-dominant progressive external ophthalmoplegia with multiple mtDNA deletions. *American Journal of Human Genetics, 85*, 290–295.

Valianpour, F., Wanders, R. J., Overnars, H., Vicken, P., Van Gennip, A. H., Baas, F., et al. (2002). Cardiolipin deficiency in X-linked cardioskeletal myopathy and neutropenia (Barth syndrome MIM 302060): A study in cultured skin fibroblasts. *Journal of Pediatrics, 141*, 729–733.

Van Goetham, G., Dermaut, B., Lofgren, A., Martin, J. J., & Van Broeckhoven, C. (2001). Mutation of POLG is associated with progressive external ophthalmoplegia characterized by mtDNA dletions. *Nature Genetics, 28*, 211–212.

Van Maldergem, L., Trijbels, F., DiMauro, S., Sindelar, P. J., Musumeci, O., Janssen, A., et al. (2002). Coenzyme Q-response Leigh's encephalopathy in two sisters. *Annals of Neurology, 52*, 750–754.

Vogel, H. (2001). Mitochondrial myopathies and the role of the pathologist in the molecular era. *Journal of Neuropathology and Experimental Neurology, 60*, 217–227.

von Kleist-Retzow, J. C., Cormier-Daire, V., Viot, G., Goldenberg, A., Mardach, B., Amiel, J., et al. (2003). Antenatal manifestations of mitochondrial respiratory chain deficiency. *Journal of Pediatrics, 143*, 208–212.

Wallace, D. C. (1999). Mitochondrial diseases in man and mouse. *Science, 283*, 482–487.

Wallace, D. C., Singh, G., Lott, M. T., Hodge, J. A., Schurr, T. G., Lezza, A. M., et al. (1988). Mitochondrial DNA mutation associated with Leber's hereditary optic neuropathy. *Science, 242*, 1427–1430.

Weiss, M. D., & Saneto, R. P. (2010). Sensory ataxic neuropathy with dysarthria and ophthalmoparesis (SANDO) in late life due to compound heterozygous POLG mutations. *Muscle and Nerve, 41*(6), 882–885.

Wolf, N. I., & Smeitink, J. A. (2002). Mitochondrial disorders: A proposal for consensus diagnostic criteria in infants and children. *Neurology, 59*, 1402–1405.

Wong, L.-J., Naviaux, R. K., Brunetti-Pierri, N., Zhang, Q., Schmitt, E. S., Truong, C., et al. (2008). Molecular and clinical genetics of mitochondrial diseases due to POLG mutations. *Human Mutation, 29*, E150–E172.

Wortmann, S. B., Rodenburg, R. J. T., Jonckheere, A., de Vries, M. C., Muizing, M., Heldt, K., et al. (2009). Biochemical and genetic analysis of 3-methylglutaconic aciduria type IV: A diagnostic strategy. *Brain, 132*, 136–146.

Zeviani, M., & Di Donato, S. (2004). Mitochondrial disorders. *Brain, 127*, 2153–2172.

CHAPTER 27

Major Structural Anomalies of the Neocortex

NANCY L. NUSSBAUM
GINA B. CHRISTOPHER
VALERIE VAN HORN KERNE

The pace and complexity of the human brain's development is nothing short of astounding; the invariable progression follows a blueprint programmed into every human being for millennia, with no intention required. When the progression is varied, it often comes at a very high cost to the individual, and the outcome can be devastating and tragic. Abnormalities in brain development may lead to a wide variety of clinical outcomes—from relatively minor consequences, such as a mild microgyria or ectopias possibly leading to subtle cognitive deficits, to the inevitable fatal outcome associated with anencephaly. In this chapter, we focus primarily on the major cortical anomalies found in the development of the human brain.

To begin, we briefly discuss the typical development of the human nervous system. It is helpful to have a basic grasp of the ontogenesis of the brain in general and the cerebral cortex in particular before further exploring structural abnormalities in development. Following this discussion, we describe a number of major structural anomalies, including schizencephaly, anencephaly, and lissencephaly. The relevant history, etiology, developmental course, prevalence, genetic and family patterns, biological and neuropsychological factors, risk factors for phenotypic expression, assessment, and treatment are covered for these cephalic disorders.

NORMAL DEVELOPMENT OF THE CEREBRAL CORTEX

Development of the nervous system begins with the development of the neural tube, commencing near the 18th day of gestation. Early in embryonic development, the ectodermal tissue thickens and forms the neural plate. The edges of the neural plate then form ridges (often referred to as *neural folds*) that curl toward each other until they fuse, forming the *neural tube* (see Figure 27.1).

Near 24 days' gestation, the anterior neural tube closes and serves as the foundation for future brain development (Clark, 2004). When the neural tube is closed, development progresses and the lateral, third, and fourth ventricles are formed. The tissue that surrounds these ventricles becomes the forebrain, the midbrain, and the hindbrain,

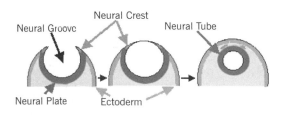

FIGURE 27.1. Neural tube development. From Chudler (2009). Used by permission of Eric H. Chudler, PhD.

respectively (Carlson, 2007). The posterior neural tube closes at approximately the 26th day of gestation and serves as the foundation for spinal cord development (Clark, 2004).

Cell proliferation, cell migration, and *cortical organization* are three stages of cerebral cortex development. Although described as discrete steps, these stages often occur simultaneously, since cell proliferation continues after neuronal migration begins (Abdel Razek, Kandell, Elsorogy, Elmongy, & Basett, 2009). Cell proliferation begins with the layer of cells that line the inside of the neural tube, referred to as the ventricular zone (VZ) (Guerrini & Marini, 2006). The VZ contains the founder cells that divide and give rise to the cells of the central nervous system (Carlson, 2007). Each founder cell first undergoes symmetrical division, producing two identical cells and thus increasing the size of the VZ. Each founder cell then undergoes asymmetrical division, producing a founder cell that remains in the VZ and another cell that is guided outward into the cerebral cortex by radial glial cell fibers. Radial glial cells were discovered by Rakic (1972, 1988), and their fibers provide the pathways for neurons to follow during their migration into the cerebral cortex (Carlson, 2007). Studies of brain development have shown that the cerebral cortex develops from the inside out. The earliest-migrating cells occupy the deepest layer of the cortex, with subsequent migrations passing through previously formed layers (Carlson, 2007). Cortical organization, the third stage of cerebral cortex development, involves formation of the cellular network and includes neuronal extensions, synaptogenesis, and maturation (Barkovich, Kuzniecky, Jackson, Guerrini, & Dobyns, 2001).

Structural anomalies of the neocortex are a heterogeneous group of disorders (Abdel Razek et al., 2009). Their numerous causes include chromosomal and genetic diseases, environmental factors, and traumas that occur at critical developmental periods. Barkovich, Kuzniecky, Jackson, Guerrini, and Dobyns (2005) proposed a classification scheme of structural anomalies of the cortex based on the stage of cerebral cortical development at which each anomaly occurs (i.e., cell proliferation, cell migration, or cortical organization). The classification scheme has evolved (Barkovich & Kuzniecky, 1996;

Barkovich et al., 2001) and is now based on the identified gene whenever possible, rather than on the clinical features associated with the disorder (Barkovich et al., 2005). Still, it is suggested that the clinical manifestations and severity of the disorders depend largely on the stage of cortical development.

Malformations due to abnormal neuronal and radial glial proliferation may result in conditions that are characterized by too many, too few, or malformed cells (Barkovich & Kuzniecky, 1996). Several conditions believed to result from a primary defect in cell proliferation include microlissencephaly, hemimegalencephaly, and focal cortical dysplasias (Abdel Razek et al., 2009). Disorders of cellular migration develop when neurons fail to reach their intended destination in the cerebral cortex early in the development of the fetal nervous system. Impairments may occur at the beginning of migration, during the ongoing process, or at the completion of migration (Gleeson & Walsh, 2000). This results in structural deformities of the cerebral hemispheres that result from undermigration, overmigration, or ectopic migration of the neurons (Menkes & Sarnat, 2000). The classic lissencephalies and heterotopias are thought to result from defects in cell migration (Abdel Razek et al., 2009). Golden (2001) reported that pachygyria (i.e., few course and wide gyri) and polymicrogyrias (i.e., many small gyri crowded in an irregular pattern) are additional neuronal migration disorders (see Figure 27.2). Malformations due to cortical organization are characterized by abnormalities in gyral formation and commonly result from prenatal ischemia or infection. Some of the associated conditions include polymicrogyrias and schizencephaly (Abdel Razek et al., 2009). Table 27.1 summarizes the structural anomalies of the neocortex.

SCHIZENCEPHALY

Schizencephaly occurs between the end of the neuronal migration period and the early phase of cortical organization (Iannetti, Spalice, Atzei, Boemi, & Trasimeni, 1996). It is a structural anomaly of the brain characterized by the presence of abnormal clefts in the cerebral hemispheres. The clefts extend from the cortical surface to the underly-

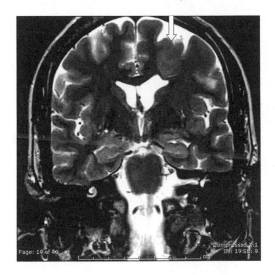

FIGURE 27.2. T2-weighted image shows migrational anomaly in a 41-year-old male with seizures. Abnormal gray matter extends from the cortex to the ventricular surface. (Courtesy of David Leake, MD, Austin, Texas.)

ing ventricular cavity, often resulting in the replacement of large portions of the cerebral hemispheres with cerebrospinal fluid (CSF) (Menkes & Sarnat, 2000). The classification of schizencephaly is based on the presence of *bilateral* clefts (i.e., clefts in both hemispheres) or *unilateral* clefts (i.e., a cleft or clefts in one hemisphere). Bilateral clefts are usually symmetrical, affecting both hemispheres of the brain (Ferrer, 1984). Schizencephaly clefts are further described as *type I* or *closed-lipped* when the cleft walls are fused, eliminating any space within the cleft for CSF; they are described as *type II* or *open-lipped* when the cleft walls are separated and filled with CSF (Clark, 2004). Type II schizencephaly is more common than type I (Guerrini, 2005), and in 70% of cases, clefts are located most frequently in the frontal and parietal lobes, typically around the sylvian fissures (Arantes, Perdigao, Pereira, & Costa, 2007; Barkovich, 1995) (see Figure 27.3).

TABLE 27.1. Structural Anomalies of the Neocortex

Structural anomaly	Pathogenesis	Characteristics	Associated anomalies disorders
Schizencephaly	Neuronal migration Cortical organization	Abnormal clefts Bilateral clefts Unilateral clefts *Type I: Closed-lipped*—cleft walls are fused *Type II: Open lipped*—cleft walls are separated and filled with cerebrospinal fluid	Agenesis of septum pellucidum Agenesis of corpus callosum Cortical dysgenesis Hydrocephalus Polymicrogyria
Anencephaly	Failure of neural tube formation Exencephaly	Partial or total absence of cerebral structures	Abnormal development of skull base
Lissencephaly	Neuronal migration Cortical organization	Deficient gyration Agyria (lack of gyri) Pachygyria (broad gyri) *Type I: Classical*—poorly defined sylvian and rolandic fissures, thickening of cerebral cortex, increased gray matter *Type II: Cobblestone*—agyria, pachygyria; abnormal migration of gray matter to cortical surface	Miller–Dieker syndrome Isolated lissencephaly sequence X-linked lissencephaly with abnormal genitalia Cerebellar hypoplasia Microlissencephaly Agenesis of corpus callosum Eye abnormalities Muscular dystrophy Walker–Warberg syndrome Muscle–eye–brain syndrome Fukuyama syndrome Hydrocephalus Encephaloceles

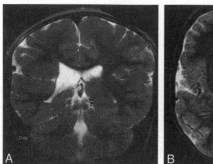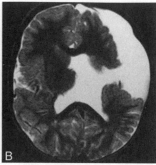

FIGURE 27.3. Schizencephaly. (A) Coronal T2-weighted image shows a closed-lipped right-sided schizencephalic defect lined by pachygyria. (Courtesy of R. Zimmerman, MD, Philadelphia, Pennsylvania.) (B) Axial T2-weighted image shows a wide CSF-filled cleft connecting the left lateral ventricle with the subarachnoid space, which is lined with gray matter parenchyma. From Abdel Rasek, Kandell, Elsorogy, Elmongy, and Bassett (2009). Copyright 2009 by the American Society of Neuroradiology. Reprinted by permission.

Schizencephaly is considered a disorder of cortical organization, since the cortex surrounding a cleft is typically polymicrogyric (Barkovich et al., 2001). In 50–90% of cases, it is associated with other brain abnormalities—agenesis of the septum pellucidum, agenesis or thinness of the corpus callosum, cortical dysgenesis, and hydrocephalus, among others (Arantes et al., 2007; Komarniski, Cyr, Mack, & Weinberger, 1990).

History

Although the first reported case of a schizencephaly cleft was identified by Kundrat in 1882 (as cited in Granata & Battaglia, 2008), the term *schizencephaly* was originated by Yakovlev and Wadsworth (1946a, 1946b). They presented case studies of five autopsied patients with severe cognitive and motor deficits, and described their morphological features (e.g., unilateral vs. bilateral and open-lipped vs. closed-lipped clefts). Prior to Yakovlev and Wadsworth's identification of the syndrome, schizencephaly had been included in the category of porencephalies (Granata & Battaglia, 2008). In 1859, Heschl coined the term *porencephaly* and used it to describe any defect that extended through the full thickness of the cerebral hemispheres (as cited in Raybaud, 1983). The term *porencephaly* is now commonly used to describe any congenital focal lesion or cavity in the brain (Raybaud, 1983).

Developmental Course

The etiology of schizencephaly is still much debated; however, the most widely accepted hypothesis is that it involves both environmental and genetic risk factors (Abdel Razek et al., 2009; Arantes et al., 2007; Granata & Battaglia, 2008). Schizencephaly may occur as a result of prenatal ischemia, exposure to toxins, viral infections, or genetic errors that occur during the cortical organization stage (Granata, Freri, Caccia, Setola, Taroni, & Battaglia, 2005). A theory suggesting that schizencephaly results from inadequate blood flow and subsequent ischemic damage to the developing cortex is supported by the frequent co-occurrence of schizencephaly with polymicrogyria. Barkovich and colleagues (2005) reported no known cases of schizencephaly without accompanying polymicrogyria. Still, *in utero* infections, toxic agents, and trauma are also implicated in the development of schizencephaly. Specifically, schizencephaly may occur with a prenatal cytomegalovirus infection (Iannetti et al., 1996). Data obtained from a study utilizing experimental animals supports the theory that clefts may be produced following *in utero* viral exposure. Specifically, the inoculation of a mumps virus strain impaired neuronal migration and produced a cleft and other brain malformations in hamsters (Takano, Takikita, & Shimada, 1999).

An alternative theory hypothesizes that schizencephaly is genetically determined. The

EMX2 gene mutation has been implicated in a minority of familial cases of schizencephaly (Granata et al., 1997), and according to Verrotti and colleagues (2010), the EMX2 gene is probably involved in controlling cortical migration and structural patterning of the developing brain. In recent studies, however, the EMX2 gene has not accounted for all cases (Menkes & Sarnat, 2000), and it has not been confirmed in follow-up studies by other researchers (Barkovich et al., 2001) or in experimental models (Granata & Battaglia, 2008). Therefore, genetic testing protocols are not currently recommended (Innes, 2008).

Prevalence

Prevalence rates for schizencephaly are not reported in the scientific literature; however, a recent epidemiological study tracing 4 million births in California from 1985 to 1991 reported that 1.54 in 100,000 births resulted in a schizencephaly diagnosis (Curry, Lammer, Nelson, & Shaw, 2005). Therefore, schizencephaly is a rare structural anomaly, and it has been reported to affect males and females equally (Granata & Battaglia, 2008).

Biological and Neuropsychological Markers

The clinical picture of schizencephaly is characterized by a range of neurological and developmental impairments, which will depend on size, location, and the unilateral or bilateral nature of the clefts. Studies by Barkovich and Kjos (1992) and Packard, Miller, and Delgado (1997) indicated that the number of lobes affected by clefts has an impact on the severity of outcome. Several studies have reported that schizencephaly clefts more often affect the frontal lobes, followed by the frontoparietal regions, and then the parietal and occipital lobes (Barkovich & Kuzniecky, 1996). The presence of associated cerebral malformations (e.g., agenesis of the septum pellucidum, agenesis of the corpus callosum, hydrocephalus) also influences developmental outcome (Arantes et al., 2007). Symptoms of schizencephaly may include developmental delay, mental retardation, speech delay, muscle weakness or paralysis, difficulties with movement, seizures, blindness, microcephaly, and emotional/behavioral disorders (Arantes et al., 2007; Packard et al., 1997). A negative prognosis is suggested when the anomaly is characterized by a large, open-lipped, bilateral cleft. There is a better prognosis in persons with unilateral forms, since cerebral plasticity may allow for reorganization of cognitive functions in the contralateral hemisphere (Al-Alawi, Al-Tawil, Al-Hathal, & Amir, 2001; Garel, 2004). Persons with small, unilateral, closed-lipped clefts have the mildest clinical features. They typically present with mild hemiparesis and seizures, but no other impairments or delays in typical developmental milestones are usually noted (Barkovich & Kjos, 1992; Barkovich & Kuzniecky, 1996; Verrotti et al., 2009). In contrast, large, bilateral, open-lipped clefts have the most severe features and typically present in early infancy (Granata et al., 2005). Bilateral clefts are typically associated with microcephaly, severe cognitive delays, and severe motor abnormalities (including spastic quadriparesis). Blindness as the result of optic nerve hypoplasia can also be common (Verrotti et al., 2009).

Motor Deficits

Overall, motor deficits are almost invariably present in children with schizencephaly, as would be expected with clefts located in the frontoparietal lobes (Granata et al., 2005; Packard et al., 1997). As mentioned previously, the severity of motor impairment will vary from apparently normal health or mild asymmetry of motor skills characteristic of unilateral clefts to spastic quadriparesis, which is often seen in patients with bilateral schizencephaly (Al-Alawi et al., 2001; Granata et al., 2005). Hypotonia (deficient muscular tone) or hemiparesis (muscular weakness or partial paralysis restricted to one side of the body) may be present (Menkes & Sarnat, 2000), and both are typically associated with a contralateral cortical cleft (Packard et al., 1997).

Cognitive Delays

The severity of cognitive and language impairments associated with schizencephaly also depends in large part on the unilateral or bilateral nature of the clefts (Granata et al., 2005). Cognitive impairments are present in approximately 50% of cases with unilateral clefts, and they are almost invariably present with bilateral clefts. Persons diagnosed with schizencephaly may display major language impairments, including a lack of speech (Verrotti et al., 2009); however, the language impairments are somewhat less severe than the motor deficits and possible seizure complications (Packard et al., 1997). Patients with unilateral, closed-lipped (type I) clefts typically have better language development than patients with bilateral, open-lipped (type II) clefts (Packard et al., 1997). In cases with unilateral clefts, the unaffected hemisphere may compensate, and cognitive functions may be completely normal. Brown, Levin, Ramsay, and Landy (1993) presented a case study of a 32-year-old, left-handed male with unilateral left-hemisphere type I (closed-lipped) schizencephaly. According to his neuropsychological test findings, the patient demonstrated average to above-average performance on all measures of language, judgment and reasoning, visual–spatial abilities, and memory function. He had completed 2 years of college education, earned an associate's degree, and managed a successful land-surveying business. He showed no evidence of cognitive or emotional dysfunction, and his only reason for seeking treatment was the onset of seizures at 26 years of age. This case example provides evidence for the compensatory mechanisms of the unaffected hemisphere in some cases of schizencephaly. Brown and colleagues raise the question about undetected cases of schizencephaly as a result of apparently normal functioning in some individuals.

Epileptic Seizures

Epilepsy may be the most serious complication associated with schizencephaly, and seizures are often the presenting symptoms (Granata et al., 2005; Menkes & Sarnat, 2000). They occur in 40–65% of cases (Granata et al., 2005), and in one large review conducted by Granata and colleagues (1997), 80% of participants reported seizures. According to Golden (2001), schizencephaly frequently co-occurs with polymicrogyria, and since most infants and children with different forms of polymicrogyria present with seizures, it is not surprising that seizures often accompany schizencephaly. Despite the high prevalence of seizures, the association between size, location, and the uni- or bilateral nature of the schizencephaly clefts on the one hand and the severity of the epilepsy on the other is still unclear (Seguti, Schappo, Sobrinho, & Ferreira, 2006). Some patients with schizencephaly present with seizures while others do not. Barkovich and Kuzniecky (1996) found that patients with unilateral schizencephaly typically have epilepsy with partial simple or complex seizures, whereas patients with bilateral schizencephaly typically present with mixed seizure disorders. In addition, Packard and colleagues (1997) reported that patients with open-lipped clefts had an earlier age of onset and less seizure control than patients with closed-lipped clefts had. Overall, various types of seizures have been reported, including generalized, tonic–clonic, partial motor, and sensory (Arantes et al., 2007). However, the seizures are mostly focal, and a single patient will typically present with a single seizure type (Granata & Battaglia, 2008). The onset of seizures occurs most frequently in early or late childhood, although many cases have had onset in either early infancy or adulthood. Patients diagnosed with bilateral clefts typically have an onset of seizures before 3 years of age (Guerrini & Marini, 2006). According to Packard and colleagues, good seizure control can be achieved in many cases.

Assessment

According to guidelines published by the American Academy of Neurology and Child Neurology Society (Shevell et al., 2003), evaluation of children who display developmental delays should include various forms of assessment. The consensus-based recommendations include obtaining a detailed family and medical history to assess for familial and prenatal risk factors; conducting a comprehensive physical exam; screening for auditory and/or visual impairments; and metabolic and electroencephalographic monitoring for individuals who present with suspected seizure activity. When assessment protocols reveal physical complications, such as motor impairments or seizures, neuroimaging is strongly recommended to rule out an underlying cortical malformation (Shevell et al., 2003).

In addition, a full neuropsychological evaluation is a valuable resource for obtaining information about a patient's cognitive, motor, behavioral, language, and executive functioning abilities. Developmental disorders require detailed assessment of cognition, academic achievement, and psychosocial adjustment for proper identification and as a guide to their management. Academic placement in special education and resource classrooms may be needed.

Neuroimaging

Prenatal ultrasound can be utilized as an initial screening exam, and one of the advantages of brain ultrasonography is that it can be used for the detection and management of neonatal disease in the preterm infant. It is a noninvasive and radiation-free procedure, and scanning technology has improved the ability to visualize cortical dysplasias in the neonatal brain (Rodriguez & Poussaint, 2007). According to Brant and Helms (2006), prenatal ultrasounds may detect only large, open-lipped schizencephaly clefts; therefore, multiple imaging planes are often necessary to optimally visualize the clefts and migrational anomalies.

Neuroimaging advancements have enhanced the ability to detect schizencephaly clefts (Clark, 2004). Magnetic resonance imaging (MRI) is preferred over x-ray computed tomography (CT), since the low-contrast resolution of the CT makes it difficult to differentiate between the gray matter of the cortex and white brain matter (Barkovich & Kuzniecky, 1996). Overall, MRI is considered superior to other imaging techniques because it provides excellent cortical detail, and it can detect with higher quality associated features such as absence of the sylvian vasculature, thinning of the corpus callosum, and absence of the septum pellucidum (Arantes et al., 2007). MRI is also preferred since it can provide contrast detail between different tissues with very similar densities, such as that between gray and white brain matter. It is the preferred imaging modality for patients with epilepsy who are suspected of having a disorder of cortical development (Barkovich & Kuzniecky, 1996). Furthermore, it has been recommended that CT not be used as a first-line neuroimaging technique for patients who have seizures (Barkovich & Kuzniecky, 1996).

The use of positron emission tomography (PET) and single-photon emission computed tomography (SPECT) to detect seizures has proven helpful, but because these functional imaging techniques lack specificity, they have not been sufficient in determining the exact location of the malformation of cortical development (Barkovich & Kuzniecky, 1996). Typically, PET and SPECT may be utilized as additional resources when possible treatments for associated seizures are being evaluated.

Treatment

Treatment for schizencephaly is primarily determined by the level of impairment caused by commonly associated conditions, such as seizures, cognitive delays, and motor deficits. The involvement of various medical and rehabilitative specialists in providing treatment and care is essential for improving a person's overall development. Occupational and physical therapy services may provide individuals with interventions focused on improving fine and gross motor skills, or assistance and training in the use of mobility devices. Speech therapy services may also be necessary when someone presents with a language delay. The implementation of an individualized educational program may be necessary for those individuals with language or cognitive deficits (Granata & Battaglia, 2008).

Treatment for seizures depends largely on their severity and responsiveness to medication or surgical interventions. According to Granata and Battaglia (2008), some individuals' seizures are unresponsive to antiepileptic drugs, and surgery should be considered. Hydrocephalus is a common condition in children who have open-lipped clefts; therefore, treatment may require the use of ventricular shunts to reduce the abnormal CSF pressure (Packard et al., 1997).

ANENCEPHALY

Anencephaly is a malformation that is characterized by partial or total absence of the cerebral structures and of the cranial vault.

It is also characterized by abnormal development of the skull base (Calzolari, Gambi, Garani, & Tamisari, 2004).

History

Anencephaly was first described by E. Geoffroy Saint-Hillare in the paleopathological literature in his descriptions of an anencephalic infant mummy (cited in Miller & Simon, 2001).

Developmental Course

Anencephaly is the most severe form of a neural tube disorder. It is also one of the most lethal congenital defects, as it comes with a 100% mortality rate in the neonatal period (Forrester & Merz, 2003). Also associated with this condition is the malformation of other organs (Calzolari et al., 2004). Studies of the pathogenesis of anencephaly suggest that the condition arises from a failure of the neural tube to close or a reopening of the neural tube after original closure (Arnold, Lang, & Sperber, 2001; Kashani & Hutchins, 2001; Matsumoto, Hatta, Moriyama, & Otani, 2002). Others suggest that the condition arises from exancephaly, a condition where the cerebral tissue is destroyed *in utero* (Cox, Rosenthal, & Holsapple, 1985; Kashani & Hutchins, 2001; Matusmoto et al., 2002).

Prevalence

The frequency of anencephaly is approximately 0.5–2 births per every 1,000 live births (Calzolari et al., 2004; Naidich, Altman, Braffman, McLone, Zimmerman, 1992). Females seem to be more susceptible, as they are affected more frequently, at a rate of 3–4:1 (Calzolari et al., 2004; Naidich et al., 1992). Survey data of parents with a prenatal diagnosis of anencephaly revealed that approximately 5% of the families affected had a family history of neural tube disorders (Jaquier, Klein, & Bolthauser, 2006).

Biological and Neuropsychological Factors

Infants born with anencephaly die quickly. Survey data of 211 pregnancies with prenatal diagnoses of anencephaly found that 28% of the sample had children who died within an hour of birth, and that by 24 hours the percentage increased to 67%. The longest survivals reported in this sample were 10, 18, and 28 days (Jaquier et al., 2006).

Risk Factors for Phenotypic Expression

The etiology of anencephaly remains unclear. Causes that have been suggested include antiepileptic drugs, mechanical insult, environmental factors, radiation, and chromosomal abnormalities (Arnold et al., 2001; Calzolari et al., 2004; Lewis, Van Dyke, Stumbo, & Berg, 1998; Volpe, 1995; Winsor, McGrath, Khalifa, & Duncan, 1997). Anencephaly is more common in whites than blacks, and is more often seen in families of lower socioeconomic status (Volpe, 1995). The risk for anencephaly increases when the mother is either especially old or young (Arnold et al., 2001; Volpe, 1995). In addition, the risk is higher for mothers with diabetes (Naidich et al., 1992).

Research has demonstrated that women with a history of miscarriage in previous pregnancies were 4.58 times more likely to have a child with anencephaly than women who did not have this history, and this finding was independent of a mother's age and number of pregnancies (Blanco-Muñoz, Lacasaña, & Borja-Aburto, 2006). This finding does not necessarily mean that miscarriage itself is the cause, but it suggests that common mechanisms could be involved in both events. Researchers suggest that environmental factors present during the multiple pregnancies, genetic factors, or a combination of both could be involved in the etiology of both events (Blanco-Muñoz et al., 2006). They additionally hypothesize that the previous miscarriages could also have involved some type of neural tube disorder, as the frequency of congenital malformations is greater in miscarriages than in live births (Blanco-Muñoz et al., 2006; Nishimura, Uwabe, & Shiota, 1987).

Finally, a lack of folic acid in the mother's diet is a risk factor that has been well documented. Folic acid assists with neural tube closure, and the U.S. government began fortification of foods with folic acid in 1998. Since this fortification process began, researchers have found an 18–30% drop in malformations of the neural tube, which include both anencephaly and spina bifida (Robbins et al., 2006).

In 1991, there was a large cluster of anencephalic births in Brownsville, Texas. In response to this event, the state of Texas established the Texas Birth Defects Registry in 1993 (Canfield et al., 2009). This has allowed for more detailed study of anencephaly in Texas. Analysis of this data suggests that prevalence is higher in Hispanics, in those who live on the Texas–Mexico border, in women with a larger number of previous live births, in women pregnant with female infants, in mothers older than 40, in women with no record of prenatal care, and among women with less than 7 years of education (Canfield et al., 2009).

Assessment

As discussed above, the mortality rate for anencephaly is high, and death occurs rapidly; therefore, there are few to no assessment data for this disorder. What data do exist come from case studies. Calzolari and colleagues (2004) completed an MRI case study of a male infant 8 hours after his birth. They found the presence of the brainstem and cerebellum, with normal development of the eyes. They suggest that these results support the theory of anencephaly as a transformation from exancephaly. MRI assessment can be helpful in distinguishing anencephaly from other disorders, as some disorders that may appear similar have anatomical conditions that are compatible with survival (Calzolari et al., 2004).

Treatment

With a 100% mortality rate and a short lifespan, treatment for anencephaly is medical and palliative in nature.

LISSENCEPHALY

General History and Description

Owen originally used the term *lissencephaly* in 1868 (cited in Hynd, Morgan, & Vaughn, 2009). Generally, the term is used to describe a brain that is deficient in gyration (Leventer, 2008) (see Figure 27.4). This deficiency can range from complete *agyria*

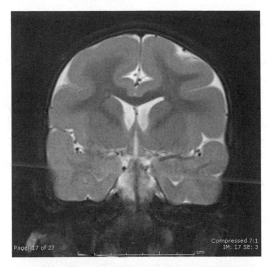

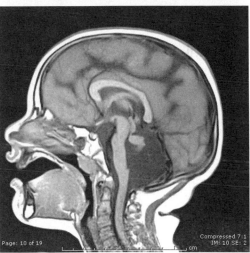

FIGURE 27.4. T2-weighted images of a 4-year-old male with lissencephaly and cerebellar hypoplasia (note diffuse pachygyria). (Courtesy of David Leake, MD, Austin, Texas.)

(lack of gyri) to *pachygyria* (broad gyri) (Takanashi, Tada, Fujii, & Barkovich, 2007). Most patients with this disorder have a combination of areas of agyria and pachygyria (Leventer, 2008). Agyria is considered more severe than pachygyria, which tends to be associated with a broader spectrum of clinical features (Liang, Lee, Young, Peng, & Shen, 2002).

There are two types of lissencephaly. Dambska, Wisniewski, and Sher (1983) were the first to divide it into *type I* and *type II* lissencephaly. Type I lissencephaly is also referred to as *classical* lissencephaly; type II lissencephaly is sometimes referred to as *cobblestone* lissencephaly. The type I–type II and classical–cobblestone distinctions are both used in current literature (Leventer, 2008). For the purposes of this chapter, the remainder of the information is presented separately for classical and cobblestone lissencephaly. Both classical and cobblestone lissencephaly are migration disorders.

Classical Lissencephaly

History

As mentioned above, lissencephaly was first described as such in 1868 by Owen. It was also the first of the human cortical malformations for which the genetic basis was identified (Leventer, 2008). In classical lissencephaly, the brain shows poorly defined sylvian and rolandic fissures and thickening of the cerebral cortex (Harding & Copp, 2002; Leventer, 2008). Severe cases can present with failure to develop the primary sulci (Harding & Copp, 2002). In addition, some areas of the brain may appear more severely affected than others, which could be due to the type of gene mutation (Dobyns et al., 1999). That is, depending on the type of gene mutation, there may be increased severity in the posterior or anterior portions of the cortex. Increased gray matter is present at a rate of 1–4 cm versus a typical 0.5 cm (Gleeson, 2001; Kuchelmeister, Bergmann, & Gullotta, 1993). Classical lissencephaly includes a range of disorders that differ in severity. These disorders include Miller–Dieker syndrome, isolated lissencephaly sequence, X-linked lissencephaly with abnormal genitalia, lissencephaly with cerebellar hypoplasia, and microlissencephaly (Clark, 2004; Gleeson, 2001; Leventer, 2008).

Developmental Course

Children born with lissencephaly tend to have a shortened lifespan, but the exact degree can vary by subtype (Garg, Sridhar, & Gulati, 2007; Leventer, 2008). These patients also present with severe to profound mental retardation (de Rijk-van Andel, Arts, & de Weerd, 1992; Gleeson, 2001; Leventer, 2008). They often have early hypotonia that can persist or evolve (Leventer, 2008); they

can also present with feeding problems (Leventer, 2008). Finally, acquired microcephaly can also be present (Gleeson, 2001).

Seizures typically begin in the first year of life and progress into intractable mixed seizure disorder as the patients grow older (de Rijk-van Andel et al., 1992; Gleeson, 2001; Leventer, 2008). There are some reports of fetal-onset seizures as well (Patante & Ghidini, 2001). Different forms of classic lissencephaly are more severe and can contribute to a shorter lifespan. These forms include Miller–Dieker, X-linked lissencephaly with abnormal genitalia, lissencephaly with complete agenesis of the corpus callosum, and lissencephaly with extreme cerebellar hypoplasia (Leventer, 2008).

Genetic and Family Patterns

The primary genes that have been identified in classical lissencephaly are the L1S1 gene and Doublecortin (Clark, 2004, Gleeson, 2001; Leventer, 2008). Within X-linked lissencephaly, the abnormalities in these genes give rise to differences in the localization of the severity of gyral abnormalities: Doublecortin mutations result in greater anterior than posterior severity, and L1S1 mutations result in the opposite pattern (Clark, 2004; Dobyns et al., 1999). Because it is X-linked, this subtype of lissencephaly occurs mostly in boys, with girls often expressing band heterotopia (Gleeson et al., 1998, 2000; Pilz et al., 1998). Women with band heterotopia are at risk for giving birth to boys with lissencephaly (Clark, 2004). Lissencephaly with cerebellar hypoplasia has been shown to be related to mutations in RELN, an important secretory extracellular protein (Hong et al., 2000). Some types of lissencephaly are passed in an autosomal recessive fashion (Clark, 2004). Other genes implicated in various types of classical lissencephaly include the 14-3-3€ gene and the ARX gene (see Leventer, 2008, for a review of gene implications).

Biological and Neuropsychological Markers

These patients present with severe to profound mental retardation (de Rijk-van Andel et al., 1992; Gleeson, 2001; Leventer, 2008). The Miller–Dieker subtype also includes facial dysmorphism, which can consist of bitemporal hollowing, upturned nares, and burying of the upper lip by the lower lip at the corners of the mouth (Clark, 2004; Leventer, 2008).

Risk Factors for Phenotypic Expression

Some research has examined group differences in clinical features. Kurul, Çakmakçi and Dirik (2004) separated patients with lissencephaly into two groups; one group had bilateral or generalized gyral malformations, and the other group had manifested local or unilateral malformations. In this study, the group with the generalized gyral malformations demonstrated a higher ratio of seizures and more frequent seizures than the other group. These patients also became symptomatic earlier than the patients with local or unilateral malformations. Moreover, this study found a high rate of family history for neurological diseases (e.g., seizure disorders and mental retardation).

Liang and colleagues (2002) found that patients in their sample with agyria, as opposed to pachygyria, tended to have worse outcomes. They also found that patients with earlier onset of seizures had worse outcomes. These researchers classified the degree of lissencephaly according to neuroimaging findings, using a system modified from de Rijk-van Andel, Arts, Barth and Loonen (1990). The system Liang and colleagues utilized ranked the patients from grade 1, which would indicate complete agyria, to grade 6, which would indicate focal pachygyria in less than 50% of the cortex. Intermediate gradations included agyria with some sulci, a mixture of agyria and pachygiria, complete pachygyria, and focal pachygyria in more than 50% of the cortex. Liang and colleagues also used neurophysiological studies to predict the neurological outcome of these patients. They found that somatosensory-evoked potential evaluation was helpful beyond neuroimaging in predicting the clinical outcome of the patients. Specifically, one child in their study was classified as having a less severe outcome based on neuroimaging alone; however, he was shown to have a worse clinical outcome than those classified by neuroimaging methods as having more severe outcomes. When the children were as-

sessed neurophysiologically, this same child was shown to have a lack of somatosensory-evoked potentials. The researchers argue that the results of the evoked potential study might explain the worse clinical outcome for this child, and suggest that this type of evaluation should be used in the future to help supplement more standard neuroimaging evaluations.

Assessment

Classical lissencephaly tends to be assessed through neuroimaging. The images can be classified by severity on a grading system such as that of de Rijk-van Andel and colleagues (1990). In addition, evaluations of cognitive and adaptive functioning are used to classify the levels of mental retardation and developmental functioning.

Treatment

With the high degree of medical complications in patients with lissencephaly, such as intractable seizures, the treatment is generally medical in nature. There is the opportunity for appropriate developmental treatments as warranted by specific deficits in motor, sensory, communicative, and cognitive functioning.

Cobblestone Lissencephaly

History

Cobblestone lissencephaly was first described by Walker (1942). This disorder is associated with eye abnormalities, muscle disease, and progressive hydrocephalus, all of which help distinguish this disorder from classical lissencephaly (Clark, 2004; Topaloglu & Taim, 2008). Krijgsman and colleagues (1980) first reported the muscular dystrophy associated with cobblestone lissencephaly. Cobblestone lissencephaly is part of a complex of symptoms that constitute muscle–eye–brain disease (Gleeson, 2001). Patients with cobblestone lissencephaly have deficient gyration and sulci, similar to those in classical lissencephaly; in addition, the cortex has a pebbled or "cobblestone" appearance, due to an abnormal migration of gray matter to the cortical surface (Clark, 2004; Gleeson, 2001; Topaloglu & Taim, 2008).

Developmental Course

Cobblestone lissencephaly is due to a defect in neuronal migration in which neurons pass their normal stopping point and erupt over the surface of the cortex into the subarachnoid spaces and the pia, causing the cobblestone appearance (Clark, 2004; Gleeson, 2001; Topaloglu & Taim, 2008). Similar to classical lissencephaly, cobblestone lissencephaly also has various subtypes; in this case, they include Walker–Warburg syndrome, muscle–eye–brain syndrome, and Fukuyama muscular dystrophy (Clark, 2004; Gleeson, 2001; Topaloglu & Taim, 2008). Fukuyama is distinguished from the other types by the severity of the muscular dystrophy associated with the condition (Clark, 2004; Fukuyama, Ohsawa, & Suzuki, 1981)

Genetic and Family Patterns

For the majority of these disorders, no genes have been isolated. The Fukuyama subtype is seen more often in Japan, and is thought to be related to a founder mutation in families of those affected (Clark, 2004). Recently, researchers identified Fukutin as a causative gene in this disorder (Kobayashi et al., 1998). It is inherited in an autosomal recessive fashion (Clark, 2004).

Biological and Neuropsychological Markers

The aforementioned muscular dystrophy is one of the main biological markers for this set of disorders (Clark, 2004; Gleeson, 2001; Topaloglu & Taim, 2008). Other abnormalities that can be seen in cobblestone lissencephaly include ocular anterior chamber abnormalities, retinal dysplasias, hydrocephalus, and encephaloceles (Clark, 2004). As in classic lissencephaly, mental retardation and epilepsy are commonly seen in these patients (Gleeson, 2001). In the Fukuyama type, there is more severe muscular dystrophy, and patients can present with evidence of hypotonia and depressed reflexes (Clark, 2004).

Assessment

Cobblestone lissencephaly also tends to be assessed through neuroimaging. As in classical lissencephaly, evaluations of cognitive and adaptive functioning are used to classify the levels of mental retardation and developmental functioning.

Treatment

The treatment for patients with cobblestone lissencephaly is often medical in nature, with physical therapy as needed to address the motor concerns. There is also the opportunity for developmental treatments as needed.

CASE EXAMPLE

Because the clinical features of these disorders can vary widely, we present a case example of structural anomalies observed in our clinic. This is not a straightforward case of lissencephaly or schizencephaly, but rather an example of structural abnormalities with a typical range of clinical features.

The patient was a European American female who was 10 years old at the time of the assessment. She had multiple congenital abnormalities, including congenital deafness that was not conducive to cochlear implant, due to dysgenesis of the cranial nerve. She also presented with a malformed right ear, submucosal cleft palate, bifid uvula, dislocated left hip, small retinal coloboma, and plagocephaly. A genetic study had been performed, and no clear genetic causative factors were found. MRI showed smaller posterior frontal and anterior temporal lobes on the left side than on the right. In addition, there was evidence of mild pachygyria in the left frontal temporal cortex. The patient had also developed feeding problems that required the insertion of a G peg; she was still using this at the time of the assessment for fluid and nutrient intake.

Neuropsychological testing results showed weaknesses in academic functioning, fine motor functioning, and executive functioning. Cognitive functioning was in the low-average range, as measured by the Test of Nonverbal Intelligence—Third Edition. These results were consistent with her frontal lobe abnormalities as seen on MRI. She had particular difficulty with language-related academic skills, including reading and written expression. These difficulties were consistent with her temporal lobe abnormalities. There was some evidence of a left-sided visual field deficit or visual neglect; there was also some evidence of strabismus.

Conclusion

Many well-deserved superlatives have been used to describe the development and functioning of the human brain. As described by Nobel laureate Eric Kandel (2007), "The brain is a complex biological organ of great computational capability that constructs our sensory experiences, regulates our thoughts and emotions, and controls our actions." Lest we take this for granted, the structural anomalies that we have discussed illustrate the complexity of this 3-pound organ that is at the center of who we are as human beings.

References

Abdel Razek, A. A. K., Kandell, A. Y., Elsorogy, L. G., Elmongy, A., & Basett, A. A. (2009). Disorders of cortical formation: MR imaging features. *American Journal of Neuroradiology, 30,* 4–11.

Al-Alawi, A. M., Al-Tawil, K. I., Al-Hathal, M. M., & Amir, I. (2001). Sporadic neonatal schizencephaly associated with brain calcification. *Annals of Tropical Paediatrics, 21,* 34–38.

Arantes, M., Perdigao, S., Pereira, J. R., & Costa, M. (2007). Atypical clinical schizencephaly. *Journal of Pediatric Neurology, 5,* 343–345.

Arnold, W. H., Lang, M., & Sperber, G. H. (2001). 3D-reconstruction of craniofacial structures of a human anencephalic fetus: Case report. *Annals of Anatomy, 183*(1), 67–71.

Barkovich, A. J. (1995). *Pediatric neuroimaging.* New York: Raven Press.

Barkovich, A. J., & Kjos, B. O. (1992). Nonlissencephalic cortical dysplasias: Correlation of imaging findings with clinical deficits. *American Journal of Neuroradiology, 13,* 95–103.

Barkovich, A. J., & Kuzniecky, R. I. (1996). Neuroimaging of focal malformations of cortical development. *Journal of Clinical Neurophysiology, 13,* 481–494.

Barkovich, A. J., Kuzniecky, R. I., Jackson, G. D., Guerrini, R., & Dobyns, W. B. (2001). Classification system for malformations of cortical development: Update 2001. *Neurology, 57,* 2168–2178.

Barkovich, A. J., Kuzniecky, R. I., Jackson, G. D., Guerrini, R., & Dobyns, W. B. (2005). A developmental and genetic classification for malformations of cortical development. *Neurology, 65,* 1873–1887.

Blanco-Muñoz, J., Lacasaña, M., & Borja-Aburto, V. (2006). Maternal miscarriage history and risk of anencephaly. *Paediatric and Perinatal Epidemiology, 20*(3), 210–218.

Brant, W. E., & Helms, C. A. (2006). *Fundamentals of diagnostic radiology.* Philadelphia: Lippincott Williams & Wilkins.

Brown, M. C., Levin, B. E., Ramsay, R. E., & Landy, H. J. (1993). Comprehensive evaluation of left hemisphere type I schizencephaly. *Archives of Neurology, 50,* 667–669.

Calzolari, F., Gambi, B., Garani, G., & Tamisari, L. (2004). Anencephaly: MRI findings and pathogenetic theories. *Pediatric Radiology, 34(12),* 1012–1016.

Canfield, M., Marengo, L., Ramadhani, T., Suarez, L., Brender, J., & Scheuerle, A. (2009). The prevalence and predictors of anencephaly and spina bifida in Texas. *Paediatric and Perinatal Epidemiology, 23(1),* 41–50.

Carlson, N. R. (2007). *Physiology of behavior* (9th ed.). Boston: Pearson Education.

Chudler, E. H. (2009). Brain development. In *Neuroscience for kids.* Retrieved April 15, 2009, from *faculty.washington.edu/chudler/dev.html*

Clark, G. D. (2004). The classification of cortical dysplasias through molecular genetics. *Brain and Development, 26*(6), 351–362.

Cox, G.G., Rosenthal, S.J., & Holsapple, J.W. (1985). Exencephaly: Sonographic findings and radiologic–pathologic correlation. *Radiology, 155*(3), 755–756.

Curry, C. J., Lammer, E. J., Nelson, V., & Shaw, G. M. (2005). Schizencephaly: Heterogeneous etiologies in a population of 4 million California births. *American Journal of Medical Genetics, 137,* 181–189.

Dambska, M., Wisniewski, K., & Sher, J. H. (1983). Lissencephaly: Two distinct clinico-pathological types. *Brain and Development, 5,* 302–310.

de Rijk-van Andel, J. F., Arts, W. F., Barth, P. G., & Loonen, M. C. (1990). Diagnostic features and clinical signs of 21 patients with lissencephaly type 1. *Developmental Medicine and Child Neurology, 32*(8), 707–717.

de Rijk-van Andel, J. F., Arts, W. F., & de Weerd, A. W. (1992). EEG and evoked potentials in a series of 21 patients with lissencephaly type I. *Neuropediatrics, 23*(1), 4–9.

Dobyns, W.B., Truwit, C.L., Ross, M.E., Matsumoto, N., Pilz, D.T., Ledbetter, D.H., et al. (1999). Differences in the gyral pattern distinguish chromosome 17-linked and X-linked lissencephaly. *Neurology, 53*(2), 270–277.

Ferrer, I. (1984). A Golgi analysis of unlayered polymicrogyria. *Acta Neuropathologica, 65,* 69–76.

Forrester, M. B., & Merz, R. D. (2003). First-year mortality rates for selected birth defects, Hawaii,

1986–1999. *American Journal of Medical Genetics. Part A, 119A*(3), 311–318.

Fukuyama, Y., Ohsawa, M., & Suzuki, H. (1981). Congenital progressive muscular dystrophy of the Fukuyama type: Clinical, genetic and pathologic considerations. *Brain and Development, 3*, 1–29.

Garel, C. (2004). *MRI of the fetal brain: Normal development and cerebral pathologies.* New York: Springer-Verlag.

Garg, A., Sridhar, M. R., & Gulati, S. (2007). Autosomal recessive type 1 lissencephaly. *Indian Journal of Pediatrics, 74*, 199–201.

Gleeson, J. G. (2001). Neuronal migration disorders. *Mental Retardation and Developmental Disabilities Research Reviews, 7*(3), 167–171.

Gleeson, J. G., Allen, K. M., Fox, J. W., Lamperti, E. D., Berkovic, S., Scheffer, I., et al. (1998). Double cortin, a brain-specific gene mutated in human X-linked lissencephaly and double cortex syndrome encodes a putative signaling protein. *Cell, 92*(1), 63–72.

Gleeson, J. G., Luo, R. F., Grant, P. E., Guerrini, R., Huttenlocher, P. R., Berg, M. J., et al. (2000). Genetic and neuroradiological heterogeneity of double cortex syndrome. *Annals of Neurology, 47*(2), 265–269.

Gleeson, J. G., & Walsh, C. A. (2000). Neuronal migration disorders: From genetic diseases to developmental mechanisms. *Trends in Neurosciences, 23*, 352–259.

Golden, J. A. (2001). Cell migration and cerebral cortical development. *Neuropathology and Applied Neurobiology, 27*, 22–28.

Granata, T., & Battaglia, G. (2008). Schizencephaly. In H. B. Sarnat & P. Curatolo (Eds.), *Handbook of clinical neurology: Vol. 87. Malformations of the nervous system* (pp. 235–246). New York: Elsevier.

Granata, T., Farina, L., Faiella, A., Cardini, R., D'Incerti, L., Boncinelli, E., et al. (1997). Familial schizencephaly associated with *EMX2* mutation. *Neurology, 48*, 1403–1406.

Granata, T., Freri, E., Caccia, C., Setola, V., Taroni, F., & Battaglia, G. (2005). Schizencephaly: Clinical spectrum, epilepsy, and pathogenesis. *Journal of Child Neurology, 20*, 313–318.

Guerrini, R. (2005). Genetic malformations of the cerebral cortex and epilepsy. *Epilepsia, 46*, 32–37.

Guerrini, R., & Marini, C. (2006). Genetic malformations of cortical development. *Experimental Brain Research, 173*, 322–333.

Harding, B., & Copp, A.J. (2002). Malformations. In J. D. Greenfield, P. L. Lantos, & D. I. Graham (Eds.), *Greenfield's neuropathology* (7th ed.). London: Arnold.

Heschl, R. (1859). Gehirndefekt und hydrocephalus. *Vierteljahresschr Prakt Heilkd (Prag), 61*, 59–74.

Hong, S., Shugart, Y., Huang, D., Shahwan, S.,

Grant, P., Hourihane, J., et al. (2000). Autosomal recessive lissencephaly with cerebellar hypoplasia is associated with human RELN mutations. *Nature Genetics, 26*(1), 93.

Hynd, G. W., Morgan, A. E., & Vaughn, M. (2009). Neurodevelopmental malformations: Etiology and clinical manifestations. In C. R. Reynolds & E. Fletcher Janzen (Eds.), *Handbook of child clinical neuropsychology* (pp. 147–168). New York: Springer.

Iannetti, P., Spalice, A., Atzei, G., Boemi, S., & Trasimeni, G. (1996). Neuronal migration disorders in children with epilepsy: MRI, interictal SPECT and EEG comparisons. *Brain and Development, 18*, 269–279.

Innes, A. M. (2008). Molecular genetic testing and genetic counseling. In H. B. Sarnat & P. Curatolo (Eds.), *Handbook of clinical neurology: Vol. 87. Malformations of the nervous system* (pp. 517–531). New York: Elsevier.

Jaquier, M., Klein, A., & Boltshauser, E. (2006). Spontaneous pregnancy outcome after prenatal diagnosis of anencephaly. *BJOG: An International Journal of Obstetrics and Gynaecology, 113*(8), 951–953.

Kandel, E. R. (2007). The new science of mind. In F. E. Bloom (Ed.), *Best of the brain from Scientific American: Mind, matter, and tomorrow's brain.* New York: Dana Press.

Kashani, A. H., & Hutchins, G. M. (2001). Meningeal–cutaneous relationships in anencephaly: Evidence for a primary mesenchymal abnormality. *Human Pathology, 32*(5), 553–558.

Kobayashi, K., Nakahori, Y., Miyake, M., Matsumura, K., Kondo-Iida, E., Nomura, Y., et al. (1998). An ancient retrotransposal insertion causes Fukuyama-type congenital muscular dystrophy. *Nature, 394*, 388.

Komarniski, C. A., Cyr, D. R., Mack, L. A., & Weinberger, E. (1990). Prenatal diagnosis of schizencephaly. *Journal of Ultrasound in Medicine, 9*, 305–307.

Kuchelmeister, K., Bergmann, M., & Gullotta, F. (1993). Neuropathology of lissencephalies. *Child's Nervous System, 9*(7), 394–399.

Kundrat, H. (1882). *Die Poroencephalie: Eine anatomische Studie.* Graz, Austria: Leuschner & Lubensky.

Kurul, S., Çakmakçi, H., & Dirik, E. (2004). Agyria–pachygyria complex: MR findings and correlation with clinical features. *Pediatric Neurology, 30*(1), 16.

Lewis, D. P., Van Dyke, D. C., Stumbo, P. J., & Berg, M. J. (1998). Drug and environmental factors associated with adverse pregnancy outcomes. Part I: Antiepileptic drugs, contraceptives, smoking, and folate. *Annals of Pharmacotherapy, 32*(7–8), 802–817.

Leventer, R. (2008). Lissenecephaly type I. In H. B. Sarnat & P. Curatolo (Eds.), *Handbook of* clinical neurology: Vol. 87. Malformations of the nervous system (pp. 205–218). New York: Elsevier.

Liang, J., Lee, W., Young, C., Peng, S., & Shen, Y. (2002). Agyria–pachygyria: Clinical, neuroimaging, and neurophysiologic correlations. Pediatric Neurology, 27(3), 171.

Matsumoto, A., Hatta, T., Moriyama, K., & Otani, H. (2002). Sequential observations of exencephaly and subsequent morphological changes by mouse exo utero development system: Analysis of the mechanism of transformation from exencephaly to anencephaly. Anatomy and Embryology, 205(1), 7–18.

Menkes, J. H., & Sarnat, H. B. (2000). Neuroembryology, genetic programming, and malformations: Part 2. Malformations of the central nervous system. In J. H. Menkes & H. B. Sarnat (Eds.), Child neurology (pp. 305–400). Philadelphia: Lippincott Williams & Wilkins.

Miller, E., & Simon, S. K. (2001). Anencephaly—something missing from the archaeological record? Paleopathology Newsletter, No. 115, 9–11.

Naidich, T. P., Altman, N. R., Braffman, B. H., McLone, D. G., & Zimmerman, R. A. (1992). Cephaloceles and related malformations. American Journal of Neuroradiology, 13(2), 655–690.

Nishimura, H., Uwabe, C., & Shiota, K. (1987). Study of human post-implantation conceptuses, normal and abnormal. Okajimas Folia Anatomica Japonica, 63(6), 337–357.

Packard, A. M., Miller, V. S., & Delgado, M. R. (1997). Schizencephaly: Correlations of clinical and radiological features. Neurology, 48, 1427–1434.

Patante, L., & Ghidini, A. (2001). Fetal seizures: Case report and literature review. Journal of Maternal Fetal Medicine, 10, 287–289.

Pilz, D. T., Matsumoto, N., Minnerath, S., Mills, P., Gleeson, J. G., Allen, K. M., et al. (1998). LIS1 and XLIS (DCX) mutations cause most classical lissencephaly, but different patterns of malformation. Human Molecular Genetics, 7(13), 2029–2037.

Rakic, P. (1972). Mode of cell migration to the superficial layers of fetal monkey neocortex. Journal of Comparative Neurology, 145, 61–83.

Rakic, P. (1988). Specification of cerebral cortical areas. Science, 241, 170–176.

Raybaud, C. (1983). Destructive lesions of the brain. Neuroradiology, 25, 265–291.

Robbins, J., Tilford, J., Bird, T., Cleves, M., Reading, J., & Hobbs, C. (2006). Hospitalizations of newborns with folate-sensitive birth defects before and after fortification of foods with folic acid. Pediatrics, 118(3), 906–915.

Rodriguez, D. P., & Poussaint, T. Y. (2007). Neuroimaging of the child with developmental delay. Topics in Magnetic Resonance Imaging, 18, 75–92.

Seguti, V. F., Schappo, A., Sobrinho, J. A. N., & Ferreira, L. S. (2006). Epilepsy secondary to schizencephaly: A comparative study. Journal of Pediatric Neurology, 4, 19–26.

Shevell, M., Ashwal, S., Donley, D., Flint, J., Gingold, M., Hirtz, D., et al. (2003). Practice parameter: Evaluation of the child with global developmental delay: Report of the quality standards subcommittee of the American Academy of Neurology and the practice committee of the Child Neurology Society. Neurology, 60, 367–380.

Takanashi, J., Tada, H., Fujii, K., & Barkovich, A. (2007). The evolving MR imaging appearance of lissencephaly: A case report. Brain and Development, 29(8), 522–524.

Takano, T., Takikita, S., & Shimada, M. (1999). Experimental schizencephaly induced by Kilham strain of mumps virus: Pathogenesis of cleft formation. NeuroReport, 10, 3149–3154.

Topaloglu, H., & Taim, B. (2008). Lissencephaly type II. In H. B. Sarnat & P. Curatolo (Eds.), Handbook of clinical neurology: Malformations of the nervous system (pp. 235–246). New York: Elsevier.

Verrotti, A., Spalice, A., Ursitti, F., Papetti, L., Mariani, R., Castronovo, A., et al. (2010). New trends in neuronal migration disorders. European Journal of Paediatric Neurology, 14(1), 1–12.

Volpe, J.J. (1995). Neurology of the newborn. Philadelphia: Saunders.

Walker, A. E. (1942). Lissencephaly. Archives of Neurology and Psychiatry, 48, 13–29.

Winsor, S. H., McGrath, M. J., Khalifa, M., & Duncan, A. M. (1997). A report of recurrent anencephaly with trisomy 2p23–2pter: Additional evidence for the involvement of 2p24 in neural tube development and evaluation of the role for cytogenetic analysis. Prenatal Diagnosis, 17(7), 665–669.

Yakovlev, P. I., & Wadsworth, R. C. (1946a). Schizencephalies: A study of the congenital clefts in the cerebral mantle: I. Clefts with fused lips. Journal of Neuropathology and Experimental Neurology, 5, 116–130.

Yakovlev, P. I., & Wadsworth, R. C. (1946b). Schizencephalies: A study of the congenital clefts in the cerebral mantle: II. Clefts with hydrocephalus and lips separated. Journal of Neuropathology and Experimental Neurology, 5, 169–206.

CHAPTER 28

Spina Bifida Myelomeningocele

ANGELA GIACOLETTI ARGENTO
SETH A. WARSCHAUSKY
LAURA SHANK
JOSEPH E. HORNYAK

This chapter is an overview of the phenotypic physical and neurocognitive profile found among children and adolescents with spina bifida myelomeningocele (SBM). Spina bifida (SB) refers to a subgroup of neural tube defects (NTDs) in which there is incomplete closure of the spinal component of the neural tube. SB can be categorized as spina bifida occulta (SBO) and spina bifida cystica (SBC). SBO is a common disorder, reported at rates as high as 5–36% in an asymptomatic population. It is the result of a failure of the posterior elements of the spinal column to close completely, with no abnormalities to the neural elements. A birthmark, tuft of hair, or dimple may overlie the defect. SBC involves a cystic structure overlying the bony defect, which may be noted intrauterine or at the time of birth. The makeup of the cystic structure may or may not cause neurological effects. A *meningocele* is a herniation of the meninges through the defect, with no neural elements. A *lipomeningocele* includes a herniation of the meninges with an accompanying lipoma, but again no neural elements. A *myelomeningocele* is the most serious form, with neural elements of the spinal cord herniating through the defect within the meningeal sac (see Figure 28.1). Prior to the 1950s, survival for SBM was only about 10%. Improved management (especially improvements in surgical repair and antibiotics) has dramatically decreased morbidity and mortality (Bowman, Boshnjaku, & McLone, 2009). The present chapter focuses exclusively on SBM and its etiology, effects, and neurological expression.

NTDs are relatively common congenital malformations, occurring at a rate of 1–2

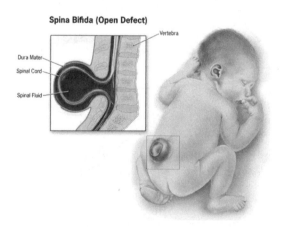

FIGURE 28.1. Spina bifida myelomeningocele (SBM). From Centers for Disease Control and Prevention, National Center on Birth Defects and Developmental Disabilities.

per 1,000 births (Copp, Greene, & Murdoch, 2003; Kibar, Capra, & Gros, 2007). There is significant temporal, geographic, and ethnic variation in prevalence. For example, there is very low prevalence among African Americans, but not among sub-Saharan Africans (Njamnshi et al., 2008). There is low prevalence among the Japanese, but very high prevalence in Shanxi Province in China (Li et al., 2006). Individuals of Celtic origin are at particularly high risk for NTDs (Gordon, 1995).

Evidence of NTDs in humans predates written history. Skeletons discovered in a cave in Morocco from 10,000 B.C.E. included split sacral vertebra (Smith, 2001). After 5000 B.C.E., skeletal evidence of SB was more common. In the 17th century, descriptions of SB include those of Nicolas Tulp (1593–1674) in his most prominent book, *Observationes Medicae* (1641); this volume included a detailed sketch, possibly by Rembrandt (Simpson, 2007). Yet SB was not widely known until the 19th century, when von Recklinghausen published a classic description of SB in 1886.

NTDs stem from partial or complete failure of neural tube closure during primary neurulation. The most common forms of NTDs are anencephaly and myelomeningocele. Etiology appears to involve environmental factors, such as geography; demographics, including socioeconomic status, maternal age, and maternal health; and teratogens. Increasing evidence of genetic influences include associations with chromosomal abnormalities, genetic syndromes, ethnicity/race, and familial distributions (Kibar et al., 2007). Heritability is estimated at 60%.

GENETIC AND ENVIRONMENTAL CAUSES OF NTDs

Recent increased understanding of the complex processes involved in neurulation has informed the search for genetic influences on NTDs. Initial steps in neurulation include formation and shaping of the neural plate. Initial elongation of the neural plate is driven by a complex process called *convergent extension* (CE). CE movements during neural tube closure are mediated by planar cell polarity pathway (PCP), or tissue polarity, signaling. Core PCP genes have been identified in animal models, and disruption of those genes in turn disrupts neurulation. However, there is not yet a precise understanding of PCP regulation of CE.

NTDs are not simple Mendelian traits—the results of a single, pathogenic dominant or recessive gene—but polygenic disorders resulting from the interaction of a number of genes with each other, as well as with environmental factors (Carter, 1969). Over the last few decades, a great deal of research has gone into trying to understand both the genetic and the environmental factors that lead to NTDs. From a genetic standpoint, the mouse has been a convenient animal to look for candidate genes. Almost 200 mutant mouse models of NTDs have been developed, with known genes in 155 models, 33 with unidentified genes, and 8 being considered multifactorial strains (Harris & Juriloff, 2007). Many of these models are knockouts, in which a single gene is switched off. Although knockouts are commonly used, they represent models of a single gene disorder, which seems to be similar to a known disease. If the disease in question is monogenic in nature, the knockout may provide an accurate model, but for polygenic traits, they may be of limited value (Koch & Britton, 2007, 2008). Currently, none of the genes identified in mouse models have been correlated with human NTDs. The mouse model genes have a high level of penetrance, while that is not the case in human NTDs. This may suggest that *if* any of these candidate genes are involved, that it may not be directly, but possibly through regulation of expression of these genes (Harris & Juriloff, 2007).

These unknown genetic factors result in an increased familial incidence. After a single NTD, the recurrence rate is reported as 2.4–5%; after a second NTD, this risk doubles (Cowchock et al., 1980). This also increases the risk in other relatives, most significantly in siblings, less so in second- and third-degree relatives (Toriello & Higgins, 1983).

A number of environmental factors have been identified that increase the risk of NTDs. These environmental factors do not always cause NTDs, but most likely are involved as the result of a susceptible genome. These include low socioeconomic class, mid-spring conception, maternal obesity, and increased intrauterine temperatures (Milunsky et al., 1992; Nevin, Johnston, & Merrett, 1981; Sandford, Kissling, & Joubert, 1992; Watkins, Scanlon, Mulinare, & Khoury, 1996). A number of medications such as the antiepileptic medications carbamazepine and valproic acid have been identified as teratogenic, increasing risk for NTDs (Lindhout, Omtzigt, & Cornel, 1992; Weinbaum et al., 1986).

Perhaps the most significant environmental factor relating to NTD has been folate and folic acid. Folic acid (pteryolmonoglatamic acid) is a synthetic vitamin, B9, with folate being its naturally occurring analog. Metabolically, folic acid plays an essential role in the transfer of single carbon units for DNA synthesis, and thus important for cell multiplication and fetal development. In addition, folic acid serves as a methyl group donor for protein methylation of some cytoskeletal proteins that are highly expressed in neural ectoderm, which eventually forms the brain and spinal cord (Moephuli, Klein, Baldwin, & Krider, 1997). A possible link between folate and NTDs was first proposed in 1976 by Richard Smithells (Smithells, Sheppard, & Schorah, 1976). This has led to numerous studies that have demonstrated the effectiveness of folic acid supplementation on decreasing the incidence of NTDs by 50–70% (Botto et al., 2005; Eskes, 2000; Habibzadeh, Schorah, Scller, Smithells, & Levene, 1993; Schorah, Habibzadeh, Wild, Smithells, & Seller, 1993; Schorah & Smithells, 1993; Schorah, Wild, Hartley, Sheppard, & Smithells, 1983; Smithells, 1982, 1989; Smithells et al., 1981a, 1981b, 1983, 1985; Smithells, Sheppard, & Wild, 1989; Smithells, Sheppard, Wild, & Schorah, 1989; Wild et al., 1986).

Thus the study of genes that predispose humans to NTDs has focused on folate-related genes, given the efficacy of prenatal folic acid in reducing incidence of NTDs. The folate-related genes of interest include those involved in transport mechanisms and those involved in metabolism. There is evidence that some mothers of children with NTDs have autoimmune responses that block uptake of folate. The most extensively studied gene involved in metabolism of folate is the MTHFR gene, which regulates the extent to which folate is available as a methyl donor for methylation of DNA and transfer RNA.

MTHFR mutations have been associated with increased risk for NTDs. Other folate-related genes have also been implicated.

In summary, NTDs are disorders resulting from the interaction of a susceptible genome (polygenic trait) with one or more environmental factors. The risk for NTDs may be associated with maternal or embryonic gene–gene and/or gene–environment interactions. The genetics of NTD risks have been studied in animal models with natural or experimentally induced mutations. To date, scores of candidate genes have been identified, typically affecting fundamental processes of neurulation, but none has been shown conclusively to play a major role in the etiology of the NTDs. Folic acid is an important environmental agent, with supplementation resulting in a markedly decreased risk of NTDs.

PHYSICAL ASPECTS OF SBM

Sensory–Motor Effects

Myelomeningoceles are typically seen at the thoracic and lumbosacral levels, as cervical lesions are usually incompatible with life. These lesions will result in motor (voluntary and autonomic) and sensory deficits at and below the level of the lesions. With the sparing of the upper extremities, this is defined as paraparesis. Paraparesis in SBM is most consistent with a lower-motor-neuron (LMN) syndrome, with occasional upper-motor-neuron (UMN) syndrome features. This is in contrast to most traumatic spinal cord injuries, which are primarily UMN syndromes. Individuals with SBM will typically have a flaccid paralysis, decreased muscle tone, areflexia, and marked muscle atrophy. UMN signs (especially spasticity) may be present with higher lesions, if there is sparing of some LMNs and sensory systems. New findings of UMN signs suggest a possible new pathological event (e.g., cord tethering, tumor), which may require further medical evaluation. Table 28.1 lists features of the UMN and LMN syndromes.

The higher the level of the lesion, the more proximal the involved muscle group will be, causing more impairment of function. Thoracic lesions will affect trunk and all muscles of legs, while low sacral lesions may only affect urinary and anal sphincters.

TABLE 28.1. Comparison of Lower-Motor-Neuron (LMN) and Upper-Motor-Neuron (UMN) Syndromes

	LMN syndromes	UMN syndromes
Weakness	Yes	Yes
Tone	Decreased (hypotonic or flaccid)	Increased (spasticity)
Tendon reflexes	Diminished or absent	Increased
Cutaneous reflexes (e.g., Babinski)	Normal or no response	Abnormal response present
Contractures	Yes, tend to be positional	Yes, tend to reflect tone patterns

It is common for there to be some asymmetry in the motor and sensory involvement between the two sides, as the malformation is a bit haphazard. Sensory loss is in a rough dermatomal pattern, again with variation based on the disorganization of the spinal cord. This loss of sensation puts a patient with SBM at risk for injuries. Pressure sores are very common in asensate areas that are exposed to pressure (e.g., buttocks, heels). Fractures can occur in the lower extremities with no pain. Individuals with SBM are also at higher risk for associated local osteopenia from poor innervation and lack of weightbearing.

Neurogenic Bowel and Bladder

Bowel and bladder control is located primarily at the sacral levels, and thus is affected in almost all cases of SBM. The bladder is typically flaccid, with relaxed sphincters. This leads to a high-capacity, low-pressure bladder, often with spontaneous leakage. If the bladder does not empty well, there may be ureteral reflux, eventually leading to hydronephrosis (dilation of the more proximal urine-collecting system) with kidney damage. At a young age, children may just use diapers. At about the time typical children are being toilet-trained, bladder catheterization via the urethra can result in adapted urinary continence. Urological surgical procedures are available to augment bladder size and create a diversionary stoma on the abdominal wall to ease self-catheterization (de Jong, Chrzan, Klijn, & Dik, 2008; Joseph, 2008). Bowel continence is also an issue. As a child approaches toilet-training age, a bowel program can be implemented to achieve adapted continence (King, Currie, & Wright, 1994; Leibold, 1991).

Orthopedic Complications

Contractures are very common in SBM, due to a lack of innervation to the muscles surrounding a joint. Contractures may be present at birth or may develop later in life. Stretching is the primary treatment for contractures, although surgical procedures may be necessary when these are severe. Kyphoscoliosis in SBM results from a number of factors. It may be present at birth or may develop later in childhood. The underlying spinal deformity provides a poor base of support for the spine above it, causing the generation of abnormal spinal curves. Abnormal curves may also develop as a result of weakness and strength imbalance of paraspinal muscles. Treatment may be observation, bracing, or surgical fusion, depending on the extent of the scoliosis and its impact on functioning (Brown, 2001).

Latex Allergy

Allergic reactions to latex and related allergenic substances (e.g., tomatoes, bananas) are very common in SBM. The cause for this is unknown; perhaps such allergies are related to early exposure to surgical procedures, though they are not as common in other disorders having similar early exposure. Reactions vary from contact dermatitis to risk of anaphylaxis. Latex and cross-reacting substances need to be avoided, though this can be quite difficult, as latex is a very commonly used substance (Eustachio, Cristina, Antonio, & Alfredo, 2003).

Sleep-Disordered Breathing

There is a 20% prevalence of moderate to severe sleep-disordered breathing (SDB) in children with SBM (Kirk, Morielli, & Brouillette, 1999). Up to 50% of individuals with the Arnold–Chiari type II malformation (see below) evidence sleep apnea, and the majority of these are children (Dauvilliers et al., 2007). Unfortunately, only a small proportion of children receive a sleep study. SDB can be associated with sudden, unexplained death during sleep, as well as cognitive impairments (e.g., in attention and memory) and mood/behavior disturbances. Thus screening for symptoms of SDB and providing appropriate treatment as indicated are important aspects of care.

NEUROPATHOLOGY IN SBM

In addition to the physical effects related to the spinal malformation and spinal cord injury, SBM is associated with characteristic malformations of key brain structures, as well as delayed maturation of gray and white matter. Ultrasound studies typically conducted by the 18th to 20th week of gestation show a characteristic "lemon-shaped" skull development. Frontally, there is a bilateral narrowing of the frontal lobes, with an associated enlargement of the ventricular atrium where the frontal, temporal, and occipital lobes converge at the lateral ventricles (Bannister, Nabiuni, Zendah, Mashayekhi, & Miyan, 2005). Posteriorally, the pons and medulla are elongated, with an accompanying deformation of the cerebellar tonsils into the cervical spinal canal and abnormalities of the fourth ventricle. Midbrain anomalies include a beaked appearance of the mesencephalic tectum. These posterior anomalies are collectively referred to as the Arnold–Chiari type II malformation (ACM). Congenital abnormalities of the corpus callosum, including the rostrum and/or splenium, are observed in over half of children with SBM. These abnormalities result from disruption of neuroembryogenesis early in gestation (approximately 7–20 weeks), during a period of rapid development of the corpus callosum (Barkovich, 2000; Hannay, 2000). The reader is referred to other sources (Bannister et al., 2005; Dennis, Hetherington, & Spiegler, 1999; Fletcher, Francis, Thompson, Davidson, & Miner, 1992; Juranek et al., 2008; Stevenson, 2004) for more detailed explanations of the brain anomalies associated with

SBM and their implications. Bannister and colleagues (2005) provide evidence from rat and human studies of the importance of cerebrospinal fluid (CSF) in neuronal development and migration. In SBM, the lack or reduction of CSF, which contains growth and signaling factors, within the subarachnoid spaces of the developing brain is proposed to lead to the observed abnormalities in cortical formation.

RISK FACTORS FOR PHENOTYPIC EXPRESSION

A number of risk factors for the phenotypic expression in SBM have been identified, including primary and secondary effects (Dennis, Landry, Barnes, & Fletcher, 2006). These effects are associated with a phenotypic neurocognitive profile that ranges from mild to severe impairment, depending on the number and extent of risk factors present for a particular individual. Risk factors include lesion level (thoracic, lumbar, sacral); shunting for hydrocephalus and number of infections or shunt revisions; seizures (see Yoshida et al., 2006); and the presence and number of oculomotor/visual deficits, such as strabismus, nystagmus, papilledema, and optic atrophy. Of particular significance are the presence and extent of characteristic central nervous system (CNS) anomalies associated with SBM.

Primary CNS Risk Factors

Higher lesion levels are associated with greater cognitive and motor impairment (Fletcher et al., 2005; Wills, 1993), and with more extensive anomalies within the cerebellum and midbrain structures, than those seen with lower lesion levels (Fletcher et al., 2005). Dennis, Landry, and colleagues (2006) found that children with lower lesion levels had greater gray matter volumes in the medial cerebellum, and white and gray matter volumes in the lateral hemispheres, than those with upper lesion levels.

The ACM, which (as noted above) includes deformation of the brainstem and cerebellum, is the most common congenital brain anomaly in SBM, occurring in the majority of cases (Barkovich, 2000). In SBM, the posterior fossa is small, and portions of the medulla, fourth ventricle, and cerebellum herniate through the foramen magnum. The pons, cerebellar vermis, and fourth ventricle thus are elongated. There is a "beaked" appearance to the mesencephalic tectum (Stevenson, 2004).

The cerebellum and basal ganglia and their interface with higher cortical systems play a role in the acquisition of motor skills, motor timing, and control of motor performance. These skills include the coordination of eye-hand movements, as well as sequencing and accommodation in response to sensory feedback (Colvin, Yeates, Enrile, & Coury, 2003; Doyon & Benali, 2005; Doyon, Penhune, & Ungerleider, 2003; Laforce & Doyon, 2001, 2002; Miall & Reckess, 2002; Salman et al., 2005; Thach, 1998). The presence of tectal beaking is associated with oculomotor impairments, including nystagmus (Tubbs et al., 2004).

Vinck, Maassen, Mullaart, and Rotteveel (2006) investigated the specific contribution of the ACM to the information processing of children with SBM. In addition, differences in phenotypic expression between children with a full range of intellect and children with IQs above 70 were examined. In the full-range group, the classic picture of deficits in perception, visual–motor integration, processing speed, verbal skills, sequential memory, and arithmetic emerged. The higher-functioning group demonstrated a different pattern of deficits in perception, verbal memory, and verbal fluency. Vinck and colleagues conclude that the higher-functioning group of children with ACM demonstrated impairments in cognitive abilities hypothesized to be mediated by the cerebellum (Leiner, Leiner, & Dow, 1993; Schmahmann & Sherman, 1998). Thus, apart from the effects of hydrocephalus and increased cranial pressures, the cerebellar abnormalities appear to make a unique contribution to the pattern of neurocognitive effects observed in SBM. Other CNS abnormalities include selective thinning of the posterior cerebral cortex (Dennis et al., 2004; Salman, Blaser, Sharpe, & Dennis, 2006). More than half of children with SBM present with agenesis or dysgenesis of the corpus callosum, which is associated with white matter dysfunction and decreased cross-hemispheric integration. Primary effects on the corpus callosum typically result in abnormalities of the splenium and rostrum, with relative preservation of the genu, and are related to prolonged disruption of neuroembryogenesis (Barkovich, 1995; Hannay, 2000). Anterior brain effects, including abnormalities of the prefrontal and frontal regions, are less well studied but have received increased attention recently.

Secondary CNS Risk Factors

A number of important secondary CNS effects are common in SBM. In particular, the presence of hydrocephalus has implications for phenotypic expression in SBM. Hydrocephalus is a common complication, affecting approximately 80–90% of individuals with SBM. It is caused by an obstruction in the normal flow of CSF, typically as a direct result of the ACM. In the newborn, the open sutures allow for the buildup of CSF, resulting in macrocephaly. In children, the ventricles become enlarged, which results in increased intracranial pressures and secondary effects on the brain. Treatment involves placement of a shunt (most commonly ventriculoperitoneal) to remove excess CSF to the peritoneum, where it is reabsorbed. As with any implant, there is a risk of failure of the shunt, as well as infection. Failure of the shunt results in increased intracranial pressure. Signs and symptoms of this include headache, visual changes, papilledema, increased motor impairments, somnolence, and irritability, among others. Shunt failure can lead to herniation, so it requires prompt medical attention, with magnetic resonance imaging (MRI) being the technology of choice to evaluate for hydrocephalus. Classically, children with early hydrocephalus demonstrate impairments in visual-perceptual and motor functions (Dennis et al., 1981; Donders, Rourke, & Canady, 1991; Fletcher et al., 1992, 1996). The neurocognitive effects associated with hydrocephalus are observed even when shunting occurs very early in life (Donders et al., 1991; Rourke, 1995). That said, other research suggests that shunt placement can improve the neuropsychological functioning of young adults with assumed arrested hydrocephalus. Specifically, improvements in verbal and visual memory, attention, and cognitive flexibility are seen (Mataro et al., 2000). Later-occurring changes in white matter tracts, including hypoplasia of the middle, posterior, or full corpus callosum, are thought to be related to hydrocephalus (Hasan, Eluvathingal, et al., 2008; Hasan, Sankar, et al., 2008).

NEUROPSYCHOLOGICAL PHENOTYPE

Intelligence

The majority of individuals with SBM have low-average to average intellectual functioning (Dennis et al., 1981; Mirzai, Ersahin, Mutluer, & Kayahan, 1998; Soare & Raimondi, 1977). Individuals with SBM and hydrocephalus demonstrate lower overall cognitive ability than those without hydrocephalus, whereas individuals with SBO or SBM but no hydrocephalus generally perform similarly to typically developing peers. Thus the associated neuropathology (in this case, hydrocephalus) is what largely affects intelligence, rather than SBM per se (Barf et al., 2003; Vinck et al., 2006).

Nonverbal Learning Disability

In efforts to organize the various neurocognitive impairments associated with SBM, the construct of nonverbal learning disability (NLD) has been widely proposed and has received some support (Fletcher, Brookshire, Bohan, Brandt, & Davidson, 1995; Fletcher, Dennis, & Northrup, 2000; Fletcher et al., 1992; Rourke, 1995; Yeates, Loss, Colvin, & Enrile, 2003), though the construct remains controversial. Several methods of classifying NLD have been proposed (Ris et al., 2007; Rourke, 1995). Typically, NLD is understood in terms of the relative strengths and weaknesses within a child's neurocognitive profile. NLD is largely characterized by relative weaknesses in visual–spatial processing, motor coordination, arithmetic, and interpersonal skills.

Risk factors for the phenotypic expression of NLD in children with SBM include white matter abnormalities such as dysgenesis of the corpus callosum (Rourke, 1995), as well as early-shunted hydrocephalus (Donders et al., 1991; Fletcher et al., 1995; Rourke, 1995); both of these are proposed to have negative effects on right-hemispheric functioning or integration of the right hemisphere with more global brain systems (Rourke, 1995).

Yeates and colleagues (2003) found NLD in 45% of their sample of children with SBM and shunted hydrocephalus, as compared with 7% of their typically developing siblings. However, a high degree of phenotypic variability was observed among the children with SBM; there were significant individual differences in their pattern of assets and deficits. These findings highlight the need for caution against overgeneralization of the NLD model for children with SBM.

Deficits in fine motor skills include slowed speed and poor dexterity and graphomotor construction (Hetherington & Dennis, 1999). Difficulties with eye–hand coordination may be attributable to deficits in perceptual and motor timing, which appear in turn to be associated with reduced cerebellar volumes (Dennis et al., 2004). Children with SBM demonstrate severe deficits in visual planning and sequencing (Snow, 1999). Consistent with the NLD profile, children with SBM demonstrate reading skills close to age expectation, but mathematics skills one standard deviation below expectation (Barnes et al., 2006). This profile persists into adulthood (Hetherington, Dennis, Barnes, Drake, & Gentili, 2006). The motor deficits associated with SBM negatively affect exploration and cognitive development (Landry, Robinson, Copeland, & Garner, 1993; Thelen & Smith, 1994).

More recent studies have sought to examine the motor performance of children with SBM in more specific terms and have observed relatively intact motor learning in children with SBM. Although children with SBM were initially slower and less accurate than typically developing children in their performance of a motor skill, with practice they were able to master this skill at a comparable performance level (Edelstein et al., 2004). Preserved motor learning was found in another study of children with SBM, despite reduced cerebellar and pericallosal gray matter volumes in these children (Dennis, Jewell, et al., 2006). These researchers distinguish between motor learning and performance and conclude that motor learning of nonreflexive tasks using hands, arms, or eyes is relatively preserved for children with SBM, even when their motor performance is impaired. In addition, aspects of spatial knowledge or way finding within a computer-simulated or "virtual" environment appear intact in children with SBM. Although route knowledge was impaired, landmark knowledge was comparable to that of typically developing children (Wiedenbauer & Jansen-Osmann, 2006). These researchers noted that behavioral measures of spatial knowledge tend to overestimate impairment in SBM because of the children's decreased mobility.

Language and Pragmatic Impairments

Although the concept of NLD suggests that the speech–language functioning of children with SBM is relatively intact, specific areas of weakness have been identified. The phrase "cocktail party syndrome" has been used to describe the pragmatic language functioning of children with SBM, particularly those with hydrocephalus. It includes hyperverbosity; fluent, well-articulated speech containing perseverations and stereotyped phrases; and an overfamiliarity of manner (Tew, 1979). Analysis of the speech samples from children with SBM suggests that although their discourse is fluent, it is not concise, fails to convey overall meaning, and lacks relevant content (Dennis & Barnes, 1993; Dennis, Jacennik, & Barnes, 1994). Motor speech deficits are also apparent in many children with SBM, including slowed speech rate and ataxic dysarthric features, which persist into adulthood (Huber-Okrainec, Dennis, Brettschneider, & Spiegler, 2002).

Children with SBM also appear to have difficulties understanding the meaning and important content of others' speech. Specifically, they are less able than their peers to understand the intended meaning of sentences in a discourse, due to their difficulties in making inferences and understanding nonliteral language in the context of a particular conversation (Barnes & Dennis, 1998). It has been suggested that these difficulties are due to impairments in their online processing of word meanings, as well as difficulties suppressing irrelevant information (Barnes, Dennis, & Hetherington, 2004). Similarly, with regard to reading, children with SBM acquire typical word knowledge, vocabulary, and decoding skills. However, their ability to understand the meaning of

what they read or make inferences based on context is impaired (Fletcher, Barnes, & Dennis, 2002). This reading pattern appears to continue into adulthood (Barnes et al., 2004). Recent research indicates that difficulties in speech and language can be found in children as young as 3 years old (Lomax-Bream, Barnes, Copeland, Taylor, & Landry, 2007).

Most of the research regarding the development of speech and language in children with SBM focuses on the impact of hydrocephalus. However, it has been suggested that hydrocephalus alone cannot account for the speech and language impairments. In a comparison of children with hydrocephalus of various etiologies, children with hydrocephalus and SBM performed worse on measures of receptive and expressive language and on word generation tasks than children with hydrocephalus of different etiologies (Brookshire et al., 1995). Vinck and colleagues (2006) found impairments in verbal fluency among children with ACM, compared to children with SBM but no ACM. These deficits were attributed to the cerebellar dysfunction rather than the associated hydrocephalus. Higher-level language skills, such as comprehension of idioms, appear related to the corpus callosal abnormalities associated with SBM (Huber-Okrainec, Blaser, & Dennis, 2005)

Attention Deficits and Executive Dysfunction

Attention deficits and impairments in other aspects of executive functioning are robust findings in populations of children and adults with SBM. These have been associated with anomalies in anterior brain (Anderson, Jacobs, & Harvey, 2005); midbrain, including the superior colliculus; and posterior brain regions (Dennis, Landry, et al., 2006; Dennis, Sinopoli, Fletcher, & Schachar, 2008). Previously, the attention deficits associated with SBM were likened to those in individuals diagnosed with attention-deficit/hyperactivity disorder. However, recent research by Dennis and colleagues suggests that attentional processes mediated by anterior brain regions tend to be relatively preserved in children with SBM, while those mediated by midbrain and posterior cortical regions are deficient. Specifically, impairments are observed in covert orienting and inhibition of return. In particular, the presence of tectal beaking, a characteristic midbrain anomaly in SBM, is associated with children's reduced ability to orient themselves in their environment—both overtly with eye movement, and covertly in the manner in which they shift attention (Dennis et al., 2005a, 2005b, 2008; Dennis, Landry, et al., 2006). The deleterious effects of hydrocephalus in particular on attention and other aspects of executive processes of children with SBM have been widely discussed (Boyer, Yeates, & Enrile, 2006; Brown et al., 2008; Burmeister et al., 2005; Dennis, Landry, et al., 2006; English, Barnes, Taylor, & Landry, 2009; Heffelfinger et al., 2008; Iddon, Morgan, Loveday, Sahakian, & Pickard, 2004; Matson, Mahone, & Zabel, 2005; Riddle, Morton, Sampson, Vachha, & Adams, 2005; Rose & Holmbeck, 2007; Swartwout et al., 2008; Tarazi, Zabel, & Mahone, 2008).

Visual-Perceptual and Motor Functioning

Children with SBM show impairment in both upper- and lower-extremity functioning (Dennis et al., 2004; Hetherington & Dennis, 1999; Jansen et al., 1991), as well as in their quality of eye movements (Biglan, 1990, 1995; Salman et al., 2005). Recent research regarding the visual-perceptual and motor functioning of children with SBM suggests that, in part due to the effects of hydrocephalus, such children demonstrate impairments relative to typically developing peers on action-based tasks including mental rotation, multistable figures, figure–ground discrimination, and route planning. In contrast, performance on spatial memory and object-based tasks such as object and face recognition, line orientation, and visual illusions is comparable to that of typical peers (Dennis, Fletcher, Rogers, Hetherington, & Francis, 2002).

Alternative Models of Neurocognitive Deficits

In response to this research describing a broadened range of more specific neurocognitive variables, Dennis, Fletcher, and colleagues have proposed an alternative model of the neuropsychological impairments associated with SBM that provides a valuable heuristic for future research. Impairments in motor coordination and timing, covert and voluntary attention, and perceptual processing, and their association with abnormalities of the cerebellar, midbrain, and parietal regions, are described. These authors posit effects of primary CNS insults on core deficits (timing, attention orienting, and movement), as well as effects of secondary CNS insults in mediating assembled and associative processes. Deficits in assembled processing and relative strengths in associative processing yield the cognitive phenotype of functional deficits and assets that has been described in the literature. These assets and deficits may be seen both within and across cognitive content domains (Dennis, Landry, et al., 2006).

ASSESSMENT

Prenatal screening tests such as alpha-fetoprotein and ultrasonography are commonly used in diagnosing SBM. Increasingly, fast and ultrafast (to decrease movement artifact, need for sedation, and imaging time) MRI is being used to confirm abnormality in equivocal cases and to identify specific CNS abnormalities, including ventriculomegaly, agenesis of the corpus callosum, migration abnormalities, and posterior fossa abnormalities; all of these can be important for management (Bekker & van Vugt, 2001; Levine, 2002; Mehta & Levine, 2005). As a child develops, serial neuropsychological evaluations are useful in identifying the child's unique profile of neurocognitive strengths and weaknesses to aid treatment planning. Neuropsychological testing can also identify changes in neurocognitive status that may signal shunt malfunction.

DEVELOPMENTAL ISSUES

The growth of children with SBM is marked by short stature. Prior to puberty, children with SBM and associated hydrocephalus demonstrate slowed linear growth and bone age. However, even after the growth spurt associated with puberty, stature is reduced. Short stature in SBM has been attributed to various factors, including shorter lower limbs and various spine deformities. In addition, it is possible that children with SBM have a growth hormone deficiency related to brain anomalies. Children with SBM are also at risk for precocious puberty, with girls developing secondary sex characteristics as early as age 8 and boys as early as age 9 (Greene, Frank, Zachmann, & Prader, 1985).

The rate of motor development in children with SBM is different from that in typically developing children. Lomax-Bream and colleagues (2007) assessed the early cognitive, motor, and language abilities of children with SB at five points in their first 3 years. Growth curve models were generated from these data. The researchers found lower levels in functioning across all domains in children with SB than in typically developing controls. Motor skills were noted to progress more quickly, while slower rates of development in cognitive and language abilities were observed. As noted earlier, speech and language impairments were found in children as young as 3 years old. The tethering of the spinal cord can also slow down motor development in children with SBM and eventually cause motor deterioration. Gross motor functioning typically deteriorates in children with SBM as they age. The majority of patients lose the ability to ambulate by the age of 10–15 years due to weight gain, making bracing difficult.

TREATMENT

Medical Treatment

Prevention efforts, including genetic counseling and folate supplementation, are critical to further reducing the incidence of SBM and other NTDs. The complex medical needs of a child with SBM are optimally managed by a multidisciplinary team. Newborns with SBM frequently require one or more surgeries within the first week of life. Initial treatment typically includes the closure of the open myelomeningocele. An additional surgery that may take place when a child with SBM is a newborn is placement of a ventriculoperitoneal shunt if necessary to treat hydrocephalus. Additional surgeries may be needed to repair shunt malfunction or infection. The two most common causes of shunt malfunction in patients with

SBM are mechanical obstruction and CSF infection. Infection occurs in 12–18% of individuals with SBM, although this rate is declining. Cognitive functioning is generally not related to the number of shunt revisions during childhood; however, in adults the number of shunt revisions is related to employment and independent living (Bowman, McLone, Grant, Tomita, & Ito, 2001; Hunt, Oakeshott, & Kerry, 1999). The herniation that characterizes the ACM may require surgical decompression. Although some patients are asymptomatic, nystagmus related to lower cranial nerve nuclei compression may be an early indicator. Surgical treatment for spinal tethering and scoliosis is also common. More than 90% of children with higher-level spinal lesions develop scoliosis in early childhood, which can cause pain, impair mobility, and affect respiratory functioning. Ongoing management of bladder and bowel incontinence is critical. The importance of bowel and bladder control in individuals with SBM goes beyond physical needs. Incontinence and lack of sphincter control are associated with less functional independence and greater social concerns (Lemelle et al., 2006; Verhoef et al., 2006). Adolescents and adults with SBM consider incontinence and toileting as primary concerns (Malone, Wheeler, & Williams, 1994), and incontinence can be a barrier to employment (Leibold, Ekmark, & Adams, 2000).

Rehabilitation Interventions

Early intervention is critical for optimal outcome in SBM. Services may be obtained through a child's school district or local hospital. A multidisciplinary team approach—including physical and occupational therapies, speech–language pathology, and rehabilitation psychology/neuropsychology, as well as early education services—is warranted. Fletcher, Ostermaier, Cirino, and Dennis (2008) review neurobehavioral outcomes and recommended interventions for use with children with SBM; they also provide a heuristic for organizing interventions targeting the cognitive and behavioral difficulties common among children with SBM on the basis of underlying neurocognitive processes. Table 28.2 summarizes key treatment targets by developmental stage

TABLE 28.2. Treatment Targets in SBM by Developmental Stage and Discipline

Stage	Target	Discipline
Infancy	Feeding and swallowing (oral hypersensitivity and gagging)	Speech–language therapy Occupational therapy
Preschool	Speech–language and pragmatic deficits Independence for feeding and dressing Fine and gross motor impairments	Speech–language therapy Occupational therapy Physical therapy Early childhood education services
School age	Learning impairments Social pragmatics Increased difficulties with mobility (secondary to tethered cord and weight gain) Precocious puberty Change in mood (depression, social isolation)	Speech–language therapy Occupational therapy Physical therapy Rehabilitation psychology/neuropsychology Special education services Medical interventions
Adolescence	Social pragmatics Executive dysfunction as demands increase Change in mood, social status (depression, social isolation) Bowel and bladder Precocious puberty	Speech–language therapy Rehabilitation psychology/neuropsychology Occupational therapy Special education services Medical/surgical intervention
Early adulthood	Transition issues Independence (transportation, employment, cooking, etc.)	Medical team Rehabilitation psychology/neuropsychology Occupational therapy

and assumes a multidisciplinary treatment approach.

CONCLUSIONS AND FUTURE DIRECTIONS

SBM, a commonly occurring NTD, results from both gene–gene and gene–environment interactions. Both physical effects related to malformation of and injury to the spinal cord, and characteristic malformations of a number of brain structures, are present. Both primary and secondary CNS processes result in the phenotypic physical and neurocognitive presentation of SBM across the lifespan. Progress in research on the genetic and environmental factors related to etiology and functional effects of SBM has provided new insights into prevention and treatment. New technologies in genetics and neuroimaging, in conjunction with neuropsychological research, will continue to contribute to our knowledge base. Continued research into rehabilitative interventions and outcome is also needed.

REFERENCES

Anderson, V., Jacobs, R., & Harvey, A. S. (2005). Prefrontal lesions and attentional skills in childhood. *Journal of International Neuropsychological Society, 11*(7), 817–831.

Bannister, C. M., Nabiuni, M., Zendah, M., Mashayekhi, F., & Miyan, J. A. (2005). Development anomalies of the cerebellar hemispheres in spina bifida aperta. In M. R. Zesta (Ed.), *Trends in spina bifida research* (pp. 31–42). Hauppage, NY: Nova Science.

Barf, H. A., Verhoef, M., Jennekens-Schinkel, A., Post, M. W., Gooskens, R. H., & Prevo, A. J. (2003). Cognitive status of young adults with spina bifida. *Developmental Medicine and Child Neurology, 45*(12), 813–820.

Barkovich, A. J. (1995). *Pediatric neuroimaging* (2nd ed.). New York: Raven Press.

Barkovich, A. J. (2000). Morphologic characteristics of subcortical heterotopia: MR imaging study. *American Journal of Neuroradiology, 21*(2), 290–295.

Barnes, M. A., & Dennis, M. (1998). Discourse after early-onset hydrocephalus: Core deficits in children of average intelligence. *Brain and Language, 61*(3), 309–334.

Barnes, M. A., Dennis, M., & Hetherington, R. (2004). Reading and writing skills in young adults with spina bifida and hydrocephalus. *Journal of International Neuropsychological Society, 10*(5), 655–663.

Barnes, M. A., Wilkinson, M., Khemani, E., Boudesquie, A., Dennis, M., & Fletcher, J. M. (2006). Arithmetic processing in children with spina bifida: Calculation accuracy, strategy use, and fact retrieval fluency. *Journal of Learning Disabilities, 39*(2), 174–187.

Bekker, M. N., & van Vugt, J. M. (2001). The role of magnetic resonance imaging in prenatal diagnosis of fetal anomalies. *European Journal of Obstetrics and Gynecology and Reproductive Biology, 96*(2), 173–178.

Biglan, A. W. (1990). Ophthalmologic complications of meningomyelocele: A longitudinal study. *Transactions of the American Ophthalmological Society, 88*, 389–462.

Biglan, A. W. (1995). Strabismus associated with meningomyelocele. *Journal of Pediatric Ophthalmology and Strabismus, 32*(5), 309–314.

Botto, L. D., Lisi, A., Robert-Gnansia, E., Erickson, J. D., Vollset, S. E., Mastroiacovo, P., et al. (2005). International retrospective cohort study of neural tube defects in relation to folic acid recommendations: Are the recommendations working? *British Medical Journal, 330*(7491), 571.

Bowman, R. M., Boshnjaku, V., & McLone, D. G. (2009). The changing incidence of myelomeningocele and its impact on pediatric neurosurgery: A review from the Children's Memorial Hospital. *Child's Nervous System, 25*(7), 801–806.

Bowman, R. M., McLone, D. G., Grant, J. A., Tomita, T., & Ito, J. A. (2001). Spina bifida outcome: A 25-year prospective. *Pediatric Neurosurgery, 34*(3), 114–120.

Boyer, K. M., Yeates, K. O., & Enrile, B. G. (2006). Working memory and information processing speed in children with myelomeningocele and shunted hydrocephalus: Analysis of the Children's Paced Auditory Serial Addition Test. *Journal of International Neuropsychological Society, 12*, 305–313.

Brookshire, B. L., Fletcher, J. M., Bohan, T. P., Landry, S. H., Davidson, K. C., & Francis, D. J. (1995). Verbal and nonverbal skill discrepancies in children with hydrocephalus: A five-year longitudinal follow-up. *Journal of Pediatric Psychology, 20*(6), 785–800.

Brown, J. P. (2001). Orthopaedic care of children with spina bifida: You've come a long way, baby! *Orthopedic Nursing, 20*(4), 51–58.

Brown, T. M., Ris, M. D., Beebe, D., Ammerman, R. T., Oppenheimer, S. G., Yeates, K. O., et al. (2008). Factors of biological risk and reserve associated with executive behaviors in children and adolescents with spina bifida myelomeningocele. *Child Neuropsychologyogy, 14*(2), 118–134.

Burmeister, R., Hannay, H. J., Copeland, K., Fletcher, J. M., Boudousquie, A., & Dennis, M. (2005). Attention problems and executive functions in children with spina bifida and hydrocephalus. *Child Neuropsychology, 11*(3), 265–283.

Carter, C. O. (1969). Spina bifida and anencephaly: A problem in genetic–environmental interaction. *Journal of Biosocial Science, 1*(1), 71–83.

Colvin, A. N., Yeates, K. O., Enrile, B. G., & Coury, D. L. (2003). Motor adaptation in children with myelomeningocele: Comparison to children with ADHD and healthy siblings. *Journal of International Neuropsychological Society, 9*(4), 642–652.

Copp, A. J., Greene, N. D. E., & Murdoch, J. N. (2003). The genetic basis of mammalian neurulation. *Nature Reviews Genetics, 4*(10), 784–793.

Cowchock, S., Ainbender, E., Prescott, G., Crandall, B., Lau, L., Heller, R., et al. (1980). The recurrence risk for neural tube defects in the United States: A collaborative study. *American Journal of Medical Genetics, 5*(3), 309–314.

Dauvilliers, Y., Stal, V., Abril, B., Coubes, P., Bobin, S., Touchon, J., et al. (2007). Chiari malformation and sleep related breathing disorders. *Journal of Neurology, Neurosurgery and Psychiatry, 78*(12), 1344–1348.

de Jong, T. P., Chrzan, R., Klijn, A. J., & Dik, P. (2008). Treatment of the neurogenic bladder in spina bifida. *Pediatric Nephrology, 23*(6), 889–896.

Dennis, M., & Barnes, M. A. (1993). Oral discourse after early-onset hydrocephalus: Linguistic ambiguity, figurative language, speech acts, and script-based inferences. *Journal of Pediatric Psychology, 18*(5), 639–652.

Dennis, M., Edelstein, K., Copeland, K., Frederick, J., Francis, D. J., Hetherington, R., et al. (2005a). Covert orienting to exogenous and endogenous cues in children with spina bifida. *Neuropsychologia, 43*(6), 976–987.

Dennis, M., Edelstein, K., Copeland, K., Frederick, J. A., Francis, D. J., Hetherington, R., et al. (2005b). Space-based inhibition of return in children with spina bifida. *Neuropsychology, 19*(4), 456–465.

Dennis, M., Edelstein, K., Hetherington, R., Copeland, K., Frederick, J., Blaser, S. E., et al. (2004). Neurobiology of perceptual and motor timing in children with spina bifida in relation to cerebellar volume. *Brain, 127*(Pt. 6), 1292–1301.

Dennis, M., Fitz, C. R., Netley, C. T., Sugar, J., Harwood-Nash, D. C., Hendrick, E. B., et al. (1981). The intelligence of hydrocephalic children. *Archives of Neurology, 38*(10), 607–615.

Dennis, M., Fletcher, J. M., Rogers, T., Hetherington, R., & Francis, D. J. (2002). Object-based and action-based visual perception in children with spina bifida and hydrocephalus. *Journal of International Neuropsychological Society, 8*(1), 95–106.

Dennis, M., Hetherington, R., & Spiegler, B. (1999). Functional consequences of congenital cerebellar dysmorphologies and acquired cerebellar lesions of childhood. In S. H. Broman & J. M. Fletcher (Eds.), *The changing nervous system: Neurobehavioural consequences of early brain disorder* (pp. 365–385). New York: Oxford University Press.

Dennis, M., Jacennik, B., & Barnes, M. A. (1994). The content of narrative discourse in children and adolescents after early-onset hydrocephalus and in normally developing age peers. *Brain and Language, 46*(1), 129–165.

Dennis, M., Jewell, D., Edelstein, K., Brandt, M. E., Hetherington, R., Blaser, S. E., et al. (2006). Motor learning in children with spina bifida: Intact learning and performance on a ballistic task. *Journal of International Neuropsychological Society, 12*(5), 598–608.

Dennis, M., Landry, S. H., Barnes, M., & Fletcher, J. M. (2006). A model of neurocognitive function in spina bifida over the life span. *Journal of International Neuropsychological Society, 12*(2), 285–296.

Dennis, M., Sinopoli, K. J., Fletcher, J. M., & Schachar, R. (2008). Puppets, robots, critics, and actors within a taxonomy of attention for developmental disorders. *Journal of International Neuropsychological Society, 14*(5), 673–690.

Donders, J., Rourke, B. P., & Canady, A. I. (1991). Neuropsychological functioning of hydrocephalic children. *Journal of Clinical and Experimental Neuropsychology, 13*(4), 607–613.

Doyon, J., & Benali, H. (2005). Reorganization and plasticity in the adult brain during learning of motor skills. *Current Opinion in Neurobiology, 15*(2), 161–167.

Doyon, J., Penhune, V., & Ungerleider, L. G. (2003). Distinct contribution of the cortico-striatal and cortico-cerebellar systems to motor skill learning. *Neuropsychologia, 41*(3), 252–262.

Edelstein, K., Dennis, M., Copeland, K., Frederick, J., Francis, D., Hetherington, R., et al. (2004). Motor learning in children with spina bifida: Dissociation between performance level and acquisition rate. *Journal of International Neuropsychological Society, 10*(6), 877–887.

English, L. H., Barnes, M. A., Taylor, H. B., & Landry, S. H. (2009). Mathematical development in spina bifida. *Developmental Disabilities Research Reviews, 15*(1), 28–34.

Eskes, T. K. (2000). From anemia to spina bifida—the story of folic acid: A tribute to Professor Richard Smithells. *European Journal of Obstetrics and Gynecology and Reproductive Biology, 90*(2), 119–123.

Eustachio, N., Cristina, C. M., Antonio, F., & Alfredo, T. (2003). A discussion of natural rubber latex allergy with special reference to children: Clinical considerations. *Current Drug Targets—Immune, Endocrine and Metabolic Disorders, 3*(3), 171–180.

Fletcher, J. M., Barnes, M., & Dennis, M. (2002). Language development in children with spina bifida. *Seminars in Pediatric Neurology, 9*(3), 201–208.

Fletcher, J. M., Brookshire, B. L., Bohan, T. P., Brandt, M. E., & Davidson, K. C. (1995). Early hydrocephalus. In B. P. Rourke (Ed.), *Syndrome of nonverbal learning disabilities* (pp. 206–238). New York: Guilford Press.

Fletcher, J. M., Copeland, K., Frederick, J. A., Blaser, S. E., Kramer, L. A., Northrup, H., et al. (2005). Spinal lesion level in spina bifida: A source of neural and cognitive heterogeneity. *Journal of Neurosurgery, 102*(3, Suppl.), 268–279.

Fletcher, J. M., Dennis, M., & Northrup, H. (2000). Hydrocephalus. In K. O. Yeates, M. D. Ris, & H. G. Taylor (Eds.), *Pediatric neuropsychology: Theory, research, and practice* (pp. 25–46). New York: Guilford Press.

Fletcher, J. M., Francis, D. J., Thompson, N. M., Davidson, K. C., & Miner, M. E. (1992). Verbal and nonverbal skill discrepancies in hydrocephalic children. *Journal of Clinical and Experimental Neuropsychology, 14*(4), 593–609.

Fletcher, J. M., McCauley, S. R., Brandt, M. E., Bohan, T. P., Kramer, L. A., Francis, D. J., et al. (1996). Regional brain tissue composition in children with hydrocephalus. Relationships with cognitive development. *Archives of Neurology, 53*(6), 549–557.

Fletcher, J. M., Ostermaier, K. K., Cirino, P. T., & Dennis, M. (2008). Neurobehavioral outcomes in spina bifida: Processes versus outcomes. *Journal of Pediatric Rehabilitation Medicine, 1*(4), 311–324.

Gordon, N. (1995). Folate metabolism and neural tube defects. *Brain and Development, 17*(5), 307–311.

Greene, S. A., Frank, M., Zachmann, M., & Prader, A. (1985). Growth and sexual development in children with meningomyelocele. *European Journal of Pediatrics, 144*(2), 146–148.

Habibzadeh, N., Schorah, C. J., Seller, M. J., Smithells, R. W., & Levene, M. I. (1993). Uptake and utilization of DL-5-[methyl-14C] tetrahydropteroylmonoglutamate by cultured cytotrophoblasts associated with neural tube defects. *Proceedings of the Society for Experimental Biology and Medicine, 203*(1), 45–54.

Hannay, H. J. (2000). Functioning of the corpus callosum in children with early hydrocephalus. *Journal of International Neuropsychological Society, 6*(3), 351–361.

Harris, M. J., & Juriloff, D. M. (2007). Mouse mutants with neural tube closure defects and their role in understanding human neural tube defects. *Birth Defects Research Part A: Clinical and Molecular Teratology, 79*(3), 187–210.

Hasan, K. M., Eluvathingal, T. J., Kramer, L. A., Ewing-Cobbs, L., Dennis, M., & Fletcher, J. M. (2008a). White matter microstructural abnormalities in children with spina bifida myelomeningocele and hydrocephalus: A diffusion tensor tractography study of the association pathways. *Journal of Magnetic Resonance Imaging, 27*(4), 700–709.

Hasan, K. M., Sankar, A., Halphen, C., Kramer, L. A., Ewing-Cobbs, L., Dennis, M., et al. (2008b). Quantitative diffusion tensor imaging and intellectual outcomes in spina bifida: Laboratory investigation. *Journal of Neurosurgery: Pediatrics, 2*(1), 75–82.

Heffelfinger, A. K., Koop, J. I., Fastenau, P. S., Brei, T. J., Conant, L., Katzenstein, J., et al. (2008). The relationship of neuropsychological functioning to adaptation outcome in adolescents with spina bifida. *Journal of International Neuropsychological Society, 14*(5), 793–804.

Hetherington, R., & Dennis, M. (1999). Motor function profile in children with early onset hydrocephalus. *Developmental Neuropsychology, 15*, 25–51.

Hetherington, R., Dennis, M., Barnes, M., Drake, J., & Gentili, F. (2006). Functional outcome in young adults with spina bifida and hydrocephalus. *Child's Nervous System, 22*(2), 117–124.

Huber-Okrainec, J., Blaser, S. E., & Dennis, M. (2005). Idiom comprehension deficits in relation to corpus callosum agenesis and hypoplasia in children with spina bifida meningomyelocele. *Brain and Language, 93*(3), 349–368.

Huber-Okrainec, J., Dennis, M., Brettschneider, J., & Spiegler, B. J. (2002). Neuromotor speech deficits in children and adults with spina bifida and hydrocephalus. *Brain and Language, 80*(3), 592–602.

Hunt, G. M., Oakeshott, P., & Kerry, S. (1999). Link between the CSF shunt and achievement in adults with spina bifida. *Journal of Neurology, Neurosurgery and Psychiatry, 67*(5), 591–595.

Iddon, J. L., Morgan, D. J., Loveday, C., Sahakian, B. J., & Pickard, J. D. (2004). Neuropsychological profile of young adults with spina bifida with or without hydrocephalus. *Journal of Neurology, Neurosurgery and Psychiatry, 75*(8), 1112–1118.

Jansen, J., Taudorf, K., Pedersen, H., Jensen, K., Scitzberg, A., & Smith, T. (1991). Upper extremity function in spina bifida. *Child's Nervous System, 7*(2), 67–71.

Joseph, D. B. (2008). Current approaches to the urologic care of children with spina bifida. *Current Urology Reports, 9*(2), 151–157.

Juranek, J., Fletcher, J. M., Hasan, K. M., Breier, J. I., Cirino, P. T., Pazo-Alvarez, P., et al. (2008). Neocortical reorganization in spina bifida. *NeuroImage, 40*(4), 1516–1522.

Kibar, Z., Capra, V., & Gros, P. (2007). Toward understanding the genetic basis of neural tube defects. *Clinical Genetics, 71*(4), 295–310.

King, J. C., Currie, D. M., & Wright, E. (1994). Bowel training in spina bifida: Importance of education, patient compliance, age, and anal reflexes. *Archives of Physical Medicine and Rehabilitation, 75*(3), 243–247.

Kirk, V. G., Morielli, A., & Brouillette, R. T. (1999). Sleep-disordered breathing in patients with myelomeningocele: The missed diagnosis. *Developmental Medicine and Child Neurology, 41*(1), 40–43.

Koch, L. G., & Britton, S. L. (2007). Evolution, atmospheric oxygen, and complex disease. *Physiological Genomics, 30*(3), 205–208.

Koch, L. G., & Britton, S. L. (2008). Development of animal models to test the fundamental basis of gene–environment interactions. *Obesity (Silver Spring), 16*(Suppl. 3), S28–S32.

Laforce, R., Jr., & Doyon, J. (2001). Distinct contribution of the striatum and cerebellum to motor learning. *Brain and Cognition, 45*(2), 189–211.

Laforce, R., Jr., & Doyon, J. (2002). Differential role for the striatum and cerebellum in response to novel movements using a motor learning paradigm. *Neuropsychologia, 40*(5), 512–517.

Landry, S. H., Robinson, S. S., Copeland, K., & Garner, P. W. (1993). Goal-directed behavior and perception of self-competence in children with spina bifida. *Journal of Pediatric Psychology, 18*, 389–396.

Leibold, S. (1991). A systematic approach to bowel continence for children with spina bifida. *European Journal of Pediatric Surgery, 1*(Suppl. 1), 23–24.

Leibold, S., Ekmark, E., & Adams, R. C. (2000). Decision-making for a successful bowel continence program. *European Journal of Pediatric Surgery, 10*(1), 26–30.

Leiner, H. C., Leiner, A. L., & Dow, R. S. (1993). Cognitive and language functions of the human cerebellum. *Trends in Neuroscience, 16*(11), 444–447.

Lemelle, J. L., Guillemin, F., Aubert, D., Guys, J. M., Lottmann, H., Lortat-Jacob, S., et al. (2006). Quality of life and continence in patients with spina bifida. *Quality of Life Research, 15*(9), 1481–1492.

Levine, D. (2002). MR imaging of fetal central nervous system abnormalities. *Brain and Cognition, 50*(3), 432–448.

Li, Z. W., Ren, A. G., Zhang, L., Ye, R. W., Li, S., Zheng, J. C., et al. (2006). Extremely high prevalence of neural tube defects in a 4–county area in Shanxi Province, China. *Birth Defects Research Part A: Clinical and Molecular Teratology, 76*(4), 237–240.

Lindhout, D., Omtzigt, J. G., & Cornel, M. C. (1992). Spectrum of neural-tube defects in 34 infants prenatally exposed to antiepileptic drugs. *Neurology, 42*(4, Suppl. 5), 111–118.

Lomax-Bream, L. E., Barnes, M., Copeland, K., Taylor, H. B., & Landry, S. H. (2007). The impact of spina bifida on development across the first 3 years. *Developmental Neuropsychology, 31*(1), 1–20.

Malone, P. S., Wheeler, R. A., & Williams, J. E. (1994). Continence in patients with spina bifida: Long term results. *Archives of Disease in Children, 70*, 107–110.

Mataro, M., Poca, M. A., Sahuquillo, J., Cuxart, A., Iborra, J., de la Calzada, M. D., et al. (2000). Cognitive changes after cerebrospinal fluid shunting in young adults with spina bifida and assumed arrested hydrocephalus. *Journal of Neurology, Neurosurgery and Psychiatry, 68*(5), 615–621.

Matson, M. A., Mahone, E. M., & Zabel, T. A. (2005). Serial neuropsychological assessment and evidence of shunt malfunction in spina bifida: A longitudinal case study. *Child Neuropsychology, 11*(4), 315–332.

Mehta, T. S., & Levine, D. (2005). Imaging of fetal cerebral ventriculomegaly: A guide to management and outcome. *Seminars in Fetal and Neonatal Medicine, 10*(5), 421–428.

Miall, R. C., & Reckess, G. Z. (2002). The cerebellum and the timing of coordinated eye and hand tracking. *Brain and Cognition, 48*(1), 212–226.

Milunsky, A., Ulcickas, M., Rothman, K. J., Willett, W., Jick, S. S., & Jick, H. (1992). Maternal heat exposure and neural tube defects. *Journal of the American Medical Association, 268*(7), 882–885.

Mirzai, H., Ersahin, Y., Mutluer, S., & Kayahan, A. (1998). Outcome of patients with meningomyelocele: The Ege University experience. *Child's Nervous System, 14*(3), 120–123.

Moephuli, S. R., Klein, N. W., Baldwin, M. T., & Krider, H. M. (1997). Effects of methionine on the cytoplasmic distribution of actin and tubulin during neural tube closure in rat embryos. *Proceedings of the National Academy of Sciences USA, 94*(2), 543–548.

Nevin, N. C., Johnston, W. P., & Merrett, J. D. (1981). Influence of social class on the risk of recurrence of anencephalus and spina bifida. *Developmental Medicine and Child Neurology, 23*(2), 155–159.

Njamnshi, A. K., Djientcheu, V. D., Lekoubou, A., Guemse, M., Obama, M. T., Mbu, R., et al. (2008). Neural tube defects are rare among black Americans but not in sub-Saharan black Africans: The case of Yaounde, Cameroon. *Journal of the Neurological Sciences, 270*(1–2), 13–17.

Riddle, R., Morton, A., Sampson, J. D., Vachha, B., & Adams, R. (2005). Performance on the NEPSY among children with spina bifida. *Archives of Clinical Neuropsychology, 20*(2), 243–248.

Ris, M. D., Ammerman, R. T., Waller, N., Walz, N., Oppenheimer, S., Maines Brown, T., et al. (2007). Taxonicity of nonverbal learning disabilities in spina bifida. *Journal of International Neuropsychological Society, 13*, 50–58.

Rose, B. M., & Holmbeck, G. N. (2007). Attention and executive functions in adolescents with spina bifida. *Journal of Pediatric Psychology, 32*(8), 983–994.

Rourke, B. P. (Ed.). (1995). *Syndrome of nonverbal learning disabilities: Neurodevelopmental manifestations.* New York: Guilford Press.

Salman, M. S., Blaser, S. E., Sharpe, J. A., & Dennis, M. (2006). Cerebellar vermis morphology in children with spina bifida and Chiari type II malformation. *Child's Nervous System, 22*(4), 385–393.

Salman, M. S., Sharpe, J. A., Eizenman, M., Lillakas, L., To, T., Westall, C., et al. (2005). Saccades in children with spina bifida and Chiari type II malformation. *Neurology, 64*(12), 2098–2101.

Sandford, M. K., Kissling, G. E., & Joubert, P. E. (1992). Neural tube defect etiology: New evidence concerning maternal hyperthermia, health and diet. *Developmental Medicine and Child Neurology, 34*(8), 661–675.

Schmahmann, J. D., & Sherman, J. C. (1998). The cerebellar cognitive affective syndrome. *Brain, 121*(Pt. 4), 561–579.

Schorah, C. J., Habibzadeh, N., Wild, J., Smithells, R. W., & Seller, M. J. (1993). Possible abnormalities of folate and vitamin B12 metabolism associated with neural tube defects. *Annals of the New York Academy of Sciences, 678*, 81–91.

Schorah, C. J., & Smithells, R. W. (1993). Primary prevention of neural tube defects with folic acid. *British Medical Journal, 306*, 1123–1124.

Schorah, C. J., Wild, J., Hartley, R., Sheppard, S., & Smithells, R. W. (1983). The effect of periconceptional supplementation on blood vitamin concentrations in women at recurrence risk for neural tube defect. *British Journal of Nutrition, 49*(2), 203–211.

Simpson, D. (2007). Nicolaes Tulp and the golden age of the Dutch Republic. *ANZ Journal of Surgery, 77*(12), 1095–1101.

Smith, G. K. (2001). The history of spina bifida, hydrocephalus, paraplegia, and incontinence. *Pediatric Surgery International, 17*(5–6), 424–432.

Smithells, R. W. (1982). Neural tube defects: Prevention by vitamin supplements. *Pediatrics, 69*(4), 498–499.

Smithells, R. W. (1989). Multivitamins for the prevention of neural tube defects: How convincing is the evidence? *Drugs, 38*(6), 849–854.

Smithells, R. W., Nevin, N. C., Seller, M. J., Sheppard, S., Harris, R., Read, A. P., et al. (1983). Further experience of vitamin supplementation for prevention of neural tube defect recurrences. *Lancet, 1*, 1027–1031.

Smithells, R. W., Sheppard, S., & Schorah, C. J.

(1976). Vitamin deficiencies and neural tube defects. *Archives of Disease in Childhood, 51*(12), 944–950.

Smithells, R. W., Sheppard, S., Schorah, C. J., Seller, M. J., Nevin, N. C., Harris, R., et al. (1981a). Apparent prevention of neural tube defects by periconceptional vitamin supplementation. *Archives of Disease in Childhood, 56*(12), 911–918.

Smithells, R. W., Sheppard, S., Schorah, C. J., Seller, M. J., Nevin, N. C., Harris, R., et al. (1981b). Vitamin supplementation and neural tube defects. *Lancet, 2,* 1425.

Smithells, R. W., Sheppard, S., & Wild, J. (1989a). Prevalence of neural tube defects in the Yorkshire region. *Community Medicine, 11*(2), 163–167.

Smithells, R. W., Sheppard, S., Wild, J., & Schorah, C. J. (1989b). Prevention of neural tube defect recurrences in Yorkshire: Final report. *Lancet, 2,* 498–499.

Smithells, R. W., Sheppard, S., Wild, J., Schorah, C. J., Fielding, D. W., Seller, M. J., et al. (1985). Neural-tube defects and vitamins: The need for a randomized clinical trial. *British Journal of Obstetrics and Gynaecology, 92*(2), 185–188.

Snow, J. H. (1999). Executive processes in children with spina bifida. *Children's Health Care, 28,* 241–253.

Soare, P. L., & Raimondi, A. J. (1977). Intellectual and perceptual–motor characteristics of treated myelomeningocele children. *American Journal of Diseases of Children, 131*(2), 199–204.

Stevenson, K. L. (2004). Chiari Type II malformation: Past, present, and future. *Neurosurgery Focus, 16*(2), E5.

Swartwout, M. D., Cirino, P. T., Hampson, A. W., Fletcher, J. M., Brandt, M. E., & Dennis, M. (2008). Sustained attention in children with two etiologies of early hydrocephalus. *Neuropsychology, 22*(6), 765–775.

Tarazi, R. A., Zabel, T. A., & Mahone, E. M. (2008). Age-related differences in executive function among children with spina bifida/hydrocephalus based on parent behavior ratings. *Clinical Neuropsychology, 22*(4), 585–602.

Tew, B. (1979). The "cocktail party syndrome" in children with hydrocephalus and spina bifida. *British Journal of Disorders of Communication, 14*(2), 89–101.

Thach, W. T. (1998). A role for the cerebellum in learning movement coordination. *Neurobiology of Learning and Memory, 70*(1–2), 177–188.

Thelen, E., & Smith, L. B. (1994). *A dynamical approach to the development of cognition and action.* Cambridge, MA: MIT Press.

Toriello, H. V., & Higgins, J. V. (1983). Occurrence of neural tube defects among first-, second-, and third-degree relatives of probands: Results of a United States study. *American Journal of Medical Genetics, 15*(4), 601–606.

Tubbs, R. S., Soleau, S., Custis, J., Wellons, J. C., Blount, J. P., & Oakes, W. J. (2004). Degree of tectal beaking correlates to the presence of nystagmus in children with Chiari II malformation. *Child's Nervous System, 20*(7), 459–461.

Verhoef, M., Barf, H. A., Post, M. W., van Asbeck, F. W., Gooskens, R. H., & Prevo, A. J. (2006). Functional independence among young adults with spina bifida, in relation to hydrocephalus and level of lesion. *Developmental Medicine and Child Neurology, 48*(2), 114–119.

Vinck, A., Maassen, B., Mullaart, R., & Rotteveel, J. (2006). Arnold–Chiari-II malformation and cognitive functioning in spina bifida. *Journal of Neurology, Neurosurgery and Psychiatry, 77*(9), 1083–1086.

Watkins, M. L., Scanlon, K. S., Mulinare, J., & Khoury, M. J. (1996). Is maternal obesity a risk factor for anencephaly and spina bifida? *Epidemiology, 7*(5), 507–512.

Weinbaum, P. J., Cassidy, S. B., Vintzileos, A. M., Campbell, W. A., Ciarleglio, L., & Nochimson, D. J. (1986). Prenatal detection of a neural tube defect after fetal exposure to valproic acid. *Obstetrics and Gynecology, 67*(3 Suppl.), 31S–33S.

Wiedenbauer, G., & Jansen-Osmann, P. (2006). Spatial knowledge of children with spina bifida in a virtual large-scale space. *Brain and Cognition, 62*(2), 120–127.

Wild, J., Read, A. P., Sheppard, S., Seller, M. J., Smithells, R. W., Nevin, N. C., et al. (1986). Recurrent neural tube defects, risk factors and vitamins. *Archives of Disease in Childhood, 61*(5), 440–444.

Wills, K. E. (1993). Neuropsychological functioning in children with spina bifida and/or hydrocephalus. *Journal of Clinical Child Psychology, 22,* 247–265.

Yeates, K. O., Loss, N., Colvin, A. N., & Enrile, B. G. (2003). Do children with myelomeningocele and hydrocephalus display nonverbal learning disabilities?: An empirical approach to classification. *Journal of International Neuropsychological Society, 9*(4), 653–662.

Yoshida, F., Morioka, T., Hashiguchi, K., Kawamura, T., Miyagi, Y., Nagata, S., et al. (2006). Epilepsy in patients with spina bifida in the lumbosacral region. *Neurosurgical Review, 29*(4), 327–332.

CHAPTER 29

Inborn Errors of Metabolism

A Brief Overview

ROBERT T. BROWN

> The topic of inborn errors of metabolism is challenging for most physicians.
> The number of known metabolic disorders is probably as large as the
> number of presenting symptoms that may indicate metabolic disturbances....
> Furthermore, physicians know they may not encounter certain rare inborn
> errors of metabolism during a lifetime of practice. Nonetheless, with a
> collective incidence of one in 1,500 persons, at least one of these disorders
> will be encountered by almost all practicing physicians.
> —RAGHUVEER, GARG, AND GRAF (2006, p. 1981)

Inborn errors of metabolism (IEMs) are genetically based disorders that interfere with normal metabolism. Metabolism occurs in sequences of biochemical reactions, called *metabolic pathways*. Each pathway involves particular enzymes that break down ingested food into usable nutrients. An IEM occurs when a defective gene results in an absent or defective enzyme in one of these pathways, blocking normal metabolism and resulting in accumulation of an abnormal substance in the body. In many cases, this abnormal substance is toxic to developing neural tissue, resulting in varying degrees of mental retardation, cerebral palsy, seizure disorders, and sensory and/or motor impairments, among other effects. Blocks of metabolism of a given substance may occur at different points in the metabolic pathway, leading to different disorders. IEMs are single-gene disorders that follow principles of Mendelian genetics. Most IEMs, such as phenylketonuria (PKU; see Waisbren, Chapter 21, this volume), are autosomal recessive

disorders, but a few, such as Lesch–Nyhan syndrome (see Wodrich & Long, Chapter 23, this volume), and adrenoleukodystrophy, are X-linked recessive disorders. Some disorders known for hundreds or thousands of years have been identified as IEMs only relatively recently, gout being perhaps the best-known and most common example. Many IEMs have been identified in the last 40 years, and some, particularly new variants, are still being discovered.

This chapter is a brief general overview of IEMs; it focuses on those with neurological consequences, including their characteristics, symptoms, diagnosis, and treatment. Readers wanting detailed information on individual IEMs other than PKU, Lesch–Nyhan syndrome, or the mucopolysaccharidoses (see M. Brown, Chapter 15, this volume) may wish to consult one of the recent books on the topic (e.g., Fernandes, Saudubray, van den Berghe, & Walter, 2005; Mayatepek, 2008; Nyhan, Barshop, & Ozand, 2005; Sarafoglou, Hoffmann, & Roth, 2009); the printed or online versions of *Mendelian Inheritance in Man* (McKusick, 1998; *www.ncbi.nlm.gov/omim*); and a series of online articles by Weiner (2009a, 2009b, 2009c, 2009d). Advanced pediatrics textbooks (e.g., Kliegman, Behrman, Jenson, & Stanton, 2007) are also useful, as indicated by citations in this chapter. In addition, the National Institute of Neurological Disorders and Stroke (NINDS) provides routinely updated webpages for many IEMs.

IEMs can be difficult to identify because they "can manifest at any time, can affect any organ system, and can mimic many common pediatric problems" (Thomas & Van Hove, 2007, p. 986). For many, even when accurately diagnosed, no effective treatment is currently available. Unfortunately, misdiagnosis, delayed diagnosis, or nondiagnosis of IEMs can lead to devastating consequences. In cases where effective treatment is available, unnecessary death or severe permanent organic damage may result. In cases where treatment is not currently available, affected individuals may not be identified and thus may be unable to participate in clinical trials of experimental treatments; accurate family histories may not be compiled; and genetic counseling may not be provided to parents. Furthermore, given that various IEMs can appear throughout infancy and into adulthood, an undiagnosed IEM may lead parents to be charged with neglect, abuse, or even Munchausen syndrome by proxy (see Pankratz, 2006).

BACKGROUND

In the late 19th century, Archibald Edward Garrod, an English physician, began to use urine with abnormal characteristics to study metabolic processes. He first studied alkaptonuria, a rare disorder whose most prominent symptom is darkening of urine after exposure to air. Affected adults typically later develop a particular form of arthritis in which brown pigment occurs in joint tissue. In his initial paper on the subject, Garrod (1902/1996) described William Bateson's description of recently rediscovered Mendelian principles of heredity and stated (p. 278): "Whether the Mendelian explanation be the true one or no there seems to be little room for doubt that the peculiarities of the incidence of alkaptonuria and of conditions which appear in a similar way are best explained by supposing that, leaving aside exceptional cases in which the character, usually recessive, assumes dominance, a peculiarity of the gametes of both parents is necessary for its production." Note that Garrod's article appeared a few years before introduction of the terms *genetics* and *genes* to the study of heredity.

Garrod subsequently presented his findings on alkaptonuria and other similar rare disorders (albinism, cystinuria, porphyrinuria [porphyria], and steatorrhea) in the Croonian Lectures (1908) and two editions of his classic monograph (Garrod, 1909, 1923), all titled with his classic phrase, *Inborn Errors of Metabolism*. Garrod described the appearance of symptoms of some of these disorders in the newborn period; he also used his other classic phrase, "one gene, one enzyme," to account for the metabolic failures. Several involved unusual bodily odors or appearance of urine and/or feces. Of interest, some forms of porphyria but not others have significant nervous system effects, including seizures and impaired mental functioning (depression, anxiety, hallucinations). Unfortunately, the importance of Garrod's findings was not appreciated for many years.

The first reported IEM associated with mental retardation was PKU, detected on the basis of mousy-smelling urine and reported by Fölling in 1934 (see Waisbren, Chapter 21). Subsequent reports of new IEMs with effects on the nervous system appeared regularly; in 1970, O'Brien described 77 separate disorders, some with numerous variants, that lead to various degrees of mental retardation. At this writing, approximately 300 of the 1,000 or so known IEMs have been found to have nervous system effects, most commonly mental retardation. Many IEMs are also now known to have variant forms, owing to involvement of other genes or different mutations on the same gene. Garrod's "one gene, one enzyme" concept is no longer applicable.

CLASSIFICATION

Several ways of classifying IEMs are available. Two quite different ones are described here—one based on the type of metabolic error, and the second based on the manner and timing of symptom manifestation.

Type of Metabolic Error

Several systems of classifying IEMs in terms of the type of metabolic error have been offered. Thomas and Van Hove (2007) divide the entire group of IEMs into seven categories. The following material is based largely on their description. For each category, major general effects and a few examples are provided.

Carbohydrate Metabolism Defects

Virtually all carbohydrate metabolism defects are associated with mental retardation, acute encephalopathy, failure to thrive, and hepatomegaly (enlarged liver). Seizures, hypotonia, vomiting, and cataracts are also common. Examples are glycogen storage diseases, galactosemia, and hereditary fructose intolerance. Untreated, all can lead to early death, but strict adherence to a diet low in the unmetabolizable substance reduces or eliminates most adverse effects.

Amino Acid Metabolism Defects

The major effects of amino acid metabolism defects are the same as those for carbohydrate metabolism defects, except for the absence of enlarged liver and inclusion of seizures, vomiting, and food aversions. In addition, hypo- and hypertonia, behavior problems, and unusual bodily odor are common. Examples are urea cycle disorders, PKU and its variants, tyrosinemia, maple syrup urine disease, and homocystinuria. Diagnosis can be made through routine newborn blood testing for abnormal metabolites. Treatment involves elimination of the unmetabolizable substance from the diet, adherence to a synthetic diet, or administration of a substance that substitutes for the missing enzyme. Without treatment, progressively severe mental retardation, seizure disorders, and other neurological disorders are predictable. With lifelong treatment beginning in the newborn period, development can be nearly normal in most cases except for specific learning problems. Effects of variants are less severe.

Organic Acid Disorders

The major and common effects of organic acid disorders are very similar to those of amino acid metabolism disorders. Diagnosis is generally made through testing for specific abnormal substances in blood or urine. Methylmalonic aciduria is an organic acid disorder with a wide range of outcomes from benign to fatal in infancy. Severity depends on the particular mutation present and on the success of treatment. It may occur with homocystinuria. Symptoms of propionic aciduria, such as poor feeding, vomiting, dehydration, acidosis, hypotonia, and seizures, appear shortly after birth. Symptoms reflect, among other conditions, encephalopathy and hyperammonia. Progression to death is often rapid. Treatment involves elimination of the unmetabolizable substance from the diet, and often large oral doses of biotin (vitamin B7) or, in the case of methylmalonic aciduria, vitamin B12.

Fatty Acid Oxidation Disorders

Considered as a group, fatty acid oxidation disorders may be among the most common IEMs (Stanley & Bennett, 2007). Major symptoms include hypoketotic hypoglycemia, hyperammonemia, hypotonia, vomiting, encephalopathy, cardiomyopathy, and hepatomegaly; these often appear after 8–12 hours of fasting, not an unusual period between dinner and breakfast. Sudden infant death may result, and rate of death in previously undiagnosed cases is high. Diagnosis is made through testing for specific abnormal substances in blood or urine. Treatment in acute episodes involves prevention of hypoglycemia by providing frequent snacks and avoiding infections. Oral carnitine is effective in some cases. Examples are three disorders associated with deficiencies in enzymes of fatty-acid ß-oxidation: very-long-chain and medium-chain acyl-coenzyme A dehydrogenase deficiency, and long-chain 3-hydroxyacyl CoA dehydrogense deficiency (e.g., Stanley & Bennett, 2007; Thomas & Van Hove, 2007).

Purine Metabolism Disorders

As with several other categories of IEMs, severity, onset, and progression of symptoms vary widely among the purine metabolism disorders. Commonly, they are associated with overproduction of uric acid. Many lead to mental retardation, seizure and movement disorders, muscle cramps, autistic and other abnormal behavior, and susceptibility to infections. Some, however, are essentially asymptomatic. The most common is gout, in which crystals of uric acid are deposited in joints, causing severe pain. Gout can develop from childhood to adulthood. Lesch–Nyhan syndrome is a well-known purine metabolism disorder (see Wodrich & Long, Chapter 23). Adenylosuccinate lyase deficiency and phosphoribosyl pyrophosphate synthetase defects are purine metabolism disorders associated with severe mental retardation, seizures, and autistic behavior. No effective treatment is available. Some reports (e.g., Page & Coleman, 2000) suggest that as many as 20% of those with autism have unusually high levels of uric acid in their urine, but the relationship between the excess uric acid and autism is unclear.

Lysosomal Storage Disorders

Lysosomes break down substrate in cells into usable materials, and each lysosomal storage disorder (LSD) is caused by a deficiency in the enzyme that deals with a specific substrate, leading to its accumulation in cells. As a group, LSDs are highly variable in severity. Characteristic symptoms include short stature, skeletal abnormalities, coarse facies, splenomegaly, neurological dysfunction, and visual and auditory impairments. Major symptoms of more severe disorders include mental retardation, developmental regression, seizures, behavior disorders, macrocephaly, and hepatomegaly. Initial diagnosis may be made through urine screening tests, but must be confirmed by appropriate enzyme analyses.

Most LSDs can be placed in one of three subgroups based on the accumulating substance: mucopolysaccharidoses, mucolipidoses, or lipidoses. Severity varies widely even within subgroup: Of the mucopolysaccharidoses (see M. Brown, Chapter 15), Hurler and Sanfilippo syndromes are associated with severe mental retardation, Hunter syndrome with mental retardation of varying degrees, and Scheie syndrome with normal intelligence. Of the mucolipidoses,

mannosidosis varies from severe symptoms, including mental retardation, to mild symptoms with near-normal intelligence. Of the lipidoses, several have different forms with different age of onset, and at least three (type 1 Gaucher, acute Niemann–Pick, and Tay–Sachs) are particularly common among Ashkenazi Jews of Eastern European descent, whereas type D Niemann–Pick is more common among those of Nova Scotian descent. Symptoms of type 1 Gaucher, the most common LSD, can appear from childhood to adulthood. Affected individuals have low blood platelets, enlarged livers and spleens, skeletal deformities, and potential lung and kidney disorders. It is non-neurological and associated with normal lifespan. Type 2 Gaucher has early infant onset of liver and spleen enlargement, with progressive brain damage and death by 2 years of age. Type 3 Gaucher has variable onset of liver and spleen enlargement, as well as brain damage reflected in seizures and motor coordination dysfunction. Death in adolescence or young adulthood is characteristic. Enzyme treatment is effective for types 1 and 3, but no effective treatment is available for type 2 (NINDS, 2009a). Niemann–Pick disease occurs in four types with different ages of onset. Type A has acute infant onset of jaundice, enlarged liver, major brain damage, and death usually by 18 months of age. Type B is non-neurological; enlarged spleen and liver occur prior to adolescence. Types C and D have childhood to adulthood onset of enlarged liver and spleen, as well as major brain damage causing motor disturbances, loss of vision and hearing, seizures, and mental retardation. Death is variable, but often in childhood. No effective treatment is available for type A, and only potentially effective ones for the others (NINDS, 2009c). Infants with Tay–Sachs appear normal at birth, but as lipids accumulate in nerve cells, mental, physical, and sensory abilities rapidly deteriorate, and seizures, severe mental retardation, and paralysis develop. No effective treatment is available, and death usually occurs by 4 years of age.

Peroxisomal Disorders

Major effects of the peroxisomal disorders include mental retardation, seizures, regressions in development, behavior abnormalities, and susceptibility to infections. These disorders involve absence or reduced levels of various *peroxisomes*—cellular organelles essential for metabolism of very-long-chain fatty acids (VLCFAs), plasmalogen production, and bile acid synthesis. "Abnormal accumulation of VLCFAs ... is the hallmark of peroxisomal disorders" (Chedrawi & Clark, 2007, paragraph 5).

Leukodystrophies, a subgroup of progressive peroxisomal disorders, lead to degeneration of white matter in the brain owing to maldevelopment of myelin sheaths. Each leukodystrophy involves a defect in one gene. In general, they appear in infancy or childhood and involve progressive declines in movement (e.g., gait, speech, and eating), vision and hearing, cognitive functioning, and physical development. Symptoms vary according to the specific type of leukodystrophy, and may be difficult to recognize in the early stages of the disease. They vary greatly in severity, with the most severe forms essentially untreatable and resulting in early death. Specific leukodystrophies include Zellweger syndrome, metachromatic leukodystrophy (MLD), X-linked adrenoleukodystrophy, and Refsum disease. Zellweger and Refsum syndromes are, respectively, perhaps the most and least severe. Several have different forms, with the early-onset version being the most severe. Zellweger syndrome involves excessive iron and copper in blood and tissue. Symptoms include enlarged liver, specific abnormal facies, mental retardation, and seizures. Affected infants may be severely hypotonic and unable to suck or swallow. Damage in severe cases may begin prenatally. Death generally occurs by 6 months of age. Late infantile MLD begins to manifest itself at 12–18 months of age with irritability and inability to walk; it progresses to muscle wasting, seizures, hypotonia, mental retardation, and death before about age 10 years (Chedrawi & Clark, 2007; NINDS, 2007, 2009b).

Timing/Manner of Symptom Manifestation

Batshaw and Tuchman (2007) described three types of IEMs in terms of their onset and progression when the disorders go unrecognized and untreated:

1. *Silent disorders* are initially asymptomatic and progress slowly, becoming apparent generally in childhood. Affected children do not show symptoms such as seizures, vomiting, or coma shortly after birth, but develop slowly and show progressive mental and other impairments. Examples include PKU and congenital hypothyroidism.

2. *Disorders presenting in acute metabolic crisis* produce severe symptoms, including seizures, vomiting, lethargy, and coma shortly after birth. As these conditions are also symptomatic of many other newborn disorders (e.g., infections; brain hemorrhage; and pulmonary, cardiac, and gastrointestinal abnormalities), immediate diagnosis and treatment are difficult if bodily fluids are not tested for specific metabolic problems. In the absence of treatment, virtually all affected individuals will die in infancy. Even with the most extreme intervention, many will die, and others show severe impairments. Examples are urea cycle disorders and organic acidemias.

3. *Disorders with progressive neurological deterioration* are, like silent disorders, asymptomatic for some time after birth. At ages ranging from a few months to years, the motor and/or cognitive skills of affected individuals begin to deteriorate. Untreated, the deterioration leads to death by childhood in severe cases. A few examples, among many, are carbohydrate metabolism defects, amino acid metabolism defects, LSDs, peroxisomal disorders, fatty acid oxidation disorders, and mitochondrial disorders.

INITIAL APPEARANCE AND DEVELOPMENT

Although onset can occur at any time in life, the most severe IEMs manifest themselves in newborns or infants who generally appear normal at birth, but develop symptoms within days or weeks (e.g., Rezvani, 2007a; Weiner, 2009c). Most of these severe disorders have neurodevelopmental effects that, unless treated immediately, can result in permanent impairments or death. For some, no effective treatment is now available, and adverse outcomes are inevitable. Tay–Sachs and late infantile MLD are two examples. In both of these, onset is in late infancy, with progressive deterioration in functioning leading to death in early childhood. Most IEMs that impair developing neural tissue are progressive, with symptoms becoming increasingly severe. Thus the longer any effective treatments are postponed, the greater the ultimate symptom severity.

Most IEMs that lead to severe symptoms in newborn or infant periods have variants that appear later, progress more slowly, and often have less severe or episodic effects. For example, MLD appears in three forms: late infantile, juvenile, and adult. In the most common, late infantile MLD (mentioned above), gait and balance problems appear, followed by hypotonia, major motor deterioration, and cognitive impairment. Progressive general deterioration leads to death by age 5–6 years. The juvenile form generally does not appear until age 5–10 years, when cognitive and motor functioning begin to decline. Overall motor control then deteriorates, frequent and difficult-to-control tonic–clonic seizures appear, and death generally occurs at about age 15–16 years. The adult form has highly variable onset, from about age 20 to 50 years; it begins with memory, personality, and psychiatric problems that slowly (perhaps over a decade or more) progress to motor disturbances, such as spasticity and seizures, and then to overall unresponsiveness (Johnston, 2007; Weiner, 2009c).

DIAGNOSIS

Because their effects overlap not only with those of other IEMs but with those of numerous other disorders, diagnosis of IEMs can be difficult. Since treatment is specific to each disorder, delayed or erroneous diagnosis can lead to delayed or erroneous treatment with potentially disastrous consequences. Many methods of identifying a disorder as a potential or specific IEM are available. Owing to the complexity of the subject, only a brief overview is given here. Much of this section, unless otherwise attributed, is based on Weiner (2009c).

Family History

Since IEMs are autosomal recessive or X-linked disorders, they virtually always appear de novo. Thus past-generation family histories are unlikely to provide clues to diagnosis. However, if one offspring has an IEM, the probability is high that others will also; thus detailed information on serious illness in siblings may be valuable. Identification of an IEM in one child may call for assessment of siblings who may also have the disorder, particularly one of the less severe variants.

Prenatal Identification

Many IEMs can be diagnosed prenatally through amniocentesis or chorionic villus sampling, but specific analyses are needed for identification of most IEMs. Therefore, diagnosis of de novo cases is unlikely.

Mandated Newborn Screening

A number of fatty acid oxidation disorders, amino acid metabolism defects, organic acid disorders, and other IEMs can be tentatively identified through mandated newborn screening using tandem mass spectroscopy. These include PKU, maple syrup urine syndrome, galactosemia, and propionic academia (see National Newborn Screening and Genetics Resource Center, 2009, for a complete list). Since the test is intentionally set to produce a low rate of false-negative results, it necessarily has high rates of false positives. Positive results therefore call for confirmation with more specialized tests.

Suggestive General Symptoms

An IEM should be expected when an otherwise normal newborn, infant, or young child shows deterioration of functioning unattributable to another disorder. Other potential symptoms include failure to thrive, abnormal physical features, skeletal malformations, major organ failure, poor feeding, vomiting, diarrhea, abnormal reflexes or movement, unusual susceptibility to illness, coma, and seizures.

In older children, adolescents, or adults, symptoms similar to those above that occur during illness, stress, or change in diet or lifestyle may reflect an undiagnosed IEM. Other potential concerns are otherwise unattributed neurological abnormalities, abnormal behavior, mental retardation, autistic behaviors, learning disabilities, anxiety disorders, seizures, motor dysfunction, and lethargy, among others.

Of particular concern in older children is partial ornithine transcarbamylase deficiency, a urea cycle defect, which may first become apparent in adolescence as "a life-threatening metabolic catastrophe … [which is] observed particularly in adolescent females with a history of protein aversion, abdominal pain, and migrainelike headaches" (Weiner, 2009c, paragraph 19).

Unusual Body Odor

Several IEMs (mainly amino acid and organic acid disorders) are associated with unusual and characteristic body or fluid odors that begin to appear at about a day after birth, when first feedings should have been metabolized. Examples (taken from Rezvani, 2007b) of amino acid disorders, with their commonly described characteristic urine odors in parentheses, are as follows: PKU (mousy), maple syrup urine syndrome (maple syrup), tyrosemia (boiled cabbage), and hawkinsinuria (swimming pool). Worth noting is the culturally specific nature of some of these terms. Those unfamiliar with maple syrup, for example, will probably have a different term to describe the odor, and I myself, although familiar with many swimming pools, am at a loss as to the nature of any single characteristic odor.

Symptoms of Sepsis

Unexplained sepsis in newborns and infants may reflect onset of an IEM: "Of term infants who develop symptoms of sepsis without known risk factors, as many as 20% may have an inborn error of metabolism" (Weiner, 2009c, paragraph 6). *Sepsis* is a widespread infection that involves the systemic inflammatory response syndrome (SIRS). SIRS is an "inflammatory cascade that … occurs when the host defense system does not recognize or clear the infection. SIRS can also occur from a number of noninfectious etiologies" (Enrione & Powell, 2007, p. 1094). Symptoms include very high temperature, tachycardia, high respiratory rate, and elevated or depressed leukocyte count. With increasing number and severity of symptoms, SIRS can progress to severe sepsis, septic shock, and death.

TREATMENT

Treatment obviously is specific to each disorder; in some cases, it is also specific to variants of the disorder and to the individual patient (Weiner, 2009d). Several have been described at other places in this chapter, although in highly condensed form. Generally, synthetic or restricted diets, medication, enzyme replacement, and bone marrow and organ transplants are useful for many IEMs. Weiner (2009d) describes acute and long-term intervention in more detail, including use of some relatively broadly effective drugs.

An important, but often neglected, aspect of treatment and intervention is consideration of the family unit's needs. Care for most individuals affected by IEMs is demanding, time-consuming, and expensive, and requires adherence to rigid protocols. Given that an affected individual may resist or resent aspects of treatment, stress on caregivers may be further increased. Unaffected siblings are also likely to suffer because care of the affected child may limit parents' time with them and because they will often have to share caretaking. Family therapy and monitoring will often be useful adjuncts to treatment of the affected individuals themselves.

CONCLUDING REMARKS

IEMs are challenging not only for physicians, as stated in the epigraph to this chapter, but for all clinicians who interact with potential or known cases. Their sheer and increasing numbers; their variants; their complex symptoms (which overlap with both those of other IEMs and those of numerous other disorders); their varied onsets, progressions, and ultimate phenotypes; and their frequent nonresponsiveness to intervention all contribute to these challenges. But as with so many other things, not knowing about them is far worse than knowing about them.

On the positive side, a great deal has changed in our understanding of IEMs since I first wrote about them almost 25 years ago (Brown, 1986). Many more have been discovered, accurately described, and effectively treated. Treatments known at that time have been refined and made more effective, and many new treatments have been developed. Many more effective treatments can be expected through stem cell replacement, enzyme replacement, and genetic modification.

REFERENCES

Batshaw, M. L., & Tuchman, M. (2007). Inborn errors of metabolism. In M. L. Batshaw, L. Pelligrino, & N. J. Roizen (Eds.), *Children with disabilities* (6th ed., pp. 285–296). Baltimore: Brookes.

Brown, R. T. (1986). Etiology and development of exceptionality. In R. T. Brown & C. R. Reynolds (Eds.), *Psychological perspectives on childhood exceptionality: A handbook* (pp. 181–225). New York: Wiley-Interscience.

Chedrawi, A., & Clark, G. D. (2007). Peroxisomal disorders: Overview. *eMedicine Specialties.* Retrieved September 20, 2009, from *emedicine. medscape.com/article/1177387-overview*

Enrione, M. A., & Powell, K. R. (2007). Sepsis, septic shock, and systemic inflammatory response syndrome. In R. M. Kliegman, R. E. Behrman, H. B. Jenson, & B. F. Stanton (Eds.), *Nelson textbook of pediatrics* (18th ed., pp. 1094–1099). Philadelphia: Saunders.

Fernandes, J., Saudubray, J.-M., van den Berghe, G., & Walter, J. H. (Eds.). (2005). *Inborn metabolic diseases: Diagnosis and treatment.* New York: Springer.

Garrod, A. E. (1996). The incidence of alkaptonuria: A study of chemical individuality. *Molecular Medicine, 2,* 274–282. (Original work published 1902)

Garrod, A. E. (1908). Croonian lectures on inborn errors of metabolism, parts I–IV. *Lancet, 2,* 1–7, 73–79, 142–148, 214–220.

Garrod, A. E. (1909). *Inborn errors of metabolism.* London: Henry Froude.

Garrod, A. E. (1923). *Inborn errors of metabolism* (2nd ed.). London: Hodder & Stoughton. (Available online at *www.esp.org/books/garrod/inborn-errors/facsimile*

Kliegman, R. M., Behrman, R. E., Jenson, H. B., & Stanton, B. F. (Eds.). (2007). *Nelson textbook of pediatrics* (18th ed). Philadelphia: Saunders.

Johnston, M. V. (2007). Neurogenerative disorders of childhood. In R. M. Kliegman, R. E. Behrman, H. B. Jenson, & B. F. Stanton (Eds.), *Nelson textbook of pediatrics* (18th ed., pp. 2499–2505). Philadelphia: Saunders.

Mayatepek, E. (2008). *Inborn errors of metabolism: Early detection, key symptoms and therapeutic options.* Bremen, Germany: UNI-MED Science.

McKusick, V.A. (1998). *Mendelian inheritance in man: A catalog of human genes and genetic disorders* (12th ed.). Baltimore: Johns Hopkins University Press.

National Institute of Neurological Disorders and Stroke (NINDS). (2007). NINDS Zellweger syndrome information page. Retrieved September 18, 2009, from *www.ninds.nih.gov/disorders/zellweger/zellweger.htm*

National Institute of Neurological Disorders and Stroke (NINDS). (2009a). NINDS Gaucher's disease information page. Retrieved September 20, 2009, from *www.ninds.nih.gov/disorders/gauchers/gauchers.htm*

National Institute of Neurological Disorders and Stroke (NINDS). (2009b). NINDS leukodystrophy information page. Retrieved September 18, 2009, from *www.ninds.nih.gov/disorders/leukodystrophy/leukodystrophy.htm*

National Institute of Neurological Disorders and Stroke (NINDS). (2009c). NINDS Niemann–Pick disease information page. Retrieved September 20, 2009, from *www.ninds.nih.gov/disorders/niemann/niemann.htm*

National Newborn Screening and Genetics Resource Center. (2009). National newborn screening status report. Retrieved October 12,2009, from *genes-r-us.uthscsa.edu/nbsdisorders.pdf*

Nyhan, W. L., Barshop, B. A., & Ozand, P. T. (Eds.). (2005). *Atlas of metabolic diseases* (2nd ed.). London: Hodder Arnold.

O'Brien, D. O. (1970). *Rare inborn errors of metabolism in children with mental retardation.* Bethesda, MD: U.S. Department of Health, Education, and Welfare.

Page, T., & Coleman, M. (2000). Purine metabolism abnormalities in a hyperuricosuric subclass of autism. *Biochimica et Biophysica Acta, 1500,* 291–296.

Pankratz, L. (2006). Persistent problems with the Munchausen syndrome by proxy label. *Journal of the American Academy of Psychiatry and Law, 34,* 90–95.

Raghuveer, T. S., Garg, U., & Graf, W. D. (2006). Inborn errors of metabolism in infancy and early childhood: An update. *American Family Physician, 73,* 1981–1990.

Rezvani, I. (2007a). An approach to inborn errors of metabolism. In R. M. Kliegman, R. E. Behrman, H. B. Jenson, & B. F. Stanton (Eds.), *Nelson textbook of pediatrics* (18th ed., pp. 527–529). Philadelphia: Saunders.

Rezvani, I. (2007b). Defects in metabolism of amino acids. In R. M. Kliegman, R. E. Behrman, H. B. Jenson, & B. F. Stanton (Eds.), *Nelson textbook of pediatrics* (18th ed., pp. 529–532). Philadelphia: Saunders.

Sarafoglou, K., Hoffmann, G., & Roth, K. (Eds.). (2009). *Pediatric endocrinology and inborn errors of metabolism.* New York: McGraw-Hill.

Stanley, C. A., & Bennett, M. J. (2007). Defects in metabolism of lipids. In R. M. Kliegman, R. E. Behrman, H. B. Jenson, & B. F. Stanton (Eds.),

Nelson textbook of pediatrics (18th ed., pp. 567–601). Philadelphia: Saunders.

Thomas, J. A., & Van Hove, J. L. K. (2007). Inborn errors of metabolism. In W. M. Hay, Jr., M. J. Levin, J. M. Sondheimer, & R. R. Deterding (Eds.), *Current diagnosis and treatment in pediatrics* (18th ed., pp. 986–1010). New York: McGraw-Hill.

Weiner, D. L. (2009a). Inborn errors of metabolism: Differential diagnoses and workup. *eMedicine Specialties.* Retrieved September 15, 2009, from *emedicine.medscape.com/article/804757-diagnosis*

Weiner, D. L. (2009b). Inborn errors of metabolism: Follow-up. *eMedicine Specialties.* Retrieved September 15, 2009, from *emedicine.medscape.com/article/804757-followup*

Weiner, D. L. (2009c). Inborn errors of metabolism: Overview. *eMedicine Specialties.* Retrieved September 15, 2009, from *emedicine.medscape.com/article/804757-overview*

Weiner, D. L. (2009d). Inborn errors of metabolism: Treatment and medication. *eMedicine Specialties.* Retrieved September 15, 2009, from *emedicine.medscape.com/article/804757-treatment*

Index

Page numbers followed by *f* indicate figure, *t* indicate table

579